Contents

Chapter 2 *Neuron–Glial Cell Cooperation*
C. Hammond

Chapter 3 *Ionic Fluxes Across the Neuronal Plasma Membrane*
C. Hammond

Chapter 4 *Basic Properties of Excitable Cells at Rest*
A. Nistri and A. Gutman

Chapter 5 *The Voltage-Gated Channels of Na⁺ Action Potentials*
C. Hammond

Chapter 6 *The Voltage-Gated Channels of Ca²⁺ Action Potentials: Generalization*
C. Hammond

Chapter 7 *The Chemical Synapses*
C. Hammond

Chapter 8 *Neurotransmitter Release*
C. Hammond

PART 2   Ionotropic and Metabotropic Receptors in Synaptic Transmission and Sensory Transduction

Chapter 9   *The Ionotropic Nicotinic Acetylcholine Receptors*
C. Hammond

Chapter 10   *The Ionotropic GABA$_A$ Receptor*
C. Hammond

Chapter 11   *The Ionotropic Glutamate Receptors*
C. Hammond

Chapter 12   *Ionotropic Mechanoreceptors: the Mechanosensitive Channels*
C. Bourque

Chapter 13 *The Metabotropic GABA$_B$ Receptors*
D. Mott

PART 3 Somato-Dendritic Processing and Plasticity of Postsynaptic Potentials

Chapter 16 *Somato-Dendritic Processing of Postsynaptic Potentials.*
I: Passive Properties of Dendrites
C. Hammond

Chapter 17 *Subliminal Voltage-Gated Currents of the Somato-Dendritic Membrane*
C. Hammond

Chapter 18 *Somato-Dendritic Processing of Postsynaptic Potentials.* *II. Role of Subliminal Depolarizing Voltage-Gated Currents*
C. Hammond

Chapter 19 *Somato-Dendritic Processing of Postsynaptic Potentials.* *III. Role of High-Voltage-Activated Depolarizing Currents*
C. Hammond

Chapter 20 *Firing Patterns of Neurons*
C. Hammond

Chapter 21 *Synaptic Plasticity*
C. Hammond

PART 4 Activity and Development of Networks: The Hippocampus as an Example

Chapter 22 *The Adult Hippocampal Network*
C. Hammond

Chapter 23 *Maturation of the Hippocampal Network*
Y. Ben Ari and C. Hammond

Contributors

Constance Hammond, (Chapters 1–3, 5–11, 15–23)
Institut de la Méditerranée, INSERM Unité 29,
Route de Luminy, BP 13, 13273 Marseille Cedex 09, France
hammond@inmed.univ-mrs.fr

Yehezkel Ben Ari (Chapter 23)
Institut de la Méditerranée, INSERM Unité 29,
Route de Luminy, BP 13, 13273 Marseille Cedex 09, France
ben-ari@inmed.univ-mrs.fr

Gautam Bhave (Chapter 14)
Division of Neuroscience, Baylor College of Medicine,
One Baylor Plaza, Houston, Texas 77030, USA

Charles Bourque (Chapter 12)
McGill University, Centre for Research in Neuroscience,
1650 Cedar avenue, Montréal PQ H3G 1A4, Québec, Canada
mdbq@musica.mcgill.ca

Monique Esclapez (Appendix 7.2)
Institut de la Méditerranée, INSERM Unité 29,
Route de Luminy, BP 13, 13273 Marseille Cedex 09, France
esclapez@inmed.univ-mrs.fr

Robert Gereau (Chapter 14)
Division of Neuroscience, Baylor College of Medicine,
One Baylor Plaza, Houston, Texas 77030, USA.
robg@cns.neusc.bcm.tmc.edu

Aron Gutman (Chapter 4)
Deceased. *Formerly of* Laboratory of Neurophysiology,
Kaunas Medical Academy, Kaunas, Lithuania

David Mott (Chapter 13)
Emory University School of Medicine, Department of Pharmacology,
Rollins Research Building, 1510 Clifton Road, Atlanta, Georgia 30322, USA
dmott@emory.edu

Andrea Nistri (Chapter 4)
International School for Advanced Studies (SISSA),
Via Beirut 4, 34014 Trieste, Italy
nistri@sissa.it

Yusuf Tan (Appendix 6.1)
Biomedical Engineering Institute, Bogazici University,
PK2 Bebek, Istanbul, Turkey
ytan@metis-tr.com

Preface

The 23 chapters of this book were written as the 23 adventures of scientists in search of a solution. I am convinced that to teach means to follow the intellectual process by which scientists elaborate an hypothesis following an observation, dissect the most appropriate way to perform experiments that will validate or invalidate the proposed novel concept and discuss their results. To solve a scientific enigma that often involves multiple parameters and possible solutions, a complicated mixture of experience, intelligence and intuition is necessary. It is a great pleasure for the teacher–narrator to reconstruct the puzzle of complementary observations and experiments made by scientists that ultimately led to the solution of the problem. Even many years after they were first performed, the elegance of certain pioneering experiments remains because their design was exactly suited to the question they addressed.

To be dogmatic in teaching, to give a set of answers without explaining how this knowledge was acquired, ignores the fact that science is in constant motion, that the solutions provided are by definition short-lasting as they generate new questions and that the process of scientific discovery, like all creative work, is enjoyable.

I thank my collaborators for having adhered to this way of teaching science and for having helped me to render this book more complete for its second edition. I am particularly grateful to Stéphane Peineau, who agreed to play the role of the naive student. This helped me to be more precise in my explanations. I wish to thank Christophe Bernard, Robert Cannon, Thierry Bal, Francis Crépel, Gyorgyi Buzsaki and J. Gerard G. Borst for their helpful comments on the new version.

Constance Hammond

Part 1

Neurons: Excitable and Secretory Cells that Establish Synapses

Neurons

By using the silver impregnation method developed by Golgi (1873), Ramon y Cajal studied neurons, and their connections, in the nervous system of numerous species. Based on his own work (1888) and that of others (for example Forel, His, Kölliker and Lenhossék) he proposed the concept that neurons are isolated units connected to each other by contacts formed by their processes: 'The terminal arborizations of neurons are free and are not joined to other terminal arborizations. They make contacts with the cell bodies and protoplasmic processes of other cellular elements'.

As proposed by Cajal, neurons are independent cells making specific contacts called *synapses*, with hundreds or thousands of other neurons sometimes greatly distant from their cell bodies. The neurons connected together form circuits, and so the nervous system is composed of neuronal networks which transmit and process information. In the nervous system there is another class of cells, the glial cells, which surround the various parts of neurons and cooperate with them. Glial cells are discussed in Chapter 2.

Neurons are *excitable* cells. Depending on the information they receive, neurons generate electrical signals and propagate them along their processes. This capacity is due to the presence of particular proteins in their plasma membrane which allow the selective passage of ions: the ion channels.

Neurons are also *secretory* cells. Their secretory product is called a *neurotransmitter*. The release of a neurotransmitter occurs only in restricted regions, the synapses. The neurotransmitter is released in the extracellular space. The synaptic secretion is highly focalized and directed specifically on cell regions to which the neuron is connected. The synaptic secretion is then different (with only a few exceptions) from other secretions, such as from hormonal cells and exocrine cells which respectively release their secretory products into the general circulation (endocrine secretion) or the external environment (exocrine secretion). Synapses are discussed in Chapter 7.

Neurons are *permanent* cells. When lesioned, most neurons cannot be replaced, since they are postmitotic cells. Thus, they renew their constituents during their entire life, involving the precise targeting of mRNAs and proteins to particular cytoplasmic domains or membrane areas.

1.1 Neurons have a cell body from which emerge two types of processes: the dendrites and the axon

Although neurons present varied morphologies, they all share features that identify them as neurons. The cell body or *soma* gives rise to processes which give the neuron the regionalization of its functions, its polarity and its capacity to connect to other neurons, to sensory cells or to effector cells.

1.1.1 The somatodendritic tree is the neuron's receptive pole

The soma of the neuron contains the nucleus and its surrounding cytoplasm (or *perikaryon*). Its shape is variable: pyramidal soma for pyramidal cells in the cerebral cortex and hippocampus; ovoid soma for Purkinje cells in the cerebellar cortex; granular soma for small multipolar cells in the cerebral cortex, cerebellar cortex and hippocampus; fusiform soma for neurons in the pallidal complex; and stellar or multipolar soma for motoneurons in the spinal cord (**Figure 1.1**).

One function of the soma is to ensure the synthesis of many of the components required for the structure and function of a neuron. Indeed, the soma contains all the organelles responsible for the synthesis of macromolecules. Most neurons in the central nervous system cannot further divide or regenerate after birth, and the cell body must maintain the structural integrity of the neuron throughout the individual's entire life. Moreover, the soma receives numerous synaptic contacts from other neurons and constitutes, with the dendrites, the

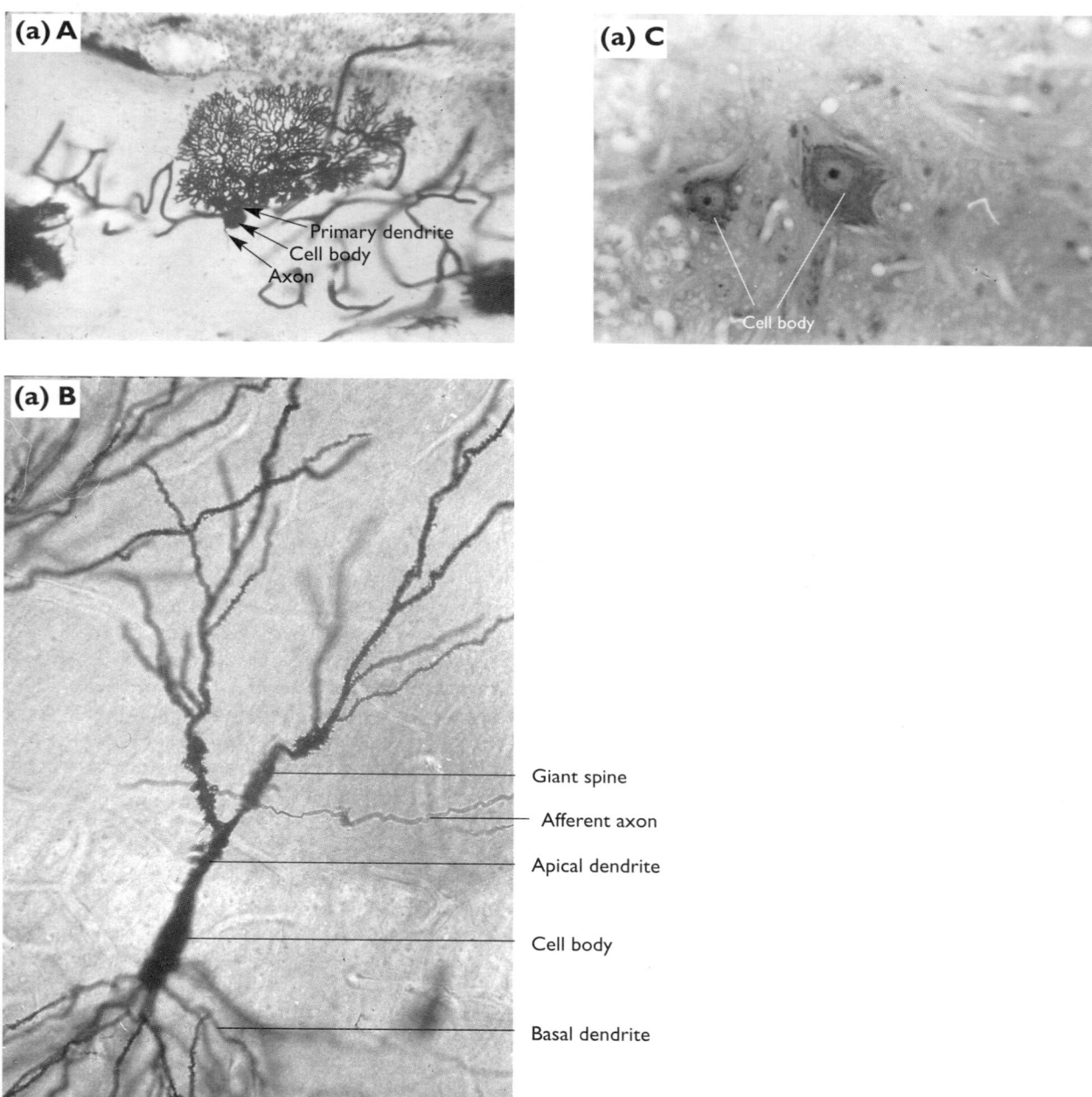

Figure 1.1 The neurons of the central nervous system present different dendritic arborizations.
(a) Photomicrographs of neurons in the central nervous system as observed under the light microscope. A – Purkinje cell of the cerebellar cortex; B – pyramidal cell of the hippocampus; C – soma of a motoneuron of the spinal cord. Golgi (A and B) and Nissl (C) staining. The Golgi technique is a silver staining which allows observation of dendrites, somas and axon emergence. The Nissl staining is a basophile staining which displays neuronal regions (soma and primary dendrites) containing Nissl bodies (parts of the rough endoplasmic reticulum). **(b)** Camera lucida drawings of neurons in the central nervous system of primates, revealed by the Golgi silver impregnation technique and reconstructed from serial sections: ST, medium spiny neuron of the striatum; GP, neurons of the globus pallidus; TH, corticothalamic neuron; STN, neuron of the subthalamic nucleus; OL, neurons of the inferior olivary complex; PU, Purkinje cell of the cerebellar cortex; SNC, dopaminergic neuron of the substantia nigra pars compacta. All these neurons are illustrated at the same magnification. Photomicrographs by Olivier Robain (aA and aB) and Paul Derer (aC). Drawings by Jérôme Yelnik, except OL and PU by Ramon Y Cajal (1911).

give a dendritic tree with specific characteristics (number of branches, volume, etc.) for each neuronal population (**Figures 1.1** and **1.2**).

The dendrites are morphologically distinguishable from axons by their irregular outline, by their diameter which decreases along their branchings, by the acute angles between the branches, and by their ultrastructural characteristics (**Figures 1.1**, **1.3** and **1.7**). The irregular outline of dendrites is related to the presence of numerous appendices of various shapes and dimensions at their surface. The most frequently observed are the dendritic spines which are lateral expansions with ovoid heads binding to the dendritic branches by a peduncle that is variable in length (**Figure 1.3**).

Some neurons are termed 'spiny' because there are between 40 000 and 100 000 spines on the surface of their dendrites (for example pyramidal neurons of the cerebral cortex and hippocampus, the medium-sized neurons of the striatum, and the Purkinje cells of the cerebellar cortex). However, other neurons with only a few spines on their dendritic surface are termed 'smooth' (for example neurons of the pallidal complex) (**Figure 1.1**).

Dendrites and soma receive numerous synaptic contacts from other neurons and constitute the main receptive area of neurons (see **Figure 1.5** and Section 7.2). In response to afferent information, they generate electrical signals such as postsynaptic potentials (EPSPs or IPSPs; see **Figure 1.5** left 1, 2) or calcium action potentials, and integrate the afferent information.

Chapters 9–11 look at the mechanisms underlying the excitatory (EPSP) and inhibitory (IPSP) postsynaptic potentials generated in the postsynaptic membrane in response to transmitter release.

Chapters 16–19 discuss how these postsynaptic responses are integrated along the somato-dendritic tree.

Although dendrites are generally a receptive zone, there are certain exceptions: some dendrites are connected with other dendrites and act as a transmitter area by releasing neurotransmitters (see **Figure 7.2d**).

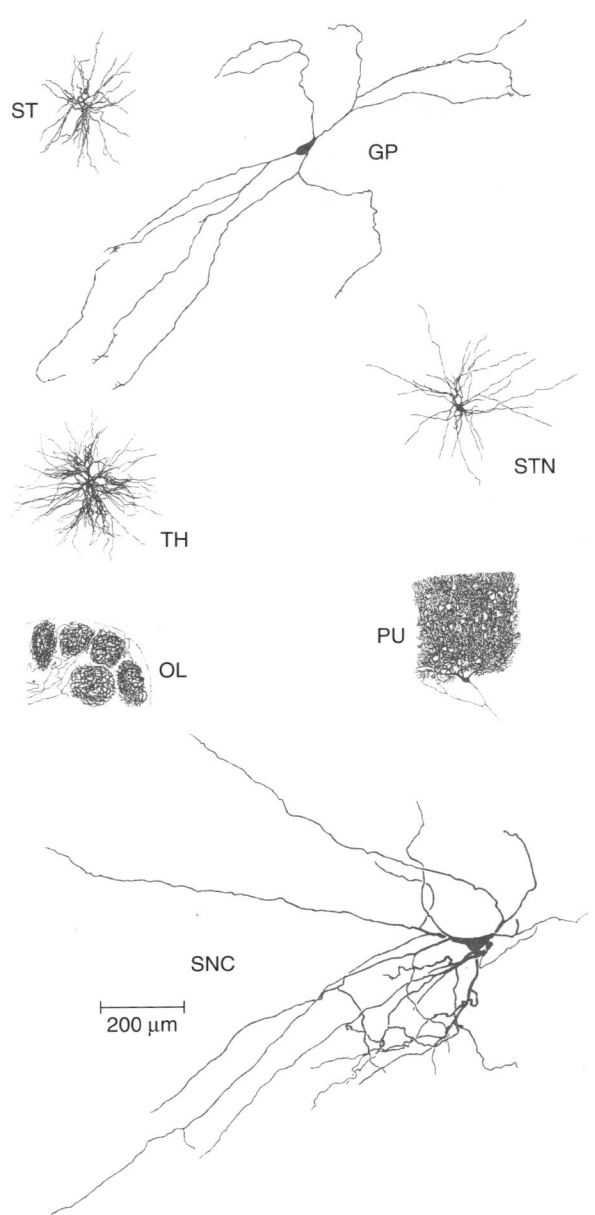

Figure 1.1(b)

main receptive area of neurons (see **Figure 1.5** and Section 7.2).

The neurons have one or several processes emerging from the cell body and arborizing more or less profusely. The two types of neuronal processes are the dendrites and the axon (**Figures 1.1** and **1.3**). This division is based on morphological, ultrastructural, biochemical and functional criteria.

The dendrites, when they emerge from the soma, are simple perikaryal extensions, the primary dendrites. On average, between one and nine primary dendrites emerge from the soma and then divide successively to

1.1.2 The axon and its collaterals are the neuron's transmitter pole

The axon is morphologically distinct from dendrites in having a smooth appearance and a uniform diameter along its entire extent, and by its ultrastructural characteristics (**Figures 1.3**, **1.6** and **1.7**). It generally emerges at the level of a conical expansion of the soma, the emerging cone, but sometimes at the level of a primary dendrite. After the emerging cone, an initial segment with a smaller diameter is observed and is followed by the true axon.

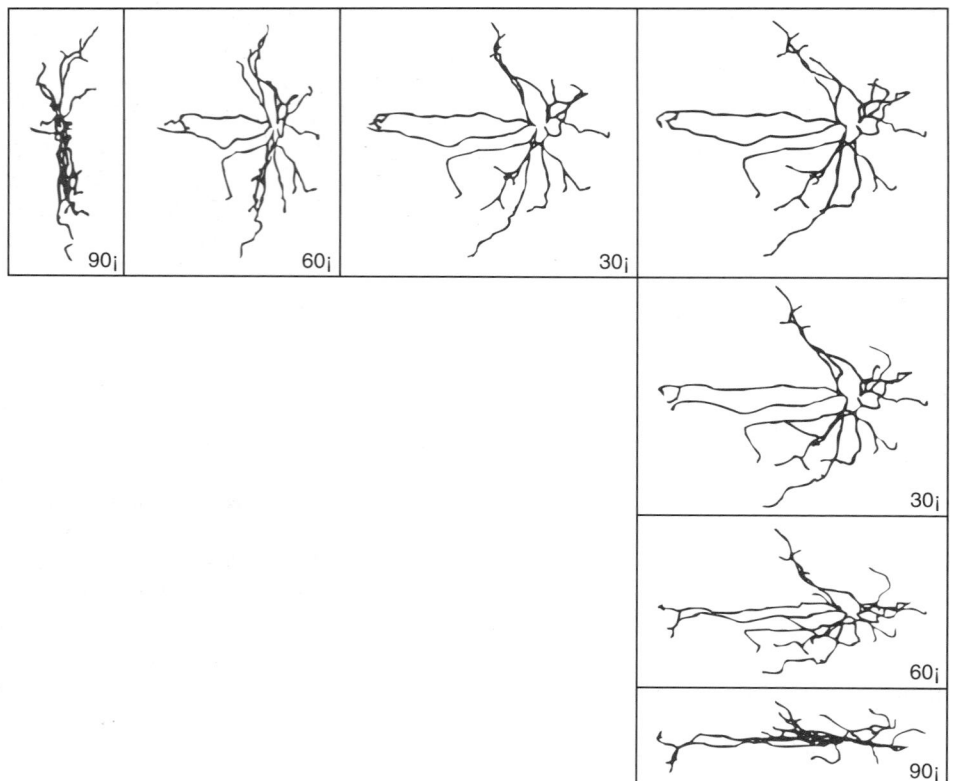

Figure 1.2 Tridimensional illustration of a dendritic arborization.
Computer drawing of a neuron of the subthalamic nucleus injected intracellularly with horseradish peroxidase (HRP) and reconstructed in three dimensions from serial sections. At 0°, the dendritic arborization of this neuron is represented in its principal plane; i.e. in the plane where it has its largest surface. In this plane, the dendritic field is almost circular (859 µm long and 804 µm wide). 30°, 60° and 90° rotations from the principal plane around the horizontal (horizontal column) and vertical (vertical column) axis show that the dendritic field has a flattened ovoidal form (230 µm thick). From Hammond C and Yelnik J (1983) Intracellular labelling of rat subthalamic nucleus with horseradish peroxidase: computer analysis of dendrites and characterization of axon arborization, *Neuroscience* **8**, 781–790, with permission.

The axon is not a single process; it is divided into one or several collaterals which form right-angles with the main axon. Some collaterals return toward the cell body area; these are recurrent axon collaterals. The axon and its collaterals may be surrounded by a sheath, the myelin sheath. Myelin is formed by glial cells (see Sections 2.2 and 2.5).

The length of an axon varies. Certain neurons in the central nervous system have axons that project to one or several structures of the central nervous system that are more or less distant from their cell bodies (**Figure 1.4**), whereas other neurons have short axons (a few microns in length) that are confined to the structure where their cell bodies are located (interneurons; see **Figure 1.13**).

Thus projection (Golgi type I) neurons and local-circuit (Golgi type II) neurons can be differentiated. In Golgi type I neurons, the length of the axon is variable: certain projection neurons are directed to one structure only (for example corticothalamic neurons; see **Figure 1.14**) whereas other projection neurons have numerous axon collaterals which project to several cerebral structures (**Figure 1.4**).

The axon and axonal collaterals in certain neurons end in a terminal arborization; i.e. numerous thin branches whose extremities, the synaptic boutons, make synaptic contacts with target cells (see **Figure 7.3**). In other neurons the axon and its collaterals have enlargements or varicosities which contact target cells along their way: these are 'boutons en passant' (see **Figures 7.12** and **7.13b**). It can be noted that both types of boutons are called *axon terminals*, although 'boutons en passant' are not the real endings of the axon.

The main characteristic of axons is their capacity to trigger sodium action potentials and to propagate them over considerable distances without any decrease in their amplitude (**Figure 1.5** left 3). Action potentials are

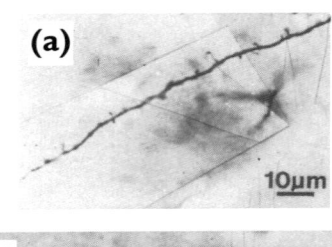

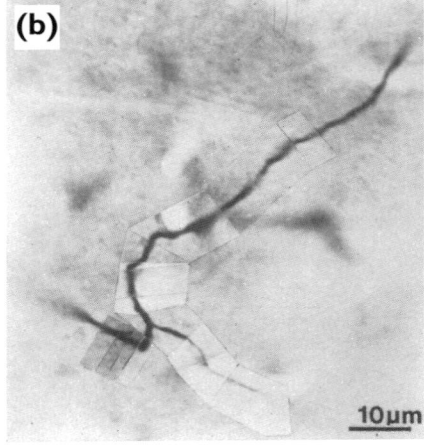

Figure 1.3 Dendrite and axon of a rat subthalamic nucleus neuron.
(a) A distal dendrite: dendritic spines of various shapes are present on its surface. (b) The axon: it has a smooth surface and gives off an axonal collateral. The processes of this neuron are stained by an intracellular injection of horseradish peroxidase. To follow the dendrites and axon along their trajectories, each figure is a photomontage of numerous photomicrographs of serial sections. From Hammond C and Yelnik J (see Figure 1.2), with permission.

generated at the initial segment level in response to synaptic information transmitted by the somato-dendritic tree. Then they propagate along the axon and its collaterals toward the axon terminals (synaptic boutons or boutons en passant). When action potentials reach the axon terminals these trigger calcium action potentials (**Figure 1.5** left 4) which may cause the release of the neurotransmitter(s) contained in axon terminals in a specific compartment, the synaptic vesicles. This secretion is localized only at the synaptic contacts. Overall, the axon is considered as the transmitter pole of the neuron.

Chapter 5 discusses the mechanisms underlying the abrupt, large and transient depolarizations called (sodium) action potentials, and how they are triggered and propogated.

Chapters 6, 7 and 8 look at how they trigger the entry of calcium in synaptic terminals and the secretion of transmitter molecules.

Certain regions – such as the initial segment, nodes of Ranvier (zones between two myelinated segments; see **Figure 1.5**) and axon terminals – can also be receptive

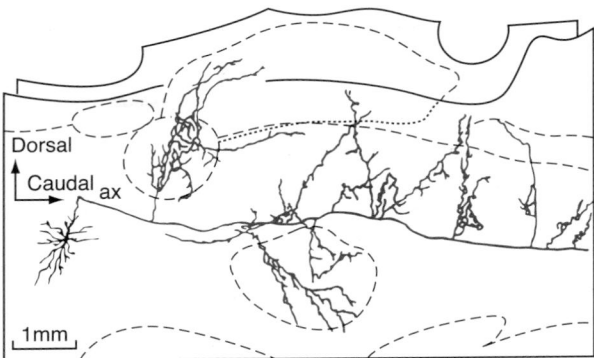

Figure 1.4 Neuron of the cat reticular formation (brain-stem) showing a complex axonal arborization.
This reticulospinal neuron has been stained by intracellular injection of peroxidase and drawn in a parasagittal plane obtained from serial sections. The axon (ax, black) gives off numerous collaterals along its rostrocaudal trajectory, making contacts with different neuronal populations (delimited by broken lines). Scale: 7 mm = 1 μm. From Grantyn A (1987) Reticulo-spinal neurons participating in the control of synergic eye and head movement during orienting in the cat, *Exp. Brain Res.* **66**, 355–377, with permission.

areas (a post-synaptic element) of synaptic contacts from other neurons (see Section 7.2).

1.2 Neurons are highly polarized cells with a differential distribution of organelles and proteins

The somatodendritic tree is the neuron's receptive pole, whereas the axon and its collaterals are the neuron's transmitter pole. Neurons are highly polarized cells. Cellular morphology and accurate organelles and protein distribution lay the basis to this polarization. The organelles and cytoplasmic elements present in neurons are the same organelles found in other cell types. However, some elements such as cytoskeletal elements are more abundant in neurons (see Appendix 1.1). The non-homogeneous distribution of organelles in their soma and processes is one of the most distinguishing characteristics of neurons.

1.2.1 The soma is the main site of macro-molecule synthesis

The soma contains the same organelles and cytoplasmic elements that exist in other cells: cellular nucleus, Golgi apparatus, mitochondria, polysomes, cytoskeletal elements and lysosomes. The soma is the main site of

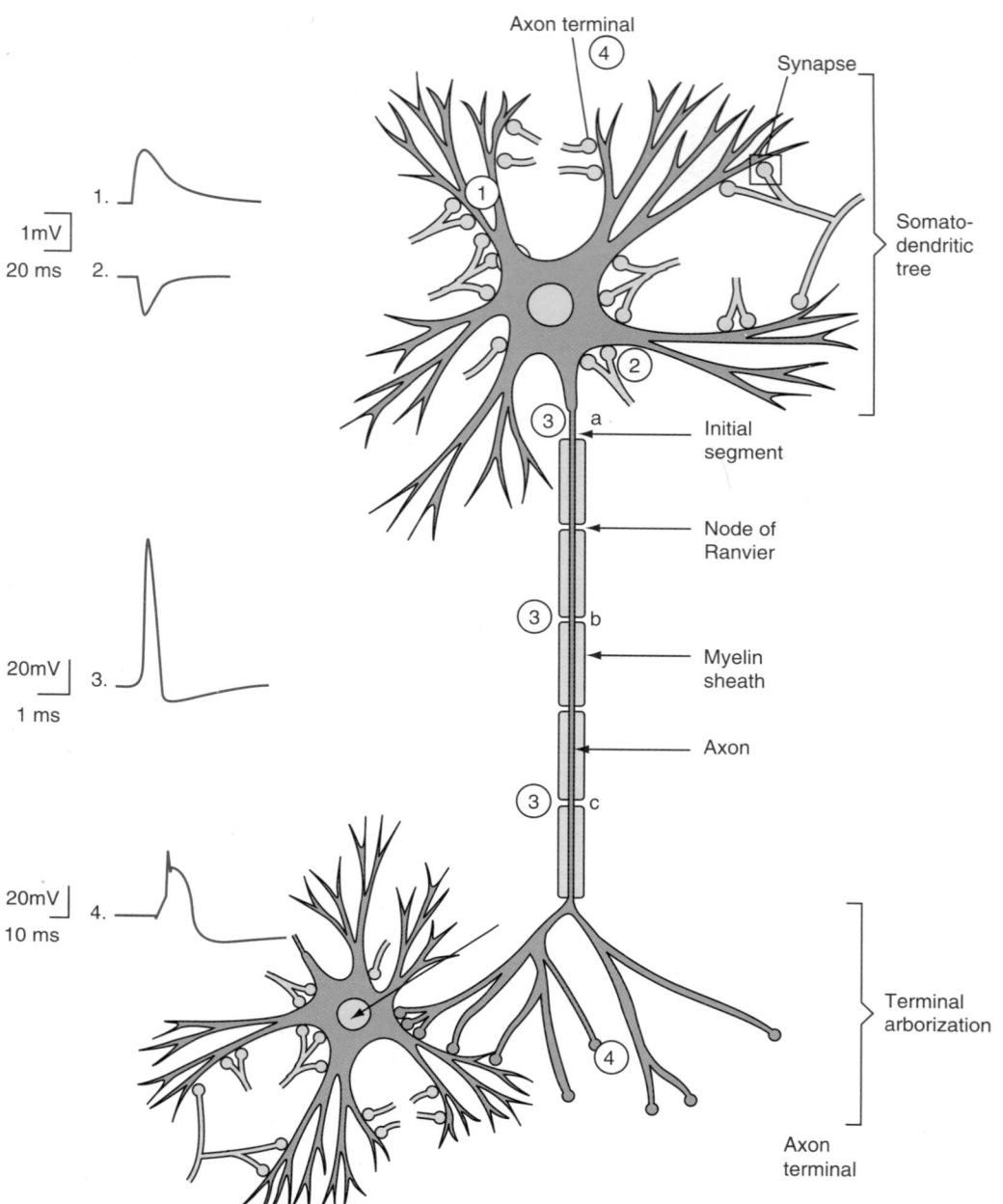

Figure 1.5 Comprehensive schematic drawing of neuron polarity.
The somatodendritic compartment of a neuron receives a large amount of information from other neurons that establish synapses with it. At each synapse level, the neuron generates postsynaptic potentials in response to the released neurotransmitter (1, EPSP; 2, IPSP). These postsynaptic potentials propagate and summate in the somatodendritic compartment, then they propagate to the initial segment of the axon where they generate (or not) action potential(s) (3a). The action potentials propagate along the axon (3b, 3c) and its collaterals up to the axon terminals where they evoke (or not) the entry of calcium (4) and neurotransmitter release. Note the different voltage and time calibrations.

synthesis of macromolecules since it is the one compartment containing all the required organelles.

Compared with other types of cells, the neuron differs at the nuclear level and more specifically at the chromatin and nucleolus levels. The chromatin is light and sparsely distributed: the nucleus is in interphase. Indeed, in humans, most neurons cannot divide after birth since they are postmitotic cells. The nucleolus is the site of ribosomal synthesis and ribosomes are essential for translating messenger RNA (mRNA) into

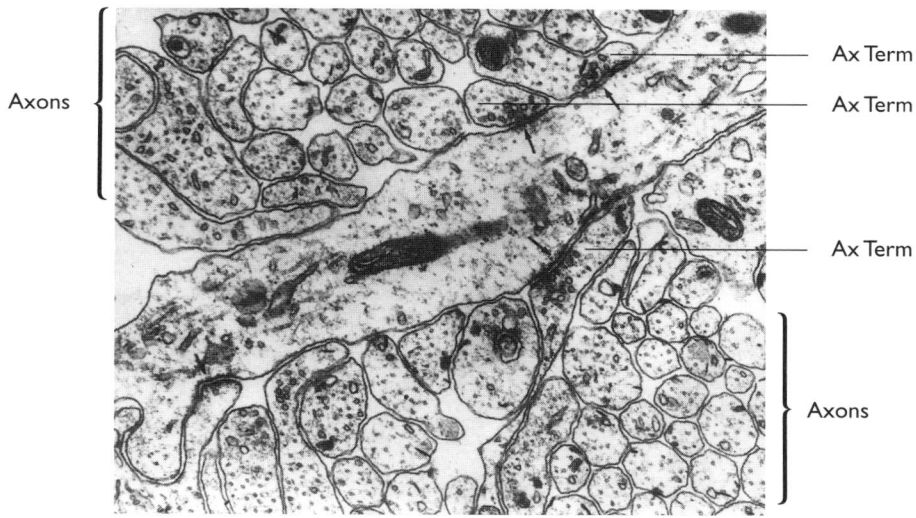

Axons

Ax Term
Ax Term

Ax Term

Axons

Figure 1.6 Photomicrograph of a tissue section of the central nervous system at the hippocampal level.
This shows the ultrastructure of a dendrite, numerous axons and their synaptic contacts (observation under the electron microscope). The apical dendrite of a pyramidal neuron contains mitochondria, microtubules, ribosomes and smooth endoplasmic reticulum. It is surrounded by fascicles of unmyelinated axons with mitochondria and microtubules but no ribosomes. The axon's trajectory is perpendicular to the section plane. Three synaptic boutons (Ax Term) with synaptic vesicles make synaptic contacts (arrows) with the dendrite. Photomicrograph by Olivier Robain.

proteins. The large size of the nucleolus indicates a high level of protein synthesis in neurons.

1.2.2 The dendrites contain free ribosomes and synthesize some of their proteins.

In dendrites can be found smooth endoplasmic reticulum, elongated mitochondria, free ribosomes or polysomes, and numerous cytoskeletal elements including microtubules which are oriented parallel to the long axis of the dendrites (see Appendix 1.1 and **Figure 1.6**).

By using the hook procedure, microtubules have been shown to have two orientations in dendrites (at least in proximal dendrites): half of them are oriented with the plus-ends distal to the cell body, and the other half have the plus-ends proximal to the cell body. This is very different from the orientation in axons, which is uniform (**Figure 1.7**). Moreover, one microtubule-associated protein (MAP), the high-molecular-weight MAP2 protein and more precisely the MAP2A and MAP2B, are more common to dendrites than to axons. For this reason MAP2A or MAP2B antibodies coupled to fluorescent molecules are useful for labelling dendrites, particularly for dendrite identification in cell cultures.

Dendritic spines contain in their neck smooth endoplasmic reticulum of a particular shape. Electron microscopy study shows that it is associated with dense material formed by neurofilaments (see Appendix 1.1).

This is the spiny apparatus and its functions are not fully understood.

mRNA trafficking and local protein synthesis in dendrites

The dendritic compartment contains ribosomes whereas an axon has considerably fewer ribosomes. One particular feature of dendrites, compared with axons, is the presence of synapse-associated polyribosome complexes (SPRCs); these are clusters of polyribosomes and associated membranous cisterns that are selectively localized beneath synapses (more precisely, beneath postsynaptic sites), at the base of dendritic spines when spines are present.

What is the origin of this selective distribution of ribosomes in neurons? This question is particularly important since this compartmentalization leads to different properties of dendrites and axons: dendrites can locally synthesize some of their proteins, whereas axons would synthesize very few of them, if any. Such a local dendritic protein synthesis requires that a particular subset of mRNAs synthesized in the nucleus is transported into the dendrites up to the polysomes where they are translated.

In cultured hippocampal neurons, RNA labelled with tritiated uridin is shown to be transported at a rate of 250–500 μm per day. This transport is blocked by

(a)

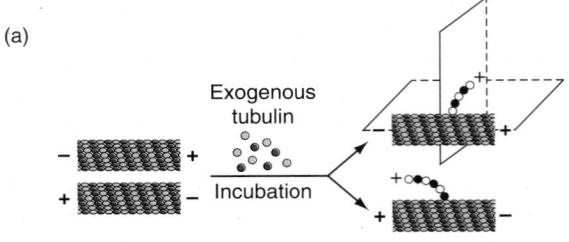

(b)

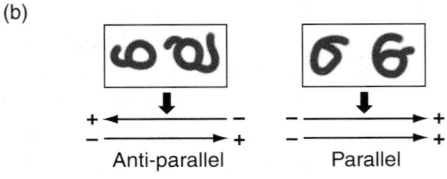

(c)

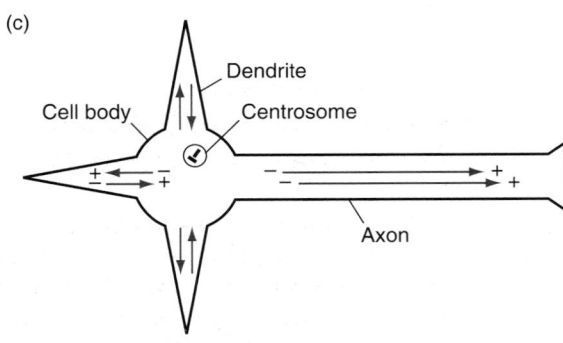

metabolic poisons and the RNA in transit appears to be bound to the cytoskeleton, since much of it remains following detergent extraction of the cells. Studies using video microscopy techniques and cell-permeant dyes which fluoresce on binding to nucleic acids have permitted observation of the movement of RNA-containing granules along microtubules in dendrites. These studies suggest that mRNAs are transported as part of a larger structure. The visualized RNA particles colocalize with poly(A) mRNA, the 60S ribosomal subunit, suggesting that the granules may represent translational units or complexes (**Figure 1.8**). Therefore, this energy-dependent transport seems to be associated with the

Figure 1.7 Microtubule polarity in neuronal processes.
(a) The polarity of microtubules is defined by the hook procedure. Neurons in culture are permeabilized in the presence of taxol to stabilize microtubules. Monomers of tubulin, purified from brain extracts, are added in the extracellular medium. Several minutes after, transversal cuts are performed at the level of dendrites or at the level of an axon. Slices are treated for electron microscopy. Hook-like structures are observed. They result from exogenous tubulin polymerization at the surface of endogenous microtubules. Hooks are always oriented toward the plus-end of microtubules. **(b)** When hooks, at the electron microscopic level, have mixed orientations (clockwise and anticlockwise), this means that endogenous microtubules are antiparallel (left). Uniformly oriented hooks (right) indicate that endogenous microtubules are parallel. **(c)** Orientation of microtubules in dendrites and the axon. Drawing (a) by Lotfi Ferhat. Drawing (b) adapted from Sharp DJ, Wenqian Yu, Ferhat L *et al.* (1997) Identification of a microtubule-associated motor protein essential for dendrite differentiation. *J. Cell. Biol.* **138**, 833–843. Drawing (c) adapted from Baas PW, Deitch JS, Black MM, Banker GA (1988) Polarity orientation of microtubules in hippocampal neurons: uniformity in the axon and nonuniformity in the dendrite, *Proc. Natl Acad. Sci. USA* **85**, 8335–8339, with permission.

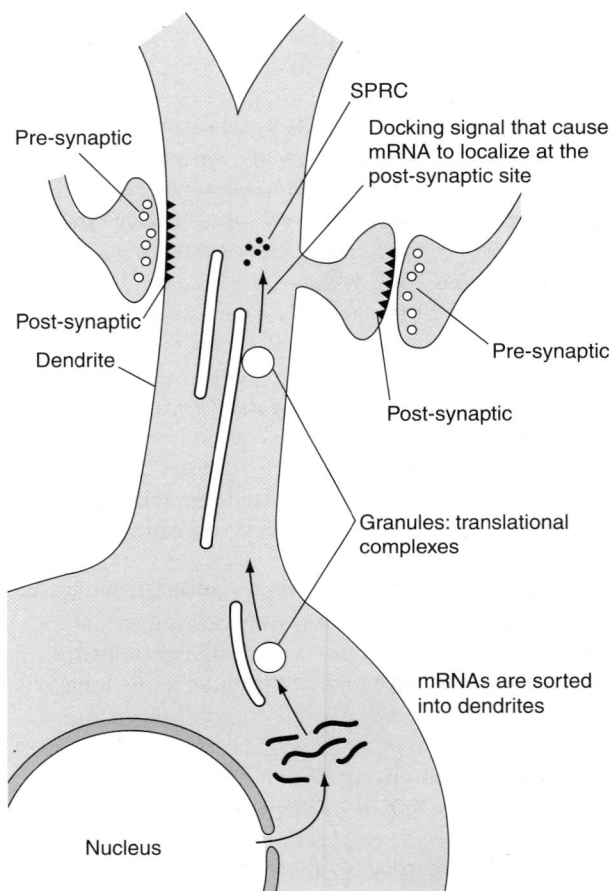

Figure 1.8 Hypothesis concerning the dendritic transport of mRNAs.
Certain mRNAs may contain some sort of signal that enmarks them for delivery into dendrites to synapse-associated polyribosome complexes (SPRCs) via an RNA granule transport system. Drawing adapted from Steward O, Wallace CS, Lyford GL, Worley PF (1998) Synaptic activation causes the mRNA for the IEG *Arc* to localize selectively near activated postsynaptic sites on dendrites. *Neuron* **21**, 741–751; and Knowles RB, Sabry JH, Martone ME *et al.* (1996) Translocation of RNA granules in living neurons, *J. Neurosci.* **16**, 7812–7820, with permission.

dendrite cytoskeleton as also shown by the delocalization of mRNA granules in response to colchicin (a drug which blocks microtubule polymerization).

However, the exact mechanisms underlying the targeting of newly synthesized mRNAs to dendrites – which includes transport (i.e. recognition of particular mRNAs within a granule and movement along microtubules) and docking (shift from a microtubule-based transport to a cytoskeletal-based anchor) – are not yet clear. Experiments performed in neurons on mRNA targeting are based on those performed in insect oocytes where the segregation of mRNAs control anterior–posterior and dorsoventral axes of the embryo.

The mRNAs present in dendrites encode proteins of different functional types. Among the mRNAs detected in dendrites by *in situ* hybridization (see Appendix 7.2) are mRNAs that encode certain cytoskeletal proteins (as the high-molecular-weight MAP2), a kinase (the α subunit of calcium/calmodulin-dependent protein kinase II), an integral membrane protein of the endoplasmic reticulum (the inositol trisphosphate receptor), calcium-binding proteins, certain units of neurotransmitter receptors (the α subunit of the glycine receptor) as well as other proteins of unknown function. Moreover, within dendrites, different mRNAs are localized in different domains and different mRNAs are localized in the dendrites of different neuron types.

The relatively large amount of RNA transported into dendrites raises the question of why neurons need this supply? Targeting of mRNAs to dendritic synthetic machinery located at the base of dendritic spines could occur, for example, in response to synaptic information and trigger local protein synthesis that would be responsible for the stability of the synaptic transmission or the modulation of it (by changing, for example, the subunits or the number of receptors to the neurotransmitter in the postsynaptic membrane).

1.2.3 The axon, to a large extent, lacks the machinery for protein synthesis

The axoplasm is devoid of ribosomes associated to the reticulum or in polysomal form. It contains thin elongated mitochondria, numerous cytoskeletal elements and transport vesicles. Axons therefore cannot restore the macromolecules from which they are made; neither can they ensure alone the synthesis of the neurotransmitter(s) that they release since they are unable to synthesize proteins (such as enzymes).

This problem is resolved by the existence of a continuous supply of macromolecules from the cell body to the axon through anterograde axonal transport (see Section 1.3). Exceptions are the olfactory neurons and the neurons of the hypothalamo-hypophyseal tract. In

the former, mRNAs for various odorant receptors, and in the latter, mRNAs encoding the neuropeptide neurotransmitters oxytocin, vasopressin and prodynorphin, are found in high abundance in their axon terminals. The significance of the localization of mRNAs in these axon terminals where ribosomes are absent remains to be resolved.

Another major difference between dendrites and axons is the orientation of microtubules. By using the hook procedure (see **Figure 1.7** and Appendix 1.1) it has been shown that the polarity of microtubules is uniform in the axon, meaning that all their plus-ends point away from the cell body, toward the axon terminals. The polarity of the microtubules is relevant for transport properties (see Section 1.3). Moreover, one MAP, the Tau protein, is more common to axons than to dendrites. Tau antibodies coupled to fluorescent molecules are useful for labelling axons, particularly for axon identification in cell cultures.

1.3 Axonal transport allows bidirectional communication between the cell body and the axon terminals

Axonal transport is the movement of subcellular structures (such as vesicles, mitochondria, etc.) and proteins (like those of the cytoskeleton) from the cell body to axonal sites (nodes of Ranvier, presynaptic release sites, etc.) and from axon terminals to the cell body.

1.3.1 Demonstration of axonal transport

Weiss and Hiscoe (1948) first demonstrated the existence of material transport in growing axons (during development) as in mature axons. Their work consisted of placing a ligature on the chicken sciatic nerve, and then examining the change in diameter of the axons over several weeks. They showed that these neurons became enlarged in their proximal part and presented degenerative signs in their distal part (**Figure 1.9**). The authors suggested that material from the cell body had accumulated above the ligature and ensured the survival of the distal part.

Later Lubinska *et al.* (1964) elaborated the concept of anterograde and retrograde transport. These authors placed two ligatures on a dog sciatic nerve, isolated part of the nerve and divided it into short segments in order to analyse their acetylcholinesterase content. This enzyme is responsible for acetylcholine degradation and was used here as a marker. They showed that it accumulates at the level of both ligatures. This result therefore suggested the existence of two types of transport: an anterograde transport (from cell body to terminals) and

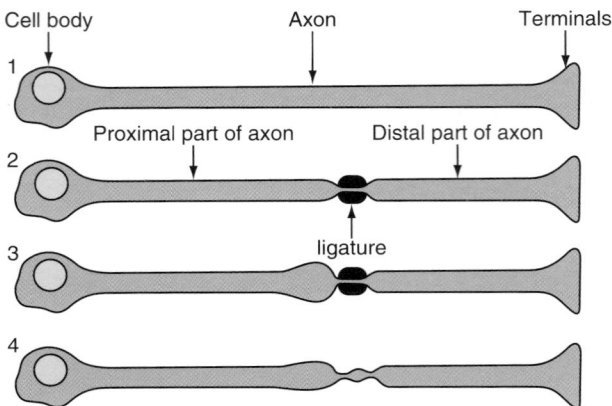

Figure 1.9 Experiment by Weiss and others demonstrating anterograde axonal transport.
Schematic of a chicken motoneuron (1). When a ligature is placed on the axon (2) an enlargement of the axon's diameter above the ligature is noted after several weeks (3). When this ligature is removed, the enlargement progressively disappears (4). From Weiss P, Hiscoe HB (1948) Experiments on the mechanism of nerve growth, *J. Exp. Zool.* **107**, 315–396, with permission.

a retrograde transport (from terminals to cell body). Moreover, it appeared that both types of transport are distributed along the entire extent of the axon.

We presently know of three types of axonal transport: fast (anterograde and retrograde), slow (anterograde) and mitochondrial.

1.3.2 Fast anterograde axonal transport is responsible for the movement of membranous organelles from cell body towards axon terminals, and allows renewal of axonal proteins

Fast anterograde axonal transport consists in the movement of vesicles along the axonal microtubules at a rate of 100–400 mm per day. These transport vesicles, which are 40–60 nm in diameter, are formed by the Golgi apparatus in the cell body (**Figure 1.10a**). They transport, among other things, proteins required to renew plasma membrane and internal axonal membranes, neurotransmitter synthesis enzymes and neurotransmitter precursors when the neurotransmitter is a peptide. This transport is independent of the type of axon (central, peripheral, etc.).

The most currently used preparation

The squid's giant axon is most commonly used for these observations since its axoplasm can easily be extruded

and a translucent cylinder of axoplasm devoid of its membrane is thus obtained. This living extruded axon keeps its transport properties for several hours. The absence of plasma membrane allows a precise control of the experimental conditions and entry into the axoplasm of several components that cannot usually pass through the membrane barrier *in vivo* (e.g. antibodies). The improvement of video techniques applied to light microscopy allowed the first observations of the movement of a multitude of small particles along the microtubules in a living extruded axon.

Identification of the moving organelles and their substrates

Analysis of the particles that accumulate on each side of the 1.0–1.5 mm long isolated frozen segments of the squid axon has permitted the identification of moving organelles in axons. Correlation between video and electron microscopy images of these axonal segments has shown that the particles moving anterogradely on video images are small vesicles (**Figure 1.10a**). Indeed, when a purified fraction of small labelled vesicles (with fluorescent dyes) is placed in an extruded axon, these vesicles and also native vesicles are transported essentially in the anterograde direction.

Evidence demonstrating the implication of microtubules in fast anterograde transport came from experiments with antimitotic agents (colchicin, vinblastin) which prevent the elongation of microtubules and block this transport. Finally, video techniques have also demonstrated that the vesicles are associated to microtubules by arms of 25–30 nm length (**Figure 1.11a**).

The role of ATP and kinesin

By analogy with actin–myosin movements in muscle cells, scientists tried to isolate in neurons an ATPase (the enzyme responsible for the hydrolysis of ATP) associated with microtubules and able to generate the movement of vesicles. To demonstrate molecular components responsible for interactions between vesicles and microtubules, the vesicle–microtubule complex system has been reconstituted *in vitro*: isolated vesicles from squid giant axons are added to a preparation of purified microtubules and placed on a glass coverslip. These vesicles occasionally move in the presence of ATP. If an extract of solubilized axoplasm is then added to this system the number of transported vesicles is considerably increased.

In order to determine the factor present in the solubilized fraction responsible for vesicle movement, a non-hydrolysable ATP analogue has been used: the

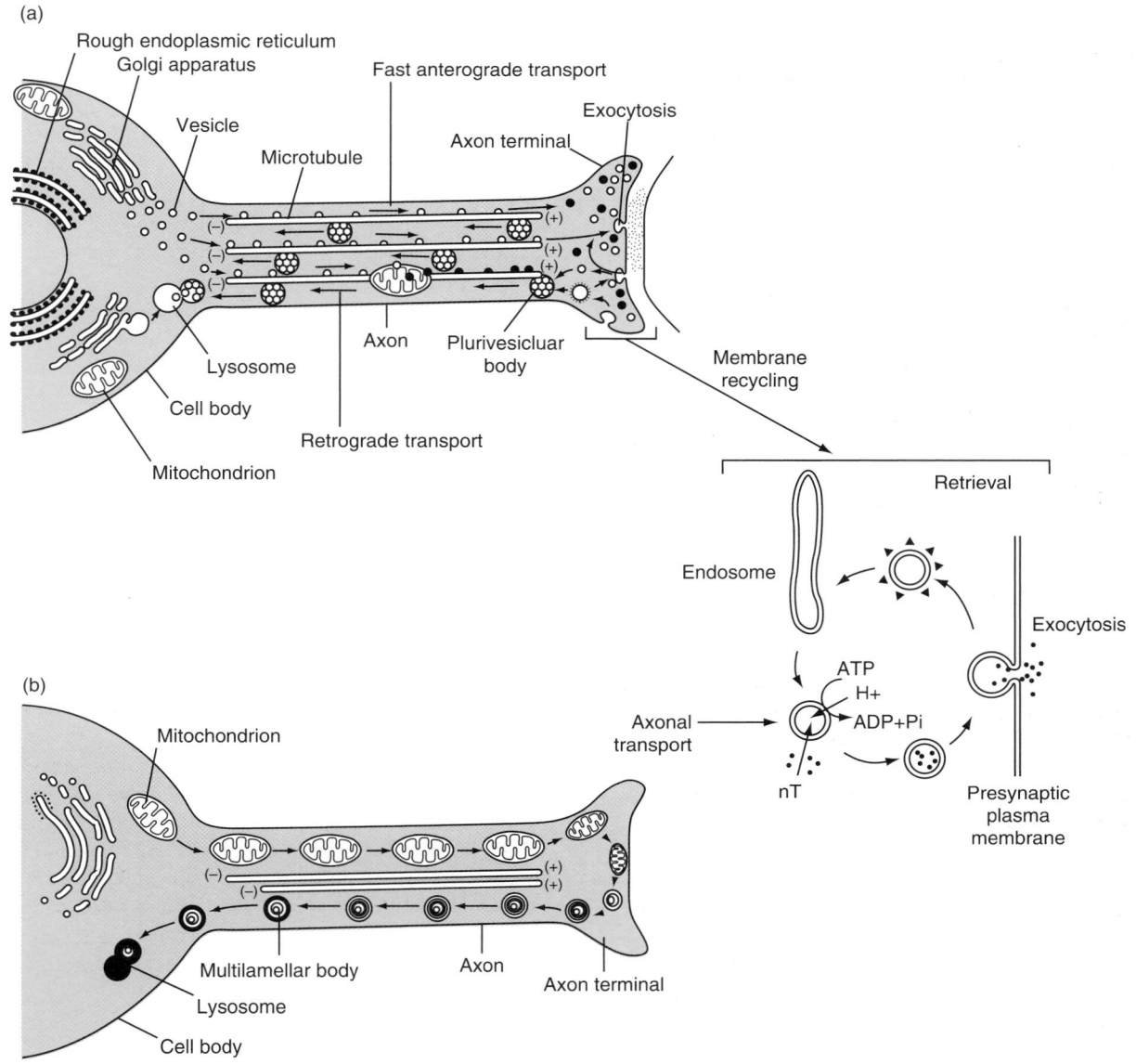

Figure 1.10 Fast axonal transport.

(a) Schematic of fast anterograde axonal transport (anterograde movement of vesicles) and retrograde axonal transport (retrograde movement of plurivesicular bodies). These two transports use microtubules as substrate. The detail shows recycling of small synaptic vesicles. Vesicles synthetized in the cell body and transported to the axon terminals are loaded with cytoplasmic neurotransmitter and targeted to the presynaptic plasma membrane. In response to Ca^{2+} entry, they fuse with the plasma membrane, release their content into the synaptic cleft (exocytosis); then they are recycled via an endosomal compartment. **(b)** Schematic of mitochondrial transport. Note that the neuron representation is extremely schematic since axons do not give off *one* axon terminal. Drawing (a) adapted from Allen R (1987) Les trottoirs roulants de la cellule, *Pour la Science*, April, 52–66; and Südhof TC, Jahn R (1991). Proteins of synaptic vesicles involved in exocytosis and membrane recycling, *Neuron* **6**, 665–77, with permission. Drawing (b) adapted from Lasek RJ, Katz M (1987) Mechanisms at the axon tip regulate metabolic processes critical to axonal elongation, *Prog. Brain Res.* **71**, 49–60, with permission.

5′-adenylyl imidophosphate (AMP-PNP). In the presence of AMP-PNP, the vesicles associate with the microtubules but then stop. In these conditions, vesicles are bound to the microtubules and also, consequently, to the transport factor. When an overdose of ATP is added to this vesicle–microtubule complex isolated by centrifugation, the AMP-PNP is removed and so vesicles are released and the transport factor is solubilized. Kinesin has been thus isolated and purified. It is a soluble microtubule-associated ATPase that couples ATP hydrolysis

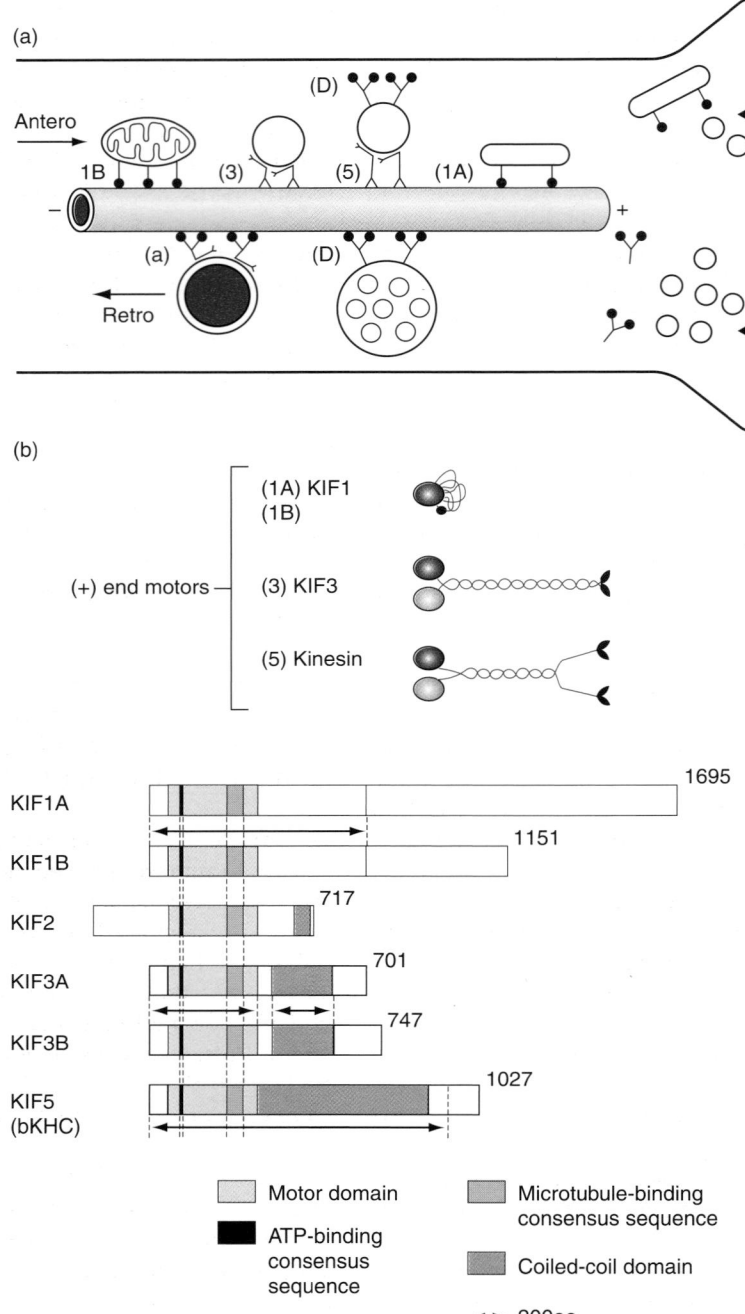

Figure 1.11 The motors of fast anterograde and retrograde axonal transport.
(a) Schematic of KIFs and their cargoes in the nerve axon. *Fast anterograde transport:* Synaptic vesicle precursors are transported by the monomeric KIF1A (1A); mitochondria are transported by monomeric KIF1B (1B); KIF3A–KIF3B heterodimers (3) and homodimer kinesin (5) convey unknown membranous organelles distinct from synaptic vesicle precursors. *Retrograde transport:* Multivesicular bodies, prelysosomal membranous organelles and endosomes are transported by brain dynein (D) and other unknown retrograde motors (U). The plus-end (fast-growing end) of the microtubule array in the axon points toward axon terminals. Insets: schematics of the KIFs, based on electron microscopy studies or predicted from analysis of primary structures. **(b)** Structure of cDNAs for murine kinesin superfamily (KIFs, plus-end motors). bKHC stands for 'brain kinesin heavy chain'. The motor domain is shown in green; KIF1, KIF3 and KIF5 are N-terminal motors whereas KIF2 is a central-motor-domain type. C-terminal motor domain types are not shown. Adapted from Hirokawa N (1996) Organelle transport along microtubules: the role of KIFs, *Trends Cell Biol.* **6**, 135–141. Insets in (a) adapted from Hirokawa N (1998) Kinesin and dynein superfamily proteins and the mechanism of organelle transport, *Science* **279**, 519–526, with permission.

to unidirectional movement of vesicles along the microtubule. As we have already seen, in axons, all microtubules are oriented, their plus-end being distally located from the cell body. It has been shown that kinesin moves vesicles in one direction only: from the minus-end toward the plus-end. All these results show that kinesin is responsible for anterograde transport. In mammals, kinesin is a homodimer composed of two identical heavy chains associated with two light chains. These form a 80 nm rod-like molecule consisting of two globular head domains (formed by the heavy chains), a stalk domain and a tail domain (formed by the light chains) (**Figure 1.11a**). Kinesin is a microtubule-associated protein (MAP) belonging to the family of mechanochemical ATPases.

In proposed mechanism models, the arms observed between vesicles and microtubules *in vitro* would be kinesin. The head transiently binds to microtubules whereas the tail would be, directly or indirectly, associated to membranous organelles. The head binds to and dissociates from a microtubule through a cycle of ATP hydrolysis.

The effects of mutations of the kinesin heavy-chain gene (*khc*) on the physiology and ultrastructure of *Drosophila* larval neurons have been studied. Motoneuron activity and corresponding synaptic (junctional) excitatory potentials of the muscle cells they innervate were recorded in control and mutant larvae in response to segmental nerve stimulation. The mutations dramatically reduced the evoked motoneuron activity and synaptic responses. The synaptic responses were reduced even when the terminals were directly stimulated. However, there was no apparent effect on the number of axons in the nerve bundle or the number of synaptic vesicles in the nerve terminal cytoplasm. These observations show that kinesin mutations impair the function of action potential propagation and neurotransmitter release at nerve terminals. Thus kinesin appears to be required for axonal transport of material other than synaptic vesicles: for example vesicles containing ion channels such as Na$^+$ channels delivered to Ranvier nodes and Ca^{2+} channels delivered to presynaptic membranes. These vesicles, called 'cargoes', are linked to kinesin. The observation that mutation of kinesin heavy chain had no effect on the number of synaptic vesicles within nerve terminals would obviously not be expected if conventional kinesin were the universal anterograde axonal transport motor.

Plus-end vesicle motors

Since the original discovery of kinesin, a large family of proteins with homology to kinesin's motor domain has been discovered. Members of the kinesin family (KIFs)

are defined by the presence of a conserved, about 350-amino-acid motor domain with ATP and putative microtubule binding sites (**Figure 1.11b**). At least 10 kinesin-related proteins are expressed primarily in postmitotic neurons. They have either a monomeric (KIF1A, KIF1B), a homodimeric (kinesin or KIF5, KIF2) or a heterodimeric (KIF3A, KIF3B) structure. They are plus-end motors that transport cargoes from the minus-end of microtubules toward their plus-end; i.e. from the cell body toward axon terminals. The motor domain is necessary and sufficient for ATP-driven movement along microtubules. The hypothesis is that each KIF member is targeted to a specific cargo population, allowing the trafficking of the different neuronal compartments to be regulated independently. Immunocytochemistry and subcellular fractionation have shown, for example, that mitochondria and precursors of synaptic vesicles have their own motors, KIF1B and KIF1A, respectively (**Figure 1.11a**). The question of how each individual motor identifies its own cargo is not yet answered.

1.3.3 Retrograde axonal transport is responsible for the movement of membranous organelles back from axon terminals to the cell body

Retrograde axonal transport allows debris elimination and could represent a feedback mechanism for controlling the metabolic activity of the soma. The vesicles or cargoes transported retrogradely are larger (100–300 nm) than those transported anterogradely. Structurally they are pre-lysosomal structures, multivesicular or multilamellar bodies (**Figures 1.10** and **1.11a**). In the squid extruded axoplasm, vesicles move on to each filament in both directions and frequently cross each other without apparent collisions or interactions.

Do filaments used for the fast transport of vesicles form a complex made up of several distinct filaments where certain filaments would be implicated in fast anterograde and others in retrograde transport? By using a monoclonal antibody raised against α-tubulin (a specific component of microtubules; see Appendix 1.1) it has been demonstrated that all the filaments implicated in anterograde or retrograde axonal transport contain α-tubulin. Moreover, by using a toxin-binding actin (and so consequently binding microfilaments) it was shown that filaments used for fast anterograde transport or retrograde transport were devoid of actin in their structure. Thus it appeared that filaments used for the movement of vesicles in both directions are microtubules.

The minus-end motor(s)

Morphometric analysis of the arms between retrograde vesicles (pluricellular bodies) and microtubules demonstrated that these are similar to arms between antero-grade vesicles and microtubules. Studies looking to find a factor different from, but homologous to, kinesin and responsible for retrograde transport were undertaken. This factor present in axoplasm homogenate might be lost during kinesin purification procedures since no retrograde vesicles movement was observed *in vitro* with kinesin. Cytoplasmic dynein (also called MAP1C) has been thus isolated. It is a microtubule-associated protein with an ATPase activity (see Figure 1.11a). Cytoplasmic dynein would have to interact with other protein(s) to bind to cargoes. Moreover, cytoplasmic dynein may not be the sole minus-end vesicle motor in neurons.

What mechanism regulates the direction of vesicle movement?

It can be hypothesized that kinesin and dynein are bound to only one type of vesicle, specific receptors present at their surface recognizing only one of the two motors. Or both motors might be located on the different vesicles, and by a regulation mechanism only one type is active and so transport takes place in only one direction. Anterogradely transported vesicle populations isolated from squid axoplasm have been shown to both carry dynein. Kinesin, in contrast, is associated only with anterogradely moving organelles. Under control conditions, the anterograde vesicles move strictly in the plus-end direction, showing that plus-end kinesin motors override the activity of dynein motors. These findings suggest that the direction of transport could be regulated via the presence or absence of tightly bound kinesin motors on the vesicle. This suggests that kinesin needs to be absent for the function of dynein to express.

Functions of retrograde transport

Retrograde axonal transport allows the return of membrane molecules to cell bodies, where they are degraded by acidic hydrolases found in lysosomes. Retrograde axonal transport is not only a means of transporting cellular debris for their elimination, but also a way of communicating information from the axon terminals to the soma. The retrogradely transported molecules would inform the cell body about activities taking place at the axon terminal level, or they may even have a neurotrophic action on the neuron. Nerve growth factor (NGF) and fibroblastic growth factor (FGF), trophic substances released by cells and taken up by endocytosis at the axon terminal level, are transported to the cell body where they have a trophic function. This uptake seems to be the major entry of NGF into neurons.

Moreover, it allows the transport of tetanus toxin or cholera toxin macromolecules that are taken up by axon terminals and have a toxic effect on the cell body. These toxins, as well as horseradish peroxidase (HRP), an enzyme taken up by the axon terminals, are used for the retrograde labelling of neuronal pathways.

In conclusion, cargoes are transported in either the antero- or retrograde direction, depending on whether plus- or minus-end motors are active on their surface. Cargoes destined for the nerve terminal, such as synaptic vesicles or their precursors, are transported by plus-end motors; while cargoes targeted for the cell body, such as vesicles containing neurotrophin-receptor complexes, are transported by minus-end motors. In axons, oriented microtubules establish a 'road map' inside the neuron to motors that are linked to particular intracellular cargoes.

1.3.4 Slow anterograde axonal transport moves cytoskeletal proteins and cytosoluble proteins

The cytoskeleton (microtubules, neurofilaments and microfilaments; see Appendix 1.1) and cytosoluble proteins (intermediate metabolic enzymes including glycolysis enzymes) are transported anterogradely at a slow rate. Slow anterograde transport is composed of:

■ the slow component 'a' (SCa) which travels at 0.1–1.0 mm per day and consists mainly of tubulin and the neurofilament subunit polypeptides;
■ the slow component 'b' (Scb) which travels at 2–8 mm per day and includes actin, regulatory proteins and metabolic enzymes.

Slow anterograde transport ensures the renewal of 80% of the total proteins present in the axon. In the elongating axon (i.e. during development or regeneration) the function of the slow transport is to supply axoplasm required for axonal growth. In mature neurons its function is to renew continuously the cytoskeleton and to act as a substrate for the anterograde and retrograde axonal transport.

In contrast to fast anterograde transport, the slow transport is specific to the axon type. For example, the nature of the transported components is different in peripheral and central axons. The mechanisms involved in slow axonal transport have remained primarily unknown. Several questions can be raised: (i) in which state are cytoskeletal proteins transported in the axons: as soluble proteins or as polymers? (ii) in which axonal region(s) is the cytoskeleton (i.e. the complex network of filaments) assembled? and (iii) how are the assembly and the interactions between different cytoskeletal elements regulated? The following are two of the hypotheses that have been proposed:

The different cytoskeletal elements may be assembled and connected by bridges in the cell body

They then progress as a whole (a matrix) in the axon. However, studies have demonstrated that crossbridges between the different cytoskeletal elements are weak and unstable. Moreover, numerous cytoskeletal discontinuities exist along the axon as seen in the nodes of Ranvier. Thus, the hypothesis of a continuous elaboration of a stable matrix of assembled cytoskeletal elements explaining the ultrastructure of the axon is very unlikely.

The cytoskeletal proteins may be transported in a soluble form or as isolated fibrils and assembled during their progression

Lasek and his colleagues proposed that the microtubules and other cytoskeletal elements in slow transport are moved as polymer by sliding. When they are assembled some become stationary and would be renewed on-site (**Figure 1.12**).

This was demonstrated by pulse-labelling studies and particularly those coupled with photobleaching experiments. Purified subunits of cytoskeletal proteins (tubulin or actin) coupled to a fluorescent dye molecule are introduced into living neurons in culture by injection into their soma. The observation with fluorescent microscopy shows that these labelled subunits are gradually incorporated into the polymer pool of the corresponding cytoskeletal proteins (microtubules and microfilaments) throughout the axon. A highly focused light source is then used to extinguish or bleach the fluorescence of the molecules contained within a discrete axonal segment. The fate of the bleached zone is followed over a period of hours. The bleached zone does not move along the axon or widen and recovers a low level of fluorescence within seconds. This latter effect is ascribed to the diffusion of free fluorescent subunits from the neighbouring fluorescent regions into the bleached region. These observations suggest that microtubules and microfilaments are essentially stationary and are exchanging subunits.

1.3.5 Axonal transport of mitochondria allows the turnover of mitochondria in axons and axon terminals

The mitochondria recently formed in the cell body are transported anterogradely in axons up to axon terminals

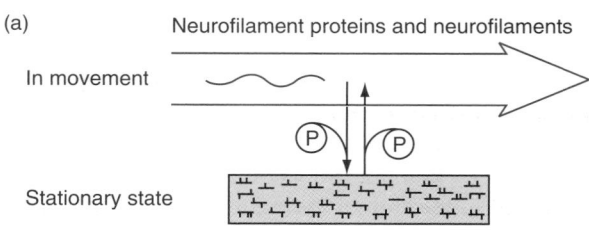

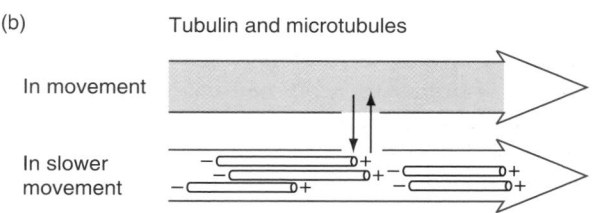

Figure 1.12 Model of slow axonal transport.
The cytoskeletal elements would be present in the axon as two forms in equilibrium with one another: a stationary (or in very slow movement) form and a form in slow movement. **(a)** Soon after their synthesis, insoluble neurofilament proteins are in polymeric or oligomeric form and move toward the axon terminals interchanging with a pool of neurofilaments in the polymeric and stationary form. The transition between both pools depends on the phosphorylation state of the neurofilament proteins. **(b)** A pool of tubulin in dimeric or insoluble oligomeric form and a pool of polymerized tubulin progress at different rates. The passage from one pool to another is made by addition of tubulin dimers at the plus-end of the microtubules. From Hollenbeck PJ (1989) The transport and assembly of the axonal cytoskeleton, *J. Cell Biol.* **108**, 223–227. Reproduced with permission of Rockfeller University Press.

at a rate of 10–40 mm per day. A retrograde movement of mitochondria showing degenerative signs is also observed (see **Figure 1.10b**). The plus-end motor KIF1B (**Figure 1.11**) has been shown to be associated with mitochondria with subcellular fractionation, and purified KIF1B can transport mitochondria along microtubules *in vitro*. This strongly suggests that KIF1B works as a motor for anterograde transport of mitochondria.

1.4 Neurons connected by synapses form networks or circuits

1.4.1 The circuit of the withdrawal medullary reflex

Sensory stimuli (including visual, auditive, tactile, gustative, olfactory, proprioceptive, and nociceptive stimuli) are detected by specific sensory receptors and transmitted to the central nervous system (encephalon and spinal cord) by networks of neurons. These stimuli are analysed at the encephalic level. They can also evoke movements such as motor reflexes on their way to higher central structures.

Thus, when a noxious stimulus (i.e. a stimulus provoking tissue damage, for example pricking or burning) is applied to the skin of the right foot, it induces a withdrawal reflex consisting of the removal of the affected foot (contraction of flexor muscles of the right inferior limb) to protect itself against this stimulus. The noxious stimulus activates nociceptors which are the peripheral endings of primary sensory neurons whose cell bodies are located, in this case, where injury is located at the body level – in dorsal root ganglia. Action potentials are then generated (or not, if the intensity of the noxious stimulus is too small) in primary sensory neurons and propagate to the central nervous system (spinal cord). Local circuit neurons of the dorsal horn of the spinal cord (**Figure 1.13a**) relay the sensory information. Sensory information is thus transmitted to motoneurons (neurons innervating skeletal striated muscles and located in the ventral horn) through a complex network of local circuit neurons (Golgi type II neurons) which have either an excitatory or an inhibitory effect. It results on the stimulus side (ipsilateral side) in an activation of the flexor motoneurons (F) and an inhibition of the extensor motoneurons (E): the right inferior limb is being withdrawn (is in flexion). The opposite limb is extended to maintain posture.

This pathway illustrates peculiarities present in numerous other circuits.

■ *Divergence of information*. Primary sensory information is distributed to several types of neurons in the medulla: local circuit neurons connected to motoneurons that innervate posterior limb muscles and also projection neurons that relay sensory informations to higher centres where they are analysed.

■ *Convergence of information*. Motoneurons receive sensory informations via local circuit neurons and also descending motor information via descending neurons whose cell bodies are located in central motor regions (motor commands elaborated at the encephalic level) (**Figure 1.13a**).

■ *Anterograde inhibition* (feedforward inhibition). A neuron inhibits another neuron by the activation of an inhibitory interneuron (**Figure 1.13b**).

■ *Recurrent inhibition* (feedback inhibition). A neuron inhibits itself by a recurrent collateral of its own axon which synapses on an inhibitory interneuron. The inhibitory interneuron establishes synapses on the motoneuron (**Figure 1.13c**). This recurrent inhibition allows for rapid cessation of the motoneuron's activity.

The last two circuits described are also called *microcircuits*, since they are included in a larger circuit or *macrocircuit*. In this selected example, all the neurons forming the microcircuit enable precise regulation of motoneuron activity.

1.4.2 The spinothalamic tract or anterolateral pathway is a somatosensory pathway

Noxious stimuli (temperature and sometimes touch) are detected at the skin level by free nerve endings, are transduced (or not) in action potentials and are conveyed to the somatosensory cortex via relay neurons. Information from the body reaches the dorsal horn neurons of the spinal cord, and information from the face reaches the trigeminal nuclei in the brainstem, via primary sensory neurons whose cell bodies are located in dorsal root ganglia or cranial ganglia, respectively. They relay on projection neurons located in dorsal horns or in trigeminal nuclei which send axons to the thalamus. These axons cross the midline, form a tract in the anterolateral part of the white matter, and terminate in nonspecific thalamic nuclei. Thalamic neurons then send the sensory information to cortical areas specializing in noxious perception (somatosensory cortex). At each level of synapses (dorsal horn or trigeminal nucleus, thalamus, cortex) the somatosensory information is not simply relayed, it is also processed through local microcircuits receiving afferent sensory information and descending information from higher centres which modulate incoming sensory information.

When superposing horizontal sections through the spinal cord (**Figures 1.13a** and **1.14**), it becomes clear that a noxious stimulus applied to the skin of the right inferior limb is transmitted to motoneurons where it can evoke a withdrawal reflex and also reaches the somatosensory cortex where it is analysed. The reflex is evoked before the consciousness of the stimulus because of the longer distance to brain areas than to the ventral horn of the spinal cord.

1.5 Summary: the neuron is an excitable and secretory cell presenting an extreme functional regionalization

This chapter has described how the various functions of neurons, such as their metabolism, excitability and secretion, are localized to specific regions of the neuron. The main neuronal compartments are the dendrites (more precisely postsynaptic sites), soma, axon and axon terminals (more precisely presynaptic sites). These regions are sometimes located at great distances from each other, and so neurons have to resolve the problems

(a)

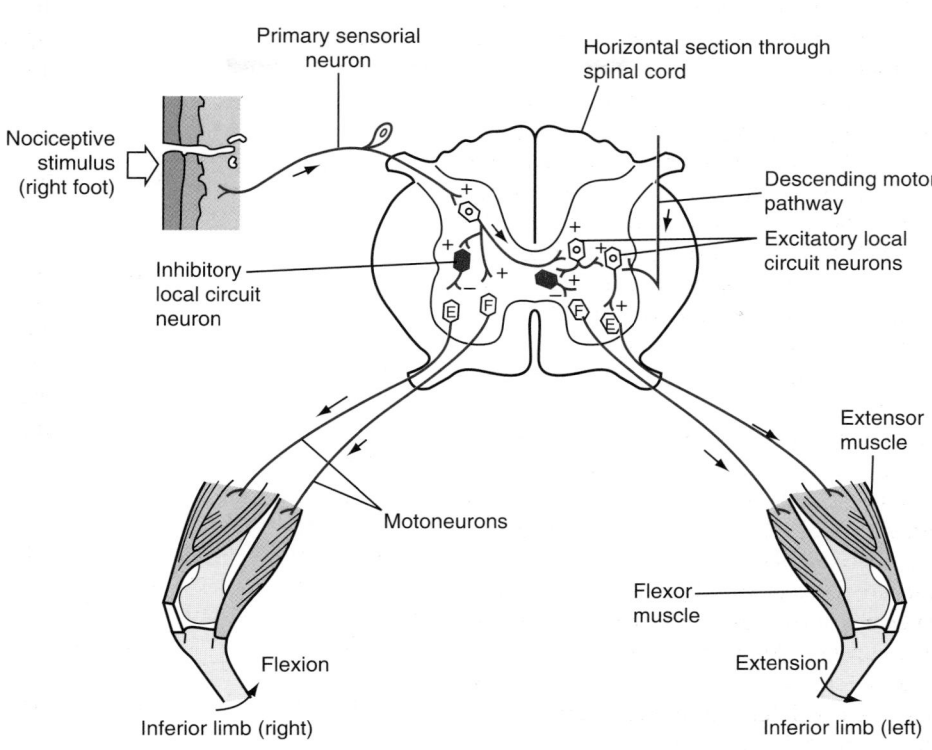

(b)   (c)

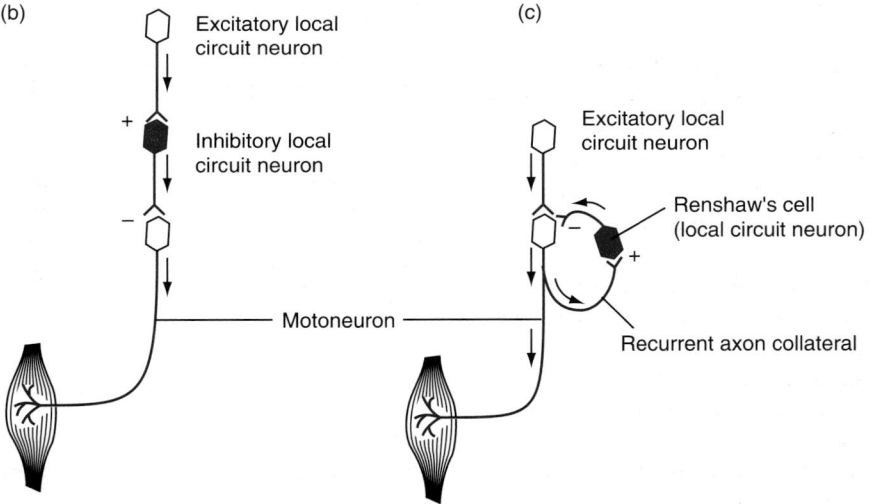

Figure 1.13 Withdrawal medullary reflex pathway.

(a) Schematic of a horizontal section through the spinal cord and of connections between a primary nociceptive sensory neuron, medullary local circuit neurons and ipsi- and contralateral motoneurons innervating inferior limb muscles. See text for details. (b) Anterograde inhibitory circuit. (c) Recurrent inhibitory circuit. Arrows show the direction of action potential propagation.

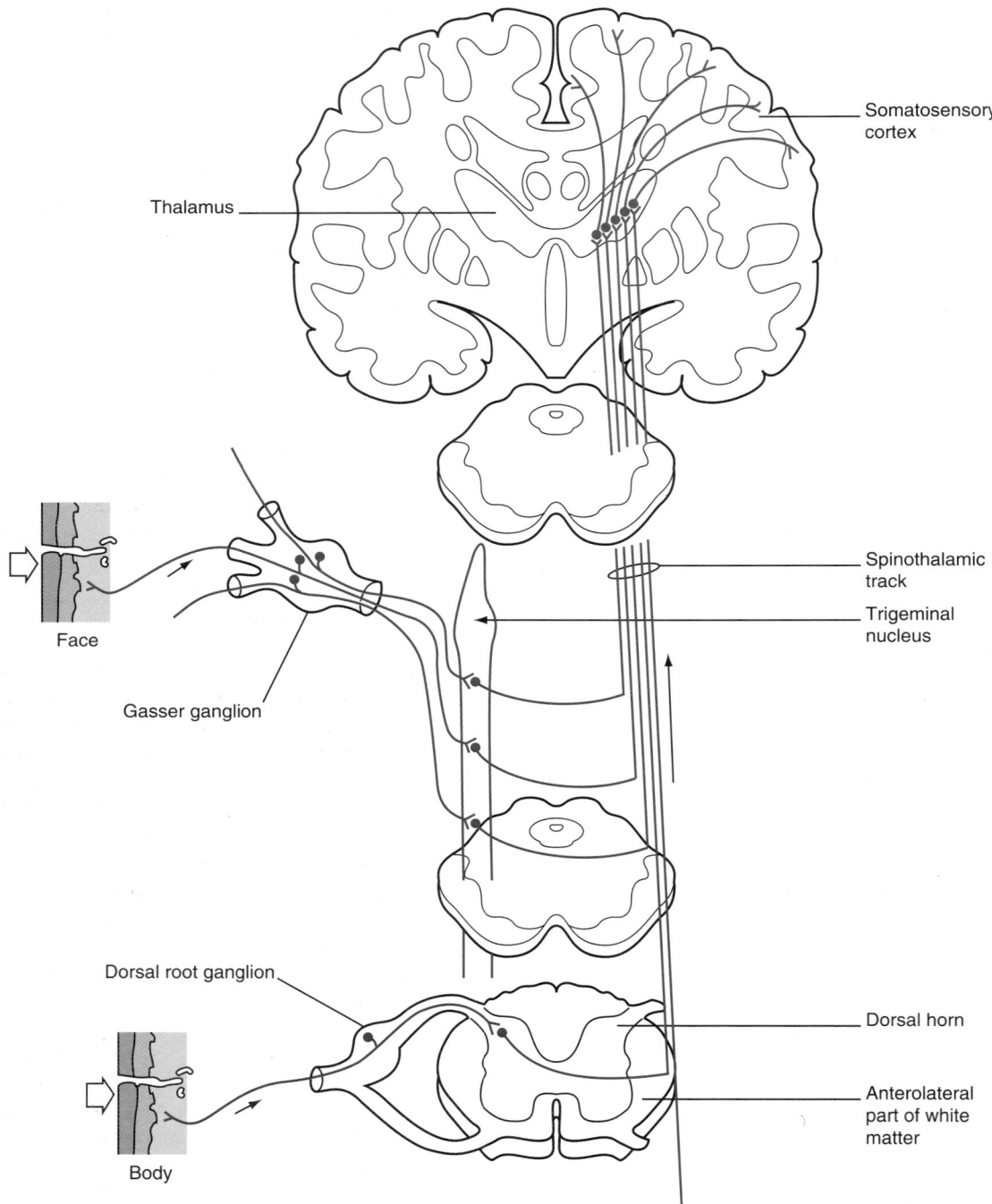

Figure 1.14 The spinothalamic tract or anterolateral ascending sensory pathway.
This pathway integrates and conveys sensory information such as nociception, temperature and some touch. Bottom to top: horizontal sections through the spinal cord, the pons and frontal section through the diencephalon. See text for explanations.

of communication between these regions and harmonization of their activities.

Regionalization of metabolic functions

The essential synthesis activity of a neuron is localized in its cell body, since dendrites can synthesize only some of their proteins, and axons are able to synthesize only a few. In this cell, where the axon's volume represents up to a thousand times the volume of the cell body, the structural and functional integrity of the axon and its terminals requires an important and continuous supply of macromolecules. This supply is ensured by anterograde axonal transport. In dendrites, RNA transport from the cell body to the polysomes has been demonstrated and would allow the synthesis of some of their proteins.

The degradation of cellular metabolism debris and non-neuronal elements taken up from the external environment by endocytosis (e.g. uptake of viruses) takes place in the lysosomes of the cell body. They are transported from axon terminals to the cell body via the retrograde axonal transport. Finally, to coordinate synthesis activity in the cell body with the needs of the axon terminals, the existence of a feedback mechanism (from terminals to cell body) seems essential. This could take place through retrograde axonal transport.

Regionalization of functions implicated in reception and transmission of electrical signals

The neuronal regions receiving synapses are mainly the dendritic (primary segments, branches and spines of dendrites) and somatic regions but also axonal regions. These receptive regions, called postsynaptic elements, have a restricted surface. They contain, within their plasma membrane, proteins specialized in the recognition of neurotransmitters: the neurotransmitter receptors (receptor channels and receptors coupled to G proteins). These proteins synthesized in the cell body are then transported toward the dendritic, somatic or axonal postsynaptic membranes to be incorporated. Similarly, the proteins specialized in the generation and propagation of action potentials (voltage-dependent channels) are synthesized in the soma and have to be transported and incorporated in the axonal membrane.

Regionalization of secretory function

This function is localized in regions making synaptic contacts and more generally in presynaptic regions such as axon terminals (and sometimes in dendritic and somatic regions). At the level of presynaptic structures, the neurotransmitter is stocked in synaptic vesicles and released. The secretory function implicates the presence of specific molecules and organelles in the presynaptic region: neurotransmitter synthesis enzymes, synaptic vesicles, microtubules and associated proteins, voltage-dependent channels, etc.

In conclusion, owing to its extreme regionalization and the extreme length and volume of its processes, the neuron has the challenge to deliver the proteins synthesized in the soma at the appropriate sites (targeting) at appropriate times.

Appendix 1.1
The cytoskeletal elements in neurons

The cytoskeletal elements present in neurons are protein polymers that form a tridimensional network, which acts as the inner structure of the entire intracellular area and forms a specialized architecture in different parts of the neuron: soma, dendrites, dendritic spines, axon and axon terminals. As in every cell, three principal types of filaments exist (**Figure A1.1**): microtubules, microfilaments and neurofilaments.

- Microtubules are hollow cylinders of approximately 25 nm diameter. Their surface is made up of a single type of globular protein, called tubulin. Tubulin is a dimer consisting of two different but homologous 55 kD polypeptides (α-tubulin and β-tubulin). Tubulin dimers bind head to tail (polymerize) to form a protofilament. In general, 13 protofilaments associate laterally to form a sheet whose closure defines the wall of the microtubule. There are particular proteins associated to microtubules, the MAPs (microtubule-associated proteins).
- Microfilaments or actin filaments are thin flexible fibres of approximately 7 nm diameter. They are polymers of actin G. Each filament has the appearance of a double-stranded helix. Because all actin G are oriented in the same direction, actin filaments have a polarity. Actin filaments assemble in bundles or networks with their associated proteins.
- Neurofilaments are a type of intermediate filament with a diameter of approximately 10 nm (they have an intermediate diameter compared with actin and microtubules). They are composed of three different fibrous proteins. They have a central α-helical rod domain, a head and a tail domain.

Microtubules and microfilaments are unstable, dynamic polymers that continuously undergo assembly and disassembly within the cell, whereas the structure of neurofilaments is more stable. Moreover, microfilaments

(a)

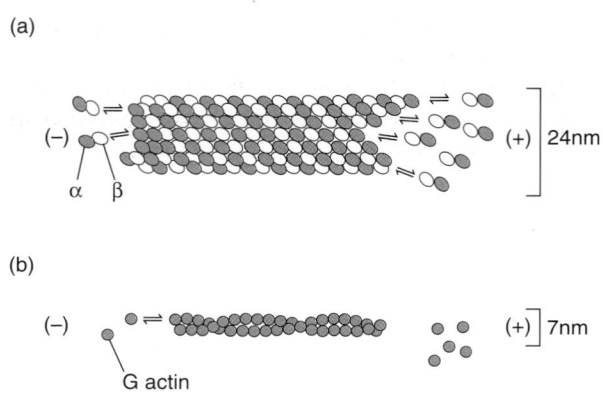

(b)

(c)

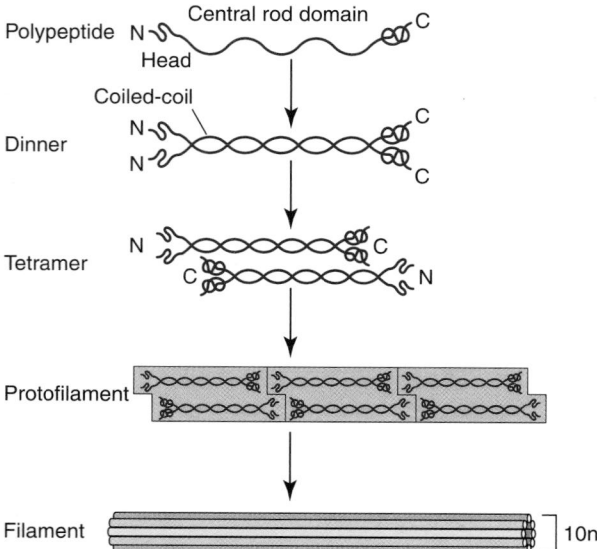

Figure A1.1 The cytoskeletal elements.

(a) The microtubules are composed of 13 rows of tubulin polymers. (b) F-actin or microfilament is formed by two-stranded helices. (c) Assembly of intermediate filaments. Drawing (a) by Lotfi Ferhat. Drawings (b) and (c) adapted from Cooper GM (1997) *The Cell: A Molecular Approach*, Washington, DC: ASM Press.

and microtubules are polarized structures. The microtubules, in the presence of guanosine triphosphate (GTP), polymerize both their ends at different rates: the end denoted 'plus' polymerizes at a higher rate than the end denoted 'minus'. The net result is a polymerization of microtubules at the plus-end that is much faster than at the minus-end (**Figure A1.1a**). Colchicin is an example of a drug that binds tubulin and inhibits microtubule polymerization.

Functions in neurons

They are the skeleton for the cell. The three types of cytoskeletal filaments are joined to each other and to mitochondria, smooth endoplasmic reticulum and vesicles by protein bridges. The network of filaments forms the neuronal skeleton, which gives the neuron its shape and a certain rigidity mostly at the level of its processes.

Cytoskeletal elements are involved in dynamic functions such as growth cone motility of developing neurites, axonal and dendrite differentiation. Indeed, the morphological and functional differences of the different neuronal compartments result in part from the differential distribution of cytoskeletal constituents. The latter have been also implicated in neurotransmitter release, motility, clustering of receptors at postsynaptic sites and synaptic plasticity. Neuronal microtubules support fast anterograde and retrograde axonal transport, and these are mediated by a class of microtubule-associated proteins called 'motor proteins'.

Further reading

Baas PW (1997) Slow axonal transport: the polymer transport model. *Trends Cell Biol.* **7**, 380–384.

Baas PW (1999) Microtubules and neuronal polarity: lessons from mitosis. *Neuron* **22**, 23–31.

Brady ST, Lasek RJ, Allen RD (1982) Fast axonal transport in extruded axoplasm from squid giant axon. *Science* **218**, 1129–1131.

Davies L, Burger B, Banker GA, Steward O (1990) Dendritic transport: quantitative analysis of the time course of somatodendritic transport of recently synthetized RNA. *J. Neurosci.* **10**, 3056–3068.

Gho M, McDonald K, Ganetzky B, Saxton WM (1992) Effects of kinesin mutations on neuronal functions. *Science* **258**, 313–316.

Goldstein LSB, Yang Z (2000) Microtubule-based transport systems in neurons: the roles of kinesins and dyneins. *Ann. Rev. Neurosci.* **23**, 39–71.

Mikami A, Paschal BM, Mazumdar M, Vallee R (1993) Molecular cloning of the retrograde transport motor cytoplasmic dynein (MAP1C). *Neuron* **10**, 787–796.

Muresan V, Godek CP, Reese TS, Schnapp BJ (1996) Plus-end motors override minus-end motors during transport of squid axon vesicles on microtubules. *J. Cell Biol.* **135**, 383–397.

Nangaku M, Sato-Yoshitake R, Okada Y, Noda Y, Takemura R, Yamazaki H, Hirokawa N (1994) KIF1B, a novel microtubule plus-end-directed monomeric motor protein for transport of mitochondria. *Cell* **79**, 1209–1220.

Schnapp BJ, Vale RD, Sheetz MP, Reese TS (1985)

Single microtubules from squid axoplasm support bidirectional movement of organelles. *Cell* **40**, 455–462.

Steward O (1997) mRNA localization in neuron: a multipurpose mechanism? *Neuron* **18**, 9–12.

St Johnston D (1995) The intracellular localization of mRNAs. *Cell* **81**, 161–170.

Vale RD, Reese TS, Sheetz MP (1985) Identification of a novel force-generating protein, kinesin, involved in microtubule-based mobility. *Cell* **42**, 39–50.

Neuron–Glial Cell Cooperation

There are roughly twice as many glial cells as there are neurons in the central nervous system. They occupy the space between neurons and neuronal processes and separate neurons from blood vessels. As a result, the extracellular space between the plasma membranes of different cells is narrow, of the order of 15–20 nm.

Virchow (1846) was the first to propose the existence of non-neuronal tissue in the central nervous system. He named it 'nevroglie' (nerve glue), because it appeared to stick the neurons together. Following this, Deiters (1865) and Golgi (1885) identified glial cells as making up the nevroglie and distinguished them from neurons.

There are several categories of glial cells. Depending on their anatomical position they are classed as follows:

- *Central glia* are found in the central nervous system, and comprise four cell types: astrocytes, oligodendrocytes, microglia (these three types are also known as interstitial glia, because they are found in interneuronal spaces) and ependymal cells which form the epithelial surface covering the walls of the cerebral ventricles and of the central canal of the spinal cord.
- *Peripheral glia* comprise a single type: Schwann cells. These cells ensheath the axons and encapsulate the cell bodies of neurons. In the latter case, they are also called satellite cells.

Glial cells, excluding microglia, have an ectodermal origin. Those of the central nervous system derive from the germinal neural epithelium (neural tube), while peripheral glia (Schwann cells) are derived from the neural crest. Microglia, in contrast, have a mesodermal origin.

Glial cells have morphological as well as functional and metabolic characteristics that distinguish them from neurons:

- They do not generate or conduct action potentials. Thus, although they extend processes, these are only of one type and are neither dendrites nor axons.
- They do not establish chemical synapses between themselves, on to neurons, or any other cell type.

- Unlike most neurons in humans, glial cells are capable of division for at least several years postnatally.

Nervous tissue is made compact by glial cells and for this reason they are often ascribed the role of supporting tissue. However, as we will see in this chapter, they have additional functions.

2.1 Astrocytes form a vast cellular network or syncytium between neurons, blood vessels and the surface of the brain

2.1.1 Astrocytes are star-shaped cells characterized by the presence of glial filaments in their cytoplasm

Astrocytes are small star-shaped cells with numerous fine, tortuous, ramified processes covered with varicosities (**Figure 2.1**). The cell body is typically 9–10 µm in diameter and the processes extend radially over 40–50 µm. These often have enlarged terminals in contact with neurons or non-neuronal tissue (like the walls of blood vessels).

Two kinds of astrocytes are recognized. Some astrocytes contain in their cytoplasm numerous glial filaments: these are fibrillary astrocytes, principally located in the white matter (**Figure 2.1**). They have numerous, radial processes which are infrequently branched and covered with 'expansions en brindilles'. Other astrocytes contain few, if any, glial filaments: these are protoplasmic astrocytes, found normally in the grey matter. They have more delicate processes, some of which are velate (veil-like). Both types of astrocytes send out processes that end on the walls of blood vessels or beneath the pial surface of the brain and spinal cord.

The principal ultrastructural characteristics of astrocytes are the glial filaments and glycogen granules

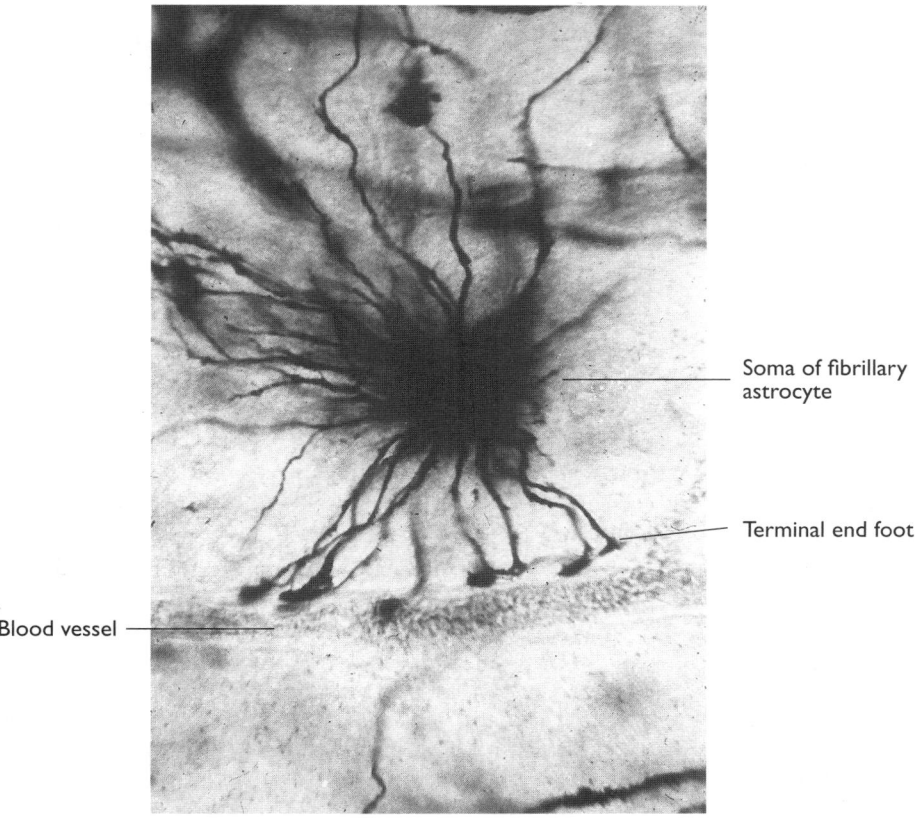

Soma of fibrillary astrocyte

Terminal end foot

Blood vessel

Figure 2.1 Fibrillary astrocyte.
Micrograph of a fibrillary astrocyte stained with a Golgi stain observed through an optical microscope. The processes of this astrocyte make contact with a blood vessel: these are the terminal end feet. Photograph by Olivier Robain.

present in the cytoplasm of their somata and processes. The filaments are 'intermediate filaments' with an average diameter of 8–10 μm. They are composed of a protein specific to astrocytes, glial fibrillary acidic protein (GFAP), consisting of a single type of subunit with a molecular weight of 50 kD, different from that of neurofilaments. This characteristic has been exploited as a method of identifying astrocytes. By using an antiserum to glial fibrillary acidic protein (anti-GFAP) linked to fluorescein, one can stain astrocytes, *in situ* or in culture, without marking either neurons or other types of glial cells.

Astrocytes, like all glial cells, do not form chemical synapses. They do, however, mutually form junctional complexes. Two types of junctions have been demonstrated: communicating junctions (or gap junctions, see **Figure 3.9**) and desmosomes (puncta adhaerentia). Coupled to each other by numerous junctional complexes, astrocytes therefore constitute a vast cellular network, or syncytium, extending from neurons to blood vessels and the external surface of the brain.

2.1.2 Astrocytes maintain the blood–brain barrier in the adult brain

The essential characteristic of astrocytic processes is their termination on the walls of blood vessels in astrocytic end feet (**Figure 2.2**). Here the end feet are joined by gap juntions and desmosomes, forming a 'palisade' between neurons and vascular endothelial cells. The space between the layer of astrocyte end feet and the endothelial cells is about 40–100 nm and is occupied by a basal lamina. Astrocytes also send processes to the external surface of the central nervous system where the astrocyte end feet, together with the basal lamina that they produce, form the 'glia limitans externa', which separates the pia mater from the nervous tissue. Astrocytes therefore constitute a barrier between neurons and the external medium (blood), preventing access of substances foreign to the central nervous system. They thus protect neurons. This barrier is not, however, totally impermeable and astrocytes are involved in selective exchange processes.

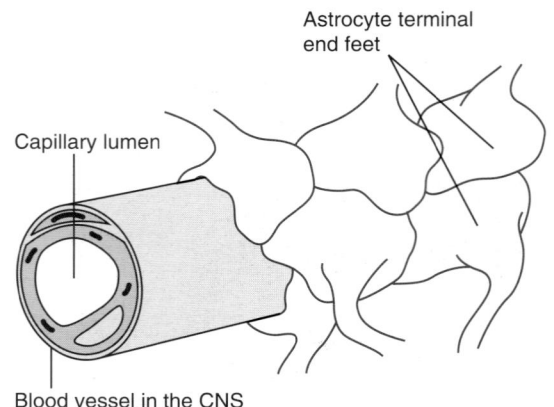

Figure 2.2 Diagram of the covering formed by astrocyte end feet around a capillary in the central nervous system (CNS). From Goldstein G, Betz L (1986) La barrière qui protège le cerveau, *Pour la Science*, November, 84–94, with permission.

Astrocyte end feet are not the blood–brain barrier. This is formed, in most regions of the central nervous system, by vascular endothelial cells joined together by tight junctions. Even though the astrocyte end feet do not form the blood–brain barrier, they have an important role in its development and maintenance. Thus, if the layer of astrocyte end feet in the adult is destroyed, by a tumour or by allergic illnesses, for example, the capillary endothelial cells immediately take on the characteristics normally observed in capillaries outside the central nervous system: they are no longer bound by tight junctions and become 'fenestrated'. In such capillaries the blood–brain barrier no longer exists.

2.1.3 Astrocytes regulate the ionic composition of the extracellular fluid

We have seen that astrocyte end feet are involved in the formation and maintenance of the blood–brain barrier, and that astrocytes thus contribute to regulation of the brain extracellular fluid. However, astrocytes have other important roles in controlling the composition of the extracellular fluid. We shall consider as an example the regulation of the extracellular potassium concentration.

The extracellular potassium concentration needs to be tightly regulated: if potassium increased it would depolarize neurons. This would first increase neuronal excitability and then inactivate action potential propagation. Regulation of the extracellular potassium concentration must occur in the face of large fluxes of potassium ions into the extracellular space during neuronal activity, when potassium ions leave neurons through voltage-activated potassium channels (see Sections 5.3 and 6.3). Astrocytes are thought to regulate extracellular potassium by the mechanism of 'spatial

buffering'. This means that astrocytes take up potassium ions in regions where the concentration rises and eventually release through their end feet an equivalent amount of potassium ions into the vicinity of blood vessels or across the glia limitans externa. The details of the process are complicated, but potassium ions are thought to enter astrocytes via channels or the sodium pump and to exit at the end feet through channels. This potassium buffering role of astrocytes is likely to be of particular importance at the nodes of Ranvier, where marked accumulation of potassium ions in the restricted extracellular space can occur, due to the conduction of action potentials.

2.1.4 Astrocytes take part in the neurotransmitter cycle

After neurotransmitters are released during synaptic transmission, they need to be removed from the extracellular space to prevent the extracellular neurotransmitter concentration from rising. Steady high concentrations of transmitter would interfere with synaptic transmission, and long-lasting activation of receptors (particularly glutamate receptors) can damage neurons. Most transmitters are removed from the extracellular space by reuptake into cells (but acetylcholine is hydrolysed; see **Figure 7.12**). Transmitters are taken up by specialized carrier molecules in the cell membrane. Although both neurons and glia express such carrier proteins, it seems that uptake into astrocytes is of particular importance. This is especially clear for the case of glutamate: astrocytes have an enormous capacity to take up this transmitter, presumably reflecting the abundance of this transmitter and the toxicity to neurons of high glutamate concentrations.

Besides their role in transmitter clearance from the synaptic cleft (by recapture), astrocytes play a role in the synthesis of transmitters and particularly glutamate and GABA. For example, thanks to the presence of glutamine synthetase in astrocytes (see **Figure 11.13**), glutamine is formed from glutamate. Glutamine is then uptaken by neurons and transformed back in glutamate.

2.2 Oligodendrocytes form the myelin sheaths of axons in the central nervous system and allow the clustering of Na+ channels at nodes of Ranvier

Two types of oligodendrocyte are recognized: interfascicular or myelinizing oligodendrocytes, found in the white matter where they make the sheaths of myelinated axons; and satellite oligodendrocytes which surround neuronal somata in the grey matter. We will deal with the former type in detail. Their major role is, by forming the myelin sheath, to electrically isolate segments of axons, induce the formation of clusters of Na^+ channels at nodes of Ranvier and therefore to allow the fast propagation of Na^+ action potentials (see Section 5.4).

2.2.1 Processes of interfascicular oligodendrocytes electrically isolate segments of central axons by forming the lipid-rich myelin sheath

The cell bodies of interfascicular oligodendrocytes are situated between bundles of axons

Interfascicular, or myelinizing, oligodendrocytes have small spherical or polyhedral cell bodies of diameter 6–8 μm and few processes. They are called interfascicular because their cell bodies are aligned between bundles (fascicles) of axons. They are distinguished from astrocytes by the sites of termination of their processes: oligodendrocyte processes enwrap axons and make no contact with blood vessels.

Observed by electron microscopy, the nucleus and perikaryon of oligodendrocytes appear dark (**Figure 2.3**), there are no glial filaments, and there are many microtubules in the somatic and dendritic cytoplasm. Because of this, oligodendrocyte processes may be confused with fine dendrites, and it is by the absence of chemical synapses that the glial processes are identified.

Oligodendrocytes can be identified by immunohistochemistry. This is done using an anti-galactoceramide immune serum (anti-gal-C), galactoceramide being a glycolipid found exclusively in the membrane of processes of myelinizing oligodendrocytes.

The myelin sheath is a compact roll of the plasmalemma of an oligodendrocyte process: this glial membrane is rich in lipids

Myelinated axons are surrounded by a succession of myelin segments, each about 1 mm long. The covered regions of axons alternate with short exposed lengths where the axonal membrane (axolemma) is not covered. These unmyelinated regions (of the order of a micron) are called nodes of Ranvier (**Figures 2.4** and **2.5a**).

A myelinated segment comprises the length of axon covered by an oligodendrocyte. One oligodendrocyte can form 20–70 myelin segments around different axons (**Figure 2.4**). Thus the degeneration or dysfunction of a single oligodendrocyte leads to the disappearance of myelin segments on several different axons.

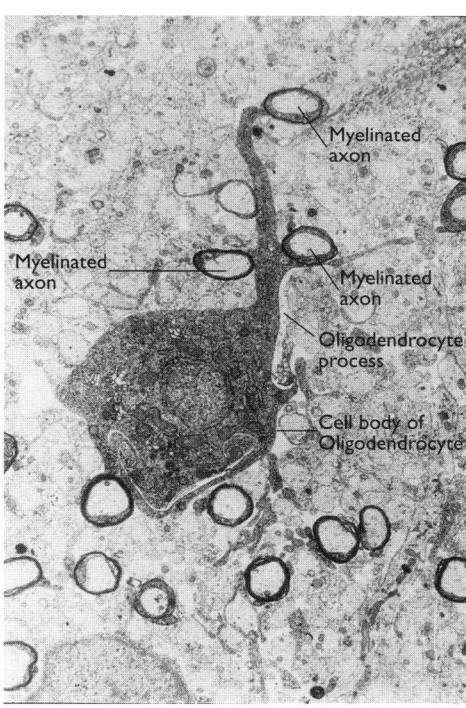

Figure 2.3 Myelinating oligodendrocyte.
Electron micrograph of an oligodendrocyte. The cell body and one of its processes enwrapping several axons can be seen. Section taken through the spinal cord. Photograph by Olivier Robain.

Formation and ultrastructure of a myelin segment

Myelinization represents a crucial stage in the ontogenesis of the nervous system. In the human at birth, myelinization is only just beginning, and in some regions is not complete even by the end of the second year of life. The first step in the process is migration of oligodendrocytes into the bundles of axons, then the myelinization of some, but not all, axons. Once contact has been made between the oligodendrocyte and axon, the initial turn of myelin around the axon is rapidly formed. Myelin is then slowly deposited over a period which in humans can reach several months. Myelinization is responsible for a large part of the increase in weight of the central nervous system following the end of neurogenesis.

In order to form the compact spiral of myelin membrane, the oligodendrocyte process must roll itself around the axon many times (up to 40 turns) (**Figure 2.5**). It is the terminal portion of the process, called the inner loop, situated at the interior of the roll, which progressively spirals around the axon. This movement necessitates the sliding of myelin sheets which are not firmly attached. During this period, the oligodendrocyte synthesizes several times its own weight of myelin membrane each day.

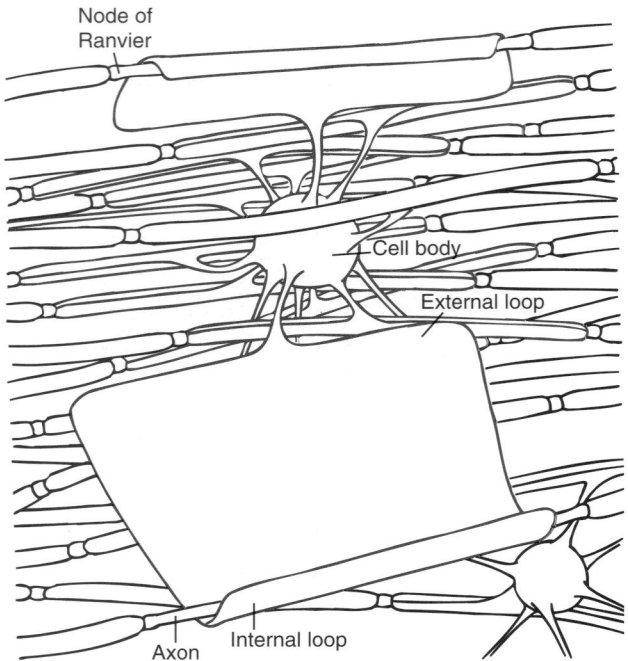

Node of Ranvier

Cell body

External loop

Axon   Internal loop

Figure 2.4 Diagram of a myelinating oligodendrocyte and its numerous processes
which each form a segment of myelin around a different axon in the central nervous system. Two myelin segments are represented, one partially unrolled, the other completely unrolled. Drawing by Tom Prentiss. In Morell P, Norton W (1980) La myéline et la sclérose en plaques, *Pour la Science* **33**, with permission.

Within the spiral the cytoplasm disappears entirely (except at the internal and external loops). The internal leaflets of the plasma membranes can thus adhere to each other. This adhesion is so intimate that the internal leaflets virtually fuse, forming the period, or major, dense line of thickness of 3 nm (**Figure 2.5b**). The extracellular space between the different turns of membrane also disappears, and the external leaflets also stick to each other. This apposition is, however, less close and a small space remains between the external leaflets. The apposed external leaflets form the minor, or interperiod, dense line (**Figure 2.5b**).

Thus, a cross-section of a myelinated axon observed by electron microscopy shows alternating dark and light lines forming a spiral around the axon. The major dense line terminates where the internal leaflets separate to enclose the cytoplasm within the external loop. The interperiod dense line disappears at the surface of the sheath at the end of the spiral (**Figure 2.5b**).

In the central nervous system there is no basal lamina around myelin segments, so myelin segments of adjacent axons may adhere to each other forming an interperiod dense line.

Myelin

Myelin consists of a compact spiral (without intracellular or extracellular space) of glial plasma membrane of a very particular composition. Lipids make up about 70% of the dry weight of myelin and proteins only 30%. Compared with the membranes of other cells, this represents an inversion of the lipid:protein ratio (**Figure 2.6**).

The lipids of myelin are divided into three groups: cholesterol, phospholipids and glycolipids. It is the high proportion of the last group, and of galactoceramide (gal-C) in particular, that characterizes the lipid composition of myelin. This glycolipid, being specific to oligodendrocytes and also very immunogenic, is, as we have already seen, often used as a marker of oligodendrocytes. Another glycolipid, sulfogalactosyl ceramide, is also present in myelin at high concentrations, but is a little less specific since it is found in other cells of the central nervous system.

We have seen that myelin has an inverted lipid:protein ratio, while the cell body membrane of the oligodendrocyte has a ratio comparable to that of other cell membranes. As the myelin of the oligodendrocyte process is in continuity with the plasma membrane of the cell body, it is necessary to postulate gradients in the composition of lipids and proteins (in opposite directions to each other) between the cell body and the various processes.

The proteins of myelin are not only less abundant than in other plasma membranes, but also less varied. Two types of protein characteristic of central myelin predominate: myelin basic proteins (MBPs), so named because they are highly charged proteins soluble in acidic solutions, and proteolipid proteins (PLP/DM20, two splicing derivatives). These, like lipids, are soluble in organic solvents. Myelin basic proteins are found on the cytoplasmic side and play a role in the adhesion of the internal leaflets of the specialized oligodendroglial plasma membrane. Proteolipid proteins are integral membrane proteins. Though they are in high abundance (they represent around 50% of the total myelin protein in the central nervous system) their exact biological role has not yet been elucidated.

Nodes of Ranvier

In the central nervous system the nodes of Ranvier, regions between myelin segments, are relatively long (several microns) compared with those in the peripheral nervous system. Here the axolemma is exposed and an accumulation of dense material is seen on the cytoplasmic side. The myelin sheath does not terminate abruptly. Successive layers of myelin membrane

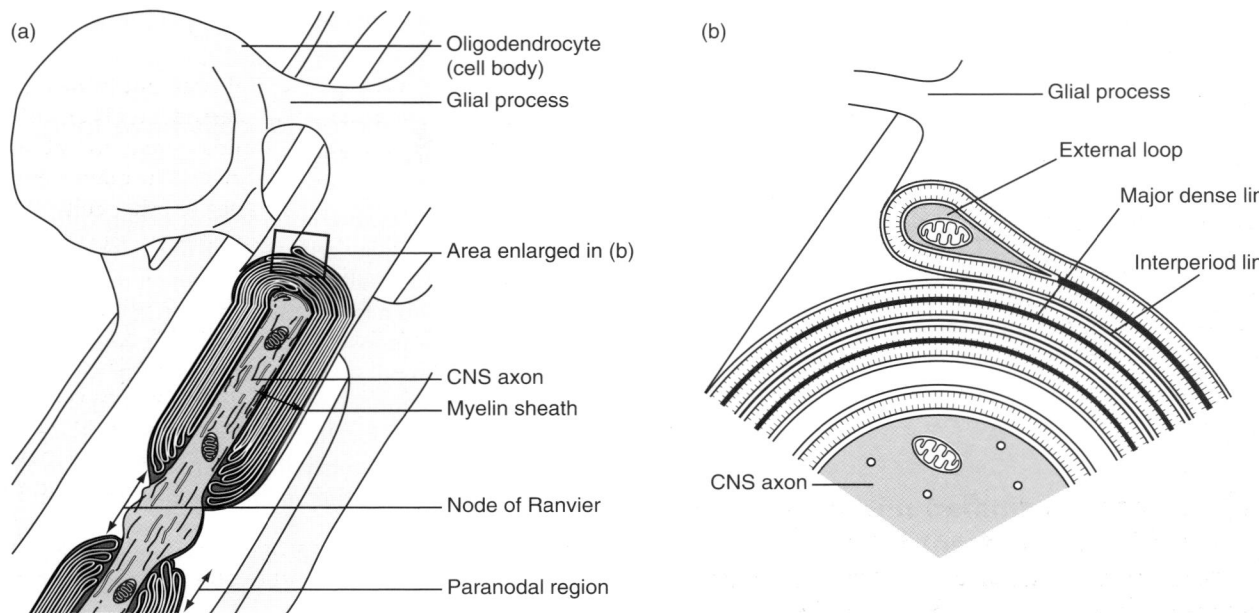

Figure 2.5 Myelin sheath of central axons.
(a) Three-dimensional diagram of the myelin sheath of an axon in the central nervous system (CNS). The sheath is formed by a succession of compact rolls of glial processes from different oligodendrocytes. **(b)** Cross-section through a myelin sheath. The dark lines, or major dense lines, and clear bands (in the middle of which are found the interperiod lines) visible with electron microscopy are accounted for by the manner in which the myelin membrane surrounds the axon, and by the composition of the membrane. The dark lines represent the adhesion of the internal leaflets of the myelin membrane while the interperiod lines represent the adhesion of the external leaflets. The lines are formed by membrane proteins while the clear bands are formed by the lipid bilayer. Drawing (a) from Bunge MB, Bunge RP, Ris H (1961) Ultrastructural study of remyelination in an experimental lesion in adult cat spinal cord, *J. Biophys. Biochem. Cytol.* **10**, 67–94, with permission of Rockerfeller University Press. Drawing (b) by Tom Prentiss. In Morell P, Norton W (1980) La myéline et la sclérose en plaques, *Pour la Science* **33**, with permission.

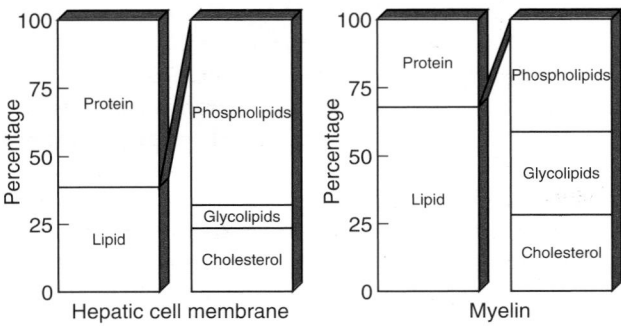

Figure 2.6 Comparison of the lipid content of plasma membrane and myelin.
The protein:lipid ratio is inverted between the two membranes. The proportions of the three groups of lipids are also different.

terminate at regularly spaced intervals along the axon, the internal layers (close to the axon) terminating first. This staggered termination of the different layers of myelin constitutes the paranodal region (**Figure 2.5a**).

2.2.2 Myelination enables rapid conduction of action potentials for two reasons

Isolation of internode axonal segments

The high lipid content and compact structure of the myelin sheath help make it impermeable to hydrophilic substances such as ions. It prevents transmembrane ion fluxes and acts as a good electrical insulator between the intracellular (i.e. intra-axonal) and extracellular media. Between the nodes of Ranvier the axon therefore behaves as an insulated cable. This permits rapid, saltatory conduction of action potentials along the axon (see Section 5.4).

Formation of Ranvier nodes with a high density of Na⁺ channels

Na⁺ channels are clustered in very high density within the nodal gap whereas voltage-dependent K⁺ channels are segregated in juxtaparanodal regions, beneath overlying myelin (see **Figure 2.5a**). To test whether oligodendrocyte contact with axon influences Na⁺ channel distribution, nodes of Ranvier in the brain of hypomyelinating mouse *Shiverer* are examined. *Shiverer* mice have oligodendrocytes that ensheath axons but do not form compact myelin and axoglial junctions. In these mutant mice, there are far fewer Na⁺ channel clusters than in control littermates and aberrant locations of Na⁺ channels are observed. If Na⁺ channel clustering depends only on the presence of oligodendrocytes and is independent of myelin and oligodendroglial contact, one would expect to find normal Na⁺ channel distribution along axons.

2.3 Microglia: ramified microglial cells represent the quiescent form of microglial cells in the central nervous system; they transform upon injury

Ramified microglial cells (**Figure 2.7b**) are small cells present throughout the whole adult central nervous system, and make up about 5–12% of central glial and neuronal cells. They are found in greater numbers in the grey matter.

2.3.1 Ramified microglial cells have long meandering processes

Microglial cells have an embryological origin different from that of other glial cells in that they derive from mesodermal (meningeal) tissue. By using a monoclonal antibody specific for a membrane glycoprotein of mouse macrophages, the mouse IgG Fc receptor, and for the myelomonocytic type 3 complement receptor and with the aid of immunocytochemical techniques (see Appendix 7.2), the localization of antibody-positive cells was observed in embryonic brains. This led to the conclusion that during the embryonic development of the central nervous system monocytes cross the brain capillaries to enter central structures and become 'ameboid' microglial cells. These cells are active macrophages phagocytosing degenerating cells and processes resulting from degeneration or remodelling of fibres in developing brain. At that stage they are endowed with a variety of hydrolytic enzymes. They then undergo a series of morphological transformations

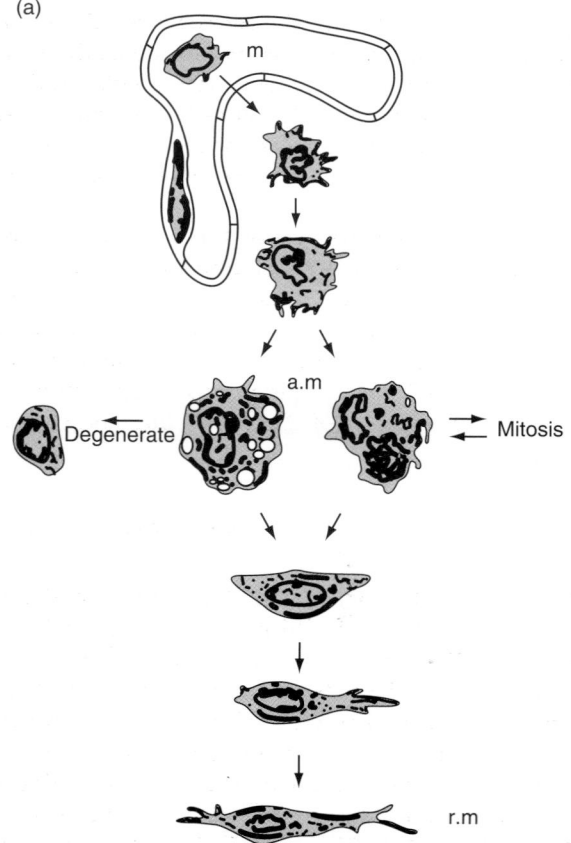

(a)

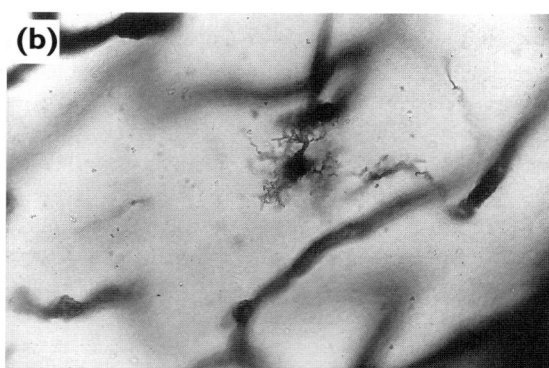

Figure 2.7 Microglial cells.
(a) Differentiation of monocytes into microglial cells during the development of the central nervous system as studied in the corpus callosum of the rat brain. Circulating monocytes (m) enter the brain parenchyma during the prenatal and early postnatal period. The cells acquire an abundant cytoplasm and become ameboid microglial cells (a.m). They show mitotic activity but many die *in situ* in the first postnatal week. The surviving cells begin to undergo morphological changes between the second and third postnatal week. They then present a branched appearance and are identified as ramified microglial cells (r.m). (b) Photograph taken using optical microscopy of an adult microglial cell (Golgi stain). Drawing adapted from Ling EA, Wong WC (1993) The origin and nature of ramified and amoeboid microglia: a historical review and current concepts, *Glia* **7**, 9–18, with permission. (b) Photograph by Olivier Robain.

and differentiate into ramified microglia during the postnatal period, a quiescent form that persists through adulthood (**Figure 2.7a**).

Ameboid microglia therefore disappear in the adult, but reappear upon injury of central nervous tissue. These microglial cells are able to move and ingest particles. In contrast, ramified microglial cells are deprived of all hydrolytic enzymes and do not ingest particles. No labelling of ramified microglial cells in young or adult rats was found after systemic injection of ³H-thymidine: these cells do not divide in normal brain. Ramified microglial cells are probably a 'resting' form of microglia, of which the function is unknown.

Ramified microglial cells have an elongated soma from which fine wavy processes carrying numerous protrusions ramify (**Figure 2.7b**). The nucleus is small and flattened or angular. It contains chromatin masses at the periphery. The endoplasmic reticulum forms very narrow, long cisternae which meander through the cytoplasm.

2.3.2 Do adult microglial cells play a role in immune processes?

Are adult microglial cells capable of phagocytosis?

Microglial activation in the brain involves a stereotypical pattern of changes including changes in cell morphology, cell number, migration to sites of neuronal activity or injury, cell surface receptor expression, increased or *de novo* expression of immunomodulators including cytokines and growth factors, and the full transformation into brain-resident phagocytes capable of clearing damaged cells and debris. Phagocytosis (the ability to ingest extracellular particles) involves immune processes. It requires the presence of Fc receptors or type 3 complement (C3) receptors. These receptors have indeed been demonstrated on microglial cells.

Are ramified glia transformed into macrophages following injury to nervous tissue?

Following injury to nervous tissue a proliferation of glial cells around the lesion is observed. Which are the glial cells capable of proliferation and of generating this reaction, called gliosis? According to Rio del Hortega, microglia present in the normal central nervous system could be transformed into reactive glial cells; i.e. divide and become macrophages capable of migration and ingestion of cellular debris. For example, in several human neurological disorders, a microglial activation characterized by proliferation, increased expression of surface antigens, migration and changes into a

macrophage-like morphology and immunophenotype is observed. However, the studies to date have been unable to provide a clear answer to this question and the problem is still not resolved. In fact, if the blood–brain barrier is damaged during injury to nervous tissue, circulating monocytes are recruited in large numbers and it becomes technically difficult to distinguish macrophages derived from monocytes from any macrophages resulting from division of 'resident' microglia.

2.4 Ependymal cells constitute an active barrier between blood and cerebrospinal fluid

2.4.1 Ependymal cells form an epithelium at the surface of the ventricles

Ependymal cells cover the walls of the cerebral ventricles (the lateral ventricles, third ventricle, cerebral aqueduct (of Sylvius) and the fourth ventricle) as well as the walls of the central canal of the spinal cord. In these cavities they form a continuous epithelium which is heterogeneous, because there are several types of ependymal cell.

All ependymal cells have a well-defined polarity: an apical, or luminal, side (in contact with the cerebrospinal fluid), site of cilia or microvilli, depending on the cell type, and a basal, or subependymal, side which rests on a basal lamina. Ependymal cells are joined to each other by junctional complexes at the edge of the apical pole. These junctions ensure the cohesion of the entire ependyma.

Ependymal cells are grouped into two main classes: ependymal cells of the choroid plexus and extrachoroidal ependymal cells which include ciliated ependymal cells and tanycytes. The distinction between these two classes is based on cytological and positional criteria. The differences used to classify ependymal cells indicate differences of function, but these remain obscure.

2.4.2 Ependymal cells of the choroid plexus

The choroid plexuses are situated in the lateral ventricles, where they stretch from the interventricular foramen (of Monro), to the tips of the inferior cornua, in the third ventricle where they cover the superior wall of the third ventricle, and on the roof of the fourth ventricle.

Ependymal cells of the choroidal plexus are characterized by a cuboidal shape. Observed in the scanning electron microscope, the luminal face has the form of a dome (**Figure 2.8**). The apical pole presents numerous

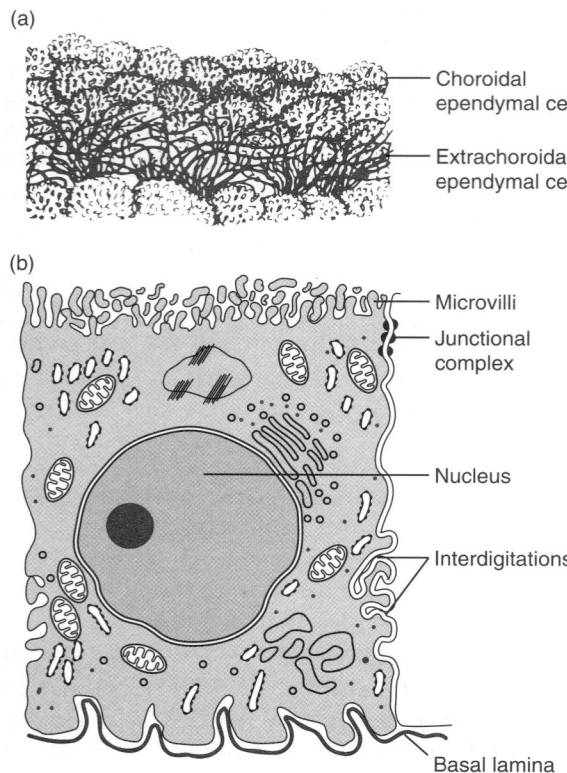

Figure 2.8 Ependymal cells.

(a) Junction between choroidal and extrachoroidal ependyma: choroidal ependymal cells with their villous surface are directly adjacent to ciliated extrachoroidal ependymal cells. **(b)** Diagram of a choroidal ependymal cell. Numerous villi and a few cilia are found at the apical pole. The lateral membranes of adjacent cells are attached near the apical pole by junctional complexes. Lower down there are numerous interdigitations between neighbouring cells. The basal pole rests on a basal lamina. Adapted from Peters A, Swan RC (1979) Choroidal epithelium, *Anat. Rec.* **194**, 325–353, with permission.

microvilli, 2–3 μm long, and occasional cilia. The spherical nucleus occupies the centre of the cell and contains relatively homogeneous chromatin. The numerous mitochondria and vesicles (30–40 nm in diameter) are largely situated towards the apical pole.

The other characteristic feature of ependymal cells of the choroidal plexus is that they are joined to each other by tight junctions (zonula occludens). These junctions, situated at the apical end of the lateral plasma membrane, form a continuous circumferential ring around each ependymal cell. At the level of the junction there is no extracellular space between the cells. This means that exchange between blood vessels (on the basal side) and the cerebrospinal fluid (apical side) can occur only via the ependymal cells. This is of considerable importance, because the capillaries in the choroidal plexuses, being

fenestrated, do not form a blood–brain barrier. Instead, the barrier here consists of the ependymal cells joined by tight junctions.

Below the tight junctions, the plasma membranes of the choroidal cells have numerous and complex interdigitations. The many (apical) microvilli, as well as the interdigitations of the basolateral region, are structures that greatly increase the area available for exchange between the cells and their environment (cerebrospinal fluid and extracellular fluid). These are, along with the presence of numerous vesicles in their cytoplasm, indicators of a large exchange of substances via secretion and absorption. Indeed, if a marker such as horseradish peroxidase (HPR) is injected into the circulation, the marker remains trapped in the region of the interdigitations and within the choroidal cells. This block of the entry of certain substances into the cerebrospinal fluid may be an important element of the active barrier between blood and cerebrospinal fluid. Conversely, tracers injected into the cerebrospinal fluid are later found in the lysosomal apparatus of the ependymal cells.

Choroidal ependymal cells occupy a special position, interposed between fenestrated blood capillaries of the choroid plexus and the cerebrospinal fluid. They constitute an active barrier between these two media (blood and cerebrospinal fluid), but also play a role in the production of cerebrospinal fluid.

2.4.3 Extrachoroidal ependymal cells

Outside the choroid plexus, the ventricles are lined by ciliated ependymal cells and by non-ciliated tanycytes. The transition between choroidal and extrachoroidal ependyma is abrupt.

Ciliated ependymal cells have numerous cilia projecting into the cavity (**Figure 2.8**). Their movements presumably aid the circulation of the cerebrospinal fluid. These cells are not joined by tight junctions.

Tanycytes are covered on their apical surface by microvilli and have characteristic long basal processes which make contact with blood capillaries, neurons or other glial cells (**Figure 2.9**). They contain numerous secretory vesicles.

The function of extrachoroidal ependymal cells seems not to be restricted solely to moving the cerebrospinal fluid with their cilia. They may also play a role in the regulation of the activity of the cells situated at their basal pole. This regulation would be controlled by signals in the cerebrospinal fluid. The discovery of the presence of various hormones and neurotransmitters in the cerebrospinal fluid suggested that ependymal cells may absorb such substances (apically) and then secrete them (basally). Such a process would permit regulation of neurons in the region of the third ventricle.

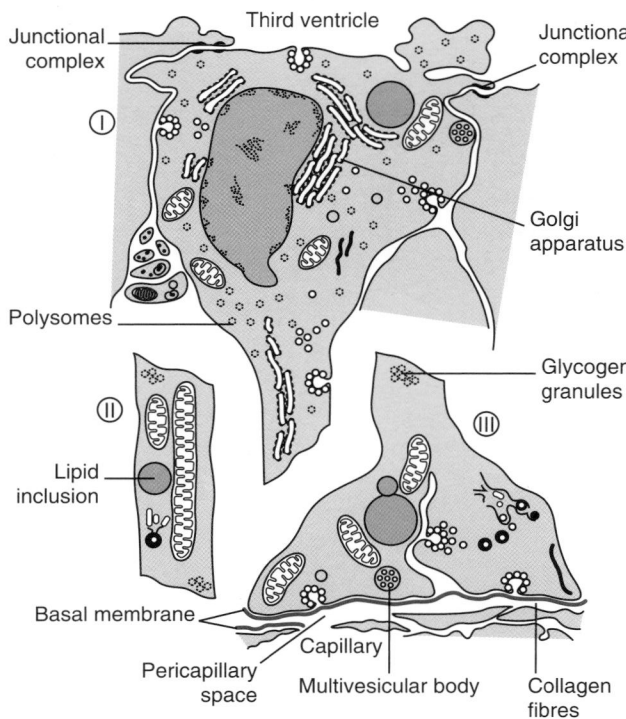

Figure 2.9 Tanycytes.
Drawing of the ultrastructure of a beta tanycyte of the rat. (I) perikaryon; (II) process; (III) termination of process. Adapted from Akmayev IG, Popov AP (1977) Morphological aspects of the hypothalamic hypophyseal system, *Cell Tiss. Res.* **180**, 263–282, with permission.

2.5 Schwann cells are the glial cells of the peripheral nervous system; they form the myelin sheath of axons or encapsulate neurons

There are three types of Schwann cell:

■ those forming the myelin sheath of peripheral myelinated axons (myelinating Schwann cells);
■ those encapsulating non-myelinated peripheral axons (non-myelinating Schwann cells);
■ those that encapsulate the bodies of ganglion cells (non-myelinating Schwann cells or satellite cells).

2.5.1 Myelinating Schwann cells make the myelin sheath of peripheral axons

Along an axon, several Schwann cells form successive segments of the myelin sheath. In contrast to oligodendrocytes, it is not a process that enwraps the peripheral axon to form the segment of myelin, but the whole Schwann cell (**Figure 2.10**). Each Schwann cell therefore forms only one myelin segment.

The composition of peripheral myelin differs from that of central myelin only in the proteins it contains. The principal protein constituents of peripheral myelin are: peripheral myelin protein 22 (PMP 22), protein zero (P0) and myelin basic proteins (MBPs). The first two proteins are specific to peripheral myelin. Peripheral myelin protein 22 is a small, hydrophobic integral membrane glycoprotein. Protein zero is a glycoprotein that has adhesive properties and is located in the inter-period line. It functions, in part, as a homotypic adhesion molecule throughout the full thickness of the myelin sheath. It is a good marker for myelinating Schwann cells.

2.5.2 Non-myelinating Schwann cells encapsulate the axons and cell bodies of peripheral neurons

Non-myelinated axons are not uncovered in the peripheral nervous system as they are in the central nervous system; they are encapsulated. A single non-myelinating Schwann cell surrounds several axons (about 5–20) for a distance of 200–500 μm in man.

In addition, spinal and cranial ganglia contain a large number of Schwann cells that do not produce myelin. These Schwann cells cover the somata of the ganglionic cells, leaving an extracellular space of about 20 nm between themselves and the surface of the covered neuron.

The lipid and protein composition of the plasma membrane of non-myelinating Schwann cells is the same as that of other eukaryotic cells (30% lipid, 70% protein).

Apart from their role in the saltatory conduction of action potentials (myelinating Schwann cells), Schwann cells also play a role in the regeneration of peripheral nerve cells. It has long been known that cut peripheral nerves can, within certain limits, regrow and reinnervate deafferented regions while central axons are not capable of this. This property of regeneration is due in large part to an enabling effect of Schwann cells on axon regrowth.

Further reading

Aldskogius H, Liu L, Svensson M (1999) Glial responses to synaptic damage and plasticity. *J. Neurosci. Res.* **58**, 33–41.
Bruce-Keller AJ (1999) Microglial–neuronal interactions in synaptic damage and recovery. *J. Neurosci. Res.* **58**, 191–201.

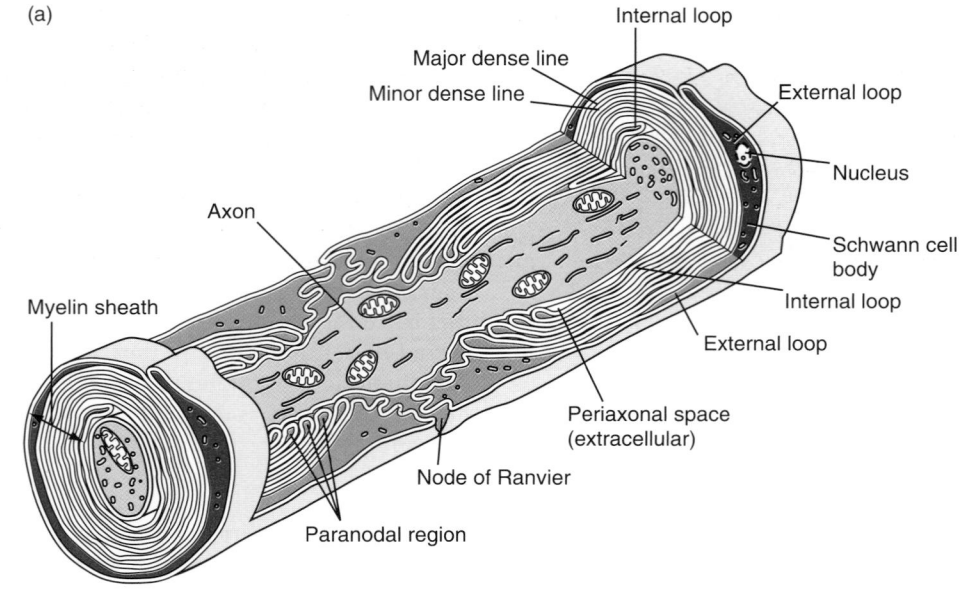

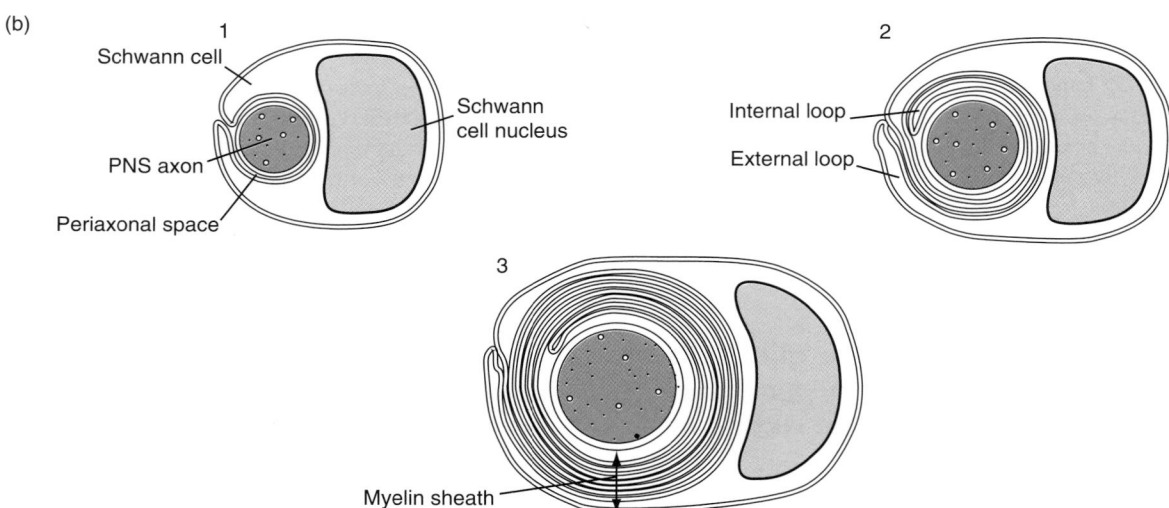

Figure 2.10 Myelin sheath of a peripheral axon.

(a) Three-dimensional diagram of the myelin sheath of an axon of the peripheral nervous system (PNS). The sheath is formed by successive rolled Schwann cells. (b) Process of myelinization. The internal loop wraps around the axon several times. During this process the axon grows and the myelin becomes compact. Contact between the Schwann cell and axon occurs only at the paranodal and nodal regions. Elsewhere an extracellular, or periaxonal, space always remains. Drawing (a) adapted from Maillet M (1977) *Le Tissue Nerveux*, Paris: Vigot, with permission. Drawing (b) by Tom Prentiss. In Morell P, Norton W (1980) La myéline et la sclérose en plaques, *Pour la Science* **33**, with permission.

Del Rio Hortega P (1932) Microglia. In: Penfield, W (ed) *Cytology and Cellular Pathology of the Nervous System*, vol. 2, pp. 481–534. New York: P.B. Hoeber.

Dupree JL, Girault JA, Popko B (1999) Axo-glial interactions regulate the localization of axonal paranodal proteins. *J. Cell Biol.* **147**, 1145–1152.

Giulian D (1987) Ameboid microglia as effectors of inflammation in the central nervous system. *J. Neurosci.* **18**, 155–171.

Kettenmann H, Ranson BR (eds) (1995) *Neuroglia*. New York: Oxford University Press.

Morell P (1984) *Myelin*, 2nd edn. New York: Plenum Press.

Palay SL, Chan-Palay V (1977) General morphology of

neurons and neuroglia. In: Brookhart JM, Mountcastle VB, Kandel ER, Geiger SR (eds) *Handbook of Physiology*, vol. 1, part 1, pp. 5–37. Bethesda, MD: American Physiological Society.

Popko B (2000) Myelin galactolipids: mediators of axon–glial interactions? *Glia* **29**, 149–153.

Rasband MN, Peles E, Trimmer JS, Levinson SR, Lux SE, Shrager P (1999) Dependence of nodal sodium channel clustering on paranodal axoglial contact in the developing CNS. *J. Neurosci.* **19**, 7516–7520.

Shapiro L, Doyle JP, Hensley P, Colman DR, Hendrickson WA (1996) Crystal structure of the extracellular domain from P0, the major structural protein of peripheral nerve myelin. *Neuron* **17**, 435–449.

Special issue on microglial cells (1993) *Glia* **7** (1).

Streit WJ (2000) Microglial response to brain injury: a brief synopsis. *Toxicol. Pathol.* **28**, 28–30.

Ionic Fluxes Across the Neuronal Plasma Membrane

The neuronal plasma membrane delimits the whole neuron, from the dendritic spines to the axon terminals. It is a barrier between the intracellular and extracellular environments. The general structure of the neuronal plasma membrane is similar to that of other plasma membranes. It is made up of proteins inserted in a lipid bilayer, forming as a whole a 'fluid mosaic' (**Figure 3.1**). However, insofar as there are functions that are exclusively neuronal, the neuronal membrane differs from other plasma membranes by the nature, density and spatial distribution of the proteins of which it is composed.

Electrical signalling in the nervous system involves the movement of ions. Among the ions present in the nervous system fluids, Na^+, K^+, Ca^{2+} and Cl^- ions seem to be responsible for almost all of the action. These ions cross the membrane through specific transmembrane proteins called *ionic channels*. These ionic fluxes are passive since they do not require energy. Ions being charged particles, ionic fluxes are ionic currents across the membrane and therefore have an immediate effect on membrane potential (electrical signalling). The aim of this chapter is to look at which proteins Na^+, K^+, Ca^{2+} and Cl^- ions passively use to cross the membrane, when and in which direction, the functional consequences of these passive ionic fluxes, and how they are maintained and controlled.

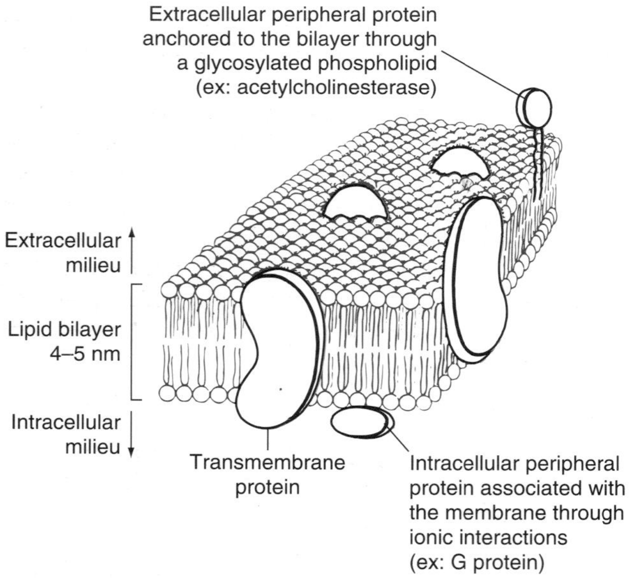

3.1 Observations and questions

3.1.1 There is an unequal distribution of ions across neuronal plasma membrane

The neuronal plasma membrane delimits the intracellular and extracellular compartments. There is an unequal distribution of ions across the plasma membrane: regardless of the animal's environment (seawater, freshwater or air), potassium (K^+) ions are the predominant cations in the intracellular fluid and sodium (Na^+) ions are the predominant cations in the extracellular fluid. The main anions of the intracellular fluid are organic molecules (P^-): negatively charged amino acids (glutamate and aspartate), proteins, nucleic acids, etc. In the extracellular fluid the predominant anions are chloride (Cl^-) ions. A marked difference between cytosolic and extracellular Ca^{2+} concentrations is also observed (**Figure 3.2**).

Spatial distribution of Ca^{2+} ions inside the cell deserves a more detailed description. Ca^{2+} ions are present in the cytosol as 'free' Ca^{2+} ions at a very low concentration (10^{-8} to 10^{-7} M) and as bound Ca^{2+} ions (bound to Ca^{2+}-binding proteins). They are also distributed in organelles able to sequester calcium, which include endoplasmic reticulum, calciosome and mitochondria, where they constitute the intracellular Ca^{2+} stores. Free intracellular Ca^{2+} ions present in the cytosol act as second messengers and transduce electrical activity in neurons into biochemical events such as

Extracellular peripheral protein anchored to the bilayer through a glycosylated phospholipid (ex: acetylcholinesterase)

Extracellular milieu

Lipid bilayer 4–5 nm

Intracellular milieu

Transmembrane protein

Intracellular peripheral protein associated with the membrane through ionic interactions (ex: G protein)

Figure 3.1 Fluid mosaic.
Transmembrane proteins and lipids are kept together by non-covalent interactions (ionic and hydrophobic).

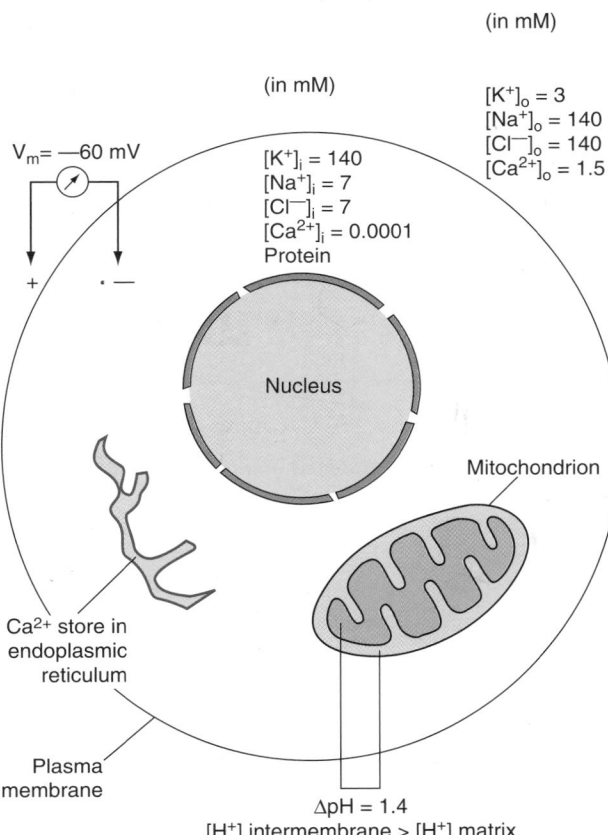

(in mM)

$[K^+]_i = 140$
$[Na^+]_i = 7$
$[Cl^-]_i = 7$
$[Ca^{2+}]_i = 0.0001$
Protein

(in mM)

$[K^+]_o = 3$
$[Na^+]_o = 140$
$[Cl^-]_o = 140$
$[Ca^{2+}]_o = 1.5$

$V_m = -60$ mV

Nucleus

Mitochondrion

Ca^{2+} store in endoplasmic reticulum

Plasma membrane

$\Delta pH = 1.4$
$[H^+]$ intermembrane > $[H^+]$ matrix

Figure 3.2 Across the plasma membrane.
Asymmetric distribution of ions across the plasma membrane (terrestrian vertebrates) and difference of potential between the two faces of the membrane at rest.

exocytosis. Ca^{2+} ions bound to cytosolic proteins or present in organelle stores are not active Ca^{2+} ions; only 'free' Ca^{2+} ions have a role.

A difference of concentration between two compartments is called a 'concentration gradient'. Measurements of Na^+, K^+, Ca^{2+} and Cl^- concentrations have shown that concentration gradients for ions are constant in the external and cytosolic compartments, at the macroscopic level, during the entire neuronal life.

How are concentration gradients kept constant?

At least two hypotheses can explain this constancy:

■ Na^+, K^+, Ca^{2+} and Cl^- ions cannot cross the plasma membrane: plasma membrane is impermeable to these inorganic ions.
■ Plasma membrane is permeable to Na^+, K^+, Ca^{2+} and Cl^- ions but there are mechanisms that continuously maintain the unequal distribution of ions.

3.1.2 Neuronal plasma membrane is permeable to ions, allowing both passive and active transport of ions

With the use of radioisotopes, it was shown that inorganic ions such as Na^+, K^+, Ca^{2+} and Cl^- can effectively cross the plasma membrane: there is a transport of Na^+, K^+, Ca^{2+} or Cl^- ions between the extracellular and cytosolic compartments. In contrast, organic ions such as proteins cannot diffuse through the membrane: the membrane is impermeable to them.

The first demonstrations of ionic fluxes across plasma membrane by Hodgkin and Keynes (1955) were based on the use of radioisotopes of K^+ or Na^+ ions. These experiments were conducted on the isolated squid giant axon. When this axon is immerged in a bath containing a control concentration of radioactive *Na^+ ($^{24}Na^+$) instead of cold Na^+ ($^{22}Na^+$), *Na^+ ions constantly appear in the cytoplasm. This *Na^+ influx is not affected by dinitrophenol (DNP), a blocker of ATP synthesis in mitochondria. It does not require energy expenditure. This is *passive* transport.

When the reverse experiment is conducted, the isolated squid giant axon is passively loaded with radioactive *Na^+ by performing the above experiment, and is then transferred to a bath containing cold Na^+. Measuring the quantity of *Na^+ that appears in the bath per unit of time ($d*Na^+/dt$, expressed in counts per minute) allows quantification of the efflux of *Na^+ (**Figure 3.3a**). In the presence of dinitrophenol (DNP) this *Na^+ efflux quickly diminishes to nearly zero. The process can be started up again by intracellular injection of ATP. Therefore the *Na^+ efflux is *active* transport. The movement of Na^+ from the cytosol to the outside (efflux) can be switched off reversibly by the use of metabolic inhibitors.

Observation of active transport of ions provides a general answer to the question: how does the cell maintain its ionic composition in the face of continuous passive exchange of all principal ions? Ionic composition of cytosol and extracellular compartments are maintained at the expense of a continuous basal metabolism that provides energy (ATP) utilized to actively transport ions and thus to compensate for their passive movements (**Figure 3.3b**).

3.1.3 There is a difference of potential between the two faces of the membrane, called membrane potential

Membrane potential (V_m) is by convention the difference between the potential of the internal and external faces of the membrane ($V_m = V_i - V_e$). Intracellular and extracellular media are neutral ionic solutions: in each

(a)

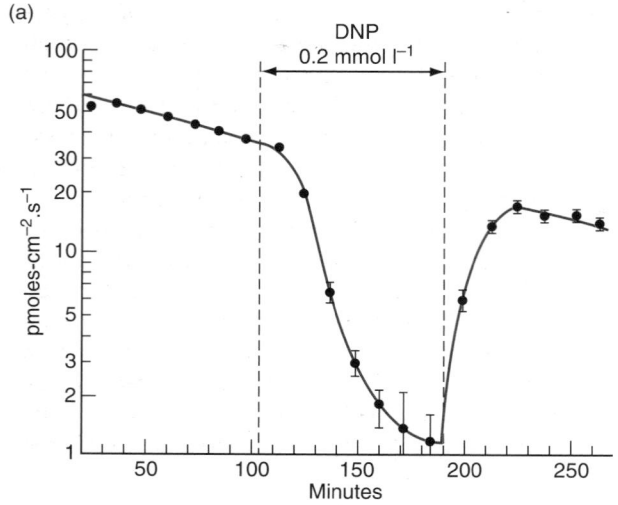

(b)

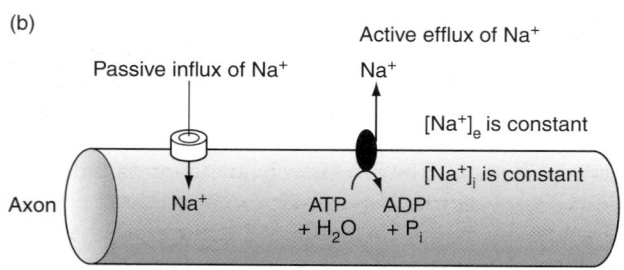

Figure 3.3 Na fluxes through the membrane of giant axons of sepia.

(a) Effect of dinitrophenol on the outflux of *Na⁺ as a function of time. The axon is previously loaded with *Na⁺. At $t = 1$, the axon is transferred in a bath devoid of *Na⁺. The ordinate (logarithmic) axis is the quantity of *Na⁺ ions that appear in the bath (that leave the axon) as a function of time. At $t = 100$ min, DNP (0.2 mM) is added to the bath for 90 min. The efflux, which previously decreased linearly with time, is totally blocked after one hour of DNP. This blockade is reversible. (b) Passive and active Na⁺ fluxes are in opposite directions. Plot (a) adapted from Hodgkin AL, Keynes RD (1955) Active transport of cations in giant axons from sepia and loligo, *J. Physiol. (Lond.)* **128**, 28–60, with permission.

medium, the concentration of positive ions is equal to that of negative ions. However, there is a very small excess of positive and negative ions accumulated on each side of the membrane. At 'rest', for example, a small excess of negative ions is accumulated at the internal side of the membrane. An equal number of positive ions is accumulated at the external side. This creates a difference of potential – the internal face is charged more negatively than the external face: V_m at rest is equal to –80 to –50 mV, depending of the neuronal type (see **Figure 3.2**).

What is particular to membrane of neurons (and of all excitable cells) is that V_m varies (**Figure 3.4**). It can be

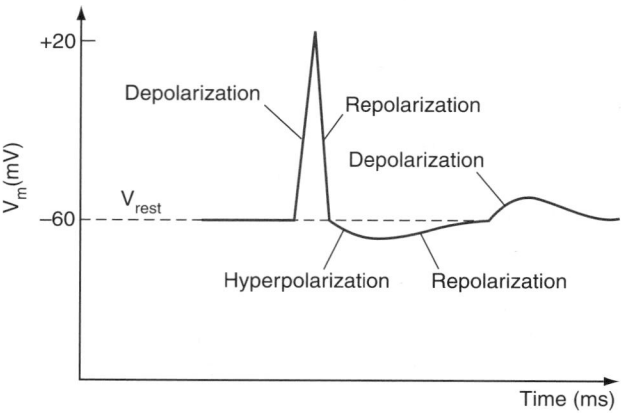

Figure 3.4 Variations of the membrane potential of neurons (V_m).

When the membrane potential is less negative than resting membrane potential (V_{rest}), the membrane is said to be depolarized. In contrast, when the membrane potential is more negative than V_{rest}, the membrane is said to be hyperpolarized. When the membrane varies from a depolarized or hyperpolarized value back to rest, the membrane repolarizes.

more negative or hyperpolarized or less negative (depolarized) or even positive (also depolarized, the internal face is positive compared to the external face). V_m varies between the extreme values –90 mV and +30 mV. The origin of the resting membrane potential is explained in Chapter 4, and variations of the membrane potential in the following chapters. Meanwhile, it is clear that a variable difference of potential exists between the two sides of the membrane, although the underlying mechanisms are not explained in this chapter.

3.1.4 Questions

In summary, we have the following facts: (i) there is an unequal distribution of ions across the neuronal plasma membrane, which stays constant during the entire neuronal life; (ii) ions move through the membrane either passively or actively; and (iii) there is a difference of potential between the two faces of the neuronal membrane. The remainder of this chapter examines the following questions:

■ Where and how do ions *passively* cross the plasma membrane? What are the respective roles of the concentration gradient and membrane potential? (Sections 3.2 and 3.3)
■ How and where do ions *actively* cross the plasma membrane and thus compensate for the passive movements? (Section 3.4)

■ What are the roles of the passive movements of ions? (Section 3.5)

3.2 Na⁺, K⁺, Ca²⁺ and Cl⁻ ions passively cross the plasma membrane through transmembrane proteins – the channels

When proteins are absent from a synthetic lipid bilayer, no movements of ions occur across this purely lipidic membrane. Owing to its central hydrophobic region, the lipid bilayer has a low permeability to hydrophilic substances such as ions, water and polar molecules; i.e. the lipid bilayer is a barrier for the diffusion of ions and most polar molecules. Therefore, Na^+, K^+, Ca^{2+} and Cl^- cross the membrane at the level of specialized transmembrane proteins. The passive transport of ions occurs through proteins, called *ionic channels* (or simply 'channels').

3.2.1 Channels are a particular class of transmembrane proteins

Transmembrane proteins span the entire width of the lipid bilayer (see **Figure 3.1**). They have hydrophobic regions containing a high fraction of non-polar amino acids and hydrophilic regions containing a high fraction of polar amino acids (see Appendix 3.1). Certain hydrophobic regions organize themselves inside the bilayer as transmembrane α-helices while more hydrophilic regions are in contact with the aqueous intracellular and extracellular environments. Interaction energies are very high between hydrophobic regions of the protein and hydrophobic regions of the lipid bilayer, as well as between hydrophilic regions of the protein and the extracellular and intracellular environments. These interactions strongly stabilize transmembrane proteins within the bilayer, thus preventing their extracellular and cytoplasmic regions from flipping back and forth.

Ionic channels have a three-dimensional structure that delimits an aqueous pore through which certain ions can pass. They provide the ions with a passage through the membrane. Each channel may be regarded as an excitable molecule as it is specifically responsive to a stimulus and can be in at least two different states: closed and open. Channel opening, a switch from the closed to the open state, is tightly controlled (see **Table 3.1**) by:

■ a change in the membrane potential – these are voltage-gated channels (Section 3.2.2);
■ the binding of an extracellular ligand, such as a neurotransmitter – these are ligand-gated channels, also called receptor channels or ionotropic receptors (Section 3.2.3);
■ the binding of an intracellular ligand such as Ca^{2+} ions or a cyclic nucleotide (Section 3.2.4);
■ mechanical stimuli such as stretch – these are mechanoreceptors (Section 3.2.5).

The channel's response to its specific stimuli, called gating, is a simple opening or closing of the pore. The pore has the important property of selective permeability, allowing some restricted class of small ions to flow passively down their electrochemical gradients (see

Table 3.1 Examples of ionic channels

Channels	Voltage-gated	Ligand-gated			Mechanically gated
Opened by	Depolarization Hyperpolarization	Extracellular ligand	Intracellular ligand		Mechanical stimuli
Localization	Plasma membrane	Plasma membrane	Plasma membrane	Organelle membrane	Plasma membrane
Examples	Na⁺ channels Ca²⁺ channels K⁺ channels Cationic channels	nAChR iGluR 5-HT₃ GABA_A GlyR	G protein-gated channels Ca²⁺-gated channels CNG channels ATP-gated channels	IP₃-gated Ca²⁺ channel Ca²⁺-gated Ca²⁺ channel	Stretch-activated channels
Closed by	Inactivation Repolarization	Desensitization Ligand recapture or degradation			Adaptation End of stimulus
Roles	Na⁺ and Ca²⁺-dependent action potentials [Ca²⁺]ᵢ increase	EPSP IPSP [Ca²⁺]ᵢ increase	EPSP IPSP Action potential repolarization Receptor potential	[Ca²⁺]ᵢ increase	Receptor potential

Section 3.3). These gated ion fluxes through pores make signals for the nervous sytem.

3.2.2 Voltage-gated channels open in response to a change in membrane potential

Channels opened by voltage changes have a three-dimensional structure which contains an aqueous pore and a voltage 'sensitive' region. Depending on the membrane potential, these channels may be in a closed state (ions cannot pass through the aqueous pore) or an open state (ions can pass through the aqueous pore); they change conformation – switching from one state to the other – depending on membrane potential changes. Most of these channels open transiently in response to membrane depolarization (**Figure 3.5a**), but some open in response to hyperpolarization. The aqueous pore of voltage-sensitive channels is essentially permeable to one ionic species. Voltage-gated channels are usually named after their most important permeant ion. However, no channel is perfectly selective. Thus, the voltage-dependent Na^+ channel is also fairly permeable to NH_4^+.

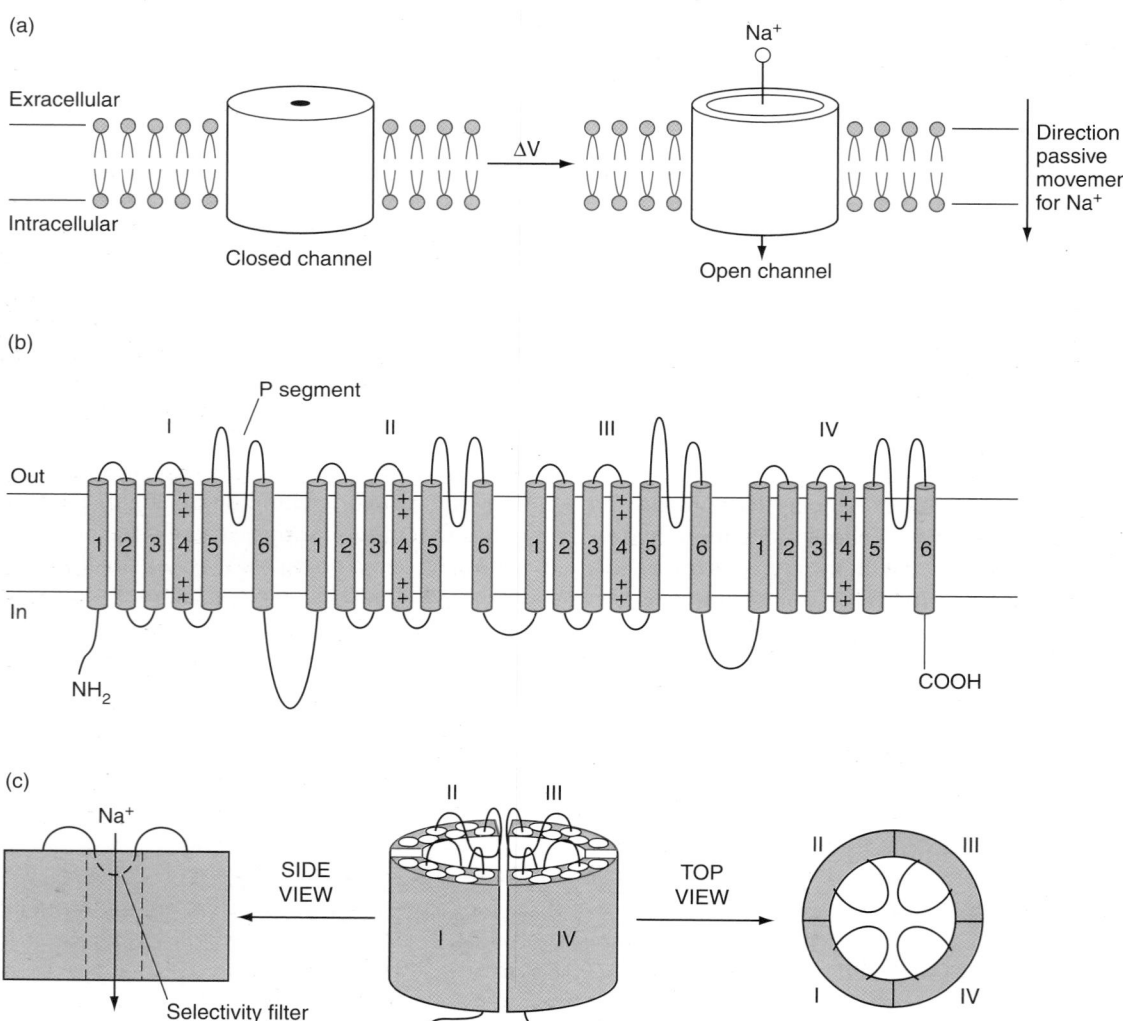

Figure 3.5 Voltage-gated channels.
(a) This channel opens as a result of changes in transmembrane potential (ΔV). (b) Putative transmembrane topology of the α-subunit of the voltage-gated Na^+ channel in the lipid bilayer. (c) Representation of the subunit as it would be seen from the side or from the top of the membrane. One can distinguish four homologous domains (labelled I to IV) each one containing six transmembrane α-helices (labelled 1 to 6). The model assumes that the four domains are arranged symmetrically around a central aqueous pore. Drawings (b) and (c) adapted from Marban E, Yamagishi T, Tomaselli G (1998) Structure and function of voltage-gated sodium channels, *J. Physiol. (Lond.)* **508**, 647–657, with permission.

The voltage-gated Na^+ channel consists of various subunits but only the principal subunit (α subunit) is required for functionality. The α subunit consists of four internally homologous domains (labelled I to IV) each of which is approximately 300 amino acids long and contains six transmembrane segments (**Figure 3.5b**). These four domains are said to be homologous because they share a high percentage of identical amino acid residues. They are separated from each other by non-homologous regions of variable lengths, of which the S5–S6 linkers form the P (pore-lining) segment. As depicted in **Figure 3.5c**, the protein wraps around a central pore. P segments of each domain come together to form the pore. They are responsible for the ionic selectivity (these regions exhibit exquisite conservation within a given channel family of like selectivity, but not among families with different selectivities). The general strategy for activation gating is the presence of a fourth transmembrane segment (S4) with positively charged residues (**Figure 3.5b**) that moves in response to a change of membrane potential (ΔV), somehow opening the channel. This structure is similar to the predicted structure of voltage-gated Ca^{2+} channels and the functional tetrameric form of K^+ channels.

The voltage-sensitive Na^+ channel is responsible for the initial inward current of Na^+ ions during the depolarizing phase of action potentials. It thus underlies the generation and propagation of Na^+ action potentials (see Chapter 5). The multiple types of voltage-sensitive Ca^{2+} channels control the entry of Ca^{2+} ions into the cell. Ca^{2+} current underlies the generation of Ca^{2+} action potentials (see Chapters 6 and 19), and intracellular Ca^{2+} triggers several Ca^{2+}-dependent intracellular processes, including the release of neurotransmitters from presynaptic terminals (see Chapter 8). The multiple types of voltage-sensitive K^+ channels do not have a single function that can be assigned to them as a group. In general, they participate in resting membrane potential and action potential repolarization (see Chapters 4, 5 and 6).

3.2.3 Ligand-gated channels opened by extracellular ligands, and receptor channels opened by neurotransmitters

These channels open as a result of the binding of an extracellular ligand (e.g. a neurotransmitter). Their common characteristic is that the receptor sites for the ligand and the ionic channel that they control are part of the *same protein*. Receptor channels are made up of several subunits (linked together by non-covalent bonds) which form the central aqueous pore. In general, the receptor sites of the neurotransmitter are present in the extracellular domains of two identical subunits. When the neurotransmitter binds to its receptor sites, the receptor channel changes conformation and transiently switches to a state in which the aqueous pore is open (**Figure 3.6a**). Thus, receptor channels ensure fast synaptic transmission by triggering a rapid increase of ionic permeability in response to the binding of a neurotransmitter. It should be noted that these channels may also present receptor sites for other endogenous molecules such as allosteric agonists which modulate their activity.

The best-known members of this group open in response to neurotransmitters (**Table 3.1**): acetylcholine (nicotinic receptors), γ-aminobutyric acid (GABA$_A$ receptors) and glutamate (NMDA and non-NMDA receptors). Nicotinic receptors (nAChR; see Chapter 9) and glutamate receptor channels (see Chapter 11) are permeable to cations Na^+, K^+ and Ca^{2+}. Conversely, GABA$_A$ receptors (see Chapter 10) are permeable to Cl^- ions.

The primary structures of the nAChR, GABA$_A$ and glutamate receptor channels show many similarities. The nAChR, for example, is a pentamer of 16 known different types of subunits α, β, γ, δ and ϵ. These different subunits show very high levels of sequence and hydrophobicity profile homologies: they contain a large N-terminal hydrophilic domain exposed to the synaptic cleft, followed by three transmembrane segments (M1–M3), a large intracellular loop and a C-terminal transmembrane segment (M4) (**Figure 3.6b**). Subunits are regularly distributed around an axis of quasi-symmetry delineating the ion channel (**Figure 3.6c**). The ion channel is lined by the M2 segment from each of the five subunits. The neurotransmitter receptor sites have been identified in the large extracellular domain of two identical subunits (the two α subunits of the nAChR receptor and the two β-subunits of the GABA$_A$ receptor).

3.2.4 Ligand-gated channels opened by intracellular ligands

These are channels gated by GTP-dependent proteins (G proteins) or by second messengers such as Ca^{2+}, IP$_3$ or cyclic nucleotides.

Channels that are directly opened by G proteins are, for example, the G protein-gated inwardly rectifying K^+ (GIRK) channels (**Figure 3.7**). GIRK channels are present in the membrane of heart cells where they are coupled to a muscarinic acetylcholine receptor (m$_2$AChR) and are involved in mediating a slowing of the heart rate (as a result of the efflux of K^+ ions) in response to acetylcholine release from the vagus nerve. They are also present in mammalian central and peripheral neurons where they are coupled via G proteins to many different neurotransmitter receptors and act to decrease firing

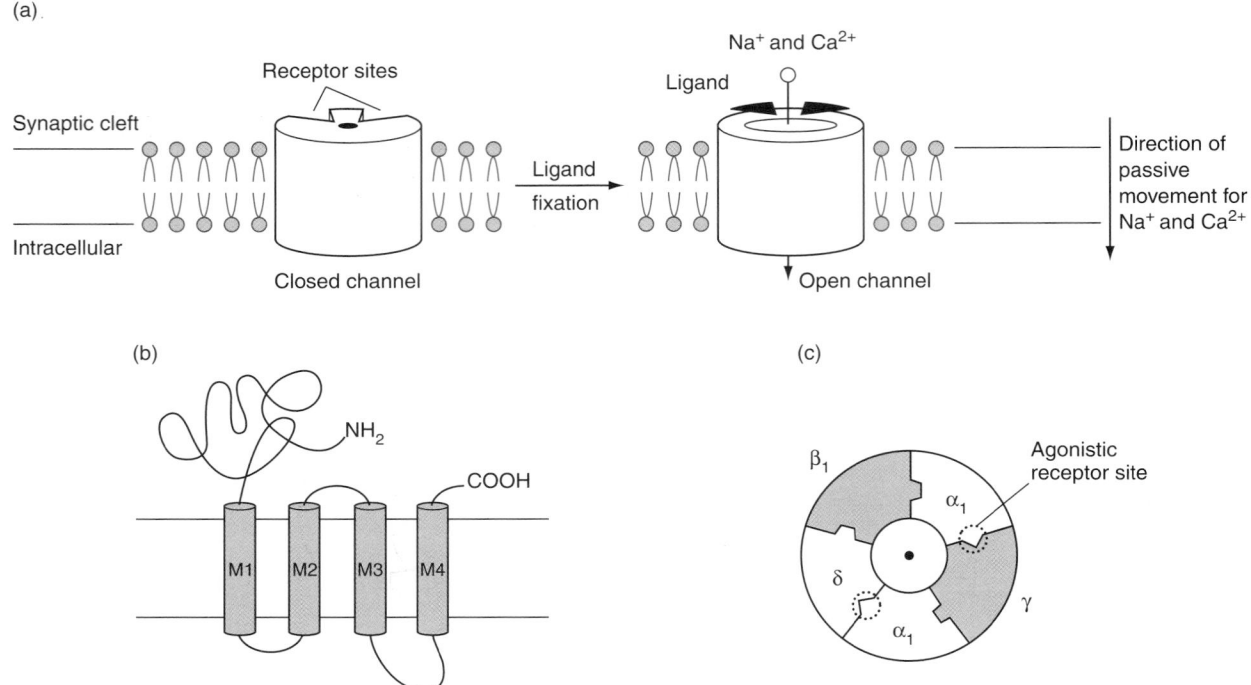

Figure 3.6 Receptor channels.
(a) Ligand-gated channel open when two molecules of a ligand are bound to the receptor sites located on the extracellular face of the protein. A neurotransmitter is an example of such a ligand. **(b)** Putative transmembrane topology of receptor channels: example of the nicotinic acetylcholine receptor (nAChR) of the muscle. This receptor is made up of two α, one β, one γ, and one δ subunit, all of which present sequence homologies and a similar transmembrane organization. The α-subunit is illustrated here in a linear representation in the membrane. **(c)** All five subunits are assembled into an $\alpha_2\beta\gamma\delta$ pentamer which forms a rosette and delimits a central aqueous pore. Both acetylcholine receptor sites are located at subunit interfaces (in their extracellular domains). Drawings (b) and (c) adapted from Changeux JP, Edelstein SJ (1998) Allosteric receptors after 30 years *Neuron* **21**, 959–980, with permission.

rate. The coupling between these G-coupled receptors (called metabotropic receptors) and GIRK channels is achieved by a high diversity of G proteins which are peripheral proteins present on the cytoplasmic side of the membrane and are formed by three different subunits (α, β, γ). Activation of the metabotropic receptor catalyses the release of the Gβγ subunit from the G protein ($G\alpha_{v/o}\beta\gamma$) and Gβγ directly interacts with GIRK channels to increase their open probability (**Figure 3.7a**).

Ca²⁺-gated channels are K⁺, Cl⁻ or cation permeable channels. A local increase in intracellular Ca²⁺ concentration favours the probability of the binding of Ca²⁺ ions to the Ca²⁺ receptor site(s) located on the cytoplasmic side of these channels. This in turn triggers the opening of the channels and the passage of ions across the membrane. Some of these channels are also voltage-gated. Their general role is to transduce a local increase in intracellular Ca²⁺ concentration in a change of membrane potential.

Cyclic nucleotide-gated (CNG) channels are cation permeable channels. Despite the fact that CNG channels are gated by the binding of a ligand, cGMP or cAMP (**Figure 3.8a**), and not by voltage, they are structurally homologous to the voltage-gated channels since their primary structure presents six hypothetic transmembrane domains (**Figure 3.8b**). Consistent with this interpretation, immunocytochemistry studies have shown that the amino terminal domain is located on the cytoplasmic side of the membrane and the beginning of the P region is located on the extracellular side of the membrane. The pore of CNG channels is permeable to both monovalent and divalent cations. The cyclic nucleotide binding site is situated near the carboxy terminus. An evolutionary connection between voltage-gated channels and CNG channels is suggested also by the presence of a cGMP-binding region in some voltage-gated channels (such as the H-channel, a hyperpolarization-activated cation channel). CNG channels may exist as tetramers (**Figure 3.8c**). The role of CNG channels of photoreceptors (cGMP-gated) and olfactory receptor cells (cAMP-gated; see Chapter 15) is to convert external sensory stimuli into changes in membrane potential.

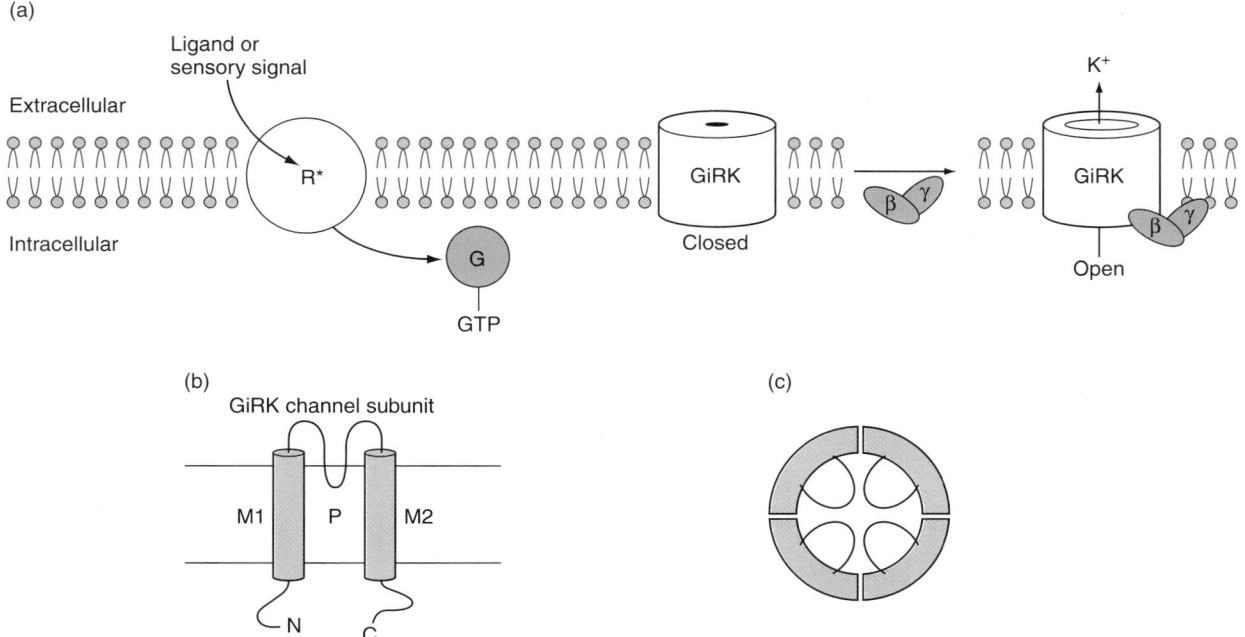

Figure 3.7 G protein-gated K channels.
(a) The opening of the G protein-gated inward rectifier K channels (GIRK) requires the binding of the G protein βγ subunits. **(b)** Putative transmembrane topology of the GIRK channel subunits with two putative transmembrane α-helices (M1 and M2) and the P region. **(c)** Top view of the putative tetrameric arrangement of the GIRK subunits around the central pore.

Consequently, sensory transduction in these cases is very rapid.

3.2.5 Mechanically gated channels opened by mechanical stimuli

Sensory receptors underlying the transduction of pressure, stretching, auditory and vestibular stimuli are ionic channels directly opened by the corresponding sensory stimulus. Consequently, transduction in these cases is very rapid.

Mechanically gated ion channels, such as stretch-activated channels, transduce mechanical stimuli into changes of membrane potential of specialized sensory cells (see Chapter 12). These channels are K+ selective, Cl− selective or non-selective cation channels. Mechanosensory transduction underlies a wide range of senses, including proprioception, touch, balance and hearing.

3.2.6 Other channels: junctional channels or gap junctions

These channels are different from all the channels mentioned so far because they are built with transmembrane proteins from two apposed plasma membranes. At the point of apposition the extracellular space is very narrow. These structures are called gap junctions

because they connect the cytoplasms of two adjacent cells. These are poorly selective channels but are more permeable to cations than to anions. They are also permeable to a number of small molecules (with molecular weights lower than 1200 D), such as the second messengers cAMP, inositol trisphosphate, but not to proteins or nucleic acids.

Junctional channels are usually open at the resting membrane potential. Their opening can be modulated by either the transjunctional potential (the voltage difference between the two internal sides of the coupled membranes), by intracellular or extracellular factors, or by second messengers. Thus, depending on the cell type they may open or close as a function of membrane potential, intracellular pH, intracellular concentration of Ca^{2+} ions and the presence of cyclic nucleotides (**Figure 3.9a**).

Connexins are the principal protein component of gap junctions. Genes coding for connexins were first sequenced from rat and human heart and liver cells and the amino acid sequences deduced. Hydrophobicity profiles and specific antibody binding to certain regions of the protein have led to a transmembrane model of the connexins. Each connexin has four putative transmembrane α-helices and both NH_2 and COOH terminals are oriented to the cytoplasmic side, accessible to intracellular regulatory elements (**Figure 3.9b**).

Junctional channels have a hexameric structure with a central aqueous pore 15 nm long, 2 nm wide at the ends

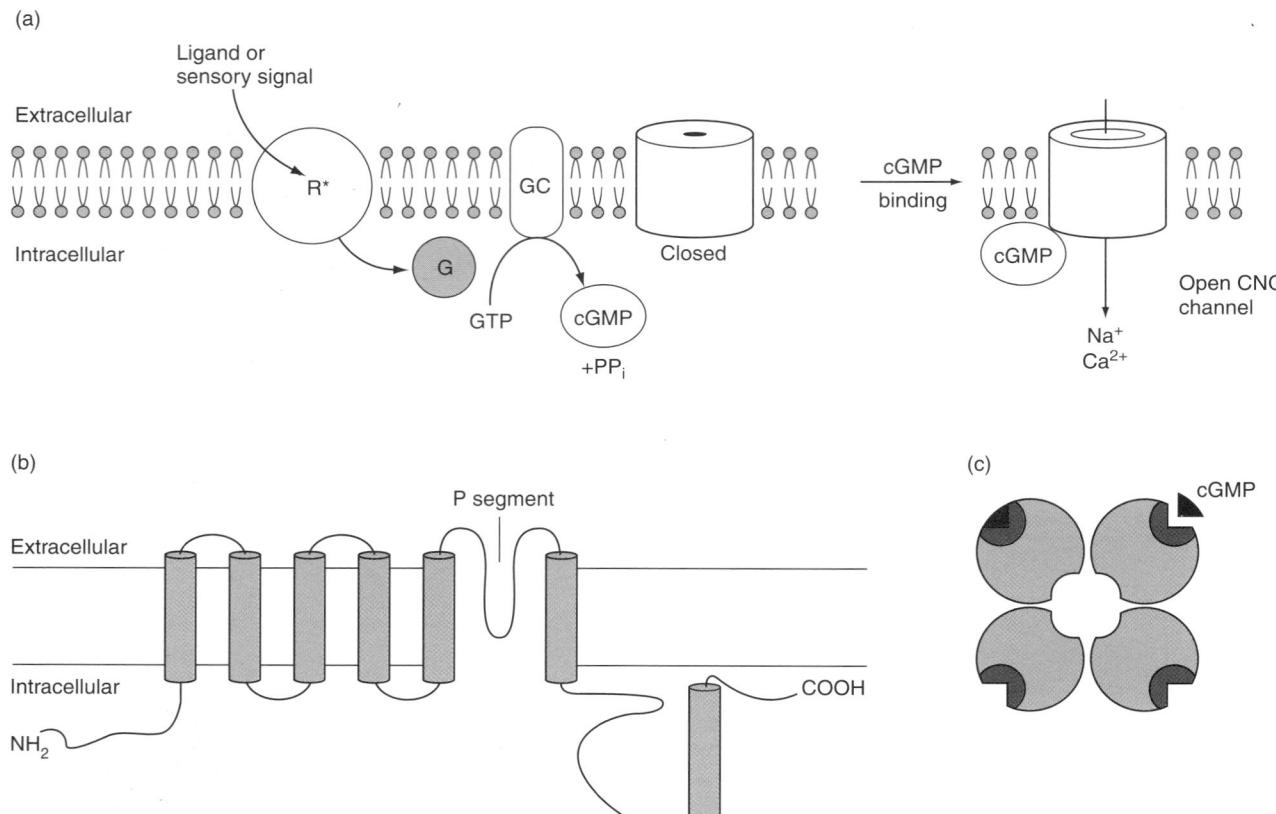

Figure 3.8 Cyclic nucleotide (CNG)-gated channels.
(a) CNG-gated channel open when four molecules of a cyclic nucleotide are bound to the receptor sites located on the intracellular face of the protein. **(b)** Putative transmembrane topology of the cGMP-gated channel of rods. The region between S5 and S6, the P segment, is thought to line the ion conducting pore. The cyclic nucleotide binding domain is shown in green. **(c)** Top view of the putative tetrameric arrangement of the subunits around the central pore. Drawings (b) and (c) adapted from Zagotta WN, Siegelbaum SA (1996) Structure and function of cyclic nucleotide-gated channels, *Ann. Rev. Neurosci.* **19**, 135–263.

and approximately 1.5 nm wide at the centre. Each hexamer belongs to the membrane of one of the coupled cells and constitutes a connexon formed by six connexins. A junctional channel is formed by the apposition of two connexons and its axis is perpendicular to the plane of the plasma membranes (**Figure 3.9c**).

There is a high density of gap junctions at electrical synapses. The function of these gap junctions is electrical and metabolic coupling as well as transfer of second messengers between the associated cells. Electrical coupling allows the rapid propagation of action potentials between neurons. This would give synchrony among a population of active neurons for the purpose of escape behaviours, for example (electrical coupling of crayfish cord neurons). In the heart, the primary function of gap junctions is to allow current flow from the pacemaker cells to ventricular muscle cells leading to their synchronized rhythmic contraction. Metabolic coupling is particularly important in the case of non-vascularized cells such as those of the eye lens. The exchange of second messengers (cyclic AMP, cyclic GMP, inositol trisphosphate, Ca^{2+}, etc.) allows the transfer of information between coupled cells.

3.2.7 Distribution of the various channels in the neuronal plasma membrane (Figure 3.10)

Voltage-sensitive Na^+ channels underlie the generation and propagation of sodium and sodium–calcium action potentials. They are present in high densities at the initial segment and nodes of Ranvier of the axon (in the case of myelinated axons) or all along the axon (in the case of non-myelinated axons). Na^+ channels are also found in the membrane of the cell body, but they are generally absent or present at a very low density in dendritic membranes. In fact, dendrites rarely generate or propagate sodium action potentials. The distribution of voltage-dependent K^+ channels will not be

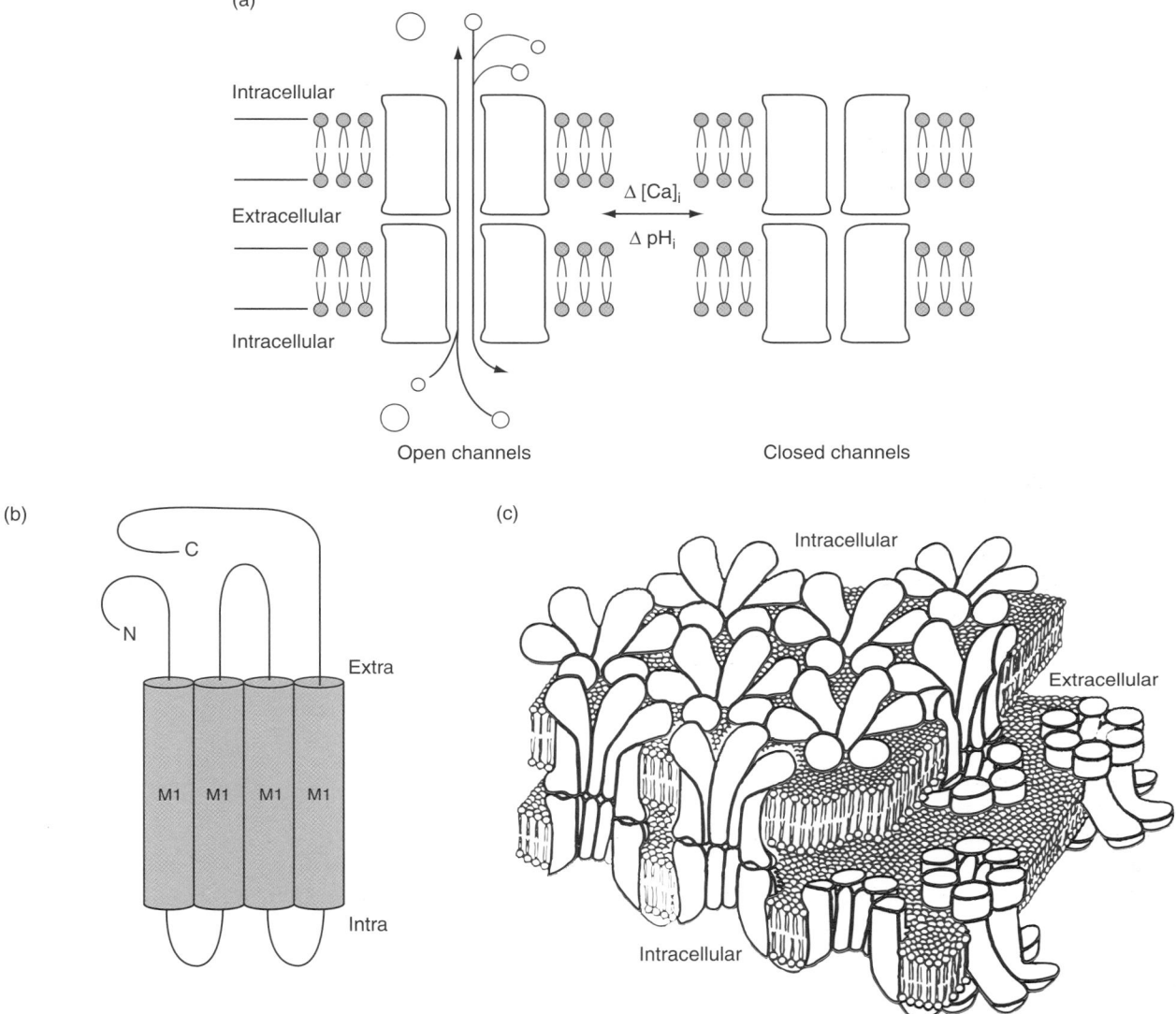

Figure 3.9 Gap junction channels.

(a) These channels allow bidirectional fluxes of ions and molecules of low molecular weight to cross them. Their opening is regulated, among other factors, by intracellular Ca^{2+} ions and pH. **(b)** Putative transmembrane organization of connexins. **(c)** Diagram of the structure of gap junctions in a lipid bilayer. These junctions are made up of 12 connexins molecules organized into two hexamers, called connexons. Each connexon has two domains, a transmembrane and a cytoplasmic domain. The aqueous pore situated at the centre of the connexon spans both plasma membranes. Drawing (b) adapted from Milks LC, Kumar NM, Houghten N *et al.* (1988) Topology of the 32-kD liver gap junction protein determined by site-directed antibody localizations, *EMBO J.* **7**, 2967–2975; (c) from Makowski L, Caspar DLD, Phillips WC *et al.* (1984) Gap junction structures: VI. Variation and conservation in connexon conformation and packing, *Biophys. J.* **45**, 208–218, with permission.

analysed here because of the large diversity of these channels.

Voltage-gated Ca^{2+} channels are located at high density at presynaptic terminals – axon terminal membranes, presynaptic dendrites or somatic presynaptic regions – where they ensure the Ca^{2+} inflow essential for the release of neurotransmitters. They can also be present in the dendritic or somatic membranes where they are the basis of the generation and propagation of calcium (dendrites) or sodium–calcium (soma) action potentials.

Neurotransmitter receptors are located at postsynaptic regions – postsynaptic membrane of the dendritic spines, the dendritic branches, the soma or the axon

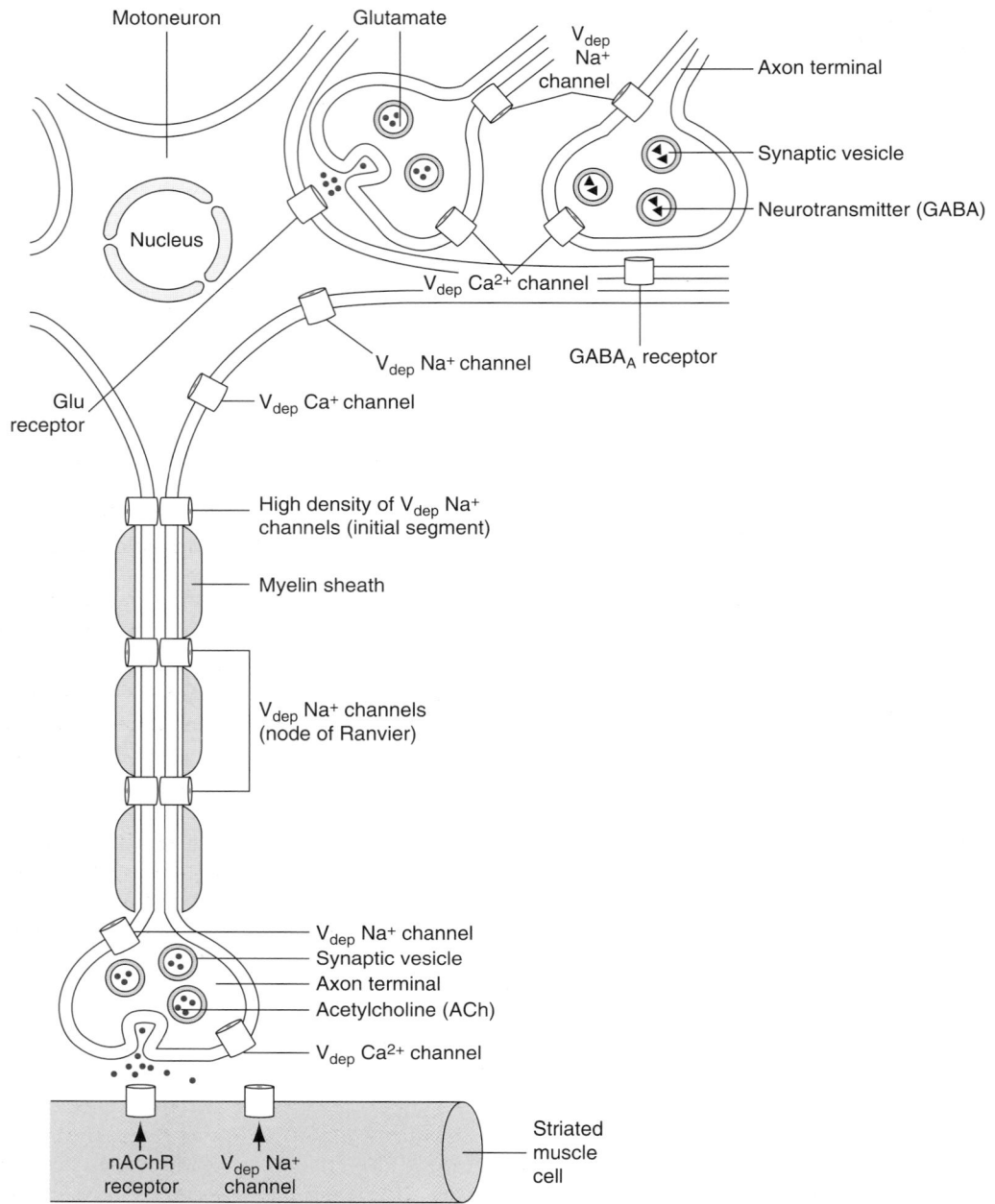

Figure 3.10 Localization of channels in the plasma membrane of neurons.

The diagram illustrates a motoneuron innervating a striated muscle cell and receiving excitatory (glutamate) and inhibitory (GABAergic) afferences originating in local circuit neurons from the spinal cord. General localization of voltage-dependent Na^+ and Ca^{2+} channels (V_{dep} channels) and receptor channels (nAChR, Glu and $GABA_A$ receptors). Voltage-gated K^+ channels and $GABA_B$ channels have been omitted. One channel symbolizes a population of channels of the illustrated type. nAChR, nicotinic acetylcholine receptor; GABA, γ-aminobutyric acid; $GABA_A$, type-A GABA receptor; Glu, glutamate.

(the latter in the case of axo-axonic synapses). They underlie synaptic transmission. They can also be found in presynaptic regions where they play a role in the control of neurotransmitter release.

Sensory receptors are located exclusively in membranes of sensory receptor cells where they underlie sensory signal transduction.

3.3 The diffusion of ions through an open channel: What is an electrochemical gradient and an ionic current?

It has been stated above that a channel is said to be in a closed state (C) when its ionic pore does not allow ions to pass. In contrast, when the channel is said to be in the open state (O), ions can diffuse through the ionic pore.

$$C \rightleftharpoons O$$

This diffusion of ions through an open channel is a passive transport since it does not require energy expenditure.

- Which type(s) of ions will move through a given open channel: cations, anions?
- In which direction will these ions move, from the external medium to the cytosol or the reverse?
- How many of these ions will move per unit of time?

3.3.1 The structure of the channel pore determines the type of ion(s) that diffuse passively through the channel

The pores of ion channels select their permeant ions. The structural basis for ion channel selectivity has been studied in a bacterial K$^+$ channel called the KcsA channel (it is a voltage-independent K$^+$ channel). All K$^+$ channels show a selectivity sequence K$^+$ = Rb$^+$ > Cs$^+$, whereas permeability for the smallest alkali metal ions Na$^+$ and Li$^+$ is extremely low. Potassium is at least 10 000 times more permeant than Na$^+$, a feature that is essential to the function of K$^+$ channels. Each subunit of the K$^+$ channel consists of an N-terminal cytoplasmic domain, followed by six transmembrane helices (or two transmembrane helices for KcsA), and a C-terminal globular domain in the cytoplasm (**Figures 3.11a,b**). The P loop (P for pore) situated between transmembrane helices 5 and 6 or 1 and 2, depending on the K$^+$ channel considered, is the region primarily responsible for ion selectivity.

The KcsA channel is overexpressed in bacteria and the three-dimensional structure of its pore is investigated by the use of X-ray crystallography. The KcsA channel is a tetramer with fourfold symmetry around a central pore. The pore is constructed of an inverted teepee with the extracellular side corresponding to the base of the teepee (**Figure 3.11c**). The overall length of the pore is 4.5 nm and its diameter varies along its distance. From inside the cell the pore begins as a water-filled tunnel of 1.8 nm length (inner pore) surrounded by predominantly non-polar side-chains pointing to the pore axis. The diameter of this region is sufficiently wide to allow the passage of fully hydrated cations. This long entry way then opens to a wider water-filled cavity (1 nm across). Beyond this vestibule is the 1.2 nm long selectivity filter. After this, the pore opens widely to the extracellular side of the membrane.

What are the respective roles of the parts of the pore?

Electrostatic calculations show that when an ion is moved along a narrow pore through a membrane it must cross an energy barrier that is maximum at the membrane centre. A K$^+$ ion can move throughout the inner pore and cavity and still remain mostly hydrated, owing to the large diameter of these regions. The role of the inner pore and the cavity is to lower the electrostatic barrier. The cavity overcomes the electrostatic destabilization from the low dielectric bilayer by simply surrounding an ion with polarizable water. Another feature that contributes to the stabilization of the cation at the bilayer centre are the four pore helices which point directly at the centre of the cavity. The amino to carboxyl orientation of these helices imposes a negative electrostatic (cation attractive) potential via the helix dipole effect. These two mechanisms (large aqueous cavity and oriented helices) serve to stabilize a cation in the hydrophobic membrane interior.

The selectivity filter that follows, in contrast, is lined exclusively by polar main-chain atoms. They create a stack of sequential carbonyl oxygen rings which provide multiple closely spaced binding sites for cations separated by 0.3–0.4 nm. This selectivity filter attracts K$^+$ ions and allows them to move.

Why are cations permeant and not anions?

As might have been anticipated for a cation channel, both the intracellular and extracellular entryways are negatively charged by acidic amino acids, an effect that would raise the local concentration of cations while lowering the concentration of anions.

Why are K$^+$ ions at least 10 000 times more permeant than Na$^+$ ions?

The selectivity filter is so narrow that a K$^+$ ion evidently dehydrates to enter into it and only a single K$^+$ ion can pass through at one time. To compensate for the energy cost of dehydration, the carbonyl oxygen atoms come in very close contact with the ion and act like surrogate water – they substitute for the hydration waters of K$^+$. This filter is too large to accommodate a Na$^+$ ion with its smaller radius (main chain oxygens are spatially

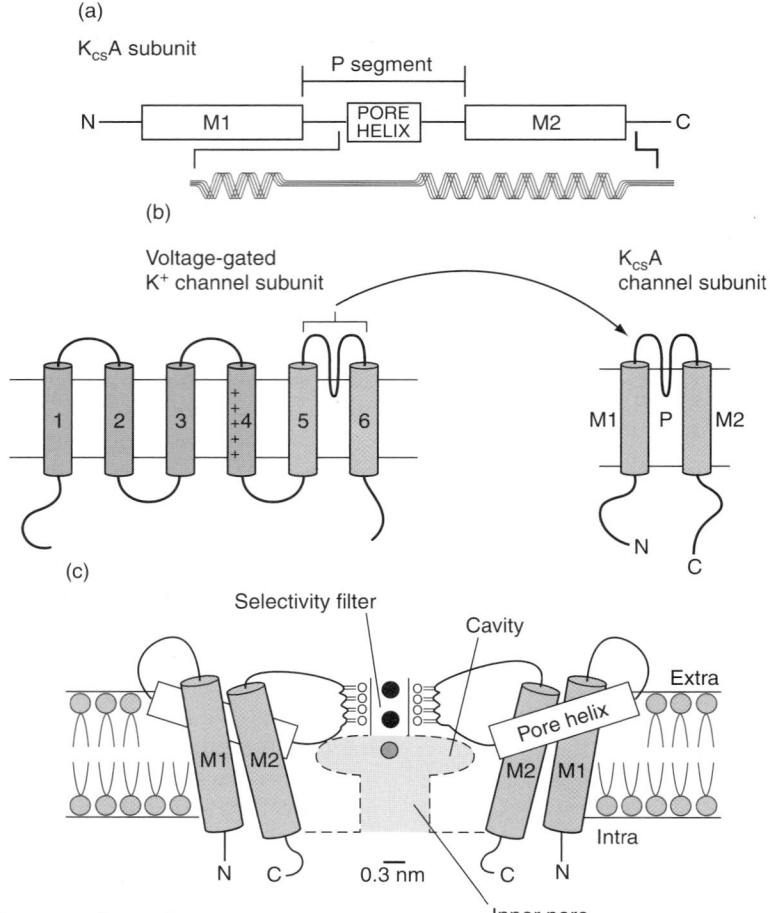

(a)

$K_{cs}A$ subunit

(b)

Voltage-gated
K+ channel subunit

$K_{cs}A$
channel subunit

(c)

Selectivity filter

Cavity

Extra

Pore helix

Intra

0.3 nm

Inner pore

Figure 3.11 Model of the KcsA channel pore.
(a) Secondary structural elements for the *Streptomyces lividans* K+ channels (KcsA). (b) Topological relationship between voltage-gated K+ channels in which six transmembrane helices from each subunit cluster around the central pore, and the KcsA channel in which two core helices, M1 and M2 and the P region, constitute each subunit of a tetrameric assembly. (c) Only two subunits of KcsA are shown for clarity. The pore axis is vertical with the extracellular side on the top. Aqueous inner pore and cavity are in green. The selectivity filter is in grey. See text for further explanations. O: oxygen. Adapted from Doyle DA, Cabral JM, Pfuetzner RA *et al.* (1998) The structure of the potassium channel: molecular basis of K+ conduction and selectivity, *Science* **280**, 69–77; and Choe S, Robinson R (1998) An ingenious filter: the structural basis for ion channel selectivity. *Neuron* **20**, 821–823.

inflexible and their relative distances to the centre of the pore cannot readily be changed). It is proposed that a K+ ion fits in the filter so precisely that the energetic costs and gains are well balanced.

What drives K+ ions to move on?

K+ ions bind simultaneously at two binding sites 0.75 nm apart near the entry and exit point of the selectivity filter. Binding at adjacent sites may provide the repulsive force for ion flow through the selectivity filter: two K+ ions at close proximity in the selectivity filter repel each other. The repulsion overcomes the strong interaction between ion and protein and allows rapid conduction in the setting of high selectivity. This leads to a rate of diffusion of around 10^8 ions per second.

3.3.2 The electrochemical gradient for a particular ion determines the direction of the passive diffusion of this ion through an open channel

To predict the direction of diffusion of ions through an open channel, both the concentration gradient of the ion and the membrane potential have to be known. The *resultant* of these two forces is called the electrochemical gradient. To understand what the electrochemical gradient is for a particular ion, the concentration gradient and membrane potential will first be explained separately.

The passive diffusion of ions down their concentration gradient

The concentration gradient of a particular ion is the difference of concentration of this ion between the two sides of the plasma membrane. A difference of concentration allows passive diffusion of ions through an open channel, since ions move from the medium where their concentration is high to the medium where their concentration is lower. Suppose that membrane potential is null ($V_m = 0$ mV); there is no difference of potential between the two faces of the membrane, so ions will diffuse according to their concentration gradient only (**Figure 3.12a**). Since the extracellular concentrations of Na^+, Ca^{2+} and Cl^- are higher than the respective intracellular ones, these ions will diffuse passively towards the intracellular medium (when Na^+, Ca^{2+} or Cl^- permeable channels are open) as a result of their concentration gradient. In contrast, K^+ will move from the intracellular medium to the extracellular one (when K^+ permeable channels are open).

The force that makes ions move down their concentration gradient is *constant* for a given ion since it depends only on the difference of concentration of this ion, which is itself continuously controlled to a constant value by active transport (pumps and transporters). However, this is not always true; during intense neuronal activity, concentration of ions may change (K^+ concentration in particular) owing to the small volume of the external medium. At the microscopic level this is not true also; intracellular Ca^{2+} concentration, for example, can increase locally by a factor of between 100 and 1000 but stay stable in the entire cytosol. However, these increases of ion concentration do not change the

direction of the concentration gradient for this ion since, as we will see, a concentration gradient cannot reverse by itself.

The passive diffusion of ions according to potential gradient

Membrane potential is a potential gradient that forces ions to move in one direction: positive ions are attracted by the 'negative' side of the membrane and negative ions by the 'positive' one. If we suppose that there is no concentration gradient for any ions (there is the same concentration of each ion in the extracellular and intracellular media), ions will diffuse according to membrane potential only. At a membrane potential $V_m = -30$ mV (**Figure 3.12b**), positively charged ions, the cations Na^+, Ca^{2+} and K^+, will move from the extracellular medium to the intracellular one according to membrane potential. In contrast, anions (Cl^-) will move from the intracellular medium to the extracellular one.

The passive diffusion of ions according to both the concentration gradient and membrane potential: the electrochemical gradient

In physiological conditions, the direction and amplitude of ion diffusion through an open channel is determined by both the concentration gradient and membrane potential. Since concentration gradient is constant for each ion, the direction and amplitude of diffusion varies with membrane potential. **Figure 3.12** shows that at a membrane potential of -30 mV, concentration gradient

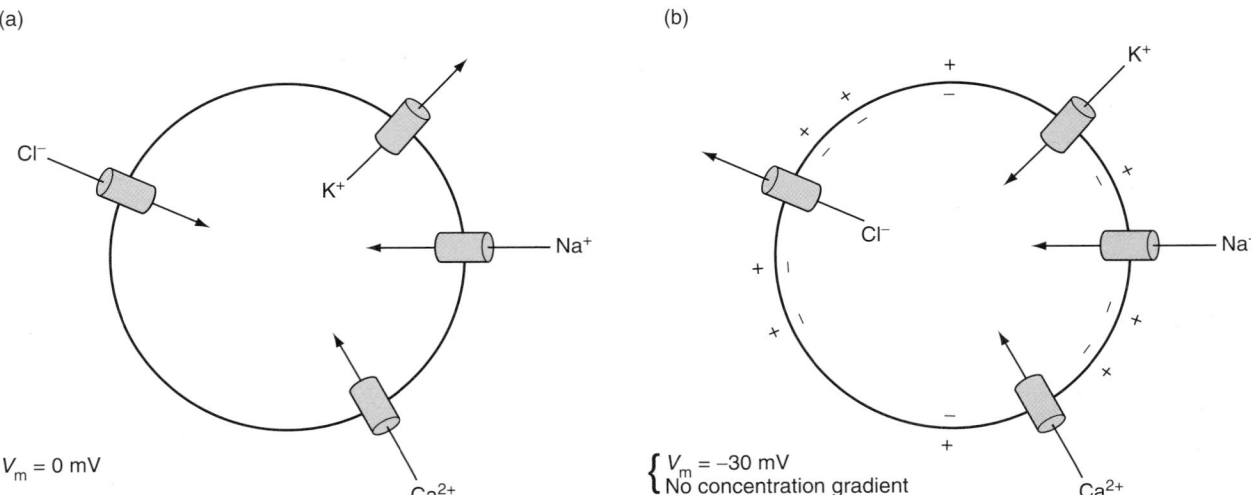

(a)

Cl^-

K^+

Na^+

$V_m = 0$ mV

Ca^{2+}

(b)

K^+

Cl^-

Na^+

$\begin{cases} V_m = -30 \text{ mV} \\ \text{No concentration gradient} \end{cases}$

Ca^{2+}

Figure 3.12 Passive diffusion.
Passive diffusion of ions according to **(a)** their concentration gradient only, or **(b)** to membrane potential only at $V_m = -30$ mV.

and membrane potential drive Na^+ and Ca^{2+} ions in the same direction, toward the intracellular medium, whereas they drive K^+ and Cl^- in reverse directions (compare the two parts of **Figure 3.12**). The resultant of these two forces, concentration and potential gradients, is the electrochemical gradient. To know how to express the electrochemical gradient, the equilibrium potential must first be explained.

The equilibrium potential, E_{ion}

All systems are moving toward equilibrium. The value of membrane potential where the concentration force that tends to move a particular ion in one direction is exactly balanced by the electrical force that tends to move the same ion in the reverse direction is called the 'equilibrium potential' of the ion (E_{ion}). The equilibrium potential for a particular ion is the membrane potential for which the net flux of this ion (f_{net}) through an open channel is null: when $V_m = E_{ion}$, $f_{net} = 0$ mol s^{-1}.

E_{ion} can be calculated using the Nernst equation (see Appendix 3.2):

$$E_{ion} = (RT/zF) \ln ([ion]_e/[ion]_i),$$

where R is the constant of an ideal gas (8.314 VCK^{-1} mol^{-1}), T is the absolute temperature in kelvins (273.16 + the temperature in °C); F is the Faraday constant (96 500 C mol^{-1}); z is the valence of the ion; and [ion] is the concentration of the ion in the extracellular or intracellular medium. This gives:

$$E_{ion} = (58/z) \log_{10} ([ion]_e/[ion]_i), \qquad (1)$$

From the equation and concentrations of **Figure 3.2**, the equilibrium potentials for each ion can be calculated:

$$E_{Na} = (58/1) \log_{10} (140/14) = +58 \text{ mV}$$
$$E_K = (58/1) \log_{10} (3/160) = -84 \text{ mV}$$
$$E_{Ca} = (58/2) \log_{10} (1/10^{-4}) = +116 \text{ mV}$$
$$E_{Cl} = (58/-1) \log_{10} (150/14) = -58 \text{ mV}.$$

These equations have the following meanings. If the channels open in a membrane are for example all permeable to K^+ ions, the efflux of K^+ ions will hyperpolarize the membrane until $V_m = E_K = -84$ mV, a potential where K^+ ions have the same tendency to diffuse towards the intracellular medium according to their concentration gradient than to move in the reverse direction according to membrane potential. At that potential the efflux of K^+ will stop and the membrane potential will stay stable if K^+ channels stay open (see Chapter 4). Now, if only Na^+ channels are open, the membrane potential will move toward $V_m = +58$ mV,

the potential at which the net flux of Na^+ is null. Similarly when $V_m = E_{Cl} = -60$ mV, Cl^- ions have the same tendency to move down their concentration gradient than to move in the reverse direction according to membrane potential; the net flux of Cl^- is null. In contrast, when V_m is different from E_{Cl}, the net flux of Cl^- is not null. This holds true for all the other ions: when V_m is different from E_{ion} there is a net flux of this ion.

The electrochemical gradient

We have seen that when $V_m = E_{ion}$ (i.e. $V_m - E_{ion} = 0$), there is no diffusion of this particular ion ($f_{net} = 0$). In contrast, when V_m is different from E_{ion} there is a passive diffusion of this ion through an open channel. The difference ($V_m - E_{ion}$) is called the electrochemical gradient. It is the force that makes the ion move through the open channel.

3.3.3 The passive diffusion of ions through an open channel is a current

To know the direction of passive diffusion of a particular ion and how many of these ions diffuse per unit of time, the direction and intensity of the net flux of ions (number of moles per second) through an open channel have to be measured. Usually the net flux (f_{net}) is not measured; the electrical counterpart of this net flux, the ionic current, is measured instead.

Passive diffusion of ions through an open channel is a movement of charges through a resistance (resistance here is a measure of the difficulty of ions moving through the channel pore). Movement of charges through a resistance is a current. Through a single channel the current is called 'single-channel current' or 'unitary current', i_{ion}. The relation between f_{net} and i_{ion} is:

$$i_{ion} = f_{net}\, z\, F.$$

The amplitude of i_{ion} is expressed in ampères (A) which are coulombs per seconds (C s^{-1}). F is the Faraday constant (96 500 C); z is the valence of the ion (+1 for Na^+ and K^+, -1 for Cl^-, $+2$ for Ca^+); and f_{net} is the net flux of the ion in mol s^{-1}.

In general, currents are expressed following Ohm's law: $U = RI$, where I is the current through a resistance R and U is the difference of potential between the two ends of the resistance. For currents carried by ions (and not by electrons as in copper wires), I is called i_{ion}, the current that passes through the resistance of the channel pore which has a resistance R (called r_{ion}). But what is U in biological systems? U is the force that makes ions move in a particular direction; it is the electrochemical gradient for the considered ion and is also called the driving force: $U = V_m - E_{ion}$ (**Figure 3.13**).

Unitary current, i_{ion}

According to Ohm's law, the current i_{ion} through a single channel is derived from $(V_m - E_{ion}) = r_{ion} \times i_{ion}$. So:

$$i_{ion} = (1/r_{ion})\,(V_m - E_{ion}) = \gamma_{ion}\,(V_m - E_{ion}).$$

γ_{ion} is the reciprocal of resistance; it is called the *conductance* of the channel, or unitary conductance. It is a measure of the ease of flow of ions (flow of current) through the channel pore. Whereas resistance is expressed in ohms (Ω), conductance is expressed in siemens (S). By convention i_{ion} is negative when it represents an inward flux of cations and positive when it represents an outward flux of cations. It is generally of the order of

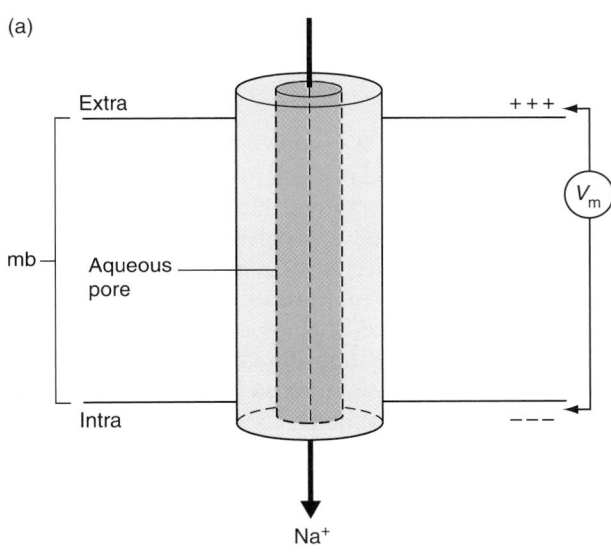

(a)

Extra

V_m

mb — Aqueous pore

Intra

Na^+

(b)

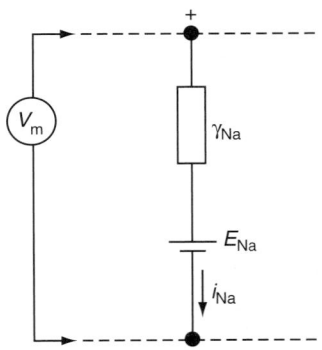

V_m

γ_{Na}

E_{Na}

i_{Na}

Figure 3.13 An Na⁺ channel.
(**a**) Schematic, and (**b**) its electrical equivalent.

pico-ampères (1 pA = 10^{-12} A). At physiological concentrations, γ_{ion} varies between 10 and 150 pico-siemens (pS), according to the channel type.

Total current, I_{ion}

In physiological situations, several channels of the same type are open at the same time in the neuronal membrane. Suppose that only one type of channel is open in the membrane, for example Na⁺ channels. The total current I_{Na} that crosses the membrane at time t is the sum of the unitary currents i_{Na} at time t:

$$I_{Na} = Np_o i_{Na},$$

where N is the number of Na⁺ channels present in the membrane; p_o is the probability of Na⁺ channels being open at time t (Np_o is therefore the number of open Na⁺ channels in the membrane at time t); and i_{Na} is the unitary Na⁺ current. More generally:

$$I_{ion} = Np_o i_{ion}.$$

By analogy, the total conductance of the membrane for a particular ion is:

$$G_{ion} = Np_o \gamma_{ion};$$

and from $i_{ion} = \gamma_{ion}(V_m - E_{ion})$ above:

$$I_{ion} = G_{ion}(V_m - E_{ion}).$$

I_{ion} and i_{ion} can be measured experimentally. The latter is the current measured from a patch of membrane where only one channel of a particular type is present. I_{ion} is the current measured from a whole cell membrane where N channels of the same type are present.

Roles of ionic currents

Ionic currents have two main functions:

■ Ionic currents change the membrane potential: either they depolarize the membrane or repolarize it or hyperpolarize it, depending on the charge carrier. These terms are in reference to resting potential (see **Figure 3.3**). A depolarization can be an action potential (see Chapters 5 and 6) or postsynaptic excitatory potentials (EPSPs; see Chapters 9, 11 and 12). These changes of membrane potential are essential to neuronal communication.
■ Ionic currents increase the concentration of a particular ion in the intracellular medium. Calcium

current, for example, is always inward. It transiently and locally increases the intracellular concentration of Ca^{2+} ions and contributes to the triggering of Ca^{2+}-dependent events such as secretion or contraction.

3.4 Active transport of Na⁺, K⁺, Ca²⁺ and Cl⁻ ions by pumps and transporters maintain the unequal distribution of ions

Passive movements of Na^+, K^+, Ca^{2+} or Cl^- ions across the membrane would normally cause concentration changes in the extracellular and intracellular compartments if they were not constantly regulated during the entire life of the neuron by transport of ions in the reverse direction, against passive diffusion; i.e. against electrochemical gradients. This type of transport is described as active since it requires energy in order to oppose the electrochemical gradient of the transported ions. Ions cross the membrane *actively* through specialized proteins known as pumps or transporters. Pumps obtain energy from the hydrolysis of ATP, whereas transporters use the energy of an ionic gradient, for example the sodium driving force.

3.4.1 Pumps are ATPases that actively transport ions

Pumps have ATPase activity (they hydrolyse ATP). This ATPase activity is generally the easiest way of identifying them. Pumps are membrane-embedded enzymes that couple the hydrolysis of ATP to active translocation of ions across the membrane. The central issue of ion motive ATPases is to couple the hydrolysis of ATP (and their auto-phosphorylation) to the translocation of ions.

The Na/K-ATPase pump

Na/K-ATPases maintain the unequal distribution of Na^+ and K^+ ions across the membrane. Na^+ and K^+ ions cross the membrane through different Na^+ and K^+ permeable channels (voltage-sensitive Na^+ and K^+ channels plus receptor channels). This pump operates continuously at a rhythm of 100 ions per second (compared with 10^6–10^8 ions per second for a channel), adjusting its activity to the electrical activity of the neuron. It actively transports three Na^+ ions towards the extracellular space for each two K^+ ions that it carries into the cell.

The energy of ATP hydrolysis is needed for the conformational changes that allow the pump to change its affinity for the ion transported, whether the binding sites are accessible from the cytoplasmic or the extracellular sides. For example, when the Na^+ binding sites are accessible from the cytoplasm, the protein is in a conformation with a high affinity (K_A = 1 mM) for intracellular Na^+ ions, and so Na^+ ions bind to the three sites. In contrast, when the three Na^+ have been translocated to the extracellular side, the protein is in a conformation with a low affinity for Na^+ ions so that the three Na^+ are released in the extracellular space.

These conformational changes are energy-dependent. The Na/K-ATPase has a catalytic α-subunit comprising about 1000 amino acids with a molecular weight of approximately 100 kDa. It comprises the catalytic site for ATP hydrolysis. It presents ten hypothetic transmembrane domains. A second β-subunit is closely associated with it. They generally form a tetramer $(\alpha\beta)_2$.

The steady unequal distribution of Na^+ and K^+ ions constitutes a reserve of energy for a cell. The neuron uses this energy to produce electric signals (action potentials, synaptic potentials) as well as to actively transport other molecules.

The Ca-ATPase pump

The function of Ca-ATPases is to maintain (with the Na–Ca transporter) the intracellular Ca^{2+} concentration at very low levels by active expulsion of Ca^{2+}. In fact, the intracellular Ca^{2+} concentration is 10 000 times lower than the extracellular concentration despite the inflow of Ca^{2+} (through receptor channels and voltage-gated Ca^{2+} channels) and the intracellular release of Ca^{2+} from intracellular stores. Maintaining a low intracellular Ca^{2+} concentration is critical since Ca^{2+} ions control several intracellular reactions and are toxic at a high concentration. Ca-ATPases are located in the plasma membrane and in the membrane of the reticulum. The former extrude Ca^{2+} from the cytoplasm whereas the latter sequester Ca^{2+} inside the reticulum (see also **Figure 8.8**).

Ca-ATPases have been isolated from the sarcoplasmic reticulum of rabbit muscle cells. They have only one subunit, called α, which presents a transmembrane organization similar to that of the α-subunit of the Na/K-ATPase. There are several sequence homologies between these two subunits. Most homologous regions are located in the large cytoplasmic domain implicated in ATP recognition and hydrolysis.

3.4.2 Transporters use the energy stored in the transmembrane electrochemical gradient of Na⁺, H⁺ or other ions

When transporters carry Na^+ or H^+ ions (along their electrochemical gradient) in the same direction as the transported ion or molecule the process is called *symport*. When the movements occur in opposite directions the process is called *antiport*. We shall study only transporters implicated in the electrical or secretory activity of neurons.

The Na–Ca transporter

This transporter uses the energy of the Na^+ gradient to actively carry Ca^{2+} ions towards the extracellular environment. It is situated in the neuronal plasma membrane and operates in synergy with the Ca-ATPase and with transport mechanisms of the smooth sarcoplasmic reticulum to maintain the intracellular Ca^{2+} concentration at a very low level. Molecular cloning, expression and deduced amino acid sequence of the Na–Ca exchanger of the cardiac sarcolemmal membrane shows that the protein has 12 hypothetic transmembrane segments.

Neurotransmitter transporters

Inactivation of most neurotransmitters present in the synaptic cleft is achieved by rapid reuptake into the presynaptic neural element and astrocytic glial cells. This is performed by specific neurotransmitter transporters, transmembrane proteins that couple neurotransmitter transport to the movement of ions down their concentration gradient. Certain neurotransmitter precursors are also taken up by this type of active transport (glutamine and choline, for instance). Once in the cytoplasm, neurotransmitters are concentrated inside synaptic vesicles by distinct transport systems driven by the H^+ concentration gradient (maintained by the vesicular H^+-ATPase).

3.5 Summary

Passage of ions through the membrane is a regulated process and the flow of ions across the neuronal plasma membrane is not a simple and anarchic diffusion through a lipid bilayer. Instead, it is restricted through transmembrane proteins whose opening (channel proteins) or activation (pumps or transporters) is tightly controlled by different factors. The following are the answers to the questions of Section 3.1.

Where and how do ions passively cross the plasma membrane?

Ions move passively across the plasma membrane through ionic channels that are specifically permeable to one or several ions. They move down their electrochemical gradient. This passive movement of charges is a current that can be recorded. Through a single channel it is a unitary current i_{ion}, and through N channels it is a macroscopic current or total current I_{ion}.

- The type of ion that moves through an open channel (ionic selectivity of the channel pore) is determined by the structure of the channel itself. This ionic selectivity gives the name to the channel. For example, a Na^+ channel is permeable to Na^+ ions; a cationic channel is permeable to cations, Na^+, K^+ and sometimes also Ca^{2+}.
- The *direction* of ion diffusion through a single channel depends on the electrochemical gradient or driving force for this particular ion ($V_m - E_{ion}$).
- The *number* of charges that diffuse through an open channel per unit of time (i_{ion}) depends on the electrochemical gradient ($V_m - E_{ion}$) but also on how easily ions move through the pore of the channel (expressed as the conductance γ_{ion} of the channel).

How and where do ions actively cross the plasma membrane and thus compensate for the passive movements?

Active movements of Na^+, K^+, Ca^{2+} or Cl^- ions across the membrane occur through pumps or transporters. Pumps obtain energy from the hydrolysis of ATP, whereas transporters use the energy of an ionic gradient, for example the sodium driving force. These transports require energy since they operate against the electrochemical gradient of the transported ions or molecules. They maintain ionic concentrations at constant values in the extracellular and intracellular compartments despite the continuous passive movements of ions across the membrane.

What are the roles of electrochemical gradients and passive movements of ions?

The electrochemical gradients of ions are a reserve of energy: they allow the existence of ionic currents and drive some active transports. Ionic currents have two main functions: (i) they evoke transient changes of membrane potential which are electrical signals of the neuron (action potentials or postsynaptic potentials or sensory potentials) essential to neuronal communication; and (ii) they locally increase the concentration of a particular ion in the intracellular medium, for example Ca^{2+} ions, and thus trigger intracellular Ca^{2+}-dependent events such as secretion or contraction.

Appendix 3.1
Hydrophobicity profile of a transmembrane protein

The hydrophobicity profile of a protein represents the degree of attraction to water of different regions of the molecule. By convention, the more hydrophilic regions are denoted – and the more hydrophobic ones are denoted +. Hydrophilicity and hydrophobicity are the two extremes of the hydrophobicity scale.

Determination of the hydrophilic and hydrophobic characters of a protein

This determination is possible when the primary structure of the protein is known. Each one of the 20 amino acids has been given a value for its hydropathic character that approximately reflects the hydrophilic or hydrophobic nature of its side-chain; i.e. its tendency to remain in contact with water (hydrophilicity) or its tendency to repel it (hydrophobicity) (**Table A3.1**). Protein segments containing a high percentage of polar or charged amino acids are hydrophilic, whereas segments containing a high percentage of non-polar amino acids (isoleucine or valine) are hydrophobic.

Table A3.1 Hydrophobicity index of the side chains of each of the 20 amino acids. From Kyte J, Doolittle RF (1982). A simple method for displaying the hydropathic character of a protein. *J. Mol. Biol.* **157**, 107–132, with permission.

Lateral chain	Hydropathy index
Isoleucine	4.5
Valine	4.2
Leucine	3.8
Phenylalanine	2.8
Cysteine/cystine	2.5
Methionine	1.9
Alanine	1.8
Glycine	−0.4
Threonine	−0.7
Tryptophane	−0.9
Serine	−0.8
Tyrosine	−1.3
Proline	−1.6
Histidine	−3.2
Glutamic acid	−3.5
Glutamine	−3.5
Aspartic acid	−3.5
Asparagine	−3.5
Lysine	−3.9
Arginine	−4.5

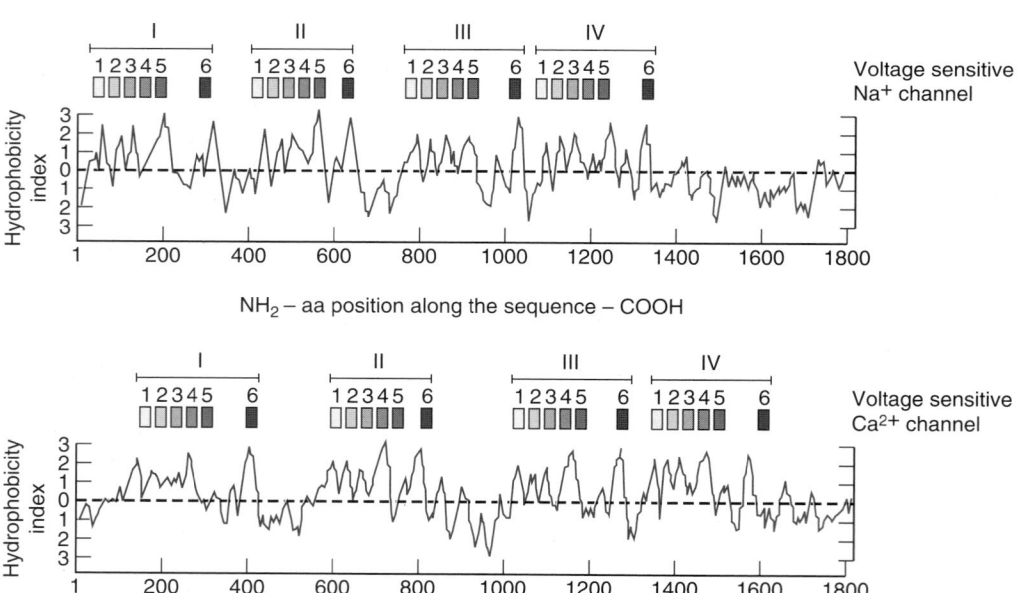

Figure A3.1 Hydrophobicity profile of the α-subunit of two voltage-sensitive channels.
The voltage-activated Na+ channel underlying the sodium action potential, and the voltage-activated dihydropyridine-sensitive Ca2+ channel. One can distinguish four hydrophobic domains (I to IV) in each protein, each composed of six segments (1 to 6). The hydrophilic COOH terminal domain of the Na+ channel is approximately twice as long as that of the Ca2+ channel. From Alsobrook JP, Stevens CF (1988) Cloning the calcium channel, *TINS* **11**, 1–2, with permission.

Computer programs exist that are capable of evaluating the hydrophilic or hydrophobic character all along a peptide sequence. By convention this analysis is performed from the NH_2 towards the COOH terminal. The length of each segment analysed is chosen by the experimenter, usually between 7 and 20 amino acids. The results can be expressed graphically: the hydrophobicity index of each segment is plotted against the position of the segment in the protein. Thus, one obtains the hydrophobicity profile (**Figure A3.1**).

Determination of the transmembrane organization of the protein

In the case of transmembrane proteins one assumes that the more hydrophobic regions, usually characterized by stretches of approximately 20 amino acids with positive values, are localized in the interior of the lipid bilayer, in the form of transmembrane α-helices. On the other hand, the more hydrophilic regions, characterized by uninterrupted negative values, are in contact with aqueous environments, thus constituting the hydrophilic extracellular or intracellular domains of the protein (see **Figures 3.5–3.8**).

Appendix 3.2
The Nernst equation

The material in this appendix is adapted from Katz B (ed) (1966) *Nerve, Muscle and Synapse* (New York: McGraw-Hill).

When $V_m = E_{ion}$, a particular ion has an equal tendency to diffuse in one direction according to its concentration gradient as to move in the reverse direction according to membrane potential. The net flux of this ion is null, so the current carried by this ion is null. $V_m = E_{ion}$ means that:

$$\text{osmotic work } (W_o) = \text{electrical work } (W_e). \quad (a)$$

The osmotic work required to move one mole of a particular ion from a compartment where its concentration is low to a compartment when its concentration is high is equal to the electrical work needed to move one mole of this ion against the membrane potential in the opposite direction. Here, active diffusion of ions is considered instead of passive diffusion.

The electrical work required to move 1 mole of an ion against a potential difference E_{ion} is:

$$W_e = zFE_{ion}, \quad (b)$$

where z is the valence of the transported ion, equal to +1

for monovalent cations such as Na^+ or K^+, to −1 for monovalent anions such as Cl^-, and to +2 for divalent cations such as Ca^{2+}.

F is the Faraday constant. F for hydrogen is the charge of one hydrogen atom: $F = Ne$. Here N is the Avogadro number, which is 6.022×10^{23} mol^{-1} (one mole of hydrogen atoms contains 6×10^{23} protons and the same number of electrons), and e is the elementary charge of a proton, which is 1.602×10^{-19} coulombs (C). So $F = 96\ 500$ C mol^{-1}.

Therefore zF with $z = 1$ is the charge of 1 mol of protons or 1 mol of monovalent cations (Na^+, K^+). The charge of one mole of monovalent anions (Cl^-) is $-F$ ($z = -1$); the charge of 1 mol of divalent cations (Ca^{2+}) is $2F$ ($z = 2$); etc.

The osmotic work required to move 1 mole of ions from a compartment where its concentration is low to a compartment where the concentration is high can be compared to the work done in compressing 1 g equivalent of an ideal gas. The gas is contained in a cylinder with a movable piston. Mechanical work to move the piston is W, calculated from force times distance of displacement of the piston (δl). The force exerted is equal to the pressure p of the gas multiplied by the surface area S of the piston. So the work δW done to displace the piston is $pS\delta l$, which equals $p\delta v$. Therefore the work done in compressing a gas from a volume v_1 to a volume v_2 is:

$$W = \int_{v_2}^{v_1} p\,dv. \quad (c)$$

The gas law tells us that $pv = RT$ (hence $p = RT/v$), with R the constant of an ideal gas ($R = 8.314$ V C K^{-1} mol^{-1}) and T is the absolute temperature.

Equation (c) can be changed to:

$$W = RT \int_{v_2}^{v_1} (1/v)dv = RT(\ln v_1 - \ln v_2)$$
$$= RT \ln (v_1/v_2). \quad (d)$$

By analogy the osmotic work is:

$$W_o = RT \ln ([ion]_e/[ion]_i). \quad (e)$$

From equation (a), $W_o = -W_e$, so from equations (b) and (e) the Nernst equation is obtained:

$$RT \ln ([ion]_e/[ion]_i) = zFE_{ion}$$

$$E_{ion} = (RT/zF) \ln ([ion]_e/[ion]_i). \quad \text{(Nernst)}$$

At 20°C, RT/F is about 25 mV, and moving from Neperian logarithms to decimal ones a factor of 2.3 is needed. Hence:

$$E_{ion} = (58/z) \log_{10} ([ion]_e/[ion]_i).$$

Further reading

Blaustein MP, Lederer WJ (1999) Sodium/calcium exchange: its physiological implications. *Physiol. Rev.* **79**, 763–854.

Carafoli E, Brini M (2000) Calcium pumps: structural basis for and mechanism of calcium transmembrane transport. *Curr. Opin. Chem. Biol.* **4**, 152–161.

Basic Properties of Excitable Cells at Rest

If a fine-tipped glass pipette (usually called a microelectrode), connected via a suitable amplifier to a recording system such as an oscilloscope, is pushed through the membrane of a living nerve cell to reach its cytoplasm, a potential difference is recorded between the cytoplasm and the extracellular compartment (**Figure 4.1a**). In fact, the cell interior shows a negative potential (typically between –60 and –80 mV) with respect to the outside, which is taken as the zero reference potential. In the absence of ongoing electrical activity, this negative potential remains stable and is therefore termed the resting membrane potential (V_{rest}). Since nerve cells communicate through rapid (milliseconds; ms) or slow (seconds; s) changes in their membrane potential, it becomes important to understand first how V_{rest} is maintained and the various mechanisms responsible for this phenomenon. It was Julius Bernstein (1902) who pioneered the theory of V_{rest} as due to selective permeability of the membrane to one ionic species only and that nerve excitation developed when such a selectivity was transiently lost. This concept leads us to consider various ways in which ions can cross a biological membrane and how these principles are applicable to the understanding of V_{rest}.

4.1 Ionic channels open at rest determine the resting membrane potential

Basically, membranes can use the following processes to shift ions across:

■ *Passive movement*. If the membrane contains permeable pores for a particular ionic species, such ions will move because of two physical causes, namely down their concentration gradient (obeying Fick's law) and according to the membrane electric field. Both processes are established by the transmembrane electrochemical gradient (i.e. they are dependent on concentration and potential). The electrochemical gradient determines the direction of movement for a particular ion, while the amount of

ionic current generated by the passage of these ions through a permeable pore depends not only on this gradient but also on the conductance (a measure of how easily ions can pass through a pore) of the pore itself. A classical theory to account for pore conductance is discussed later.

■ *Facilitated diffusion*. This process relies on carrier molecules residing in the cell membrane to help the translocation of ions without expenditure of external energy, while the concentration and electrical gradients remain the factors controlling the direction of movement and the final distribution attained.

(a)

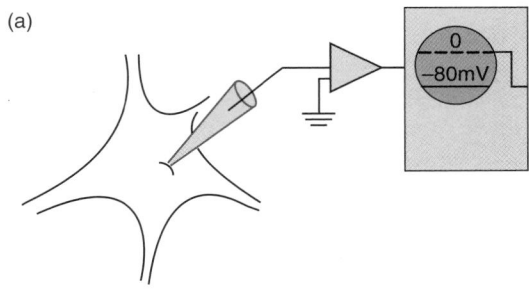

(b)

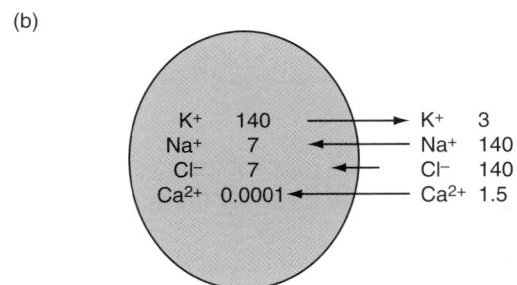

Figure 4.1 Resting membrane potential and ion concentrations.
(a) Schematic representation of microelectrode impalement of a nerve cell with a resting membrane potential of –80 mV.
(b) Idealized nerve cell (depicted as a sphere) with relative concentrations of intra- and extracellular ions. Direction of arrows indicates the direction of ion movement through open channels. Ion concentrations are expressed in millimoles.

■ *Active transport*. This requires selective transporter molecules plus energy expenditure (for example, obtained from hydrolysis of ATP or from movement of Na$^+$ down its electrochemical gradient). In this way, ions can be transported against electrochemical gradients. Often two (or more) ionic species are coupled to a single carrier molecule: if there is no net charge transfer (for example, one positive ion is moved out while a similarly charged ion enters into the cell), then the process is said to be electroneutral. However, the *stoichiometry* (i.e. the relative number of individual ions bound to a carrier molecule) of the carrier-mediated transport is often more complex (for instance three Na$^+$ are counter transported with one Ca^{2+}) so that there is a net gain or loss of charges in the cell and a resultant change in V_{rest}, as discussed in a subsequent section.

Of the three mechanisms introduced above, passive diffusion is by far the most important process for the immediate control of the membrane potential of nerve cells and thus their V_{rest}. The chief factor is the permeability of the membrane through specific pores of *ionic channels*, a phenomenon that depends on:

■ the conductance of single channels;
■ the probability of the channels opening;
■ the density of channels in the neuronal membrane.

If the channels are open, then the movement of a particular ionic species will depend on the electrochemical gradient. However, the crucial point is the mechanism that opens (or *gates*) channels: in the case of ligand-gated channels the signal is a chemical substance interacting with a specific receptor site of the channel; in the case of voltage-gated channels a rapid change in membrane potential will open them. Furthermore, some channels appear to be persistently open and are thus important in determining the actual value of V_{rest}. The principal ionic mechanisms of V_{rest} will thus be examined.

4.1.1 The plasma membrane separates two media of different ionic composition

The cytoplasm of a nerve cell is rich in K$^+$ (approximately 140 mM) while it is relatively poor in Na$^+$ (approximately 7 mM). The internal concentration of Cl$^-$ is also usually low (assume about 7 mM, though this value differs considerably depending on the cell considered) while the intracellular free Ca^{2+} is only about 0.1 µM. The cell inside is also rich in anions such as proteins and phosphates which have a large molecular weight and do not permeate through membrane channels. The cell membrane (with its lipoprotein composition) can be equated to an insulator separating two electrically conductive media (intracellular and extracellular electrolytes): it thus plays the role of a dielectric in a capacitor and it can be assigned an average capacity (C) value of 1 µF cm^{-2}.

The composition of the extracellular solution (in mM) is the opposite of the internal one: for example, Na$^+$ is about 140, K$^+$ is only about 3, Cl$^-$ is about 140 and Ca^{2+} is around 1.5 (**Figure 4.1b**). The extracellular concentration of large anions is very low. These large asymmetries in ion distribution imply a dynamic state through which cell-to-cell signalling is made possible.

4.1.2 At rest most of the channels open are K$^+$ channels

According to the original theory of Bernstein, under resting conditions the cell membrane permeability is minimal to Na$^+$, Cl$^-$ and Ca^{2+} while it is high to K$^+$. This condition can be verified experimentally by measuring ionic fluxes with radioactive tracers or by electrophysiological tests (as explained later). K$^+$ will therefore move outwards following its concentration gradient: in doing so it will subtract negative charges from the cell interior and will induce a relatively negative internal potential. Such a negativity will oppose further outward movements of K$^+$ until an equilibrium is reached when the concentration gradient for K$^+$ cancels the drive exerted by the electrical gradient. In other words, an *equilibrium potential* (E_{rev}) is obtained. Hence, at a membrane potential corresponding to E_{rev}, although K$^+$ keeps moving in and out of the cell, there is no net change in its concentration across the membrane (**Figure 4.2**).

E_{rev} is given by the Nernst equation, which for excitable cells according to Bernstein's theory related to K$^+$ is:

$$E_{rev} = (RT/zF) \ln ([K^+]_o/[K^+]_i),   (1)$$

where R is the gas constant, T is absolute temperature, z is valency, F is the Faraday number and $[K^+]_o$ and $[K^+]_i$ indicate extra- and intracellular potassium ion concentrations, respectively. Equation (1) is a particular case of Boltzmann's Law, relating molecular concentration at some place to potential energy of the molecule in that place.

At 20°C, $RT/zF = 25$ mV. This value can be multiplied by 2.3 to convert the natural logarithm into base 10 (log), thus giving 58 mV (at 37°C this value is 61 mV). Taking the K$^+$ concentration values indicated above means that E_{rev} for K$^+$ is −97 mV; i.e. the value at which there is no net transfer of K$^+$ across the cell membrane. Of course, this description of the K$^+$ potential is entirely based on a physical theory of passive ion movements. Its

(a)

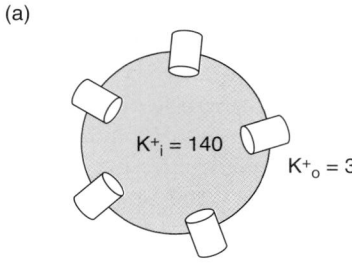

(b)

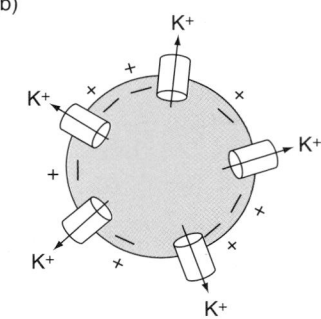

(c)

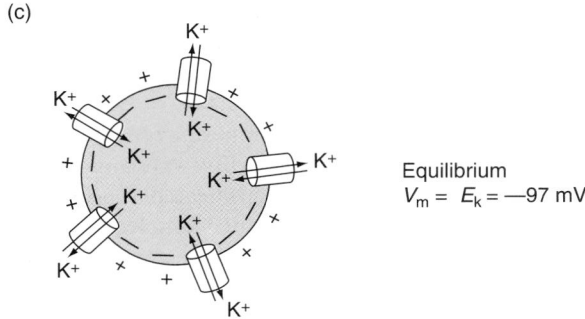

Equilibrium
$V_m = E_k = -97$ mV

Figure 4.2 Establishment of V_{rest} in a cell where most of the channels open are K⁺ channels.
Suppose that at $t = 0$ and cell potential = 0 mV (a), K⁺ will move outwards due to its concentration gradient (b). Loss of intracellular K⁺ induces a negative potential (V_m) as $V_m = E_K$ (c).

Table 4.1 Examples of ionic concentrations in the extracellular and intracellular media and the resulting Nernst potential for each ion

Ion	Intracellular concentration (mM)	Extracellular concentration (mM)	Nernst reversal potential (mV)
K⁺	140	3	–97
Na⁺	7	140	+75
Cl⁻	7	140	–75
Ca²⁺	0.0001	1.5	+129

a scheme of ion distribution across the cell membrane at rest, while **Table 4.1** summarizes these values.

4.1.3 In muscle cells, K⁺ and Cl⁻ ion movements participate equally in resting membrane potential

Some excitable cells, notably skeletal muscle fibres, have a demonstrably high resting permeability not only to K⁺ but also to Cl⁻. This condition can be equated to that of a semipermeable membrane separating two water solutions containing permeable ions (K⁺ and Cl⁻ in this case) but with an impermeable large ionic species (e.g. proteins) present on one side only. It is also necessary to suppose that the semipermeable membrane can withstand considerable hydrostatic pressure. In this system the non-permeable negatively charged ions will attract K⁺ while repelling Cl⁻. At equilibrium the following relation is established:

$$(RT/zF) \ln ([K^+]_o/[K^+]_i) = - (RT/zF) \ln ([Cl^-]_o/[Cl^-]_i), \quad (2)$$

since $z = 1$ for K⁺ and $z = -1$ for Cl⁻. Equation (2) can be simplified to:

$$[K^+]_o [Cl^-]_o = [K^+]_i [Cl^-]_i, \quad (3)$$

which is an example of the *Donnan equilibrium* applied to a cell. Note that one side of the membrane (corresponding to the intracellular compartment) will have a total concentration of ions larger than on the opposite side. This situation will tend to attract water molecules (which are considered to move freely across the membrane) until the larger hydrostatic pressure resulting from water accumulation prevents further movement of water molecules, thus yielding an equilibrium condition. Donnan equilibrium is a process whereby some cells can establish asymmetrical ion gradients at rest without the need of an active transport system.

transmembrane flux, however, involves active transport of ions as well.

Note that, in the case of central neurons with a strongly asymmetrical distribution of Cl⁻ between the extracellular and intracellular compartments, the Nernst equation for Cl⁻ (based on the concentrations stated above) yields an E_{rev} for this anion of –75 mV, since $E_{rev} = -58 \log ([Cl^-]_o/[Cl^-]_i)$ (owing to the negative value of z in equation (1)), which transforms into $E_{rev} = 58 \log ([Cl^-]_i/[Cl^-]_o)$. The Nernst equation applied to Na⁺ predicts an E_{rev} value of +75 mV. However, the gradients for Na⁺ and, in particular, for Ca²⁺ are regulated by complex mechanisms relying on transporters and intracellular sequestration so that the possibility of predicting the precise reversal potential of responses mediated by rises in Na⁺ or Ca²⁺ permeability on the basis of their apparent transmembrane concentrations is limited. **Figure 4.1b** presents

4.1.4 In central neurons, K⁺, Cl⁻ and Na⁺ ion movements participate in resting membrane potential: the Goldman–Hodgkin–Katz equation

Unlike muscle fibres, the value of V_{rest} of central neurons is not as negative as the predicted E_{rev} for K⁺, nor can it be adequately accounted for by the Donnan equilibrium for K⁺ and Cl⁻. Furthermore, inspection of the Nernst equation applied to K⁺ indicates that a 10-fold change in the concentration ratio should alter the membrane potential of a neuron by 58 mV (**Figure 4.3**).

This relation can be tested in experiments in which the extracellular (or intracellular) concentration of this ion is altered and the resulting membrane potential measured with a sharp or patch microelectrode. A semi-log plot of the extracellular K⁺ concentration (abscissa) against the membrane potential (ordinate) should thus have a slope of 58 mV per 10-fold change in K⁺; this condition is rarely encountered in neurons but it seems to be more common for glial cells (which sometimes are termed K⁺ electrodes because their membrane potential is linearly dependent on K⁺). In the case of neurons, non-linearity of this plot is frequently seen, particularly at low levels of extracellular K⁺.

These observations confirm that K⁺ is a very important ion for setting the value of neuronal V_{rest} but that other ionic mechanisms must also play a significant role. Since the intracellular concentration of Na⁺ is not negligible, this implies that this ionic species can accumulate inside the cytoplasm, presumably because its rather positive E_{rev} (+75 mV) versus a very negative V_{rest} creates an electrochemical gradient extremely favourable to Na⁺ entry. Equally, the asymmetric distribution of Cl⁻ suggests its possible role in determining V_{rest}. In order to take into account various ionic species it was useful to introduce what is commonly called the *Goldman–Hodgkin–Katz equation* (GHK):

$$V_{rest} = 58 \log \times \frac{p_K[K^+]_o + p_{Na}[Na^+]_o + p_{Cl}[Cl^-]_i}{p_K[K^+]_i + p_{Na}[Na^+]_i + p_{Cl}[Cl^-]_o} \quad (4)$$

where p is the permeability coefficient (cm s⁻¹) for each ionic species as explained in Section 4.1.5.

Note that if the resting permeability to Na⁺ and Cl⁻ is very low, the GHK equation closely resembles the Nernst equation for K⁺.

In applying the GHK equation to nerve cells, the following assumptions must be made:

- The voltage gradient across the membrane is uniform in the sense that it changes linearly within the membrane. This assumption has led to the GHK equation being called the *constant field equation*.
- The overall net current flow across the membrane is zero as the currents generated by individual ionic species are balanced out.
- The membrane is in a steady state since there is no time-dependent change in ionic flux or channel density. This is obviously not applicable to non-steady state conditions of rapidly changing membrane potential as produced when a nerve cell fires action potentials.
- Any role of active transport mechanisms is ignored. However, as discussed later, there is evidence for this transport of various ionic species.
- The ionic species are monovalent cations or anions which do not interact among themselves or with water molecules. This point does not hold true if there is a measurable permeability to divalent cations such as Ca²⁺. Furthermore, it has been reported that ions can interact among themselves within the same channel.
- The role of membrane surface charges is ignored. This is a relatively major limitation because the cell membrane contains negative charges on its inner and outer layers (amino acid residues of membrane proteins which are typically negatively charged). The electric field generated by these charges is able to influence the kinetic properties of ionic channels (gating, activation and inactivation). Adding divalent cations such as Ca²⁺ or Mg²⁺ leads to screening of these charges and consequent changes in channel properties.
- The mobility of each ionic species and its diffusion coefficient (D) within the membrane of thickness (δ) is constant.

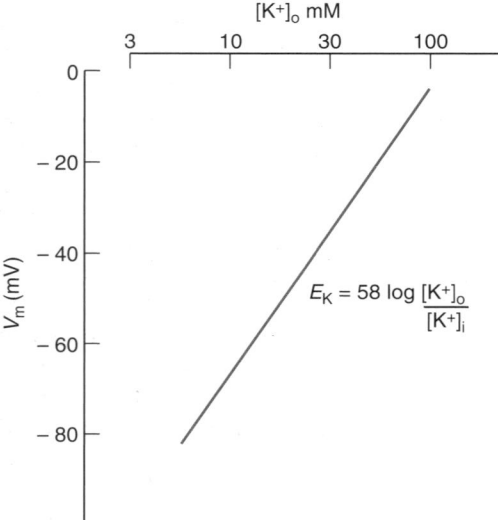

Figure 4.3 Theoretical diagram of E_K versus the external concentration of K⁺ ions ([K⁺]$_o$).
$E_K = (RT/zF)\,2.3 \times \log\,([K^+]_o/[K^+]_i)$.

- The ions do not bind to specific sites in the membrane and their concentration (C) can be expressed by a linear partition coefficient ($\beta = C_{membrane}/C_{solution}$). However, there is evidence that ions can bind to sites inside channels and influence channel kinetics.
- The ionic activities (a) can be replaced by their concentrations.

In summary, according to the GHK equation, the cell membrane potential is considered as a tridimensional space through which ions move, whereas in real terms the membrane contains distinct narrow pores for different ions.

4.1.5 Some principles related to the derivation of the GHK equation

In spite of the fact that several of these assumptions do not appear to be applicable to nerve cells, the GHK model can be a useful tool to describe the behaviour of an excitable membrane. It is of interest to understand the basic principles behind the derivation of this equation because they have important implications for the basic neurophysiological properties of excitable cells. The starting point is the Nernst–Planck diffusion equation which describes the dependence of the ionic flux across the membrane on the electrochemical and concentration gradients of a given ion. This can be represented by:

$$j = uc\left[RT\frac{d(\ln a)}{dx} + zF\frac{dV}{dx}\right],$$ (5)

where j is the net ionic flux of a given ionic species, u is the absolute mobility of the ion (cm s^{-1} per unit force) through the membrane, c is the ion concentration at a point x in the membrane, R and T have the same meanings as in equation (1), a is the ionic activity, and dV/dx is the potential gradient.

For the GHK equation the permeability coefficient for an ionic species can be calculated as $p = \beta^*D/\delta$ (these terms are explained in 4.1.4). If only one ionic species permeates across the nerve cell membrane the Nernst–Planck flux equation (5) can then be rewritten as:

$$j = \frac{pzFV}{RT}\left[\frac{C_o - C_i \exp\left(\frac{zFV}{RT}\right)}{1 - \exp\left(\frac{zFV}{RT}\right)}\right],$$ (6)

where C_o and C_i are the concentrations of the ion outside and inside the cell, respectively (all the other terms have been described earlier in the text). It is clear that membrane permeability to more than one ionic species will be described by the sum of similar equations for each ion considered. It was mentioned earlier that in order to measure the permeability coefficient (p) of an ion it is possible to perform radioactive tracer experiments, although a major limitation of this approach is the difficulty of resolving ion fluxes on a timescale of a few seconds or even milliseconds. An alternative approach of high temporal resolution is to use electrophysiological techniques working on the principle that movement of ions through the membrane will generate an ionic current (I). This phenomenon is described by:

$$I = jFz.$$ (7)

The term I is the current density expressed in A cm^{-2}, while F is the Faraday number in C mol^{-1} and j is the net ionic flux density in (mol s^{-1})/cm^2. If the terms of equation (6) are multiplied by zF, and expressing ion movements as current (I), for the case of a single ionic species the following is obtained:

$$I = \frac{p(zF)^2 V}{RT} \cdot \frac{C_o - C_i \exp\left(\frac{zFV}{RI}\right)}{1 - \exp\left(\frac{zFV}{RT}\right)}.$$ (8)

4.2 Membrane pumps are responsible for keeping constant the concentration gradients across membranes

Expressions such as the GHK or Nernst equations ((4) or (1)) describe the behaviour of ions in purely physical terms and, in doing so, they cannot take into account biological processes influencing ionic gradients. It was already noted at the beginning of the twentieth century that heart muscle cells, which fire Na$^+$ and K$^+$ dependent action potentials through the lifetime of the individual, should gradually lose their intracellular concentration of K$^+$ and replace it with Na$^+$; yet, the K$^+$ content of these cells is virtually the same in young and old animals, suggesting that an ion redistribution process is continuously taking place. Later work suggested that skeletal muscle fibres probably use a transport mechanism to restore their ionic gradients after fatigue and proposed the existence of a 'sodium pump'; namely a system able to exchange Na$^+$ for K$^+$ across the cell membrane using intracellular ATP. The sodium pump, which appears to be a ubiquitous characteristic of cells, exerts the fundamental role of exchanging intracellularly accumulated Na$^+$ for extracellular K$^+$ in order to preserve the correct ionic gradients.

The pump is a protein with enzymatic function, located in the cell membrane and comprising four subunits (two α and two β; see Section 3.4) of which several isoforms are known. One important feature of the pump activity is its stoichiometry whereby three Na+ are exchanged for two K+: in practice, this means that for each cycle of pump activity one extra positive charge is subtracted from the cell cytoplasm, thus generating a hyperpolarization (i.e. making the intracellular compartment more negative as a result of positive current outflow). This phenomenon is shown in **Figure 4.4**. Consequently, not only is the sodium pump necessary to re-establish ionic gradients after intense nerve cell activity, but it also helps the membrane potential to return to the initial V_{rest} value or to be even more negative, thus providing temporary inhibition against further excitation.

The operation of the pump is thought to be triggered by binding of intracellular Na+ and ATP to internal facing sites of this protein. Transformation of ATP into ADP releases a phospho group which leads to a conformational change in the pump with trapping of three Na+ which are released into the outside compartment. K+ then binds to the pump outer sites and releases the phospho group into the extracellular water: removal of the phospho residues induces a conformational change in the pump with translocation and release of K+ to the cell inside.

Pharmacological block of the sodium pump is produced by cardiac glycosides (e.g. ouabain) or oligomycin; a K+-free extracellular solution is a useful experimental tool to block the pump activity of cells *in*

vitro. Lowering the ambient temperature will also depress the sodium pump activity.

While the sodium pump is probably the main representative of membrane transporters for ions, other mechanisms also exist. In particular, extracellular Na+ is exchanged for intracellular Ca^{2+} with a 3:1 stoichiometry; such a mechanism is again electrogenic (because it is based on a net inflow of positive charges) and has the role of keeping the intracellular concentration of Ca^{2+} low (**Figure 4.5**). Since Na+ moves according to its gradient, the system does not require energy in the form of ATP hydrolysis. It uses the energy of Na+ in the extracellular space and it relies on the operation of the sodium pump to maintain a low intracellular level of Na+. Intracellular Ca^{2+} at rest is also kept at submicromolar level by sequestration into cell organelles via distinct pump mechanisms (see also **Figure 8.8**).

Finally, in mature brain neurons the intracellular concentration of Cl- is usually found to be very low because various pumps actively extrude this anion (coupling its transport with that of Na+, K+ or bicarbonate). When inhibitory neurotransmitters such as GABA (or glycine) activate Cl- permeable channels, the gradient caused by pumps allows an influx of Cl- to hyperpolarize (and thus inhibit) neuronal membranes (see Chapter 10).

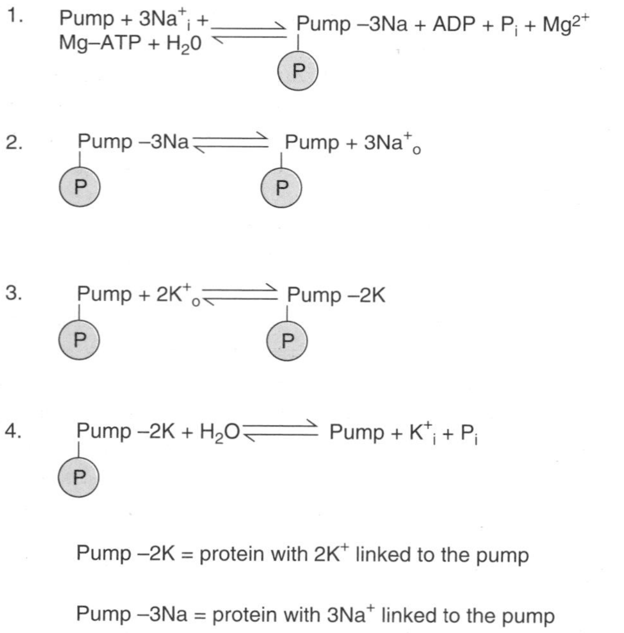

4.3 A simple equivalent electrical circuit for resting membrane properties

4.3.1 Membrane potential has an ohmic behaviour at rest

A convenient description of the electrical behaviour of nerve cells is provided by formally applying to them Ohm's Law, which establishes the relation between current (I) and potential (V): thus $I = V/R$, where V is the cell membrane potential and R is the cell resistance. Taking $1/R$ as the conductance (g), $I = gV$. One can then relate I to V with a simple plot (usually called the I/V

1.   Pump + 3Na+$_i$ + Mg–ATP + H_2O $\longrightarrow$ Pump –3Na + ADP + P_i + Mg^{2+}
        (P)

2.   Pump –3Na $\rightleftharpoons$ Pump + 3Na+$_o$
        (P)   (P)

3.   Pump + 2K+$_o$ $\rightleftharpoons$ Pump –2K
        (P)   (P)

4.   Pump –2K + H_2O $\rightleftharpoons$ Pump + K+$_i$ + P_i
        (P)

Pump –2K = protein with 2K+ linked to the pump

Pump –3Na = protein with 3Na+ linked to the pump

Figure 4.4 Different states of the sodium–potassium pump to shift Na+ and K+ across the cell membrane.
P, phospho group.

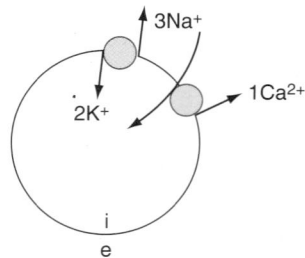

Figure 4.5 Schematic of the Na/K ATPase and Na/Ca pumps.

(a)

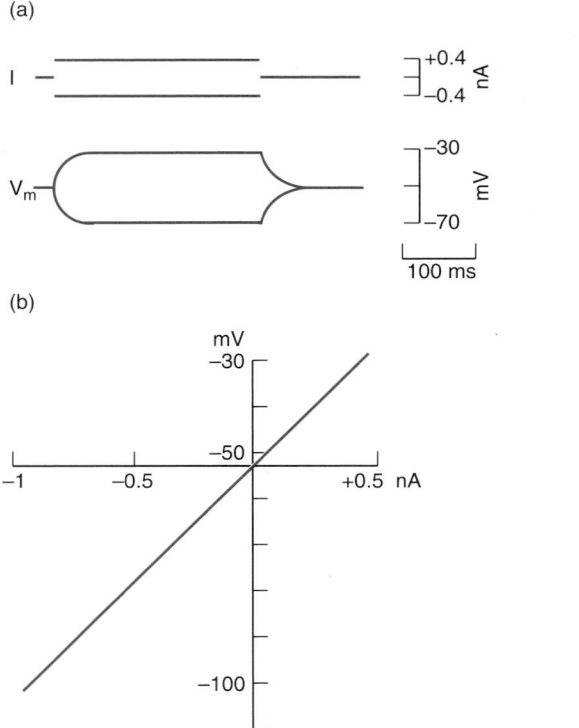

(b)

Figure 4.6 **Ohmic behaviour of the membrane potential around the resting potential.**

(a) Time-dependent responses to ± 0.4 nA current injected for 300 ms. Upper traces, current *I*; lower traces, membrane potential changes V_m. (b) Membrane potential at the end of the current pulse (i.e. at 300 ms) plotted against current intensity. From Adams PR, Brown DA, Constanti A (1982) M-currents and other potassium currents in bullfrog sympathetic neurones. *J. Physiol. (Lond.)* **330**, 537–572, with permission.

curve), the slope of which will be a measure of g (**Figure 4.6**). If the I/V curve is linear, this is said to display *ohmic* behaviour. Conversely, if diffusion is involved in the ionic current flow, the I/V curve becomes nonlinear because g becomes a function of membrane potential.

The Nernst equation (1) predicts that the net ion flow across the cell membrane ceases when the transmembrane potential (V_m) is the same as the Nernst E_{rev} of the ion. One may instead adopt a simple electrical circuit to represent this phenomenon so that the transmembrane gradient for a given ion concentration produces an electromotive force (E) which is equal to the Nernst potential (see **Table 4.1**). In other words, there is an electrochemical current source for each ion. The current source is characterized by its internal conductance, g, in addition to E_{ion}. The current is then described as:

$$i = g(V_m - E_{ion}) \qquad (9)$$

for unitary current, or

$$I = g(V_m - E_{ion})$$

for macroscopic current, with $I = N p_o i$. N is the total number of channels, g is the macroscopic conductance and p_o is the probability of these channels being in the open state.

Note that the microscopic conductance of a single channel is often termed γ. Since the present chapter is not concerned with distinct species of single channels responsible for V_{rest}, for the sake of simplicity the notation g will be used here for the micro as well as the macroscopic conductance.

By electrophysiological convention, the current leaving the cell has a positive sign while the one entering the cell has a negative one. The same equation may be adopted for a single ionic channel, in spite of the possibility of interaction of ions within the channel itself. Indeed, every channel may be characterized by a potential, E_{ion}, at which the current stops flowing through it. Obviously, one may not *a priori* assume that the value of g for each channel is a constant which does not depend on V; i.e. that i/V is a linear function according to Ohm's Law. However, the use of Ohm's Law for a description of channel current is an approximation justified by its simplicity and, to a certain extent, by experimental evidence. In fact, the current through the open pore of many types of ionic channel is actually found to be linearly dependent on the membrane potential while g always depends on the concentration of the current-carrying ions (g is an empirical measure of how easily and quickly ions can go through a pore of the membrane). Important functional consequences are that the channel conductance is switched on and off by neurotransmitters or variations in membrane potential (and the speed of such a change) as described elsewhere.

Equation (9) may be used to describe many electrical events in the nerve cell, including its resting state. One should expect that there must be a V_{rest} value at which the sum of all membrane currents (active pump currents included) is equal to zero. This value represents a condition of electrical equilibrium for the membrane since the current does not change the total charge and hence the potential is also not changing. The equilibrium value of the potential, or resting potential V_{rest}, is thus given by:

$$g_K(V_{rest} - E_K) + g_{Na}(V_{rest} - E_{Na}) + g_{Ca}(V_{rest} - E_{Ca})$$
$$+ g_{Cl}(V_{rest} - E_{Cl}) + \dots i_{Na/K} + i_{Ca} + \dots = 0, \qquad (10)$$

where i is the current generated by operation of the various ionic pumps, and it may depend upon V, ion concentrations, etc. The ellipses indicate possible addition of other channels and pumps. It should also be noted that for each ion there are often several different types of channel with distinct conductance and gating properties, but that, in the present simplified scheme, these are all lumped together into a single species.

4.3.2 Stability, bistability and instability of resting membrane potential

At this point, it is of utmost importance to discuss the notion of equilibrium stability. V_{rest} is stable whenever any small deviation of it (ΔV_{rest}) elicits a current of same polarity which restores V_{rest} to its normal value. Let us consider, for example, a slight depolarization ($\Delta V_{rest} > 0$). Then, a positive current will be generated to cancel membrane depolarization. Similarly, a hyperpolarization ($\Delta V_{rest} > 0$) will evoke a negative current which again restores V_{rest}. This situation occurs, for example, in ohmic systems. A steady resting potential (**Figure 4.7a**) is therefore a characteristic of most excitable and all non-excitable cells. Of course, very large signals (depolarizations or hyperpolarizations) will not be cancelled out by currents of the same polarity and regenerative membrane responses may appear (for instance action potentials are triggered when membrane depolarization reaches a certain threshold, as discussed in Chapter 2).

Some nerve cells (e.g. motoneurons) have an additional stable level of electrical equilibrium. This stable point corresponds to a steady depolarization generated by a voltage-activated slow inward current. Such cells are called *bistable* and their steady depolarization level may be considered as a *metastable* point. It only exists until such a time when slow changes in ion concentration, conductance and/or pump current changes make the second stable solution of equation (10) impossible. Thus, a short excitatory input is sufficient to shift the cell from the stable state, V_{rest}, to the metastable steady depolarization; and vice versa, a short inhibitory process is enough to return the cell to V_{rest} (**Figure 4.7b**).

In pacemaker cells (for example, some cells present in the heart or in certain brainstem or hypothalamic nuclei) V_{rest} is intrinsically *unstable* and, as such, it cannot be reliably measured. Any deviation (ΔV_{rest}) of membrane potential generates membrane currents that further enhance it; i.e. depolarization activates a negative (depolarizing) current, while hyperpolarization activates a positive one. This situation results in membrane potential oscillations around a 'resting' level (**Figure 4.7c**), which are precisely what a pacemaker cell should spontaneously express to drive the activity of nearby cells.

4.3.3 An electrical model of resting membrane potential

Let us simplify equation (10) by reducing the currents to the passive movement of K^+, Na^+ and Cl^-, which substantially determine V_{rest}. **Figure 4.8a** presents an electrical equivalent for such simplification. Pump currents may be neglected since the main current through the Na/K ATPase is a counterflow of K^+ and Na^+. By transforming the simplified equation (10), we obtain:

$$V_{rest} = \frac{g_K E_K + g_{Na} E_{Na} + g_{Cl} E_{Cl}}{g_K + g_{Na} + g_{Cl}}. \tag{11}$$

The meaning of this is as follows. In **Figure 4.8b**, instead of three parallel current sources for K^+, Na^+ and Cl^-, we have lumped them together into only one source with driving (electromotive) force E equal to V_{rest} and an inward conductance g_m equal to the sum of the specific ionic (channel) conductances $g_K + g_{Na} + g_{Cl}$. One may consider, instead of the absolute value of membrane potential, only its deviation from V_{rest}. In this case the equivalent electromotive force becomes equal to zero and the equivalent scheme of the cell membrane simplifies to an *RC*-circuit (**Figure 4.8c**). If one includes more

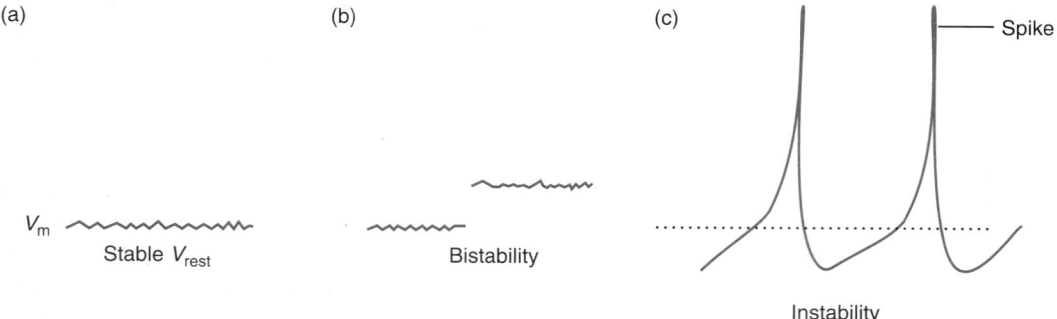

(a)   (b)   (c)   ——— Spike

V_m ~~~~~~~~~~
        Stable V_{rest} Bistability   Instability

Figure 4.7 **Schematic of a stable (a), a bistable (b) and an unstable (c) resting membrane potential.**

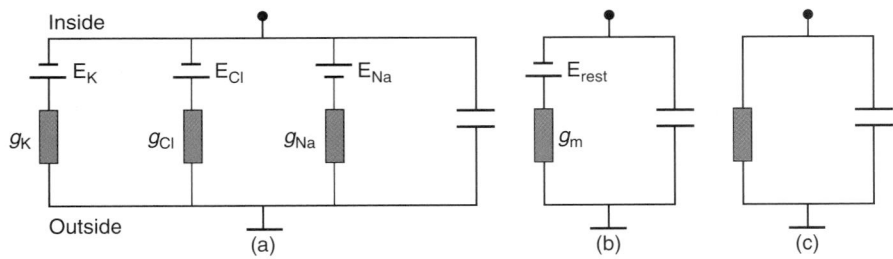

Figure 4.8 Simplified equivalent scheme to account for membrane electrical characteristics near the resting potential.
(a) Three main ionic current sources. Note: E_K and E_{Cl} are negative while E_{Na} is positive. **(b)** An equivalent current source for the resting potential. **(c)** Electrical scheme for below-threshold potential changes (passive de- and hyperpolarizations) relative to the resting potential. Battery symbols indicate electromotive forces, boxes represent conductances and parallel plates indicate membrane capacitors.

channel types, then the notion of resting current still holds true. The equivalent scheme of **Figure 4.8c** is applicable only to depolarizations and hyperpolarizations characterized by linear (ohmic) current–voltage relations.

In standard excitable cells it means that these potential changes from V_{rest} are not activating voltage-gated currents; e.g. they are below the threshold for spike generation. For bistable cells, instead of Ohm's Law one must consider an N-shaped current–voltage relation as shown in **Figure 4.9**. In pacemaker cells approximately

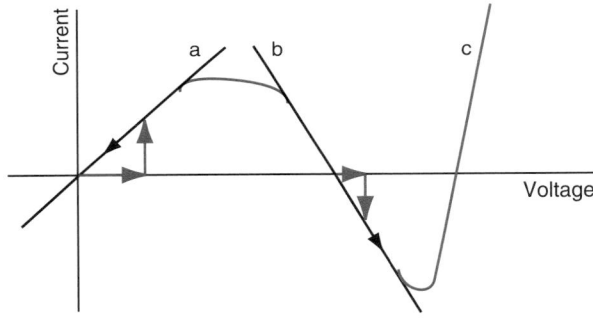

Figure 4.9 Theoretical current–voltage curves.
This example shows the case of a cell with one stable resting potential (line 'a') or with an unstable resting potential (line 'b'). The example of a bistable cell current–voltage relation is presented by the green line ('c', partly including also the black lines 'a' and 'b'). The arrows along the horizontal voltage axis indicate the direction of membrane potential change (ΔV_{rest}) which in the case of the stable cell (a) evokes an outward (positive) current (see vertical arrow) which forces (small arrowhead) the membrane potential to return to resting level. When the signs of potential and current change are the same, as in (a), the conductance (given by the slope of the line) is positive and V_{rest} is stable; if these signs are different, as in the case of (b) (note negative conductance), V_{rest} becomes unstable as an inward (negative) current depolarizes the membrane potential. In bistable cells both extreme zero-current points (V_{rest} and steady depolarization) are stable while the middle one is unstable.

ohmic current–voltage relations with *negative* membrane conductance exist. The direction of the current–voltage relation when crossing the voltage axis determines the stability of the corresponding equilibrium (zero-current) point.

From the scheme of **Figure 4.1** and equations (10) and (11), the resting potential should be very close to the electromotive force for the ion with largest membrane conductance. As a rule, g_K is the largest one. (Note: It may seem that (10) and (11) for V_{rest} have little in common with the Donnan equilibrium – see (3). Nonetheless, this is not so. The principal small inorganic permeable cation that is screening non-permeable organic anions in the cytoplasm is K^+. Its electromotive force is the closest to the Donnan equilibrium because considerable additional energy would otherwise be needed to maintain the cell potential and the concentration gradients at resting state.) This is why the V_{rest} is so susceptible to E_K changes. The high intracellular K^+ concentration actually does not change much during electrical activity, while the low extracellular concentration can do so markedly. During sustained convulsive activity a considerable amount of K^+ leaves the cell; hence, the extracellular concentration of this ion increases and, consequently, E_K and V_{rest} are shifted toward less negative values.

4.4 Advantages and disadvantages of sharp (intracellular) versus patch electrodes for measuring the resting membrane potential

In order to measure membrane potential, optical and electrophysiological techniques can be employed. The optical techniques make use of membrane-soluble substances whose light absorption or luminescence is a function of the electric field applied. The transmembrane electric field is strong enough, approximately

$20\,MV\,m^{-1}$, to produce such effects. At the present time optical techniques are in the process of further development and their sensitivity is increasing, although they are used by just a few laboratories. It is still unclear to what extent the molecules used for optical measurements affect cell properties. Furthermore, optical techniques are used to measure potentials, not currents.

Membrane potentials and currents (under voltage clamp) are measured by employing methods of cellular electrophysiology. Nerve cell impalement with a tapered, sharp saline-filled pipette has been used for almost half a century. However, this technique entails some problems.

- Firstly, in order to provide the pipette with the necessary ability to pass current, the filling salt solution has to be more concentrated (by one order of magnitude) than the cytoplasm. Leakage of ions from the pipette into the cell shifts their physiological concentration in the cytoplasm and might therefore affect the normal performance of cellular organelles, enzymes, pumps and channels with consequent changes in membrane potential.
- Secondly, it is possible that the impalement itself (in addition to any alterations in the cytoplasm composition) may introduce considerable artefactual leakage (often termed *shunt*) of the membrane, which corresponds to a parasitic membrane conductance.
- Thirdly, the pipette might destroy the cytoskeleton and subcellular structures.

The cell is not always able to compensate for all these factors. Indeed, some cells, particularly smaller ones, cannot survive the impalement. Major signs of cell deterioration are high membrane conductance and low V_{rest}, which can be present even in those neurons that do survive.

- Fourthly, the electrode resistance and capacitance are often large and thus difficult to compensate.
- Finally, a junctional current may arise at the interface between pipette orifice and cytoplasm owing to the differences in electrolyte composition and concentration.

Whole-cell patch clamp is another electrophysiological technique to measure the cell potential and current. In this case negative pressure is applied to a pipette (usually of larger orifice than the ones used for intracellular recording) in order to establish a tight contact (*seal*) with the nerve cell membrane. A small area (*patch*) of the cell is thus forced inside the pipette orifice and eventually ruptured so that the cytoplasm is in direct continuity with the pipette interior (see Appendix 5.3). The tight seal ensures reliable insulation of the inside of the electrode from the extracellular medium, thereby excluding the possibility of membrane shunting. Electrical currents originating from the cell are thus unable to escape at the interface between membrane and electrode tip. When there is a loose contact between membrane and electrode (e.g because of damage to the cell) signals are largely attenuated or even lost (this phenomenon is called *shunting*). Indeed, in certain cases (e.g. neurons in hippocampal slices), the cell apparent conductance decreases several times compared with that measured with a sharp intracellular microelectrode. The whole cell patch clamp thus enables one to record more reliably potential and current signals from small cells and even from fine processes such as dendrites. Furthermore, the mechanical stability of recording is much improved over conventional intracellular methods.

Nonetheless, the method is not devoid of shortcomings. First of all, the suction effect caused by the initial negative pressure may remove small molecules of biological importance from the cytoplasm. This phenomenon might alter the activity of membrane channels which are controlled by intracellular chemical messengers (e.g. cAMP or cGMP). Gradual replacement of the cell cytoplasm by the pipette internal solution (*intracellular dialysis*) during prolonged recording might compound this effect. Hence, it is feasible that the very low cell conductance observed with whole-cell patch clamping may be, at least in part, artefactual. The negative pressure applied to the cell might disturb the membrane structure and even open stretch-activated channels. Still unresolved are the problems associated with compensation of electrode capacitance and resistance and with the contact between pipette electrolyte and cytoplasm.

In an attempt to reduce the problems caused by intracellular dialysis and washout, a modification of the whole-cell patch clamp technique has been introduced whereby chemical perforation (*perforated patch*) of the membrane patch beneath the pipette is used. This effect is achieved by adding to the pipette solution a *channel-forming* substance, such as the antibiotics nystatin or amphotericin. Such substances create artificial pores in the patch of membrane under the electrode tip through which only small monovalent ions can pass. However, one still faces the problem of high and unstable resistance of the clamped membrane patch which, in the case of *in situ* neurons, is not dissimilar to the situation obtained with an intracellular sharp microelectrode. Furthermore, the perforating molecules endow the membrane with a selective ion permeability, thereby affecting the membrane electrical properties and turning on an artefactual electromotive force.

From this discussion it is clear that an ideal electrophysiological method to study membrane potential and current is not yet available. The present techniques are useful but impose several experimental constraints. The shortcomings inherent in electrophysiological measurements are well described by Niels Bohr's famous statement that any biological measurement entails interference with the object's life activities and, hence, a bias in the values obtained. Choosing the method of measurement most appropriate for a given objective is an arduous task for a neuroscientist who must be able not only to measure the resting potential and apparent cell conductance but also to detect the presence of an injury shunt.

4.5 Background currents which flow through voltage-gated channels open at resting membrane potential also participate in V_{rest}

Under resting conditions many nerve cells normally display a stable V_{rest} as a result of the combined action of the so-called *leak* conductance (measured as the linearity of the I/V curve according to Ohm's Law) caused by passive permeability mainly to K^+ (and, to a smaller extent, to other ions), and a variable degree of shunt conductance generated by the presence of the recording electrode itself. In certain neurons this picture is complicated by the overlapping presence of other currents caused by flow of ions through specific membrane channels which are permanently open at or around V_{rest}. In this case such channels are persistently activated by either intracellular (or extracellular) chemicals or the actual level of V_{rest}. A necessary property of these channels is that they do not undergo significant inactivation (i.e. spontaneous closure despite the continuous presence of the gating signal): under these circumstances the current flowing through these channels is termed *background* current.

The interest in background currents stems from the fact that they may be the target for the action of neurotransmitters or drugs which can change the membrane potential and the excitability of neurons by selective up- or down-regulation of channels already open at rest. This situation may be exemplified by the action of some endogenously occurring neuropeptides, of which substance P and TRH are notable representatives. Let us suppose that one is recording from a brain neuron that has an apparently stable V_{rest} which (assuming ideal experimental conditions of minimal conductance shunt by the electrode) is actually due to two mechanisms: passive permeability to various ions (K^+, Na^+, Cl^- and Ca^{2+}) and selective permeability to K^+ through membrane channels that are activated by hyperpolarization. The relatively negative membrane potential ensures constant opening of these channels which will tend to hyperpolarize the cell towards the value of E_K, an action opposed by the leak channel activity (with reversal potential less negative than E_K). Binding of substance P to specific receptors (coupled to G-proteins) will activate a series of intracellular biochemical reactions leading to closure of the hyperpolarization-activated K^+ channels (called *inward rectifier* channels). The result will be a depolarization of the cell with a *decrease* in conductance (because channels have been closed). The depolarization will thus bring the membrane nearer the threshold for action potential generation; at the same time, the conductance decrease will make the membrane more sensitive to signals coming from other cells because (according to Ohm's Law) synaptic currents generated by various transmitters now evoke larger variations in membrane potential. In this fashion substance P can produce a sustained up-regulation of the excitability of a neuron. The action of TRH is similar (though not identical) to that of substance P since it also involves suppression of a background K^+ current apparently distinct from the inward rectifier current.

Other background currents that operate at V_{rest} are also known to exist in brain neurons with different degrees of expression depending on the cell type considered: some are selectively mediated by K^+, such as the *M-current* (so-called because it is blocked by acetylcholine acting via muscarinic receptors; see Section 17.3.4); others are generated by channels permeable to Na^+ and K^+ (with a reversal potential positive to V_{rest}, such as I_Q or I_h; see Section 17.2.3); or to Cl^- especially when cells contain a high concentration of this anion owing its efflux from the recording electrode.

Further reading

Adams PR, Brown DA, Constanti A (1982) Pharmacological inhibition of the M-current. *J. Physiol.* **332**, 223–262.

Baginskas A, Gutman A, Svirskis G (1993) Bi-stable dendrite in constant electric field: a model analysis. *Neuroscience* **53**, 595–603.

Glynn IM (1993) All hands to the sodium pump. *J. Physiol.* **462**, 1–30.

Hamill OP, Marty A, Neher E, Sakmann B, Takahashi T (1981) Improved patch-clamp techniques for high resolution current recording from cells and cell-free membrane patches. *Pflugers Arch.* **391**, 85–100.

Hultborn H, Kiehn O (1992) Neuromodulation of vertebrate motor neuron membrane properties. *Curr. Opin. Neurobiol.* **2**, 770–775.

Nistri A, Fisher ND, Gurnell M (1990) Block by the neuropeptide TRH of an apparently novel K$^+$ conductance of rat motoneurones. *Neurosci. Lett.* **120**, 25–30.

Staley K (1994) The role of an inwardly rectifying chloride conductance in postsynaptic inhibition. *J.* *Neurophysiol.* **72**, 273–284.

Yamaguchi K, Nakajima Y, Nakajima S, Stanfield PR (1990) Modulation of inwardly rectifying channels by substance P in cholinergic neurones from rat brain in culture. *J. Physiol.* **426**, 499–520.

The Voltage-Gated Channels of Na⁺ Action Potentials

The ionic basis for nerve excitation was first elucidated in the squid giant axon by Hodgkin and Huxley (1952) using the voltage clamp technique. They made the key observation that two separate, voltage-dependent currents underlie the action potential: an early transient inward Na⁺ current which depolarizes the membrane, and a delayed outward K⁺ current largely responsible for repolarization. This led to a series of experiments that resulted in a quantitative description of impulse generation and propagation in the squid axon.

Nearly 30 years later, Sakmann and Neher, using the patch clamp technique, recorded the activity of the voltage-gated Na⁺ and K⁺ channels responsible for action potential initiation and propagation. Taking history backwards, action potentials will be explained from the single channel level to the membrane level.

5.1 Properties of action potentials

5.1.1 The different types of action potentials

The action potential is a sudden and transient depolarization of the membrane. The cells that initiate action potentials are called 'excitable cells'. Action potentials can have different shapes; i.e. different amplitudes and durations. In neuronal somas and axons, action potentials have a large amplitude and a small duration: these are the Na⁺-dependent action potentials (**Figures 5.1 and 5.2a**). In other neuronal cell bodies, heart ventricular cells and axon terminals, the action potentials have a longer duration with a plateau following the initial peak: these are the Na⁺/Ca²⁺-dependent action potentials (**Figure 5.2b–d**). Finally, in some neuronal dendrites and some endocrine cells, action potentials have a small amplitude and a long duration: these are the Ca²⁺-dependent action potentials.

Action potentials have common properties; for example they are all initiated in response to a membrane depolarization. They also have differences; for example in the type of ions involved, their amplitude, duration, etc.

5.1.2 Na⁺ and K⁺ ions participate in the action potential of axons

The activity of the giant axon of the squid is recorded with an intracellular electrode (in current clamp; see **Appendix 5.1**) in the presence of seawater as the external solution.

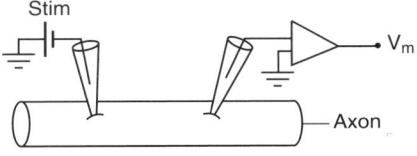

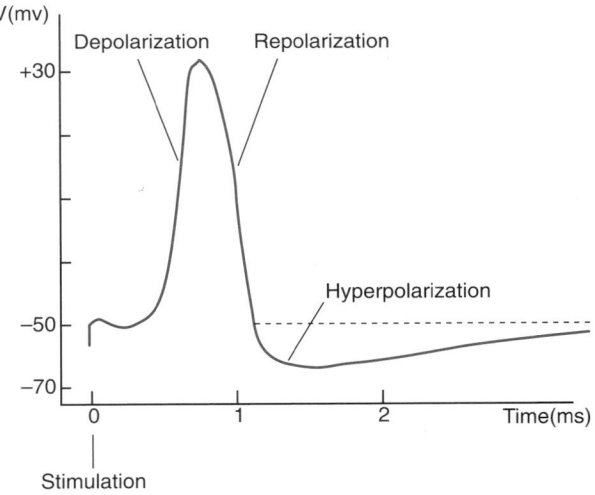

Figure 5.1 Action potential of the giant axon of the squid. Action potential recorded intracellularly in the giant axon of the squid at resting membrane potential in response to a depolarizing current pulse (the extracellular solution is seawater). The different phases of the action potential are indicated. Adapted from Hodgkin AL, Katz B (1949) The effect of sodium ions on the electrical activity of the giant axon of the squid, *J. Physiol.* **108**, 37–77, with permission.

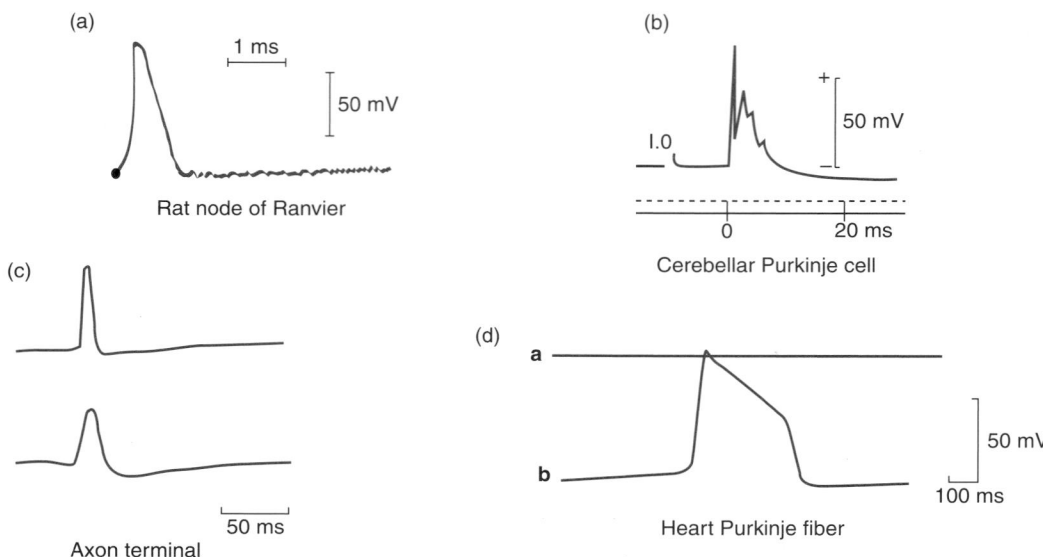

Figure 5.2 Different types of action potentials recorded in excitable cells.

(a) Sodium-dependent action potential recorded intracellularly in a node of Ranvier of a rat nerve fibre. Note the absence of a hyperpolarization phase. **(b)–(d)** Sodium–calcium-dependent action potentials. Intracellular recording of the complex spike in a cerebellar Purkinje cell in response to climbing fibre stimulation: an initial Na$^+$-dependent action potential and a later larger slow potential on which are superimposed several small Ca^{2+}-dependent action potentials. The total duration of this complex spike is 5–7 ms **(b)**. Action potential recorded from axon terminals of *Xenopus* hypothalamic neurons (these axon terminals are located in the neurohypophysis) in control conditions (top) and after adding blockers of Na$^+$ and K$^+$ channels (TTX and TEA, bottom) in order to unmask the Ca^{2+} component of the spike (this component has a larger duration due to the blockade of some of the K$^+$ channels) **(c)**. Intracellular recording of an action potential from an acutely dissociated dog heart cell (Purkinje fibre). Trace 'a' is recorded when the electrode is outside the cell and represents the trace 0 mV. Trace 'b' is recorded when the electrode is inside the cell. The peak amplitude of the action potential is 75 mV and the total duration 400 ms **(d)**. All these action potentials are recorded in response to an intracellular depolarizing pulse or to the stimulation of afferents. Note the differences in their durations. Part (a) adapted from Brismar T (1980) Potential clamp analysis of membrane currents in rat myelinated nerve fibres, *J. Physiol.* **298**, 171–184, with permission. Parts (b)–(d) adapted from Coraboeuf E, Weidmann S (1949) Potentiel de repos et potentiels d'action du muscle cardiaque, mesurés à l'aide d'électrodes internes, *C. R. Soc. Biol.* **143**, 1329–1331; and Eccles JC, Llinas R, Sasaki K (1966) The excitatory synaptic action of climbing fibres on the Purkinje cells of the cerebellum, *J. Physiol.* **182**, 268–296; and Obaid AL, Flores R, Salzberg BM (1989) Calcium channels that are required for secretion from intact nerve terminals of vertebrates are sensitive to ω-conotoxin and relatively insensitive to dihydropyridines, *J. Gen. Physiol.* **93**, 715–730; with permission.

Na$^+$ ions participate in the depolarization phase of the action potential

When the extracellular solution is changed from seawater to a Na$^+$-free solution, the amplitude and rise time of the depolarization phase of the action potential gradually and rapidly decreases, until after 8 s the current pulse can no longer evoke an action potential (**Figure 5.3**). Moreover, in control seawater, tetrodotoxin (TTX), a specific blocker of voltage-gated Na$^+$ channels, completely blocks action potential initiation (**Figures 5.4a,c**), thus confirming a major role of Na$^+$ ions.

K$^+$ ions participate in the repolarization phase of the action potential

Application of tetraethylammonium chloride (TEA), a blocker of K$^+$ channels, greatly prolongs the duration of the action potential of the squid giant axon without changing the resting membrane potential. The action potential treated with TEA has an initial peak followed by a plateau (**Figures 5.4a,b**) and the prolongation is sometimes 100-fold or more.

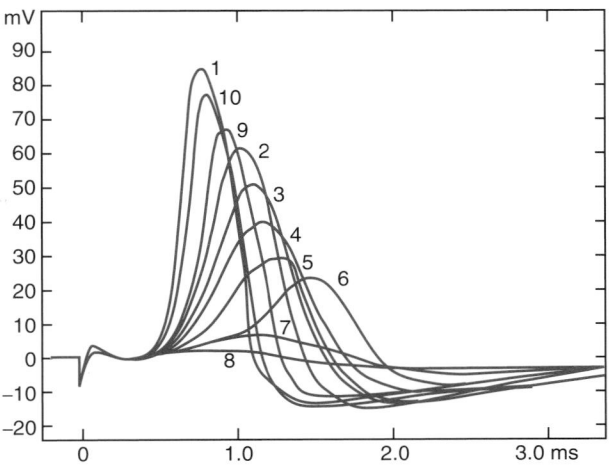

Figure 5.3 The action potential of the squid giant axon is abolished in an Na⁺-free external solution.
(1) Control action potential recorded in sea water; (2)–(8) recordings taken at the following times after the application of a dextrose solution (Na-free solution): 2.30, 4.62, 5.86, 6.10, 7.10 and 8.11 s; (9) recording taken 9 s after reapplication of seawater; (10) recording taken at 90 and 150 s after reapplication of seawater; traces are superimposed. From Hodgkin AL, Katz B (1949) The effect of sodium ions on the electrical activity of the giant axon of the squid, *J. Physiol.* **108**, 37–77, with permission.

5.1.3 Na⁺-dependent action potentials are all or none and propagate along the axon with the same amplitude

Depolarizing current pulses are applied through the intracellular recording electrode, at the level of a neuronal soma or axon. We observe that (i) to a certain level of membrane depolarization called the threshold potential, only an ohmic passive response is recorded (**Figure 5.5a,** right); (ii) when the membrane is depolarized just above threshold, an action potential is recorded. Then, increasing the intensity of the stimulating current pulse does not increase the amplitude of the action potential (**Figure 5.5a,** left). The action potential is all or none.

Once initiated, the action potential propagates along the axon with a speed varying from 1 to 100 m s⁻¹ according to the type of axon. Intracellular recordings at varying distances from the soma show that the amplitude of the action potential does not attenuate: the action potential propagates without decrement (**Figure 5.5b**).

5.1.4 Questions about the Na⁺-dependent action potential

■ What are the structural and functional properties of the Na⁺ and K⁺ channels of the action potential? (Sections 5.2 and 5.3)

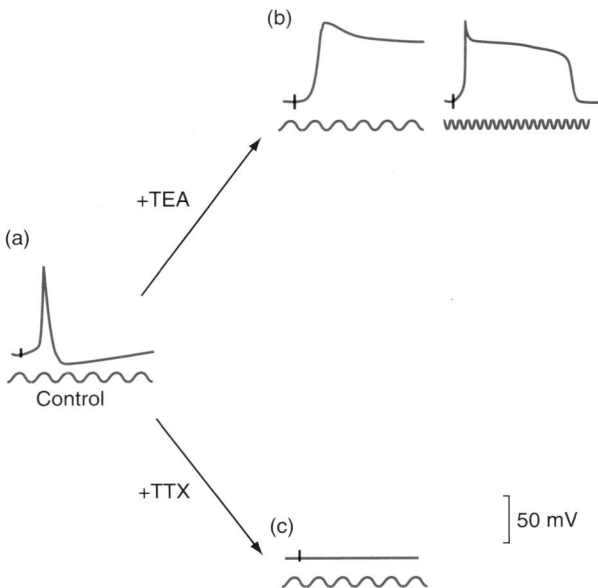

Figure 5.4 Effects of tetrodotoxin (TTX) and tetraethylammonium chloride (TEA) on the action potential of the squid giant axon.
(a) Control action potential. (b) TEA application lengthens the action potential (left), which then has to be observed on a different time scale (right). (c) TTX totally abolishes the initiation of the action potential. Adapted from Tasaki I, Hagiwara S (1957) Demonstration of two stable potential states in the squid giant axon under tetraethylammonium chloride, *J. Gen. Physiol.* **40**, 859–885, with permission.

■ What represents the threshold potential for action potential initiation? (Section 5.4)
■ Why is the action potential all or none? (Section 5.4)
■ What are the mechanisms of action potential propagation? (Section 5.4)

5.2 The depolarization phase of Na⁺-dependent action potentials results from the transient entry of Na⁺ ions through voltage-gated Na⁺ channels

5.2.1 The Na⁺ channel consists of a principal large α-subunit with four internal homologous repeats and auxiliary β-subunits

The primary structures of the *Electrophorus* electroplax Na⁺ channel, the three distinct Na⁺ channels from rat brain (designated types I, II and III) and the Na⁺ channel from skeletal and heart muscle cells have been elucidated by cloning and sequence analysis of the

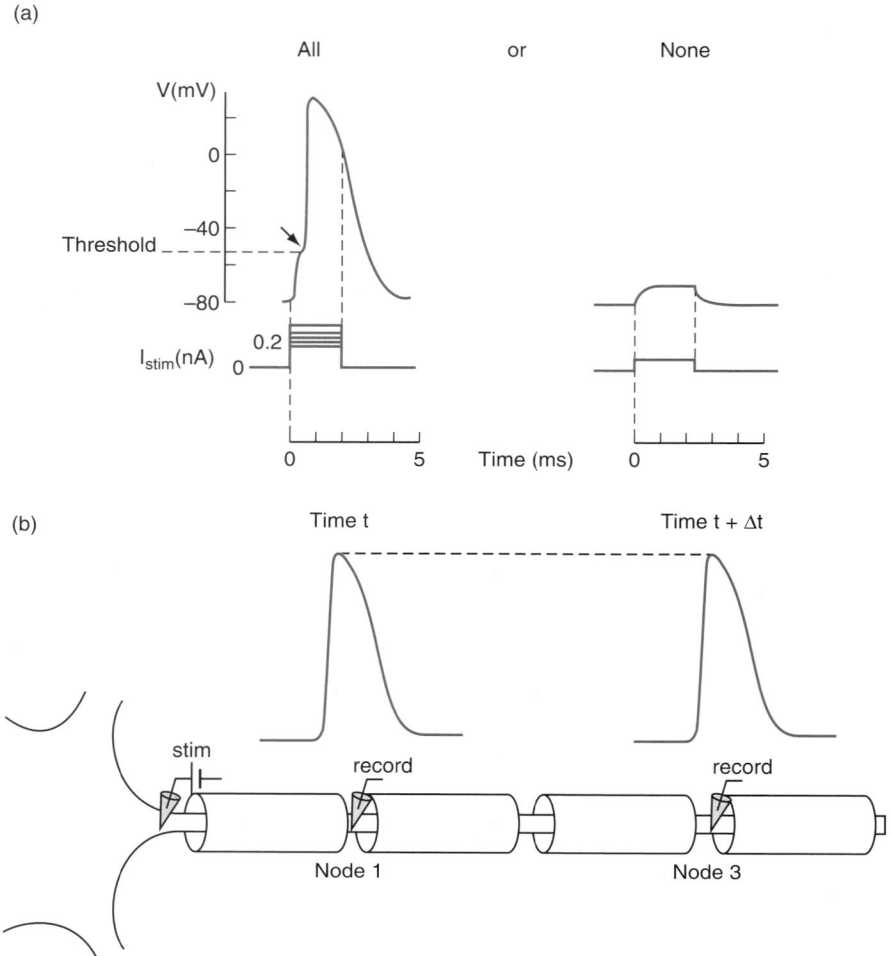

Figure 5.5 Properties of the Na⁺-dependent action potential.

(a) The response of the membrane to depolarizing current pulses of different amplitudes is recorded with an intracellular electrode. Upper traces are the voltage traces, bottom traces are the current traces. Above 0.2 nA an axon potential is initiated. Increasing the current pulse amplitude does not increase the action potential amplitude (left). With current pulses of smaller amplitudes, no action potential is initiated. (b) An action potential is initiated in the soma–initial segment by a depolarizing current pulse (stim). Intracellular recording electrodes inserted along the axon record the action potential at successive nodes at successive times. See text for further explanations.

complementary DNAs. The Na⁺ channel in all these structures is composed of a large polypeptide consisting of about 2000 amino acid residues, the principal α-subunit. It exhibits four homologous internal repeats (I to IV) each of which has six putative membrane-spanning segments (S1 to S6) (**Figure 5.6**). The four homologous domains are presumably oriented in a pseudosymmetric fashion across the membrane in order to form a central pore (see **Figure 3.5**).

Each homology unit contains a unique segment, the S4 segment, with positively charged residues: an arginine or a lysine residue at every third position with mostly non-polar residues intervening between the basic residues (see **Figure 5.15a**). The structure of the S4 segment is strikingly well conserved in all the types of Na⁺ channels analysed so far. It has been proposed that the positive charges in this segment represent the voltage sensor (see Section 5.2.7).

The brain Na⁺ channels have two auxiliary subunits designated β1 and β2. They are small proteins of about 200 amino acid residues, with a substantial N-terminal extracellular domain, a single putative membrane-spanning segment and a small C-terminal intracellular domain (**Figure 5.6**). The β2-subunit is covalently attached to the α-subunit by disulphide linkage, whereas the β1-subunit is non-covalently associated. The Na⁺

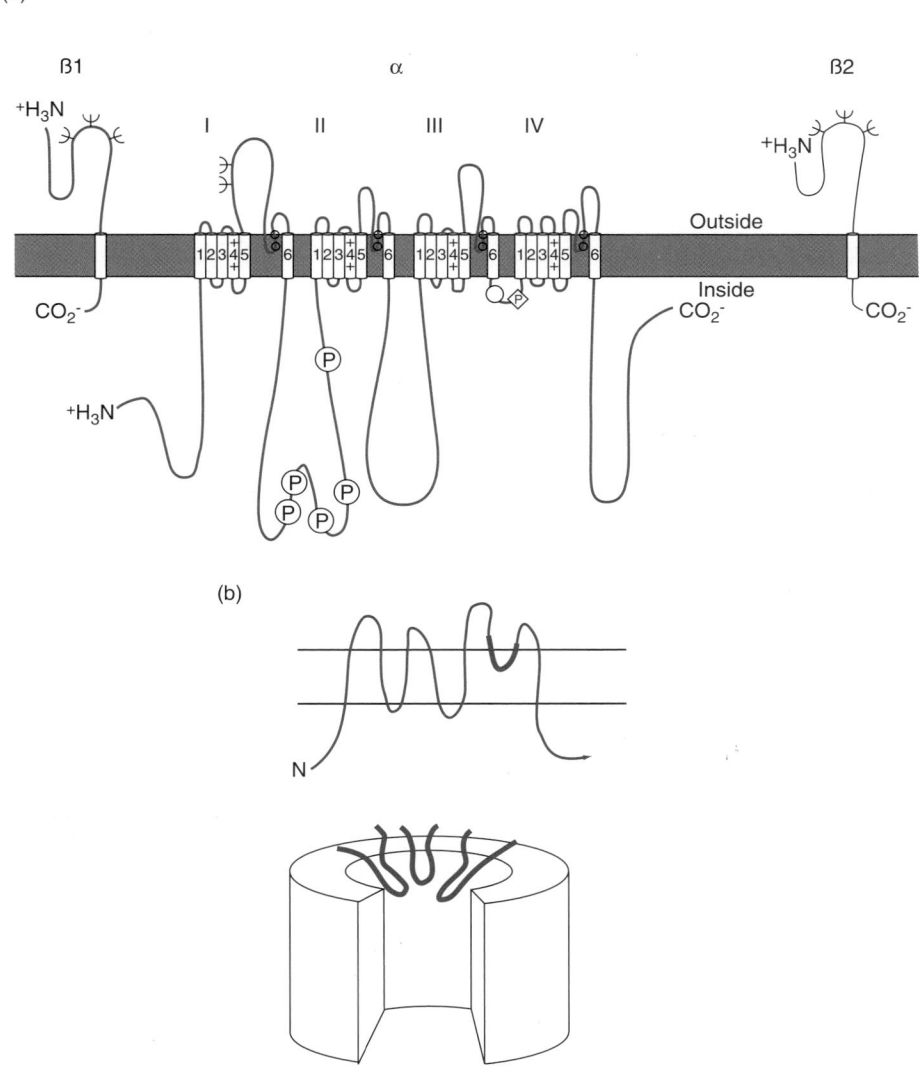

Figure 5.6 Putative transmembrane organization of the α and β subunits of the voltage-gated Na+ channel.
(a) Cylinders represent putative membrane-spanning segments, ψ sites of probable N-linked glycosylation and P sites of demonstrated protein phosphorylation. **(b)** Each of the four domains has a region linking segments S5 and S6 that forms a pore loop (upper trace). Diagram of a voltage-activated channel arranged to form a central pore (lower trace). Pore loops enter into the pore to form an active site where ion selectivity occurs (one quarter of the channel is omitted). Drawing (a) from Isom LL, De Jongh KS, Caterall WA (1994) Auxiliary subunits of voltage-gated ion channels, *Neuron* **12**, 1183–1194, with permission. Drawing (b) adapted from MacKinnon R (1995) Pore loops: an emerging theme in ion channel structure, *Neuron* **14**, 889–892, with permission.

channel from skeletal muscle sarcolemma contains a non-covalently associated β-subunit similar to brain β1.

The α-subunit mRNA isolated from rat brain or the α-subunit RNAs transcribed from cloned cDNAs from rat brain are sufficient to direct the synthesis of functional Na+ channels when injected into oocytes. These results establish that the protein structures necessary for voltage gating and ion conductance are contained within the α-subunit itself. However, the properties of these channels are not identical to native Na+ channels and it has been shown that the auxiliary β-subunits play a role in the targeting and stabilization of the α-subunit in the plasma membrane, its sensitivity to voltage and rate of inactivation.

5.2.2 Membrane depolarization favours conformational change of the Na⁺ channel towards the open state; the Na⁺ channel then quickly inactivates

The function of the Na⁺ channel is to transduce *rapidly* membrane depolarization into an entry of Na⁺ ions. The activity of a single Na⁺ channel was first recorded by Sigworth and Neher in 1980 from rat muscle cells with the patch clamp technique (cell-attached patch; see Appendix 5.3).

It must be first explained that the experimenter does not know before recording it, which type of channel(s) is in the patch of membrane isolated under the tip of the pipette. He or she can only increase the chance of recording a Na⁺ channel, for example, by studying a membrane where this type of channel is frequently expressed and by pharmacologically blocking the other types of channels that could be activated together with the Na⁺ channels (voltage-gated K⁺ channels are blocked by TEA). The recorded channel is then identified by its voltage dependence, reversal potential, unitary conductance, ionic permeability, mean open time, etc. Finally, the number of Na⁺ channels in the patch of membrane cannot be predicted. Even when pipettes with small tips are used, the probability of recording more than one channel can be high because of the type of membrane patched. For this reason, very few recordings of single native Na⁺ channels have been performed. (The number of Na⁺ channels in a patch is known from recordings where the membrane is strongly depolarized in order to increase to a maximum the probability of opening the voltage-gated channels present in the patch.)

Voltage-gated Na⁺ channels of the skeletal muscle fibre

A series of recordings obtained from a single Na⁺ channel in response to a 40 mV depolarizing step given every second is shown in **Figures 5.7a and c**. The holding potential is around −70 mV (remember that in the cell-attached patch, the membrane potential can only be estimated). A physiological extracellular concentration of Na⁺ ions is present in the pipette.

At holding potential, no variations in the current traces are recorded. After the onset of the depolarizing step, unitary Na⁺ currents of varying durations but of the same amplitude are recorded (lines 1, 2, 4, 5, 7 and 8) or not recorded (lines 3, 6 and 9). This means that six times out of nine, the Na⁺ channel has opened in response to the depolarization. The Na⁺ current has a rectangular shape and is downward. By convention, inward currents of + ions are represented as downward (inward means that + ions enter the cell; see Section 3.3.3). The histogram

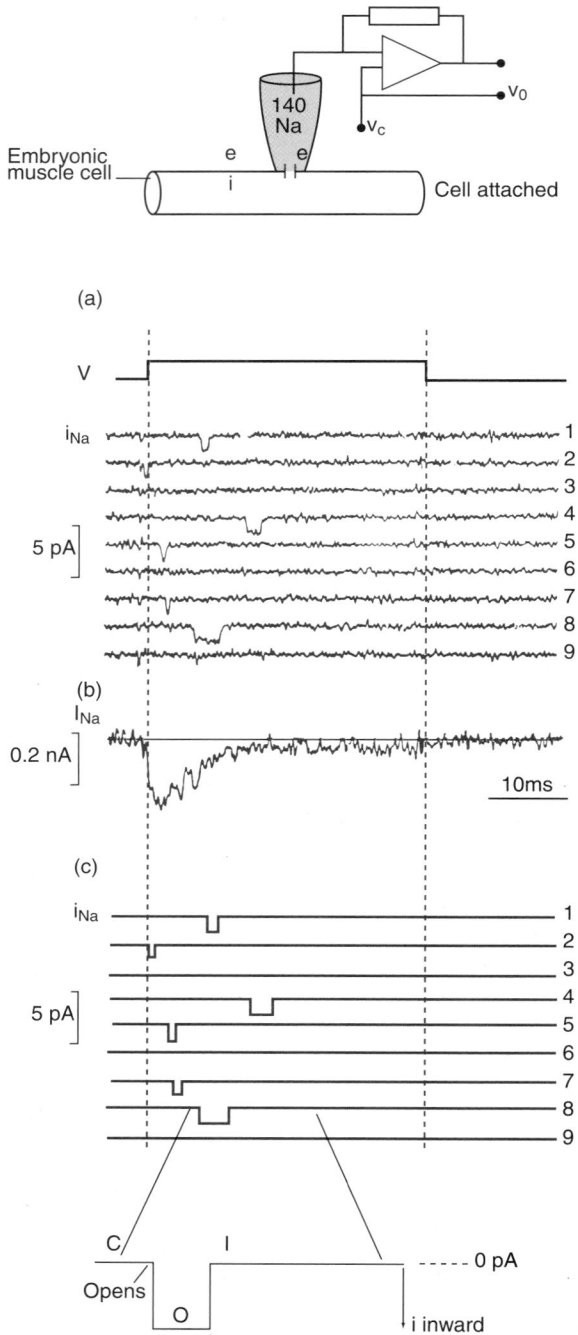

Figure 5.7 Single Na⁺ channel openings in response to a depolarizing step (muscle cell).

The activity of the Na⁺ channel is recorded in patch clamp (cell-attached patch) from an embryonic muscle cell. **(a)** Nine successive recordings of single channel openings (i_{Na}) in response to a 40 mV depolarizing pulse (V trace) given at 1 s intervals from a holding potential 10 mV more hyperpolarized than the resting membrane potential. **(b)** Averaged inward Na⁺ current from 300 elementary Na⁺ currents as in (a). **(c)** The same recordings as in (a) are redrawn in order to explain more clearly the different states of of the Na⁺ current amplitude recorded in response to a 40 mV depolarizing step gives a mean amplitude for i_{Na} of around –1.6 pA (see Appendix 5.3).

It is interesting to note that once the channel has opened, there is a low probability that it will reopen during the depolarization period. Moreover, even when the channel does not open at the beginning of the step, the frequency of appearance of Na⁺ currents later in the depolarization is very low; i.e. the Na⁺ channel inactivates.

Rat brain Na⁺ channels

The activity of rat brain Na⁺ channels has been studied in cerebellar Purkinje cells in culture. Each trace of **Figures 5.8a and c** shows the unitary Na⁺ currents (i_{Na}) recorded during a 20 ms membrane depolarization to –40 mV (test potential) from a holding potential of –90 mV. Rectangular inward currents occur most frequently at the beginning of the depolarizing step but can also be found at later times (**Figure 5.8a**, line 2). The histogram of the Na⁺ current amplitudes recorded at –40 mV test potential gives a mean amplitude for i_{Na} of around –2 pA (**Figure 5.8d**). Events near –4 pA correspond to double openings (at least two channels are present in the patch).

The unitary current has a rectangular shape

The rectangular shape of the unitary current means that when the Na⁺ channel opens, the unitary current is nearly immediately maximal. The unitary current then stays constant: the channel stays open for a time which varies; finally the unitary current goes back to zero though the membrane is still depolarized. The channel may not reopen (**Figures 5.7a,c**) since it is in an inactivated state (**Figure 5.7c**, bottom trace). After being opened by a depolarization, the channel does not go back to the closed state but inactivates. In that state, the pore of the channel is closed (no Na⁺ ions flow through the pore) as in the closed state but the channel cannot reopen immediately (which differs from the closed state). The inactivated channel is refractory to opening

the channel. On the bottom line one opening is enlarged. C, closed state; O, open state; I, inactivated state. The solution bathing the extracellular side of the patch or intrapipette solution contains (in mм): 140 NaCl, 1.4 KCl, 2.0 MgCl₂, 1 CaCl₂ and 20 HEPES at pH 7.4. TEA 5 mм is added to block K⁺ channels and bungarotoxin to block acetylcholine receptors. Adapted from Sigworth FJ, Neher E (1980) Single Na⁺ channel currents observed in rat muscle cells, *Nature* **287**, 447–449, with permission.

unless the membrane repolarizes to allow it to return to the closed (resting) state.

In other recordings, such as that of **Figures 5.8a and c,** the Na⁺ channel seems to reopen once or twice before inactivating. This may result from the presence of two (as here) or more channels in the patch so that the unitary currents recorded do not correspond to the same channel. It may also result from a slower inactivation rate of the channel recorded, which in fact opens, closes, reopens and then inactivates.

The unitary current is carried by a few Na⁺ ions

How many Na⁺ ions enter through a single channel? Knowing that in the preceding example, the unitary Na⁺ current has a mean amplitude of –1.6 pA for 1 ms, the number of Na⁺ ions flowing through one channel during 1 ms is $1.6 \times 10^{-12}/(1.6 \times 10^{-19} \times 10^3) = 10\,000$ Na⁺ ions (since 1 pA = 1 pC s⁻¹ and the elementary charge of one electron is 1.6×10^{-19} C). This number, 10^4 ions, is negligible compared with the number of Na⁺ ions in the intracellular medium: if $[Na^+]_i = 14$ mM, knowing that 1 mole represents 6×10^{23} ions, the number of Na⁺ ions per litre is $6 \times 10^{23} \times 14 \times 10^{-3} = 10^{22}$ ions l⁻¹. In a neuronal cell body or a section of axon, the volume is of the order of 10^{-12} to 10^{-13} litres. Then the number of Na⁺ ions is around 10^9 to 10^{10}.

The Na⁺ channel fluctuates between the closed, open and inactivated states

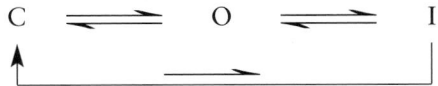

where C is the channel in the closed state, O in the open state and I in the inactivated state. Both C and I states are non-conducting states. The C to O transition is triggered by membrane depolarization. The O to I transition is due to an intrinsic property of the Na⁺ channel. The I to C transition occurs when the membrane repolarizes or is already repolarized. In summary, the Na⁺ channel opens when the membrane is depolarized, stays open during a mean open time of less than 1 ms, and then usually inactivates.

5.2.3 The time during which the Na⁺ channel stays open varies around an average value, τ_o, called the mean open time

In **Figures 5.7a** and **5.8a** we can observe that the periods during which the channel stays open, t_o, are variable.

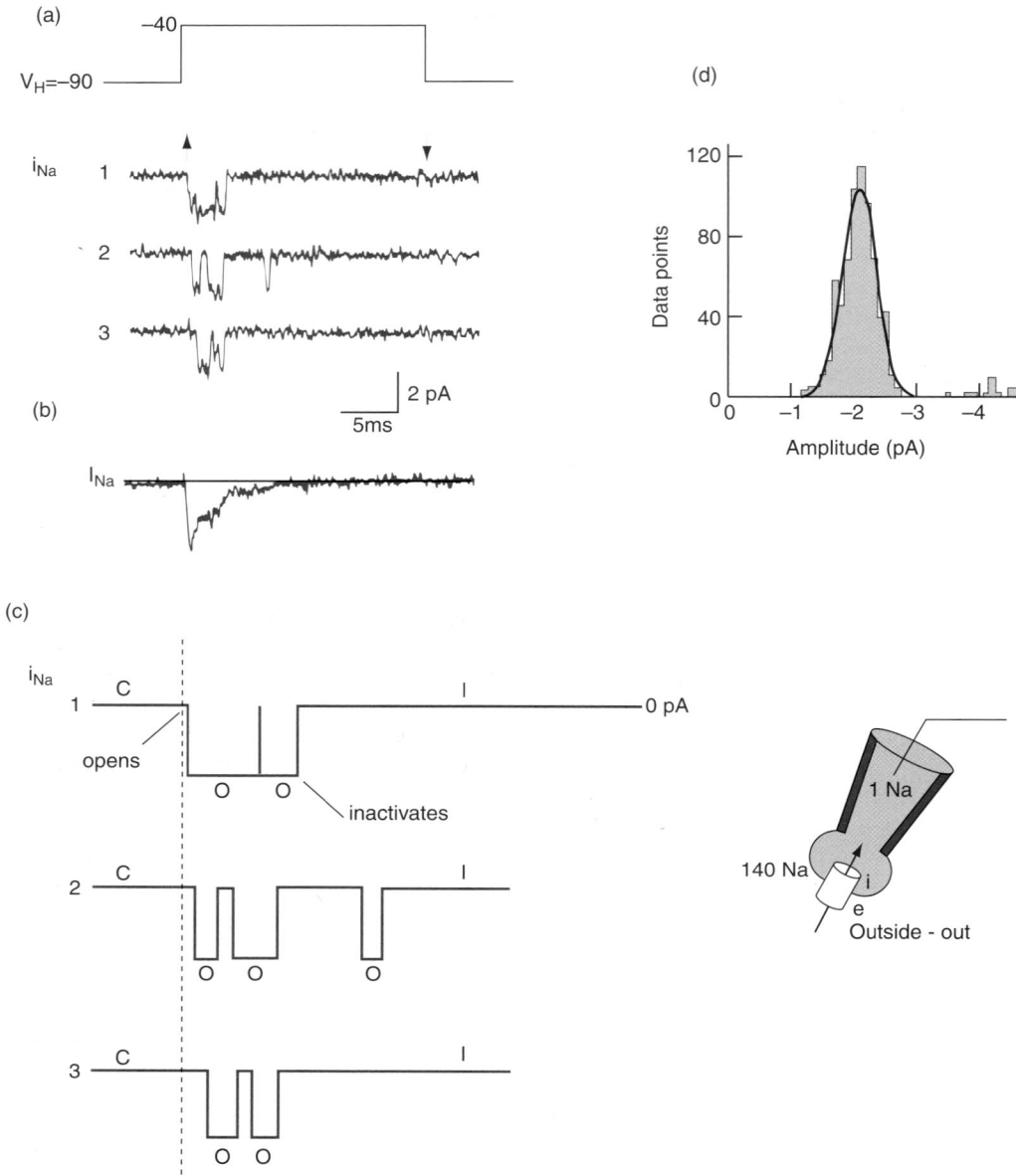

Figure 5.8 Single-channel activity of a voltage-gated Na⁺ channel from rat brain neurons.

The activity of a Na⁺ channel of a cerebellar Purkinje cell in culture is recorded in patch clamp (outside-out patch) in response to successive depolarizing steps to –40 mV from a holding potential of –90 mV. **(a)** The 20 ms step (upper trace) evokes rectangular inward unitary currents (i_{Na}). **(b)** Average current calculated from all the sweeps which had active Na⁺ channels within a set of 25 depolarizations. **(c)** Interpretative drawing on an enlarged scale of the recordings in (a). **(d)** Histogram of elementary amplitudes for recordings as in (a). The continuous line corresponds to the best fit of the data to a single Gaussian distribution. C, closed state; O, open state; I, inactivated state. The solution bathing the outside face of the patch contains (in mM): 140 NaCl, 2.5 KCl, 1 CaCl², 1 MgCl², 10 HEPES. The solution bathing the inside of the patch or intrapipette solution contains (in mM): 120 CsF, 10 CsCl, 1 NaCl, 10 EGTA-Cs⁺, 10 HEPES-Cs⁺. Cs⁺ ions are in the pipette instead of K⁺ ions in order to block K⁺ channels. Adapted from Gähwiler BH, Llano I (1989) Sodium and potassium conductances in somatic membranes of rat Purkinje cells from organotypic cerebellar cultures, *J. Physiol.* **417**, 105–122, with permission.

The mean open time of the channel, τ_o, at a given potential is obtained from the frequency histogram of the different t_o at this potential. When this distribution can be fitted by a single exponential, its time constant provides the value of τ_o (see Appendix 5.3). The functional significance of this value is the following: during a time equal to τ_o the channel has a high probability of staying open.

For example, the Na⁺ channel of the skeletal muscle fibre stays open during a mean open time of 0.7 ms. For the rat brain Na⁺ channel of cerebellar Purkinje cells, the distribution of the durations of the unitary currents recorded at –32 mV can be fitted with a single exponential with a time constant of 0.43 ms (τ_o = 0.43 ms).

5.2.4 The i_{Na}–V relation is linear: the Na⁺ channel has a constant unitary conductance γ_{Na}

When the activity of a single Na⁺ channel is now recorded at different test potentials, we observe that the amplitude of the inward unitary current diminishes as the membrane is further and further depolarized (see **Figure 5.10a**). In other words, the net entry of Na⁺ ions through a single channel diminishes as the membrane depolarizes. The i_{Na}–V relation is obtained by plotting the amplitude of the unitary current (i_{Na}) versus membrane potential (V_m). It is linear between –50 mV and 0 mV (**Figure 5.9a**). For membrane potentials more hyperpolarized than –50 mV, there are no values of i_{Na} since the channel rarely opens or does not open at all. Quantitative data for potentials more depolarized than 0 mV are not available.

The critical point of the current–voltage relation is the membrane potential for which the current is zero; i.e. the reversal potential of the current (E_{rev}). If only Na⁺ ions flow through the Na⁺ channel, the reversal potential is equal to E_{Na}. From –50 mV to E_{rev}, i_{Na} is inward and its amplitude decreases. This results from the decrease of the Na⁺ driving force ($V_m - E_{Na}$) as the membrane approaches the reversal potential for Na⁺ ions (see Sections 3.3.2 and 3.3.3). For membrane potentials more depolarized than E_{rev}, i_{Na} is now outward. Above E_{rev}, the amplitude of the outward Na⁺ current increases as the driving force for the exit of Na⁺ ions increases.

The linear i_{Na}–V relation is described by the equation $i_{Na} = \gamma_{Na}(V_m - E_{Na})$, where V_m is the test potential, E_{Na} is the reversal potential of the Na⁺ current, and γ_{Na} is the conductance of a single Na⁺ channel (unitary conductance). The value of γ_{Na} is given by the slope of the linear i_{Na}–V curve. It has a constant value at any given membrane potential. This value varies between 5 and 18 pS depending on the preparation.

5.2.5 The probability of the Na⁺ channel being in the open state increases with depolarization to a maximal level

An important observation at the single channel level is that the more the membrane is depolarized, the higher is the probability that the Na⁺ channel will open. This observation can be made from two types of experiments:

- The activity of a single Na⁺ channel is recorded in patch clamp (cell-attached patch). Each depolarizing step is repeated several times and the number of times the Na⁺ channel opens is observed (**Figure 5.10a**). With depolarizing steps to –70 mV from a holding potential of –120 mV, the channel very rarely opens; and if it does, the time spent in the open state is very short. In contrast, with depolarizing steps to –40 mV, the Na⁺ channels open for each trial.
- The activity of two or three Na⁺ channels is recorded in patch clamp (cell-attached patch). In response to depolarizing steps of small amplitude, Na⁺ channels do not open or only one Na⁺ channel opens at a time. With larger depolarizing steps, the overlapping currents of two or three Na⁺ channels can be observed, meaning that this number of Na⁺ channels open with close delays in response to the step (not shown).

From the recordings of **Figure 5.10a**, we can observe that the probability of the Na⁺ channel being in the open state varies with the value of the test potential. It also varies with time during the depolarizing step: openings occur more frequently at the beginning of the step. The open probability of Na⁺ channels is voltage- and time-dependent. By averaging a large number of records obtained at each test potential, the open probability (p_t) of the Na⁺ channel recorded can be obtained at each time t of the step (**Figure 5.10b**). We observe from these curves that after 4–6 ms the probability of the Na⁺ channel being in the open state is very low, even with large depolarizing steps: the Na⁺ channel inactivates in 4–6 ms. When we compare now the open probabilities at the different test potentials, we observe that the probability of the Na⁺ channel being in the open state at time t = 2 ms increases with the amplitude of the depolarizing step.

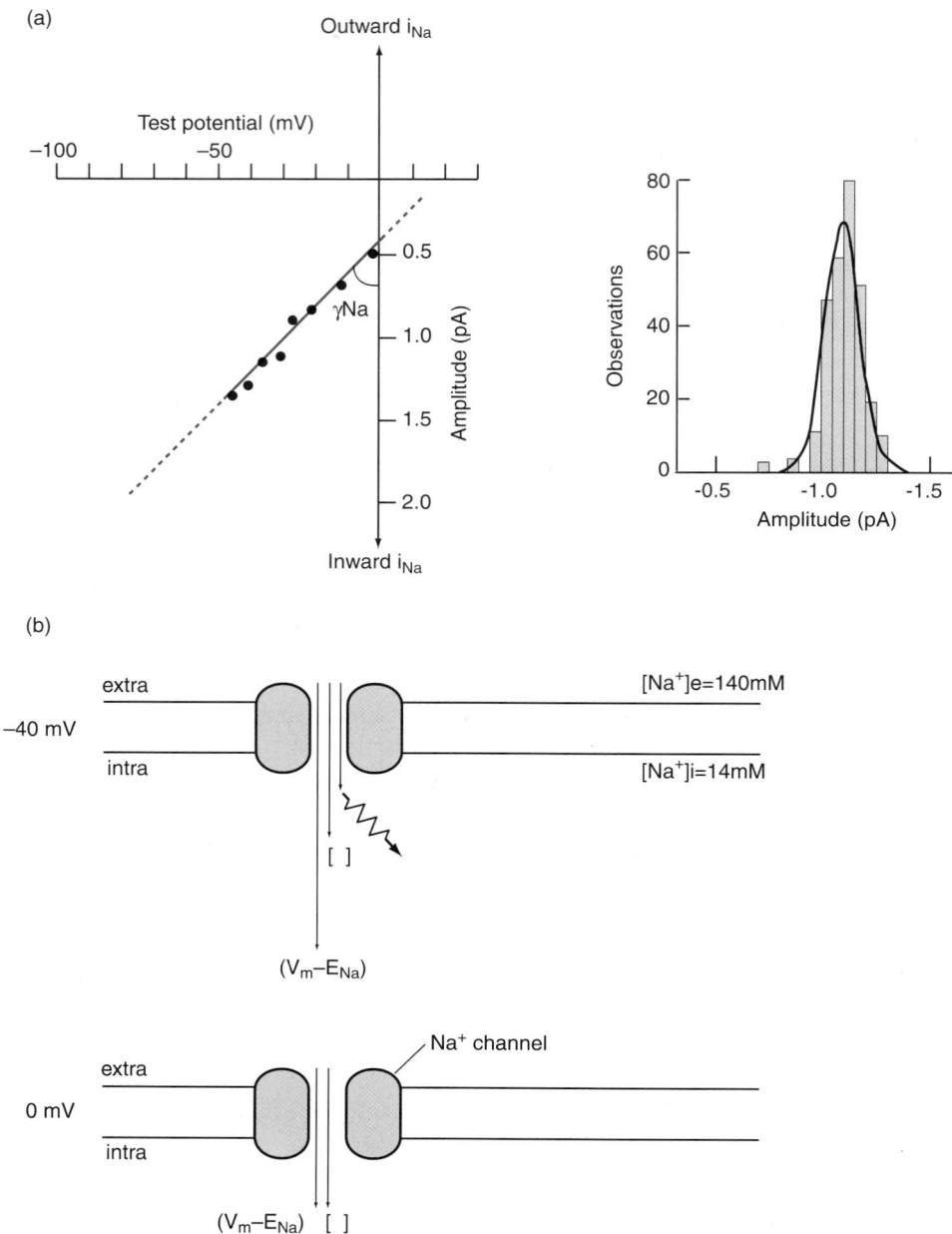

Figure 5.9 The single-channel current/voltage (i_{Na}/V) relation is linear.
(a) The activity of the rat type II Na$^+$ channel expressed in *Xenopus* oocytes from cDNA is recorded in patch clamp (cell-attached patch). Plot of the unitary current amplitude versus test potential: each point represents the mean of 20–200 unitary current amplitudes measured at one potential (left) as shown at –32 mV (right). The relation is linear between test potentials –50 and 0 mV (holding potential = –90 mV). The slope is γ_{Na} = 19 pS. (b) Drawings of an open voltage-gated Na$^+$ channel to explain the direction and amplitude of the net flux of Na$^+$ ions at two test potentials (–40 and 0 mV). [], force due to the concentration gradient across the membrane; ∿, force due to the electric gradient; V_m–E_{Na}, driving force. The solution bathing the extracellular side of the patch or intrapipette solution contains (in mM): 115 NaCl, 2.5 KCl, 1.8 CaCl$_2$, 10 HEPES. Plot (a) adapted from Stühmer W, Methfessel C, Sakmann B *et al.* (1987) Patch clamp characterization of sodium channels expressed from rat brain cDNA, *Eur. Biophys. J.* **14**, 131–138, with permission.

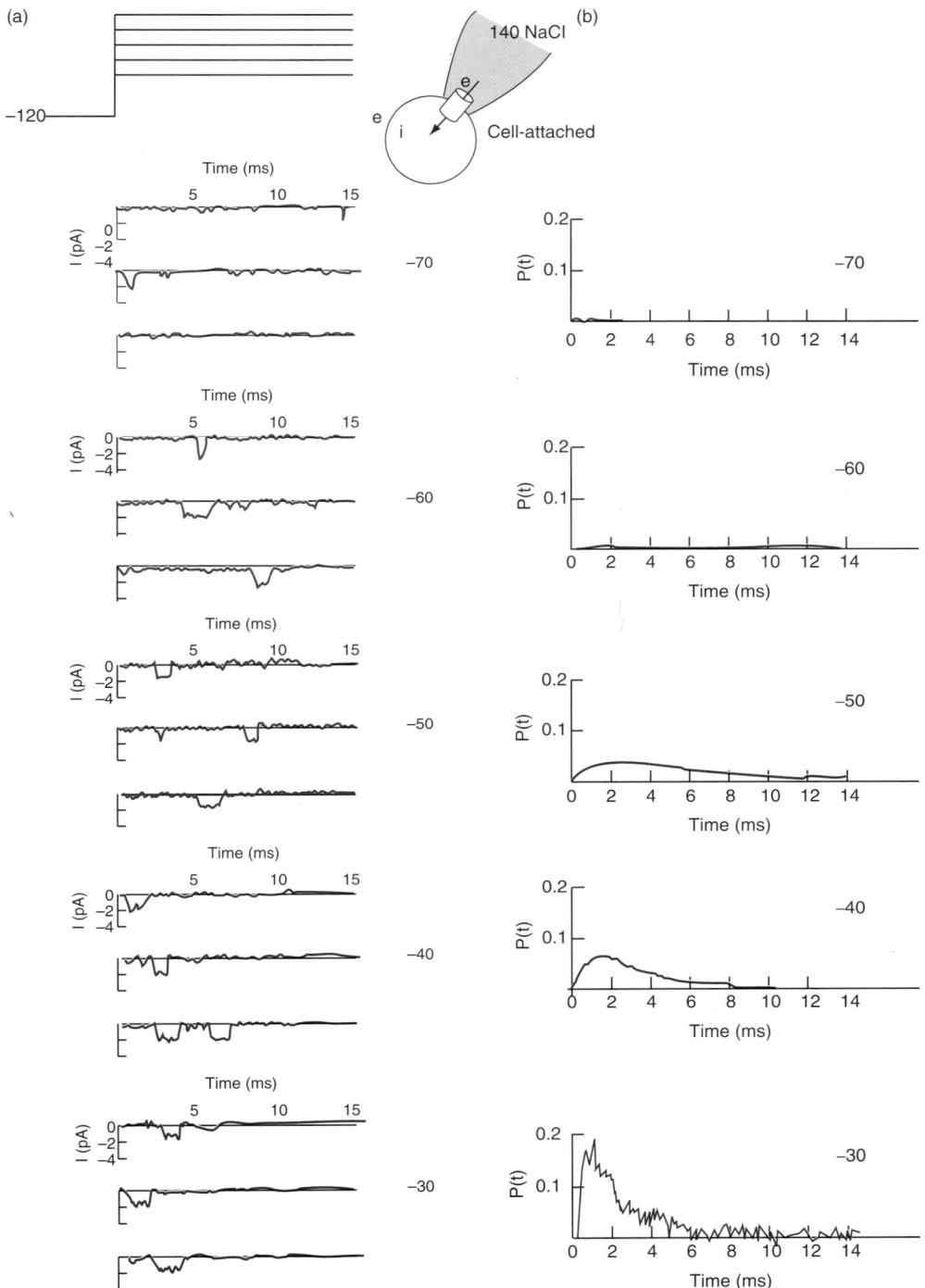

Figure 5.10 The open probability of the voltage-gated Na+ channel is voltage- and time-dependent.
Single Na+ channel activity recorded in a mammalian neuroblastoma cell in patch clamp (cell-attached patch). **(a)** In response to a depolarizing step to the indicated potentials from a holding potential of –120 mV, unitary inward currents are recorded. (b) Ensemble of averages of single-channel openings at the indicated voltages; 64 to 2000 traces are averaged at each voltage to obtain the time-dependent open probability of a channel ($p_{(t)}$) in response to a depolarization. The open probability at time t is calculated according to the equation: $p_{(t)} = I_{Na(t)}/Ni_{Na}$, where $I_{Na(t)}$ is the average current at time t at a given voltage, N is the number of channels (i.e. the number of averaged recordings of single channel activity) and i_{Na} is the unitary current at a given voltage. At –30 mV the open probability is maximum. The channels inactivate in 4 ms. Adapted from Aldrich RW, Steven CF (1987) Voltage-dependent gating of sodium channels from mammalian neuroblastoma cells, *J. Neurosci.* **7**, 418–431, with permission.

5.2.6 The macroscopic Na⁺ current (I_{Na}) has a steep voltage dependence of activation and inactivates within a few milliseconds

The macroscopic Na⁺ current, I_{Na}, is the sum of the unitary currents, i_{Na}, flowing through all the open Na⁺ channels of the recorded membrane

At the axon initial segment or at nodes of Ranvier, there are N Na⁺ channels that can be activated. We have seen that the unitary Na⁺ current flowing through a single Na⁺ channel has a rectangular shape. What is the time course of the macroscopic Na⁺ current, I_{Na}?

If we assume that the Na⁺ channels in one cell are identical and function independently, the sum of many recordings from the same Na⁺ channel should show the same properties as the macroscopic Na⁺ current measured from thousands of channels with the voltage clamp technique. In **Figure 5.7b**, an average of 300 unitary Na⁺ currents elicited by a 40 mV depolarizing pulse is shown. For a given potential, the 'averaged' inward Na⁺ current has a fast rising phase and presents a peak at the time $t = 1.5$ ms. The peak corresponds to the time when most of the Na⁺ channels open at each trial. Then the averaged current decays with time because the Na⁺ channel has a low probability of being in the open state later in the step (owing to the inactivation of the Na⁺ channel). At each trial, the Na⁺ channel does not inactivate exactly at the same time, which explains the progressive decay of the averaged macroscopic Na⁺ current. A similar averaged Na⁺ current is shown in **Figure 5.8b**. The averaged current does not have a rectangular shape because the Na⁺ channel does not open with the same delay and does not inactivate at the same time at each trial.

The *averaged* macroscopic Na⁺ current has a similar time course to the *recorded* macroscopic Na⁺ current from the same type of cell at the same potential. However, the averaged current from 300 Na⁺ channels still presents some angles in its time course. In contrast, the macroscopic recorded Na⁺ current is smooth. The more numerous are the Na⁺ channels opened by the depolarizing step, the smoother is the total Na⁺ current. The value of I_{Na} at each time t at a given potential is:

$$I_{Na} = N p_{(t)} i_{Na},$$

where N is the number of Na⁺ channels in the recorded membrane and $p_{(t)}$ is the open probability at time t of the Na⁺ channel; it depends on the membrane potential and on the channel opening and inactivating rate constants. i_{Na} is the unitary Na⁺ current and $N p_{(t)}$ is the number of Na⁺ channels open at time t.

The I_{Na}–V relation is bell-shaped though the i_{Na}–V relation is linear

We have seen that the amplitude of the unitary Na⁺ current decreases linearly with depolarization (see **Figure 5.9a**). In contrast, the I_{Na}–V relation is not linear. The macroscopic Na⁺ current is recorded from a myelinated rabbit nerve with the double electrode voltage clamp technique. When the amplitude of the peak Na⁺ current is plotted against membrane potential, it has a clear bell-shape (**Figures 5.11 and 5.12a**).

Analysis of each trace from the smallest depolarizing step to the largest shows that:

- For small steps, the peak current has a small amplitude (0.2 nA) and a slow time to peak (1 ms). At these potentials the Na⁺ driving force is strong but the Na⁺ channels have a low probability of opening (**Figure 5.11a**). Therefore, I_{Na} represents the current through a small number of open Na⁺ channels. Moreover, the small number of activated Na⁺ channels open with a delay since the depolarization is just *subliminal*. This explains the slow time to peak.
- As the depolarizing steps increase in amplitude (to –42/–35 mV), the amplitude of I_{Na} increases to a maximum (–3 nA) and the time to peak decreases to a minimum (0.2 ms). Larger depolarizations increase the probability of the Na⁺ channel being in the open state and shorten the delay of opening (see **Figure 5.10**). Therefore, though the amplitude of i_{Na} decreases between –63 and –35 mV, the amplitude of I_{Na} increases owing to the large increase of open Na⁺ channels.
- After this peak, the amplitude of I_{Na} decreases to zero since the open probability does not increase enough to compensate for the decrease of i_{Na}. The reversal potential of I_{Na} is the same as that of i_{Na} since it depends only on the extracellular and intracellular concentrations of Na⁺ ions.
- I_{Na} changes polarity after E_{rev}: it is now an outward current whose amplitude increases with the depolarization.

It is important to note that membrane potentials more depolarized than +20 mV are non-physiological.

Activation and inactivation curves: the threshold potential

Activation is the rate at which a macroscopic current turns on in response to a depolarizing voltage step. The Na⁺ current is recorded in voltage clamp from a node of rabbit nerve. Depolarizing steps from –70 mV to +20 mV are applied from a holding potential of –80 mV. When the ratio of the peak current at each test potential

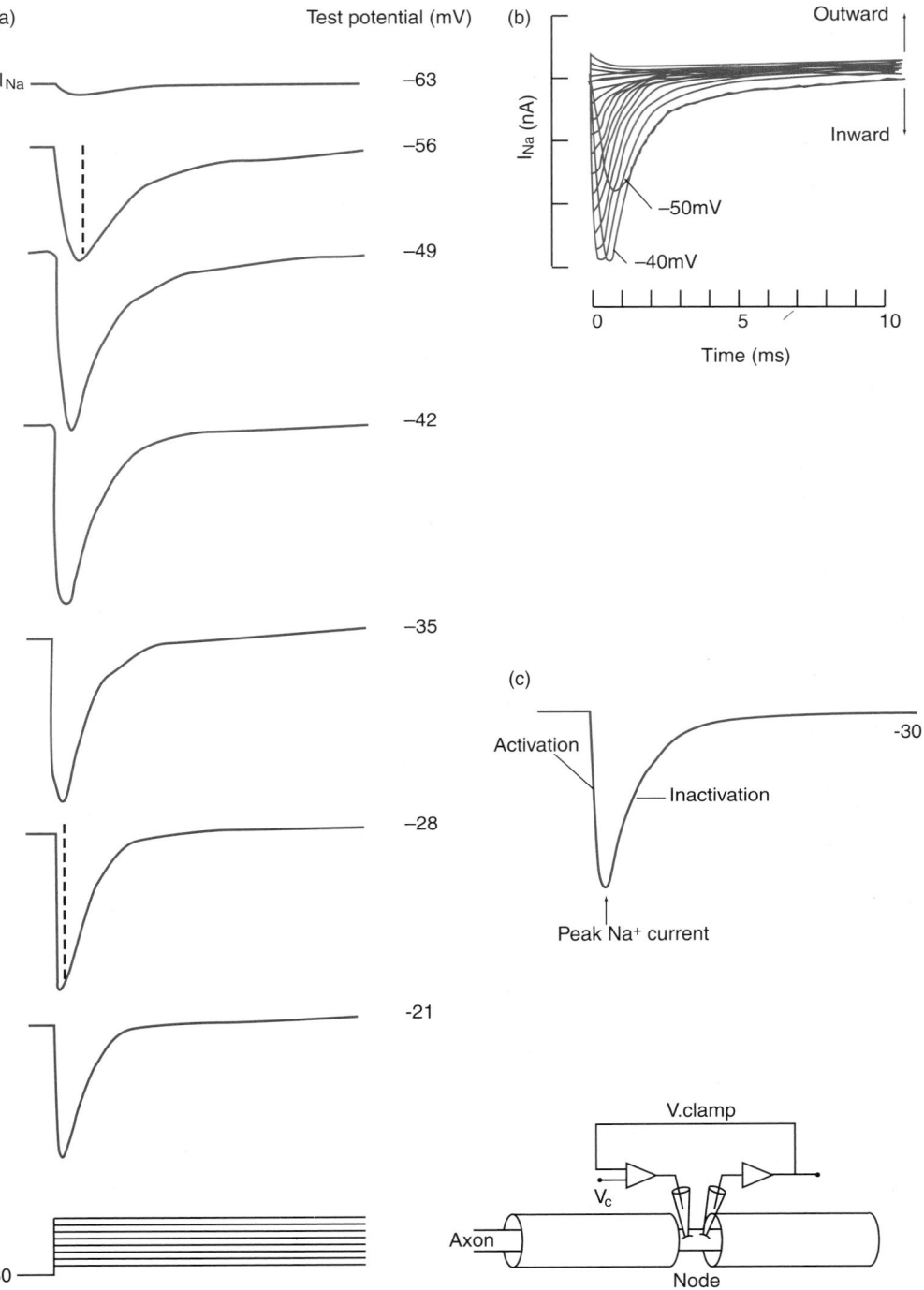

Figure 5.11 Voltage dependence of the macroscopic voltage-gated Na⁺ current.
The macroscopic voltage-gated Na⁺ current recorded in a node of a rabbit myelinated nerve in voltage clamp conditions. **(a)** Depolarizing steps from −70 mV to −21 mV from a holding potential of −80 mV evoke macroscopic Na⁺ currents (I_{Na}) with different time courses and peak amplitudes. The test potential is on the right. Bottom trace is the voltage trace. **(b)** The traces in (a) are superimposed and current responses to depolarizing steps from −14 to +55 mV are added. The outward current traces are recorded when the test potential is beyond the reversal potential (+30 mV in this preparation). **(c)** I_{Na} recorded at −30 mV. The rising phase of I_{Na} corresponds to activation of the Na⁺ channels and the decrease of I_{Na} corresponds to progressive inactivation of the open Na⁺ channels. The extracellular solution contains (in mM): 154 NaCl, 2.2 CaCl₂, 5.6 KCl; pH 7.4. Adapted from Chiu SY, Ritchie JM, Bogart RB, Stagg D (1979) A quantitative description of membrane currents from a rabbit myelinated nerve, *J. Physiol.* **292**, 149–166, with permission.

to the maximal peak current ($I_{Na}/I_{Na\ max}$) is plotted against test potential, the activation curve of I_{Na} can be visualized. The distribution is fitted by a sigmoidal curve (**Figure 5.12b**). In this preparation, the threshold of Na$^+$ channel activation is –60 mV. At –40 mV, I_{Na} is already maximal ($I_{Na}/I_{Na\ max} = 1$). This steepness of activation is a characteristic of the voltage-gated Na$^+$ channels.

Inactivation of a current is the decay of this current during a maintained depolarization. To study inactivation, the membrane is held at varying holding potentials and a depolarizing step to a fixed value is applied where I_{Na} is maximal (0 mV for example). The amplitude of the peak Na$^+$ current is plotted against the holding potential. I_{Na} begins to inactivate at –90 mV and is fully inactivated at –50 mV. Knowing that the resting membrane potential in this preparation is around –80 mV, some of the Na$^+$ channels are already inactivated at rest.

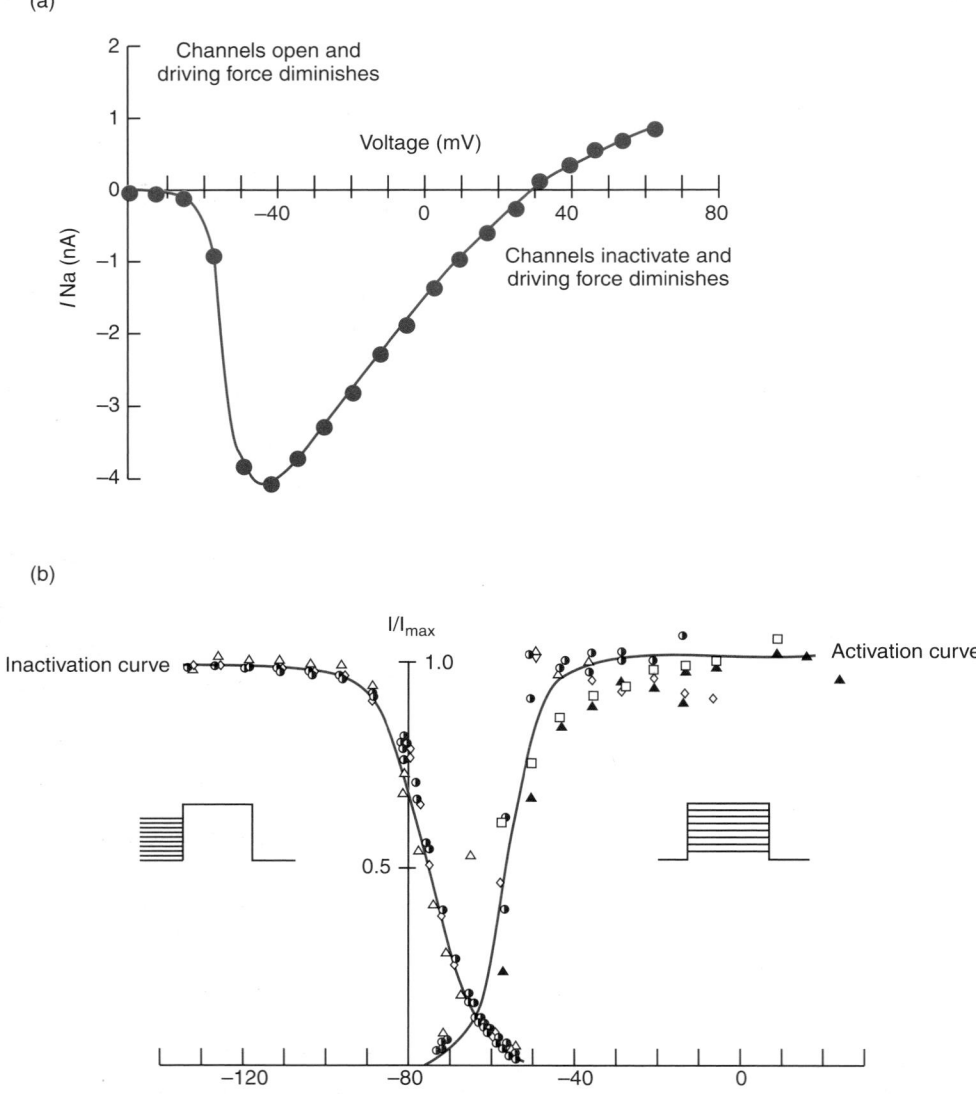

Figure 5.12 Activation–inactivation properties of the macroscopic voltage-gated Na$^+$ current.

(a) The I_{Na}–V relation has a bell shape with a peak at –40 mV and a reversal potential at +30 mV (the average E_{Na} in the rabbit node is +27 mV). (b) Activation (right curve) and inactivation (left curve) curves obtained from nine different experiments. The voltage protocols used are shown in insets. In the ordinates, I/I_{max} represents the ratio of the peak Na$^+$ current (I) recorded at the tested potential of the abscissae and the maximal peak Na$^+$ current (I_{max}) recorded in this experiment. It corresponds in the activation curve to the peak current recorded at –40 mV in Figure 5.11. From Chiu SY, Ritchie JM, Bogart RB, Stagg D (1979) A quantitative description of membrane currents from a rabbit myelinated nerve, *J. Physiol.* **292**, 149–166, with permission.

Ionic selectivity of the Na⁺ channel

To compare the permeability of the Na⁺ channel to several monovalent cations, the macroscopic current is recorded at different membrane potentials in the presence of external Na⁺ ions and when all the external Na⁺ are replaced by a test cation. Lithium is as permeant as sodium but K⁺ ions are weakly permeant (P_K/P_{Na} = 0.048). Therefore, Na⁺ channels are highly selective for Na⁺ ions and only 4% of the current is carried by K⁺ ions (**Figure 5.13**).

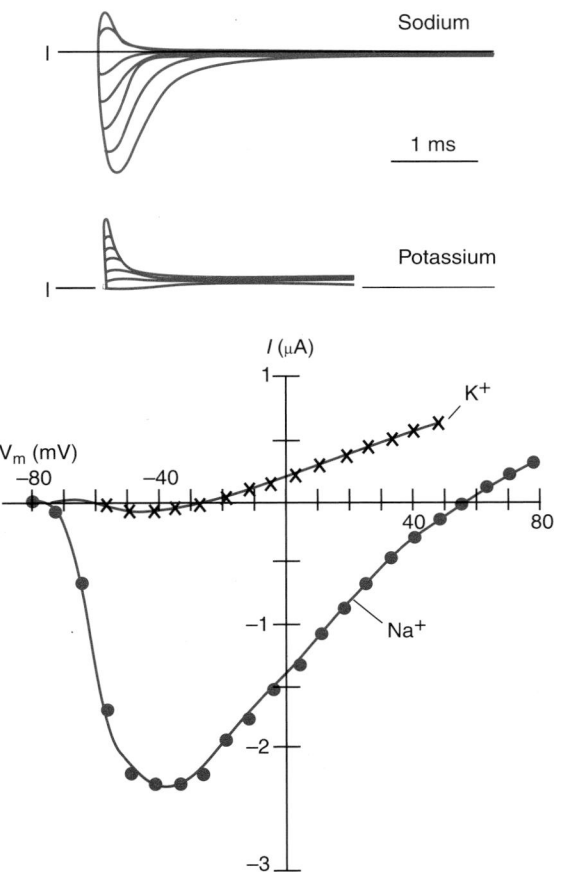

Figure 5.13 Ionic selectivity of the Na⁺ channel.
The macroscopic Na⁺ current is recorded with the double electrode voltage clamp technique in a mammalian skeletal muscle fibre at different test membrane potentials (from –70 to +80 mV) from a holding potential of –80 mV. **(a)** Inward currents in normal Na⁺–Ringer (sodium) and in a solution where all Na⁺ ions are replaced by K⁺ ions (potassium). The other voltage-gated currents are blocked. **(b)** I–V relation of the currents recorded in (a). I is the amplitude of the peak current at each tested potential. Adapted from Pappone PA (1980) Voltage clamp experiments in normal and denervated mammalian skeletal muscle fibers, J Physiol. **306**, 377–410, with permission.

Tetrodotoxin is a selective open Na⁺ channel blocker

A large number of biological toxins can modify the properties of the Na⁺ channel. One of these, tetrodotoxin (TTX), which is found in the liver and ovaries of the fish tetrodon, has a binding site supposed to be located near the extracellular mouth of the pore. A single point mutation of the rat brain Na⁺ channel type II, which changes the glutamic acid residue 387 to glutamine (E387Q) in the repeat I, renders the channel insensitive to concentrations of TTX up to tens of micromolars. *Xenopus* oocytes are injected with the wild-type mRNA or the mutant mRNA and the whole cell Na⁺ currents are recorded with the double-electrode voltage clamp technique. TTX sensitivity is assessed by perfusing TTX-containing external solutions and by measuring the peak of the whole-cell inward Na⁺ current (the peak means the maximal amplitude of the inward Na⁺ current measured on the I_{Na}/V relation). The dose–response curves of **Figure 5.14** show that 1 μM of TTX completely abolishes the wild-type Na⁺ current, but has no effect on the mutant Na⁺ current. The other characteristics of the Na⁺ channel are not significantly affected, except for a reduction in the amplitude of the inward current at all potentials tested. All these results suggest that the link between segments S5 and S6 in repeat I of the rat brain Na⁺ channel is in close proximity to the channel mouth (see **Figures 3.5** and **5.6**).

5.2.7 Segment S4, the region between segments S5 and S6, and the region between domains III and IV play a significant role in activation, ion permeation and inactivation, respectively

The major questions about a voltage-gated ionic channel and particularly the Na⁺ channel are the following:

■ How does the channel open in response to a voltage change?
■ How is the permeation pathway designed to define single-channel conductance and ion selectivity? (see also Section 3.3.1)
■ How does the channel inactivate?

In order to identify regions of the Na⁺ channels involved in these functions, site-directed mutagenesis experiments were performed. The activity of each type of mutated Na⁺ channel is analysed with patch clamp recording techniques.

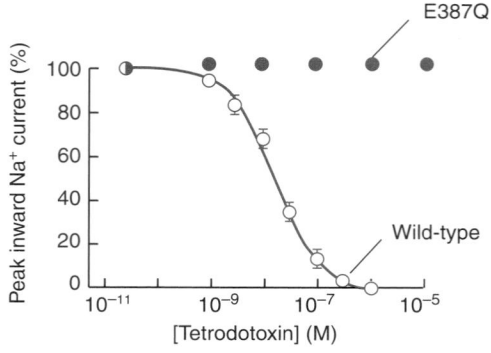

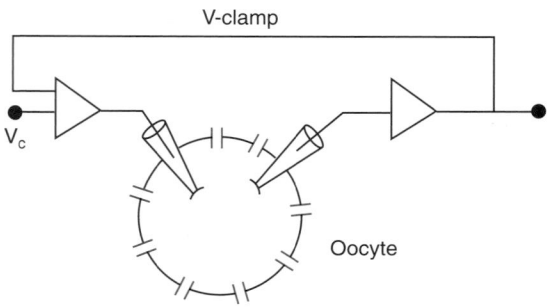

Figure 5.14 A single mutation close to the S6 segment of repeat I completely suppresses the sensitivity of the Na⁺ channel to TTX.

A mutation of the glutamic acid residue 387 to glutamine (E387Q) is introduced in the rat Na⁺ channel type II. *Xenopus* oocytes are injected with either the wild-type mRNA or the mutant mRNA. The macroscopic Na⁺ currents are recorded 4–7 days later with the double electrode voltage clamp technique. Dose–response curves for the wild-type (open circles) and the mutant E387Q (filled circles) to tetrodotoxin (TTX). TTX sensitivity is determined by perfusing TTX-containing external solutions and by measuring the macroscopic peak inward current. The TTX concentration that reduces the wild-type Na⁺ current by 50% (IC_{50}) is 18 nM. Data are averaged from 7–8 experiments. From Noda M, Suzuki H, Numa S, Stühmer W (1989) A single point mutation confers tetrodotoxin and saxitoxin insensitivity on the sodium channel II, *FEBS Lett.* **259**, 213–216, with permission.

The short segments between putative membrane-spanning segments S5 and S6 are membrane associated and contribute to pore formation

The Na⁺ channels are highly selective for Na⁺ ions. This selectivity presumably results from negatively charged amino acid residues located in the channel pore. Moreover, these amino acids must be specific to Na⁺ channels (i.e. different from the other members of voltage-gated cationic channels such as K⁺ and Ca²⁺ channels) to explain their weak permeability to K⁺ or Ca²⁺ ions.

Studies using mutagenesis to alter ion channel function have shown that the region connecting the S5 and S6 segments forms part of the channel lining (see **Figure 5.6**). A single amino acid substitution in these regions, in repeats III and IV, alters the ion selectivity of the Na⁺ channel to resemble that of Ca²⁺ channels. These residues would constitute part of the selectivity filter of the channel. There is now a general agreement that the selectivity filter is formed by pore loops; i.e. relatively short polypeptide segments that extend into the aqueous pore from the extracellular side of the membrane. Rather than extending completely across the lipid bilayer, a large portion of the pore loop is near the extracellular face of the channel. Only a short region extends into the membrane to form the selectivity filter. In the case of the voltage-gated Na⁺ channel, each of the four homologous domains contributes a loop to the ion conducting pore (**Figure 5.6b**).

The S4 segment is the voltage sensor

The S4 segments are positively charged and hydrophobic (**Figure 5.15a**). Moreover, the typical amino acid sequence of S4 is conserved among the different voltage-gated channels. These observations led to the suggestion that S4 segments have a transmembrane orientation and are voltage sensors. To test this proposed role, positively charged amino acid residues are replaced by neutral or negatively charged residues in the S4 segment of a rat brain Na⁺ channel type II. The mutated channels are expressed in *Xenopus* oocytes. When more than three positive residues are mutated in the S4 segments of repeat I or II, no appreciable expression of the mutated channel is obtained. The replacement of only one arginine or lysine residue in segment S4 of repeat I by a glutamine residue shifts the activation curve to more positive potentials (**Figures 5.15b and c**).

It is hypothesized that the positive charges in S4 form ion pairs with negative charges in other transmembrane regions, thereby stabilizing the channel in the non-conducting closed conformation. With a change in the electric field across the membrane, these ion pairs would break as the S4 charges move and new ion pairs would form to stabilize the conducting, open conformation of the channel.

The cytoplasmic loop between domains III and IV contains the inactivation particle which, in a voltage-dependent manner, enters the mouth of the Na⁺ channel pore and inactivates the channel

The results obtained from three different types of experiments strongly suggest that the short cytoplasmic loop

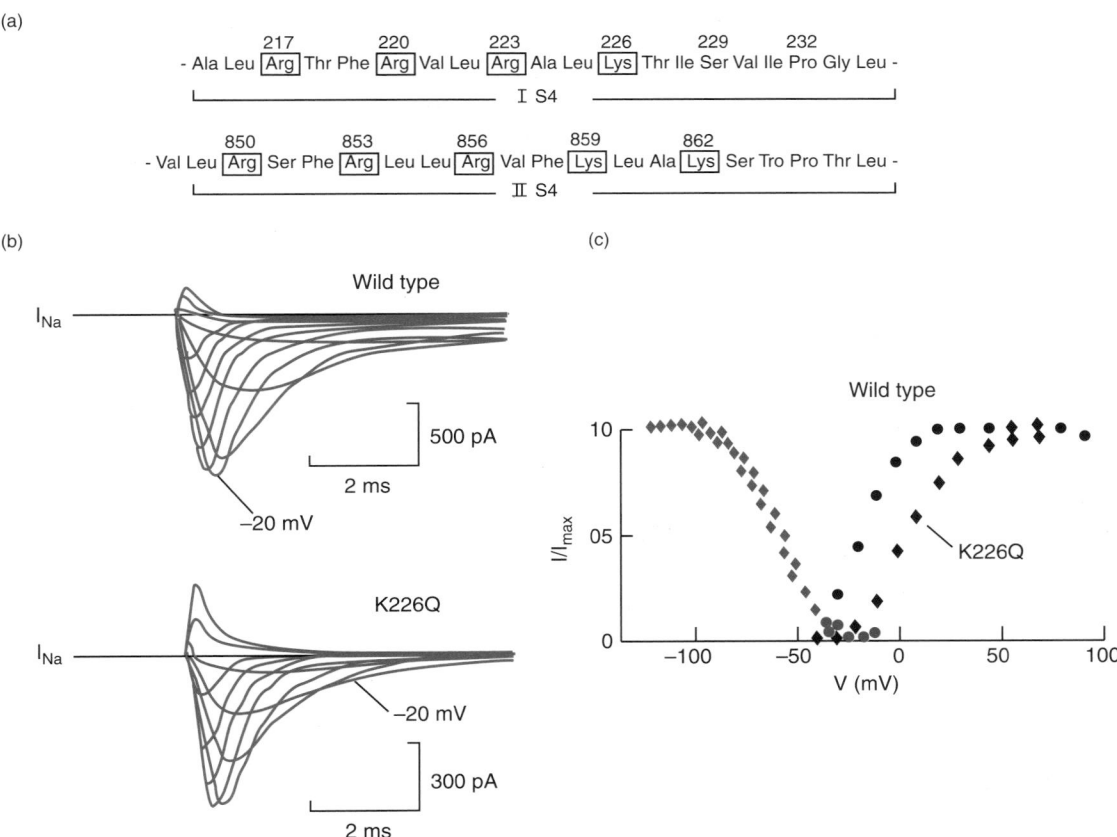

Figure 5.15 Effect of mutations in the S4 segment on Na⁺ current activation.
Oocytes are injected with the wild-type rat brain Na⁺ channel or with Na⁺ channels mutated on the S4 segment. The activity of a population of Na⁺ channels is recorded in patch clamp (cell-attached macropatches). **(a)** Amino acid sequences of segment S4 of the internal repeats I (I S4) and II (II S4) of the wild-type rat Na⁺ channel. Positively charged amino acids are boxed with solid lines and the numbers of the relevant residues are given. In the mutated channel studied here the lysine residue in position 226 is replaced by a glutamine residue (K226Q). **(b)** In response to step depolarizations ranging from −60 to +70 mV from a holding potential of −120 mV, a family of macroscopic Na⁺ currents is recorded for each type of Na⁺ channel. The arrow indicates the reponse to the test potential −20 mV. Note that at −20 mV the amplitude of the Na⁺ current is at its maximum for the wild-type and less than half maximum for the mutated channel. **(c)** Steady-state activation (right) and inactivation (left) curves for the wild-type (circles) and the mutant (diamonds) Na⁺ channels. Adapted from Stühmer W, Conti F, Suzuki H *et al.* (1989) Structural parts involved in activation and inactivation of the sodium channel, *Nature* **339**, 597–603, with permission.

connecting homologous domains III and IV, L_III–IV loop (see **Figures 5.6a** and **5.16a**), is involved in inactivation: (i) cytoplasmic application of endopeptidases; (ii) cytoplasmic injection of antibodies directed against a peptide sequence in the region between repeats III and IV; and (iii) cleavage of the region between repeats III and IV (**Figures 5.16a–c**); all strongly reduce or block inactivation. Moreover, in some human pathology where the Na⁺ channels poorly inactivate (as shown with single-channel recordings from biopsies), this region is mutated.

Positively charged amino acid residues of this L_III–IV loop are not required for inactivation since only the mutation of a hydrophobic sequence, isoleucine-phenylalanine-methionine (IFM), to glutamine completely blocks inactivation. The critical residue of the IFM motif is phenylalanine since its mutation to glutamine slows inactivation 5000-fold. It is proposed that this IFM sequence is directly involved in the conformational change leading to inactivation. It would enter the mouth of the pore, thus occluding it during the process of inactivation. In order to test this hypothesis, the ability of

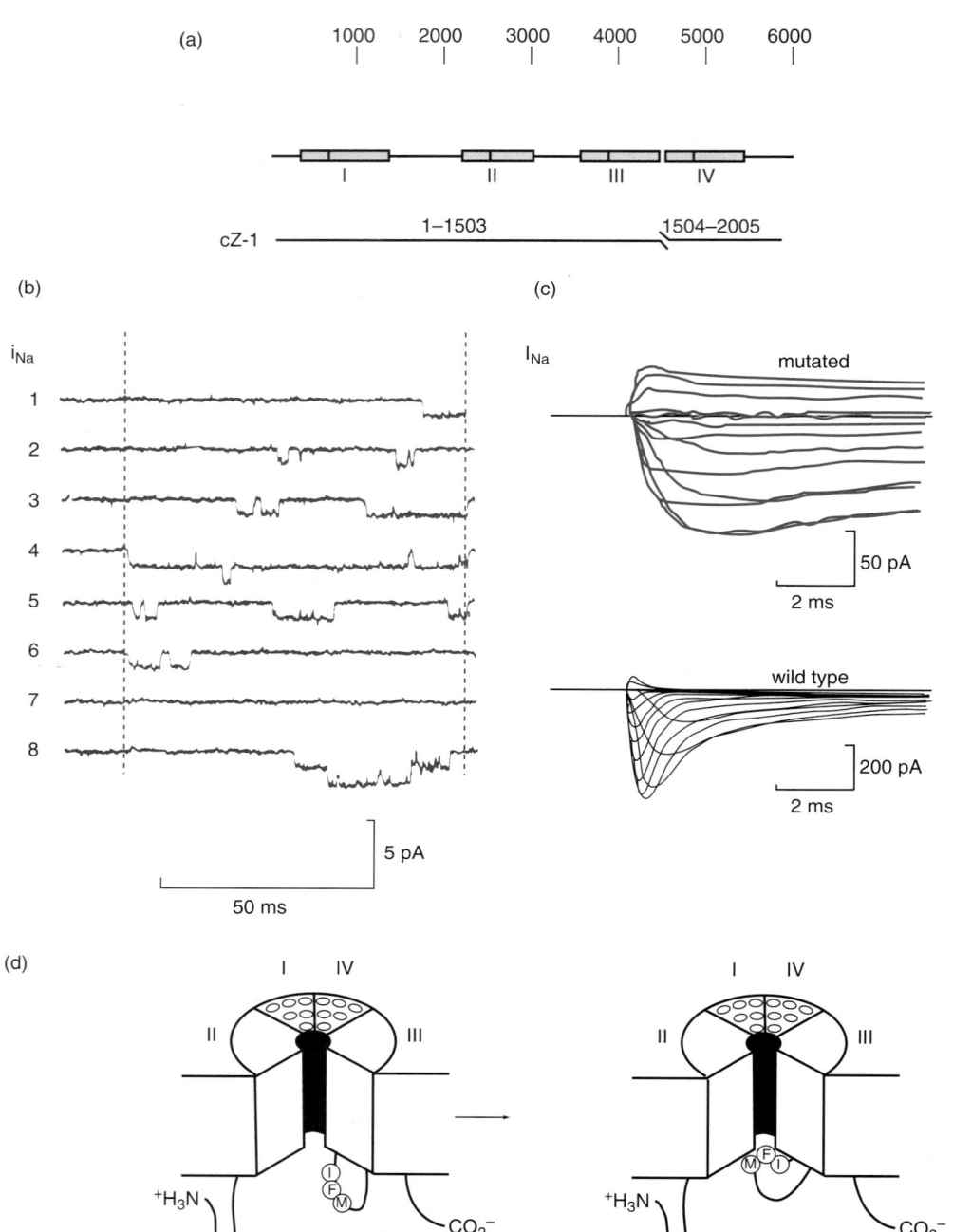

Figure 5.16 Effects of mutations in the region between repeats III and IV on Na+ current inactivation.
(a) Linear representation of the wild-type Na+ channel (upper trace) and the mutated Na+ channel (bottom trace). The mutation consists of a cut with an addition of four to eight residues at each end of the cut. An equimolar mixture of the two mRNAs encoding the adjacent fragments of the Na+ channel protein separated with a cut is injected in oocytes. (b) Single-channel recordings of the activity of the mutated Na+ channel in response to a depolarizing step to –20 mV from a holding potential of –100 mV. Note that late single or double openings (line 8) are often recorded. The mean open time τ_o is 5.8 ms and the elementary conductance γ_{Na} is 17.3 pS. (c) Macroscopic Na+ currents recorded from the mutated (upper trace) and the wild-type (bottom trace) Na+ channels. (d) Model for inactivation of the voltage-gated Na+ channels. The region linking repeats III and IV is depicted as a hinged lid that occludes the transmembrane pore of the Na+ channel during inactivation. Parts (a)–(c) from Pappone PA (1980) Voltage clamp experiments in normal and denervated mammalian skeletal muscle fibers, *J Physiol.* **306**, 377–410, with permission. Drawing (d) from West JW, Patton DE, Scheuer T *et al.* (1992) A cluster of hydrophobic amino acid residues required for fast sodium channel inactivation, *Proc. Natl Acad. Sci. USA* **89**, 10910–10914, with permission.

synthetic peptides containing the IFM motif to restore fast inactivation to non-inactivating rat brain Na⁺ channels expressed in kidney carcinoma cells is examined. The intrinsic inactivation of Na⁺ channels is first made non-functional by a mutation of the IFM motif. When the recording is now performed with a patch pipette containing the synthetic peptide with an IFM motif, the non-inactivating whole cell Na⁺ current now inactivates. Since the restored inactivation has the rapid, voltage-dependent time course characteristic of inactivation of the wild-type Na⁺ channels, it is proposed that the IFM motif serves as an inactivation particle (**Figure 5.16d**).

5.2.8 Conclusion: the consequence of the opening of a population of N Na⁺ channels is a transient entry of Na⁺ ions which depolarizes the membrane above 0 mV

The function of the population of N Na⁺ channels at the axon initial segment or at nodes of Ranvier is to ensure a *sudden* and *brief* depolarization of the membrane above 0 mV.

Rapid activation of Na⁺ channels makes the depolarization phase sudden

In response to a depolarization to the threshold potential, the closed Na⁺ channels (**Figure 5.17a**) of the axon initial segment begin to open (b). The flux of Na⁺ ions through the few open Na⁺ channels depolarizes the membrane more and thus triggers the opening of other Na⁺ channels (c). In consequence, the flux of Na⁺ ions increases, depolarizes the membrane more and opens other Na⁺ channels until all the N Na⁺ channels of the segment of membrane are opened (d). In (d) the depolarization phase is at its peak. Na⁺ channels are opened by depolarization and once opened they contribute to the membrane depolarization and therefore to their activation: it is a self-maintained process.

Rapid inactivation of Na⁺ channels makes the depolarization phase brief

Once the Na⁺ channels have opened, they begin to inactivate (e). Therefore, though the membrane is depolarized, the influx of Na⁺ ions diminishes quickly. Therefore the Na⁺-dependent action potential is a spike and does not present a plateau phase. Inactivation is a very important protective mechanism since it prevents potentially toxic persistent depolarization.

5.3 The repolarization phase of the sodium-dependent action potential results from Na⁺ channel inactivation and partly from K⁺ channel activation

The participation of a voltage-gated K⁺ current in action potential repolarization differs from one preparation to another. For example, in the squid axon the voltage-gated K⁺ current plays an important role in spike repolarization, though in mammalian peripheral nerves this current is almost absent. However, the action potentials of the squid axon and that of mammalian nerves have the same duration. This is because the Na⁺ current in mammalian axons inactivates two to three times faster than that of the frog axon. Moreover, the leak K⁺ currents are important in mammalian axons (see below).

This section will explain the structure and activity of the voltage-gated, delayed rectifier K⁺ channels responsible for action potential repolarization in the squid or frog nerves. Then Section 5.4 will explain the other mode of repolarization observed in mammalian nerves, in which the delayed rectifier current does not play a significant role.

5.3.1 The K⁺ channel consists of an α-subunit with a single repeat and auxiliary β-subunits

K⁺ channels represent an extremely diverse ion channel type. They all consist of an α-subunit with a single repeat made of six putative membrane-spanning segments (S1 to S6) and a typical sequence between S5 and S6 probably tucked into the membrane (**Figure 5.18**). The hydropathy profile of this single repeat is similar to each of the internal repeats of the Na⁺ channel, suggesting similar transmembrane topologies for these voltage-gated channels. K⁺ channels are therefore generally believed to form homotetramers in the cell membrane. As for the Na⁺ channel, the region linking segments S5 and S6 contributes substantially to the formation of the pore. In this example of a probably homotetrameric channel, four identical loops, one from each subunit, would extend into the pore to form the selectivity filter (see **Figure 5.6b**).

Purified neuronal K⁺ channels from mammalian brain have auxiliary small β-subunits considered intracellularly located and associated with the α-subunit. As for Na⁺ channels, these auxiliary subunits play an important role in the inactivation properties of the K⁺ channels.

Voltage-gated K⁺ channels can be classified into two major groups based on physiological properties:

■ delayed rectifiers which activate after a delay

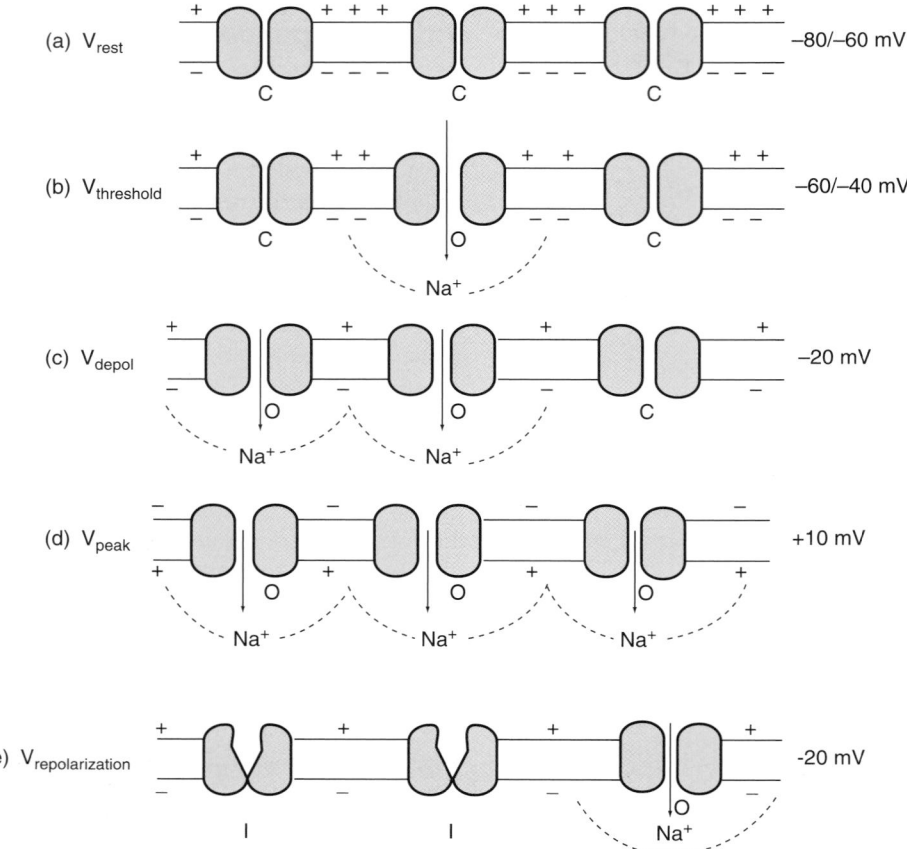

Figure 5.17 Different states of voltage-gated Na⁺ channels in relation to the different phases of the Na⁺-dependent action potential.

C, closed state; O, open state; I, inactivated state; →, driving force for Na⁺ ions.

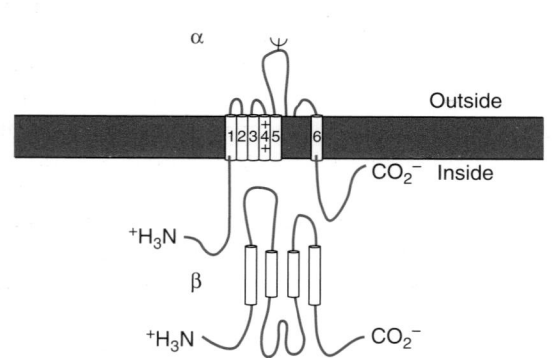

Figure 5.18 Putative transmembrane organization of the α-subunit of the delayed rectifier, voltage-gated K⁺ channel and its associated cytoplasmic β-subunit.

Cylinders represent putative α-helical segments, ψ sites of probable N-linked glycosylation. Adapted from Isom LL, De Jongh KS, Caterall WA (1994) Auxiliary subunits of voltage-gated ion channels, *Neuron* **12**, 1183–1194, with permission.

following membrane depolarization and inactivate slowly;

■ A-type channels which are fast activating and fast inactivating.

The first type, the delayed rectifier K⁺ channels, plays a role in action potential repolarization. The A-types inactivate too quickly to do so.

5.3.2 Membrane depolarization favours the conformational change of the delayed rectifier channel towards the open state

The function of the delayed rectifier channel is to transduce, with a delay, membrane depolarization into an exit of K⁺ ions

Single-channel recordings were obtained by Conti and Neher in 1980 from the squid axon. We shall, however, look at recordings obtained from K⁺ channels expressed

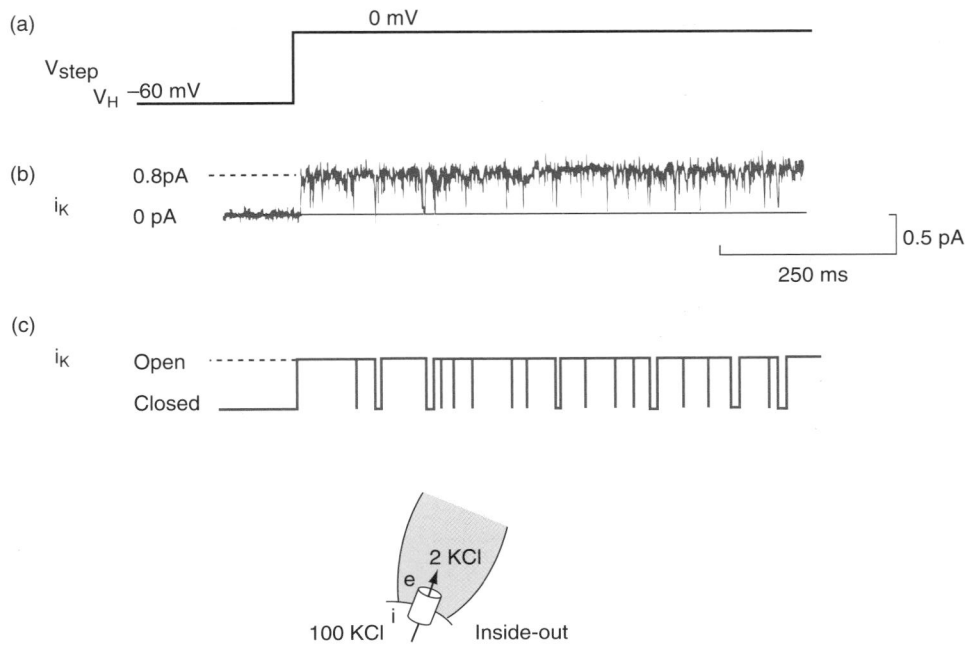

Figure 5.19 Single K⁺ channel openings in response to a depolarizing step.
The activity of a single delayed rectifier channel expressed from rat brain cDNA in a *Xenopus* oocyte is recorded in patch clamp (inside-out patch). A depolarizing step to 0 mV from a holding potential of –60 mV evokes the opening of the channel. The elementary current is outward. The channel then closes briefly and reopens several times during the depolarization, as shown in the drawing (bottom line) that interprets the current trace. Bathing solution or intracellular solution (in mM): 100 KCl, 10 EGTA, 10 HEPES. Pipette solution or extracellular solution (in mM): 115 NaCl, 2 KCl, 1.8 CaCl₂, 10 HEPES. Adapted from Stühmer W, Stocker M, Sakmann B *et al.* (1988) Potassium channels expressed from rat brain cDNA have delayed rectifier properties, *FEBS Lett.* **242**, 199–206, with permission.

in oocytes or in mammalian cell lines from cDNA encoding a delayed rectifier channel of rat brain. Since the macroscopic currents mediated by these channels have time courses and ionic selectivity resembling those of the classical delayed outward currents described in nerve and muscle, these single-channel recordings are good examples for describing the properties of a delayed rectifier current.

Figure 5.19 shows a current trace obtained from patch clamp recordings (inside-out patch) of a rat brain K⁺ channel (RCK1) expressed in a *Xenopus* oocyte. In the presence of physiological extracellular and intracellular K⁺ concentrations, a depolarizing voltage step to 0 mV from a holding potential of –60 mV is applied. After the onset of the step, a rectangular pulse of elementary current, upwardly directed, appears. It means that the current is outward; K⁺ ions leave the cell. In fact, the driving force for K⁺ ions is outward at 0 mV.

It is immediately striking that the gating behaviour of the delayed rectifier channel is different from that of the Na⁺ channel (compare **Figures 5.7a** or **5.8a** and **5.19**). Here, the rectangular pulse of current lasts the whole depolarizing step with short interruptions during which the current goes back to zero. It indicates that the delayed rectifier channel opens, closes briefly and

reopens many times during the depolarizing pulse: the delayed rectifier channel does not inactivate within seconds. Another difference is that the delay of opening of the delayed rectifier is much longer than that of the Na⁺ channel, even for large membrane depolarizations (mean delay 4 ms in **Figure 5.20a**).

When the same depolarizing pulse is now applied every 1–2 s, we observe that the delay of channel opening is variable (1–10 ms) but gating properties are the same in all recordings: the channel opens, closes briefly and reopens during the entire depolarizing step (**Figure 5.20a**). Amplitude histograms collected at 0 mV membrane potential from current recordings, such as those shown in **Figure 5.20a**, give a mean amplitude of the unitary currents of +0.8 pA (**Figure 5.20c**). This means that the most frequently occurring main amplitude is +0.8 pA.

5.3.3 The open probability of the delayed rectifier channel is stable during a depolarization in the range of seconds

The average open time τ_o measured in the patch illustrated in **Figure 5.19** is 4.6 ms. The mean closed time is

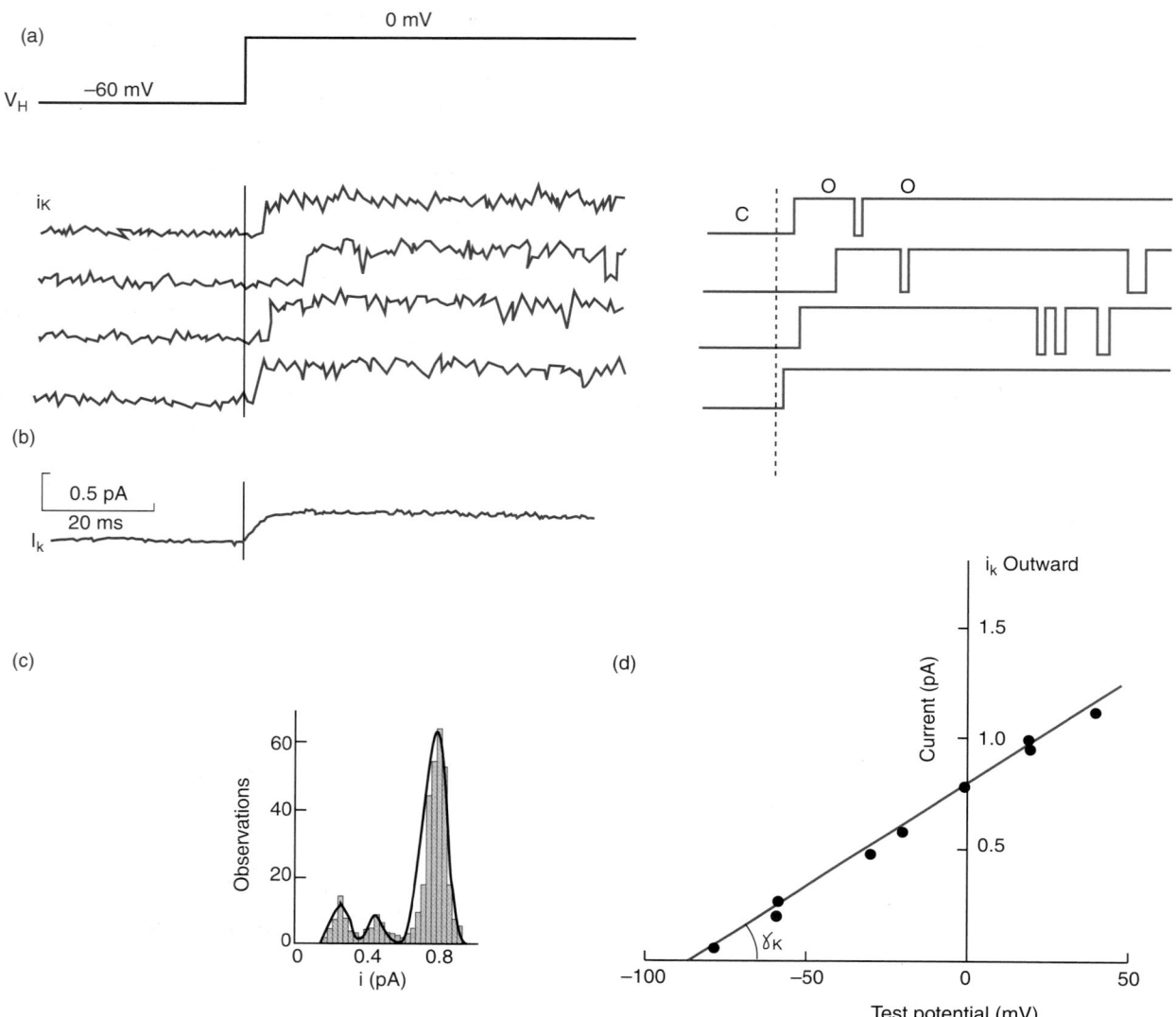

Figure 5.20 Characteristics of the elementary delayed rectifier current.
Same experimental design as in Figure 5.19. The patch of membrane contains a single delayed rectifier channel. **(a)** Successive sweeps of outward current reponses to depolarizing steps from −60 mV to 0 mV (C for closed state, O for open state of the channel). **(b)** Averaged current from 70 elementary currents as in (a). **(c)** Amplitude histogram of the elementary outward currents recorded at test potential 0 mV. The mean elementary current amplitude observed most frequently is 0.8 pA. **(d)** Single channel current–voltage relation (i_K–V). Each point represents the mean amplitude of at least 20 determinations. The slope is γ_K = 9.3 pS. The reversal potential E_{rev} = −89 mV. From Stühmer W, Stocker M, Sakmann B *et al.* (1988) Potassium channels expressed from rat brain cDNA have delayed rectifier properties, *FEBS Lett.* **242**, 199–206, with permission.

1.5 ms. As seen in **Figures 5.19** and **5.20a**, during a depolarizing pulse to 0 mV the delayed rectifier channel spends much more time in the open state than in the closed state: at 0 mV its average open probability is high (p_o = 0.76).

In order to test whether the delayed rectifier channels show some inactivation, long-lasting recordings are performed. Though no significant inactivation is apparent during test pulses in the range of seconds, during long test depolarizations (in the range of minutes) the chan-

nel shows steady-state inactivation at positive holding potentials (not shown). Therefore, in the range of seconds, the inactivation of the delayed rectifier channel can be omitted: the channel fluctuates between the closed and open states:

$$C \rightleftharpoons O$$

The transition from the closed (C) state to the open (O) state is triggered by membrane depolarization with a delay. The delayed rectifier channel activates in the range of milliseconds. In comparison, the Na+ channel activates in the range of submilliseconds. The O to C transitions frequently happen though the membrane is still depolarized. It happens also when membrane repolarizes.

5.3.4 The K+ channel has a constant unitary conductance γ_K

In **Figure 5.21a**, unitary currents are shown in response to increasing depolarizing steps from −50 to +20 mV from a holding potential of −80 mV. We observe that both the amplitude of the unitary current and the time spent by the channel in the open state increase with depolarization.

When the mean amplitude of the unitary K+ current is plotted versus membrane test potential, a linear i_K/V

relation is obtained (**Figures 5.20d** and **5.21b**). This linear i_K/V relation (between −50 and +20 mV) is described by the equation $i_K = \gamma_K (V_m - E_K)$, where V_m is the membrane potential, E_K is the reversal potential of the K+ current, and γ_K is the conductance of the single delayed rectifier K+ channel, or unitary conductance. Linear back-extrapolation gives a reversal potential value around −90/−80 mV, a value close to E_K calculated from the Nernst equation. This means that from −80 mV to more depolarized potentials, which correspond to the physiological conditions, the K+ current is outward. For more hyperpolarized potentials, the K+ current is inward.

The value of γ_K is given by the slope of the linear i_K/V curve. It has a constant value at any given membrane potential. This value varies between 10 and 15 pS depending on the preparation (**Figures 5.20d** and **5.21b**).

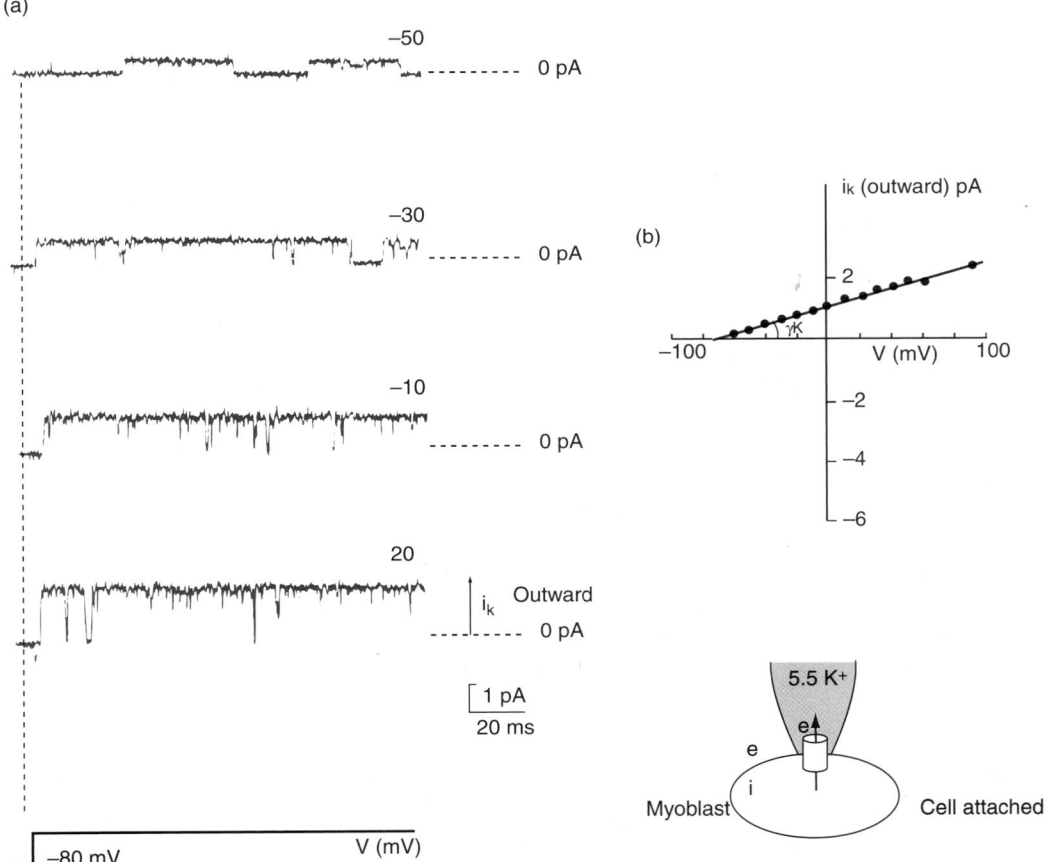

Figure 5.21 The single-channel current/voltage (i_K/V) relation is linear.
Delayed rectifier K+ channels from rat brain are expressed in a myoblast cell line. **(a)** The activity of a single channel is recorded in patch clamp (cell-attached patch). Unitary currents are recorded at different test potentials (from −50 mV to +20 mV) from a holding potential at −80 mV. Bottom trace is the voltage trace. **(b)** i_K–V relation obtained by plotting the mean amplitude of i_K at the different test potentials tested. i_K reverses at $V = -75$ mV and $\gamma_K = 14$ pS. Intrapipette solution (in mM): 145 NaCl, 5.5 KCl, 2 CaCl$_2$, 2 MgCl$_2$, 10 HEPES. Adapted from Koren G, Liman ER, Logothetis DE *et al.* (1990) Gating mechanism of a cloned potassium channel expressed in frog oocytes and mammalian cells, *Neuron* **2**, 39–51, with permission.

5.3.5 The macroscopic delayed rectifier K+ current (I_K) has a delayed voltage dependence of activation and inactivates within tens of seconds

Whole cell currents in *Xenopus* oocytes expressing delayed rectifier channels start to activate at potentials positive to –30 mV and their amplitude is clearly voltage-dependent. When unitary currents recorded from 70 successive depolarizing steps to 0 mV are averaged (**Figure 5.20b**), the macroscopic outward current obtained has a slow time to peak (4 ms) and lasts the entire depolarizing step. It closely resembles the whole cell current recorded with two electrode voltage clamps in the same preparation (rat brain delayed rectifier channels expressed in oocytes; see **Figure 5.22a**). The whole cell current amplitude at steady state (once it has reached its maximal amplitude) for a given potential is:

$$I_K = Np_o i_K,$$

where N is the number of delayed rectifier channels in the membrane recorded, p_o the open probability at steady state and i_K the elementary current. The number of open channels Np_o increases with depolarization (to a maximal value) and so does I_K.

The I_K/V relation shows that the whole cell current varies linearly with voltage from a threshold potential which in this preparation is around –40 mV (**Figure 5.22b**). When the membrane is more hyperpolarized than the threshold potential, very few channels are open and I_K is equal to zero. For membrane potentials more depolarized than the threshold potential, I_K depends on p_o and the driving force state ($V_m - E_K$) which augments with depolarization. Once p_o is maximal, I_K augments linearly with depolarization since it depends only on the driving force.

The delayed rectifier channels are selective to K+ ions

Ion substitution experiments indicate that the reversal potential of I_K depends on the external K+ ions concentration as expected for a selective K+ channel. The

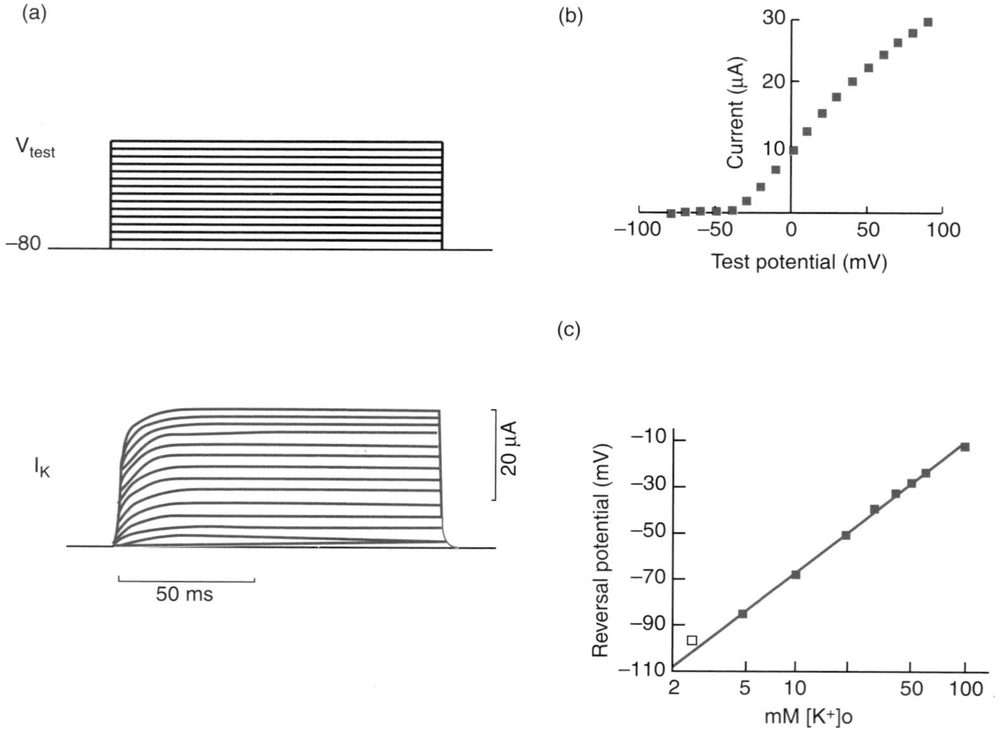

Figure 5.22 Characteristics of the macroscopic delayed rectifier K+ current.
The activity of N delayed rectifier channels expressed from rat brain cDNA in oocytes recorded in double electrode voltage clamp. **(a)** In response to depolarizing steps of increasing amplitude (given every 2 s) from a holding potential of –80 mV (upper traces), a non-inactivating outward current of increasing amplitude is recorded (lower traces). **(b)** The amplitude of the current at steady state is plotted against test potential. The potential threshold for its activation is –40 mV. **(c)** The value of the reversal potentials of the macroscopic current is plotted against the extracellular concentration of K+ ions on a semi-logarithmic scale. The slope is –55 mV. From Stühmer W, Stocker M, Sakmann B *et al.* (1988) Potassium channels expressed from rat brain cDNA have delayed rectifier properties, *FEBS Lett.* **242**, 199–206, with permission.

reversal potential of the whole cell current is measured as in **Figure 5.22b** in the presence of different external concentrations of K+ ions. These experimental values are plotted against the external K+ concentration, $[K^+]_o$, on a semi-logarithmic scale. For concentrations ranging from 2.5 (normal frog Ringer) to 100 mM, a linear relation with a slope of 55 mV for a 10-fold change in $[K^+]_o$ is obtained (**Figure 5.22c**). These data are well fitted by the Nernst equation. It indicates that the channel has a higher selectivity for K+ ions over Na+ and Cl− ions.

The delayed rectifier channels are blocked by millimolar concentrations of tetraethylammonium (TEA) and by Cs+ ions.

Ammonium ions can pass through most K+ channels, whereas its quaternary derivative TEA cannot, resulting in the blockade of most of the voltage-gated K+ chan-

nels: TEA is a small open channel blocker. Amino acids in the carboxyl half of the region linking segments S5 and S6 (i.e. adjacent to S6) influence the sensitivity to pore blockers such as TEA.

5.3.6 Conclusion: during an action potential the consequence of the delayed opening of K+ channels is an exit of K+ ions which repolarizes the membrane to resting potential

Owing to their delay of opening, delayed rectifier channels open when the membrane is already depolarized by the entry of Na+ ions through open voltage-gated Na+ channels (**Figure 5.23**). Therefore, the exit of K+ ions

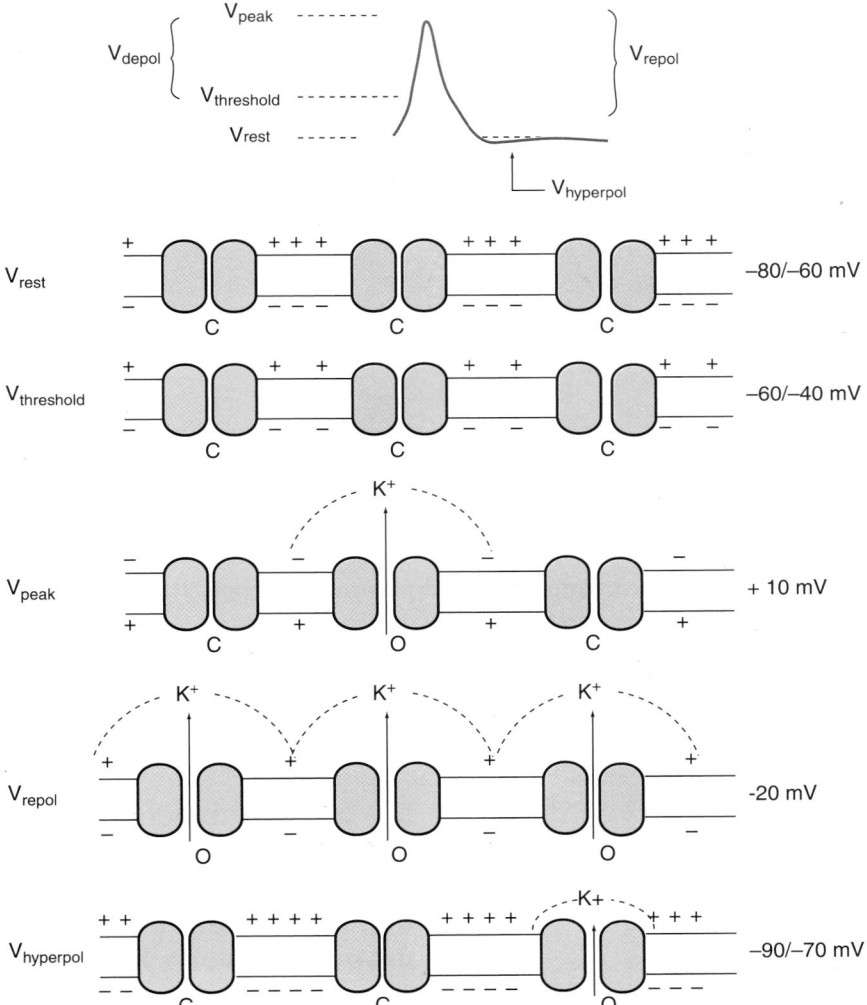

Figure 5.23 States of the delayed rectifier K+ channels in relation to the different phases of the Na+-dependent action potential.
C, closed state; O, open state; ↑, driving force for K+ ions.

(a)

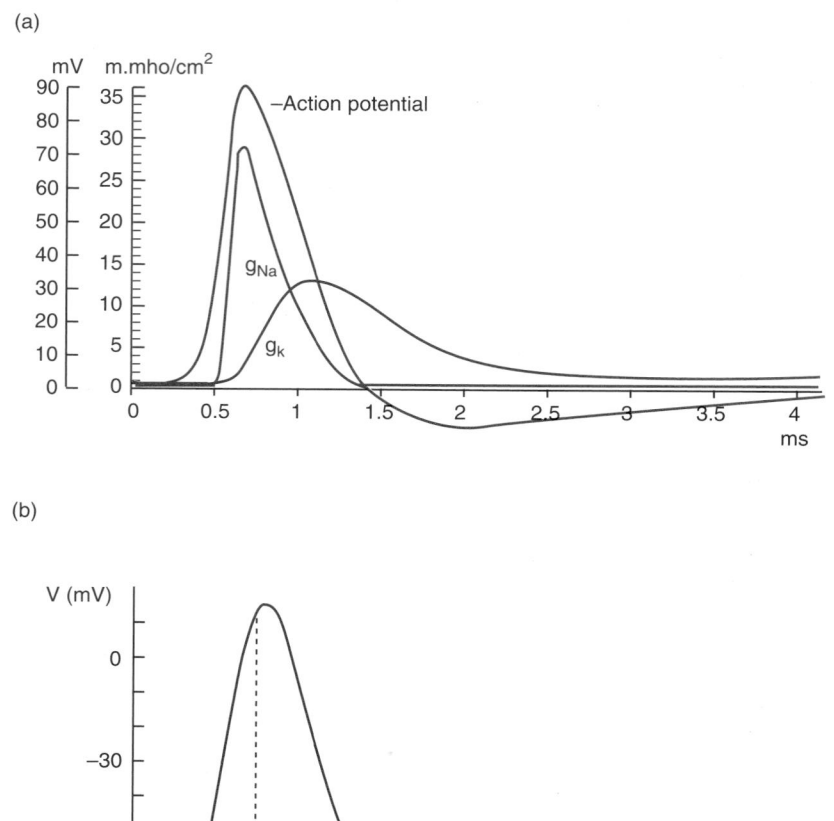

(b)

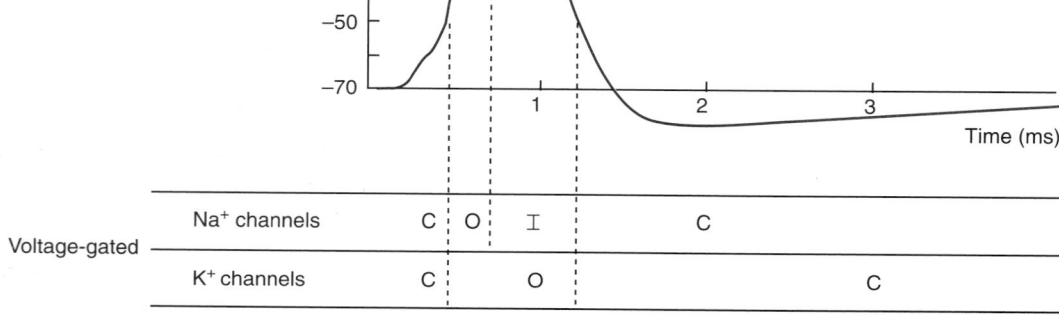

Figure 5.24 Gating of Na⁺ and K⁺ channels during the Na⁺-dependent action potential.
(a) Interpretation of the manner in which the conductances to Na⁺ (γ_{Na}) and K⁺ (γ_{K}) contribute to the action potential. (b) State of the Na⁺ and K⁺ voltage-gated channels during the course of the action potential. O, channels open; I, channels inactivate; C, channels close or are closed. Trace (a) adapted from Hodgkin AL, Huxley AF (1952) A quantitative description of membrane current and its application to conduction and excitation in nerve, *J. Physiol.* **117**, 500–544, with permission.

does not occur at the same time as the entry of Na⁺ ions (see also **Figure 5.24**). This allows the membrane to first depolarize in response to the entry of Na⁺ ions and then to repolarize as a consequence of the exit of K⁺ ions.

5.4 Sodium-dependent action potentials are initiated at the axon initial segment in response to a membrane depolarization and then actively propagate along the axon

Na⁺-dependent action potentials, because of their short duration (1–5 ms), are also named spikes. Na⁺ spikes, for a given cell, have a stable amplitude and duration; they all look alike, and are binary, all-or-none. The pattern of discharge (which is often different from the frequency of discharge) and not individual spikes, carries significant information.

5.4.1 Summary of the Na⁺-dependent action potential

The depolarization phase of Na⁺ spikes is due to the rapid time to peak inward Na⁺ current which flows into the axon initial segment or node. This depolarization is brief because the inward Na⁺ current inactivates in milliseconds (**Figure 5.24b**).

In the squid giant axon or frog axon, spike repolarization is associated with an outward K⁺ current (**Figures 5.24 and 5.25**) through delayed rectifier channels since TEA application dramatically prolongs the action potential (see **Figure 5.4b**). As pointed out by Hodgkin and Huxley: 'The rapid rise is due almost entirely to Na⁺ conductance, but after the peak the K⁺ conductance takes a progressively larger share until, by the beginning of the hyperpolarized phase, the Na⁺ conductance has become negligible. The tail of raised conductance that falls away gradually during the positive phase is due solely to K⁺ conductance, the small constant leak conductance being of course present throughout.'

In contrast, in rat or rabbit myelinated axons the action potential is very little affected by the application of TEA. The repolarization phase in these preparations is largely associated with a leak K⁺ current. Voltage clamp studies confirm this observation. When the leak current is subtracted, almost no outward current is recorded in rabbit node (**Figure 5.25b**).

However, squid and rabbit nerve action potentials have the same duration (**Figure 5.25a**). In this preparation, the normal resting membrane potential is around −80 mV, which suggests the presence of a large leak K⁺ current. Moreover, test depolarizations evoke large outward K⁺ currents insensitive to TEA (**Figure 5.26**). How does the action potential repolarize in such preparations? First the Na⁺ currents in the rabbit node inactivate two to three times faster than those in the frog node. Second, the large leak K⁺ current present at depolarized membrane potentials repolarizes the membrane. The amplitude of the leak K⁺ current augments linearly with depolarization, depending only on the K⁺ driving force.

5.4.2 Depolarization of the membrane to the threshold for voltage-gated Na⁺ channel activation has two origins

The inward current which depolarizes the membrane of the initial segment to the threshold potential for voltage-gated Na⁺ channel opening is one of the following:

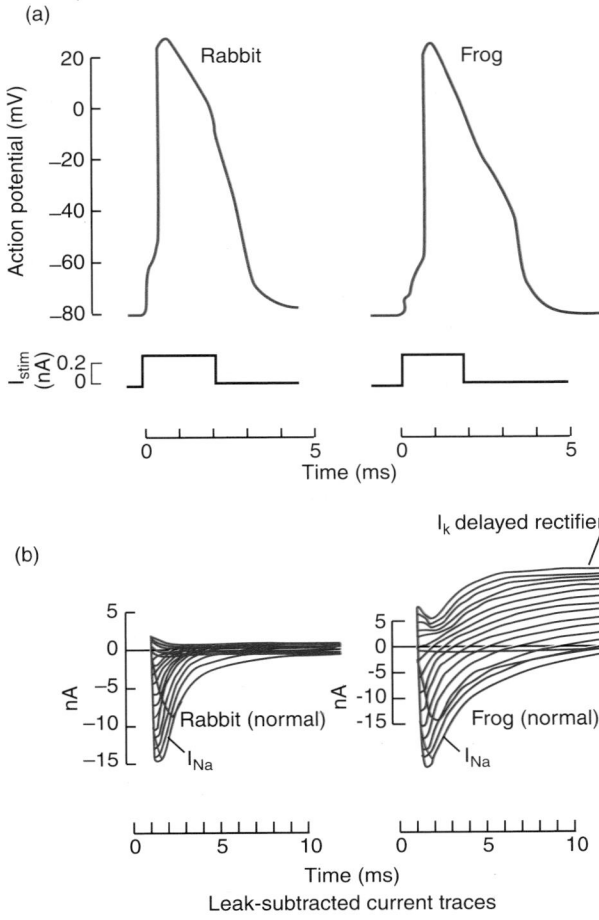

Figure 5.25 The currents underlying the action potentials of the rabbit and frog nerves.

(a) The action potentials are recorded intracellularly at 14°C. Bottom trace is the current of stimulation injected in order to depolarize the membrane to initiate an action potential. (b) The currents flowing through the membrane at different voltages recorded in voltage clamp. In the rabbit node, very little outward current is recorded after the large inward Na⁺ current. In the frog nerve, a large outward K⁺ current is recorded after the large inward Na⁺ current. Leak current is subtracted from each trace and does not appear in these recordings. Adapted from Chiu SY, Ritchie JM, Bogart RB, Stagg D (1979) A quantitative description of membrane currents in rabbit myelinated nerve, *J. Physiol.* **292**, 149–166, with permission.

■ A depolarizing current resulting from the activity of excitatory afferent synapses (see Chapters 9 and 11) or afferent sensory stimuli (see Chapters 12 and 15). In the first case, the synaptic currents generated at post-synaptic sites in response to synaptic activity summate, and when the resulting current is inward it can depolarize the membrane to the threshold for

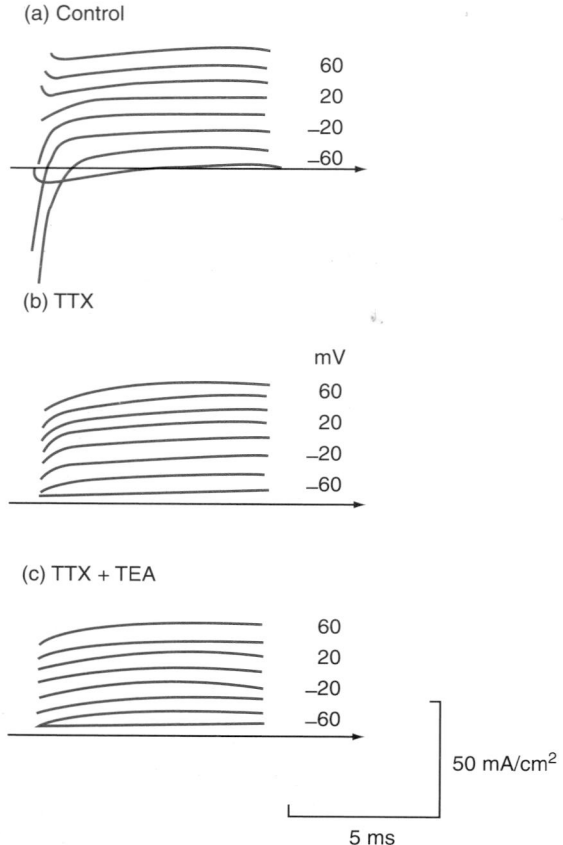

(a) Control

60
20
−20
−60

(b) TTX

mV
60
20
−20
−60

(c) TTX + TEA

60
20
−20
−60

50 mA/cm²

5 ms

Figure 5.26 TEA-resistant outward current in a mammalian nerve.
The currents evoked by depolarizing steps from −60 to +60 mV from a holding potential of −80 mV are recorded in voltage clamp in a node of Ranvier of an isolated rat nerve fibre. Control inward and outward currents (a), after TTX 25 nM (b), and after TTX 25 nM and TEA 5 mM (c) are added to the extracellular solution. The outward current recorded in (c) is the leak K^+ current. The delayed outward K^+ current is taken as the difference between the steady state outward current in (b) and the leak current in (c). Adapted from Brismar T (1980) Potential clamp analysis of membrane currents in rat myelinated nerve fibres, *J. Physiol.* **298**, 171–184, with permission.

spike initiation. In the second case, sensory stimuli are transduced in inward currents that can depolarize the membrane to the threshold for spike initiation.

■ An intrinsic regenerative depolarizing current such as, for example, in heart cells or invertebrate neurons.

5.4.3 The site of initiation of Na⁺-dependent action potentials is the axon initial segment

The site of initiation was suggested long ago to occur in the axon initial segment since the threshold for spike initiation was the lowest at this level. However, this has only recently been directly demonstrated with the double patch clamp technique. First the dendrites and soma belonging to the same Purkinje neuron of the cerebellum are visualized in a rat brain slice. Then the activity is recorded simultaneously at both these sites with two patch electrodes (whole-cell patches). To verify that somatic and dendritic recordings are made from the same cell, the Purkinje cell is filled with two differently coloured fluorescent dyes: Cascade blue at the soma and Lucifer yellow at the dendrite. To determine the site of action potential initiation during synaptic activation of Purkinje cells, action potentials are evoked by

(a)

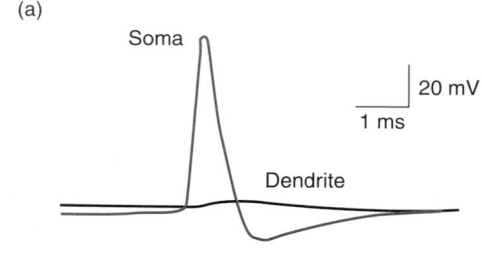

Soma

20 mV
1 ms

Dendrite

(b)

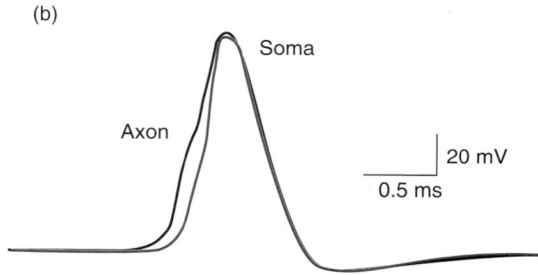

Soma

Axon

20 mV
0.5 ms

Figure 5.27 The Na⁺-dependent action potential is initiated in the axon initial segment in Purkinje cells of the cerebellum.
The activity of a Purkinje cell recorded simultaneously at the level of the soma and (a) 117 μm away from the soma at the level of a dendrite, or (b) 7 μm away from the soma at the level of the axon initial segment, with the double patch clamp technique (whole-cell patches). Afferent parallel fibres are stimulated by applying brief voltage pulses to an extracellular patch pipette. In response to the synaptic excitation, an action potential is evoked in the Purkinje cell and recorded at the two different neuronal sites: soma and dendrite (a) or soma and axon (b). Adapted from Stuart G, Hauser M (1994) Initiation and spread of sodium action potentials in cerebellar Purkinje cells, *Neuron* **13**, 703–712, with permission.

stimulation of afferent parallel fibres which make synapses on distal dendrites of Purkinje cells (see **Figures 7.8** and **7.9**).

In all Purkinje cells tested, the evoked action potential recorded from the soma has a shorter delay and a greater amplitude than that recorded from a dendrite (**Figure 5.27a**). Moreover, the delay and the difference in amplitude between the somatic spike and the dendritic spike both augment when the distance between the two patch electrodes is increased. This suggests that the site of initiation is proximal to the soma.

Simultaneous whole cell recordings from the soma and the axon initial segment were performed to establish whether action potential initiation is somatic or axonal in origin. The action potential clearly occurs first in the axon initial segment (**Figure 5.27b**). These results suggest that the actual site of Na⁺-dependent action potential initiation is in the axon initial segment of Purkinje cells. Experiments carried out by Sakmann *et al.* in other brain regions give the same conclusion for all the neurons tested. This may be due to a higher density of sodium channels in the membrane of the axon initial segment.

The action potential, once initiated, spreads passively back into the dendritic tree of Purkinje cells (passively means that it propagates with attenuation since it is not reinitiated in dendrites). Simultaneously it actively propagates into the axon (not shown here; see below). In some neurons, for example the pyramidal cells of the neocortex, the action potential actively back-propagates into the dendrites, but this is not a general rule.

5.4.4 The Na⁺-dependent action potential actively propagates along the axon to axon terminals

Voltage-gated Na⁺ channels are present all along the axon at a sufficient density to allow firing of axon potentials.

The propagation is active

Active means that the action potential is reinitiated at each node of Ranvier for a myelinated axon or at each point for a non-myelinated axon. The flow of Na⁺ ions through the open Na⁺ voltage-gated channels of the axon initial segment creates a current that spreads passively along the length of the axon to the first node of Ranvier (**Figure 5.28**). It depolarizes the membrane of the first node to the threshold for action potential initiation. The action potential is now at the level of the first node. The entry of Na⁺ ions at this level will depolarize the membrane of the second node and open the closed

Na⁺ channels. The action potential is now at the level of the second node.

The propagation is unidirectional owing to Na⁺ channel inactivation

When the axon potential is, for example, at the level of the second node, the voltage-gated Na⁺ channels of the first node are in the inactivated state since they have just been activated or are still in the open state (**Figure 5.28**). These Na⁺ channels cannot be activated. The current lines flowing from the second node will therefore activate only the voltage-gated Na⁺ channels of the third node towards axon terminals, where the voltage-gated Na⁺ channels are in the closed state (**Figure 5.28**). In the axon, under physiological conditions, the action potential cannot back-propagate.

The refractory periods between two action potentials

After one action potential has been initiated, there is a period of time during which a second action potential cannot be initiated or is initiated but has a smaller amplitude (**Figure 5.29**): this period is called the 'refractory period' of the membrane. It results from Na⁺ channel inactivation. Since the Na⁺ channels do not immediately recover from inactivation, they cannot reopen immediately. This means that once the preceding action potential has reached its maximum amplitude, Na⁺ channels will not reopen before a certain period of time needed for their de-inactivation (**Figure 5.24b**). This represents the absolute refractory period which lasts in the order of milliseconds.

Then, progressively, the Na⁺ channels will recover from inactivation and some will reopen in response to a second depolarization: this is the relative refractory period. This period finishes when all the Na⁺ channel at the initial axonal segment or at a node are de-inactivated. This actually protects the membrane from being depolarized all the time and enables the initiation of separate action potentials.

5.4.5 Do the Na⁺ and K⁺ concentrations change in the extracellular or intracellular media during firing?

Over a small time scale, the external or internal Na⁺ or K⁺ concentrations do not change during the emission of action potentials. A small number of ions are in fact flowing through the channels during an action potential and the Na–K pump re-establishes continuously the extracellular and intracellular Na⁺ and K⁺

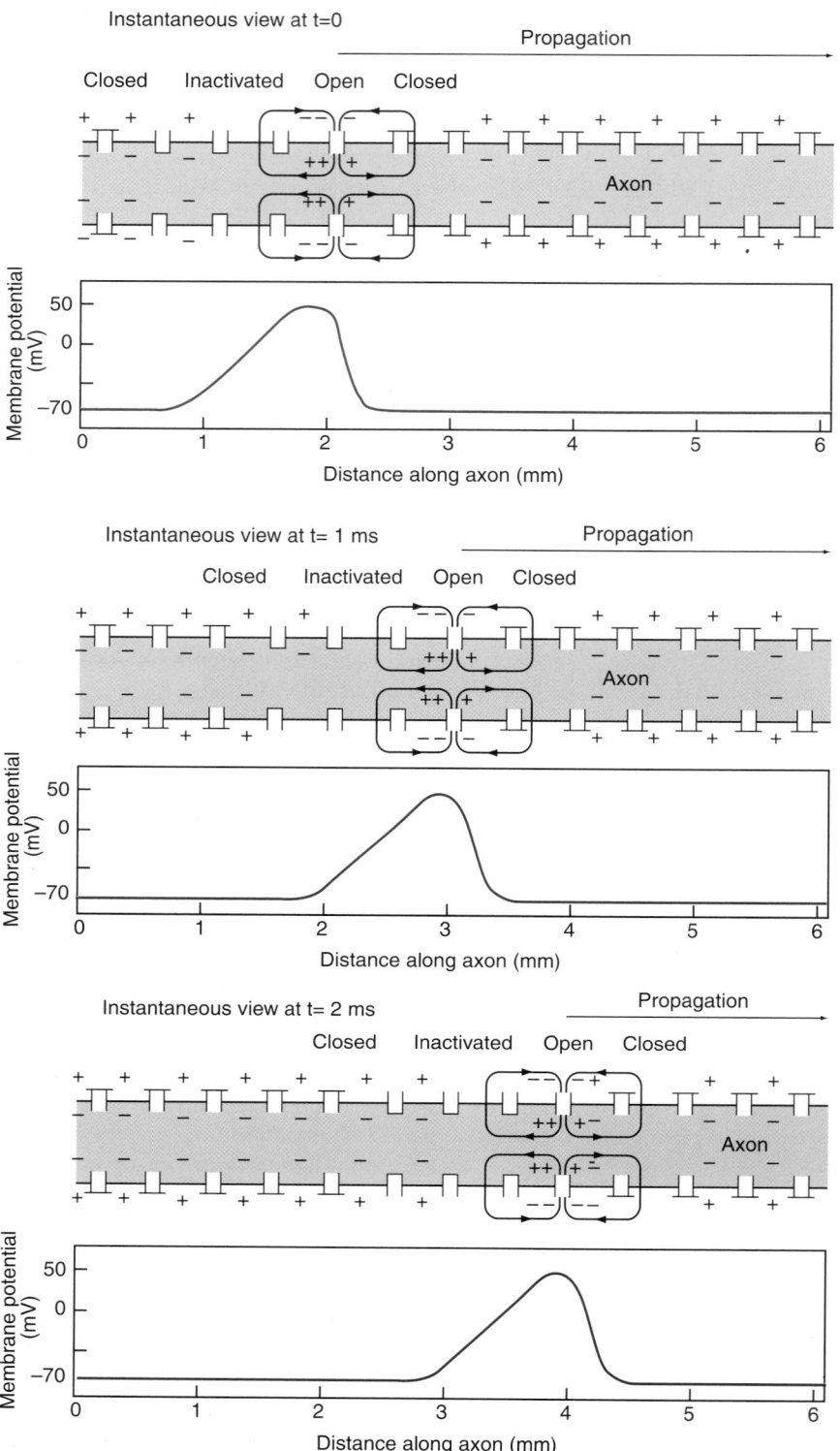

Figure 5.28 Active propagation of the Na⁺-dependent action potential in the axon and axon collaterals.
Scheme provided by Alberts B, Bray D, Lewis J *et al.* (1983) *Molecular Biology of the Cell*, New York: Garland Publishing.

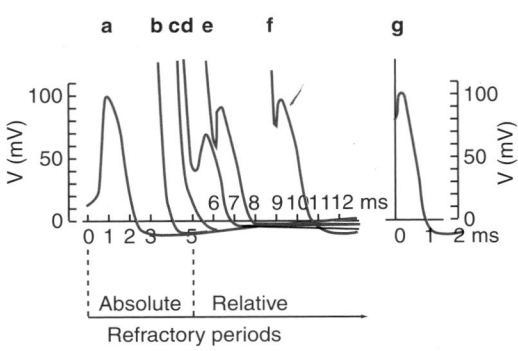

Figure 5.29 The refractory periods.

A first action potential is recorded intracellularly in the squid axon *in vitro* in response to a small depolarizing stimulus (a). Then a second stimulus with an intensity six times greater than that of the first is applied 4, 5, 6 or 9 ms after. The evoked spike is either absent (b and c; only the stimulation artifact is recorded) or has a smaller amplitude (d to f). Finally, when the membrane is back in the resting state, the evoked action potential has the control amplitude (g). Adapted from Hodgkin AL, Huxley AF (1952) A quantitative description of membrane current and its application to conduction and excitation in nerve, *J. Physiol.* **117**, 500–544, with permission.

concentrations at the expense of ATP hydrolysis. Over a longer time scale, during high-frequency trains of action potentials, the K⁺ concentration can significantly increase in the external medium. This is due to the very small volume of the extracellular medium surrounding neurons and the limited speed of the Na–K pump. This excess of K⁺ ions is buffered by glial cells which are highly permeable to K⁺ ions (see Section 2.1.3).

5.4.6 The role of the Na⁺-dependent action potential is to evoke neurotransmitter release

The role of the Na⁺-dependent action potential is to propagate, without attenuation, a strong depolarization to the membrane of the axon terminals. There, this depolarization opens the high-threshold voltage-gated Ca²⁺ channels. The resulting entry of Ca²⁺ ions into axon terminals triggers exocytosis and neurotransmitter release. The probability value of all these phenomena is not 1. This means that the action potential can fail to invade an axon terminal, the Ca²⁺ entry can fail to trigger exocytosis, etc. Neurotransmitter release is explained in Chapter 8.

5.4.7 Characteristics of the Na⁺-dependent action potential are explained by the properties of the voltage-gated Na⁺ channel

The *threshold* for Na⁺-dependent action potential initiation results from the fact that voltage-gated Na⁺ channels open in response to a depolarization positive to $-50/-40$ mV. The Na⁺-dependent action potential is *all-or-none* because voltage-gated Na⁺ channels self-activate (see **Figure 5.17**). It propagates *without attenuation* since the density of voltage-gated Na⁺ channels is constant along the axon or at nodes of Ranvier. It propagates *unidirectionally* because of the rapid inactivation of voltage-gated Na⁺ channels. The instantaneous frequency of Na⁺-dependent action potentials is limited by the *refractory periods*, which also results from voltage-gated Na⁺ channel inactivation.

Appendix 5.1
Current clamp recording

The current clamp technique, or intracellular recording in current clamp mode, is the traditional method for recording membrane potential: resting membrane potential and membrane potential changes such as action potentials and postsynaptic potentials. Membrane potential changes result from intrinsic or extrinsic currents. Intrinsic currents are synaptic or autorhythmic currents. Extrinsic currents are currents of known amplitude and duration applied by the experimenter through the intracellular recording electrode, in order to mimic currents produced by synaptic inputs.

Current clamp means that the *current applied* through the intracellular electrode is clamped to a constant value by the experimenter. It does not mean that the *current flowing through the membrane* is clamped to a constant value.

How to record membrane potential

The intracellular electrode (or the patch pipette) is connected to a unity-gain amplifier that has an input resistance many orders of magnitude greater than that of the micropipette plus the input resistance of the cell membrane ($R_p + R_m$). The output of the amplifier follows the voltage at the tip of the intracellular electrode (V_p) (**Figure A5.1**). By definition, membrane potential V_m is equal to $V_i - V_e$ (i for intracellular and e for extracellular). In **Figure A5.1**, $V_i - V_e = V_p - V_{bath} = V_p - V_{ground} = V_p - 0 = V_p$. When a current I is simultaneously passed through the electrode, $V_p = V_m$ as long as the current I is very small in order not to cause a significant voltage drop across R_p (see the last section of this appendix).

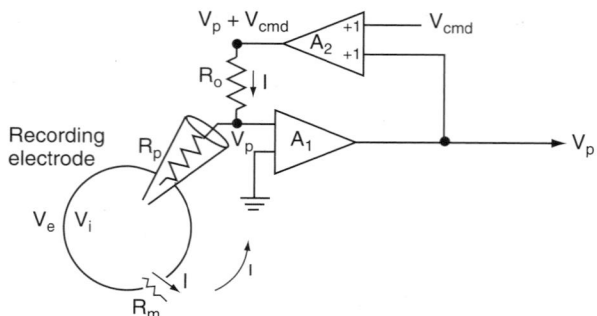

Figure A5.1 A unity gain amplifier A1 and a current source made by adding a second amplifier A2.

The micropipette voltage V_p is measured by A1. The command voltage V_{cmd} and V_p are the inputs of A2 (V_p and V_{cmd} are added). The current I applied by the experimenter in order to induce V_m changes, flows through R_o and is equal to $I = V_p/R_o$ since the voltage across the output resistor R_o is equal to V_{cmd} regardless of V_p. I flows through the micropipette into the cell then out through the cell membrane into the bath grounding electrode. I is here an outward current. Capacitances are ignored. Adapted from *The Axon Guide*, Axon Instruments Inc., 1993.

How to inject current through the intracellular electrode

If a current injection circuit is connected to the input node, the current injected (I) flows down the electrode into the cell (**Figure A5.1**). This current source allows a constant (DC) current to be injected, either outward to depolarize the membrane or inward to hyperpolarize the membrane (**Figure A5.2**). When the recording electrode is filled with KCl, a current that expells K^+ ions into the cell interior depolarizes the membrane (V_m becomes less negative) (**Figure A5.2a**), whereas a current that expels Cl^- ions into the cell interior hyperpolarizes the membrane (V_m becomes more negative) (**Figure A5.2b**).

Outward means that the current is flowing through the membrane from the inside of the cell to the bath; inward is the opposite

The current source can also be used to inject a short-duration pulse of current: a depolarizing current pulse above threshold to evoke action potential(s) or a low-amplitude depolarizing (**Figure A5.3**) or hyperpolarizing current pulse to measure the input membrane resistance R_m since $\Delta V_m = R_m \times \Delta I$.

How to measure the membrane potential when a current is passed down the electrode

The injected current (I) causes a corresponding voltage drop (IR_p) across the resistance of the pipette (R_p). It is therefore difficult to separate the potential at the tip of the electrode ($V_p = V_m$) from the total potential ($V_p + IR_p$). For example, if $R_p = 50\ M\Omega$ and $I = 0.5\ nA$, $IR_p = 25\ mV$, a value in the V_m range. A special compensation

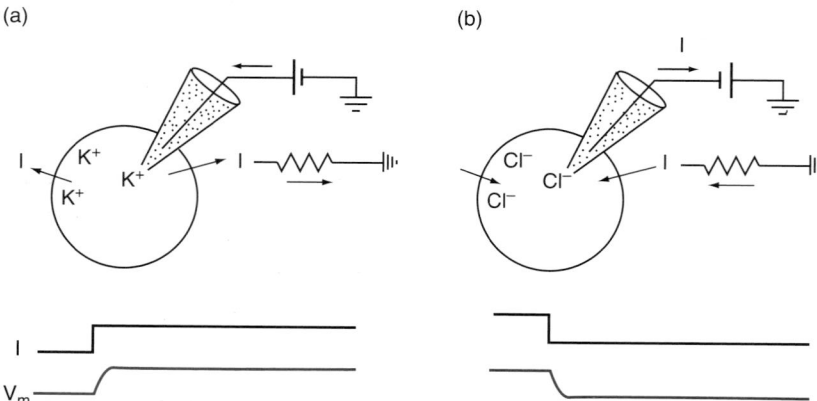

Figure A5.2

(a) When the recording electrode is filled with KCl, a current expels K^+ ions into the cell interior to depolarize the membrane (V_m becomes less negative). **(b)** A current expels Cl^- ions into the cell interior to hyperpolarize the membrane (V_m becomes more negative).

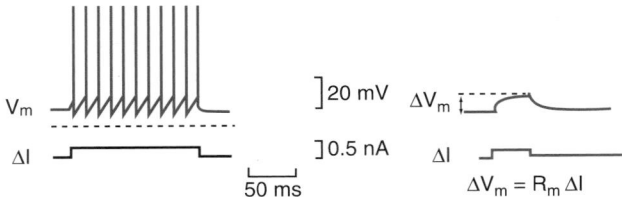

$$\Delta V_m = R_m \Delta I$$

Figure A5.3 Injection of a suprathreshold (left) **and sub-threshold** (right) **depolarizing pulse.**

circuitry can be used to eliminate the micropipette voltage drop IR_p.

Appendix 5.2
Voltage clamp recording

The voltage clamp technique (or intracellular recording in voltage clamp mode) is a method for recording the current flowing through the cell membrane while the membrane potential is held (clamped) at a constant value by the experimenter. In contrast to the current clamp technique (see Appendix 5.1), voltage clamp does not mimic a process found in nature. However, there are several reasons for performing voltage clamp experiments:

■ When studying voltage-gated channels, voltage clamp allows control of a variable (voltage) that determines the opening and closing of these channels.
■ By holding the membrane potential constant, the experimenter ensures that the current flowing though the membrane is linearly proportional to the conductance G ($G = 1/R$) being studied. To study, for example, the conductance G_{Na} of the total number (N) of voltage-gated Na+ channels present in the membrane, K+ and Ca2+ voltage-gated channels are blocked by pharmacological agents, and the current I_{Na} flowing through the membrane, recorded in voltage clamp, is proportional to G_{Na}:

$$I_{Na} = V_m G_{Na} = kG_{Na}, \text{ since } V_m \text{ is constant.}$$

How to clamp the membrane potential at a known and constant value

The aim of the voltage clamp technique is to adjust continuously the membrane potential V_m to the command potential V_{cmd} fixed by the experimenter. To do so, V_m is continuously measured *and* a current I is passed through the cell membrane to keep V_m at the desired value or command potential (V_{cmd}). Two voltage clamp

techniques are commonly used. With the two-electrode voltage clamp method, one electrode is used for membrane potential measurement and the other for passing current (**Figure A5.4**). The other method uses just one electrode, in one of the following ways:

■ The same electrode is used part time for membrane potential measurement and part time for current injection (also called the discontinuous single-electrode voltage clamp technique, or dSEVC). This is used for cells that are too small to be impaled with two electrodes; it will not be explained here.
■ In the patch clamp technique the same electrode is used full time for simultaneously measuring membrane potential and passing current (see Appendix 5.3).

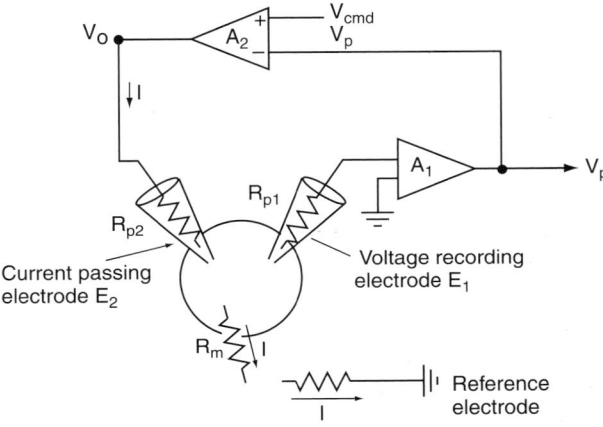

Figure A5.4 Two-electrode voltage clamp.
Adapted from *The Axon Guide*, Axon Instruments Inc., 1993.

In the two-electrode voltage clamp technique, the membrane potential is recorded by a unity gain amplifier A1 connected to the voltage-recording electrode E1. The membrane potential measured, V_m (or V_p; see Appendix 5.1) is compared with the command potential V_{cmd} in a high-gain differential amplifier A2. It sends a voltage output V_o proportional to the difference between V_m and V_{cmd}. V_o forces a current I to flow through the current-passing electrode E2 in order to obtain $V_m - V_{cmd} = 0$. The current I represents the total current that flows through the membrane. It is the same at every point of the circuit.

Example of a voltage-clamp recording experiment

Two electrodes are placed intracellularly into a neuronal soma (an invertebrate neuron for example) (**Figure A5.5**). The membrane potential is first held at −80 mV. In

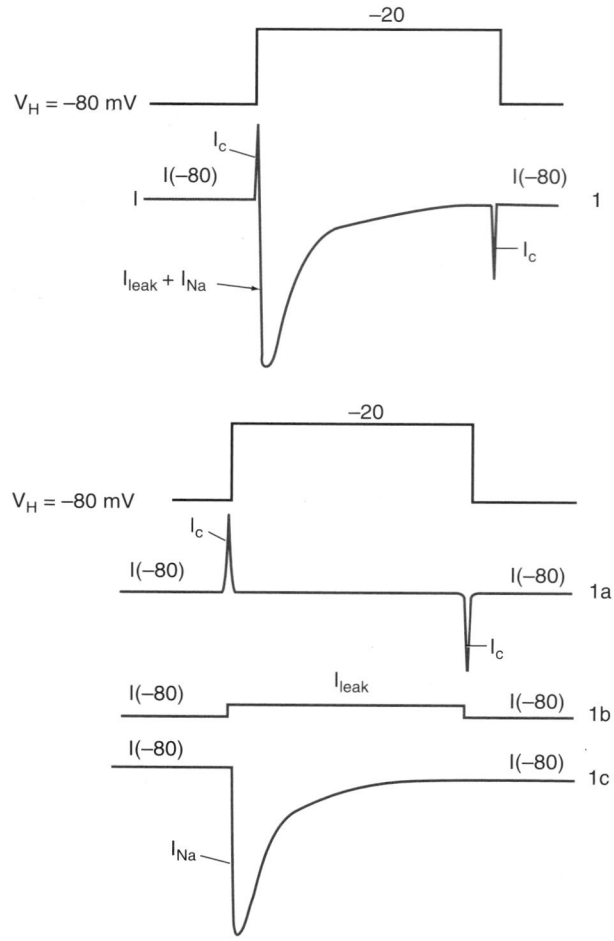

Figure A5.5 Various currents.
(1 = 1a + 1b + 1c) evoked by a voltage step to –20 mV (V_H = –80 mV) in the presence of K$^+$ and Ca^{2+} channel blockers.

this condition an outward current flows through the membrane in order to maintain the membrane potential at a value more hyperpolarized than V_{rest}. This stable outward current I_{-80} flows through the membrane as long as V_{cmd} = –80 mV.

A voltage step to –20 mV is then applied for 100 ms. This depolarizing step opens voltage-gated channels. In the presence of K$^+$ and Ca^{2+} channel blockers, only a voltage-gated Na$^+$ current is recorded. To clamp the membrane at the new V_{cmd} = –20 mV, a current $I_{(-20)}$ is sent by the amplifier A2. On the rising phase of the step this current is equal to the capacitive current I_c necessary to charge the membrane capacitance to its new value plus the leak current I_L flowing through leak channels (lines 1a and 1b). Since the depolarizing step opens Na$^+$ voltage-gated channels, an inward current I_{Na} flowing through open Na$^+$ channels will appear after a small

delay (line 1c). Normally, this inward current flowing through the open Na$^+$ channels, I_{Na}, should depolarize the membrane but in voltage clamp experiments it does not: a current constantly equal to I_{Na} but of opposite direction is continuously sent (in the microsecond range) in the circuit to compensate I_{Na} and to clamp the membrane to V_{cmd}. Therefore, once the membrane capacitance is charged, $I_{(-20)} = I_L + I_{Na}$. Usually on recordings, I_C is absent owing to the possibility of compensating for it with the voltage clamp amplifier.

Once the membrane capacitance is charged, the total current flowing through the circuit is $I = I_L + I_{Na}$ (I_c = 0). Therefore, in all measures of I_{Na}, the leak current I_L must be deduced. To do so, small-amplitude hyperpolarizing or depolarizing steps (ΔV_m = ±5 to ±20 mV) are applied at the beginning and at the end of the experiment. These voltage steps are too small to open voltage-gated channels in order to have I_{Na} = 0 and $I = I_L$. If we suppose that I_L is linearly proportional to ΔV_m, then I_L for a ΔV_m of +80 mV (from –80 to 0 mV) is eight times the value of I_L for ΔV_m = +10 mV (see **Figure 4.6**).

Is all the membrane surface clamped?

In small and round cells such as pituitary cells, the membrane potential is clamped on all the surface. In contrast, in neurons, because of their geometry, the voltage clamp is not achieved on all the membrane surface: the distal dendritic and axonal membranes are out of control because of their distance from the soma where the intracellular electrodes are usually placed. Such space clamp problems have to be taken into account by the experimenter in the analysis of the results. In the giant axon of the squid, this problem is overcome by inserting two long axial intracellular electrodes into a segment of axon in order to control the membrane potential all along this segment.

Appendix 5.3
Patch clamp recording

The patch clamp technique is a variation of the voltage clamp technique. It allows the recording of current flowing through the membrane: either the current flowing through all the channels open in the whole cell membrane or the current flowing through a single channel in a patch of membrane. In this technique, only one electrode is used full time for both voltage recording and passing current (it is a continuous single-electrode voltage clamp technique, or cSEVC). The patch clamp technique was developed by Neher and Sakmann. By applying very low doses of acetylcholine to a patch of muscle membrane they recorded for the first time, in

1976, the current flowing through a single nicotinic cholinergic receptor channel (nAChR), the unitary nicotinic current.

Some of the advantages of the patch clamp technique are that (i) with all but one configuration (cell-attached configuration) the investigator has access to the intracellular environment (**Figure A5.6**); (ii) it allows the recording of currents from cells too small to be impaled with intracellular microelectrodes, and (iii) it allows the recording of unitary currents (current through a single channel).

A5.3.1 The various patch clamp recording configurations

First a tight seal between the membrane and the tip of the pipette must be obtained. The tip of a micropipette that has been fire polished to a diameter of about 1 μm is advanced towards a cell until it makes contact with its membrane. Under appropriate conditions, a gentle suction applied to the inside of the pipette causes the formation of a very tight seal between the membrane and the tip of the pipette. This is the cell-attached

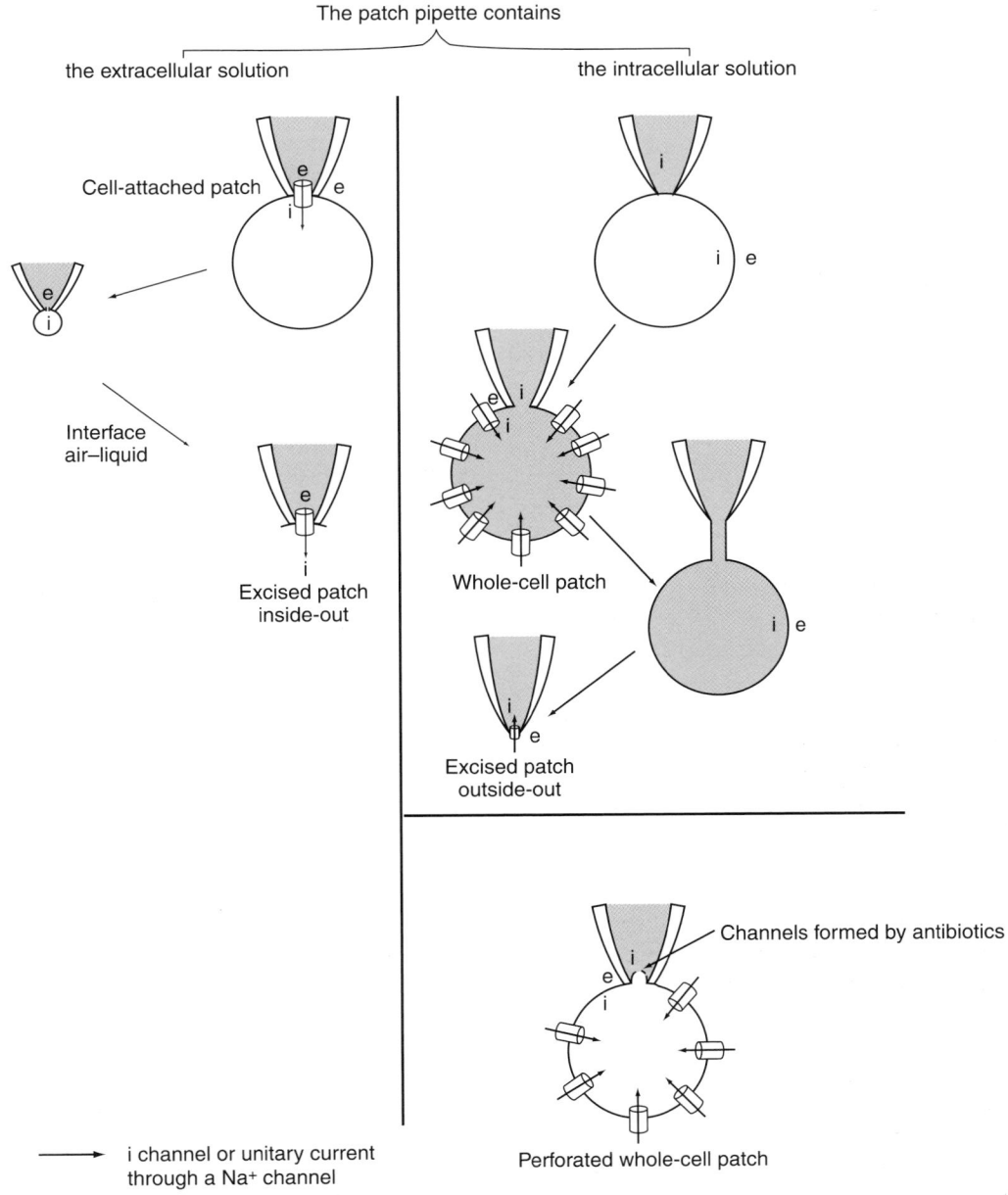

Figure A5.6 **Configurations of patch clamp recording.**

configuration (**Figure A5.6**). The resistance between the interior of the pipette and the external solution can be very large, of the order of $10\,G\Omega$ ($10^9\,\Omega$) or more. It means that the interior of the pipette is isolated from the extracellular solution by the seal that is formed.

This very large resistance is necessary for two reasons (**Figure A5.7**):

■ It allows the electrical isolation of the membrane patch under the tip of the pipette since practically no current can flow through the seal. This is important because if a fraction of the current passing through the membrane patch leaks out through the seal, it is not measured by the electrode.

■ It augments the signal-to-noise ratio since thermal movement of the charges through a bad seal is a source of additional noise in the recording. A good seal thus enables the measurement of the current flowing through one single channel (unitary current) which is of the order of picoampères.

From the 'cell-attached' configuration (the last to be explained), one can obtain other recording configurations. In total, three of them are used to record unitary currents, and one (whole-cell) to record the current flowing through all the open channels of the whole cell membrane.

Whole-cell configuration

This configuration is obtained from the cell-attached configuration. If a little suction is applied to the interior of the pipette, it may cause the rupture of the membrane patch under the pipette. Consequently, the patch pipette now records the activity of the whole cell membrane (minus the small ruptured patch of membrane). Rapidly, the intracellular solution equilibrates with that of the pipette, the volume of the latter being many times larger. This is especially true for inorganic ions.

This configuration enables the recording of the current flowing through the N channels open over the entire surface of the cell membrane. Under conditions where all the open channels are of the same type (with the opening of other channels being blocked by pharmacological agents or the voltage conditions), the total current flowing through a population of identical channels can be recorded, such that at steady state:

$$I = Np_oi,$$

where N is the number of identical channels, p_o the probability that these channels are in the open state, Np_o the number of identical channels in the open state, and i the unitary current.

The advantages of this technique over the two-electrode voltage clamp technique are: (i) the recording under voltage clamp from cell bodies too small to be impaled with two electrodes and even one; and (ii) there is a certain control over the composition of the internal environment and a better signal-to-noise ratio. The limitation of this technique is the gradual loss of intracellular components (such as second messengers), which will cause the eventual disappearance of the responses dependent on those components.

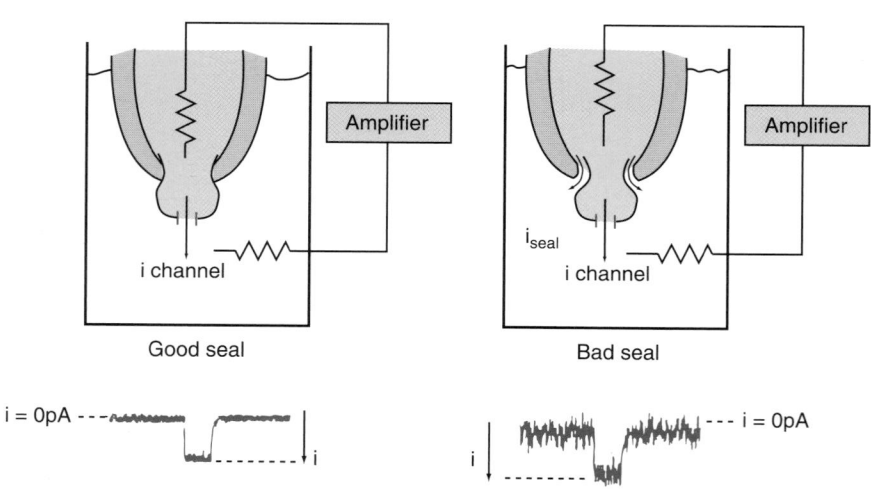

Good seal   Bad seal

i = 0pA

Unitary inward currents

Figure A5.7 Good and bad seals.
From *The Axon Guide*, Axon Instruments Inc., 1993.

Perforated whole-cell configuration

This is a variation of the whole-cell configuration, and also allows the recording of current flowing through the N channels open in the whole membrane but avoids washout of the intracellular solution. This configuration is obtained by introducing into the recording pipette a molecule such as nystatin, amphotericin or gramicidin, which will form channels in the patch of membrane under the tip of the electrode. To record in this configuration, first the cell-attached configuration is obtained and then the experimenter waits for the nystatin channels (or amphotericin or gramicidin channels) to form without applying any suction to the electrode. The channels formed by these molecules are mainly permeable to monovalent ions and thus allow electrical access to the cell's interior. Since these channels are not permeant to molecules as large or larger than glucose, whole cell recording can be performed without removing the intracellular environment. This is particularly useful when the modulation of ionic channels by second messengers is studied.

In order to evaluate this problem of 'washout', we can calculate the ratio between the cell body volume and the volume of solution at the very end of a pipette. For example, for a cell of 20 μm diameter the volume is: $(4/3)\pi(10 \times 10^{-6})^3 = 4 \times 10^{-15}$ litres. If we consider 1 mm of the tip of the pipette, it contains a volume of the solution approximately equal to 10^{-13} l, which is 100 times larger than the volume of the cell body.

Excised patch configurations

If one wants to record the unitary current *i* flowing through a single channel and to control simultaneously the composition of the intracellular environment, the so-called excised or cell-free patch configurations have to be used. The *outside-out configuration* is obtained from the whole-cell configuration by gently pulling the pipette away from the cell. This causes the membrane patch to be torn away from the rest of the cell at the same time that its free ends reseal together. In this case the intracellular environment is that of the pipette, and the extracellular environment is that of the bath. This configuration is used when rapid changes of the extracellular solution are required to test the effects of different ions or pharmacological agents when applied to the extracellular side of the membrane.

The *inside-out configuration* is obtained from the cell-attached configuration by gently pulling the pipette away from the cell, lifting the tip of the pipette from the bath in the air and putting it back into the solution (interface of air–liquid). In this case, the intracellular environment is that of the bath and the extracellular one is that of the pipette (the pipette is filled with a pseudo-extracellular solution). This configuration is used when rapid changes in the composition of the intracellular environment are necessary to test, for example, the effects of different ions, second messengers and pharmacological agents in that environment.

Cell-attached configuration

The intracellular environment is that of the cell itself, and the extracellular environment of the recorded membrane patch is the pipette solution. This configuration enables the recording of current flowing through the channel or channels present in the patch of membrane that is under the pipette and is electrically isolated from the rest of the cell. If one channel opens at a time, then the unitary current *i* flowing through that channel can be recorded. The recordings in cell-attached mode present two limitations: (i) the composition of the intracellular environment is not controlled; and (ii) the value of the membrane potential is not known and can only be estimated.

Let us assume that the voltage in the interior of the patch pipette is maintained at a known value V_p (p = pipette). Since the voltage across the membrane patch is $V_m = V_i - V_e = V_i - V_p$, it will not be known unless V_i, the voltage at the internal side of the membrane, is also known. V_i cannot be measured directly. One way to estimate this value is to measure the resting potential of several identical cells under similar conditions (with intracellular or whole-cell recordings), and to calculate an average V_i from the individual values. Sometimes, however, V_i can be measured when the cell is large enough to allow a two-electrode voltage clamp recording to be made simultaneously with the patch clamp recording (with a *Xenopus* oocyte, for example). Another method consists of replacing the extracellular medium with isotonic K^+ (120–150 mM). The membrane potential under these conditions will be close to 0 mV.

To leave the intracellular composition intact while recording the activity of a single channel is particularly useful for studies of the modulation of an ionic channel by second messengers.

A5.3.2 Principles of the patch clamp recording technique

In the patch clamp technique, as in all voltage clamp techniques, the membrane potential is held constant (i.e. clamped) while the current flowing through a single open channel or many open channels (Np_o) is measured (**Figure A5.8**). In the patch clamp technique only one micropipette is used full time for both voltage clamping

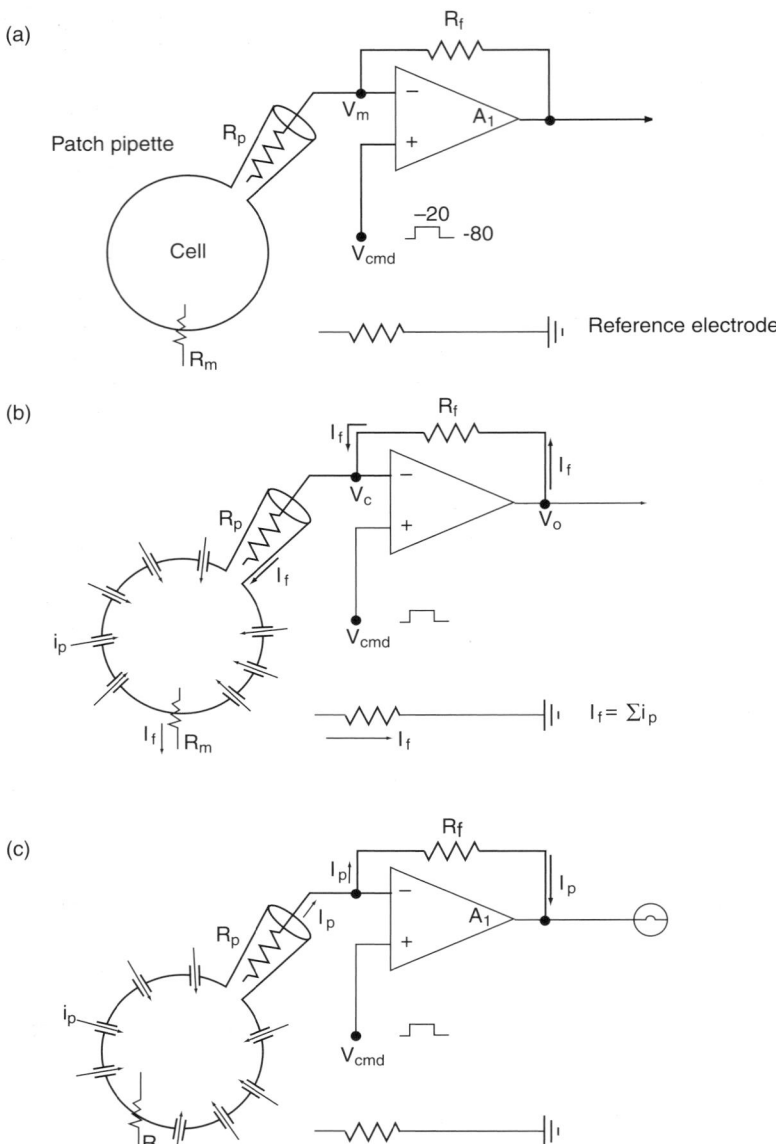

Figure A5.8 Example of a patch clamp recording in the whole-cell configuration.
(a) The amplifier compares V_m to the new $V_{cmd} = -20$ mV. (b) The amplifier sends V_o so that $V_m = V_{cmd} = -20$ mV. Owing to the depolarization to -20 mV, the Na$^+$ channels open and unitary inward currents i_p flow through the N open channels ($Ni_p = I_p$). (c) The whole-cell current I_p flows through the circuit and is measured as a voltage change.

and current recording. How at the same time via the same pipette can the voltage of the membrane be controlled and the current flowing through the membrane be measured?

When an operational amplifier A1 is connected as shown in **Figure A5.8a** with a high megohm resistor R_f (f = feedback), a current-to-voltage converter is obtained. The patch pipette is connected to the negative input and the command voltage (V_{cmd}) to the positive one. The resistor R_f can have two values: $R_f = 1$ GΩ in

the whole-cell configuration and 10 GΩ in the excised patch configurations.

How the membrane is clamped at a voltage equal to V_{cmd}

R_p represents the electrode resistance and R_m the membrane input resistance (**Figure A5.8a**). Suppose that the membrane potential is first clamped to -80 mV ($V_{cmd} =$

–80 mV), then a voltage step to –20 mV is applied for 100 ms (V_{cmd} = –20 mV for 100 ms). The membrane potential (V_m) has to be clamped quickly to –20 mV ($V_m = V_{cmd}$ = –20 mV) whatever happens to the channels in the membrane (they open or close). The operational amplifier A1 is able to minimize the voltage difference between two inputs to a very small value (0.1 µV or so). A1 compares the value of V_{cmd} (entry +) to that of V_m (entry –). It then sends a voltage output (V_o) in order to obtain $V_m = V_{cmd}$ = –20 mV (**Figure A5.8b**).

What is this value of V_o? Suppose that at the time t of its peak the Na⁺ current evoked by the voltage step to –20 mV is I_{Na} = 1 nA. V_o will force a current I = –1 nA to flow through $R_f = 10^9 \, \Omega$ in order to clamp the membrane potential: $V_o = R_f I = 10^9 \times 10^{-9}$ = 1 V. It is said that V_o = 1 V/nA or 1 mV/pA.

The limits of V_o in patch clamp amplifiers are +15 V and –15 V. This means that V_o cannot be bigger than these values, which is largely compatible with biological experiments where currents through the membrane do not exceed 15 nA.

The amplifier A1 compares V_m with V_{cmd} and sends V_o at a very high speed. This speed has to be very high in order to correct V_m according to V_{cmd} very quickly. The ideal clamp is obtained at the output of the circuit via R_f (black dot V_c on the scheme of Figure A5.8b). As in the voltage clamp technique, a capacitive current is present at the beginning and at the end of the voltage step on the current trace and a leak current during the step, but they are not re-explained here.

A5.3.3 The unitary current i is a rectangular step of current (see Figures 5.8a and c)

We record, for example, in the outside-out patch clamp configuration the activity of a single voltage sensitive Na⁺ channel. When a positive membrane potential step is applied to depolarize the patch of membrane from –90 mV to –40 mV, an inward current i_{Na} flowing through the open Na⁺ channel is recorded (inward current means a current that flows across the membrane from the outside to inside). By convention, inward currents are represented as downward deflections and outward currents as upward deflections.

The membrane depolarization causes activation of the voltage-dependent Na⁺ channel, and induces its transition from the closed (C) state (or conformation) to the open (O) state, a transition symbolized by:

$$C \rightleftharpoons O,$$

where C is the closed state of the channel (at –90 mV) and O is the open state of the channel (at –40 mV).

While the channel is in the O conformation (at –40 mV), Na⁺ ions flow through the channel and an inward current caused by the net influx of Na⁺ ions is recorded. This current reaches its maximum value very rapidly. Thus, the maximal net ion flux is established almost instantaneously given the time scale of the recording (of the order of microseconds). The development of the inward current thus appears as a vertical downward deflection.

A delay between the onset of the voltage step and the onset of the current i is observed. This delay has a duration that varies from one depolarizing test pulse to another and also according to the channel under study. This delay is due to the conformational change or changes of the channel protein. In fact, such changes previous to opening can be multiple:

$$C_1 \rightleftharpoons C_2 \rightleftharpoons C_3 \rightleftharpoons O$$

Notice that the opening delay does not correspond to the intrinsic duration of the process of conformational change, which is extremely short. It corresponds to the statistical nature of the equilibrium between the 2, 3, N closed and open conformations. The opening delay therefore depends on the time spent in each of the different closed states (C_1, C_2, C_3).

The return of the current value to zero corresponds to the closing of the channel. This closure is the result of the transition of the channel protein from the open state (O) to a state in which the channel no longer conducts (state in which the aqueous pore is closed). It can be either a closed state (C), an inactivated state (I) or a desensitized state (D). In the case of the Na⁺ channel, the return of the current value to zero is due mainly to the transition of the protein from the open state to the inactivated state (O → I). Before closing for a long time, the channel can also flicker between the open and closed state (C ⇌ O):

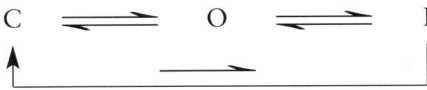

Just as the current reaches its maximum value instantaneously during opening, it also returns instantaneously to its zero value during closing of the pore. Because of this, the unitary current i has a step-like rectangular shape.

A5.3.4 Determination of the conductance of a channel

If we repeat several times the experiment shown in **Figure 5.8a**, we observe that for a given voltage step ΔV, i varies around an average value. The current fluctuations are measured at regular intervals before, during and immediately after the depolarizing voltage pulse. The distribution of the different i values during the voltage pulse describes a Gaussian curve in which the peak corresponds to the average i value (**Figure 5.8d**). There is also a peak around $0\,pA$ (not shown on the figure) which corresponds to the different values of i when the channel is closed. Since the channel is in the closed state most of the time, where i has values around $0\,pA$, this peak is higher than the one corresponding to $i_{channel}$ (around $-2\,pA$). The width of the peak around $0\,pA$ gives the mean value of the fluctuations resulting from noise. Therefore, the two main reasons for these fluctuations of $i_{channel}$ are: the variations in the noise of the recording system and the changes in the number of ions that cross the channel during a unit of time Δt.

Knowing the average value of i and the reversal potential value of the current (E_{rev}), the average conductance value of the channel under study, γ, can be calculated: $\gamma = i/(V_m - E_{rev})$.

However, there are cases in which the distribution of i for a given membrane potential shows several peaks. Different possibilities should be considered:

- Only one channel is being recorded from but it presents several open conformational states, each one with different conductances. The peaks correspond to the current flowing through these different substates.
- Two or more channels of the *same* type are present in the patch and their activity recorded. The peaks represent the multiples of i ($2i$, $3i$, etc.).
- Two or more channels of *different* types are present in the patch and their activity is simultaneously recorded. The peaks correspond to the current through different channel types.

A5.3.5 Mean open time of a channel

An ionic channel fluctuates between a closed state (C) and an open state (O):

$$C \underset{\alpha}{\overset{\beta}{\rightleftharpoons}} O$$

where α is the closing rate constant or, more exactly, the number of channel closures per unit of time spent in the open state O. β is the opening rate constant or the number of openings per unit of time spent in the closed state R (α and β are expressed in s^{-1}).

Once activated, the channel remains in the O state for a time t_o, called open time. When the channel opens, the unitary current i is recorded for a certain time t_o. t_o for a given channel studied under identical conditions varies from one recording to another (**Figure A5.9**). t_o is an

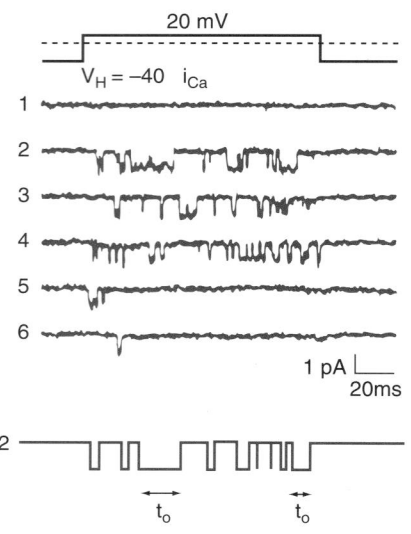

Figure A5.9 Example of the patch clamp recording of a single voltage-dependent Ca+ channel.

In response to a voltage step to +20 mV from a holding potential of −40 mV, the channel opens and closes several times during each of the six trials. Adapted from Fox AP, Nowyky MC, Tsien RW (1987) Single-channel recordings of three types of calcium channels in chick sensory neurones, *J. Physiol. (Lond.)* **394**, 173–200, with permission.

aleatory variable of an observed duration. When the number of times a value of t_o (in the order of milli- or microseconds) is plotted against the values of t_o, one obtains the open time histogram; i.e. the distribution of the different values of t_o (**Figure A5.10**). This distribution declines and the shorter open times are more frequent than the longer ones.

Why does the distribution of t_o decrease?

The histogram is constructed as follows. At time $t = 0$, all the channels are open (the delay of opening is ignored, all the openings are aligned at time 0; **Figure A5.10**). As time t increases, the number of channels that remain open can only decrease since channels progressively close. This can also be expressed as follows: the longer the observation time, the lower the probability that the channel is still in the open state. Or, alternatively, the longer the observation time, the closer the probability will be to 1 that the channel will shut (1 is the maximum value used to express a probability). It is not a Gaussian curve because the delay of opening is ignored and all the openings begin at $t = 0$.

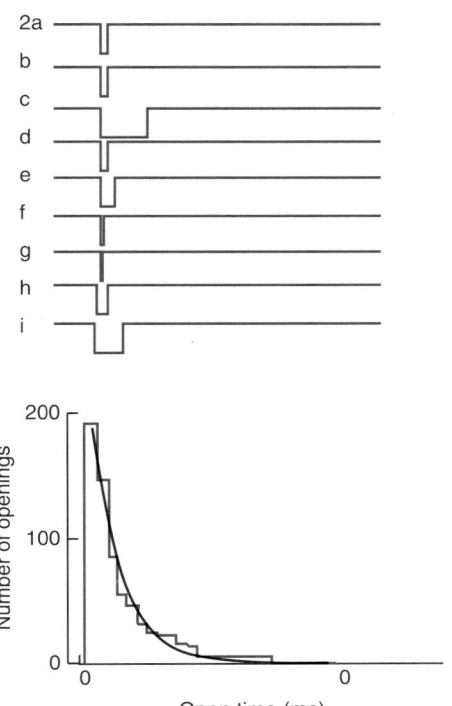

Figure A5.10 Determination of the mean open time of a channel.

Trial 2 of Figure A5.9 is selected and all the openings are aligned at time 0. τ_o = 1.2 ms.

Why is the decrementing distribution of t_o exponential?

A channel open at $t = 0$ has a probability of closing at $t+\Delta t$. It has the same probability of closing if it is still open at the beginning of any subsequent observation interval Δt. This type of probability is described mathematically as an exponential function of the observation time. Thus, when the openings of a homogeneous population of channels are studied, the decrease in the number of events is described by a single exponential.

Experimental determination of τ_o, the mean open time of a channel

The mean open time τ_o is the time during which a channel has the highest probability of being in the open state: it corresponds to the sum of all the values that t_o may take, weighted by their corresponding probability values. This value is easy to calculate if the distribution is described by a single exponential. In order to verify that the histogram is actually described by a single exponential, one has to first build the histogram by plotting the number of times a value of t_o is observed as a function of t_o; i.e. number of events = $f(t_o)$.

The exponential that describes the histogram has the form $y = y_o e^{-t/\tau_o}$, where y is the number of events observed at each time t. This curve will be linear on semi-logarithmic coordinates if it is described by a single exponential. The slope can be measured with a regression analysis. It corresponds to the mean open time τ_o of the channel. τ_o is the value of t_o for a number of events equal to $1/e$. It is the 'expected value' of t_o. The expected value of t_o is the sum of all the values of t_o weighted by their corresponding probabilities.

In the case of the conformational changes C $\rightleftharpoons$ O, the value of τ_o provides an estimate of the closure rate constant α, because at steady state $\tau_o = 1/\alpha$. For example, from the open time histogram of the nicotinic receptor channel, we can determine its mean open time τ_o. Knowing that in conditions where the desensitization of the channel is negligible $\tau_o = 1/\alpha$, we can calculate from τ_o the closing rate constant of the channel. If τ_o = 1.1 ms, α = 900 s⁻¹. The channel closes 900 times for each second spent in the open state. In other words there is an average of 900 transitions of the channel to the closed state for each second spent in the open state.

Further reading

Caterall WA (2000) From ionic currents to molecular mechanisms: the structure and function of voltage-gated sodium channels. *Neuron* **26**, 13–25.

Eaholtz G, Scheuer T, Catterall WA (1994) Restoration of inactivation and block of open sodium channels by an inactivation gate peptide. *Neuron* **12**, 1041–1048.

Hamill OP, Marty A, Neher E *et al.* (1981) Improved patch damp technique for high resolution current recording from cells and cell-free membrane patches. *Pflügers Archiv.* **391**, 85–100.

Hodgkin AL, Huxley AF (1952) A quantitative description of membrane current and its application to conduction and excitation in nerve. *J. Physiol.* (Lond) **117**, 500–544.

Korn SI, Marty A, Connor JA, Horn R (1991) Perforated patch recording. *Methods Neurosci.* **4**, 264–373.

McCormick KA, Srinivasan J, White K, Scheuer T, Caterall WA (1999) The extracellular domain of the beta1 subunit is both necessary and sufficient for beta1-like modulation of sodium channel gating. *J. Biol. Chem.* **274**, 32638–32646.

Neher E, Sakmann B (1976) Single channel currents recorded from membrane of denervated frog muscle fibres. *Nature* **260**, 779–802.

Noda M, Ikeda T, Suzuki H *et al.* (1986) Expression of functional sodium channels from cloned cDNA. *Nature* **322**, 826–828.

Numann K, Caterall WA, Scheuer T (1991) Functional

modulation of brain sodium channels by protein kinase C phosphorylation. *Science* **254**, 115–118.

Qu Y, Rogers JC, Chen SF, McCormick KA, Scheuer T, Catterall WA (1999) Functional roles of the extracellular segments of the sodium channel alpha subunit in voltage-dependent gating and modulation by beta1 subunits. *J. Biol. Chem.* **274**, 32647–32654.

Stuart G, Häuser M (1994) Initiation and spread of sodium action potentials in cerebellar purkinje cells. *Neuron* **13**, 703–712.

Vassilev PM, Scheuer T, Catterall WA (1988) Identification of an intracellular peptide segment involved in sodium channel inactivation. *Science* **241**, 1658–1661.

The Voltage-Gated Channels of Ca²⁺ Action Potentials: Generalization

Chapter 5 explained the Na^+-dependent action potential propagated by axons. There are two other types of action potentials: (i) the Na^+/Ca^{2+}-dependent action potential present in axon terminals or heart muscle cells (**Figure 5.2d**), for example, where it is responsible for Ca^{2+} entry and an increase of intracellular Ca^{2+} concentration, a necessary prerequisite for neurotransmitter release (secretion) or muscle fibre contraction; and (ii) the Ca^{2+}-dependent action potential present in, for example, the dendrites of cerebellar Purkinje cells and in endocrine cells (**Figure 6.1a**). In Purkinje cell dendrites, it depolarizes the membrane and thus modulates neuronal integration; in endocrine cells it provides a Ca^{2+} entry to trigger hormone secretion.

6.1 Properties of Ca²⁺-dependent action potentials

In some neuronal cell bodies, in heart ventricular muscle cells and in axon terminals, the action potentials have a longer duration than Na^+ spikes, with a plateau following the initial peak: these are the Na^+/Ca^{2+}-dependent action potentials (see **Figures 5.2b–d**). In some neuronal dendrites and some endocrine cells, action potentials have a small amplitude and a long duration: these are the Ca^{2+}-dependent action potentials (**Figure 6.1**). All action potentials are initiated in response to a membrane depolarization. Na^+, Na^+/Ca^{2+} and Ca^{2+}-dependent action potentials differ in the type of voltage-gated channels responsible for their depolarization and repolarization phases. We will examine the properties of a Ca^{2+}-dependent action potential.

6.1.1 Ca²⁺ and K⁺ ions participate in the action potential of endocrine cells

The activity of pituitary endocrine cells that release growth hormone is recorded in the perforated whole-cell configuration (current clamp mode; see Appendix 5.1). They display a spontaneous activity. When these cells are previously loaded with the Ca^{2+}-sensitive dye Fura-2, changes of intracellular Ca^{2+} concentration can be also quantified (see **Appendix 6.1**). Simultaneous recording of potential and $[Ca^{2+}]_i$ changes shows that for each action potential there is a corresponding $[Ca^{2+}]_i$ increase (**Figure 6.1a**). This strongly suggests that Ca^{2+} ions are entering the cell during action potentials.

Ca²⁺ ions participate in the depolarization phase of the action potential

When the extracellular solution is changed from control Krebs to a Ca^{2+}-free solution, or when nifedipin, an L-type Ca^{2+} channel blocker, is added to the external medium (**Figure 6.1b**), the amplitude and rise time of the depolarization phase of the action potential gradually and rapidly decreases until action potentials are no longer evoked.

K⁺ ions participate in the repolarization phase of the action potential

Application of charybdotoxin (CTX) or apamin, blockers of Ca^{2+}-activated K^+ channels, increases the peak amplitude and prolongs the duration of action potentials (**Figure 6.1c**). Note that apamin also blocks the after-spike hyperpolarization (**Figure 6.1c**, right).

6.1.2 Questions about the Ca²⁺-dependent action potential

■ What are the structural and functional properties of the Ca^{2+} and K^+ channels involved? (Sections 6.2 and 6.3)
■ What represents the threshold potential for Ca^{2+}-dependent action potential initiation. Where are Ca^{2+}-dependent action potentials initiated? (Section 6.4)

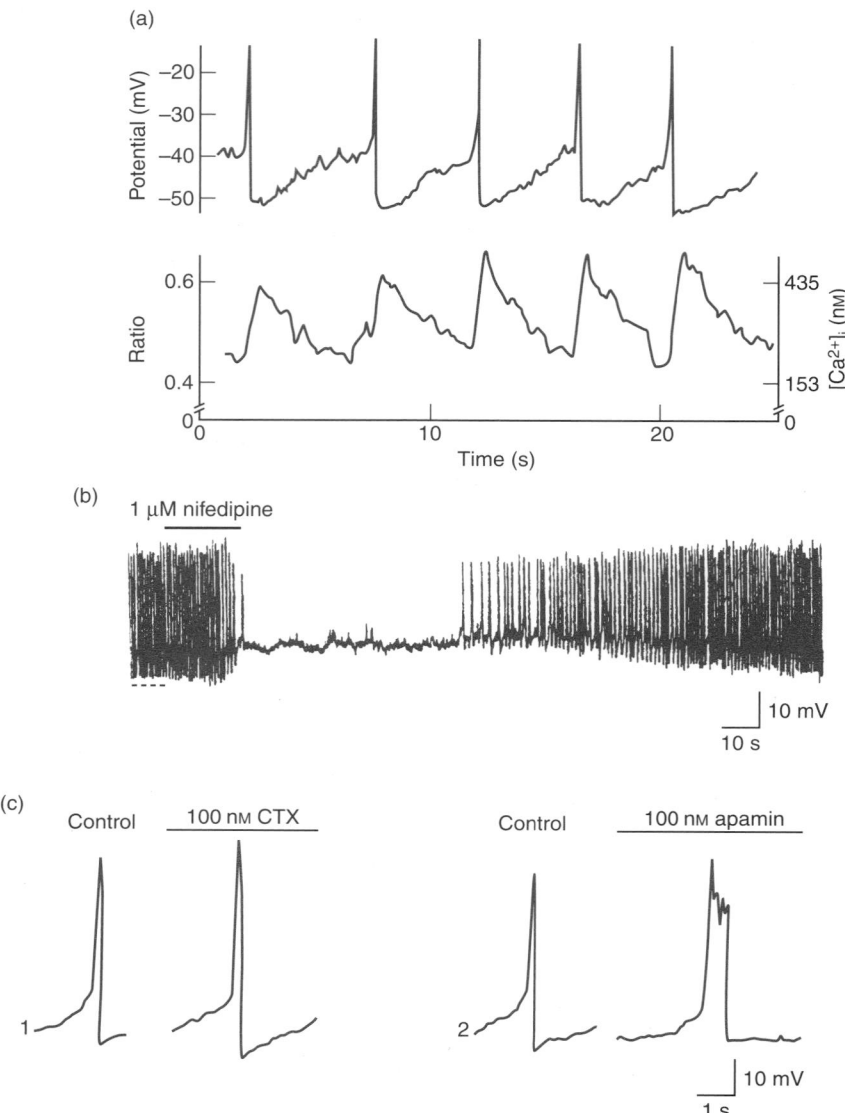

Figure 6.1 The Ca²⁺-dependent action potential of an endocrine cell.
Growth-hormone secreting cells of the anterior pituitary in culture are loaded with the Ca²⁺-sensitive dye Fura-2 and their activity is recorded in perforated whole-cell patch configuration (current clamp mode). **(a)** Simultaneous recordings of action potentials (top trace) and cytosolic [Ca²⁺] oscillations (bottom trace) in control conditions. **(b)** Nifedipin, an L-type Ca²⁺ channel blocker, is applied for 20 s. **(c)** Action potential in the absence and presence of blockers of Ca²⁺-activated K⁺ channels, charybdotoxin (CTX, 1) and apamin (2). Adapted from Kwiecien R, Robert C, Cannon R *et al.* (1998) Endogenous pacemaker activity of rat tumour somatotrophs, *J. Physiol.* **508**, 883–905, with permission.

6.2 The depolarizing or plateau phase of Ca²⁺-dependent action potentials results from the transient entry of Ca²⁺ ions through voltage-gated Ca²⁺ channels

The voltage-gated Ca²⁺ channels involved in these action potentials are high threshold-activated (HVA)

Ca²⁺ channels. There are three main types of such channels: the L-type (L for long lasting), the N-type (N for neuronal or for neither L nor T) and the P-type (P for Purkinje cells where they have been first described).

6.2.1 The voltage-gated Ca²⁺ channels are a diverse group of multisubunit proteins

They are composed of a typical central α-subunit (named α_1) and different auxiliary subunits which include an intracellular β subunit (**Figure 6.2a**) and a transmembrane, disulphide-linked $\alpha_2\delta$-subunit complex. The α_1-subunit of 190–250 kD is the largest subunit with four internal homologous repeats (I to IV), and it incorporates the conduction pore, the voltage sensor and gating apparatus and the known sites of channel regulation by second messengers, drugs and toxins. Depending on the tissue of origin, a γ-subunit may also form part of the channel complex. At present, at least ten isoforms of the α_1-subunit have been cloned. The pharmacological and electrophysiological diversity of Ca²⁺ channels arises pri-marily from the existence of these multiple forms of α_1-subunits. Their nomenclature as forming an L, N or P channel is still under discussion (**Figure 6.2b**).

How to record the activity of Ca²⁺ channels in isolation?

This needs to block the voltage-gated channels that are not permeable to Ca²⁺ ions. Different strategies can be used: in whole-cell or intracellular recordings, TTX and TEA are added to the extracellular solution and K⁺ ions are replaced by Cs⁺ in the intra-pipette solution, in order to block voltage-gated Na⁺ and K⁺ channels. In cell-attached recordings the patch pipette is filled with a solution containing Ca²⁺ or Ba²⁺ ions as the charge

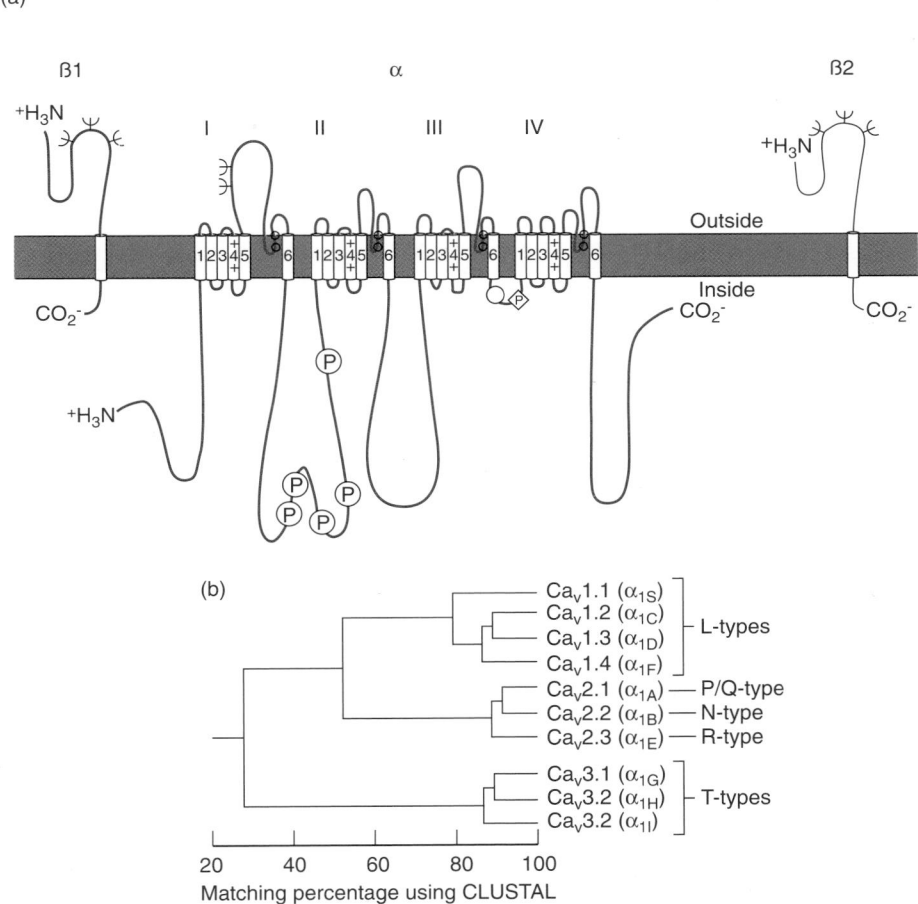

Figure 6.2 Subunits of voltage-gated Ca²⁺ channels.
(a) Putative transmembrane organization of the α_1 and auxiliary β subunits of the voltage-gated Ca²⁺ channels. Cylinders represent putative membrane-spanning segments, Ψ sites of probable N-linked glycosylation. (b) Phylogeny of the α_1 subunits and their two nomenclatures. Only the membrane-spanning segments and the pore loops (around 350 amino acids) are compared, which clearly defines three families. Drawing (a) from Isom LL, De Jongh KS, Caterall WA (1994) Auxiliary subunits of voltage-gated ion channels, *Neuron* **12**, 1183–1194, with permission. Drawing (b) adapted from Ertel EA, Campbell KP, Harpold MM *et al.* (2000) Nomenclature of voltage-gated calcium channels, *Neuron* **25**, 533–535, with permission.

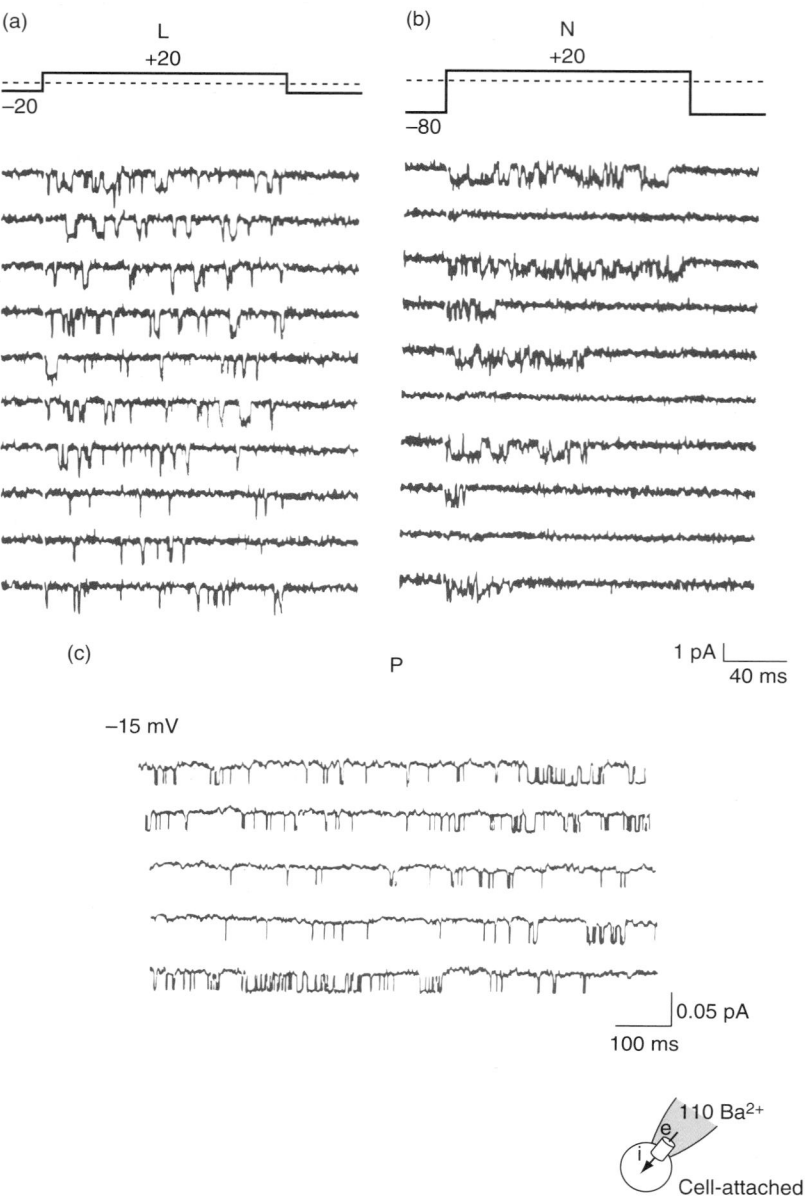

Figure 6.3 Single-channel recordings of the high-threshold Ca^{2+} channels: the L, N and P channels.

The activity of **(a)** single L and **(b)** N Ca^{2+} channels is recorded in patch clamp (cell-attached patches) from dorsal root ganglion cells and that of a single P channel **(c)** is recorded from a lipid bilayer in which a P channel isolated from cerebellum has been incorporated. All recordings are performed with Ba^{2+} (110 or 80 mM) as the charge carrier. In response to a test depolarizing step to +20 mV (a, b) or at a depolarized holding potential of –15 mV (c), unitary inward currents are recorded. Upper traces are voltage and the corresponding unitary current traces are the bottom traces (5–10 trials). V_H = –20 mV in (a), –80 mV in (b) and –15 mV in (c). In (a) and (b) the intra-pipette solution contains: 110 mM $BaCl_2$, 10 mM HEPES and 200 μM TTX. The extracellular solution bathing the membrane outside the patch contains (in mM): 140 K aspartate, 10 K-EGTA, 10 HEPES, 1 $MgCl_2$ in order to zero the cell resting membrane potential. In (c) the solution bathing the extracellular side of the bilayer contains (in mM): 80 $BaCl_2$, 10 HEPES. The solution bathing the intracellular side of the bilayer in (c) contains (in mM): 120 CsCl, 1 $MgCl_2$, 10 HEPES. Parts (a) and (b) adapted from Nowycky MC, Fox AP, Tsien RW (1985) Three types of neuronal calcium channel with different calcium agonist sensitivity, *Nature* **316**, 440–443, with permission. Part (c) adapted from Llinas R, Sugimori M, Lin JW, Cherksey B (1989) Blocking and isolation of a calcium channel from neurons in mammals and cephalopods utilizing a toxin fraction (FTX) from funnel-web spider poison, *Proc. Natl Acad. Sci. USA* **86**, 1689–1693, with permission.

carrier. When Ba^{2+} substitutes for Ca^{2+} in the extracellular solution, the inward currents recorded in response to a depolarizing step are Ba^{2+} currents. Ba^{2+} is often preferred to Ca^{2+} since it carries current twice as effectively as Ca^{2+} and poorly inactivates Ca^{2+} channels (see Section 6.2.3). As a consequence, unitary Ba^{2+} currents are larger than Ca^{2+} ones and can be studied more easily.

Another challenge is to separate the various types of Ca^{2+} channels in order to record the activity of only one type (since in most of the cells they are co-expressed). These different Ca^{2+} channels are the high voltage-activated L, N and P channels (this chapter) and the low-threshold T channel. T-type Ca^{2+} channels are low threshold-activated channels, also called subliminal Ca^{2+} channels, that can be identified by their low threshold of activation and their rapid inactivation. They are studied with other subliminal channels in Section 17.2.2.

HVA Ca^{2+} channels can be separated into L and non-L channels but the best way to characterize the three types of channels is by their selective sensitivity to toxins or dihydropyridine derivatives. L-type channels are, for example, selectively opened by Bay K 8644 and blocked by nimodipine, both 1,4-dihydropyridine compounds; N-type channels are blocked by a toxin from the marine snail *Conus geographus*, the ω-conotoxin; and P-type channels are selectively blocked by a purified polyamine fraction of the funnel-web spider (*Agelenopsis aperta*) venom (FTX) and a peptide component of the same venom, ω-agatoxin IVA (ω-Aga-IVA).

6.2.2 The L, N and P-type Ca^{2+} channels open at membrane potentials positive to −20 mV; they are high-threshold Ca^{2+} channels

The L-type Ca^{2+} channel has a large conductance and inactivates very slowly with depolarization

The activity of single L-type Ca^{2+} channels is recorded in sensory neurons of the chick dorsal root ganglion in patch clamp (cell-attached patch with Ba^{2+} as the charge carrier). In response to a test depolarization to +20 mV from a *depolarized* holding potential (−40 to 0 mV), unitary inward Ba^{2+} currents are evoked and recorded throughout the duration of the depolarizing step (**Figure 6.3a**).

The voltage-dependence of activation is studied with depolarizations to various test potentials from a holding potential of −40 mV (**Figure 6.4**). With test depolarizations up to +10 mV, openings are rare and of short duration. Activation of the channel becomes significant at

+10 mV: openings are more frequent and of longer duration. At all potentials tested, openings are distributed relatively evenly throughout the duration of the depolarizing step (**Figures 6.3a** and **6.4a**). At −20 mV, the mean single-channel amplitude of the L current (i_L) is around −2 pA. i_L amplitude diminishes linearly with depolarization: the i_L/V relation is linear between −20 and +20 mV. Between these membrane potentials, the unitary conductance, γ_L, is constant and equal to 20–25 pS in 110 mM Ba^{2+} (**Figure 6.4c**).

The main characteristics of L-type channels are (i) their very slow inactivation during a depolarizing step; (ii) their sensitivity to dihydropyridines; and (iii) their loss of activity in excised patches.

Bay K 8644 is a dihydropyridine compound that increases dramatically the mean open time of an L-type channel without changing its unitary conductance (**Figure 6.5**). It has no effect on the other Ca^{2+} channel types (see **Figure 6.9**). Bay K 8644 binds to a specific site on the α_1-subunit of L channels and changes the gating mode from brief openings to long-lasting openings even at weakly depolarized potentials (V_{step} = −30 mV). Other dihydropyridine derivatives such as nifedipine, nimodipine and nitrendipine selectively block L channels (see **Figure 6.16**).

The loss of activity of an L channel in excised patch can be observed in outside-out patches. In response to a test depolarization to +10 mV the activity of an L channel rapidly disappears (**Figure 6.6**). To determine the nature of the cytoplasmic constituent(s) necessary to restore the activity of the L channel, inside-out patches are performed, a configuration that allows a change of the medium bathing the intracellular side of the membrane.

The activity of a single L channel is first recorded in cell-attached configuration in response to a test depolarization to 0 mV (**Figure 6.7**). Then the membrane is pulled out in order to obtain an inside-out patch. The L-type activity rapidly disappears and is not restored by adding ATP–Mg to the intracellular solution. In contrast, when the catalytic subunit of the cAMP-dependent protein kinase (PKA) is added, the L-channel activity reappears (the catalytic subunit of PKA does not need the presence of cAMP to be active). This suggests that PKA directly phosphorylates the L channel thus allowing its activation by the depolarization. It means that, in physiological conditions, the activity of L channels requires the activation of the following cascade: the activation of adenylate cyclase by the α_s-subunit of the G_s protein, the formation of cAMP and the subsequent activation of protein kinase A. Other kinases might also play a role.

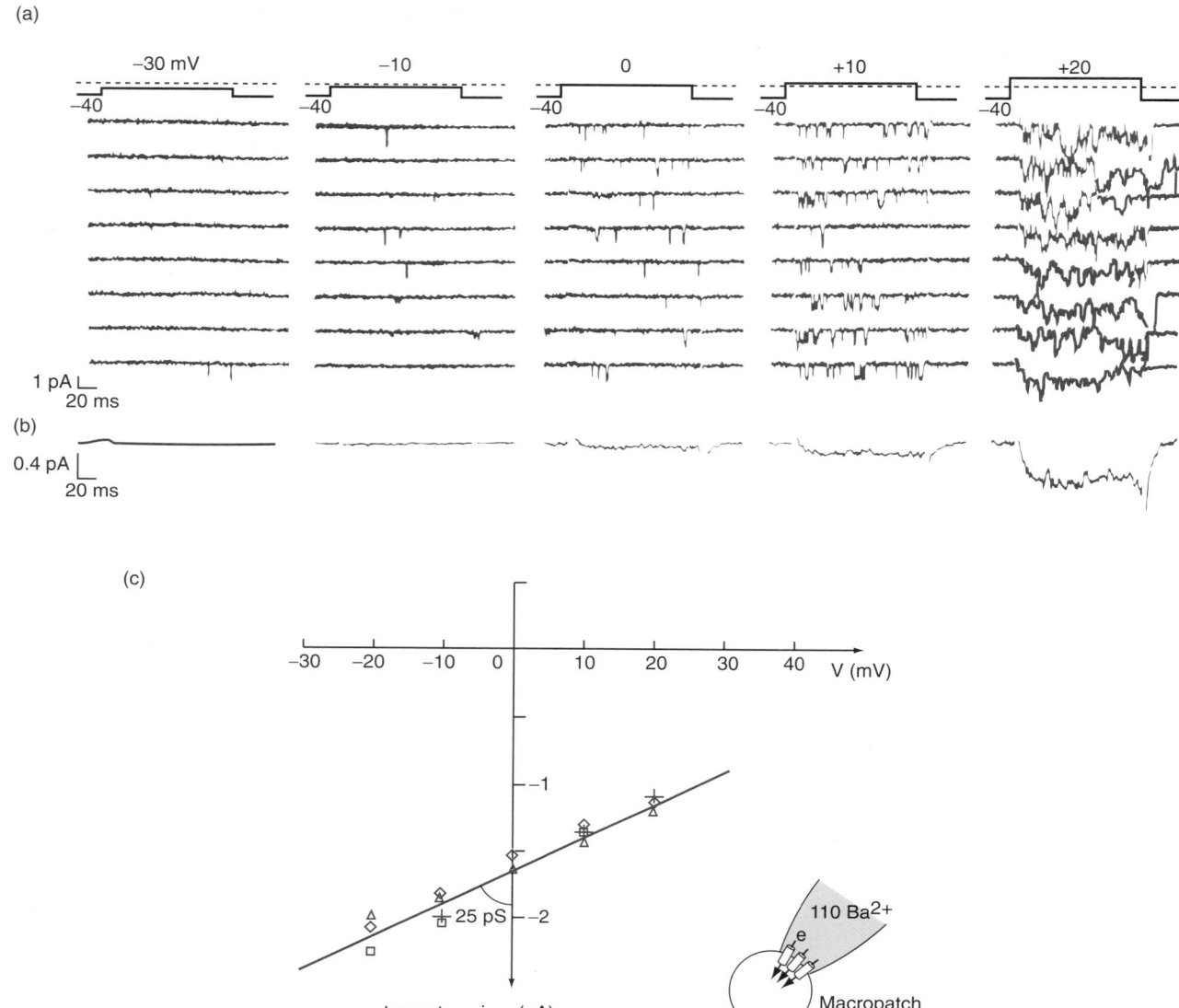

Figure 6.4 Voltage dependence of the unitary L-type Ca²⁺ current.

(a) The activity of L channels (the patch of membrane contains more than one L channel) is recorded in patch clamp (cell-attached patch) in a sensory dorsal root ganglion neuron. The patch is depolarized to −30, −10, 0, +10 and +20 mV from a holding potential of −40 mV. **(b)** Macroscopic current traces obtained by averaging at least 80 corresponding unitary current recordings such as those in (a). The probability of the L channels being in the open state increases with the test depolarization so that at +20 mV, openings of the 4–5 channels present in the patch overlap, leading to a sudden increase in the corresponding macroscopic current. **(c)** The unitary L current amplitude (i_L) is plotted against membrane potential (from −20 to +20 mV) in the absence (+, square) or presence (Δ, lozange) of Bay K8644 in the patch pipette. The amplitude of i_L decreases linearly with depolarization between −20 and +20 mV with a slope $\gamma_L = 25$ pS. The intrapipette solution contains (in mM): 110 BaCl$_2$, 10 HEPES. The extracellular solution bathing the extracellular side of the membrane outside of the recording pipette contains (in mM): 140 K-aspartate, 10 K-EGTA, 1 MgCl$_2$, 10 HEPES. A symmetric K⁺ solution is applied in order to zero the cell resting potential. Adapted from Fox AF, Nowycky MC, Tsien RW (1987) Single-channel recordings of three types of calcium channels in chick sensory neurons, *J. Physiol.* **394**, 173–200, with permission.

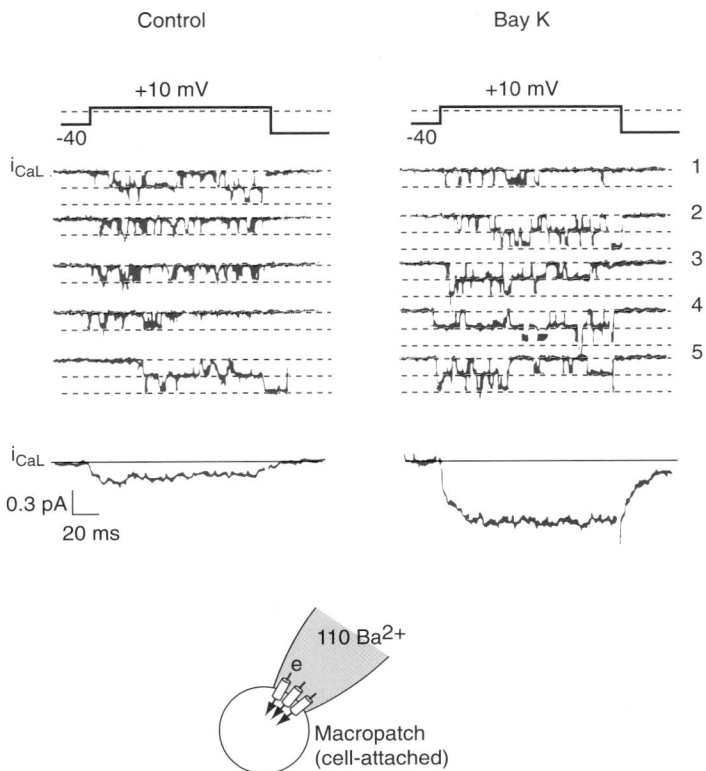

Figure 6.5 Bay K8644 promotes long-lasting openings of L-type Ca²⁺ channels.
The activity of three L channels is recorded in patch clamp (cell-attached patch). Top traces: a depolarizing step to +10 mV from a holding potential of –40 mV is applied at a low frequency. Middle traces (1 to 5): five consecutive unitary current traces recorded in the absence (left) and presence (right) of 5 μM Bay K8644 in the bathing solution. Recordings are obtained from the same cell. Dashed line indicates the mean amplitude of the unitary current (–1.28 pA) which is unchanged in the presence of Bay K. Bottom traces: macroscopic current traces obtained by averaging at least 80 corresponding unitary current recordings. Adapted from Fox AP, Nowycky MC, Tsien RW (1987) Single channel recordings of three types of calcium channels in chick sensory neurones, *J. Physiol.* **394**, 173–200, with permission.

The N-type Ca²⁺ channel inactivates with depolarization in the tens of milliseconds range and has a smaller unitary conductance than the L-type channel

The activity of single N-type channels is recorded in the same preparation in patch clamp (cell-attached patch, with Ba²⁺ as the charge carrier). In contrast to the L channels, N channels inactivate with depolarization. Therefore their activity has to be recorded in response to a test depolarization from a *hyperpolarized* holding potential (–80 to –60 mV) (**Figure 6.3b**). At holding potentials positive to –40 mV (e.g. –20 mV; **Figure 6.3a**), the N channel(s) is inactivated and its activity is absent on the recordings.

N-channel activity differs from that of the L channel in several aspects:

■ N channels often open in bursts and inactivate with time and voltage (see Section 6.2.3).

■ Measured at the same test potential, the mean amplitude of the N unitary current is smaller than that of L (e.g. $i_N = -1.22 \pm 0.03$ pA and $i_L = 2.07 \pm 0.09$ at –20 mV; **Figures 6.3a and b**) which makes its mean unitary conductance also smaller ($\gamma_N = 13$ pS in 110 mM Ba²⁺; **Figure 6.8b**).

■ N channels are insensitive to dihydropyridines but are selectively blocked by ω-conotoxin GUIA.

■ They do not need to be phosphorylated to open (**Figure 6.6**).

The P-type Ca²⁺ channel differs from the N channel by its pharmacology

The activity of a single P-type channel is recorded from lipid bilayers in which purified P channels from cerebellar Purkinje cells have been incorporated. Ba²⁺ ions are used as the charge carrier. The activity of the P channel is recorded at different steady holding potentials. At

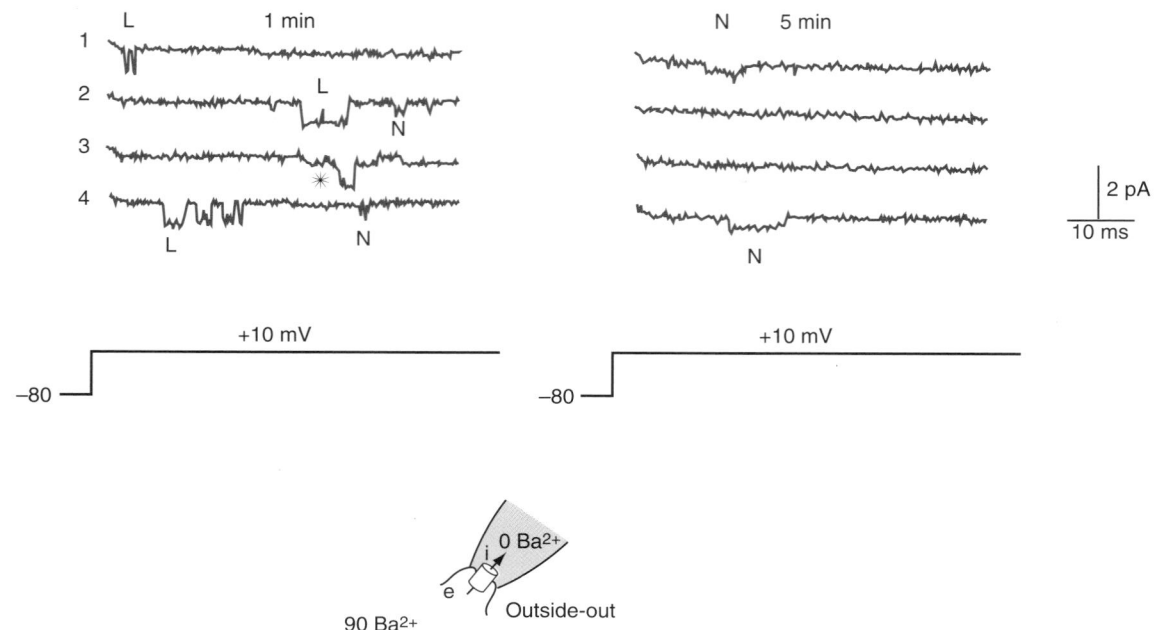

Figure 6.6 In excised patches, the activity of L channels disappears within minutes.
The activity of an L and N channel is recorded in patch clamp (outside-out patches from a pituitary cell line in culture) in response to a depolarizing pulse to +10 mV from a holding potential of −80 mV. Left: One minute after forming the excised patch, the two types of channels open one at a time or their openings overlap (line 3, *). Five minutes after, only the activity of the N-type is still present. The activity of the L-type will not reappear spontaneously. The extracellular solution contains (in mM): 90 BaCl₂, 15 TEACl, 2×10^{-3} TTX, 10 HEPES. The intra-pipette solution contains (in mM): 120 CsCl, 40 HEPES. Adapted from Armstrong D, Eckert R (1987) Voltage-activated calcium channels that must be phosphorylated to respond to membrane depolarization, *Proc. Natl Acad. Sci. USA* **84**, 2518–2522, with permission.

−15 mV, the channel opens, closes and reopens during the entire depolarization, showing little time-dependent inactivation (**Figure 6.3c**). The mean unitary conductance, γ_P, is 10–15 pS in 80 mM Ba²⁺. Recordings performed in dendrites or the soma of cerebellar Purkinje cells with patch clamp techniques (cell-attached patches) gave similar values of the unitary conductance ($\gamma_P = 9$–19 pS in 110 mM Ba²⁺), but for undetermined reasons the threshold for activation is at a more depolarized potential (−15 mV) than for isolated P channels inserted in lipid bilayers (−45 mV). When the funnel web toxin fraction (FTX) is added to the recording patch pipette (the intra-pipette solution bathes the extracellular side of the patch), only rare high-threshold unitary currents are recorded from Purkinje cell dendrites or soma at all potentials tested (Bay K 8644 or ω-conotoxin have no effect). These results suggest that the P channel is the predominant high-threshold Ca²⁺ channel expressed by Purkinje cells. They also show that the use of selective toxins allows the differentiation between P, N and L channels.

6.2.3 Macroscopic L, N and P-type Ca²⁺ currents activate at a high threshold and inactivate with different time courses

The macroscopic L, N and P-type Ca²⁺ currents (I_{Ca}), at time t during a depolarizing voltage step, are equal to: $I_{Ca} = Np_t i_{Ca}$ where N is number of L, N or P channels in the membrane, p_t is their probability of being open at time t during the depolarizing step, Np_t is the number of open channels at time t during the depolarizing step and i_{Ca} is the unitary L, N or P current. At steady state, $I_{Ca} = Np_o i_{Ca}$, where p_o is the probability of the channel being open at steady state.

The I/V relations for L, N and P-type Ca²⁺ currents have a bell shape with a peak amplitude at positive potentials

The *I/V* relation of the different types of high threshold Ca²⁺ currents is studied in whole cell recordings in the presence of external Ca²⁺ as the charge carrier. To separate the L, N and P currents, specific blockers are added

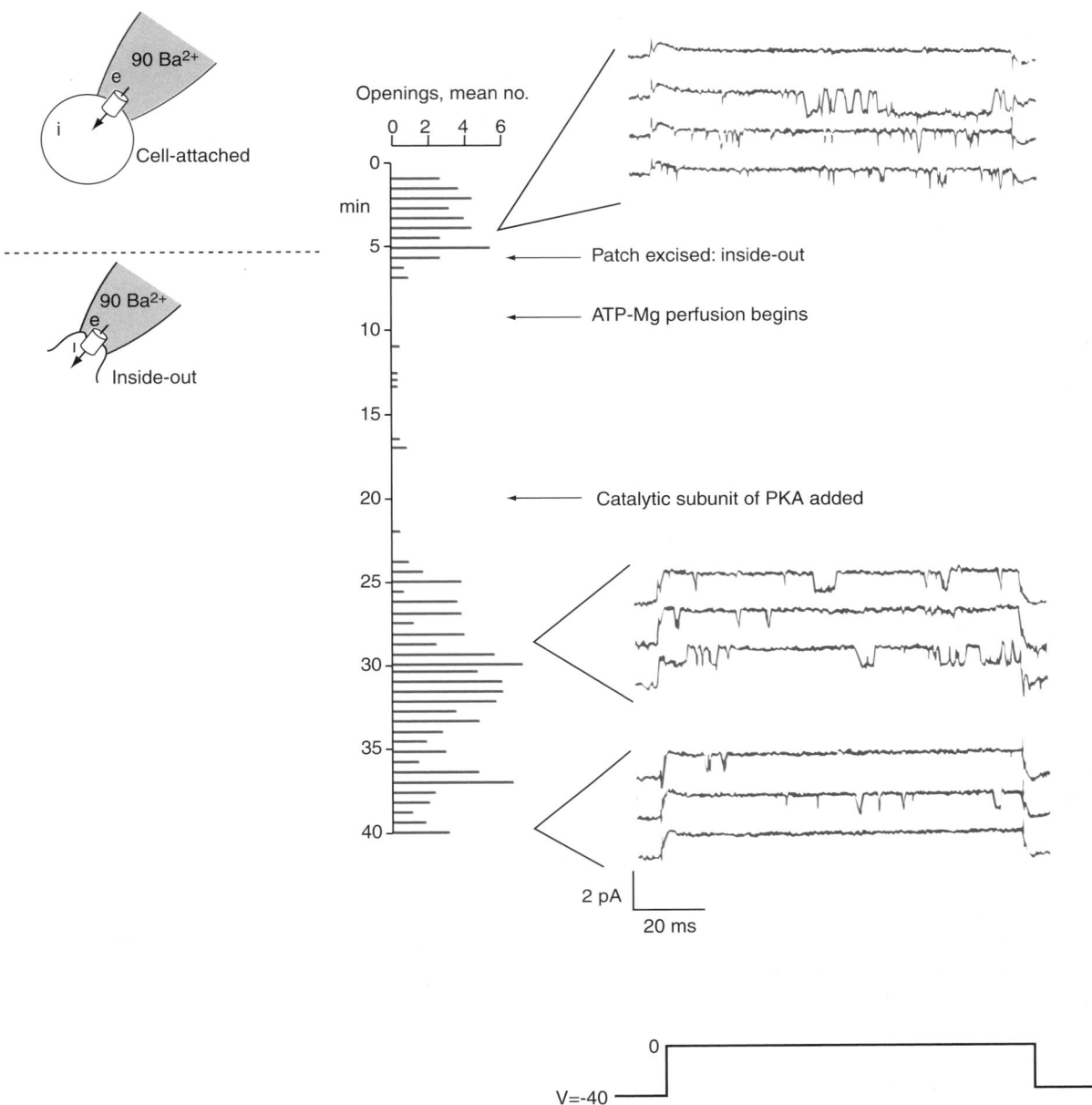

Figure 6.7 Phosphorylation reverses the loss of activity of the L channels in an inside-out patch.
The activity of an L-type channel is recorded in patch clamp (inside-out patch from a pituitary cell line in culture) in response to a depolarizing pulse to 0 mV from a holding potential of –40 mV. The horizontal traces are the unitary current traces and the vertical histogram represents the average number of channel openings per trace, determined over 30 s intervals and plotted versus time of the experiment (0–40 min). After 5 min of recording in the cell-attached configuration, the activity of the channel is recorded in the inside-out configuration. See text for further explanations. The intra-pipette solution contains (in mM): 90 BaCl$_2$, 15 TEACl, 2 x 10^{-3} TTX, 10 HEPES. The solution bathing the intracellular side of the patch contains (in mM): 120 CsCl, 40 HEPES. From Armstrong D, Eckert R (1987) Voltage-activated calcium channels that must be phosphorylated to respond to membrane depolarization, *Proc. Natl Acad. Sci. USA* **84**, 2518–2522, with permission.

to the external medium or the membrane potential is clamped at different holding potentials. With this last procedure, the L current can be separated from other Ca^{2+} currents since it can be evoked from depolarized holding potentials. As shown in **Figure 6.9**, the L and N currents averaged from the corresponding unitary currents recorded in 110 mM Ba^{2+} clearly differ in their time course. The averaged N current decays to zero level in 40 ms while the averaged L current remains constant during the 120 ms depolarizing step to +10 mV. As

(a)

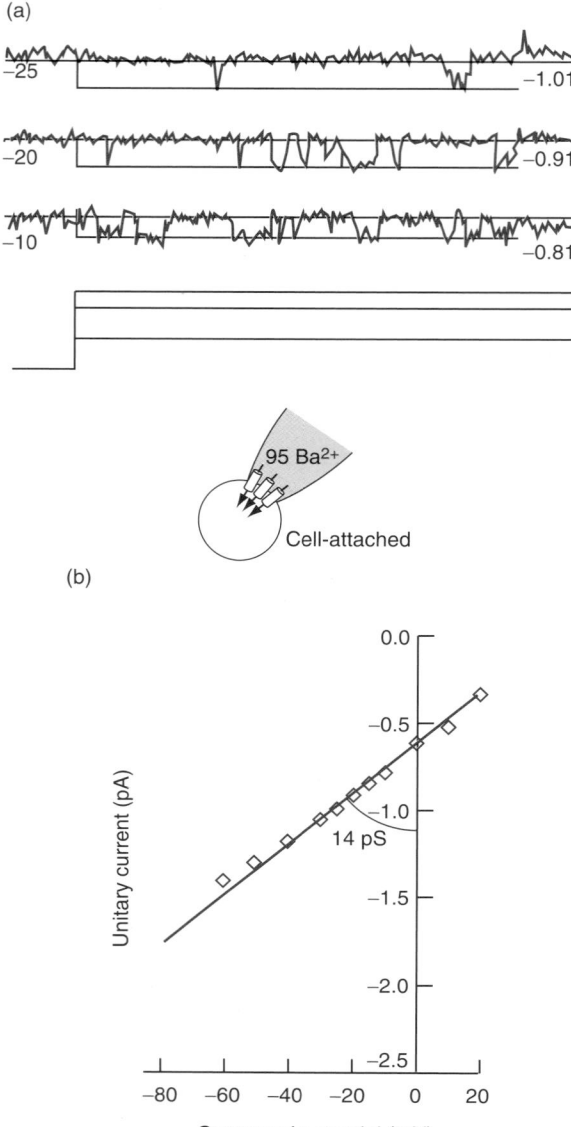

(b)

Unitary current (pA)

0.0

−0.5

14 pS

−1.0

−1.5

−2.0

−2.5

−80   −60   −40   −20   0   20

Command potential (mV)

Figure 6.8 Voltage dependence of the unitary N current, i_N.
(a) The activity of an N channel is recorded in patch clamp (cell-attached patch) in a granule cell of the hippocampus. The patch is depolarized to −25, −20 and −10 mV from a holding potential of −80 mV. The amplitude of the unitary current at these voltages is indicated at the end of each recording. (b) The unitary N current amplitude (i_N) is plotted against membrane potential (from −60 to +20 mV). The amplitude of i_N decreases linearly with depolarization between −60 and +20 mV with a slope $\gamma_N = 14$ pS ($n = 14$ patches). Adapted from Fisher RE, Gray R, Johnston D (1990) Properties and distribution of single voltage-gated calcium channels in adult hippocampal neurons, *J. Neurophysiol.* **64**, 91–104, with permission.

already observed (**Figures 6.3a and b**), by holding the membrane at a depolarized potential, the N current inactivates and the L current can be studied in isolation.

The macroscopic N- and L-type Ca^{2+} currents are studied in spinal motoneurons of the chick in patch clamp (whole cell patch) in the presence of Na^+ and K^+ channel blockers and in the presence of a T-type Ca^{2+} channel blocker. In response to a depolarizing voltage step to +20 mV from a holding potential of −80 mV, a mixed N and L whole cell current is recorded (**Figure 6.10a**). When the holding potential is depolarized to 0 mV, a voltage step to +20 mV now only evokes the L current (**Figure 6.10b**). The difference current obtained by subtracting the L current from the mixed N and L current gives the N current (**Figure 6.10c**). The I/V relations of these two Ca^{2+} currents have a bell shape with a peak around +20 mV (**Figures 6.10d and e**). For comparison the peak amplitude of the macroscopic Na^+ current is around −40 mV (see **Figure 5.12a**).

The macroscopic P-type Ca^{2+} current is studied in cerebellar Purkinje cells. These neurons express T, P and few L-type Ca^{2+} channels. In presence of Na^+ and K^+ channel blockers and by choosing a holding potential where the low threshold T current is inactivated, the macroscopic P current can be studied. The I_P/V relation has a bell shape. The maximal amplitude is recorded around −10 mV (**Figure 6.11**).

The bell shape of all the I_{Ca}/V relations is explained by the gating properties of the Ca^{2+} channels and the driving force for Ca^{2+} ions. The peak amplitude of I_{Ca} increases from the threshold potential to a maximal amplitude (**Figures 6.10d,e, 6.11b and 6.12a**) as a result of two opposite factors: the probability of opening which strongly increases with depolarization (**Figure 6.12b**) and the driving force for Ca^{2+} which linearly decreases with depolarization (i_{Ca} linearly diminishes). After a maximum, the peak amplitude of I_{Ca} decreases owing to the progressive decrease of the driving force for Ca^{2+} ions and the increase of the number of inactivated channels. Above +30/+40 mV, the probability of opening (p_o) no longer plays a role since it is maximal (**Figure 6.12b**). I_{Ca} reverses polarity between +50 mV and +100 mV, depending on the preparation studied. This value is well below the theoretical E_{Ca}.

This discrepancy is partly due to the strong asymmetrical concentrations of Ca^{2+} ions. To measure the reversal potential of I_{Ca}, the outward current through Ca^{2+} channels must be measured. This outward current, caused by the extremely small intracellular concentration of Ca^{2+} ions, is carried by Ca^{2+} ions but also by internal K^+ ions, which are around 10^6 times more concentrated than internal Ca^{2+} ions. This permeability of Ca^{2+} channels to K^+ ions 'pulls down' the reversal potential of I_{Ca} towards E_K.

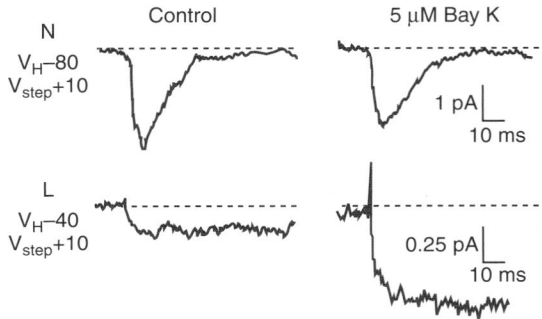

N
V_H−80
V_{step}+10

Control

5 µM Bay K

1 pA
10 ms

L
V_H−40
V_{step}+10

0.25 pA
10 ms

Figure 6.9 Averaged N- and L-type Ca²⁺ currents.
Single-channel N current averages (top traces) and L current averages (bottom traces) from cell-attached recordings of dorsal root ganglion cells with Ba²⁺ as the charge carrier (see also Figure 6.3a,b). Currents are averaged before (left) and after (right) exposure to 5 µM Bay K8644. Voltage steps from −80 mV to +10 mV (top traces) and from −40 to +10 mV (bottom traces). From Nowycky MC, Fox AP, Tsien RW (1985) Three types of neuronal calcium channel with different calcium agonist sensitivity, *Nature* **316**, 440–443, with permission.

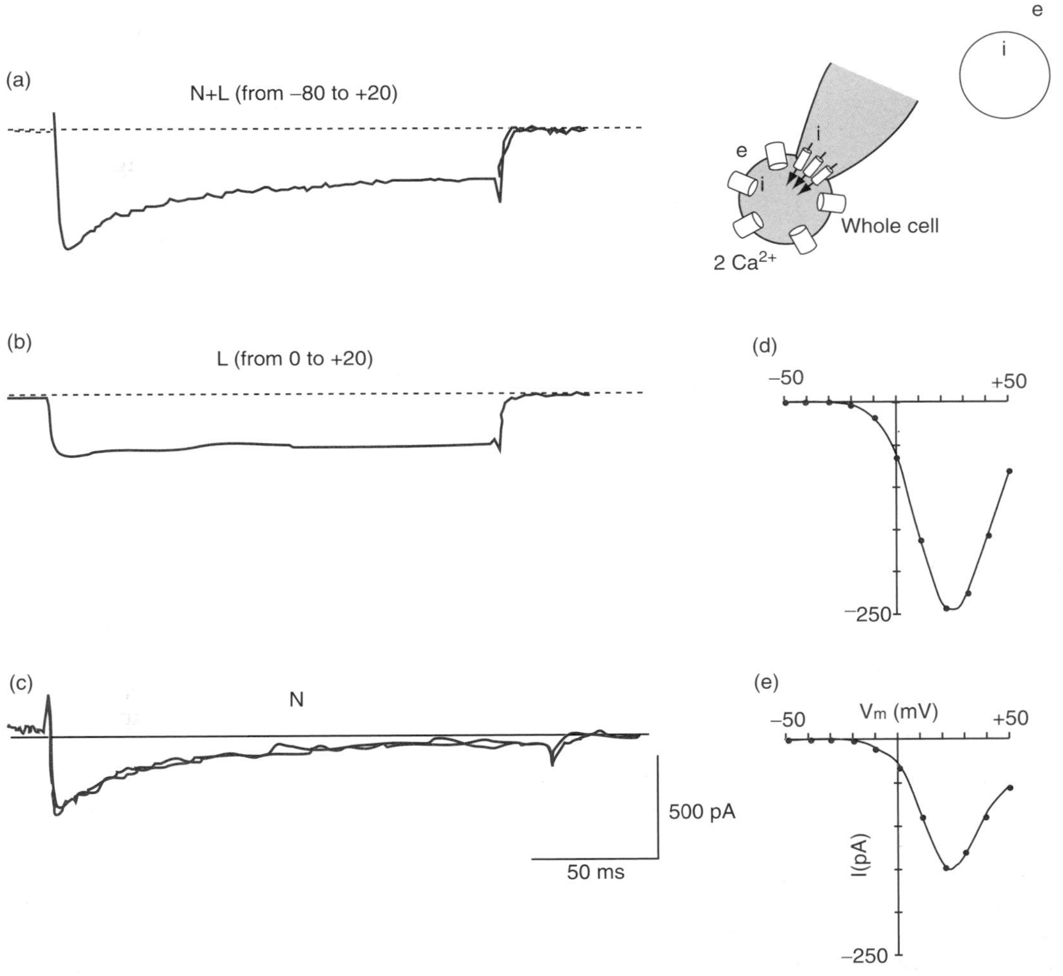

(a)

N+L (from −80 to +20)

e

i

e

i

Whole cell

2 Ca²⁺

(b)

L (from 0 to +20)

(d)

−50   +50

−250

(c)

N

500 pA

50 ms

(e)

−50 V_m (mV)   +50

I(pA)

−250

Figure 6.10 N- and L-type macroscopic Ca²⁺ currents.
(a) The mixed N and L macroscopic current is recorded with Ca²⁺ as the charge carrier (whole-cell patch) from chick limb motoneurons in culture in response to a voltage step from −80 to +20 mV. (b) The macroscopic L current is recorded in isolation by changing the holding potential to 0 mV. (c) The difference current obtained by subtracting the L current (b) from the N and L current (a) is the N current. (d) I/V relation for the L current recorded as in (b). (e) I/V relation for the N current obtained as the difference current. The intrapipette solution contains (in mM): 140 Cs aspartate, 5 MgCl₂, 10 Cs EGTA, 10 HEPES, 0.1 Li₂GTP, 1 MgATP. The bathing solution contains (in mM): 146 NaCl, 2 CaCl₂, 5 KCl, 1 MgCl₂, 10 HEPES. Adapted from McCobb DP, Best PM, Beam KG (1989) Development alters the expression of calcium currents in chick limb motoneurons, *Neuron* **2**, 1633–1643, with permission.

(a)

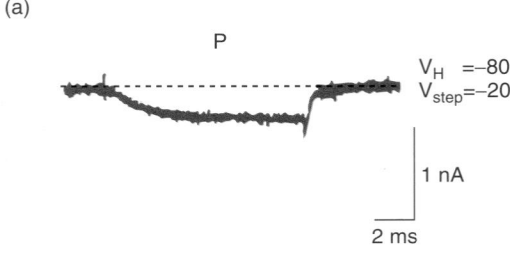

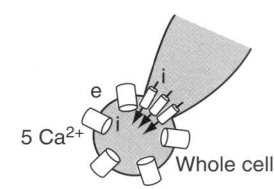

(b)

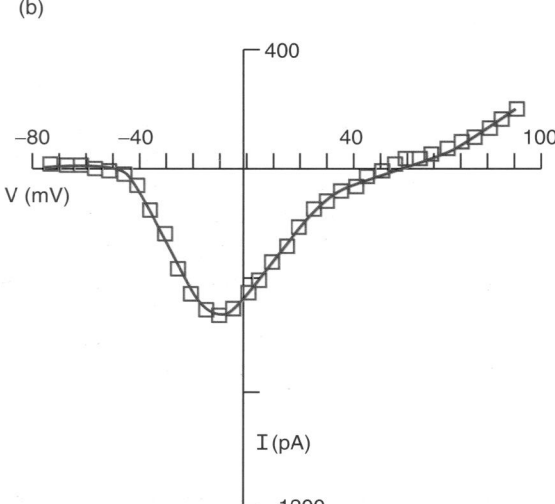

Figure 6.11 P-type macroscopic Ca²⁺ current.
The whole-cell P current recorded from acutely dissociated Purkinje cells (whole-cell patch) with Ca^{2+} as the charge carrier. **(a)** Whole-cell P current recorded in response to a depolarizing pulse to –20 mV from a holding potential of –80 mV. **(b)** I/V relation of the P current. In the recordings the low threshold T-type Ca^{2+} current was either absent, inactivated or subtracted. The intra-pipette solution contains (in mM): 120 TEA glutamate, 9 EGTA, 4.5 $MgCl_2$ 9 HEPES. The bathing solution contains (in mM): 5 $CaCl_2$, 154 TEACl, 0.2 $MgCl_2$, 10 glucose, 10 HEPES. Adapted from Reagan LJ (1991) Voltage-dependent calcium currents in Purkinje cells from rat cerebellar vermis, *J. Neurosci.* **7**, 2259–2269, with permission.

Activation–inactivation properties

Activation properties are analysed by recording the macroscopic L, N or P currents in response to increasing test depolarizations from a fixed hyperpolarized holding potential (–80 mV, **Figures 6.13b, 6.14b** and **6.15b**). In dorsal ganglion neurons, the L and N currents are half activated around 0 mV (**Figures 6.13c** and **6.14c**) while in Purkinje cells the P current is half activated around –20 mV (**Figure 6.15c**).

Voltage-gated Ca²⁺ channels show varying degrees of inactivation

Inactivation properties are analysed by recording the macroscopic L, N or P-type Ca^{2+} currents evoked by a voltage step to a fixed potential from various holding potentials (with Ca^{2+} as the charge carrier). The L current is half inactivated around –40 mV (**Figures 6.13a and c**), the N current around –60 mV (**Figures 6.14a and c**) and the P current around –45 mV (**Figures 6.15a and c**).

In summary, L channels generate a large Ca^{2+} current that is activated by large depolarizations to 0/+10 mV and inactivates with a very slow time course during a step. N and P channels generate smaller Ca^{2+} currents that are activated with depolarization to –30/0 mV and inactivate or not during a depolarizing step.

The inactivation process of Ca^{2+} channels can be voltage-dependent, time-dependent *and* calcium-dependent. Voltage-dependent inactivation is observed by changing the holding potential (see **Figures 6.13a, 6.14a** and **6.15a**). Time-dependent inactivation is observed during a long depolarizing step, in presence of Ba^{2+} as the change carrier (**Figure 6.16**). Ca^{2+}-dependent inactivation depends on the amount of Ca^{2+} influx through open Ca^{2+} channels. It can be considered as a negative feedback control of Ca^{2+} channels by Ca^{2+} channels.

Calcium-dependent inactivation

Several lines of evidence point to the existence of a Ca^{2+}-induced inactivation of Ca^{2+} currents:

■ The degree of inactivation is proportional to the amplitude and frequency of the Ca^{2+} current.
■ Intracellular injection of Ca^{2+} ions into neurons produces inactivation.
■ Intracellular injection of Ca^{2+} chelators such as EGTA or BAPTA reduces inactivation (**Figure 6.17**).
■ Substitution of Ca^{2+} ions with Sr^{2+} or Ba^{2+} reduces inactivation.
■ Very large depolarizations to near E_{Ca}, where the entry of Ca^{2+} ions is small, produce little inactivation.

Recordings of L and N channels in **Figures 6.13** and **6.14** were obtained with Ca^{2+} as the charge carrier and that of

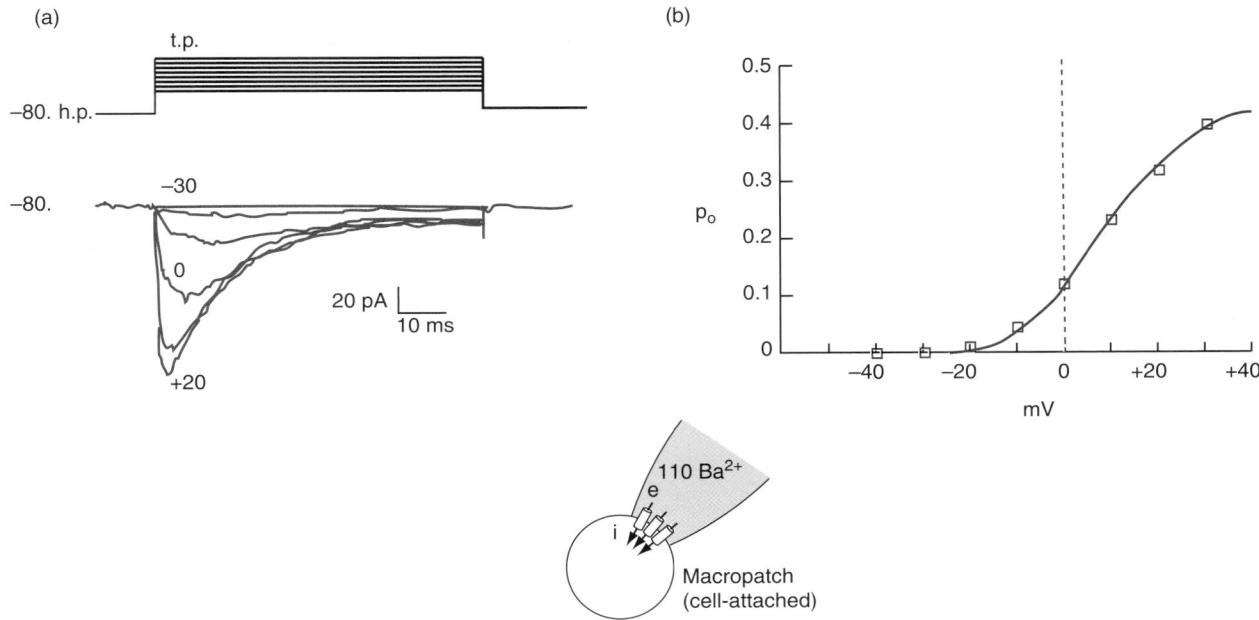

Figure 6.12 The peak opening probability of the N current.
The macroscopic N current is recorded in a dorsal root ganglion neuron from a cell-attached patch containing hundreds of N channels (macropatch). **(a)** Current recordings (bottom traces) in response to test potentials (t.p.) ranging from –30 mV to +20 mV from a holding potential (h.p.) of –80 mV (upper traces). **(b)** Voltage-dependence of the peak opening probability (p_o) from data obtained in (a). Values of p_o are obtained by dividing the peak current I by the unitary current i_N obtained at each test potential and by an estimate of the number of channels in the patch (599): $p_o = I/Ni_N$. N was determined by comparison with the single-channel experiment in Figure 6.3b, which shows that in response to a depolarization to +20 mV from a holding potential of –80 mV, $p_o = 0.32$ and $i_N = 0.76$ pA. I, the peak current evoked by the same voltage protocol, is 145 pA. $N = I/p_o i_N = 145/(0.32 \times 0.76) = 599$ channels. The intra-pipette solution contains (in mM): 100 CsCl, 10 Cs-EGTA, 5 MgCl$_2$, 40 HEPES, 2 ATP, 0.25 cAMP; pH = 7.3. The extracellular solution contains (in mM): 10 CaCl$_2$, 135 TEACl, 10 HEPES, 0.2 × 10^{-3} TTX; pH = 7.3. From Nowycky MC, Fox AP, Tsien RW (1985) Three types of neuronal calcium channel with different calcium agonist sensitivity, *Nature* **316**, 440–443, with permission.

P channels in **Figure 6.15** with Ba^{2+} as the charge carrier. Therefore, the inactivation seen in **Figures 6.13** and **6.14** results from voltage, time and the increase of intracellular Ca^{2+} ions. In contrast, the inactivation of the P current observed in **Figure 6.15** is a voltage- and time-dependent process.

The macroscopic Ca^{2+} current of *Aplysia* neurons is recorded in voltage clamp. During depolarizing voltage steps, the Ca^{2+} current increases to a peak and then declines to a steady state Ca^{2+} current (a non-inactivating component of current). The buffering of cytoplasmic free Ca^{2+} ions with EGTA increases the amplitude of the peak current and that of the steady-state current (**Figure 6.17**). This shows that the increase of intracellular Ca^{2+} ions resulting from Ca^{2+} entry through Ca^{2+} channels causes Ca^{2+} current inactivation. It also shows that the peak current is probably already decreased in amplitude owing to early development of inactivation.

In L-type Ca^{2+} channels of cardiac muscle cells, a Ca^{2+}-binding motif located in the COOH terminus of the α_{1C}-subunit provides the Ca^{2+} binding site that initiates

Ca^{2+}-sensitive inactivation. L channels are transiently expressed in HEK 293 cells from cDNA encoding the native α_{1C} or α_{1E} subunits or from a chimeric cDNA encoding an α-subunit where the entire COOH terminus of α_{1E} is substituted into α_{1C} (α_{1E} forms a neuronal Ca^{2+} channel lacking Ca^{2+} inactivation). All these α subunits are co-expressed with a β-subunit (β_{2a}) in order to ensure robust expression. Ca^{2+} and Ba^{2+} currents are recorded from the chimeric Ca^{2+} channel. Since no Ca^{2+}-dependent inactivation is recorded from the chimeric Ca^{2+} channel, the α_{1C} COOH terminus appears essential for the initiation of Ca^{2+} inactivation in this α-subunit.

6.3 The repolarization phase of Ca^{2+}-dependent action potentials results from the activation of K$^+$ currents I_K and $I_{K(Ca)}$

The K$^+$ currents involved in calcium spike repolarization are the delayed rectifier (I_K) studied above and the Ca^{2+}-activated K$^+$ currents ($I_{K(Ca)}$). Meech and

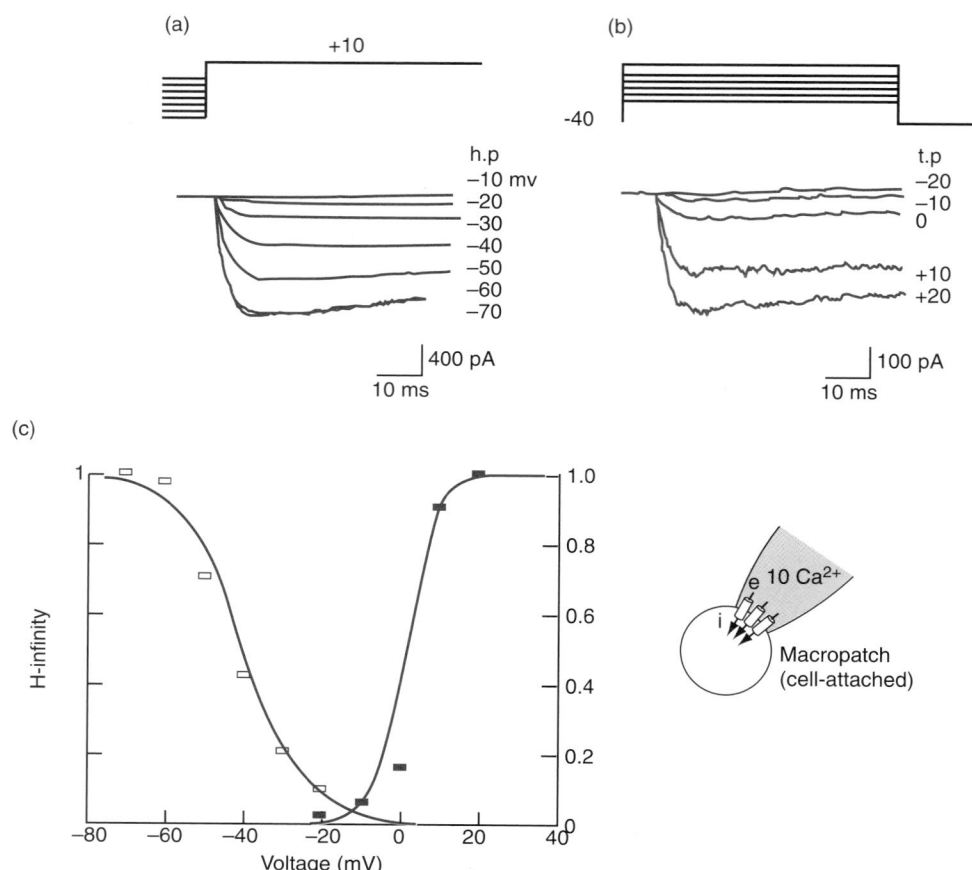

Figure 6.13 Voltage dependence of activation and inactivation of the L-type Ca²⁺ current.
The macroscopic L current is recorded in a cell with very little T or N current. **(a)** Inactivation of the L current with holding potential: a test depolarization to +10 mV is applied from holding potentials (h.p.) varying from −70 to −10 mV. **(b)** Activation of the L current with depolarization: test depolarizations (t.p.) to −30, −20, −10, 0, +10 and +20 mV are applied from a holding potential of −40 mV. **(c)** Activation–inactivation curves obtained from the data in (b) and (a), respectively. The peak Ca²⁺ current amplitudes (I) are normalized to the maximal current ($I_{max} = 1$) obtained in each set of experiments and plotted against the holding (inactivation curve, □) or test potential (activation curve, ●). For the activation curve, data are plotted as $I = I_{max}\{1 + \exp[(V_{1/2} - V)/k]\}^{-1}$ and for the inactivation curve as $I = I_{max}\{1 + \exp[(V - V_{1/2})/k]\}^{-1}$. $V_{1/2}$ is the voltage at which the current I is half-activated ($I = I_{max}/2$ when $V_{1/2} = 2$ mV) or half-inactivated ($I = I_{max}/2$ when $V_{1/2} = -40$ mV). All the recordings are performed in the presence of 10 mM Ca²⁺ in the recording pipette solution which bathes the extracellular side of the channels. Adapted from Fox AP, Nowycky M, Tsien RW (1987) Kinetic and pharmacological properties distinguishing three types of calcium currents in chick sensory neurones, *J. Physiol.* **394**, 149–172, with permission.

Strumwasser in 1970 were the first to describe that a microinjection of Ca²⁺ ions into *Aplysia* neurons activates a K⁺ conductance and hyperpolarizes the membrane. On the basis of these results, the authors postulated the existence of a Ca²⁺-activated K⁺ conductance. The amount of participation of Ca²⁺-activated K⁺ currents in spike repolarization depends on the cell type.

6.3.1 The Ca²⁺-activated K⁺ currents are classified as big K (BK) channels and small K (SK) channels

Big K channels have a high conductance (100–250 pS depending on K⁺ concentrations) and are sensitive to both voltage *and* Ca²⁺ ions so that their apparent sensitivity to Ca²⁺ ions is increased when the membrane is depolarized. Their activity is blocked by TEA and charybdotoxin, a toxin from scorpion venom. Small K channels have a smaller conductance (10–80 pS depending on K⁺ concentrations) and are insensitive to TEA and

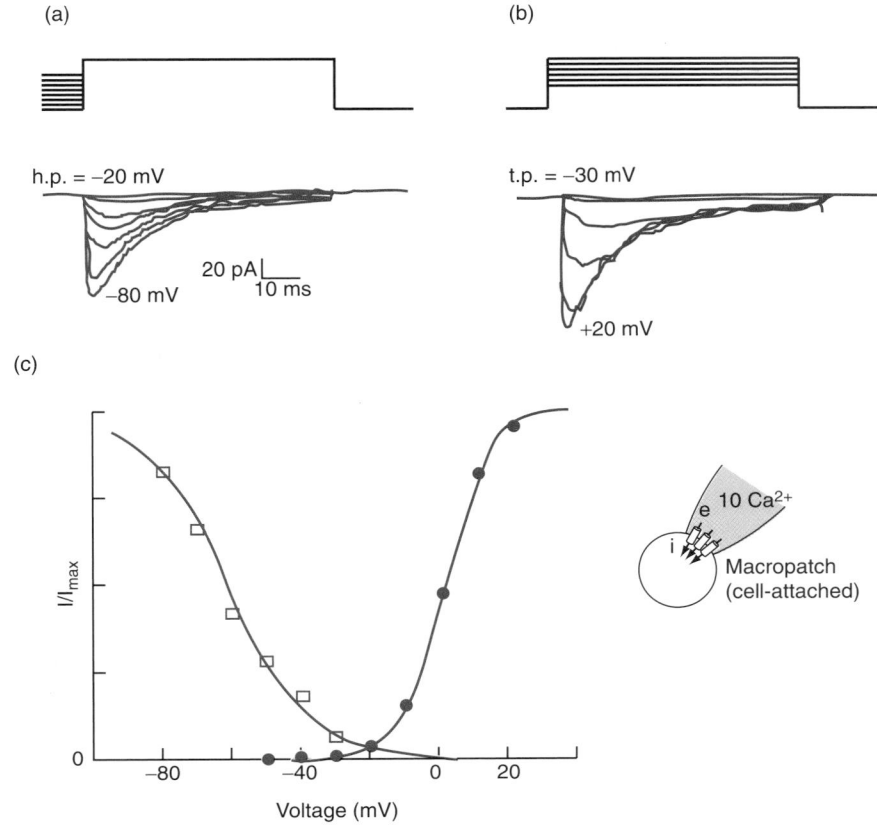

Figure 6.14 Voltage dependence of activation and inactivation of the N-type Ca²⁺ current.
The macroscopic N current is recorded in cell-attached patches containing hundreds of channels (macropatch). **(a)** Inactivation of the N current with holding potential: test depolarization to +10 mV is applied from holding potentials (h.p.) varying from −70 to −10 mV. **(b)** Activation of the N current with depolarization: test depolarizations (t.p.) to −30, −20, −10, 0, +10 and +20 mV are applied from a holding potential of −80 mV. **(c)** Activation–inactivation curves obtained from the data in (b) and (a), respectively. The peak Ca²⁺ current amplitudes (I) are normalized to the maximal current (I_{max} = 1) obtained in each set of experiments and plotted against the holding (inactivation curve, □) or test potential (activation curve, ●). For the activation curve, data are plotted as $I = I_{max}\{1 + \exp[(V_{1/2} = V)/k)]\}^{-1}$ and for the inactivation curve as $I = I_{max}\{1 + \exp[(V - V_{1/2}/k)]\}^{-1}$. $V_{1/2}$ is the voltage at which the current I is half-activated ($I = I_{max}/2$ when $V_{1/2}$ = 1.5 mV) or half-inactivated ($I = I_{max}/2$ when $V_{1/2}$ = −61.5 mV). The number of channels is estimated as in Figure 6.12. Adapted from Fox AP, Nowycky MC, Tsien RW (1987) Single-channel recordings of three types of calcium channels in chick sensory neurones, *J. Physiol.* **394**, 173–200, with permission.

charybdotoxin but sensitive to apamin, a toxin from bee venom. It is a heterogeneous class containing both voltage-dependent and voltage-independent channels. Big K and small K channels are very selective for K⁺ ions over Na⁺ ions and are activated by increases in the concentration of cytoplasmic Ca²⁺ ions.

Biochemical purification of big K channels from mammalian smooth muscle shows that they are composed of two structurally distinct subunits, α and β. The β-subunits are encoded by a single gene that undergoes alternative splicing. The primary structure of the α-subunits of big K channels reveals a core domain similar to that of other voltage-gated channels that has six putative transmembrane segments (S1 to S6), a string of regularly spaced positive charges in S4 and a highly conserved region between S5 and S6 defining the pore. The primary sequence is approximately twice the length of that of other voltage-gated K⁺ channels. This additional length is due to an appended sequence on the carboxyl side of the core domain. This raises the possibility that the additional C-terminal sequence may participate in functions particular to big K channels such as Ca²⁺-dependent gating. The smaller β-subunit shows no homology with other ion channel subunits.

Although expression of the α-subunit alone in *Xenopus* oocytes is sufficient to generate K⁺ channels that are gated by voltage and Ca²⁺, these properties are quantitatively different from the native ones. Currents from cells expressing α/β heteromultimers more closely resemble those of native channels. Immunoprecipitation

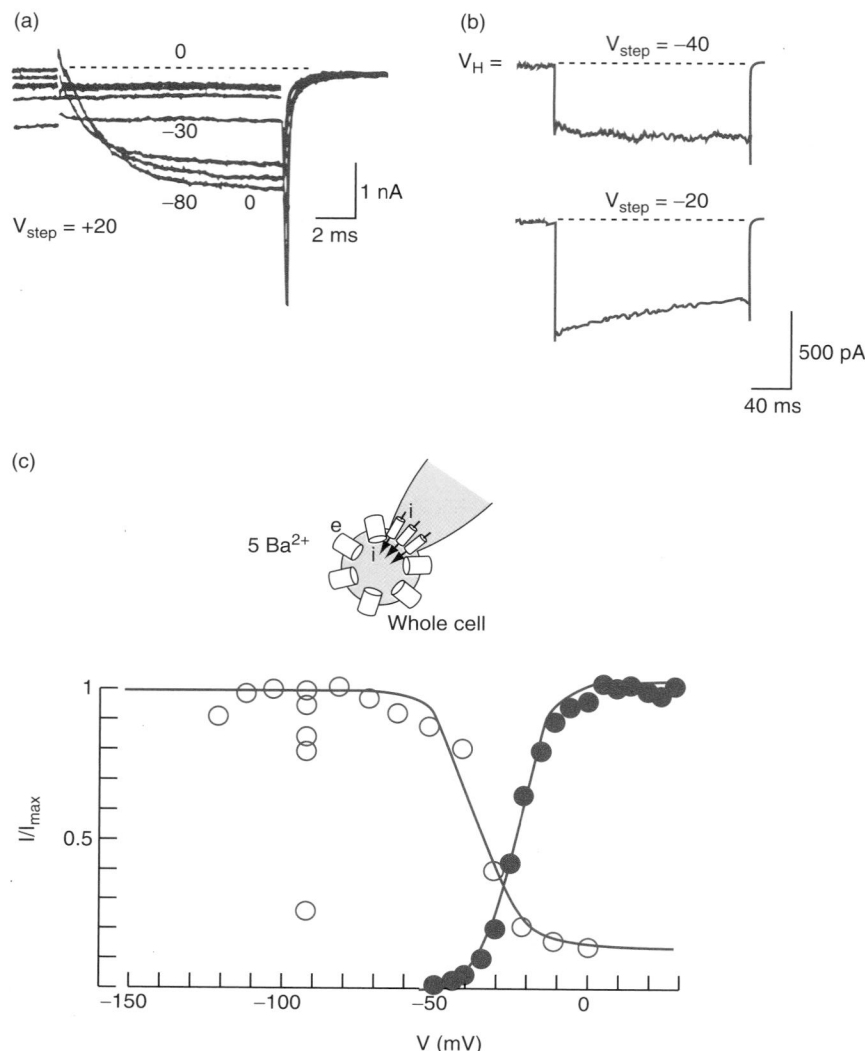

Figure 6.15 Voltage dependence of activation and inactivation of the P-type Ca²⁺ current.
The macroscopic P current is recorded in Purkinje cells (whole-cell patch). The T-type Ca^{2+} current present in these cells is either absent or subtracted. **(a)** Inactivation of the P current with holding potential: a test depolarization to +20 mV is applied from holding potentials varying from –80 to 0 mV. **(b)** Activation of the P current with depolarization: test depolarizations (V_{step}) to –40 and –20 mV are applied from a holding potential of –110 mV. **(c)** Activation–inactivation curves obtained from the data obtained in (b) and (a), respectively. The peak Ca^{2+} current amplitudes (I) are normalized to the maximal current ($I_{max} = 1$) obtained in each set of experiments and plotted against the holding (inactivation curve, ○) or test potential (activation curve, ●). For the activation curve, data are plotted as $I = I_{max}\{1 + \exp [(V_{1/2} - V)/k)]\}^{-1}$ and for the inactivation curve as $I = I_{max}\{1 + \exp [(V - V_{1/2})/k)]\}^{-1}$. $V_{1/2}$ is the voltage at which the current I is half-activated ($I = I_{max}/2$ when $V_{1/2} = -22$ mV) or half-inactivated ($I = I_{max}/2$ when $V_{1/2} = -34$ mV). In all recordings, the extracellular solution contains 5 mM Ba²⁺. Adapted from Regan L (1991) Voltage-dependent calcium currents in Purkinje cells from rat cerebellar vermis, *J. Neurosci.* **11**, 2259–2269, with permission.

experiments indicate that the two subunits are tightly associated since antibodies directed against one subunit can precipitate both subunits. These data suggest that both α and β subunits contribute to the functional properties of big K channels and that the α-subunit forms part of the transduction machinery of the channels.

6.3.2 Ca²⁺ entering during the depolarization or the plateau phase of Ca²⁺-dependent action potentials activates K_(Ca) channels

To study Ca²⁺-activated K⁺ channels from rat brain neurons, plasma membrane vesicle preparation is

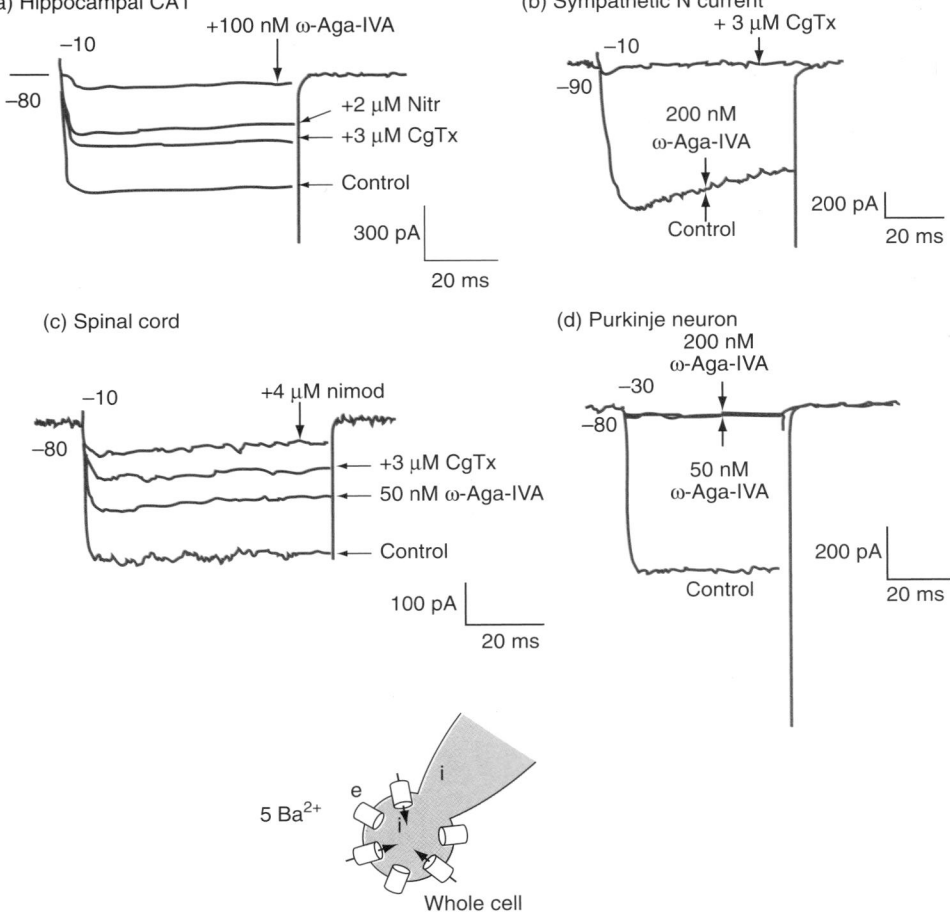

Figure 6.16 Pharmacology of L-, N- and P-type Ca²⁺ channels.
The macroscopic mixed Ca²⁺ currents are recorded in different neurons with Ba²⁺ as the charge carrier (whole-cell patch). High threshold Ca²⁺ currents are evoked by depolarizations to −30 or −10 mV from a holding potential of −90 or −80 mV. Various blockers or toxins are applied in order to block selectively one type of high-threshold Ca²⁺ current at a time: ω-conotoxin (CgTx, 3 μM) selectively blocks N current, nitrendipine or nimodipine (nitr., nimod., 2–4 μM) selectively blocks L current, and ω-agatoxin (ω-Aga-IVA, 50–200 nM) selectively blocks P current. In hippocampal cells of the CA1 region and in spinal cord interneurons, the high-threshold Ca²⁺ current is a mixed N, L and P current. In sympathetic neurons it is almost exclusively N and in Purkinje cells almost exclusively P. The intra-pipette solution contains (in mM): 108 Cs methanesulphonate, 4 MgCl₂, 9 EGTA, 9 HEPES, 4 MgATP, 14 creatine phosphate, 1 GTP; pH = 7.4. The extracellular solution contains (in mM): 5 BaCl₂, 160 TEACl, 0.1 EGTA, 10 HEPES; pH = 7.4. Adapted from Mintz IM, Adams ME, Bean B (1992) P-type calcium channels in rat central and peripheral neurons, *Neuron* **9**, 85–95, with permission.

incorporated into planar lipid bilayers. In such conditions, the activity of four distinct types of Ca²⁺-activated K⁺ channels is recorded. We will look at one example of a big K and one example of a small K channel. This preparation allows the recording of single-channel activity (**Figure 6.18**).

The current–voltage relations obtained in the presence of two different extracellular K⁺ concentrations show that the current reverses at E_K, the theoretical reversal potential for K⁺ ions as expected for a purely K⁺-selective channel. The Ca²⁺-dependence is studied by raising the

intracellular Ca²⁺ concentration in the range of 0.1–10 μM. Channels are activated by micromolar concentrations of Ca²⁺. The open probabilities of the big K and small K channels are largely increased when the medium bathing the intracellular side of the membrane contains 0.4 μM Ca²⁺ instead of 0.1 μM (**Figures 6.19a and b**). For comparison the Ca²⁺-sensitivity of big K channels from cultured rat skeletal muscle is shown in **Figure 6.19c**. The rat brain big K channels are sensitive to nanomolar concentrations of charybdotoxin (CTX) and millimolar concentrations of extracellular TEA ions (**Figure 6.20**).

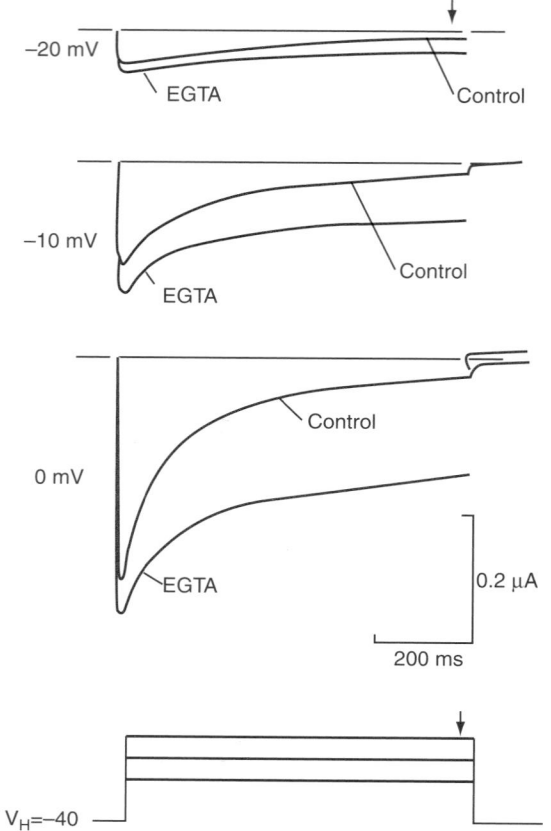

Figure 6.17 Intracellular EGTA slows Ca²⁺-dependent inactivation of Ca²⁺ channels.

The macroscopic Ca²⁺ current is recorded in axotomized *Aplysia* neurons in double-electrode voltage clamp (axotomy is performed in order to improve space clamp). Control Ca²⁺ currents are recorded in response to step depolarizations to –20, –10 and 0 mV from a holding potential of –40 mV (control traces). Iontophoretic ejection of EGTA (300–500 nA for 4–8 min) increases the peak amplitude of the Ca²⁺ current and slows its inactivation at all potentials tested (EGTA traces). The amplitude of the non-inactivating component of the current is measured at the end of the steps (arrow). Adapted from Chad J, Eckert R, Ewald D (1984) Kinetics of calcium-dependent inactivation of calcium current in voltage-clamped neurones in *Aplysia californica*, J. *Physiol. (Lond.)* **347**, 279–300, with permission.

The macroscopic Ca²⁺-activated K⁺ currents are recorded from a bullfrog sympathetic neuron in a single-electrode voltage clamp (V_H = –28 mV). The iontophoretic injection of Ca²⁺ ions through the intracellular recording electrode triggers an outward current (**Figure 6.21a**). Its amplitude increases when the iontophoretic current is increased ; i.e. the amount of Ca²⁺ ions injected is increased. To study the voltage-dependence and the kinetics of activation of this Ca²⁺-activated outward current, depolarizing steps from a holding potential of –50 mV are applied in the presence

of 2 mM of Ca²⁺ in the extracellular medium (**Figure 6.21b**, 2 Ca). Suppression of Ca²⁺ entry by removal of Ca²⁺ ions from the extracellular medium (0 Ca) eliminates an early Ca²⁺-activated outward current. In the Ca-free medium, only the sigmoidal delayed rectifier K⁺ current I_K is recorded. In the presence of external Ca²⁺ ions, both I_K and a $I_{K(Ca)}$ are recorded (**Figure 6.21b**, right). The recorded $I_{K(Ca)}$ corresponds to a big K current also called I_C in some preparations. It has activation kinetics sufficiently rapid to play a role in spike repolarization (**Figure 6.22**).

In nerve terminals at the motor end plate, big K channels are co-localized with voltage-dependent Ca²⁺ channels. They play an important role in repolarizing the plasma membrane following each action potential. This repolarization resulting from the increased activity of Ca²⁺-activated K⁺ channels closes voltage-dependent Ca²⁺ channels and constitutes an important feedback mechanism for the regulation of voltage-dependent Ca²⁺ entry. $K_{(Ca)}$ current thereby lowers intracellular Ca²⁺ concentration and dampens neurotransmitter secretion. Conversely when it is strongly reduced by TEA or apamin, transmitter release is increased.

6.4 Calcium-dependent action potentials are initiated in axon terminals as in dendrites

6.4.1 Depolarization of the membrane to the threshold for the activation of L-, N- and P-type Ca⁺ channels has two origins

L-, N- and P-type Ca²⁺ channels are high-threshold Ca²⁺ channels. This means that they are activated in response to a relatively large membrane depolarization. In cells (e.g. neurons, heart muscle cells) where the resting membrane potential is around –80/–60 mV, a 40–60 mV depolarization is therefore needed to activate the high-threshold Ca²⁺ channels. Such a membrane depolarization is too large to result directly from the summation of excitatory postsynaptic potentials (EPSPs). This depolarization usually results from a Na⁺ spike. In heart Purkinje cells, Na⁺ entry during the sudden depolarization phase of the action potential depolarizes the membrane to the threshold for L-type Ca²⁺ channel activation: the Na⁺-dependent depolarization phase is immediately followed by a Ca²⁺-dependent plateau (see **Figure 5.2d**). In axon terminals, the situation is similar: the Na⁺-dependent action potential actively propagates to axon terminals where it depolarizes the membrane to the threshold potential for N- or P-type Ca²⁺ channel activation: a Na⁺/Ca²⁺-dependent action potential is initiated (see **Figure 5.2c**).

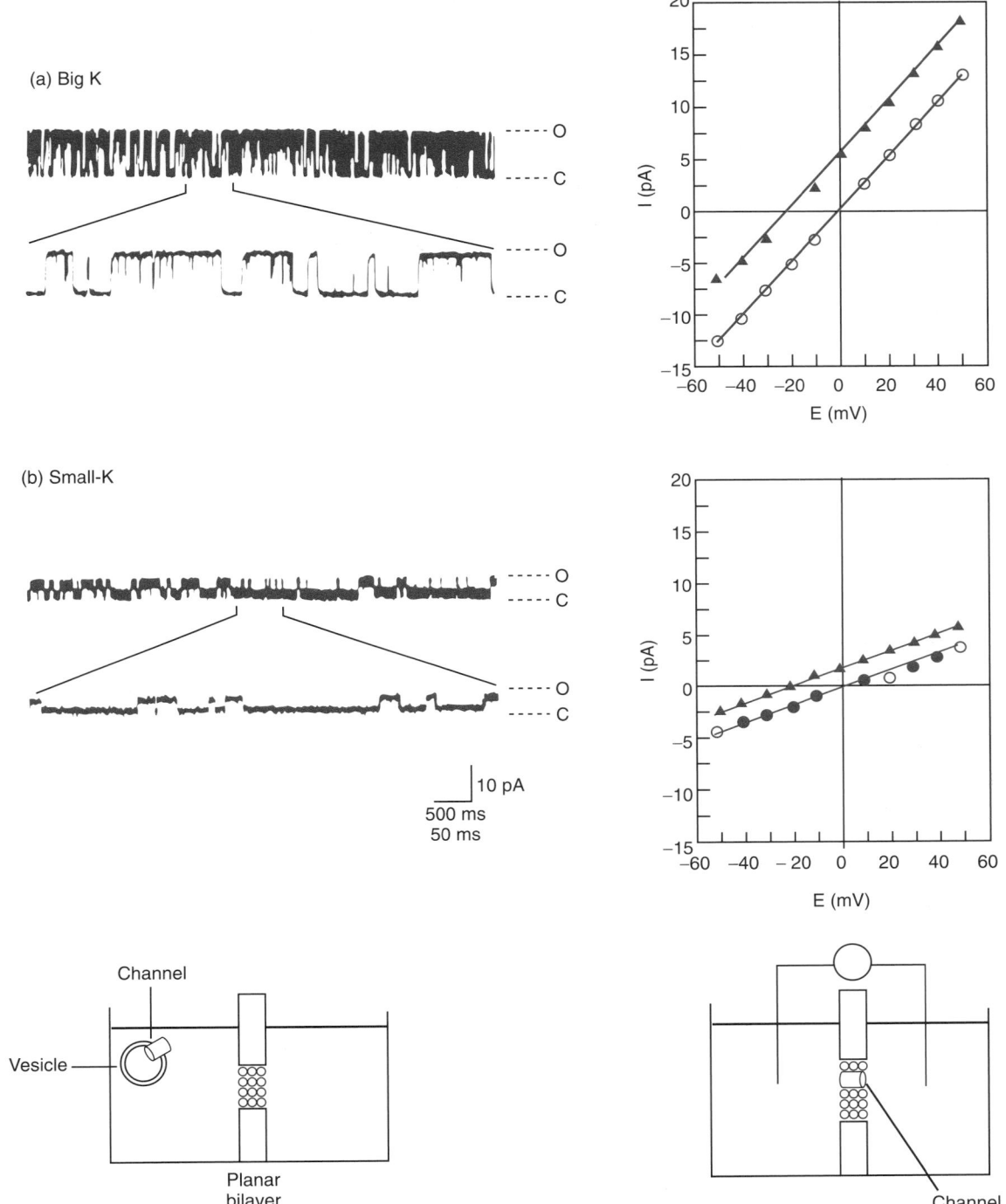

Figure 6.18 Two types of rat brain Ca^{2+}-activated K$^+$ channels incorporated into lipid bilayers.
(a, b) Left: Single-channel recordings in symmetrical K$^+$ (the extracellular and intracellular solutions contain 150 mM KCl) at V_H = 40 mV. For all traces channel openings correspond to upward deflections. The recording length of upper traces is 6.4 s and each lower trace is expanded to show a 640 ms recording. Right: I/V relations for the big K channel and the small K channel in symmetrical K$^+$ (150 mM, circles) and 150 mM KCl inside, 50 mM KCl outside (triangles). The slope conductance for each of these channels in symmetrical 150 mM KCl is 232 pS (big K channel) and 77 pS (small K channel). All the recordings are performed in the presence of 1.05 mM CaCl$_2$ in the intracellular solution. Adapted from Reinhart PH, Chung S, Levitan IB (1989) A family of calcium-dependent potassium channels from rat brain, *Neuron* **2**, 1031–1041, with permission.

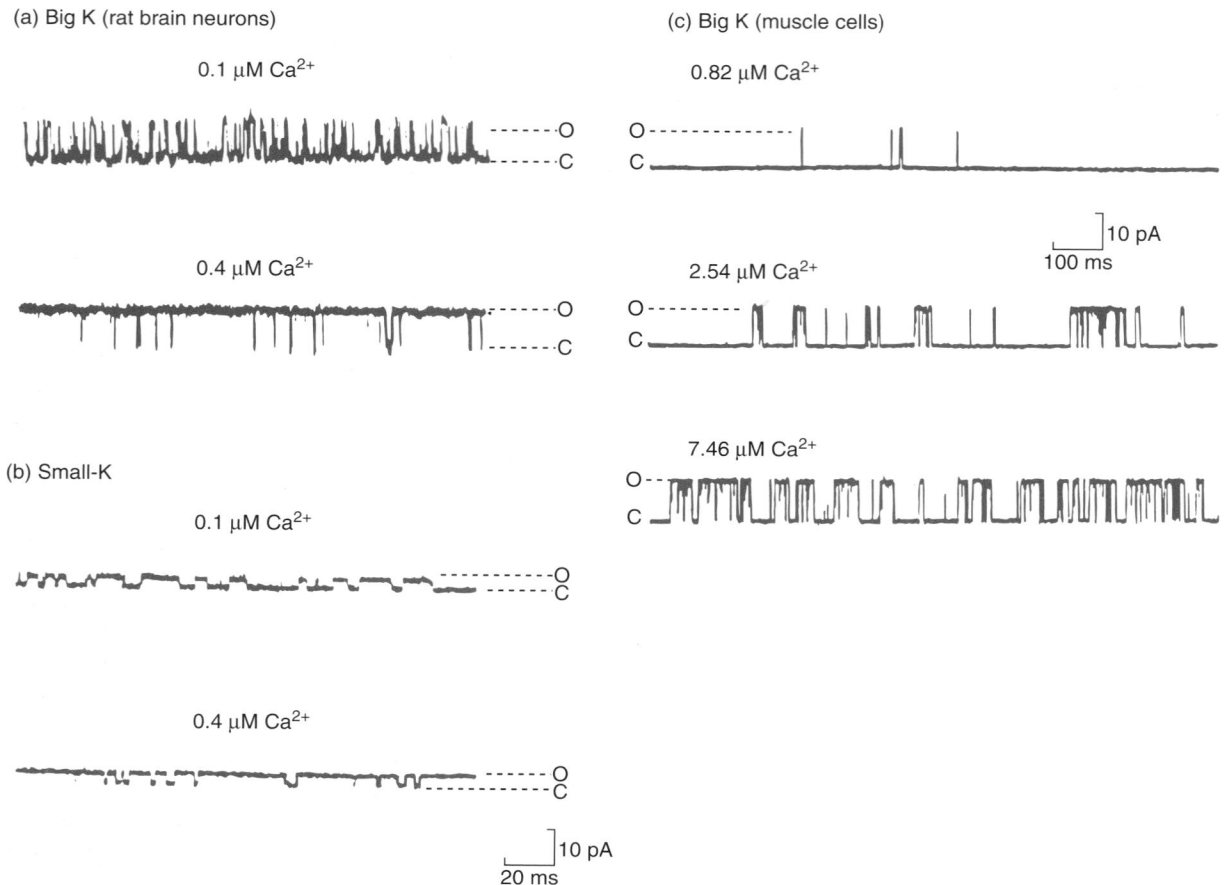

Figure 6.19 Ca²⁺-dependence of Ca²⁺-activated K⁺ channels.

(a, b) Single-channel activity of Ca²⁺-activated channels from the rat brain. The activity of the 232 pS big K channel and that of the 77 pS small K channel is recorded in the presence of 0.1 μM Ca²⁺ (upper traces) and 0.4 μM Ca²⁺ (lower traces) in symmetrical 150 mM KCl (V_H = +20 mV). **(c)** Single-channel activity of a big K channel from rat skeletal muscle recorded at three different Ca²⁺ concentrations in symmetrical 140 mM KCl (V_H = +30 mV). O, open state; C, closed state. Part (a) from Chad J, Eckert R, Ewald D (1984) Kinetics of calcium-dependent inactivation of calcium current in voltage-clamped neurones in *Aplysia californica, J. Physiol. (Lond.)* **347**, 279–300, with permission. Part (b) adapted from McManus OB, Magleby KL (1991) Accounting for the calcium-dependent kinetics of single large-conductance Ca²⁺-activated K⁺ channels in rat skeletal muscle, *J. Physiol.* **443**: 739–777, with permission.

In cerebellar Purkinje neurons the situation is somehow different: dendritic P-type Ca²⁺ channels are opened by the large EPSP resulting from climbing fibre EPSP. As a result, Ca²⁺-dependent action potentials are initiated and actively propagate in dendrites (see **Figure 5.2b**; also see Sections 19.2 and 20.3).

The cells that do not express voltage-gated Na⁺ channels and initiate Ca²⁺-dependent action potentials (endocrine cells for example; see **Figure 6.1**) usually present a depolarized resting membrane potential (–50/ –40 mV) close to the threshold for L-type Ca²⁺ channel activation. In such cells, the activation of high-threshold Ca²⁺ channels results from a depolarizing current generated by receptor activation or from an intrinsic pacemaker current (for example, activation of the T-type Ca²⁺ current – see Section 17.2.2 – or the turning off of a leak K⁺ current).

6.4.2 The role of the calcium-dependent action potentials is to provide a local and transient increase of [Ca²⁺]ᵢ to trigger secretion, contraction and other Ca²⁺-gated processes

In some neurons, Ca²⁺ entry through high-threshold Ca²⁺ channels participates in the generation of various forms of electrical activity such as dendritic Ca²⁺ spikes

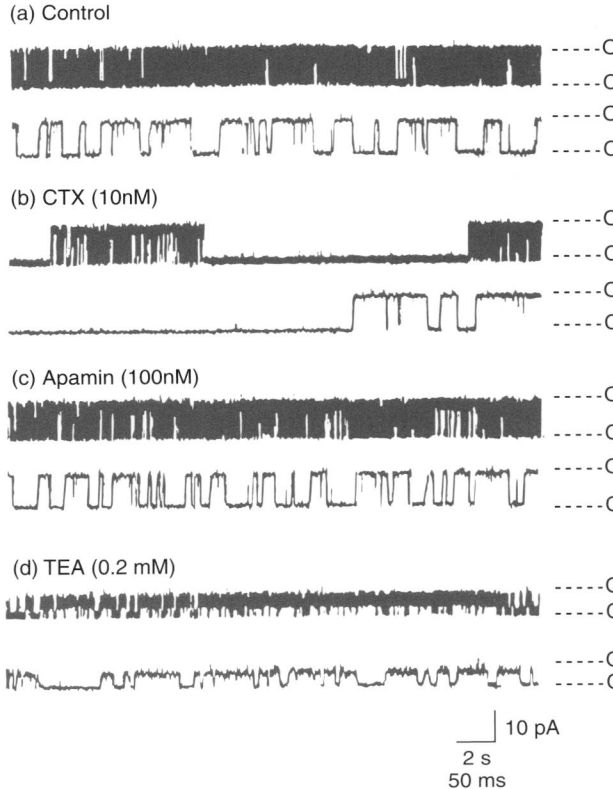

(a) Control

----O
----C
----O
----C

(b) CTX (10nM)

----O
----C
----O
----C

(c) Apamin (100nM)

----O
----C
----O
----C

(d) TEA (0.2 mM)

----O
----C
----O
----C

| 10 pA
2 s
50 ms

Figure 6.20 Pharmacology of the big K channel.
Single-channel activity of the big K channel (232 pS channel) in symmetrical 150 mM KCl at two different time bases (V_H = +40 mV). **(a)** Control conditions. **(b–d)** In the presence in the extracellular solution of, respectively, 10 nM charybdotoxin (CTX), 100 nM apamin, and 0.2 mM tetraethylammonium chloride (TEA). All the recordings are performed in the presence of 1.05 mM Ca^{2+} in the intracellular solution. From Chad J, Eckert R, Ewald D (1984) Kinetics of calcium-dependent inactivation of calcium current in voltage-clamped neurones in *Aplysia californica, J. Physiol. (Lond.)* **347**, 279–300, with permission.

(Purkinje cell dendrites) and activation of Ca^{2+}-sensitive channels such as Ca^{2+}-activated K^+ or Cl^- channels. However, the general role of Ca^{2+}-dependent action potentials is to provide a local and transient increase of intracellular Ca^{2+} concentration. Under normal conditions, the intracellular Ca^{2+} concentration is very low, less than 10^{-7} M. The entry of Ca^{2+} ions through Ca^{2+} channels locally and transiently increases the intracellular Ca^{2+} concentration up to 10^{-4} M. This local $[Ca^{2+}]_i$ increase can trigger Ca^{2+}-dependent intracellular events such as exocytosis of synaptic vesicles, granules or sliding of the myofilaments actin and myosin. It thus couples action potentials (excitation) to secretion (neurons and other excitable secretory cells, see Chapter 8) or it couples action potentials to contraction (heart muscle

cells). The influx of Ca^{2+} also couples neuronal activity to metabolic processes and induces long-term changes in neuronal and synaptic activity. During development, Ca^{2+} entry regulates outgrowth of axons and dendrites and the retraction of axonal branches during synapse elimination and neuronal cell death.

6.5 A note on voltage-gated channels and action potentials

Voltage-gated Na^+, K^+ and Ca^{2+} channels of action potentials share a similar structure and are all activated by membrane depolarization. The Na^+, Na^+/Ca^{2+} and Ca^{2+} action potentials have a similar pattern: the depolarization phase results from the influx of cations, Na^+ and/or Ca^{2+}, and the repolarization phase results from the inactivation of Na^+ or Ca^{2+} channels together with the efflux of K^+ ions. However, action potentials have at least one important difference. The Na^+-dependent action potential is all-or-none. In contrast the Ca^{2+}-dependent action potential is gradual. This reflects different functions. The Na^+-dependent action potential propagates over long distances *without attenuation* in order to transmit information from soma-initial segment to axon terminals where they trigger Ca^{2+}-dependent action potentials. Ca^{2+}-dependent action potentials have the general role of providing a local, *gradual* and transient Ca^{2+} entry.

Appendix 6.1
Fluorescence measurements of intracellular Ca^{2+} concentration

A6.1.1 The interaction of light with matter

Light is electromagnetic radiation that oscillates both in space and time, and has electric and magnetic field components that are perpendicular to each other. If for the sake of simplicity one focuses only on the electromagnetic component, it can be seen that the molecule, which is much smaller than the wavelength of light, will be perturbed by light because its electronic charge distribution will be altered by the oscillating electric field component of the light. Without resorting to complicated quantum mechanical calculations we can say that light will interact with matter via a resonance phenomenon; i.e. the matter will absorb light only if the energy of the incoming photon is exactly equal to the difference between the potential energy of the lowest vibrational level of the ground state and that of one of the vibrational levels of the first excited state (**Figure A6.1**). The absorption of light therefore occurs in discrete amounts

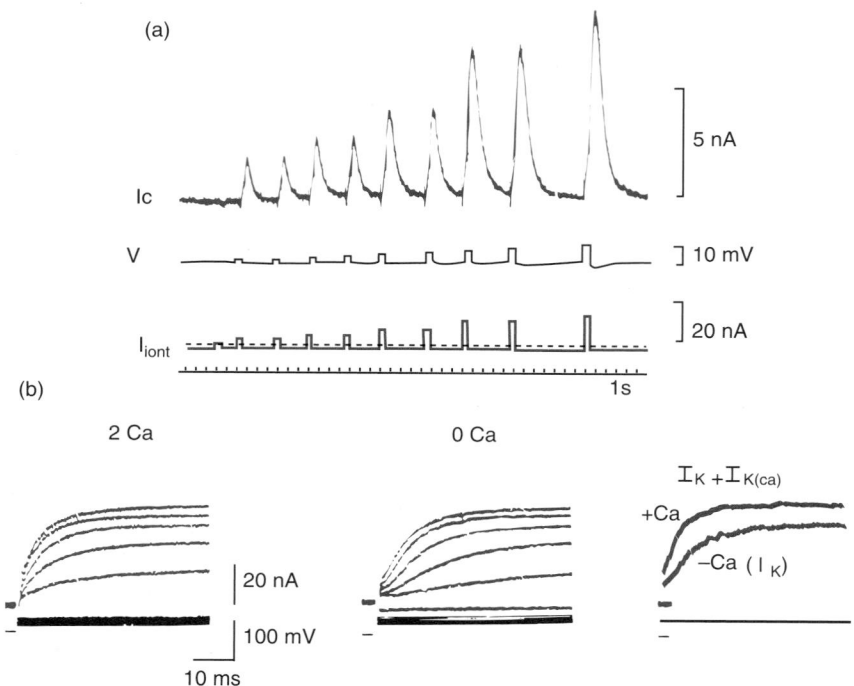

Figure 6.21 The macroscopic Ca²⁺-activated K⁺ current of bullfrog sympathetic neurons.
(a) Outward currents recorded in single-electrode voltage clamp at a holding potential of –28 mV. In response to increasing 0.4 s intracellular iontophoretic injections of Ca²⁺ from a microelectrode containing 200 mM CaCl₂, increasing outward currents are recorded. **(b)** Outward currents recorded during voltage steps to –20, –10, 0 and +20 mV from a holding potential of –50 mV in the presence of 2 mM external Ca²⁺ (2 Ca) and a Ca-free external medium (0 Ca). The leak current is subtracted. The two superimposed current traces recorded at the same potential in the presence (+ Ca) or absence (– Ca) of external Ca²⁺ ions show that an early component of the outward current is present ($I_{K(Ca)}$) in the presence of Ca²⁺ ions. Adapted from Brown DA, Constanti A, Adams PR (1983) Ca²⁺-activated potassium current in vertebrate sympathetic neurons, *Cell Calcium* **4**, 407–420, with permission.

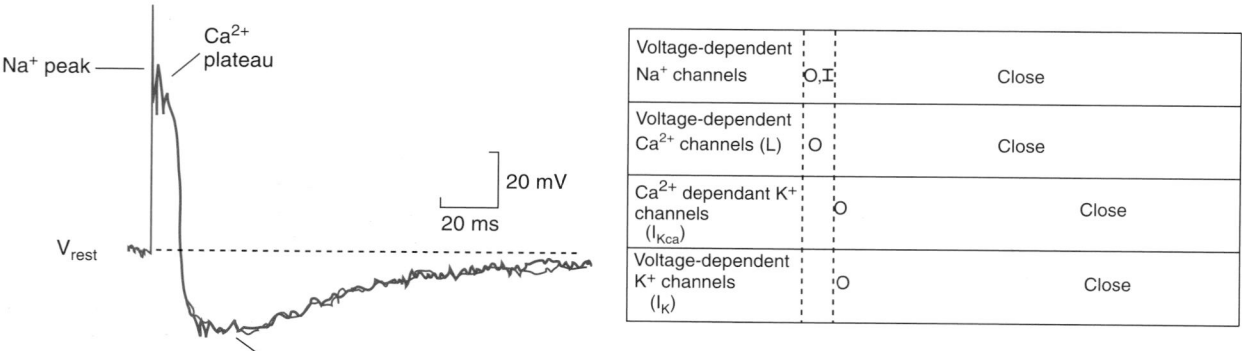

Figure 6.22 States of voltage-gated Na⁺, Ca²⁺ and K⁺ channels.
Different states in relation to the various phases of the Na⁺/Ca²⁺-dependent action potential. Example of the action potential recorded in olivary neurons of the cerebellum.

termed quanta. The energy E in a quantum of light (a photon) is given by:

$$E = h\nu = hc/\lambda,$$

where h is Planck's constant, ν and λ are the frequency and wavelength of the incoming light, and c is the speed of light in a vacuum. When a quantum of light is absorbed by a molecule, a valence electron will be boosted into a higher energy orbit, called *the excited state*. This phenomenon will take place in 10^{-15} s, resulting in conservation of the molecular coordinates. For the sake of simplicity the rotational energy levels are not taken into account and it is assumed that at room temperature the electrons will be at their lowest vibrational energy level.

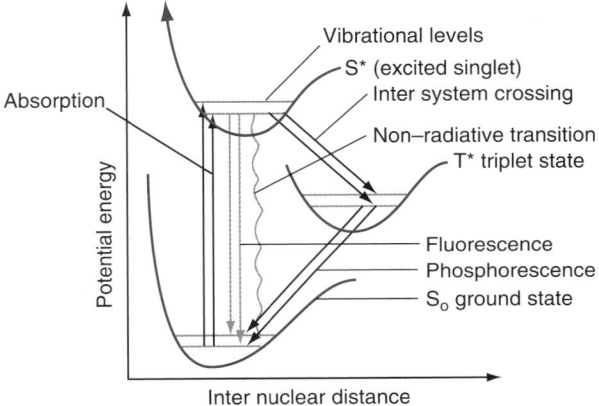

Figure A6.1 Pathways to excitation and de-excitation of an electron.

The rotational levels between the vibrational levels and higher excited states are not shown for the sake of simplicity.

The difference of energy between the vibrational levels being typically in the order of 10 kcal mol^{-1}, there is not enough thermal energy to excite a transition to higher vibrational levels at room temperature. One might thus assume that most of the electrons will lie at the lowest vibrational level of the ground state $S_{v=0}$ (S for singlet, as the electrons spins are antiparallel). Because absorptive transitions occur to one of the vibrational levels of the excited state, had there been no interaction with the solvent molecules one could have measured the energy difference between the ground state and each of the vibrational levels of the excited state. This type of spectra can only be obtained for chemical compounds in the gaseous state. The absorption spectra under those circumstances would resemble narrowly separated bands; however, the interaction of the orbital electrons with solvent molecules will broaden those peaks, producing the absorption spectra of the more familiar form.

A6.1.2 The return from the excited state

The electrons that have been promoted to one of the vibrational levels of the excited state will lose their vibrational energy through interaction with solvent molecules by a process known as *vibrational relaxation*. This process has a time scale much shorter than the lifetime of the electrons in the excited state (10^{-9} to 10^{-7}s for aromatic molecules). The electrons that have been promoted to the excited state will return to the ground state from the lowest lying excited vibrational state, by one of the following ways.

Fluorescence emission

Some of the electrons in the excited state will return to one of the vibrational levels of the ground state by a radiative transition, whose frequency will be a function of the energy difference separating these levels. If one simply assumes that the energy spacing the vibrational levels of the excited and ground states are similar, one expects the fluorescence emission spectrum to be a mirror image of the absorption spectrum (**Figure A6.2**).

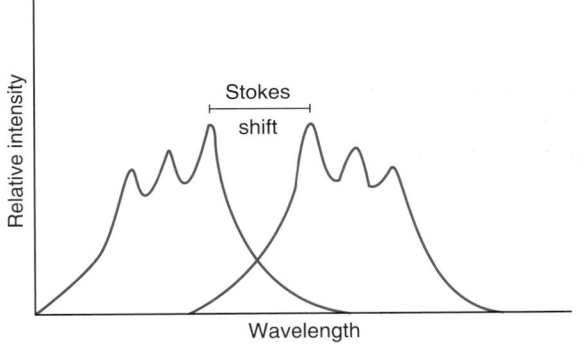

Figure A6.2 Excitation (left) **and emission** (right) **spectra of a hypothetical molecule.**

The excitation spectrum has the same peaks as the absorption spectrum; the separation between the individual peaks reflects the potential energy differences between the vibrational levels.

A further expectation will be that the $S_{v=0}$ to $S^*_{v=0}$ absorption will be at the same frequency as the $S^*_{v=0}$ to $S_{v=0}$ emission; however, this is rarely the case, as the absorption process takes place in about 10^{-15} s. The orientation of the solvent molecules with respect to the electronic states will be conserved as well as the quantum coordinates of the molecule; however, as the excited level lifetimes are rather long, the solvent molecules will reorient favourably about the electronic levels, resulting in a difference in the zero—zero frequencies. This difference between $S_{v=0}$ to $S^*_{v=0}$ absorption and $S^*_{v=0}$ to $S_{v=0}$ emission is termed the *Stoke's shift*.

Non-radiative transition

In this process the excitation energy will be lost mainly by interactions with solvent molecules, resulting in some of the electrons of the excited state returning to the ground state with a non-radiative transition. This process is favoured by an increase in temperature, and can explain why increasing the temperature causes a decrease in fluorescence intensities.

Quenching of the excited state

The excitation energy might be lost through interactions, in the form of collisions of quenchers with the electrons in the excited orbital. Typical quenchers such as O_2, I^- and Mn^{2+} ions will quench every time they collide with an excited singlet.

Intersystem crossing

Intersystem crossing is a mechanically forbidden quantum process that occurs by a spin exchange of the electron of the excited singlet state, resulting in an excited triplet state T^*. As this process involves a forbidden transition its probability of occurrence will be extremely low; nevertheless it will occur because the potential energy of the excited triplet is usually lower than that of the excited singlet state. The electron in the excited triplet state can then become de-excited by a non-radiative transition, quenching, or by a radiative transition called *phosphorescence* (the light emitted will be of longer wavelength than fluorescence because of the lower potential energy of the excited triplet). One should note that the return to the ground state necessitates a novel forbidden transition $T^*_{v=0}$ to $S_{v=x}$ (x for any vibrational level of the ground state). The probability of this transition will be extremely low, for the same reasons given above, resulting in a long lifetime of the excited triplet state (seconds to days). This long-lived triplet state will result in a very weak intensity of radiation, will be prone to quenching by collisions with quenchers, and the non-radiative processes will compete well with the phosphorescence. Phosphorescence in solution will rarely be observed. In order to observe phosphorescence at all, one must rigorously remove oxygen from the medium, and should use rigid glasses at very low temperatures, in order to minimize the competing non-radiative processes.

Some of the electrons that have undergone intersystem crossing, and therefore are in the $T^*_{v=0}$ state, may undergo a novel intersystem crossing to the S^* level by the thermal energy provided by the solution, provided the energy difference between the T^* and S^* states is small; the return from the $S^*_{v=0}$ to $S^*_{v=x}$ level by fluorescence emission is called *delayed fluorescence* and has the effect of lengthening the fluorescence lifetime of the molecule beyond what is expected in normal fluorescence emissions.

Photolysis

The molecules in the excited state will undergo certain chemical reactions which will result in the loss of fluorescence ; this is called *photobleaching*. It is estimated that the fluorescein molecule can be excited about 1000 times before it bleaches. Some of the reaction products might be damaging for the cell, resulting in phototoxicity. In order to keep the photobleaching and phototoxicity to a bare minimum it is advisable to use the minimal intensity levels and the minimal exposure times appropriate for the measurement.

A6.1.3 Fluorescence measurements: general points

Advantages

When comparing the sensitivity of fluorescence with that of other techniques, it is notable that in the absence of a chromophore, provided there is no background fluorescence, the level of the signal will be zero, so even a very small change in concentration of the chromophore can be detected by a large amplification, limited by the noise level of the amplifier chain. In the case of an absorption measurement, however, the absence of the chromophore will result in zero absorption (i.e. 100% transmission), giving the maximum expected signal. The amplification factor will therefore be limited by the saturation of the amplifiers, and a small change in concentration of the chromophore will result in a small percentage change over the maximum signal level, which may not be detected. This difficulty can be overcome to some extent by the use of differential detection techniques, but even under these conditions the need for an extremely good match between the differential amplification chains will limit the sensitivity of detection. With absorption measurements, changes of the order of 1 ppm (parts per million) can be detected; with fluorescence techniques, changes of 10^{-4} to 10^{-5} ppm can be detected, a sensitivity that is comparable to radioactive tracers.

Observation of fluorescence emission

The fundamental principle underlying a fluorimeter is to maximize collection of the fluorescence emission and to minimize collection of excitation light. This is usually accomplished by selecting a band of excitation wavelength that will not be present in the emission spectrum, by the use of filters (interference or combination filters), or by using a monochromator on the excitation side and highpass or bandpass filters on the emission side. The emission-side filters will pass wavelengths longer than the excitation wavelength (remember the Stoke's shift). For the measurement of fluorescence from individual cells, the epi-illuminated fluorescence microscope is used, which is described below.

Epiluminescence microscope

Most modern fluorescence microscopes use the epiluminescence technique, which means that both the excitation and emission light have a common optical path through the objective. The key element of epi-illumination is the dichroic mirror; it is an interference mirror formed by successive depositions of dielectric layers on a transparent substrate. The dichroic mirror will reflect the wavelengths below its cutoff frequency and transmit those that are above the cutoff. This cutoff frequency should be chosen so that it reflects all of the excitation wavelength, and transmits most of the emission wavelength. The Stoke's shift is an aid in this respect.

Dichroic mirrors are far from being ideal: they may have bandpass characteristics at a different wavelength, and they are very sensitive to the angle of incidence of the light beam. It is now possible to find polychroic mirrors that allow the simultaneous detection of many chromophores (**Figure A6.3**).

A6.1.4 Fluorescence imaging hardware

Owing to the competing processes that cause a non-radiative transition, the fluorescence quantum yield is rather low, for some molecules of the order of 50% or lower. The main loss of fluorescence emission is from the collection optics. Because the fluorescence is emitted in all directions, the light collection efficiency of the best microscope objectives cannot be more than 15%. The detector photocathodes (usually poly-metal alkali) will have quantum yields of the order of 20%. Even with this highly optimistic approach, it can be seen that for 100 molecules excited, one can expect at most one photon reaching the detector. In reality this figure is much lower.

To cope with such low levels of light, intensified CCD cameras have been used. Kodak developed a CCD array with a quantum efficiency of 80%; cooling the microchip reduces the thermal noise to very low levels and allows one to measure very low fluorescence intensities. The measurements will, however, be limited by the readout noise of the amplifiers which are of the order of 15 electrons. For measurement of even lower fluorescence intensities the avalanche photodiode APD remains the detector of choice but requires laser scanning hardware and suffers from the 'dead time effect' at larger photon fluxes.

The choice of photodetector therefore depends largely on the fluorescence emission intensity. For very low intensities the APD is the detector of choice; at larger intensities the cooled CCD array gives the best signal-to-noise ratio.

A6.1.5 Methods of calcium measurement by fluorescence

The main requirement for an indicator to report the concentration of an ion is a change in its optical properties, and at the same time it should be highly specific for the ion in question, at physiological pH values. Furthermore its binding and release from the ion must be faster than the kinetics of the intracellular ionic changes. One can therefore envisage the production of probes that will change their absorption, bioluminescence (such as aequorin) or fluorescence properties. Fluorescence is the technique of choice because of its higher sensitivity. In fluorescence measurements, the change in optical property sought to report an ionic concentration might be a change in quantum yield, excitation spectra or emission spectra.

This seemingly formidable task has been resolved by Tsien and colleagues, who have developed many probes sensitive to the free Ca^{2+} concentration. The common property of these probes is that they are all a fluorescent

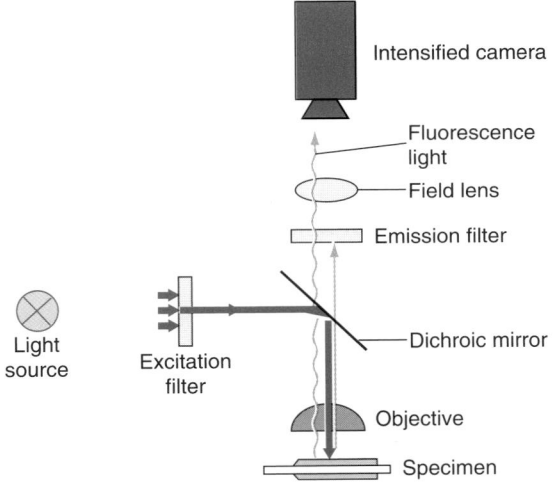

Figure A6.3 Epi-illumination microscopy.

derivative of the calcium chelator BAPTA, which in turn is an aromatic analogue of the commonly used calcium chelator (EGTA, ethyleneglycol bis (13-aminoether) -N,N,N′,N′ tetra-acetic acid) (**Figure A6.4**). The probes form an octahedral complex, with the calcium ion at the centre of the plane formed by the COO⁻ groups of the carboxylic acid. The binding and unbinding of the ion induces a strain or relaxation on the electron cloud of the aromatic groups, which in turn results in changes of the spectral properties of the reporter chromophore.

Three such reporter chromophores have found much use in the measurement of intracellular free calcium

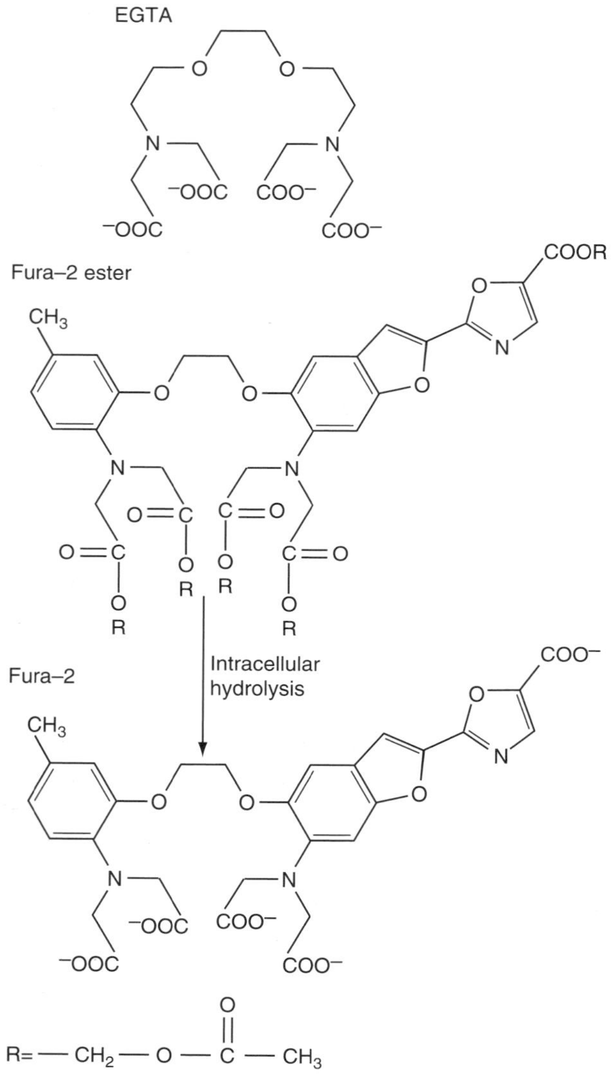

concentrations, namely INDO, Fura-2, and FLUO-3. Each of these probes has a certain number of advantages over the others, depending on the measurement technique sought. INDO and Fura-2 are ratiometric probes; i.e. the change in spectral properties will occur at two different wavelengths, and by measuring the fluorescence intensities at these two wavelengths and taking their ratio one can calculate the absolute value of the free calcium concentration within the cytosol, given by the following formula (see Grynkiewicz et al., 1985):

$$[Ca] = K_i\{(R - R_{min})/(R_{max} - R)\},$$

where R_{min} is the ratio at two wavelengths at zero ion concentration, R_{max} is the ratio at 'infinite' ion concentration, R is the ratio of the measurements, and K_i is an instrumental constant unifying instrumental parameters together with the K_D of the chromophore for calcium.

The major advantage of ratiometric probes is the fact that they are insensitive to the intensity of the emitted light, which changes from the centre to the periphery of most of the cells. This is because of differences in thickness at the centre and towards the edges, so there are more chromophores in the centre than at the edges.

INDO's emission properties at 405 nm and 480 nm change upon binding to Ca^{2+} (λ_{exc} = 350 nm). The two emission intensities can easily be measured by using a beam splitter, two interference filters and two photomultipliers; it is fairly difficult to envisage the use of two intensified cameras to form an image unless one uses a specifically split CCD array. Therefore INDO has been applied in processes that require either rapid determination of the free calcium concentration (i.e. cell sorting), or where the kinetics of the free calcium change are fast.

Fura-2, upon binding to calcium, undergoes a change in its absorption spectrum and therefore in its excitation spectrum; namely the emission intensity (collected at λ_{em} = 510 nm and higher) increases at λ_{exc} = 340 nm and decreases at λ_{exc} = 380 nm (**Figure A6.5**). A typical property of all the indicators that undergo either an excitation or emission shift is the presence of an 'isosbestic point', namely the presence of a 'unique point' in the spectrum when the parameter sought is changed (calcium in the case of Fura-2). The isosbestic point will be present only when two species are in equilibrium (in our case calcium-bound and free forms of Fura-2 or of INDO). The absence of this point can be taken as an indication of contamination by another ion. This point appears at 360 nm for Fura-2.

As Fura-2 undergoes a change in its absorption properties, alternating the excitation filters at the two chosen wavelengths, mostly at 340 and 380 nm, and collecting the emission above 510 nm with an intensified camera, one can construct the free calcium image, or the time

Figure A6.4 Chemical structure of Fura-2.
Note the similarities between Fura-2 and the acetoxymethylester variety Fura-2AM and EGTA. The AM variety is membrane permeant, and is de-esterified by intracellular esterases, liberating Fura-2, formaldehyde and acetate ions.

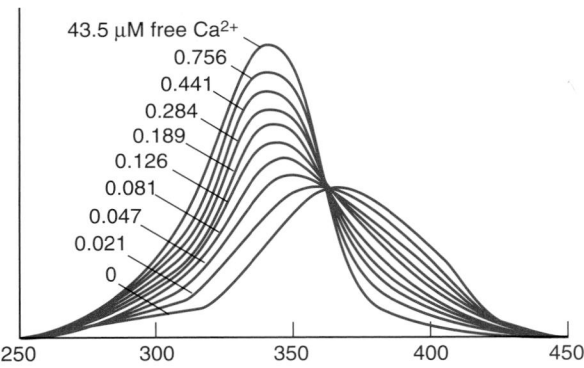

Figure A6.5 Excitation spectral changes of Fura-2 as a function of Ca²⁺ concentration.
Each curve represents the intensity of fluorescence emitted by Fura-2 (at $\lambda = 510$ nm) as a function of the wavelength of excitation (from 250 to 450 mm) and for a given Ca²⁺ concentration (from 0 to 43.5 µM). Knowing that Fura-2 + Ca²⁺ ⇌ Fura-2-Ca, the curve obtained in the presence of the maximal Ca²⁺ concentration (43.5 µM) represents the excitation spectrum of the bound form of Fura (Fura-2-Ca). In contrast, the curve obtained for the minimal Ca²⁺ concentration (0 µM) represents the excitation spectrum of the free form of Fura (Fura-2). It appears clearly that measured at $\lambda = 340/350$ nm and at $\lambda = 380$ nm, the intensity of fluorescence emitted by Fura-2 varies with the ratio free/bound forms of Fura; i.e. with Ca²⁺ concentration.

series of the changing free calcium in a living cell, by calculating the free calcium concentration at each pixel (picture element). One is not limited to these two wavelengths; it might even be advantageous to take the images at longer wavelengths than 340 nm as most of the old fluorescence microscopes are opaque to this wavelength. In cases where the kinetics of the intracellular calcium change are fast, one might use the property of the isosbestic point, and take an image at this point before stimulating the calcium increase and an image at the end of the experiment; taking the other images at 380 nm will allow the experimenter to follow calcium changes at video rates. These properties together with the high quantum efficiency and low bleaching made the Fura-2 the indicator of choice for imaging purposes.

With the advent of confocal microscopy, an indicator with absorption properties in the visible part of the spectrum was needed (confocal microscopes use laser scanning, and ultraviolet lasers are rather expensive). FLUO-3 Calcium Green and Oregon Green were developed to respond to this need. The main disadvantage of these probes is that their quantum efficiency changes at one wavelength only (~530 nm, when excited at the 488 nm line of the argon laser) upon binding to calcium. It is therefore not possible to measure absolute values of

calcium directly; nevertheless, if the resting levels of the free calcium concentration in the cell are known, the values obtained before stimulation can be used to calculate an approximate value of free calcium concentration as calcium increase is stimulated.

A6.1.6 Two-photon absorption

In 1931, Maria Goeppert-Mayer predicted the possibility of simultaneous absorption by a molecule of two photons of long wavelength, combining their energies to cause the transition to the excited state. This can be viewed as two IR (near infrared) photons being absorbed simultaneously by a molecule which will normally be excited at UV wavelengths (**Figure A6.6a**). This technique, however, did not find practical use until the advent of very short pulse-width lasers for the reasons outlined below.

The probability of two-photon absorption is ~10^{31} times lower (10^{-16} cm² additional cross-section for the second photon and 10^{-15} s for simultaneity of the two) than the probability of one-photon absorption, and therefore will not occur under normal illumination conditions. Typical cross-sections for one-photon absorption are of the order of 10^{-16} cm²; for the two-photon case they are 10^{-48} cm⁴ s⁻¹. The two-photon cross-sections are cited in GM (Goeppert-Mayer) units, with 1 GM being 10^{-50} cm⁴ s⁻¹.

In order for this absorption to occur one needs very high photon fluxes confined to a small volume. This was made possible by the advent of pulsed lasers, which typically generate pulses of 70 fs width at average power levels of 1–2 W at repetition rates of 80 MHz. For fluorescence measurements of biological samples one will typically use 10 mW of laser intensity of ~800 nm at the specimen plane. Under those conditions the excitation will be confined to the focal volume only, as the necessary photon flux can only be reached at this plane. This has two very important implications. As the excitation is limited to the focal plane, the emission will be limited to this plane also (**Figure A6.6b**) and this results in a confocal image. Other chromophores in the light cone will not be excited, so photodamage and phototoxicity resulting from photolysis of the chromophore is greatly reduced. Light at long wavelengths will be less prone to scattering and so have greater penetration in biological tissue, enabling researchers to measure Ca²⁺ dynamics in a non-invasive fashion from deeper locations. It has been possible to measure Ca²⁺ signals from rat brain at a depth of 500 µm from the surface.

Absorption is not limited to two photons only. Triple-photon absorption by nucleic acids with cross-sections as large as 10^{-75} cm⁶ s⁻² have been reported.

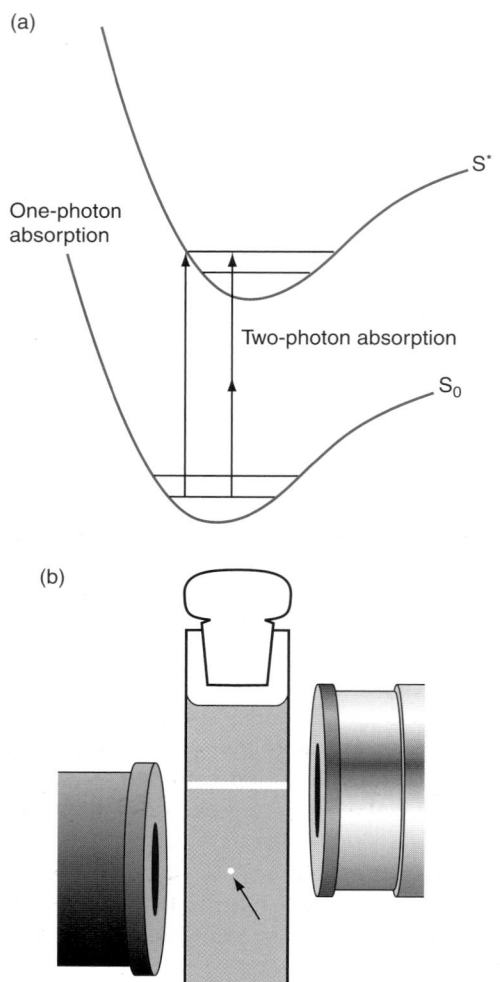

Figure A6.6 Comparison of one-photon and two-photon absorption.

(a) Two photons in the red (right) combine their energies to get absorbed as a one blue photon (left). The energies of the photons can be thought as equal to the amplitude of the vectors. The two photons that get absorbed need not have equal energies. **(b)** Fluorescence emission profile produced by one-photon absorption occurs throughout the laser beam focused in a fluorescent solution by the objective on the right. With two-photon scheme, excitation is limited to the focal point of the objective on the left (shown by the arrow) providing inherent 3-dimensional resolution.

This technique currently has the drawback of requiring rather expensive lasers, but one can expect prices to come down in the future, allowing their routine use.

Experience shows that there will never be enough light and there is the temptation to increase the concentration of the reporter molecule within the cell. In the case of calcium measurements this will have the adverse effect of buffering the calcium and preventing its rise (all the molecules of interest were synthesized taking

BAPTA as a model, which is a high-affinity chelator for calcium, which has the same backbone as EGTA). It is necessary to find a compromise between the signal-to-noise level and the buffering of the molecule in general, the best approach being to use the least amount of indicator required for the job.

A6.1.7 Measurement of other ions by fluorescence techniques

Indicators for Mg^{2+} and other divalents

Mag-Fura and Magnesium Green are Mg^{2+} indicators. They are designed around the same EGTA chelator structure as for Ca^{2+} indicators. Mg^{2+} indicators are designed to respond maximally to the Mg^{2+} concentrations commonly found in cells – typically 0.1–6 mM. They also bind Ca^{2+} with a low affinity. Typical physiological Ca^{2+} concentrations (10 nM–1 µM) do not usually interfere with Mg^{2+} measurements. Although Ca^{2+} binding by Mg^{2+} indicators can be a complicating factor in Mg^{2+} measurements, this property can also be exploited for measuring high Ca^{2+} concentrations (1–100 µM) such as those seen in the mitochondria. Mag-Fura and Magnesium Green do have similar spectral properties as their calcium counterparts.

Most of the reporter molecules synthesized for Ca^{2+} or Mg^{2+} will also interact with other polyvalent ions such as Tb^{3+}, Cd^{2+}, Hg^{2+}, Ni^{2+} and Ba^{2+} and in some cases with better quantum yields. This annoying property can be turned to advantage to measure changes in the concentrations of those ions.

Indicators for Na^+ and K^+

SBFI and PBFI are designed around a crown ether chelator to which benzofuranyl chromophores are linked, conferring to those molecules the same spectroscopic properties as Fura. Hence the same filter sets can be used as for Fura. The cavity size of the crown ether is the factor which determines the specificity of the molecule to Na^+ or K^+. The specificities of both SBFI and PBFI for their respective ions is much smaller than that of Fura for Ca^{2+}, and the K_D changes as a function of the concentration of the other ion, the ionic strength, pH and temperature.

Sodium Green is designed around a crown ether chelator to which two dichlorofluorescein chromophores are linked, resulting in similar spectroscopic properties as Calcium Green (i.e. excited at 488 nm). The cavity size of the crown ether results in a greater selectivity for Na^+ over K^+ compared with SBFI – 41 versus 18 times, respectively. The spectral properties, however, result in emission changes at one wavelength only, so ratiometric measurements with this reporter molecule are not possible.

All of the cation reporter molecules suffer K_D changes as a result of intracellular interactions as mentioned above, so they need to be calibrated *in situ* using pore-forming antibiotics like gramicidin and loading the cells with known ionic conditions. Another point which must be borne in mind is the fact that protein dye interactions might dampen or completely eliminate the signals.

Indicators for Cl⁻

All of the chloride indicators are based on methoxy-quinolinium derivatives and report the chloride by the diffusion-limited collisional quenching of the chromophore in the excited state interacting with the halide ion. The quenching is not accompanied by spectral shifts, so ratiometric measurements are not possible. As the quenching depends on collisional encounters of the halide ion, it is very sensitive to intracellular viscosity and temperature. The quenching efficiency is greater for the other halides such as Br⁻ and I⁻.

Appendix 6.2
Tail currents

Tail currents are observed in voltage or patch clamp experiments. 'Tail' means that the voltage-gated current is observed at the end of a depolarizing voltage step, upon sudden removal of the depolarization of the membrane. Tail currents do not exist in physiological conditions; they are 'experimental artifacts'. However, there are several reasons for studying tail currents: they are tools for determining characteristics of currents such as reversal potential and inactivation rate constants. Tail currents were first described by Hodgkin and Huxley (1952) in the squid giant axon.

Single-channel tail current

In patch clamp recordings of the activity of a single voltage-gated channel, a unitary current of much larger amplitude is occasionally observed at the end of the voltage step (**Figure A6.7**). It corresponds to the current flowing through a channel that is not yet closed at the end of the depolarizing step. Therefore tail currents are recorded for voltage-gated channels that do not rapidly close or inactivate during a depolarizing step, such as delayed rectifier K⁺ or L-type Ca²⁺ channels.

The activity of an L-type Ca²⁺ channel is recorded in patch clamp (cell-attached patch) in the presence of the

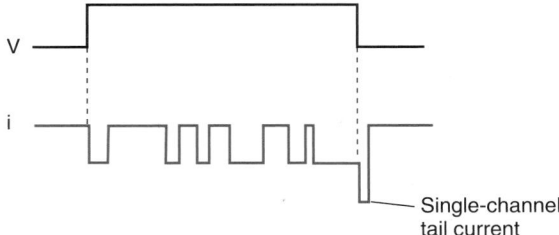

Figure A6.7 Activity of an L-type Ca²⁺ channel.
Recorded in patch clamp (cell-attached patch) in the presence of 110 mM external Ba²⁺. In response to a depolarizing step in the presence of 5 μM Bay K8644, a single-channel current of larger amplitude is recorded upon repolarization. It is a single-channel Ca²⁺ tail current.

selective agonist Bay K8644. On stepping back the membrane to the holding potential, the L-type Ca²⁺ channel opened by the preceding depolarization does not immediately close since the transition O ⇌ C is not immediate. The inward unitary Ca²⁺ current recorded at this moment is larger (**Figure A6.7**) because of the larger driving force upon removal of depolarization than during the depolarizing step: during the depolarizing step to 0 mV, $i_{Ca} = \gamma_{Ca}(V_m - E_{Ca}) = \gamma_{Ca}(0 - 50) = -50\gamma_{Ca}$; upon removal of depolarization $i_{Ca} = \gamma_{Ca}(V_m - E_{Ca}) = \gamma_{Ca}(-60 - 50) = -110\gamma_{Ca}$.

Then, after a few milliseconds, owing to closing of the channel, the tail current returns to zero (the voltage-gated channel closes in response to the repolarization of the membrane).

Whole-cell tail current

In voltage or whole-cell patch clamp recordings (in the presence of Na⁺ and K⁺ channel blockers), a voltage step to 0 mV from a holding potential of –40 mV activates a number N of L-type Ca²⁺ channels and an inward Ca²⁺ current is recorded. At the end of the voltage step a Ca²⁺ current of larger amplitude and small duration is always recorded: the tail Ca²⁺ current (**Figure A6.8**). Then the amplitude of this tail current progressively diminishes. The peak of the whole-cell tail current has a larger amplitude than that of the whole-cell current recorded during the voltage step since the driving force for Ca²⁺ ions is larger upon removal of depolarization than during the depolarization, as explained above.

The tail current diminishes progressively owing to the progressive closure of the N open Ca²⁺ channels: the channels do not all close at the same time once the membrane is repolarized. The whole-cell tail current of **Figure A6.8** represents the summation of hundreds to thousands of recordings of single-channel tail currents.

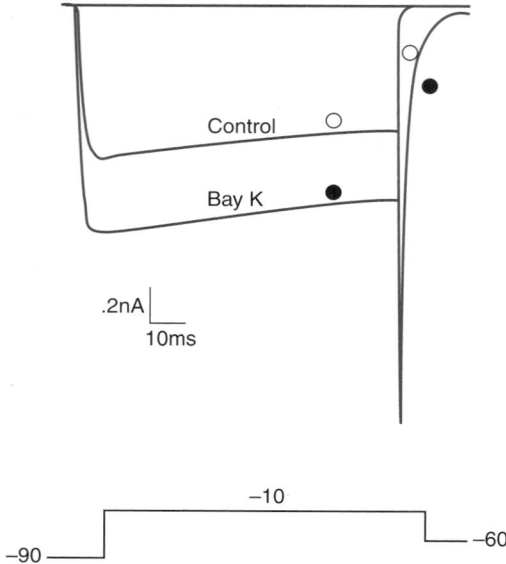

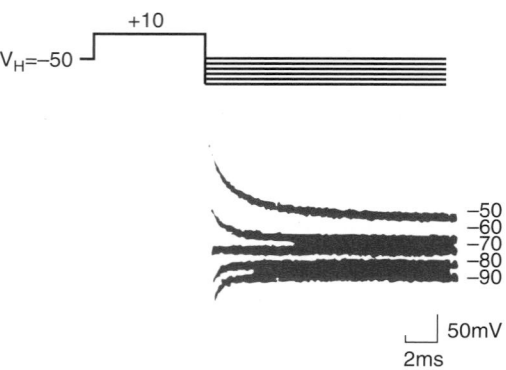

Figure A6.8 Activity of a dorsal root ganglion neuron.
Recorded in single-electrode voltage clamp in the presence of Na[+] and K[+] channel blockers and 2 mM external Ba[2+]. A depolarization to −10 mV followed by a repolarization to −60 mV is applied to the membrane from a holding potential V_H = −90 mV. The depolarizing step evokes an inward Ba[2+] current followed by an inward Ba[2+] tail current (control, open circle). The presence of 1 μM Bay K 8644 increases the amplitude of the Ba[2+] current during the step. It also prolongs the Ba[2+] tail current (black circle). Adapted from Carbone E, Formenti A, Pollo A (1990) Multiple actions of Bay K 8644 on high-threshold Ca channels in adult rat sensory neurons, *Neurosci. Lett.* **111**, 315–320, with permission.

Figure A6.9 Activity of a chick dorsal root ganglion cell.
Recorded in single-electrode voltage clamp, in the presence of 1 μM TTX and 10 mM Co[2+] to block, respectively, Ca[2+] and Na[+] channels. Depolarizations to +10 mV from a holding potential of −50 mV followed by successive repolarizations to −50, −60, −70, −80 and −90 mV are applied (*V* traces). Bottom *I* traces show the K[+] tail currents at the corresponding membrane potentials (the outward K[+] current during the step is not shown). The reversal potential of the K[+] tail current is −70 mV. It indicates the value of E_K in these cells. To separate the ionic tail current from the capacitive current, the latter was subtracted from the total current by digital summation of the currents elicited with identical depolarizing and hyperpolarizing test pulses. Adapted from Dunlap K, Fischbach GD (1981) Neurotransmitters decrease the calcium conductance activated by depolarization of embryonic chick sensory neurones, *J. Physiol. (Lond.)* **317**, 519–535, with permission.

In **Figures A6.7** and **A6.8**, the tail currents are inward. The direction of a tail current (as for any type of current) depends on the sign of the driving force; i.e. the value of membrane potential upon repolarization (V_H) and that of the reversal potential of the current (E_{rev}) which depends on the ions flowing through the open channels. By varying the voltage at the end of the depolarizing step the tail current varies in amplitude and direction (inward to outward or the reverse) and it is possible to determine the reversal potential of the tail current under study: when $V_H = E_{rev}$ the tail current is equal to zero (**Figure A6.9**). This value of E_{rev} is the same for the tail current and the current recorded during the voltage step since it concerns the same channels.

The voltage protocol of **Figure A6.9** allows the determination of E_{rev} and consequently identification of the type of ions that carry the current. E_{rev} can also be determined directly by changing the voltage-step value. However, for K[+] channels for example, E_{rev} is near −100 mV, a membrane potential where the open probability of voltage-gated channels is very low. By using tail currents, this problem is overcome.

Further reading

Bertolino M, Llinas RR (1992) The central role of voltage-activated and receptor-operated calcium channels in neuronal cells. *Ann. Rev. Pharmacol. Toxicol.* **32**, 399–421.

Caterall WA (1998) Structure and function of neuronal Ca[2+] channels and their role in transmitter release. *Cell Calcium* **24**, 307–323.

De Leon M, Wang Y, Jones J *et al.* (1995) Essential Ca[2+]-binding motif for Ca[2+]-sensitive inactivation of L-type Ca[2+] channels. *Science* **270**, 1502–1506.

Denk W, Piston DW, Webb WW (1995) Two-photon molecular excitation in laser-scanning microscopy. In Pawley, JB (ed) *Handbook of Biological Microscopy.* New York: Plenum Press.

Felix R (1999) Voltage-dependent Ca[2+] channel alpha$_2$-delta auxiliary subunit: structure, function and regulation. *Recept. Chann.* **6**, 351–362.

Grynkiewicz G, Poenie M, Tsien RY (1985) A new generation of calcium indicators with greatly improved fluorescence properties. *J. Biol. Chem.* **260**:3440–3448.

Hodgkin AL, Huxley AF (1952) A quantitative description of membrane current and its application to conduction and excitation in nerve. *J. Physiol.* (Lond) **117**, 500–544.

Hofmann F, Lacinova L, Klugbauer N (1999) Voltage-dependent calcium channels: from structure to function. *Rev. Physiol. Biochem. Pharmacol.* **139**, 33–87.

Miller C (1995) The charybdotoxin family of K+ channel-blocking peptides. *Neuron* **15**, 5–10.

Neher E, Augustine GJ (1992) Calcium gradients and buffers in bovine chromaffin cells. *J. Physiol. Lond.* **450**, 273–301.

Randall A, Benham CD (1999) Recent advances in the molecular understanding of voltage-gated Ca2+ channels. *Cell Neurosci.* **14**, 255–272.

Stea A, Soong TW, Snutch TP (1995) Determinants of

PKC-dependent modulation of a family of neuronal calcium channels. *Neuron* **15**, 929–940.

Tan YP, Llano I, Hopt A, Wuerrihausen F, Neher E (1999) Fast scanning and efficient photodetection in a simple two-photon microscope. *J. Neurosci. Meth.* **92**, 123–135.

Tsien RY (1989) Fluorescent probes of cell signalling. *Ann. Rev. Neurobiol.* **12**, 221–253.

Varadi G, Mori Y, Mikala G, Schwartz A (1995) Molecular determinants of Ca2+ channels function and drug action. *Trend. Pharmacol. Sci.* **16**, 43–49.

Zamponi GW, Bourinet E, Nelson D, Nargeot J, Snutch TP (1997) Crosstalk between G proteins and protein kinase C mediated by the calcium channel alpha₁ subunit. *Nature* **385**, 442–446.

The Chemical Synapses

In 1888, Ramon y Cajal suggested that the contacts between the axon terminals of a neuron and the dendrites or the perikaryon of another neuron are the points at which information flows from one neuron to the other: 'Les articulations ou contacts utiles et efficaces entre neurones ne s'effectuent qu'entre cylindre-axiles, collatérales ou terminales d'un neurone et les prolongements ou le corps cellulaire d'un autre neurone.' The term *synapse* was introduced by Sherrington (1897) to describe these zones of contact between neurons, specialized in the transmission of information.

In fact, the term 'synapse' is not used exclusively to describe connections between neurons (interneuronal connections) but also those between neurons and effector cells such as muscular and glandular cells (neuro-effector synapses) and those between receptive cells and neurons (**Figure 7.1**). These contacts are the points where the information is transmitted from one cell to the other: synaptic transmission.

According to morphological and functional criteria, there are various types of synapses, including chemical, electrical and mixed types.

Chemical synapses

These are characterized morphologically by the existence of a space between the plasma membranes of the connected cells. These spaces are called *synaptic clefts*. In this case, a molecule – the neurotransmitter – conveys information between the presynaptic cell and the postsynaptic cell. Chemical synapses will be described in this chapter (**Figure 7.2a**). Some of the chemical synapses have particular characteristics:

- *Reciprocal synapses* are formed by the juxtaposition of two chemical synapses oriented in the reverse direction to each other (**Figure 7.2d**).
- *Glomeruli* are formed by a group of chemical synapses. In some cases a group of dendrites form chemical synapses with the axon they surround (**Figure 7.2e**). In other cases, numerous axon terminals form synapses with the dendrite they surround.
- *Electrical synapses* or gap junctions are characterized

by the apposition of the plasma membranes of the connected cells. In this case the ions flow directly from one cell to the other without the use of a chemical transmitter. Gap junctions also allow the exchange of small-diameter intracellular molecules such as second messengers and metabolites. The gap junctions are described in more detail in Section 3.2.6 (**Figure 7.2b**). These synapses are common between glial cells in the mammalian central nervous system.

- *Mixed synapses* are formed by the juxtaposition of a chemical synapse and a gap junction (**Figure 7.2c**). In mammals, between neurons, these synapses are more common than the electrical synapses.

7.1 The synaptic complex's three components: presynaptic element, synaptic cleft and postsynaptic element

This section takes as an example the interneuronal chemical synapses. Under an electron microscope, a section of brain tissue taken from a region of the central nervous system rich in cell bodies and dendrites (grey matter) reveals many synaptic contacts at the surface of a dendritic shaft or of a dendritic spine (**Figure 7.3**, arrows). One of these synaptic contacts represents a synaptic complex (**Figure 7.4a**). The synaptic complex includes three components: the presynaptic element, the synaptic cleft and the postsynaptic element. The synaptic complex is *the non-reducible basic unit* of each chemical synapse since it includes the minimal requirement for efficient chemical synaptic transmission.

7.1.1 The pre- and postsynaptic elements are morphologically and functionally specialized

The presynaptic element is characterized by the presence of numerous mitochondria and synaptic vesicles which store the neurotransmitter (**Figures 7.3** and **7.4**). Two types of synaptic vesicles are described: the clear

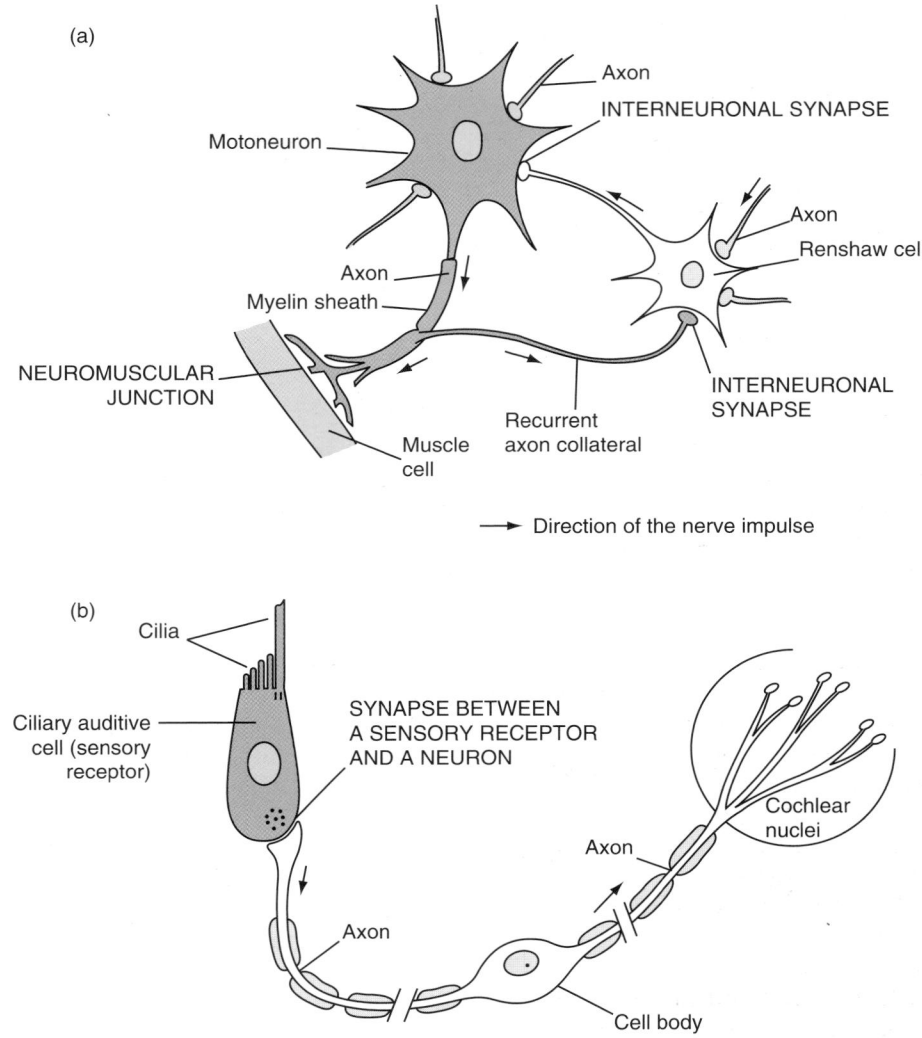

Figure 7.1 Types of cells connected by chemical synapses.
(a) Interneuronal synapses and neuromuscular junction. Example of synapses between a motoneuron (Golgi type I neuron that innervates striated muscle fibres) and a Renshaw cell (a Golgi type II neuron in the spinal cord) and between a motoneuron and a striated muscle cell. (b) Synapse between a sensory receptor and a neuron. Example of synapses between an auditory receptive cell (ciliary cell in the cochlea) and a primary sensory neuron whose cell body is located in the spiral ganglion. This neuron is free of dendrites and has a T-shaped axon that drives sensory information from the periphery to the central nervous system. Drawing (a) from Eckert R, Randall D, Augustine G (1988) *Animal Physiology*, New York: W. A. Freeman, with permission.

vesicles (40–50 nm in diameter) and the dense-core vesicles or dense granules, which have an electron-dense core (40–60 nm in diameter). Occasionally, under the presynaptic membrane can be seen an electron-dense zone with a geometry more or less distinguishable, the presynaptic grid (see **Figure 7.10**). It corresponds to a particular organization of the cytoskeleton which is related to the exocytotic machinery.

The postsynaptic element in the interneuronal synapses is characterized by a sub-membranous electron-dense zone, which most probably corresponds to the region where the postsynaptic receptors are anchored. In cases where the postsynaptic element is non-neuronal, we shall see that various other postsynaptic specializations exist.

The synaptic complex displays a particular asymmetric structure, the synaptic vesicles being present only in the presynaptic element. This structural asymmetry suggests a functional asymmetry.

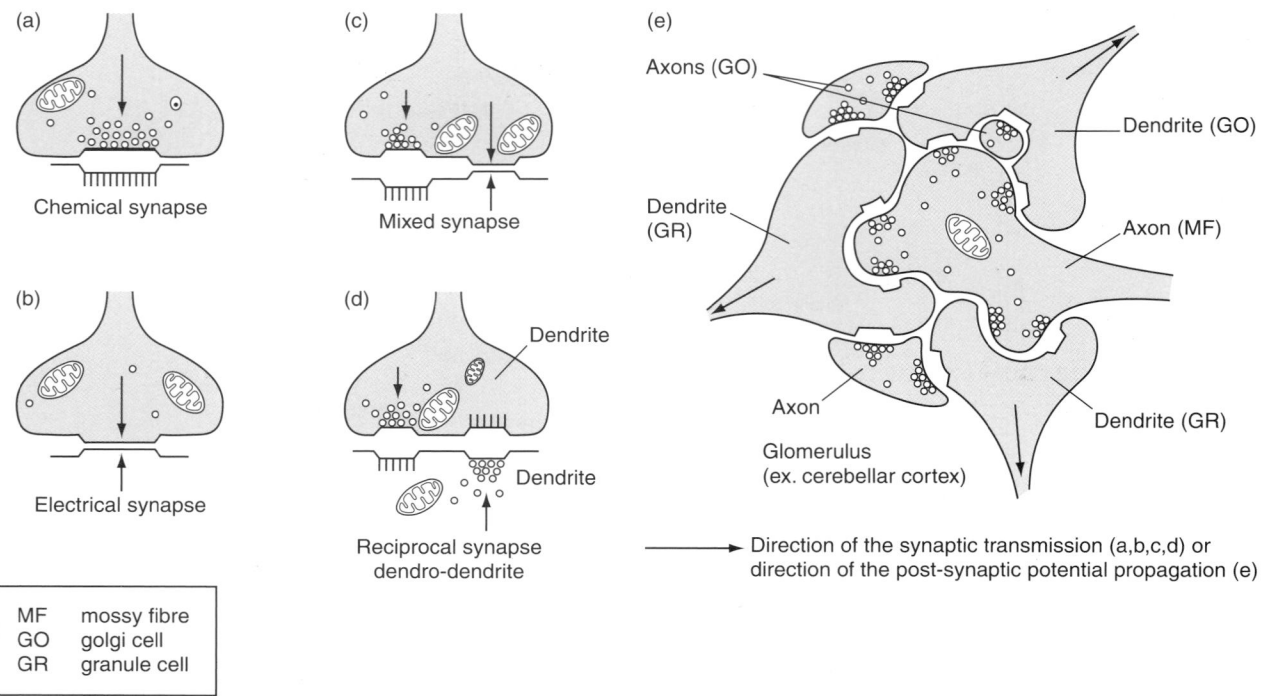

(a) Chemical synapse

(b) Electrical synapse

(c) Mixed synapse

(d) Reciprocal synapse dendro-dendrite

Dendrite

Dendrite

(e)
Axons (GO)

Dendrite (GO)

Dendrite (GR)

Axon (MF)

Axon

Dendrite (GR)

Glomerulus (ex. cerebellar cortex)

⟶ Direction of the synaptic transmission (a,b,c,d) or direction of the post-synaptic potential propagation (e)

MF	mossy fibre
GO	golgi cell
GR	granule cell

Figure 7.2 Types of synapses.

See text for explanations. MF, mossy fibre; GO, Golgi cell; GR, granule cell. Parts (a)–(d) from Bodian D (1972) Neuronal junctions: a revolutionary decade, *Anat. Rec*, **174**, 73–82, with permission. Drawing (e) from Steiger U (1967) Uber den Feinbau des Neuropils im Corpus pedunculatum des Waldaneise, *Z. Zelforsch.* **81**, 511–536, with permission.

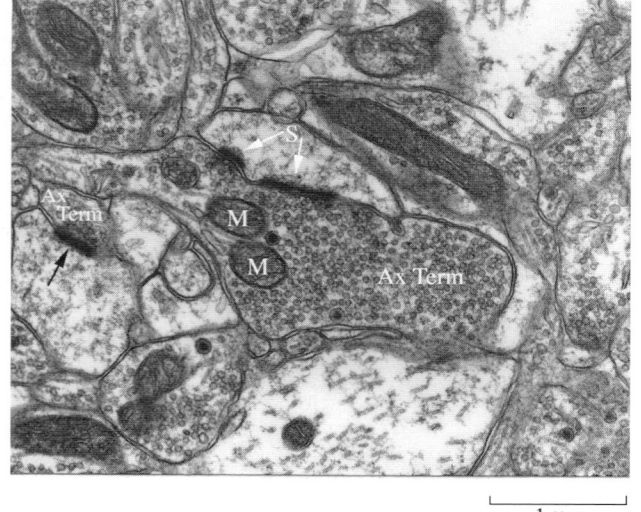

1 µm

Figure 7.3 Axo-spinous synapses.

One of which (centre) is a 'perforated' synapse. Microphotography of a section of the hippocampus (molecular layer of the fascia dentata) observed under the electron microscope. Two synaptic boutons (Ax Term.) filled with synaptic vesicles and forming one or two asymmetric synaptic contacts (arrows) with dendritic spines (S) of pyramidal neurons can be visualized. M: mitochondria, Bar: 1 micrometre (Microphotography Alfonso Represa).

7.1.2 General functional model of the synaptic complex

A general functional model of chemical synaptic transmission is as follows. The newly synthesized neurotransmitter molecules are stored in the synaptic vesicles present in the presynaptic element. In a non-depolarized presynaptic element, the voltage-sensitive Ca^{2+} channels are closed and Ca^{2+} ions cannot enter the intracellular space. The exocytosis of synaptic vesicles is normally triggered by an increase of the intracellular Ca^{2+} concentration. Then, while the presynaptic membrane is at rest (i.e. as long as it is not depolarized by the arrival of an action potential), the probability of exocytosis of a synaptic vesicle and the release of its content into the synaptic cleft is very low: the neurotransmitter molecules are not released in significant quantities into the synaptic cleft. There is no synaptic transmission.

Now, when Na^+-dependent action potentials (AP) propagate to axon terminals, they induce a depolarization of the presynaptic membrane (**Figure 7.4a**, 1). This results in opening of the voltage-sensitive Ca^{2+} channels present in the presynaptic membrane (2). Ca^{2+} entry through the opened channels evokes an increase of the intracellular Ca^{2+} concentration ($[Ca^{2+}]_i$) a factor required for triggering exocytosis of synaptic vesicles.

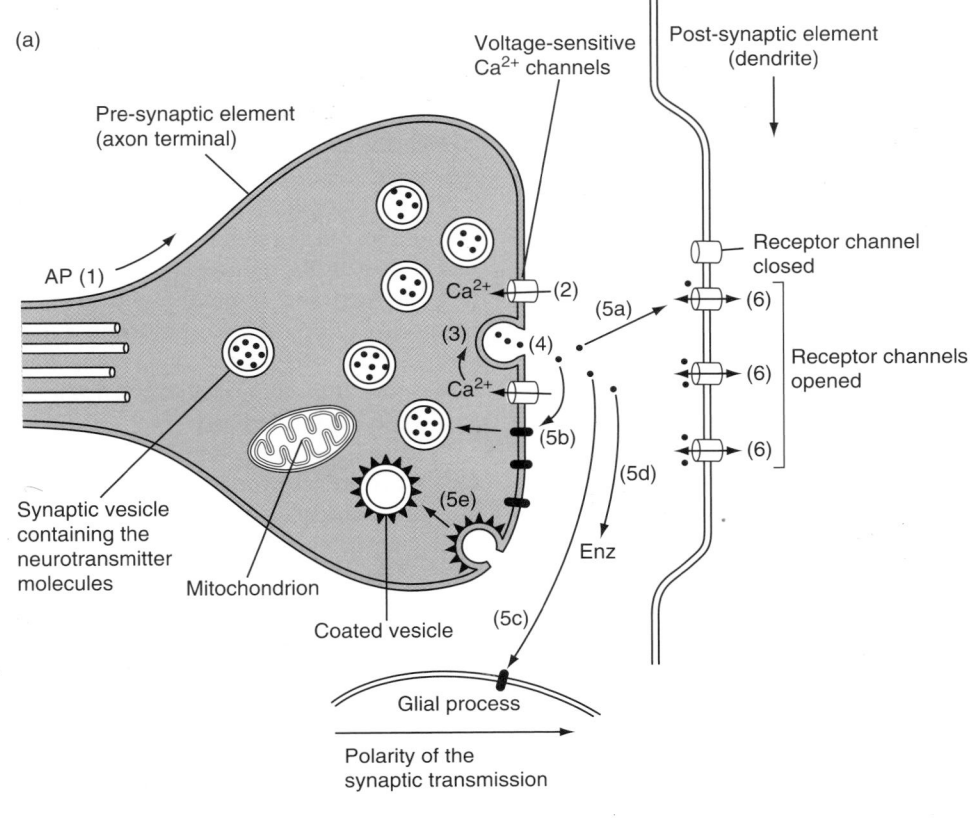

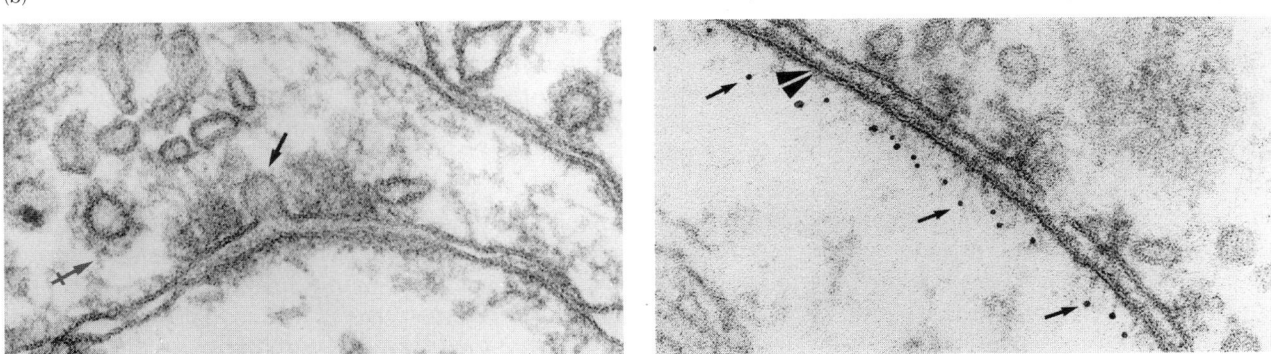

Figure 7.4 Pre- and post-synaptic specializations.

(a) Schematic of the synaptic transmission (AP, action potential; see text for explanation). (b) Electron photomicrographs of transverse sections at the level of synaptic complexes. Left: A figure of exocytosis (long arrow) between two dense presynaptic projections. A coated vesicle (crossed arrow) characteristic of the recycling of the membrane is also seen (inhibitory synapse afferent to the Mauthner cell in the fish). Right: Postsynaptic localization of the glycine receptors, visualized with gold particles associated to a specific monoclonal antibody (single arrow). These are lined up at distance from the membrane; this space originates mainly from the aggregation of the antibodies used to label indirectly the receptors (inhibitory synapse afferent to a motoneuron in the spinal cord of the rat). Part (b, left) from Triller A, Korn H (1985) Activity-dependent deformations of pre-synaptic grids at central synapses. *J. Neurocytol.* **14**, 177–192, with permission. Part (b, right) from Triller A, Cluzeaud F, Pfeiffer F, Korn H (1986) Distribution and transmembrane organization of glycine receptor at central synapses: an immunocytochemical touch. In Levi-Montalcini R *et al.* (eds) *Molecular Aspects of Neurobiology*, Berlin: Springer Verlag, with permission.

Thus, the probability of exocytosis of synaptic vesicles is strongly increased. This results in fusion of a docked vesicle(s) with the presynaptic plasma membrane (3) and release of the neurotransmitter molecules in the synaptic cleft (extracellular medium; 4). Once released into the synaptic cleft, neurotransmitter molecules bind to an ensemble of receptors: postsynaptic receptors (5a; receptor-channels and G-protein coupled receptors), presynaptic receptors (G-protein coupled receptors, 5b neurotransmitter transporters), glial receptors (5c; neurotransmitter transporters), and in some synapses enzymes (5d) that degrade the neurotransmitter molecules present in the synaptic cleft. All these receptors are proteins that bear specific receptor sites to the neurotransmitter. By binding to postsynaptic receptor-channels (5a) or to postsynaptic receptors coupled to G-proteins, the neurotransmitter will induce the movement of ions through postsynaptic channels (6) and a postsynaptic current. At that stage, the synaptic transmission is completed. By binding to transporters present in the neuronal and glial membranes or in the cleft, the neurotransmitter is rapidly eliminated from the synaptic cleft. In the presynaptic element, the neurotransmitter is taken back into vesicles or degraded. The membrane is recycled by an endocytotic process (5e). All the events here called (5) are simultaneous.

To refill the synaptic vesicles, the neurotransmitter has also to be synthesized *de novo*. Neurotransmitters are generally synthesized in axon terminals from a precursor present in the axon terminals or taken up from blood. The enzymes necessary for its synthesis are synthesized in the soma and carried via the anterograde axonal transport to the axon terminals (see Section 1.3.2). However, neurotransmitter peptides are synthesized as an inactive precursor form in the neuronal soma, and are carried to the axonal terminals via anterograde axonal transport (see **Figure A7.1**). The factors involved in regulation of neurotransmitter synthesis (i.e. how the terminals or the soma are instructed to synthesize more or fewer neurotransmitter molecules) is still under study.

This general scheme is of course oversimplified. For example, the presynaptic element can contain more than a single neurotransmitter; the intracellular concentration of Ca^{2+} ions can be increased also by the release of such ions from intracellular stores; and the role of presynaptic receptors has been ignored, for which there is evidence in the majority of synapses.

As we have seen, the *presynaptic element* contains the machinery for the synthesis, storage, release and inactivation of neurotransmitter(s). The presynaptic active zone is the complex formed by the synaptic vesicles and the region of the presynaptic membrane where exocytosis occurs (**Figure 7.4b**). Various methods can be used to characterize the neurotransmitter(s) present in a presynaptic element: immunohistochemical methods that identify the synthesis enzyme of the neurotransmitter in various parts

of the neuron, and the *in situ* hybridization technique that identifies the mRNA coding for the synthesis enzyme of the neurotransmitter (see **Appendix 7.2**). However, identification of a substance as a neurotransmitter requires experimental proof of a number of other criteria (see **Appendix 7.1**). If these criteria have not been satisfied, the substance is called a *putative* neurotransmitter.

The *postsynaptic element* is specialized to receive information. Its plasma membrane contains proteins that are receptors for the neurotransmitter: receptor channels (**Figure 7.4c**) and G-protein linked receptors. Various methods can be used to characterize the receptors present in the postsynaptic membrane: radioautographic techniques with monoclonal antibodies, or more rarely anti-idiotype antibodies.

In most cases synaptic transmission is unidirectional (or polarized): it propagates only from the presynaptic element, which contains the neurotransmitter, to the postsynaptic element at the surface of which are receptors for the neurotransmitter (**Figure 7.4a**). In the case of dendro-dendritic synapses (olfactory bulb of the rat), we recognize two juxtaposed synaptic complexes that work in opposite polarities; these are the reciprocal synapses (**Figure 7.2d**). However, it is worth noting that, here also, the synaptic transmission is polarized in each of the synaptic complexes.

7.1.3 Complementarity between the neurotransmitter stored and released by the presynaptic element and the nature of receptors in the postsynaptic membrane

In all synapses, receptors present in the postsynaptic membrane are those that specifically recognize the neurotransmitter released from the corresponding presynaptic element. For example, in glutamatergic synapses, glutamate receptors are found highly concentrated in the membrane of the corresponding postsynaptic element. Efficient synaptic transmission requires, in fact, specific localization of receptors on the postsynaptic membrane apposed to the transmitter release site. This is the case even in synapses where the pre- and postsynaptic cells have different embryonic origin (as in a nerve–muscle junction, for example). This pre–post complementarity requires, at least, the following steps to be completed: targeting, anchoring and clustering of postsynaptic receptors.

Targeting of receptors to a specific postsynaptic membrane

How do neurons target specific proteins to specialized neuronal subdomains? We shall take the example of metabotropic glutamate receptors (G-protein linked receptors of glutamate). They are a homologous family of differentially targeted receptors. Among mGluRs (see Chapter 14), mGluR1a and mGluR2 are targeted to dendrites and excluded from axons, whereas mGluR7 is targeted to dendrites and axons. In order to study the peptide sequence that could be responsible for this differential targeting, native or chimeric mGluRs are expressed, one at a time, in cultured hippocampal neurons, from viral vectors. The distribution of these expressed mGluRs is then checked by labelling mGluR with a specific antibody coupled to a fluorescent marker (Texas Red) and by labelling axon with a tau antibody (green) or dendrites with a MAP2 antibody (green).

First, the distribution of expressed mGluRs is checked. The selective distribution of endogenous mGluRs is reproduced for expressed mGluRs: axon exclusion of mGluR1a and mGluR2 and axon targeting for mGluR7 (all three are also targeted to dendrites). What mediates the axon exclusion of mGluR1a and mGluR2? The working hypothesis is that, since the C-terminal cytoplasmic domain of these receptors is the most divergent region of the primary sequence of mGluRs, it is involved in targeting. To answer this question, the distribution of chimeric mGluRs, such as mGluR2tail7 and mGluR7tail2 constructs is studied (**Figure 7.5a**). To be sure that tails are intact in the constructs, antibodies against tail2 or tail7 are tested. As they still recognize the tails, the C-terminal epitope of chimeric mGluR forms correctly from the transfected chimeric cDNA.

Analysis of these chimeric constructs reveals that the C-terminal cytoplasmic domain of mGluRs contains the axon/dendrite targeting information. The mGluR2tail7 – containing the backbone of mGluR2 up to and including the seventh transmembrane domain followed by the C-terminal 65-amino-acid domain of mGluR7 – is targeted to axons (**Figure 7.5b**, left column). The reciprocal chimera mGluR7tail2 is present in dendrites but excluded from axons (**Figure 7.5b**, right column). To more narrowly define the targeting signal only the 30-amino-acid distal part of the C-terminal domain between mGluR2 and mGluR7 is swapped. These constructs are not as efficiently targeted as the first ones, showing that axon exclusion of mGluR7 versus mGluR2 is dependent on the 65-amino-acid C-terminal sequences primarily and not exclusively on the more distal amino acids. The mGluR2 C-terminus is required for axon exclusion and the mGluR7 C-terminus is required for axon targeting of the native proteins. These are 'axon exclusion' and 'axon targeting' signals. The mGluR targeting signals may function at any stage in targeting: sorting into specific vesicles from the *trans*-Golgi network, transport by association with specific motors, selection of plasma membrane addition sites,

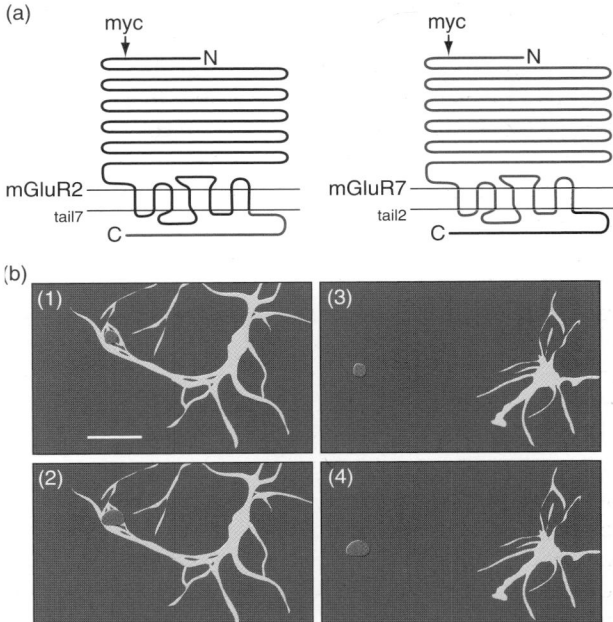

Figure 7.5 Differential targeting of mGluR chimera.
(a) Schematics of mGluR chimera (mGluR2tail7 and mGluR7tail2) primary structures with mGluR2 structure shown in black and mGluR7 structure shown in green. The *myc* ten aminoacid epitope tag (arrow) is inserted in the N-terminal extracellular domains, three amino acids past the signal sequence. **(b)** Left: Expressed *myc*-mGluR2tail7 recognized by surface labelling with the *myc* antibody (1) and labelling after permeabilization with an antibody against the C-terminus of mGluR7 (2). Both epitopes give the same distribution pattern, with labelling the full extent of the transfected neuron on the right and the axon of the transfected neuron in contact with a non-transfected neuron on the left. Right: expressed *myc*-mGluR7tail2 was recognized by surface labelling with the *myc* antibody (3) and labelling after permeabilization with an antibody against the C-terminus of mGluR2 (4). Again, both epitopes give the same distribution pattern, with labelling of the somatodendritic domain of the transfected neuron on the right. Scale bar, 50 mm. From Nash Stowell J, Craig AM (1999). Axon/dendrite targeting of metabotropic glutamate receptors by their cytoplasmic carboxy-terminal domains. *Neuron* **22**, 525–536, with permission.

etc. When mGluR1a and mGluR2 are not detected at the surface of the axon, they are also not detected in the axoplasm. Therefore, the mGluR targeting signals such as 'axon exclusion' may act at an early stage, such as sorting out into vesicles directly targeted to dendrites.

Anchoring and clustering of receptors in the postsynaptic membrane

A single neuron may receive input from thousands of synaptic connections on its cell body and dendrites. To

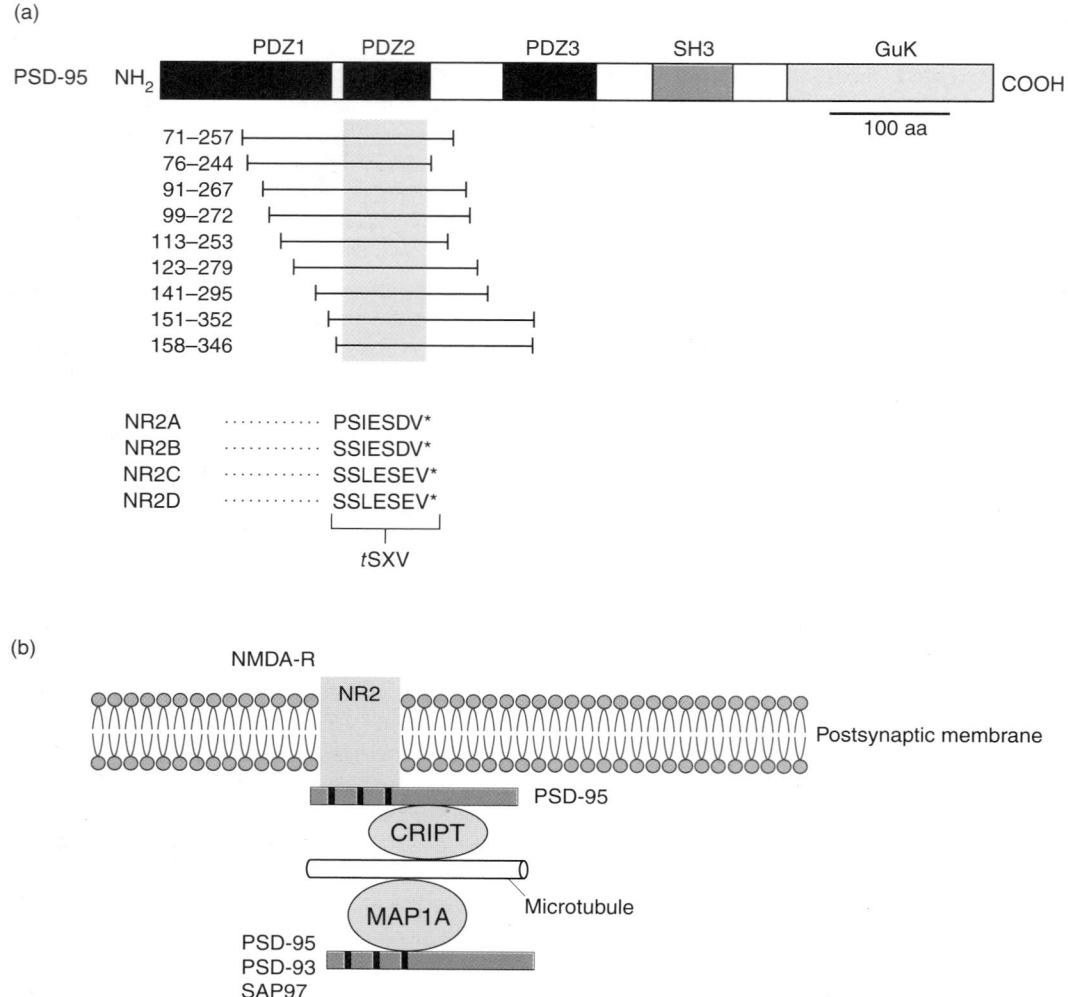

Figure 7.6 PDZ-containing proteins and anchoring of NMDA receptor subunits.
(a) Schematic of the PSD-95 protein (GuK, guanylate-kinase-like domain). The *t*SXV domain of NR2B subunit situated in the C-terminal region (bottom) interacts with the second PDZ domain in PSD95. Randomly generated PSD95 sequences interacting in the yeast two-hybrid system with the C-terminal *t*SXV sequence of NR2B are aligned to the domain map and identified by amino acid numbers. **(b)** Schematic of possible interactions in the postsynaptic element between the NR2 subunit of the NMDA receptor (NMDA-R), anchor proteins (PSD 95, PSD 93, SAP 97), cytoskeletal proteins and microtubule-associated proteins (CRIPT for cysteine rich-interactor of PDZ three; MAP 1A). Part (a) from Kornau HC, Schenker LT, Kennedy MB, Seeburg PH (1995) Domain interaction between NMDA receptor subunits and the postsynaptic density protein PSD-95. *Science* **269**, 1737–1740, with permission. Part (b) drawing by Lotfi Ferhat.

integrate these signals rapidly and specifically, the neuron anchors a high concentration of receptors at postsynaptic sites, matching the correct receptor with the neurotransmitter released from the presynaptic terminal. The mechanism of site-specific receptor clustering has been most thoroughly investigated at the neuromuscular junction (a cholinergic synapse; see Section 7.3). Rapsyn is believed to be one of the molecules responsible for nicotinic cholinergic receptors (nAChR) clustering. For glycine receptors (GlyR), postsynaptic clustering is dependent on gephyrin, a 93 kD channel-

associated protein, that is totally unrelated to rapsyn. We shall take here the example of the identification of anchor proteins for an ionotropic glutamatergic receptor, the NMDA (*N*-methyl-D-aspartate) receptor (see Chapter 11).

NMDA receptors are formed by assembly of the principal subunit NR1 with different NR2 subunits (NR2A to D). A conspicuous feature of the NR2 subunits is their extended, intracellular C-terminal sequence distal to the last transmembrane region. The working hypothesis is that this region participates in anchoring. In an attempt to identify molecules that can mediate the association between NMDA receptors and cytoskeleton, the yeast two-hybrid system is used to search for such gene products that bind to the intracellular C-terminal tails of NR2 subunits at synapses. The NR2 subunits are found to interact specifically with a family of membrane-associated synaptic proteins. In mammals, this family to date includes PSD-93, PSD-95/SAP90, SAP97, SAP102 (PSD for postsynaptic density, SAP for synapse-associated protein). In their N-terminal half, this family of proteins is characterized by the presence of three domains with a length of approximately 90 amino acids, termed PDZ domains (1–3); they are therefore called PDZ-containing proteins (P for PSD-95, D for *dlg* and Z for ZO-1, the first proteins to be identified with these domains) (**Figure 7.6a**). PDZ repeats are protein-binding sites that recognize a short consensus peptide sequence of NR2 subunits (**Figure 7.6b**).

PDZ domains also bind to intracellular proteins such as microtubule-associated proteins (MAPs) (**Figure 7.6b**). For example PSD-93, PSD-95 and SAP97 bind to MAP1A. PSD-95 also interacts with microtubules via another microtubule-associated protein. This suggests that interactions of NR2 subunits with PDZ-containing proteins link NMDA receptors to cytoskeletal proteins and cross-link NMDA receptors to each other.

7.2 The interneuronal synapses

7.2.1 In the CNS the most common synapses are those where an axon terminal is the presynaptic element

As described in Section 1.1.2, the axon terminals are either *terminal boutons* (**Figure 7.3**) which are terminals of axonal branches, or *boutons en passant* (**Figure 7.15**) which appear as swellings located along the non-myelinated axons and at the nodes of Ranvier along myelinated axons. These two types of axon terminals form synaptic contacts with various neuronal postsynaptic elements: a dendrite (axo-dendritic synapse), a soma (axo-somatic synapse) or an axon (axo-axonic synapse) (**Figure 7.7**). More rarely, there are synapses in which the presynaptic element is a dendrite (dendro-dendritic synapse; see **Figure 7.2d**) or a soma (soma-somatic or soma-dendritic synapses).

7.2.2 At low magnification, the axo-dendritic synaptic contacts display features implying various functions

We will consider as an example the cerebellar cortex, a layered structure in which the cells and their afferents are well characterized. The Purkinje cells are the single 'output' cells of the cerebellar cortex (Golgi type I neurons, **Figure 7.8a**) which send their axons to the deep cerebellar nuclei. They have a cell body with a large diameter (20–30 μm) from which emerges a single dendritic trunk that gives rise to numerous spiny dendritic branches which arborize in the molecular layer. The dendritic tree is planar, and the dendritic branches extend mainly in the transverse plane. The neurotransmitter of Purkinje cells is γ-aminobutyric acid (GABA).

Purkinje cells receive two types of excitatory afferents: the climbing fibres (axons of the neurons in the inferior olivary nucleus) and the parallel fibres (axons of the granule cells in the cerebellar cortex). The inhibitory afferents arise mainly from the numerous local circuit neurons in this structure: the basket cells, the stellate cells and the Golgi cells (**Figure 7.8b**).

A single climbing fibre innervates each single Purkinje cell. The climbing fibre gives rise to numerous axon collaterals that 'fit' the shape of the postsynaptic dendritic tree: the axon collaterals 'climb' along the dendrites (**Figures 7.8a** and **7.9a,b**) forming numerous synaptic contacts with the soma and the dendrites of the Purkinje cell. These contacts are axo-dendritic or axo-spinous, the presynaptic element being a terminal bouton. Such a synaptic organization implies that this excitatory afferent is very efficient: a single action potential along the climbing fibre can in fact induce a response in the Purkinje cell.

The axons of the granule cells form very different synaptic contacts with the Purkinje cells. The axons enter the molecular layer where they bifurcate and extend for 2 mm in a plane perpendicular to the plane of the dendritic tree of the Purkinje cell and form what are called parallel fibres (**Figure 7.8**). Parallel fibres form a few 'en passant' synapses (axo-spinous synapses between axonal varicosities and distal dendritic spines), with the numerous Purkinje cells (about 50). Therefore, each Purkinje cell receives synaptic contacts from about 200 000 parallel fibres. The consequence of such a synaptic organization is as follows. Activation of a parallel fibre cannot induce a Purkinje cell response since the activation of one or a few of these excitatory synapses cannot trigger postsynaptic action potentials; numerous parallel fibres converging on to a single Purkinje cell must be activated to induce a response in this cell.

The basket cells are local circuit neurons (Golgi type II neurons) which inhibit the activity of Purkinje cells. The axons of these neurons project to a large number of Purkinje cells and give rise to numerous axon collaterals which form 'baskets' around the soma of Purkinje cells. The axonal branches extend further and terminate 'en pinceau' around the initial segment of the Purkinje cells' axon (**Figures 7.8** and **7.9a,c**). Such an organization allows inhibition of the Purkinje cells at a strategic point

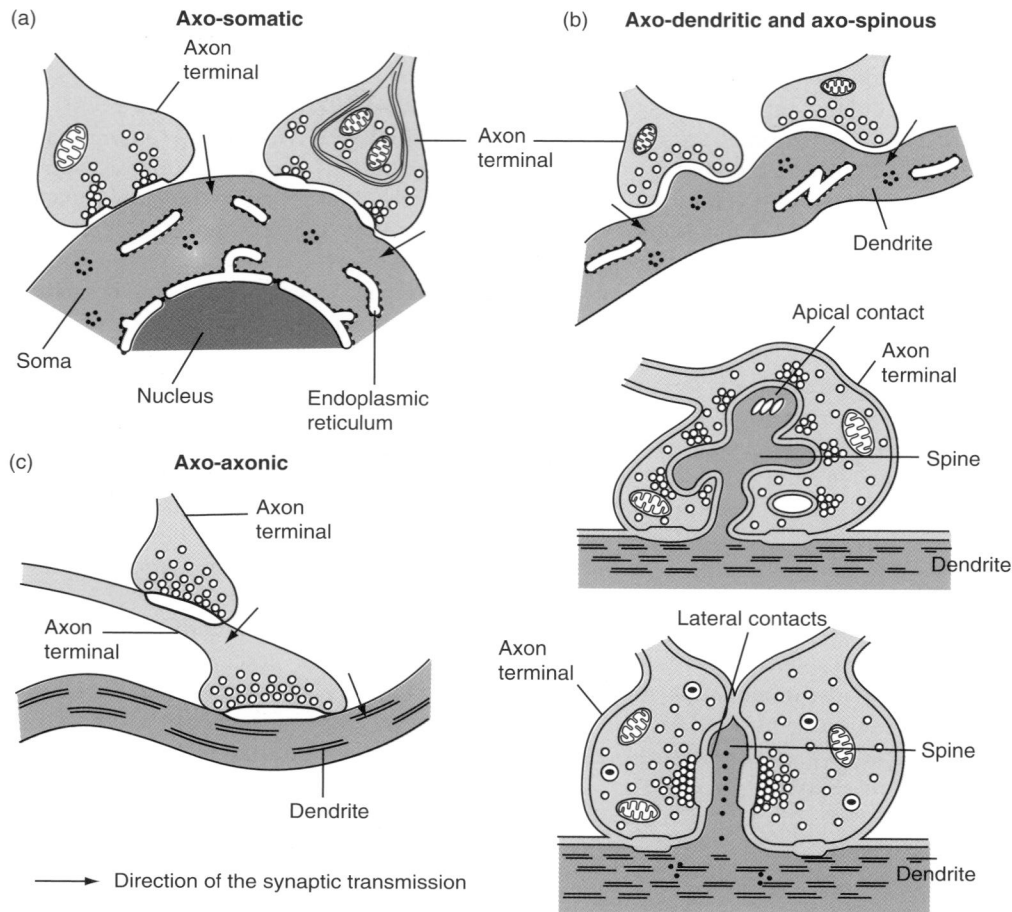

Figure 7.7 Types of interneuronal synapses.
(a) Terminal boutons forming axo-somatic synapses. (b) Top to bottom: Synapses between terminal boutons and a smooth dendritic branch (axo-dendritic synapse) and two examples of indented synapses between terminal boutons and a dendritic spine (axo-spinous synapses). (c) Synapse between an axon terminal and a terminal axon collateral (axo-axonic synapse). The 'postsynaptic' axon terminal is itself 'presynaptic' to a dendrite. From Hamlyn LH (1972) The fine structure of the mossy fiber endings in the hippocampus of the rabbit, *J. Anat.* **96**, 112–120, with permission.

where the sodium action potentials arise. This represents an efficient way of counteracting the excitatory potentials propagating along the dendritic branches to the initial axonal segment.

7.2.3 Interneuronal synapses display ultrastructural characteristics that vary between two extremes: types 1 and 2

A classification of the synapses on the basis of the form of their synaptic complex was proposed by Gray (1959). This author described two types of synaptic complexes in the cerebral cortex which he named types 1 and 2 (**Figure 7.10**).

■ Type 1 synapses are asymmetrical because they have a prominent accumulation of electron-dense material on the postsynaptic side. These synapses are found more often on dendritic spines or distal dendritic branches. The presynaptic element contains round vesicles and the synaptic cleft is about 30 nm wide.

■ Type 2 synapses are symmetrical because they have electron-dense zones of the same size in both the pre- and postsynaptic elements. The presynaptic element contains oval-shaped vesicles and the synaptic cleft is narrow. These synapses are more commonly found at the surface of dendritic trunks and soma.

(a)

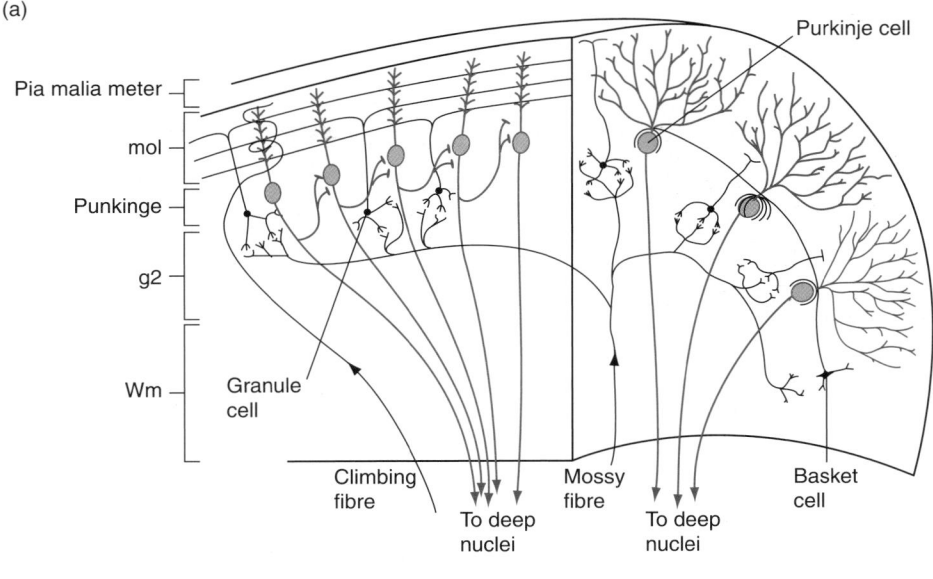

Pia malia meter

mol

Punkinge

g2

Wm — Granule cell

Purkinje cell

Climbing fibre

Mossy fibre

Basket cell

To deep nuclei

To deep nuclei

(b)

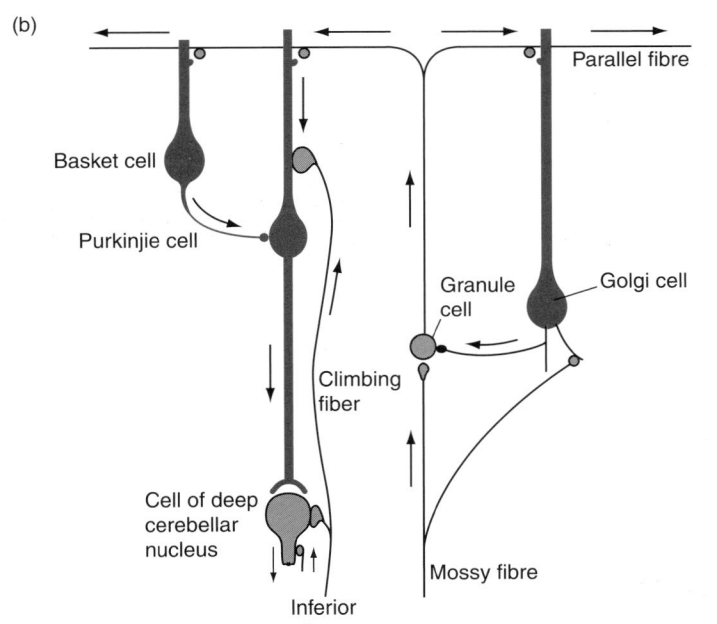

Parallel fibre

Basket cell

Purkinjie cell

Granule cell

Golgi cell

Climbing fiber

Cell of deep cerebellar nucleus

Mossy fibre

Inferior olive

Figure 7.8 Synaptic connections in the cerebellar cortex.

(a) Diagram of cells in a folium of the cerebellum. The layers are depicted: from the surface (pia-mater) to the depth, the molecular layer (mol), the layer of Purkinje cells (Pc), the granular layer (gr) and the white matter (wm). By comparing the drawings of the Purkinje cells in the sagittal plane with those in the transverse plane, notice that the dendritic tree of the Purkinje cells is planar. A climbing fibre which arborizes along the dendrites of one of the Purkinje cells is shown. It synapses directly with one Purkinje cell. Mossy fibres synapse with many granule cells. The axons of the granule cells enter the molecular layer and bifurcate in a T to form the parallel fibres running lengthwise in the folium. Granule cell axons synapse with Purkinje cells and basket cells. **(b)** Schematic representation of the principal synaptic connections within the cerebellar cortex. Inhibitory GABAergic Purkinje cells are in green; inhibitory GABAergic interneurons are in black; excitatory neurons are stippled. Drawing (a) from Gardner E (1975) *Fundamentals of Neurology*, Philadelphia: W. B. Saunders. Drawing (b) from Eccles JC (1973) *J. Physiol. (Lond.)* **299**, 1–3, with permission.

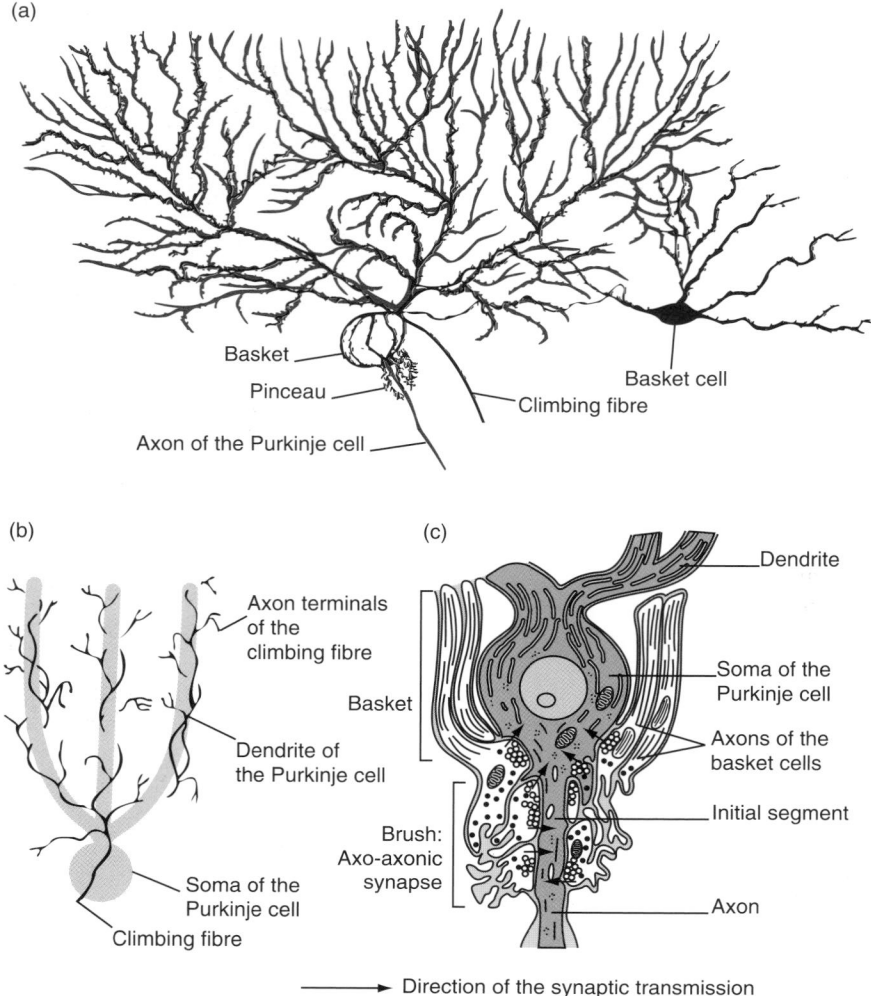

(a)

Basket
Pinceau
Axon of the Purkinje cell
Basket cell
Climbing fibre

(b)

Axon terminals of the climbing fibre
Basket
Dendrite of the Purkinje cell
Soma of the Purkinje cell
Climbing fibre

(c)

Dendrite
Soma of the Purkinje cell
Axons of the basket cells
Initial segment
Brush: Axo-axonic synapse
Axon

→ Direction of the synaptic transmission

Figure 7.9 Varieties of synaptic arrangements at the level of a Purkinje cell.
Representation on a single drawing **(a)** and in two separated schematic drawings **(b and c)** of the synaptic arrangements between a climbing fibre and a Purkinje cell (a and b) and between a basket cell and a Purkinje cell (a and c). Part (a) from Chan-Palay V, Palay S (1974) *Cerebellar Cortex: Cytology and Organization*, Berlin: Springer Verlag, with permission. Part (b) from Scheibel ME, Scheibel AB (1958) *Electroenceph. Clin. Neurophysiol.* **Suppl. 10**, 43–50, with permission. Part (c) from Hamori J, Szentagothai J (1965) The Purkinje cell baskets: ultrastructure of an inhibitory synapse, *Acad. Biol. Hung.* **15**, 465–479, with permission.

On the basis of correlations between physiological and morphological data obtained in the cerebellar cortex, Gray proposed that type 1 synapses are excitatory whereas type 2 synapses are inhibitory.

In the central nervous system (CNS), types 1 and 2 synapses are the extremes of a morphological continuum since synaptic complexes may have intermediate forms and display features that characterize both types of synapse; e.g. a large synaptic cleft (type 1) and a narrow postsynaptic density (type 2). In addition, it has been shown that the form of the synaptic vesicles is dependent on the fixation technique used.

7.3 The neuromuscular junction is the group of synaptic contacts between the terminal arborization of a motor axon and a striated muscle fibre

The motoneurons or motor neurons have their cell body located in motor nuclei of the brainstem or in the ventral horn of the spinal cord. The axons of these neurons are myelinated and form the cranial and spinal nerves that innervate the skeletal striated muscles (see Section 1.4.1). In general, a single striated muscle fibre is innervated by one motoneuron but a single motoneuron can innervate many muscle fibres. The myelin sheath of

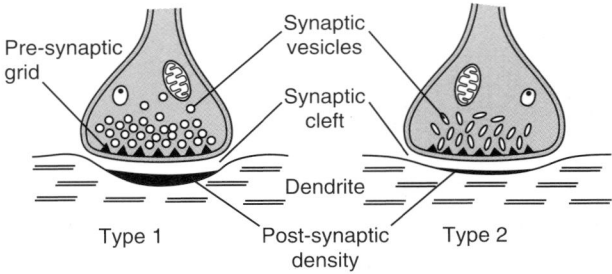

Figure 7.10 Schematic representation of type 1 (asymmetric) and type 2 (symmetric) synapses according to Gray.

each axon is interrupted at the zone where the axon arborizes at the surface of the muscle fibre. At this point, the thin non-myelinated axonal branches possess numerous varicosities which are located in the depression at the surface of the muscle fibre: the synaptic gutter. The axon terminals are covered by the non-myelinating Schwann cells (Figure 7.11; see also Section 2.5.2).

7.3.1 In the axon terminals, the synaptic vesicles are concentrated at the level of the electron-dense bars; they contain acetylcholine

The neuromuscular junction is formed by the juxtaposition of the terminals of a motor axon and the corresponding sub-synaptic domains of a striated muscle fibre, these two elements being separated by a 50–100 nm wide cleft. In a transverse section of a neuromuscular junction observed under electron microscopy (Figure 7.12a) the vesicles in the presynaptic element are small (40–60 nm diameter), clear and contain acetylcholine, the neurotransmitter of all the neuromuscular junctions. Larger vesicles (80–120 nm diameter) that contain an electron-dense material are also present but in a much lower proportion (1% of the total population). The vesicles are aggregated in the presynaptic zones where an electron-dense material is present, the dense bars. These dense bars are functionally homologous to the presynaptic grid of interneuronal synapses. They are 100 nm wide and are located perpendicularly to the largest axis of each axonal branch. The vesicles are aligned along each side of these bars. The complex of dense bars and synaptic vesicles forms a presynaptic active zone (Couteaux 1960). There are many active zones per varicosity. They are located opposite to the folds of the postsynaptic plasma membrane. Each active zone with the folds of the sarcolemma in front of them forms a synaptic complex. Therefore, the neuromuscular junction contains numerous synaptic complexes.

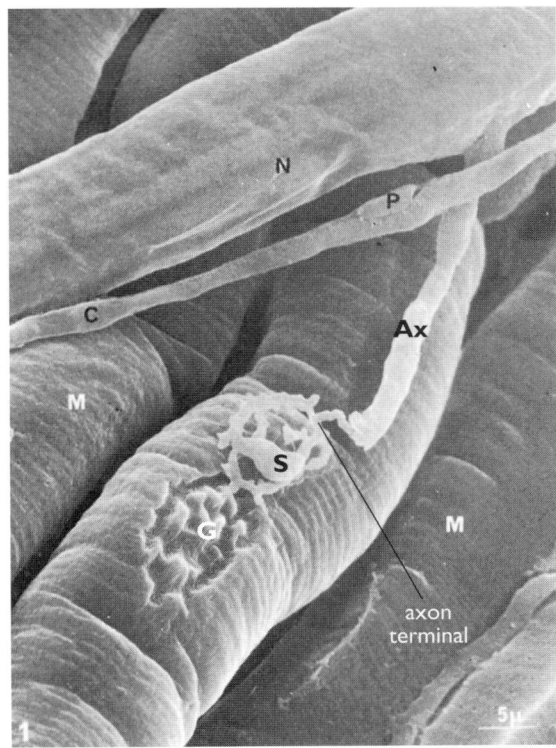

Figure 7.11 The neuromuscular junction.
Photograph of a rat neuromuscular junction observed under the scanning electron microscope. The terminal part of the axon (ax) is detached from the muscle cell (M) in order to show the synaptic gutter (G); c, capillary; N, motor nerve; S, nucleus of a Schwann cell. From Matsuda Y et al. (1988) Scanning electron microscopic study of denervated and reinnervated neuromuscular junction, Muscle Nerve 11, 1266–1271, with permission.

Synthesis of acetylcholine takes place in the cytoplasm of the presynaptic element from two precursors: choline and acetylcoenzyme A (acetyl CoA). The reaction is catalysed by choline acetyltransferase (CAT). Acetylcholine is transported actively into synaptic vesicles where it is stored (see Figure 9.20a). The protein responsible for this active transport is a transporter which uses the energy of the proton (H^+) gradient. This gradient of protons is established by active transport of H^+ ions from the cytoplasm towards the interior of the vesicles by a H^+-ATPase pump.

7.3.2 The synaptic cleft is narrow and occupied by a basal lamina which contains acetylcholinesterase

The postsynaptic muscular membrane (sarcolemma) is covered, on the extracellular surface, with a layer of electron-dense material, the basal lamina (Figures 7.12a and c). This lamina, which follows the folds of the

(a)

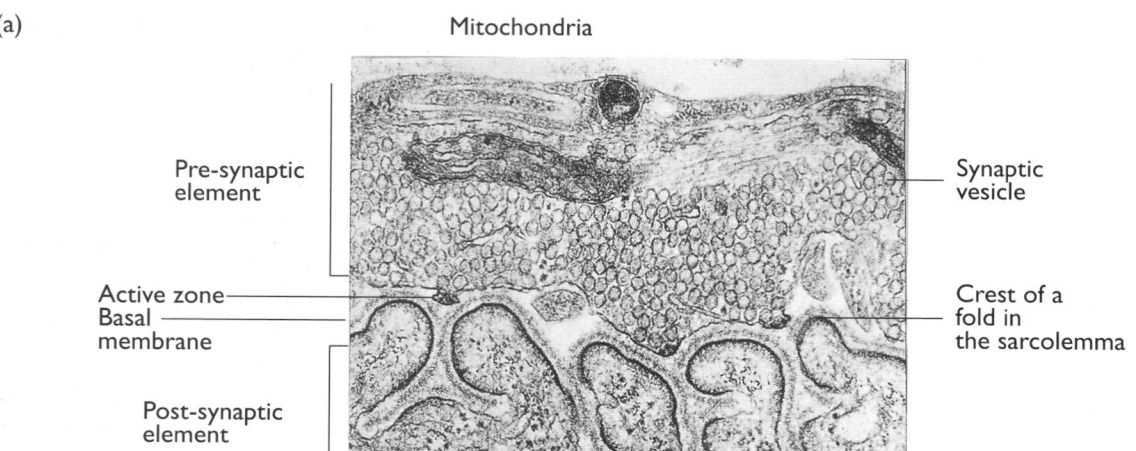

Mitochondria

Pre-synaptic element

Synaptic vesicle

Active zone

Basal membrane

Crest of a fold in the sarcolemma

Post-synaptic element

(b)

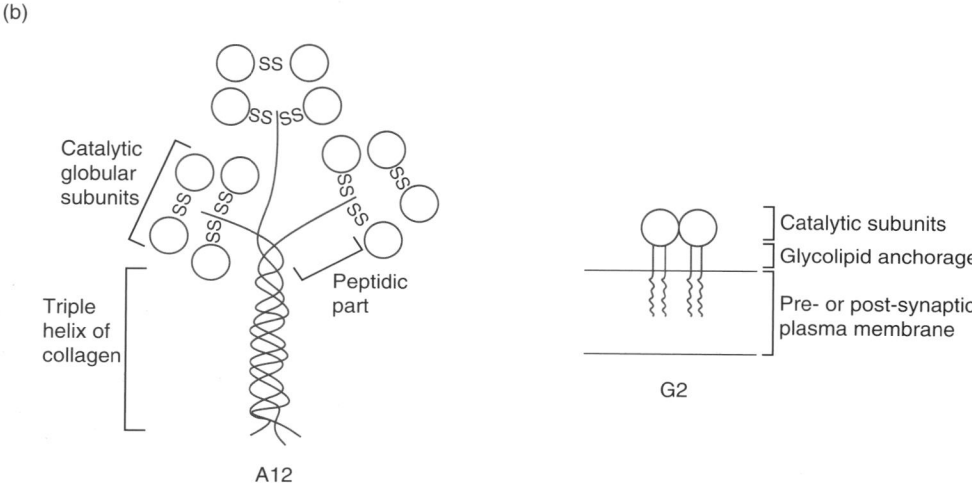

Catalytic globular subunits

SS

SS SS

SS

SS SS

SS SS

SS

Peptidic part

Triple helix of collagen

A12

Catalytic subunits

Glycolipid anchorage

Pre- or post-synaptic plasma membrane

G2

(c)

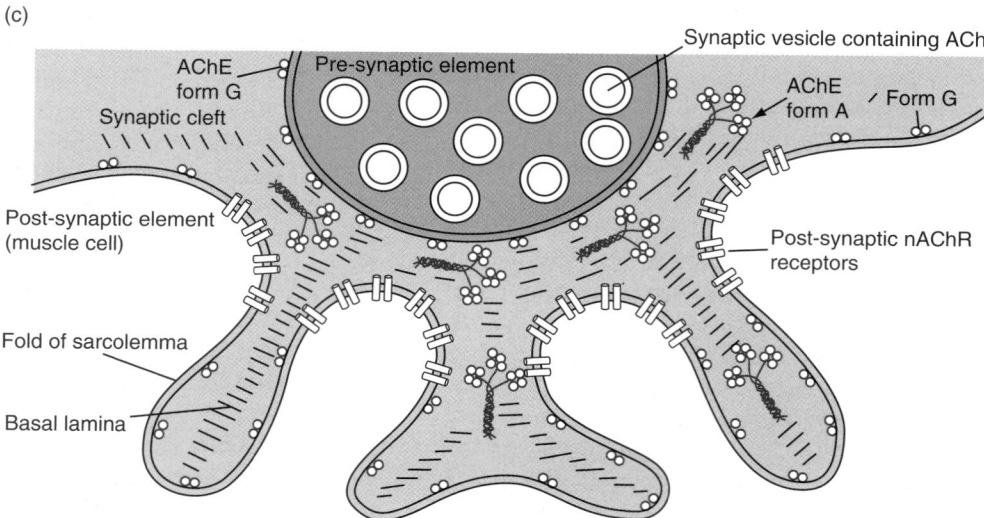

Synaptic vesicle containing ACh

AChE form G

Pre-synaptic element

Synaptic cleft

AChE form A

Form G

Post-synaptic element (muscle cell)

Post-synaptic nAChR receptors

Fold of sarcolemma

Basal lamina

sarcolemma, is a conjunctive tissue secreted by the non-myelinating Schwann cells covering the axon terminals. It contains, *inter alia*, collagene, proteoglycans and laminin.

Acetylcholinesterases are glycoproteins synthesized in the soma and carried to the terminals via anterograde axonal transport. They are inserted into the presynaptic membrane and the basal lamina. They display an important structural polymorphism (**Figure 7.12b**): they have a globular form (G) or an asymmetric form (A). These different forms have distinct localizations. Globular forms (G) are anchored in the pre- or postsynaptic membrane (these are ectoenzymes) and are secreted as a soluble protein into the synaptic cleft. Asymmetric forms (A) are anchored in the basal lamina (**Figure 7.12c**). The molecules of acetylcholine, released in the synaptic cleft, when the neuromuscular junction is activated, cross the basal lamina which comprises loose stitches, and a part of these acetylcholine molecules is thus degraded before being fixed to postsynaptic receptors. The other part is quickly degraded after its fixation. Acetylcholinesterases hydrolyse acetylcholine into acetic acid and choline. Choline is taken up by presynaptic terminals for the synthesis of new molecules of acetylcholine. This degradation system of acetylcholine is a very efficient system for inactivation of a neurotransmitter.

Figure 7.12 Ultrastructure of a neuromuscular junction and the location of acetylcholinesterases.

(a) Microphotography of the neuromuscular junction of a batrachian observed under the electron microscope. In the axon terminal can be seen mitochondria and numerous vesicles. The axonal plasma membrane displays signs of exocytosis (active zones). The basal lamina is located in the synaptic cleft. The postsynaptic muscle cell membrane has numerous folds. **(b)** Schematic of the asymmetric (A12) and globular (G2) forms of acetylcholinesterase (AChE) (top). The index number of A or G indicates the number of catalytic subunits. The asymmetric forms consist of a collagen tail, three peptide parts and catalytic subunits. The globular forms consist of one or more catalytic subunits (hydrophilic domain) and a glycolipid part (hydrophobic domain) which permits their insertion in the lipid bilayer. **(c)** Location of acetylcholinesterase in the neuromuscular junction. The A forms are synthesized in the motoneurons and secreted into the synaptic cleft where they are associated with the basal lamina. The globular forms are synthesized in the motoneurons and inserted into the presynaptic plasma membrane or secreted into the synaptic cleft. Microphotograph (a) by Pécot-Dechavassine. Drawings (b) and (c) from Berkaloff A, Naquet R, Demaille J (eds) (1987) *Biologie 1990: Enjeux et Problématiques*, Paris: CNRS, with permission.

7.3.3 Nicotinic receptors for acetylcholine are abundant in the crests of the folds in the postsynaptic membrane

The plasma membrane of muscle cells, the sarcolemma, presents numerous folds in mammalian neuromuscular junctions. By using a radioactive ligand for a type of acetylcholine nicotinic receptor, α-bungarotoxin labelled with a radioactive isotope or a fluorescent molecule, it has been shown that the radioactive material accumulates predominantly in the crests of the folds in the sarcolemma. Immunocytochemical techniques produce similar results. Other studies have shown that they are anchored to the underlying cytoskeleton (see the following section).

The nicotinic receptor is a transmembrane glycoprotein comprising four homologous subunits assembled into a heterologous $\alpha_2\beta\gamma\delta$ pentamer. It is a receptor channel permeable to cations whose activation results in the net entry of positively charged ions and in depolarization of the postsynaptic membrane. The structure and functional characteristics of the muscular nicotinic receptors are given in Chapter 9.

7.3.4 Mechanisms involved in the accumulation of postsynaptic receptors in the folds of the postsynaptic muscular membrane

The acetylcholine nicotinic receptors are, in the adult neuromuscular junction, present in high density (about 10 000 molecules per µm) in the postsynaptic regions and occur in a much lower density in the non-synaptic membrane (extrajunctional membrane). Under the nerve terminal, the muscle cell is free of the myofilaments actin and myosin. At this level, four to eight cell nuclei are found, the fundamental nuclei (Ranvier 1875). The myonuclei located outside the postsynaptic region (extrasynaptic) are the sarcoplasmic nuclei. The formation of this well organized sub-synaptic domain – which concerns not only the nicotinic receptors but also the Golgi apparatus and the cytoskeleton (it also comprises the organization of the basal lamina and the distribution of the asymmetric form of acetylcholinesterase in the synaptic cleft) – occurs in numerous steps during maturation of the neuromuscular junction (**Figure 7.13a**):

■ There is an increase in the number of nicotinic receptors (1 and 2) during fusion of the myoblasts to form myotubes, owing to the neosynthesis of these receptors. They have an even distribution over the membrane surface. This phenomenon is independent of the neuromuscular activity since it is not affected by the injection *in ovo* of nicotinic antagonists such as curare.

- There is formation of aggregates of nicotinic receptors under the nerve terminal (3–5) and disappearance of extrajunctional receptors (5). Upon innervation, nAChR rapidly accumulates under the nerve endings. *In situ* hybridization experiments with a genomic coding probe (see **Appendix 7.2**) have shown that in innervated 15-day-old chick muscle, the nAChR α-subunit mRNAs accumulate under the nerve endings. More precisely, accumulation of the mRNAs increases around the sub-synaptic (fundamental) nuclei and decreases around the sarcoplasmic nuclei. This can be interpreted as a differential expression of the nAChR α-subunit gene in the fundamental and sarcoplasmic nuclei. The presence of motor nerve and muscle activity are both crucial for the regulation of nAChR mRNA levels in the developing fibre.

- Distribution of the Golgi apparatus, studied by using a monoclonal antibody directed against it, shows a similar evolution. In cultured myotubes, the Golgi apparatus is associated with every nucleus. Conversely, in 15-day-old innervated chick muscle, the Golgi apparatus is now restricted to discrete, highly focused regions that appear to co-distribute with endplates (revealed by fluorescein isothiocyanate conjugated α-bungarotoxin, a labelled ligand of nAChR).

- There is stabilization of nicotinic receptors in the postsynaptic membrane (5).

These observations raise questions about the nature of the signalling pathways which underlie such a reorganization. Is there activation of second messengers by anterograde signals from the nerve endings that would lead to positive regulation of the expression of the nicotinic receptor in the junctional regions and negative regulation in the extrajunctional regions? Are there retrograde signals too?

Aggregation of proteins at the nerve–muscle contact depends, in fact, on instructive signals that are released by the motor axon. More than 20 years ago, McMahan and colleagues identified the basal lamina as the carrier of the information necessary to induce pre- and postsynaptic specializations during neuromuscular regeneration. A protein, agrin, was purified from basal lamina extracts of the cholinergic synapse of the electric organ of *Torpedo californica* (see **Figure 9.1**). When added to cultured myotubes, soluble agrin induces the aggregation of acetylcholine receptors. This led McMahan to formulate the following hypothesis: 'Agrin is released from motor neurons, binds to a receptor on the muscle cell surface and induces postsynaptic specializations.

Subsequent binding of agrin to synaptic basal lamina will then immobilize agrin.'

The fact that neural agrin is necessary and sufficient for postsynaptic differentiation is confirmed by the following experiment. Agrin is a protein of 225 kD, consisting of domains found in other basal lamina proteins. The region of agrin necessary and sufficient to bind to the basal lamina (it binds in fact to laminins) maps to the amino-terminus end of the molecule. The most carboxy-terminus is necessary and sufficient for its nAChR-aggregating activity. Agrin mRNA undergoes alternative splicing at several sites, two of which modulate agrin's ability to induce nAChR clustering in cultured muscle cells. In innervated adult rat muscle, injection of expression constructs that encode full-length chick neural agrin is sufficient to induce postsynaptic specializations: after 4–6 weeks, staining with anti-chick agrin fluorescent antibodies reveals the deposit of neural agrin in basal lamina at the ectopic site of injection (**Figure 7.13b**). In this area, aggregation of nAChRs is observed with immunocytochemistry. Therefore, ectopic expression of recombinant agrin in adult muscle *in vivo* induces the formation of postsynaptic-like structures that closely resemble the muscle endplate.

Which molecule is the agrin receptor(s) and what are the second messengers activated by agrin and responsible for postsynaptic differentiation? Agrin initiates a signalling cascade which is still under study. Interestingly, voltage-dependent Na^+ channels are also concentrated at the synapse where they are restricted to the depth of postjunctional folds. This clustering pathway also involves agrin.

7.4 The synapse between the vegetative postganglionic neuron and the smooth muscle cell

Smooth muscle cells are present in most of the visceral organs (digestive system, uterus, bladder, etc.) but also in the wall of blood vessels and around the hair follicles. They are innervated by postganglionic neurons of the autonomic nervous system (orthosympathetic neurons and parasympathetic neurons) (**Figure 7.14**).

7.4.1 The presynaptic element is a varicosity of the postganglionic axon

The axons of the postganglionic neurons are not myelinated. Before contacting the smooth muscles, the axons divide into numerous thin filaments 0.1–0.5 μm in diameter which travel alone or in fascicles over long distances along the smooth muscle cells (**Figures 7.14** and **7.15a**). Each of these filaments has swellings or

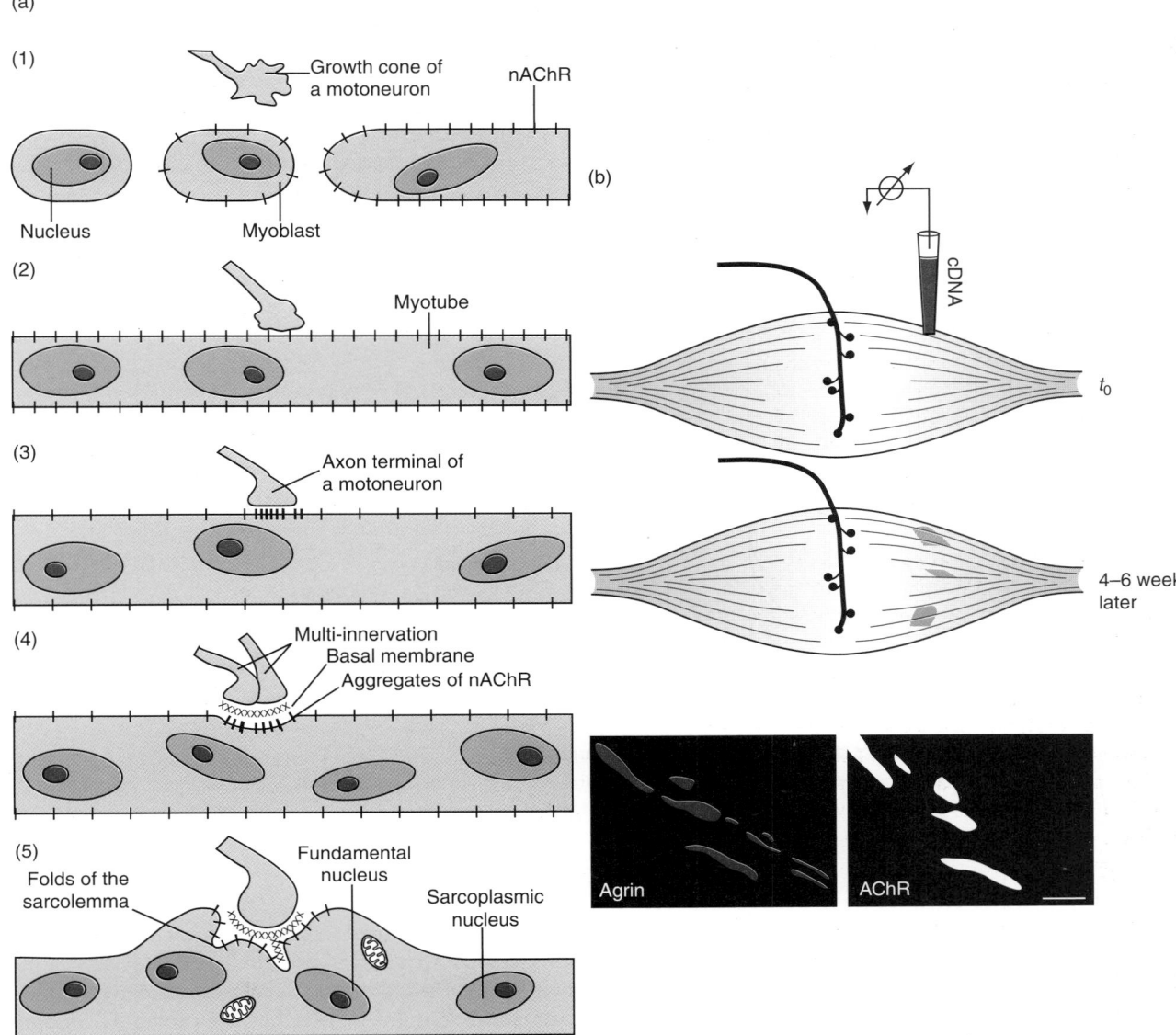

Figure 7.13 Postsynaptic differentiation at the neuromuscular junction.
(a) The different steps in postsynaptic differentiation. The black thin bars indicate the nicotinic receptor (nAChR). (1, 2) Fusion of myoblasts to form myotubes and approach of the axon growth cone; (3) the growth cone forms contact with the myotube and induces the clustering of nicotinic receptors at this level; (4) numerous motor terminals converge towards a single aggregate of nicotinic receptors; but (5) a single terminal stabilizes and the folds of the sarcolemma develop. **(b)** Injection of expression constructs that encode full-length neural agrin into single muscle fibres *in vivo* (t_0). After 4–6 weeks, muscle fibres have a deposit of chick neural agrin in muscle basal lamina at ectopic sites. Staining of the muscle anti-chick agrin antibodies reveals the depositing of neural agrin as visualized in optical longitudinal sections through ectopic sites (Agrin). In this area, ectopic neural agrin induces aggregation of nAChRs (AChR) as visualized by *in situ* hybridization. Scale bar, 15 μm. Drawing (a) from Laufer R, Changeux JP (1989) Activity-dependent regulation of gene expression in muscle and neuronal cells, *Mol. Neurobiol.* **3**, 1–53, with permission. Part (b) from Ruegg MA, Bixby JL (1998) Agrin orchestrates synaptic differentiation at the vertebrate neuromuscular junction, *Trend. Neurosci.* **21**, 22–27, with permission.

varicosities 0.5–2.0 μm in diameter spaced 3–5 μm apart. The varicosities contain mitochondria and numerous synaptic vesicles, whereas the intervaricose segments contain mainly elements of the cytoskeleton (**Figure 7.15b**). The varicosities are the presynaptic elements. There are no electron-dense regions in the presynaptic membrane, which suggests the absence of a preferential zone for exocytosis (active zone) in these synapses.

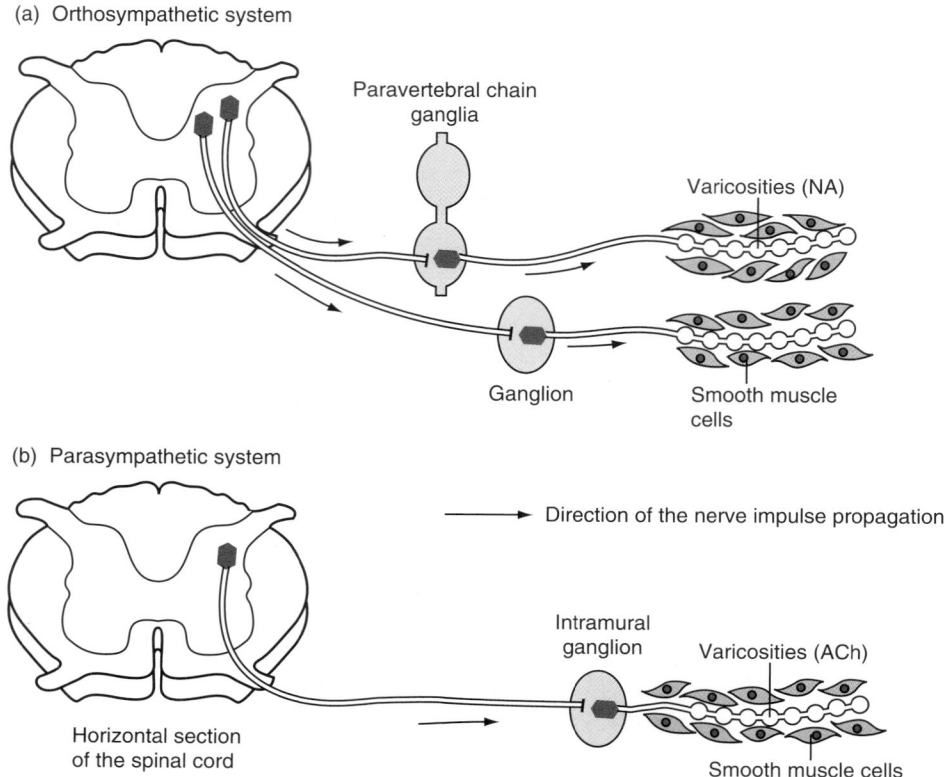

(a) Orthosympathetic system

Paravertebral chain ganglia

Varicosities (NA)

Ganglion

Smooth muscle cells

(b) Parasympathetic system

Direction of the nerve impulse propagation

Intramural ganglion

Varicosities (ACh)

Horizontal section of the spinal cord

Smooth muscle cells

Figure 7.14 The orthosympathetic and parasympathetic systems.
The synapses between postganglionic neurons and smooth muscle fibres are shown. The axon terminals of postganglionic neurons are varicosities and the synaptic contacts are of the 'boutons en passant' type. ACh, acetylcholine; NA, noradrenaline; arrows show the direction of action potential propagation.

The axonal varicosities contain a large number of small granular synaptic vesicles with an electron-dense central core (30–50 nm diameter), but also some large granular vesicles (60–120 nm diameter) and small agranular vesicles. The neurotransmitter of the orthosympathetic postganglionic neurons is noradrenaline (NA) (**Figure 7.14a**). It is stored in small and large granular vesicles. Noradrenaline is a catecholamine (as dopamine and adrenaline) synthesized from the amino acid tyrosine.

The noradrenaline receptors present in the postsynaptic membrane of smooth muscle cells are G-protein-coupled receptors. The inactivation of noradrenaline released from nerve terminals is, to a large extent, achieved by reuptake by the catecholaminergic neurons or the nearby glial cells. It is recycled into the synaptic vesicles or degraded by specific enzymes such as the monoamine oxidase (MAO). Some of the catecholamines are degraded in the synaptic cleft by the catechol-O-methyl-transferase (COMT).

Acetylcholine (ACh) is the neurotransmitter of the parasympathetic postganglionic neurons (**Figure 7.14b**). The varicosities of these axons contain mainly small

agranular vesicles but also large granular vesicles. Acetylcholine is stored in small agranular vesicles. The acetylcholine receptors present in the postsynaptic membrane of smooth muscle cells are cholinergic muscarinic receptors (mAChR); they are protein-G coupled receptors.

7.4.2 The width of the synaptic cleft is very variable

Where the synaptic cleft is narrowest, in the vas deferens or in the pupil for example, it measures between 15 and 20 nm. However, in the wall of blood vessels, the closest contacts are spaced 50–100 nm apart.

7.4.3 The autonomous postganglionic synapse is specialized to ensure a widespread effect of the neurotransmitter

The large width of the synaptic cleft results in a widespread effect of the neurotransmitter on the

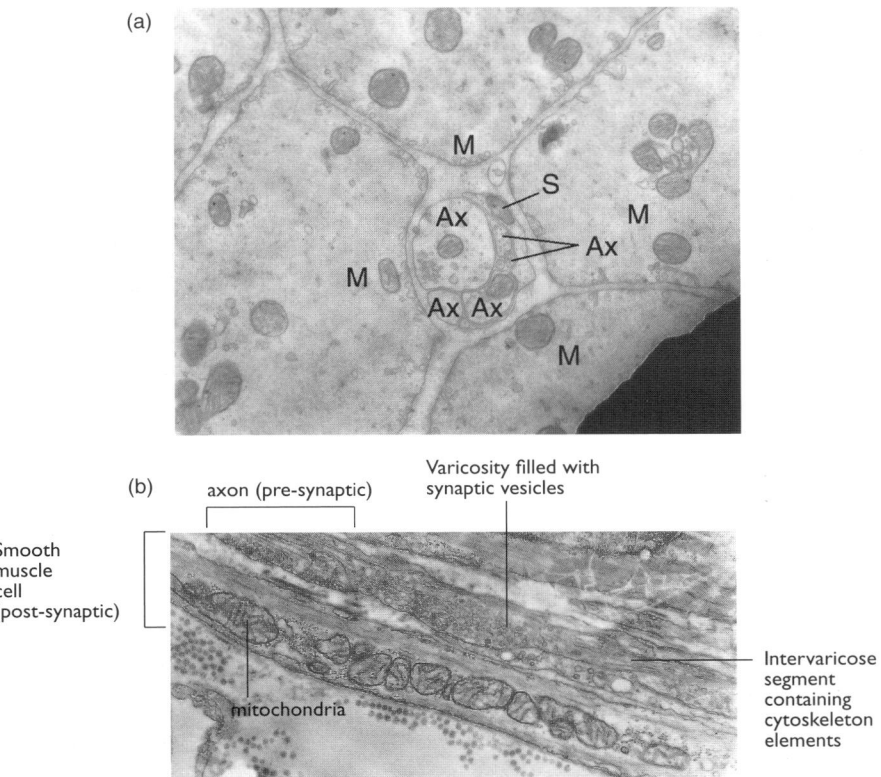

Figure 7.15 A nerve–smooth muscle synapse.

(a) Microphotograph of smooth muscle cells of the intestine (M) and postganglionic axon fascicles (parasympathetic nervous system, Ax) which are half-covered by a Schwann cell (S), sectioned in the transverse plane and observed under the electron microscope. Note the width of the synaptic cleft. **(b)** Longitudinal section of a postganglionic axon showing a varicosity filled with vesicles and an intervaricose region. The postsynaptic smooth muscle cell contains numerous mitochondria. Microphotography by Jacques Taxi.

postsynaptic membrane compared with the neuromuscular junction or central synapses, where secretion of the neurotransmitter is focused on a small postsynaptic region. Moreover, in some autonomous synapses, there is no distinguishable specialization of the presynaptic membrane, which suggests that the vesicles have no preferential site for exocytosis. Formation of a dense plexus by the postganglionic axons also contributes to the extended diffusion of presynaptic messages. Therefore, activation of a postganglionic neuron results in activation of numerous postsynaptic cells. Finally, the presence of numerous gap junctions which connect smooth muscle cells permits spread of the synaptic response to neighbouring muscle cells, even to those not innervated.

7.5 Example of a neuroglandular synapse

This section considers the synapse between an orthosympathetic preganglionic neuron and the chromaffin cell of the adrenal medulla (**Figure 7.16**).

The adrenal medulla is the central part of the adrenal gland, the endocrine gland located above each kidney. It is formed by secretory cells, which are called chromaffin cells since they are coloured by chromium salts. The adrenal medulla is innervated by orthosympathetic preganglionic neurons which have axons that form the splanchnic nerve. When this nerve is stimulated, the chromaffin cells secrete essentially adrenaline but also noradrenaline and enkephalins (endogenous opioid peptides). These hormones are then transported via the blood to numerous target tissues and mainly the heart and blood vessels.

The *presynaptic element* of this synapse is the axon terminal of the splanchnic orthosympathetic preganglionic neurons. Their cell bodies are located in the intermediate horn of the spinal cord. Most of the axons are non-myelinated and are surrounded by the extensions of the non-myelinating Schwann cells. This glial sheath is present until the axon collaterals penetrate the junctional space. The axon terminals are mainly terminal boutons with a diameter ranging between 1 and 3 µm. They contain clear vesicles (10–60 nm diameter) as well as some

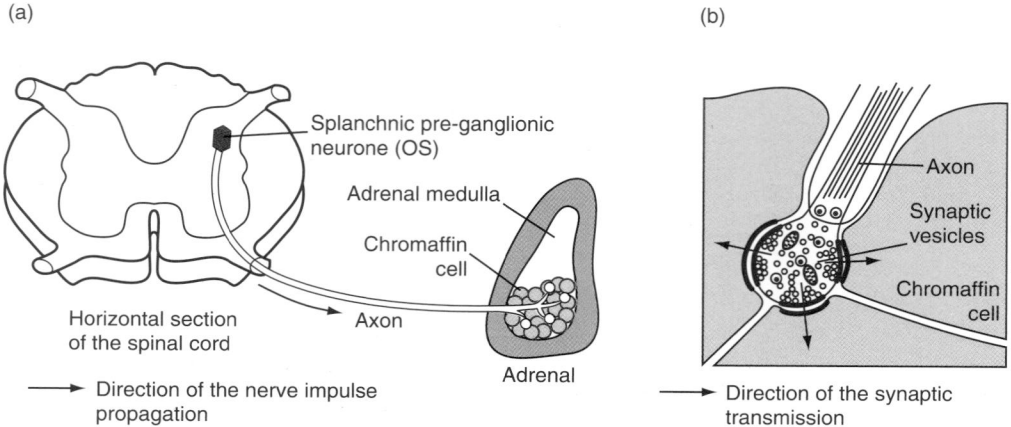

Figure 7.16 Synapses between an orthosympathetic preganglionic neuron and chromaffin cells in the adrenal medulla.
(a) The cell bodies of preganglionic neurons are localized in the spinal cord and their axons form the orthosympathetic splanchnic nerve. These neurons innervate the chromaffin cells. **(b)** Postganglionic axon terminal forming numerous contacts with chromaffin cells. Drawing (b) from Coupland RE (1965) Electron microscopic observations on the structure of the rat adrenal medulla: II. Normal innervation, *J. Anat. (Lond.)* **99**, 255–272, with permission.

dense-core and granular vesicles (25–115 nm diameter). Acetylcholine is the neurotransmitter of this synapse. The terminal boutons form a large variety of synaptic contacts with the chromaffin cells. They are characterized by a narrow synaptic cleft (15–20 nm) and the presence of electron-dense pre- and postsynaptic zones similar to those observed at the level of the central interneuronal synapses.

In the *postsynaptic region*, the cytoplasm of the chromaffin cells is free of chromaffin granules, organelles that store hormones in the adrenal medulla. The acetylcholine receptors present in the postsynaptic membrane are cholinergic nicotinic receptor channels. In the rest of the chromaffin cell cytoplasm there are numerous chromaffin granules. These granules are coloured by chromium salts which react with adrenaline to form a yellow–brown precipitate.

7.6 Summary

Chemical synapses are connections between two neurons or between a neuron and a non-neuronal cell (muscle cell, glandular cell, sensory cell). The synaptic complex is the non-reducible basic unit of each chemical synapse as it represents the minimal requirement for an efficient chemical synaptic transmission. It includes three elements: the presynaptic element (such as an axon terminal), a synaptic cleft, and a postsynaptic element (such as a dendritic spine).

The *presynaptic element* is characterized by (i) an active zone (i.e. a specialized presynaptic membrane area) where the density of Ca^{2+} channels is high and where

occurs the fusion of synaptic vesicles (exocytosis), and (ii) a nearby cytoplasmic region where the synaptic vesicles are found close to the presynaptic membrane, with a particular cytoskeletal arrangement. The regulated release of neurotransmitter occurs at active zones. However, the active zone is not a characteristic of all synapses. A few monoaminergic synapses and peptidergic synapses do not have discernible active zones. The presence of an active zone would be a clue to focal neurotransmitter release.

The *postsynaptic element* is characterized, in interneuronal synapses, by a sub-membranous electron-dense zone (postsynaptic density), which most probably corresponds to the region where the postsynaptic receptors are anchored. There is a strict complementarity between the neurotransmitter released by the presynaptic element and the postsynaptic receptors inserted in the postsynaptic membrane. This includes specific targeting, anchoring and clustering of postsynaptic receptors.

The ultrastructure of chemical synapses is asymmetric, synaptic vesicles that contain the neurotransmitter(s) being present only in the presynaptic element. Synaptic transmission is unidirectional – it always occurs from the presynaptic element to the postsynaptic one.

Appendix 7.1
Neurotransmitters, agonists and antagonists

Neurotransmitters are molecules of varied nature: quaternary amines, amino acids, catecholamines or peptides, which are released by neurons at chemical synapses. They transmit a message from a neuron to another neuron, or to an effector cell, or a message from a sensory cell to a neuron.

A7.1.1 Criteria to be satisfied before a molecule can be identified as a neurotransmitter

Identification of a substance as a neurotransmitter requires the experimental proof of several criteria. If these are not satisfied, the term *putative* neurotransmitter is used. The criteria are:

- The putative neurotransmitter must be present in the presynaptic element.
- The precursors and enzymes necessary for *synthesis* of the putative neurotransmitter must be present in the presynaptic neuron.
- The putative neurotransmitter must be released in response to activation of the presynaptic neuron and in a quantity sufficient to produce a postsynaptic response. This release should be dependent on Ca^{2+} ions.
- There should be *binding to specific postsynaptic receptors*: (i) specific receptors of the neurotransmitter are present in the postsynaptic membrane; (ii) application of the substance at the level of the postsynaptic element reproduces the response obtained by stimulation of the presynaptic neuron; and (iii) drugs, which specifically block or potentiate the postsynaptic response, have the same effects on the response induced by the application of the putative neurotransmitter.
- The elements of the synaptic nervous tissue (pre- or postsynaptic elements, glial cells, basal membrane) must possess one or several mechanisms for *inactivation* of the putative neurotransmitter.

Currently few molecules have satisfied all these criteria to be firmly identified as a neurotransmitter at a particular synapse. In most cases there is no more than fragmentary evidence owing to technical limitations.

A7.1.2 Types of neurotransmitter

Acetylcholine: a quaternary amine

In the peripheral nervous system, acetylcholine is the neurotransmitter of all the synapses between motoneurons and striated muscle cells, of all the synapses between preganglionic and postganglionic neurons of the para- and orthosympathetic systems, and of all the synapses between parasympathetic postganglionic neurons and effector cells (see **Figures 7.12, 7.14** and **7.16**). It is also a neurotransmitter in the central nervous system. Choline acetyltransferase (CAT), the enzyme required for acetylcholine synthesis, is a specific marker of cholinergic neurons. Using immunocytochemical or *in situ* hybridization techniques (see **Appendix 7.2**), one can visualize cholinergic neuronal pathways by labelling choline acetyltransferase or its mRNA. At the same time, the acetylcholine receptors can be localized.

Amino acids: glutamate, GABA (γ-aminobutyric acid) and glycine

In contrast to other neurotransmitters, glutamate also plays an important role in cellular metabolism (in intermediary metabolism, in the synthesis of proteins and as precursor of GABA). It is, therefore, present in all neurons and its identification as a neurotransmitter poses several problems.

In fact, evidence for the enzymes of its synthesis or degradation cannot represent a valid criterion for the identification of glutamatergic neurons. These difficulties can be overcome as glutamate is present in much higher concentrations in neurons where it plays a neurotransmitter role. In addition, these neurons have the property of recapturing selectively glutamate with the help of a high-affinity transport system, and localization of this transport system can be used to identify glutamate neurons. Glutamic acid decarboxylase, the enzyme required for GABA synthesis, is a good marker of GABAergic neurons. In the CNS, two isoforms of glutamic acid decarboxylase (GAD67 and GAD65), each encoded by a different gene and highly conserved among vertebrates, are co-expressed in most GABA neurons. Thus GABAergic neurons (cell bodies, axon terminals and fibres) can be visualized by the localization of these two forms of GADs or their mRNAs by immunocytochemistry and *in situ* hybridization, respectively, or by immunohistochemical detection of GABA itself.

Monoamines

These are classified as catecholamines (adrenaline, noradrenaline, dopamine), indolamine (serotonin) and imidazole (histamine). Adrenaline, noradrenaline and dopamine are all catecholamines. Their structure has a common part, the catechol nucleus (a benzene ring with two adjacent substituted hydroxyl groups). They are synthesized from a common precursor, tyrosine. Serotonin or 5-hydroxytryptamine (5HT) is synthesized from tryptophan, a neutral amino acid.

Neuropeptides

Peptides that are present in neurons with a supposed role in synaptic transmission are called neuropeptides. They are, for example, opioid peptides (enkephalins, dynorphin, β-endorphin) or they are peptides that have already been identified in the gastrointestinal tract (substance P, cholecystokinin, vasoactive intestinal peptide (VIP)) or in the hypothalamo-hypophyseal complex (luteinizing hormone releasing hormone (LHRH), somatostatin, adrenocorticotropic hormone (ACTH), vasopressin) or they are also circulating hormones (corticotropin or ACTH, insulin), before they were suggested as neurotransmitters in the central nervous system. It seems reasonable that other neuropeptides await discovery. These peptides were proposed to be neurotransmitters on the basis of their presence and synthesis in the neurons as well as by their release from axonal terminals by a Ca^{2+}-dependent mechanism. For some peptides other criteria have also been demonstrated.

The differences in the chemical nature of neurotransmitters have a fundamental consequence. Non-peptidic neurotransmitters are synthesized in axonal terminals: a precursor (or precursors) synthesized by the neuron or taken up from the extracellular medium is transformed into a neurotransmitter via an enzymatic reaction in axon terminals. The synthesis enzyme(s) is (are) synthesized in the cell body and transported to axon terminals via axonal transport. The newly synthesized neurotransmitter is then actively transported inside the synaptic vesicles (**Figure A7.1a**). Peptidic neurotransmitters are synthesized in the cell body since axon terminals, being deprived of the organelles responsible for protein synthesis, cannot themselves synthesize neuropeptides (**Figure A7.1b**). These are synthesized in cell bodies in the form of larger peptides called *precursors*. These precursors are then transported to the axon terminals by fast axonal transport. Cleavage of the precursors into neuroactive peptides is carried out by vesicular peptidases during anterograde axonal transport. Since these precursors have no biological activity, regulation of peptidase activity seems to be an important factor in the regulation of the synthesis of peptidic neurotransmitters.

Concerning their mode of inactivation, most of the neurotransmitters are taken up by axon terminals or glial cells via specific transporters. The major exception is acetylcholine, which is degraded in the synaptic cleft by acetylcholinesterases. Since enzymatic degradation is more rapid than a transporter reaction, acetylcholine is much more rapidly inactivated than the other neurotransmitters.

A7.1.3 Agonists and antagonists of a receptor

An *agonist* is a molecule (drug, neurotransmitter, hormone) that binds to a specific receptor, activates the receptor and thus elicits a physiological response:

$$A + R \underset{k_{-1}}{\overset{k_{+1}}{\rightleftharpoons}} AR \rightleftharpoons AR^* ---\rightarrow \text{physiological response,}$$

where A is the agonist, R is the free receptor, AR is the agonist–receptor complex and AR^* is the activated state of the receptor bound to the agonist. k_{+1} and k_{-1} measure the rate at which association and dissociation occur. An agonist (and an antagonist) is defined in relation to a receptor and not to a neurotransmitter. For example, an agonist of nicotinic acetylcholine receptors such as nicotine is not an agonist of muscarinic acetylcholine receptors though both receptors are activated by acetylcholine.

An *antagonist* is a molecule that prevents the effect of the agonist. A *competitive antagonist* (C) is a receptor antagonist that acts by binding reversibly to agonist receptor site (R). It does not activate the receptor and thus does not elicit a physiological response:

$$B + R \underset{k_{-1B}}{\overset{k_{+1B}}{\rightleftharpoons}} BR ---\rightarrow \text{no physiological response.}$$

The effect of a *reversible competitive antagonist* can be reversed when the agonist concentration is increased since the agonist (A) and the reversible competitive antagonist (B) compete for the same receptor site (R). Competition means that the receptor can bind only one molecule (A or B) at a time. An *irreversible competitive antagonist* is a receptor antagonist that dissociates from the receptor slowly or not at all. For this reason its effect cannot be reversed when the agonist concentration is increased.

Appendix 7.2
Identification and localization of neurotransmitters and their receptors

A7.2.1 Immunocytochemistry

Principle and definitions

Immunocytochemical techniques are based on the high specificity of the antigen–antibody reaction. They consist of the detection of an antigen present in histological or cellular structures by application on tissues or cells of its specific antibody or antiserum. The complex antigen–antibody formed is then visualized under light or electron microscopy by means of various methods of detection described below.

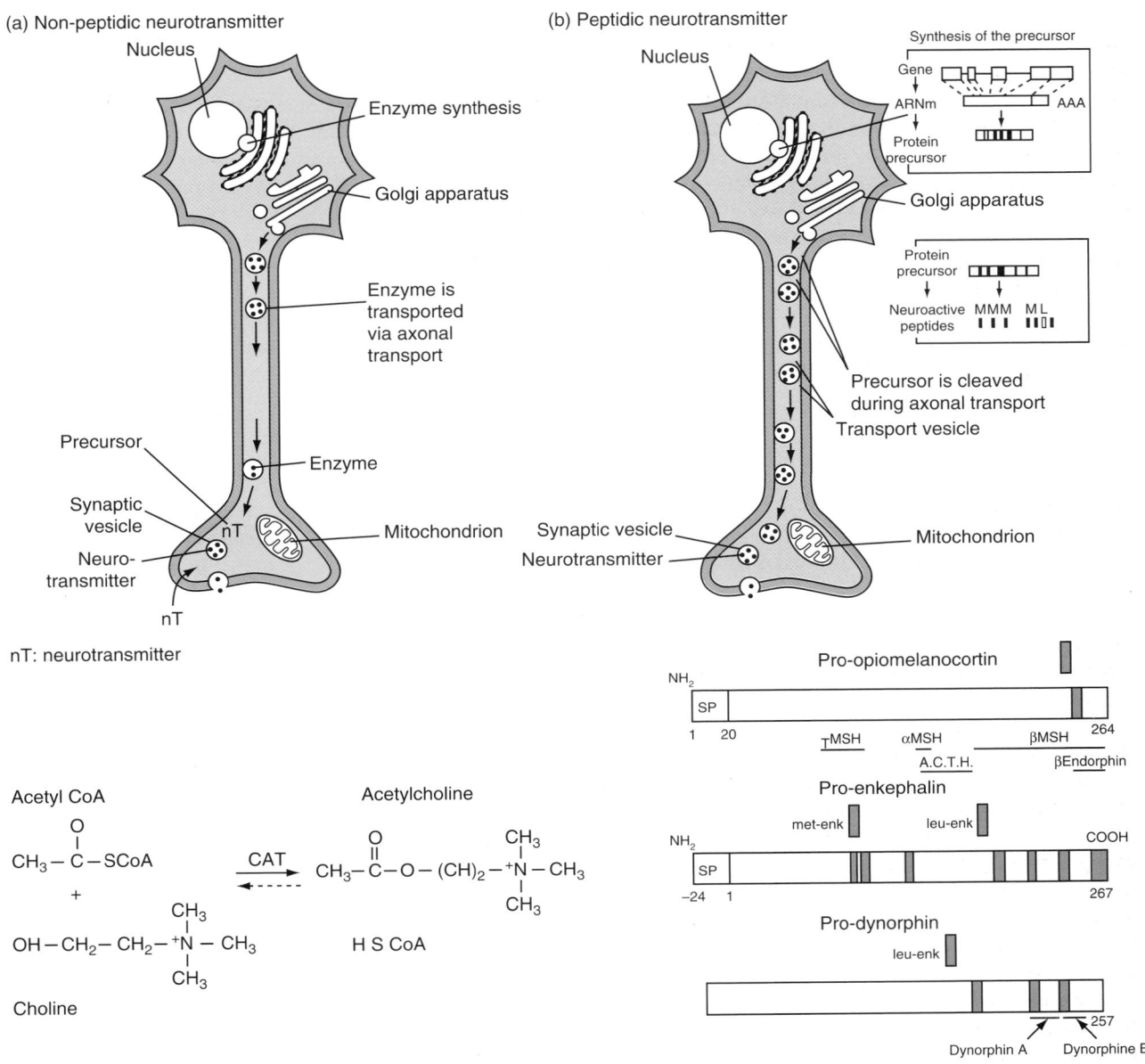

Figure A7.1 Synthesis of non-peptidic and peptidic neurotransmitters.
(a) Non-peptidic type (example, acetylcholine). (b) Peptidic type (example, opioid peptides). Bottom left: The synthesis reaction of acetylcholine from acetylcoenzyme A. Bottom right: Precursors of endorphines are pro-opiomelanocortin, pro-enkephalin A and pro-dynorphin. The peptides they contain are shown. The numbers indicate the position of the peptides along the protein. CAT, choline acetyltransferase; HSCOA, coenzyme A; MSH, melanocyte stimulating hormone; ACTH, corticotropin; enk, enkephalin; SP, substance P.

The antigen is an endogenous molecule able to induce the formation of antibodies when injected into a foreign body. The antigen will be recognized specifically by these antibodies. Antigens are endogenous particles such as synthesis enzymes or receptors for neurotransmitters. Neuroactive peptides or amino acid neurotransmitters can become antigenic after being conjugated to a carrier protein or a polysaccharide.

The antibodies are immunoglobulins of type G (IgG) or type M (IgM), Y-shaped molecules that display a minimum of two binding sites for the antigen. These two binding sites recognize a very short amino acid sequence of the antigen. This sequence is called an antigenic determinant. The term 'hapten' is used to described an amino acid sequence that binds specifically to the binding site of the antibody but cannot induce on its own an immune response (example: an amino acid neurotransmitter like GABA).

Two families of antibodies are commonly used in immunocytochemistry: polyclonal antibodies (or anti-serum) and monoclonal antibodies. A *monoclonal antibody* is the product of a single B lymphocyte clone (**Figure A7.2a**). It is made of a population of identical antibody molecules, each of them recognizing the same antigenic determinant (or hapten) on the antigen. A *polyclonal antibody* consists of a heterogeneous family of antibodies that recognize different antigenic determinants on the same antigen. They are generated in a host animal (usually a rabbit) after its immunization by injec-

tion of the antigen. The antibody (polyclonal or monoclonal) used to recognize an antigen into the tissues is called the *primary antibody*.

Antibodies are themselves antigenic, so it is possible to produce antibodies that will recognize antigenic determinants on various regions of an antibody. Antibodies directed against 'primary antibodies' are called *secondary antibodies*. They are anti-IgG or anti-IgM antibodies. These secondary antibodies can be labelled and are then used to detect the antigen/primary-antibody complex.

Among the different antigenic determinants of an antibody those that are associated with the antigen-

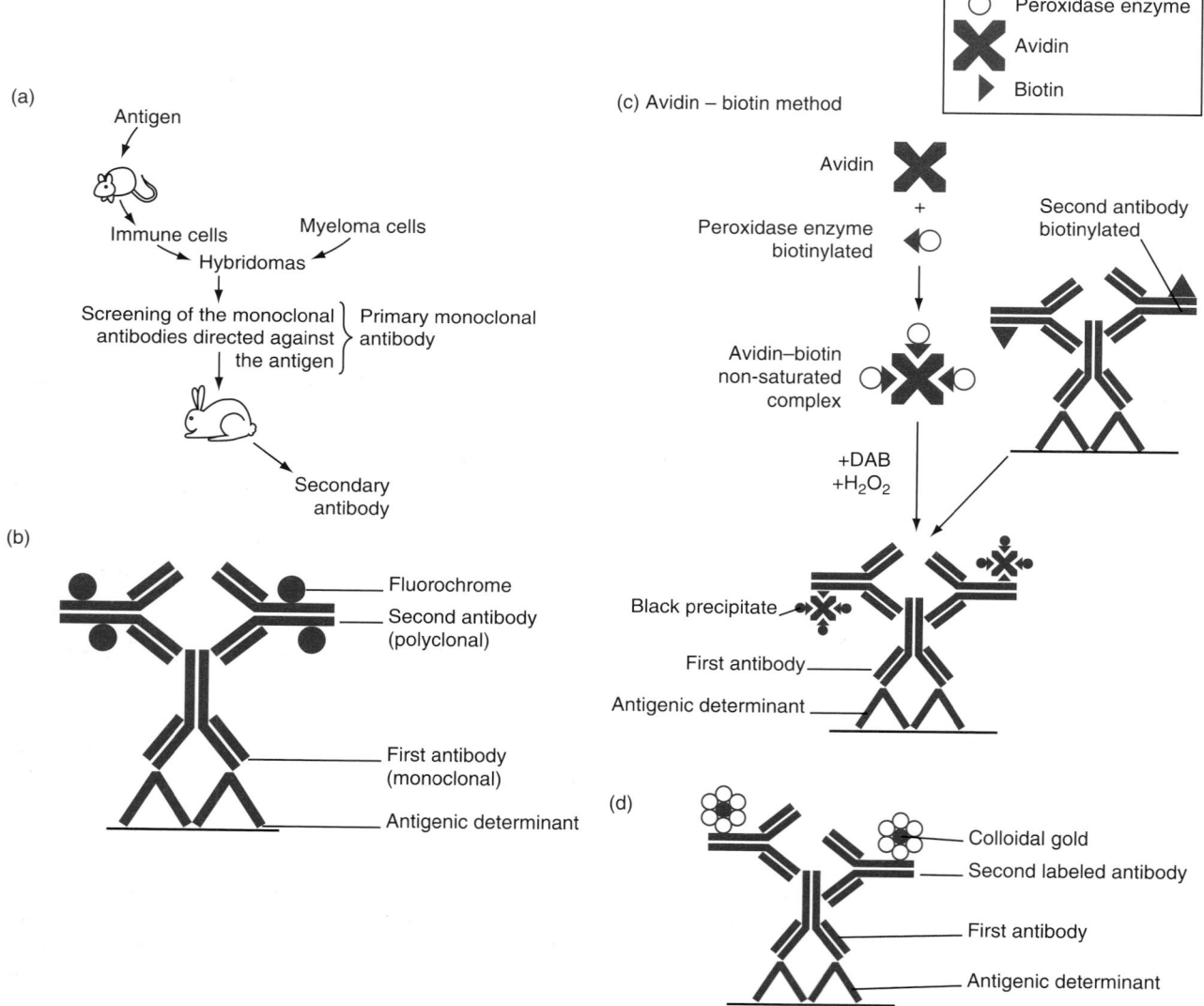

Figure A7.2 Synthesis and labelling of secondary antibodies raised against monoclonal antibodies specific to a neuronal antigen.

binding site are called *idiotypes*. Secondary antibodies directed against the specific antigen-binding sites (idiotypes) of a primary antibody are called *anti-idiotype antibodies*. These anti-idiotype antibodies are also useful tools for the localization of receptors.

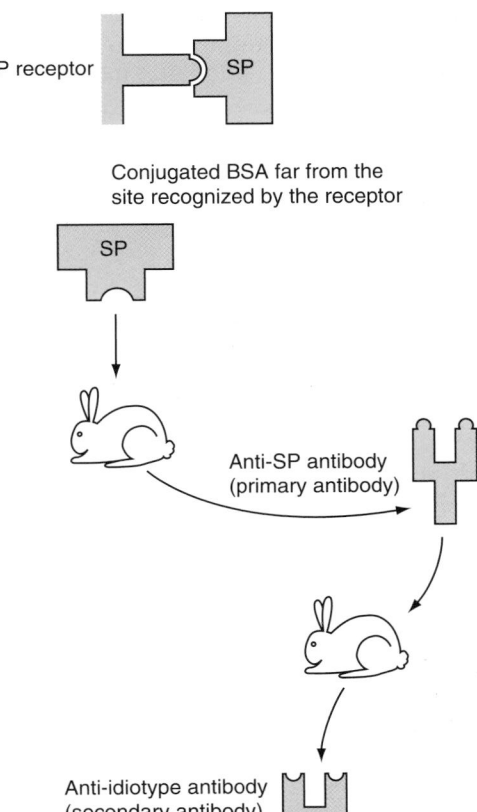

Figure A7.3 **Synthesis of anti-idiotype antibodies for substance P (SP).**

Applications

Localization of neurons synthesizing a specific neurotransmitter

If we want to localize, for example, the cholinergic neurons in a section of brain tissue, the approach is to reveal the neurons that contain the synthesis enzyme for acetylcholine, choline acetyltransferase (ChAT). Sections of brain tissue are incubated with a primary antibody directed against ChAT. The antibodies will bind specifically to the antigen into sections and a stable complex antigen–antibody will be formed only in the neurons that contain ChAT. After washing the sections to remove the antibodies that did not link with the antigen, the complex antigen–antibody is detected according to one of the methods described below (detection).

Localization of receptors of a neurotransmitter

Primary antibodies directed against a purified receptor can be used to localize a specific type of receptor on sections of brain tissue, similarly to the localization of synthesis enzymes of neurons.

A second method for localization of receptors use the anti-idiotype antibodies (**Figure A7.3**). Anti-idiotype antibodies are generated against primary antibodies specific to the ligand of the receptor. For example, for the localization of substance P receptors, anti-idiotype antibodies are generated against the antibody specific to substance P. Anti-idiotype antibodies are used since their antigen-binding sites have structural similarities with the ligand itself, of which they constitute a sort of 'molecular image'. This property allows them to bind the biological receptor. This method displays the advantage to enable receptor antibodies to be obtained without a pre-purification of the receptor. The receptor can therefore be localized and its stereospecificity studied.

Detection of the antigen–antibody complex

Most of the detection methods use markers (labels). The marker is bound to the secondary antibody to obtain *labelled secondary antibodies* which, by reacting with the *antigen–primary antibody complex,* will allow the visualization of the antigen under light or electron microscopy. The markers used for light microscopy are (i) fluorochromes that can be detected with a microscope equipped with an epifluorescence system, or (ii)

enzymes (such as peroxidase) that will induce a chromogen reaction in presence of its substrate (such as the diaminobenzide). For electron microscopy, electron dense compounds such as colloidal gold particles are used (**Figure A7.2d**).

Why use labelling of secondary antibodies and not primary ones?

Labelling of antibodies (markers are directly conjugated to the primary antibodies) displays many disadvantages. The labelling of the antibody reduces significantly its capacity to recognize the antigen, thus its specificity. Moreover there is only one molecule of marker for a single antigen–antibody complex. Therefore this technique is poorly sensitive and cannot be used to localize antigens that are present in small quantity in neurons. In addition, for each antigen studied, it is necessary to label the corresponding antibody. For these reasons indirect labelling methods have been developed to increase the sensitivity of detection by amplification of the labelling. All of them use as a first step an unlabelled primary antibody that binds to its antigen into the section. In the following step the primary antibody is recognized by a secondary antibody raised in another species. The secondary antibody is a serum anti-heterologous IgG (or IgM) that binds to many antigenic sites on the primary antibody.

Three main methods commonly used

In the first method (**Figure A7.2b and d**), the secondary antibody is labelled with one of the markers previously described. Since many labelled secondary antibodies bind to a single primary antibody molecule, this technique allows an increase in the labelling and consequently a better visualization of the antigen.

In the peroxidase anti-peroxidase (PAP) detection method, the molecules of secondary antibody are unlabelled and applied in excess, allowing one of their antigen binding sites to be left free. A third step consists in incubating the tissue in a solution containing the peroxidase–antiperoxidase complex formed by several molecules of peroxidase and antibodies directed against those molecules. The antibodies of the PAP complex are raised in the same species as the primary antibody and thus are recognized by the free antigen-binding sites of the secondary antibody.

The avidin (or streptavidin) biotin method (**Figure A7.2c**) uses the very high affinity of a little hydrosoluble vitamin, biotin, for the protein avidin. The tissue is incubated in the presence of the secondary antibody previously conjugated to biotin molecules (biotinylated secondary antibodies), then in the presence of the preformed complex consisting of molecules of biotin and avidin covalently bound with markers such as peroxidase or fluorochromes.

Both PAP and avidin–biotin methods allow a strong amplification of the labelling and are the most sensitive immunocytochemical techniques.

A7.2.2 In situ hybridization

Principle

The aim of these techniques is the detection of a specific nucleic acid sequence in cells on histological sections or in cultured cells. *In situ* hybridization techniques are based on the capacity of all nucleic or ribonucleic acids sequences (ADN or ARN) to bind to a complementary sequence. The sequence of nucleic acids to recognize may correspond to chromosomal DNA, called 'hybridization on chromosomes'. But in general the term '*in situ* hybridization' relates to the detection of messenger RNA (mRNA). This detection or recognition is made possible by the use of a probe that corresponds

to a sequence of nucleic acids complementary to the DNA or RNA that is to be detected. The probe is labelled with a marker. When they are in the presence of each other, the specific labelled probe and the endogenous RNA (or DNA) recognized by the probe, hybridize (because of the complementary sequences). The hybrids thus formed are detected by means of the marker linked to the probe.

Application

The *in situ* hybridization technique allows visualization of gene transcripts and, therefore, localization of the potential site of synthesis for the protein or the peptide coded by this gene. In the case of nerve cells, this technique can localize neurons that express a gene coding for a neurotransmitter (if it is a peptide), for a synthesis or degradative enzyme of a specific neurotransmitter, or for a receptor for a neurotransmitter. For example, it has been used to localize neurons that contain the mRNA coding for the precursors of the enkephalins. Moreover, the role of various factors that regulate the expression of these peptides can be studied because this technique can be used to analyse variations in the level of transcripted mRNA in relation to the activity of the neuron, the presence of hormonal factors, etc.

Probes

The most commonly used types are double-stranded DNA, single-stranded DNA, single-stranded RNA and oligodeoxyribonucleotides. The latter three, which include only complementary strands (antisense) to the targeted sequence (cellular mRNA), provide the highest sensitivity. The labelling of the probe is performed in general during probe synthesis by incorporation of markers into the probe.

Double-stranded DNA probes are cDNAs (complementary DNA to cellular mRNA). They are obtained by reverse transcription of cellular RNAs by means of a reverse transcriptase, an enzyme which is able to make complementary single-stranded DNA chains from RNA templates. This is followed by second-strand synthesis using a DNA polymerase. cDNAs are inserted into plasmid vectors, this cDNA library is then screened to identify and isolate the cDNA of interest. This cDNA is then amplified in bacteria or by the polymerase chain reaction (PCR) using oligoprimers on opposite strands. The double-stranded DNA probe can be labelled by different techniques: the nick-translation method consists to induce cuts in the double strand DNA with a DNAse and to repair these cuts by incorporation of labelled and unlabelled desoxynucleotides in the presence of DNA polymerase; the random primed method use, after denaturation of the two strands of cDNA, the ability of the fragment of DNA polymerase to copy single-stranded DNA templates primed with random hexanucleotide mixture. Finally the probes can be labelled during the PCR reaction in the presence of labelled nucleotides. Random priming and PCR give the highest efficiency of labelling.

Double-stranded DNA probes need to be denatured before use for hybridization. These probes are less sensitive than the single-stranded type because many of the two strands can reappariate during the hybridization reaction instead of hybridizing with the target.

Single-stranded DNA probes are preferentially obtained by PCR-based methods using a specific primer from the complementary strand of the RNA transcript and a mixture of labelled and unlabelled desoxynucleotides. Probes which do not reappariate with themselves are thus more sensitive and produce less background noise than double-stranded DNA probes.

Single-stranded RNA probes are produced by *in vitro* transcription of specific cDNAs sub-cloned into a transcription vector (plasmid containing the appropriate polymerase initiation site), by means of an RNAse polymerase. Before this transcription step, the plasmid is linearized with a restriction enzyme to avoid the transcription of plasmid sequences that will cause high backgrounds. The labelling is performed during the transcription by incorporation of labelled nucleotides. The labelled transcript is in general hydrolysed to obtain probes of approximately 150–200 nucleotides in length.

Among the different types of probe, RNA probes are the most sensitive. Since RNA–RNA hybrids are more stable than DNA–RNA ones, strong specific staining with low background can be achieved with RNA probes by using post-hybridization treatment with RNAse and high-temperature washes.

Oligonucleotides are obtained through automated chemical synthesis. They are small (typically 20–30 bases in length) single-stranded DNA probes. Labelling of the probes is performed during synthesis or by adding a tail of labelled nucleotides. Their small size gives them good access to the targeted nucleic acid sequence but limits their sensitivity. However, they are useful when target abundance is high, when gene-specific probes cannot be obtained otherwise, or when only protein sequence information is available.

Markers

Two major families of markers are used for probe labelling: radioactive labels which are detected by autoradiography, and non-radioactive labels which are detected by immunocytochemistry. For many years radioisotopes have been the only markers available to label nucleotides. Among the different radioisotopes used to label probes, ^{35}S is the most commonly used for radioactive *in situ* hybridization. ^{35}S-labelled probes give a resolution of about one cell diameter and relatively rapid results (the time exposure for detection of hybrids is about one week). Despite their high sensitivity, radiolabelled probes have disadvantages such as safety measures required during experimental procedures, limited utilization time, and limited spatial resolution due to scattering of emitted radiation.

More recently non-radioactive *in situ* hybridization techniques have been introduced with the development of hapten-labelled nucleotides that can be well incorporated during probe synthesis. Biotin- or dioxigenin-labelled probes are the most commonly used for cellular mRNA detection. Fluorescent labelling is successfully used for chromosomal *in situ* hybridization. Non-radioactive labelled probes are stable, give rapid results and display high levels of cellular resolution comparable to that obtained with immunocytochemistry. Furthermore, they open up new opportunities with the possibility of using different labels for simultaneous detection of different sequences in the same tissue.

Detection of the hybrids

For radioactive probes, a low-resolution signal can be obtained by placing the tissue or cells mounted on slides in contact with X-ray film for overnight exposure. This step allows one to control the efficiency of the reaction. If satisfactory, a greater resolution is obtained by dipping the slides in a liquid photographic emulsion, exposed for one or several weeks and developed. In general, a nuclear stain of cells is performed (for example, with Toluidine Blue) before observation under a microscope with brightfield or darkfield illumination.

Detection of hybrids labelled with non-radioactive probes is performed by immunocytochemistry using specific antibody conjugated with enzyme such as peroxidase or alkaline phosphatase that will give a colour precipitate in the presence of their substrates.

Further reading

Betz H (1999) Structure and functions of inhibitory and excitatory glycine receptors. *Ann. NY Acad. Sci.* **868**, 667.

Brenman JE, Topinka JR, Cooper EC *et al.* (1998) Localization of postsynaptic density-93 to dendritic microtubules and interaction with microtubule-associated protein 1A. *J. Neurosci.* **18**, 8805–8813.

Cohen I, Rimer M, Lomo T, McMahan UJ (1997) Agrin-induced postsynaptic-like apparatus in skeletal muscle fibers in vivo. *Mol. Cell. Neurosci.* **9**, 237–253.

Couteaux R (1998) Early days in the research to localize skeletal muscle acetylcholinesterases. *J. Physiol. (Paris)* **92**, 59–62.

Massoulie J, Anselmet A, Bon S *et al.* (1998) Acetylcholinesterase: C-terminal domains, molecular forms and functional localization. *J. Physiol. (Paris)* **92**, 183–190.

Niethammer M, Sheng M (1998) Identification of ion channel-associated proteins using the yeast two-hybrid system. *Meth. Enzymol.* **293**, 104–122.

Nitkin RM, Smith MA, Magill C *et al.* (1987) Identification of agrin, a synaptic organizing protein from Torpedo electric organ. *J. Cell Biol.* **105**, 2471–2478.

Sanes JR (1998) Agrin receptors at the skeletal neuromuscular junction. *Ann. NY Acad. Sci.* **841**, 1–13.

Wang ZZ, Mathias A, Gautam M, Hall ZW (1999) Metabolic stabilization of muscle nicotinic acetylcholine receptor by rapsyn. *J. Neurosci.* **19**, 1998–2007.

Neurotransmitter Release

The neuron is a secretory cell. The secretory product, the neurotransmitter, is released at the level of chemical synapses (see Chapter 7 and Appendix 7.1). Neurotransmitters achieve the transmission of information at the level of chemical synapses between neurons, neurons and muscle cells, neurons and glandular cells and sensory receptors and neurons.

Neurotransmitters synthesized by the neuron are stored in the presynaptic element, inside the synaptic vesicles. In the absence of presynaptic activity, the probability of a neurotransmitter being released in the synaptic cleft is very low. This probability increases strongly when the presynaptic element is depolarized by an action potential. The vesicle hypothesis of neurotransmitter release, first formulated by Del Castillo and Katz (1954), is the generally accepted theory of neurotransmitter release (see Appendix 8.1). It states that the neurotransmitter molecules released in the synaptic cleft are those stored in synaptic vesicles (see **Figure 7.4a**). Many recent studies have confirmed the existence of vesicular release, such as data obtained with combined capacitance measurements and amperometry or optical analysis of labelled synaptic vesicles.

Many presynaptic elements contain small synaptic vesicles as well as large dense core vesicles (see Section 7.1.1). Demonstration at the frog neuromuscular junction that exocytosis of small and large dense core vesicles can be dissociated pharmacologically strongly suggests the existence of differences in the mechanisms that regulate exocytosis of the two types of secretory vesicles. However, the two systems share at least some common mechanisms for final fusion since both are sensitive to botulinum toxins. This chapter focuses on Ca^{2+}-regulated release of neurotransmitter from small synaptic vesicles.

Among the events coupling presynaptic membrane depolarization to neurotransmitter release, local rise of intracellular Ca^{2+} concentration has been clearly established as one of the prerequisites. The molecular mechanisms responsible for the coupling between Ca^{2+} ion influx and exocytosis are being elucidated. This includes the identification of the proteins involved in exocytosis, the steps regulating exocytosis and their order of appearance in the phenomenon. It is noteworthy that even when all the proper conditions come together (a presynaptic spike, opening of Ca^{2+} channels, Ca^{2+} entry), the existence of exocytosis of a synaptic vesicle is still not guaranteed (see Appendix 8.2).

The examples in this chapter will be taken mainly from studies on the glutamatergic synapses of the mammalian central nervous system (**Figures 8.1a and b**), and on other synapses that have been examined owing to the large diameter of their presynaptic element, such as the squid giant synapse (**Figure 8.1c**) and the neuromuscular junction (see **Figures 7.11** and **7.12a**).

8.1 Observations and questions

8.1.1 Quantitative data on synapse morphology and synaptic transmission

The regulated release of neurotransmitter occurs at the active zone of a synaptic complex. Synapses of the mammalian central nervous system generally exhibit one or two active zones (or release sites) per bouton (**Figures 8.2a and b**); but there are exceptions, such as the perforated synapse of the hippocampus (see **Figure 7.3**) or the calyx of Held in the medial trapezoid body of the brainstem (**Figure 8.1b**) that contain more than one active zone (**Figure 8.2c**) (around 4–5 for the former and at least 200 for the latter). Giant synapses such as in the squid (**Figure 8.1c**) comprise around 4400 active zones and the neuromuscular junction (see **Figure 7.12a**) from 300 to 1000 active zones.

Synapses of the mammalian central nervous system have small dimensions. In the hippocampus, synaptic terminals are rarely more than 1–5 μm wide, but there are exceptions. Vesicle have diameters of 25–60 nm. Cleft diameter ranges from 0.1 to 1 μm and pre- and postsynaptic elements are distant by 10–30 nm (cleft width). Postsynaptic density areas range from 0.01 to 0.5 μm². In three dimensions, the surfaces of presynaptic

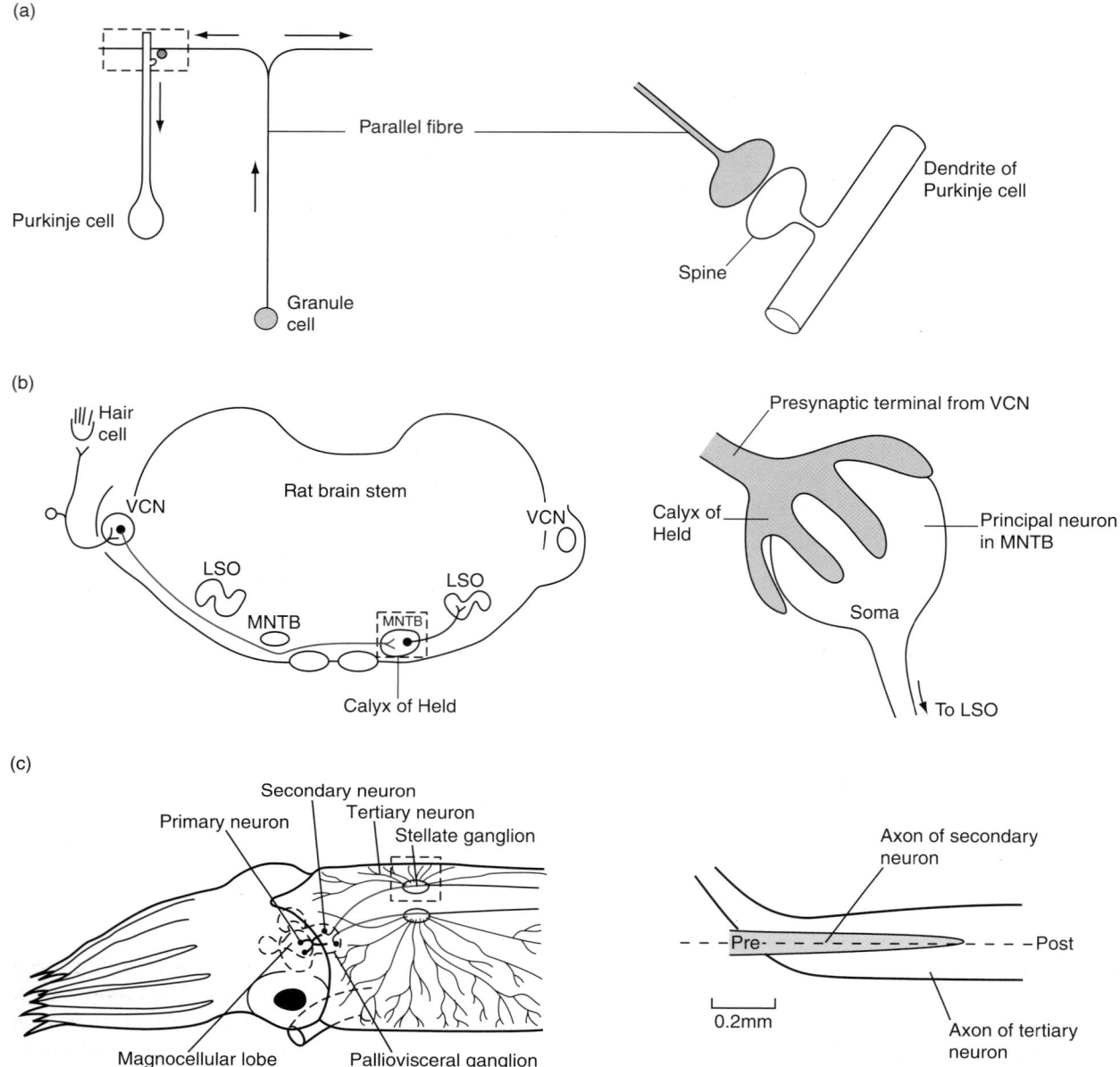

Figure 8.1 Three examples of preparations in which synaptic transmission has been studied.
(a) *The cerebellar cortex*. Left: Schematic showing the connections between a granular cell axon (parallel fibre) and a Purkinje cell. These synapses are axo-spinous (right). **(b)** *The calyx of Held*. Left: Frontal section of the brainstem drawn at the level of the 8th nerve. The axon collaterals of the globular cells of the ventral cochlear nucleus (VCN) project to the neurons of the contralateral medial nucleus of the trapezoid body (MNTB). This synapse is axo-somatic and each MNTB neuron receives only one axon terminal that forms the calyx of Held (right). **(c)** *Squid giant synapse*. Secondary neurons, that receive sensory information from the primary ones (left), establish giant axo-axonic synapses with tertiary neurons (right). The tertiary neurons are responsible for contraction of the mantle muscles thus permitting expulsion of water and propelling the animal out of the danger zone. The dotted square indicates the region enlarged on the right of the figures. LSO, lateral superior olive. Drawing (b) adapted from Forsythe ID, Barnes-Davies M, Brew HM (1995) The calyx of Held: a model for transmission at mammalian glutamatergic synapses. In: *Excitatory Aminoacids and Synaptic Transmission*, 2nd edn, New York: Academic Press. Drawing (c) from Llinas R (1982) Calcium in synaptic transmission, *Sci. Amer.* **247**, 56–65, with permission.

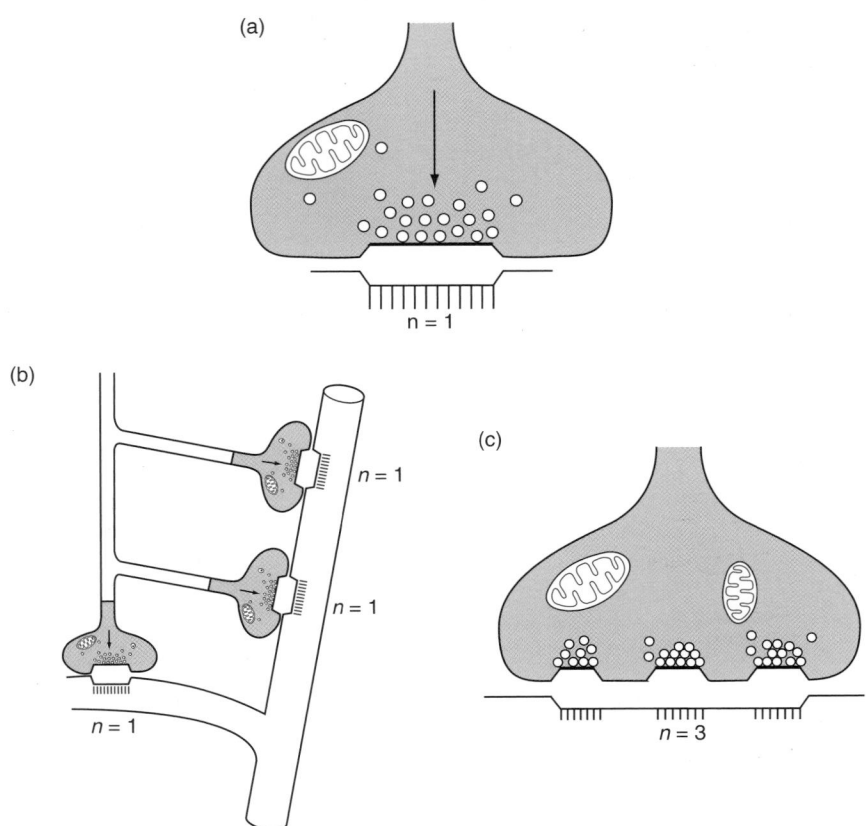

Figure 8.2 Number *n* of active zones per presynaptic terminal.
Drawings of synaptic boutons of the central nervous system with presynaptic active zone(s) and postsynaptic membranes. The active zones are represented as a black bar with adjacent synaptic vesicles. The number of active zones per bouton is $n = 1$ in **(a)** and **(b)** but $n = 3$ in **(c)**. The synaptic connections are such that a single presynaptic spike will activate a maximum of one active zone in (a), and a maximum of three in (b) and (c). Adapted from Korn H (1984) *Exp. Brain Res.* **Suppl. 9**, 201–224, with permission.

and postsynaptic membranes have the shape of two plates facing one another.

Postsynaptic responses are either a depolarization or a hyperpolarization of the postsynaptic membrane. The former is called the *excitatory postsynaptic potential* (EPSP; **Figure 8.3a**) since it brings the membrane potential closer to the spike threshold, and the latter is called the *inhibitory postsynaptic potential* (IPSP) since it does the opposite. These responses, being voltage changes, are recorded in current clamp. The underlying currents can be recorded in voltage clamp; they are the *excitatory or inward* (EPSC; **Figure 8.3b**) and the *inhibitory or outward* (IPSC) postsynaptic currents. In this chapter, only excitatory responses are studied.

In response to a single spike in the presynaptic axon, a small-amplitude EPSP (or EPSC) is recorded; it is called 'single-spike EPSP' (or EPSC). It has the following characteristics: the synaptic delay ranges from 200 µs to 1 ms (**Figure 8.3b**); the amplitude of the single-spike EPSP ranges from 200 µV to 1 mV (**Figure 8.3a**) depend-

ing on the number of boutons and active zones activated by the presynaptic spike (**Figure 8.2**). The half-duration of a single-spike EPSP is in the order of milliseconds to tens of milliseconds. Each single presynaptic spike does not necessarily evoke a postsynaptic potential – there are failures of synaptic transmission (**Figure 8.3a**).

In summary, the synapse is an electrochemical unit specialized to function on a distance scale of micrometres and a time scale of submilliseconds.

8.1.2 Ways of estimating neurotransmitter release in central mammalian synapses

Recording of the postsynaptic response

If one considers the schematic representation of synaptic transmission in **Figure 7.4a**, neurotransmitter release corresponds to steps 2, 3 and 4. One way to estimate neurotransmitter release is to measure the postsynaptic

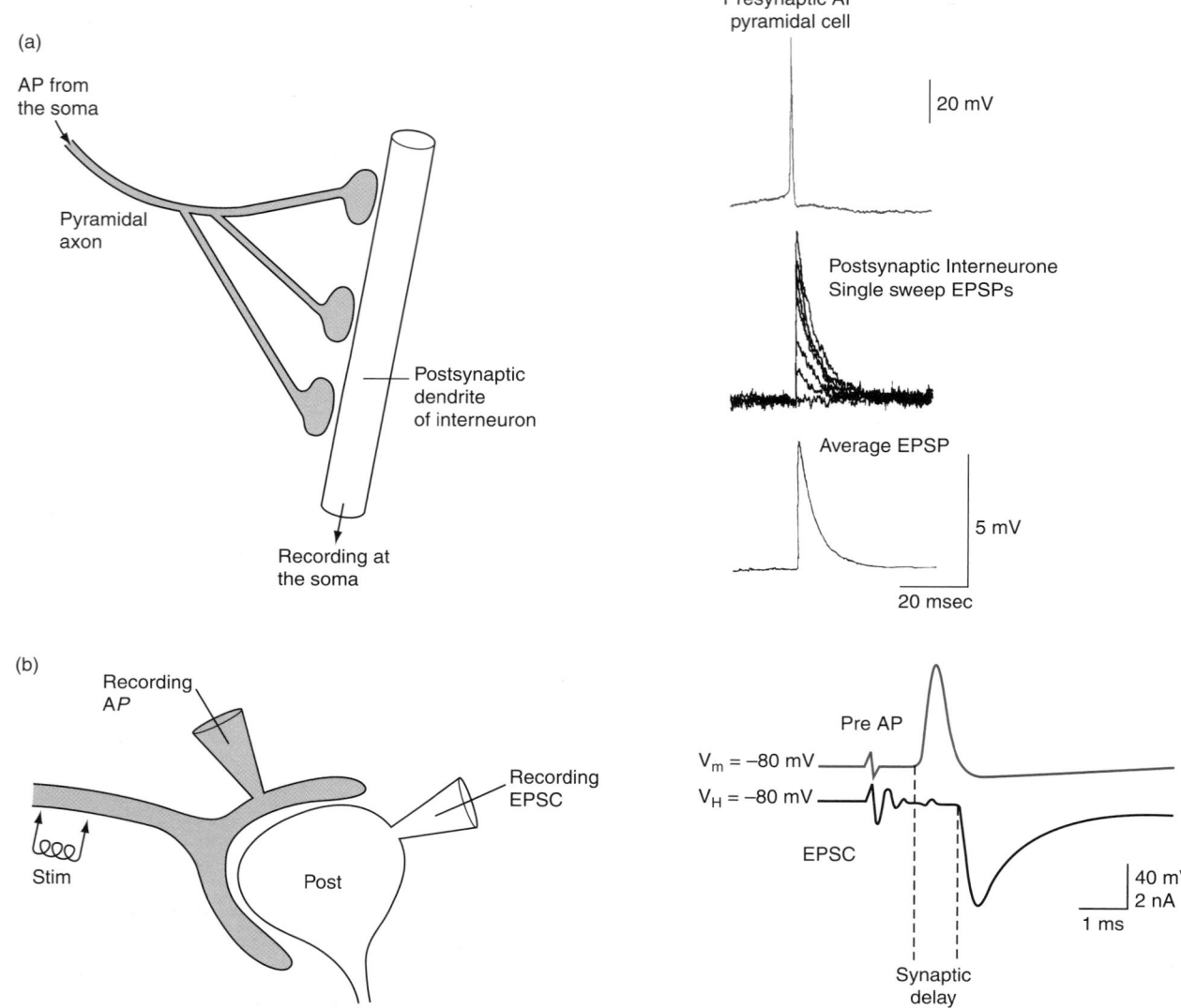

Figure 8.3 Basic properties of synaptic transmission.
(a) In the neocortex, pyramidal neurons are Golgi type I neurons, whose main axons leave the cortex after giving off collaterals. Left: These collaterals establish excitatory synapses with dendrites of local interneurons (Golgi type II neurons). Three synapses are represented but their exact number in the experiment performed at right were not determined. Right: In response to each presynaptic action potential (AP) evoked in the pyramidal neuron (top trace), a single-spike EPSP is recorded in the postsynaptic interneuron: it fluctuates in amplitude from 0 mV (failure) to 5 mV (middle traces); EPSPs recorded in response to four successive presynaptic spikes are superimposed (bottom traces). $V_m = -75$ mV in middle and bottom traces. **(b)** The synaptic delay between a presynaptic action potential (AP) evoked by stimulation of the afferent axon and recorded in the calyx of Held, and the postsynaptic response (excitatory postsynaptic current, EPSC) recorded in the postsynaptic soma varies from 500 µs to 1 ms. Drawing (a) from Thomson AM personal communication. Drawing (b) from Borst JGG, Helmchen F, Sakmann B (1995) Pre- and postsynaptic whole-cell recordings in the medial nucleus of the trapezoid body of the rat. *J. Physiol.* **489**, 825–840, with permission.

response that it evokes. It is an *indirect measure* since it includes events following release, such as neurotransmitter diffusion from the pre- to the postsynaptic element, binding of neurotransmitter molecules to postsynaptic receptors (step 5a), and induction of the postsynaptic cur-

rent (step 6). In addition, to be a reliable detector of release events the postsynaptic responses (EPSP or IPSP) should not activate postsynaptic voltage-dependent currents that would amplify or decrease them. Most of the data on neurotransmitter release explained here have

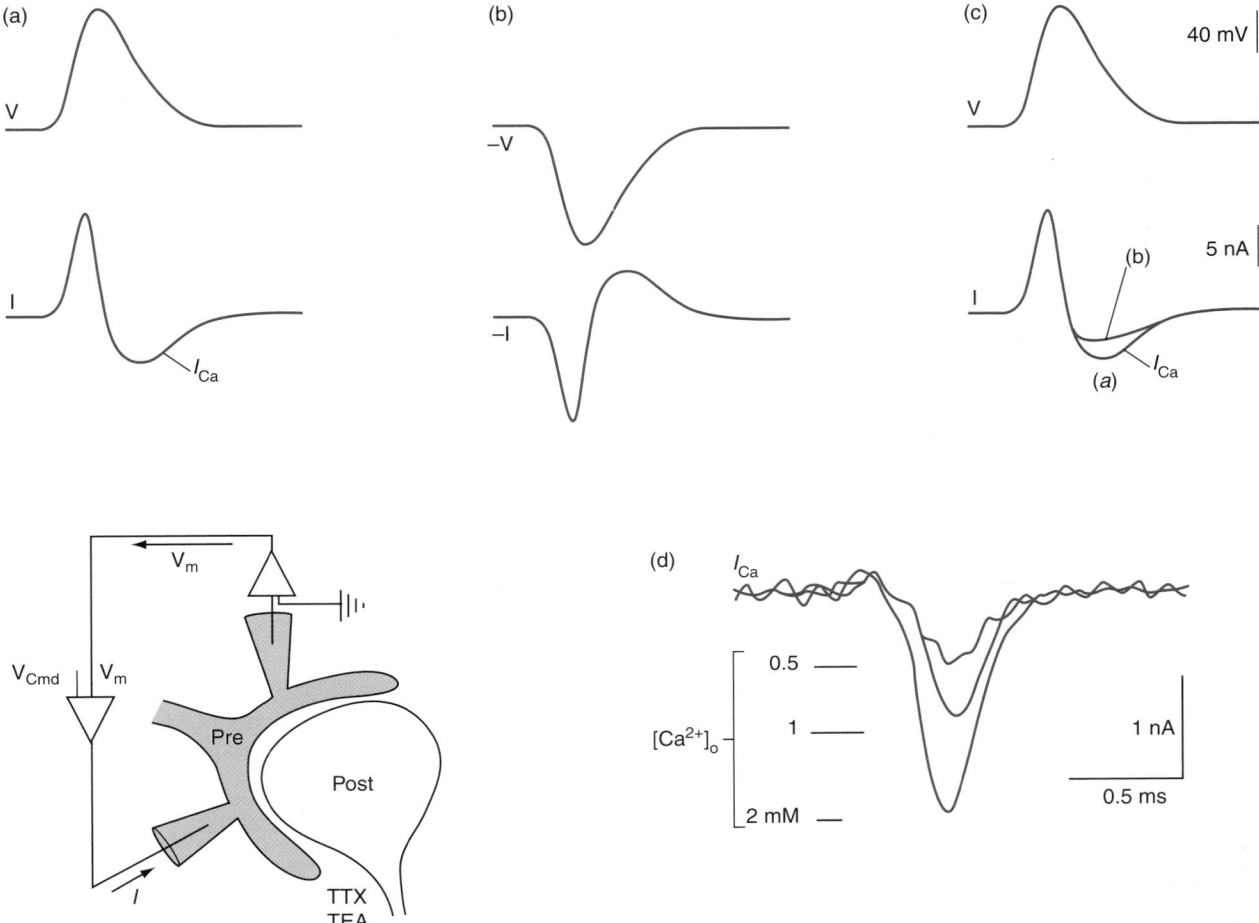

Figure 8.4 Ca²⁺ current flows into presynaptic terminal during the repolarizing phase of the presynaptic spike.
Two whole-cell electrodes are positioned in the calyx of Held; one measures the membrane potential (V) and the other one injects current (I). It is a two-electrode voltage clamp configuration. The preparation is bathed in 2 mM external Ca^{2+} with TTX and TEA to block the voltage-gated Na^+ and K^+ currents. **(a)** The voltage clamp command is an action potential waveform (V) from a holding potential of −80 mV. The current that flows through the membrane is shown on the bottom trace (I). **(b)** The action potential waveform command is inverted (−V) and so is the current that flows through the membrane (−I). In **(c)** both signals are superimposed (those in (b) have been inverted for superimposition). It shows that the current needed for the action potential is similar in (a) and (b) during the depolarization phase of the action potential. In contrast, the (a) current is larger during the repolarization phase of the action potential. **(d)** The difference between the (a) and (b) currents (I_{Ca}). This current is reduced in 1 or 0.5 mM external Ca^{2+} ($[Ca^{2+}]_o$). To perform the experiments in (b), the voltage command (i.e. the action potential waveform injected) is reduced to avoid a large signal in the negative direction (from −80 mV it would hyperpolarize the membrane to −200 mV). Then the currents are scaled up. Adapted from Borst JGG, Sakmann B (1996) Calcium influx and transmitter release in a fast CNS synapse, *Nature* **383**, 431–434, with permission.

been obtained from recordings of postsynaptic responses to a single presynaptic action potential.

Other techniques

Other techniques can be used to monitor transmitter release from peripheral synapses, large synaptosomes or endocrine cells; they are the patch clamp capacitance technique and amperometry.

The first consists of measuring the membrane capacitance that is directly proportional to the membrane surface area. Upon fusion of a secretory vesicle, membrane area and therefore capacitance increases stepwise by an amount equal to the vesicle or granule membrane area.

Amperometry monitors the release of secretory products by measuring the oxidation of electroactive substances (serotonin, catecholamines, dopamine) with a carbon fibre microelectrode placed near the cell.

8.1.3 Questions

Considering the general functional model of synaptic transmission which states that exocytosis of synaptic vesicles is triggered by an increase of the intracellular Ca^{2+} concentration in the presynaptic element ($[Ca^{2+}]_i$) (in **Figure 7.4a**), the following questions can be asked:

- Is $[Ca^{2+}]_i$ increase a prerequisite for transmitter release? Which type of Ca^{2+} channels are present in the presynaptic membrane and in response to which signal do they open (step 2)?
- Is the presynaptic $[Ca^{2+}]_i$ increase local and transient in response to a presynaptic spike (step 3)?
- How does $[Ca^{2+}]_i$ increase trigger exocytosis? Why is it so rapid (step 3)?
- How many vesicles fuse with the presynaptic membrane in response to a single presynaptic spike (step 4)?
- How much neurotransmitter is released into the synaptic cleft from a single vesicle (step 4)? What is the neurotransmitter lifetime in the cleft?
- What is the mechanism underlying the clearance of the transmitter from the synaptic cleft (steps 5)?

To answer the above questions, we will study the processes of transmitter release in chronological order, from depolarization of the presynaptic membrane by an action potential to the release of transmitter from synaptic vesicles (presynaptic processes I and II; Sections 8.2 and 8.3). Processes occurring in the synaptic cleft, just after transmitter release, are studied in Section 8.4. Details on the quantal and probabilistic nature of neurotransmitter release are given in Appendices 8.1 and 8.2.

8.2 Presynaptic processes I: From presynaptic spike to $[Ca^{2+}]_i$ increase

8.2.1 The presynaptic Na^+-dependent spike depolarizes the presynaptic membrane, opens presynaptic Ca^{2+} channels and triggers Ca^{2+} entry

In a resting presynaptic element, Ca^{2+} ions are present at a very low concentration, 10^{-8} to 10^{-7} M. This intracellular Ca^{2+} concentration, $[Ca^{2+}]_i$, is at least 10 000 times smaller than the extracellular one (see **Figure 3.2**). It is maintained at this resting level by various Ca^{2+} clearance mechanisms (see Section 8.2.4). In response to a presynaptic action potential it suddenly increases in the presynaptic element (**Figure 7.4a**, step 1, and **Figure 8.6**).

What is the origin of $[Ca^{2+}]_i$ increase in the presynaptic element? Is $[Ca^{2+}]_i$ increase a prerequisite for transmitter release?

In an extracellular medium deprived of Ca^{2+} ions or containing Ca^{2+} channel blockers such as Co^{2+} or Cd^{2+} ions, presynaptic $[Ca^{2+}]_i$ increase and postsynaptic response are no longer observed although presynaptic action potentials are unchanged. This suggests that external Ca^{2+} ions enter the presynaptic element through voltage-gated Ca^{2+} channels (that are blocked by Co^{2+} and Cd^{2+}; see Section 6.1). It also shows that presynaptic $[Ca^{2+}]_i$ increase is a prerequisite for synaptic transmission. This has been shown to be valid for all chemical synapses that have been studied.

What triggers the opening of voltage-gated Ca^{2+} channels?

The following hypothesis has been proposed. The brief membrane depolarization that occurs in the ascending phase of each Na^+-dependent presynaptic spike triggers the opening of voltage-dependent Ca^{2+} channels and allows subsequent Ca^{2+} influx into the presynaptic element.

In order to check that a presynaptic depolarization can trigger Ca^{2+} entry, Llinas and coworkers (1966) performed the following experiment in the squid giant synapse. They introduced two microelectrodes, one in the presynaptic element to inject a depolarizing current and one in the postsynaptic element to record its activity, and blocked Na^+-dependent spikes with TTX. In such conditions, direct depolarization of the presynaptic membrane, though it fails to evoke a presynaptic spike (because of TTX), evokes a presynaptic $[Ca^{2+}]_i$ increase and a postsynaptic response. A presynaptic membrane depolarization can thus trigger Ca^{2+} channel opening and neurotransmitter release.

8.2.2 Ca^{2+} enters the presynaptic bouton during the time course of the presynaptic spike through high-voltage-activated Ca^{2+} channels (N- and P/Q-types)

The calyx of Held is an axo-somatic synapse located in the rat brainstem, in the medial nucleus of the trapezoid body (MNTB), a nucleus that participates in sound localization. It is the largest synapse in the mammalian central nervous system. The presynaptic axon originates in the contralateral cochlear nucleus and each MNTB postsynaptic neuron receives only one calyx (see **Figure 8.1b**). Synaptic transmission is glutamatergic.

When does Ca²⁺ enter the presynaptic element in response to a presynaptic spike?

In order to record the presynaptic Ca^{2+} current, the presynaptic membrane is clamped at $V_H = -80$ mV by means of two whole-cell electrodes. To isolate the presynaptic Ca^{2+} current, voltage-dependent Na^+ and K^+ currents are blocked with TTX and TEA, respectively. An action potential waveform is injected into the presynaptic terminal through one of the whole-cell electrodes. It evokes a presynaptic Ca^{2+} current that is recorded by the second whole-cell electrode. Recordings show that Ca^{2+} influx is tightly associated with the repolarizing phase of the action potential (**Figure 8.4**): it is essentially a tail current (see Appendix 6.2) that activates shortly after the peak of the action potential and ends before repolarization is complete. It has a peak amplitude of 2.6 ± 0.2 nA and a half-width of about 350 ms. The delay between the beginning of the action potential and that of Ca^{2+} current is about 500 µs at 23–24°C.

Which types of Ca²⁺ channels are involved in transmitter release?

This has been first investigated in the frog neuromuscular junction and then in different other preparations. Antibodies against ω-conotoxin GVIA that selectively bind to N-type Ca^{2+} channels were seen to label active zones on the terminals of motoneurons. In central synapses, to examine the Ca^{2+} channels responsible for Ca^{2+} influx and transmitter release, pharmacological agents that selectively block a type of Ca^{2+} channel have been tested on the amplitude of the presynaptic Ca^{2+} increase and the postsynaptic response.

Consider the example of the glutamatergic synapse between the axons of granule cells (parallel fibres) and Purkinje cells in the rat cerebellum (see **Figures 7.8** and **8.1a**). The presynaptic Ca^{2+} concentration is determined with the Ca^{2+}-sensitive dye magfura, a low-affinity Ca^{2+}-sensitive dye, that emits light in the presence of free Ca^{2+} with a sensitivity of 10^{-4} M (see Appendix 6.1). The transmitter release is estimated from the postsynaptic excitatory current recorded in voltage clamp (whole-cell configuration) from the Purkinje soma. Parallel fibres are excited by a stimulating electrode placed in the molecular layer (**Figure 8.5a**). Ca^{2+} entry in response to presynaptic stimulation is measured as a fluorescence signal.

A single stimulus produces an abrupt change in fluorescence (a fluorescence transient) which returns to resting levels within a few hundreds of milliseconds. At saturating concentration, ω-conotoxin GVIA (0.5 µM) inhibits by $27.0 \pm 1.7\%$ the fluorescence transient elicited by the stimulation (**Figure 8.5b**, top traces). In compari-

son, ω-agatoxin IVA (200 nM) reduces the amplitude of the transient by $50.1 \pm 0.9\%$ (**Figure 8.5c**, top traces) and nimodipine (5 µM), an L-type channel blocker, has no effect. Simultaneous application of the two toxins has an additive effect and inhibits Ca^{2+} influx by $77 \pm 3\%$ (**Figure 8.5d**). In conclusion, at this cerebellar synapse, the ω-conotoxin-sensitive N-type and the ω-agatoxin-sensitive P/Q-type Ca^{2+} channels are both present in the presynaptic membrane and allow around 80% of Ca^{2+} entry in response to a presynaptic spike.

For all synapses studied so far, Ca^{2+} enters presynaptic terminals mainly through N- and/or P/Q-type Ca^{2+} channels. The functional properties of these channels impose at least one constraint: since N and P/Q-type Ca^{2+} channels are high-voltage-activated channels, Ca^{2+} enters presynaptic terminals only in response to a *large* membrane depolarization (such as the depolarizing phase of the Na^+ action potential).

8.2.3 Presynaptic [Ca²⁺]ᵢ increase is transient and restricted to micro- or nanodomains close to docked vesicles

How does Ca²⁺ rise in a presynaptic terminal, uniformly or in domains?

This has been studied in the squid giant synapse (see **Figure 8.1c**) with Ca^{2+} imaging techniques. A low affinity Ca^{2+}-sensitive dye (*n*-aequorin J, a protein that emits light in the presence of free Ca^{2+} with a minimum sensitivity of 10^{-4} M; see Appendix 6.1) is injected into the presynaptic terminal in order to visualize only zones where Ca^{2+} concentration is high. Then the presynaptic axon is stimulated at 10 Hz. Multiple fluorescent domains, equally spaced, with a mean size of 0.250 to 0.375 µm² (mean 0.313 µm²) are seen in the presynaptic terminal (**Figure 8.6**). Their number 4500 is quite close to the average number of release sites in this terminal (4400). These microdomains are located at active zones of the presynaptic plasma membrane. This observation is evidence for the fact that voltage-dependent Ca^{2+} channels are clustered at active zones. Since the presynaptic stimulation used in this experiment is not an action potential, it does not allow to apprehend the physiological Ca^{2+} concentration in presynaptic microdomains.

Where are presynaptic Ca²⁺ channels located?

The rapidity with which neurotransmitter release can be triggered after Ca^{2+} influx (within 200 µs) makes it likely that Ca^{2+} ions act at a very short distance from the Ca^{2+} channels. This suggested that: (i) Ca^{2+} channels

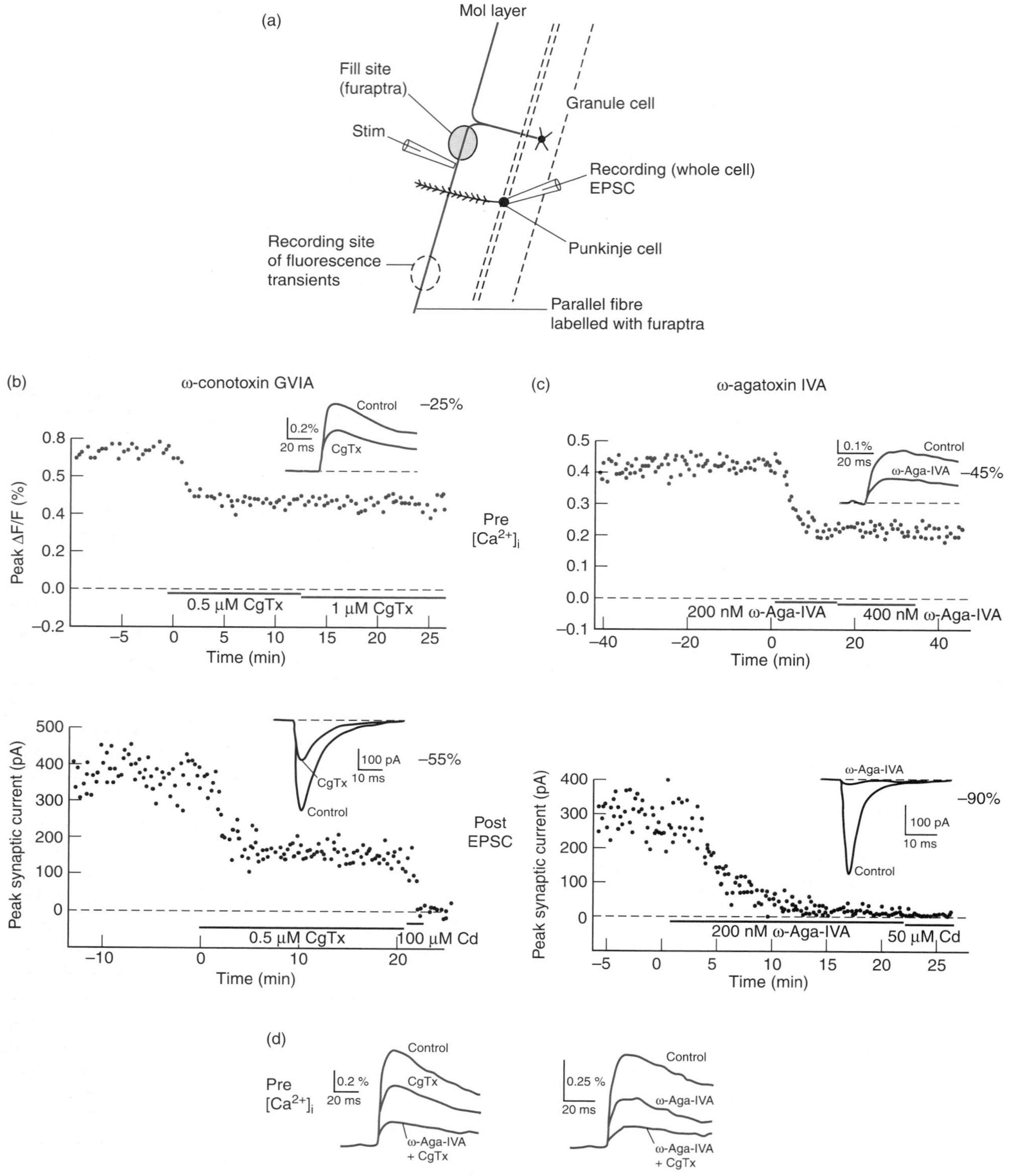

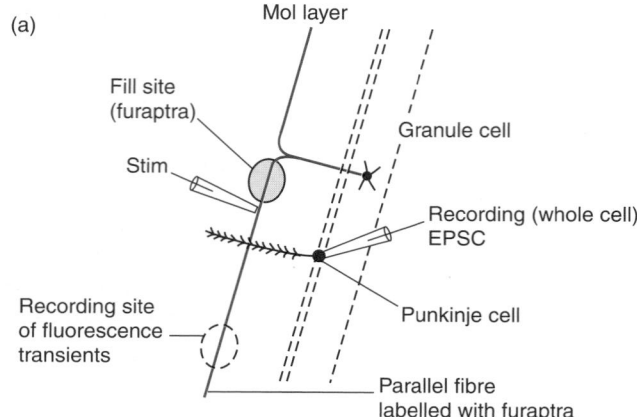

(a)

Mol layer

Fill site
(furaptra)

Stim

Granule cell

Recording (whole cell)
EPSC

Punkinje cell

Recording site
of fluorescence
transients

Parallel fibre
labelled with furaptra

(b)

ω-conotoxin GVIA

Peak ΔF/F (%)

Control
−25%
0.2%
20 ms
CgTx

0.5 μM CgTx   1 μM CgTx

Time (min)

Pre
$[Ca^{2+}]_i$

Peak synaptic current (pA)

−55%
100 pA
10 ms
CgTx
Control

0.5 μM CgTx   100 μM Cd

Time (min)

(c)

ω-agatoxin IVA

0.1%
20 ms
Control
ω-Aga-IVA
−45%

200 nM ω-Aga-IVA   400 nM ω-Aga-IVA

Time (min)

Post
EPSC

Peak synaptic current (pA)

ω-Aga-IVA
−90%
100 pA
10 ms
Control

200 nM ω-Aga-IVA   50 μM Cd

Time (min)

(d)

Pre
$[Ca^{2+}]_i$

0.2 %
20 ms
Control
CgTx
ω-Aga-IVA
+ CgTx

0.25 %
20 ms
Control
ω-Aga-IVA
ω-Aga-IVA
+ CgTx

Figure 8.5 (left) N- and P/Q-type Ca²⁺ channel blockers reduce presynaptic Ca²⁺ influx and synaptic transmission at a cerebellar synapse.

(a) In a transverse cerebellar slice, the relative locations of labelling with the dye furaptra (fill site), stimulus electrode and recording sites (whole-cell recording of EPSC from a Purkinje soma and recording of presynaptic fluorescence transients in the molecular layer). (b) Amplitude of furaptra fluorescence transients ($\Delta F/F$) in the presence of increasing concentrations of ω-conotoxin GVIA (CgTx) to block the N-type Ca²⁺ current (top traces). Concomitant recording of the postsynaptic current is shown in the bottom trace. Each furaptra transient is elicited by a single stimulus of the parallel fibre tract and is a measure of the presynaptic Ca²⁺ influx. The inset shows superimposed fluorescence transients in control conditions and after addition of 0.5 and 1 μM CgTx. (c) The same experiment as in (b) but in the presence of increasing concentrations of ω-agatoxin IVA (ω-Aga IVA) to block the P/Q-type Ca²⁺ current. The inset shows superimposed fluorescence transients in control conditions and after addition of 200 and 400 nM ω-Aga IVA. Concomitant recording of the postsynaptic current is shown in the bottom trace. (d) Additive effects of the sequential application of saturating concentrations of the toxins on the furaptra transients. Adapted from Mintz I, Sabatini BL, Regehr WG (1995) Calcium control of transmitter release at a cerebellar synapse, *Neuron* **15**, 675–688, with permission.

and release sites are located at a close distance; and (ii) there exists a stable complex between synaptic vesicles and plasma membrane, preassembled in the resting state, before $[Ca^{2+}]_i$ increases – Ca²⁺ diffusion is too restricted and delay of exocytosis too short to allow for vesicle movement before fusion with the plasmamem-

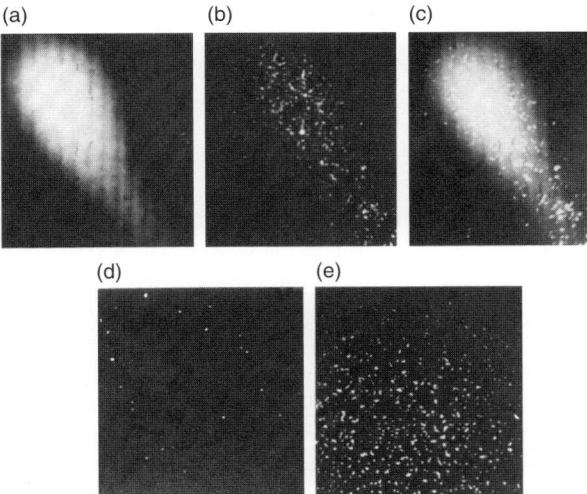

Figure 8.6 Microdomains of Ca²⁺ increase in the presynaptic terminal of the squid giant synapse.

(a) Fluorescence image of a presynaptic terminal injected with n-aequorin-J. When the presynaptic fibre is fully loaded, it is continuously stimulated at 10 Hz for 10 s. (b) The acquisition during these 10 s of tetanic stimulation reveals stable quantum emission domains that appear as white spots. The background fluorescence shown in (a) disappears in (b) due to subtraction. (c) Superposition of the fluorescent images in (a) and (b) reveals that the distribution of the microdomains of high calcium coincides with the presynaptic terminal. Emission domains in an unstimulated terminal (d) and in the same terminal during tetanic stimulation (e) are shown at high magnification. Adapted from Llinas R, Sugimori M, Silver RB (1992) Microdomains of high calcium concentration in a presynaptic terminal, *Science* **256**, 677–679, with permission.

brane (Ca²⁺ ions diffuse no more than a few vesicle diameters into the cytoplasm). In other words, presumably synaptic vesicle available for rapid transmitter release must be predocked in the vicinity of Ca²⁺ channels.

The localization of Ca²⁺ channels relative to the position of transmitter release sites was first investigated with imaging (**Figure 8.7a**) and immunocytochemical (**Figure 8.7b**) techniques. In the frog neuromuscular junction, the presynaptic nerve terminal is a long structure (several hundreds of micrometres) characterized by the presence of neurotransmitter release sites or active zones spaced at regular 1 μm intervals. Directly across the synaptic cleft just facing active zones are clusters of nicotinic acetylcholine receptors (nAChR) located on the edge of the post junctional folds (see **Figure 7.12a**). The preparation is double-labelled to disclose both postsynaptic nAChR and presynaptic N-type Ca²⁺ channels. The idea is that the localization of postsynaptic nAChRs indicates exactly the localization of presynaptic active zones. Ca²⁺ channels are labelled with biotinylated ω-conotoxin, a specific and irreversible blocker of N-type Ca²⁺ channels and of synaptic transmission at the frog neuromuscular junction. To reveal ω-conotoxin-sensitive Ca²⁺ channel labelling, preparations are then incubated with streptavidin Texas Red (see Appendix 7.2) which fluoresces red. When nerve terminals are removed by pulling off branches of the motor nerve, the Ca²⁺ channel labelling totally disappears, indicating that ω-conotoxin binding sites are strictly located on presynaptic terminals. Postsynaptic nicotinic receptors nAChR are labelled with α-bungarotoxin coupled to boron dipyrromethane difluoride which fluoresces green. Under the light microscope, each fluorescent band of presynaptic Ca²⁺ channels is matched by a fluorescent stain of postsynaptic nAChR (**Figure 8.7b**). Bands of labelled Ca²⁺ channels and labelled nAChRs are thus almost perfectly aligned, suggesting that Ca²⁺ channels are clustered in the membrane of presynaptic active zones, opposite the postjunctional folds.

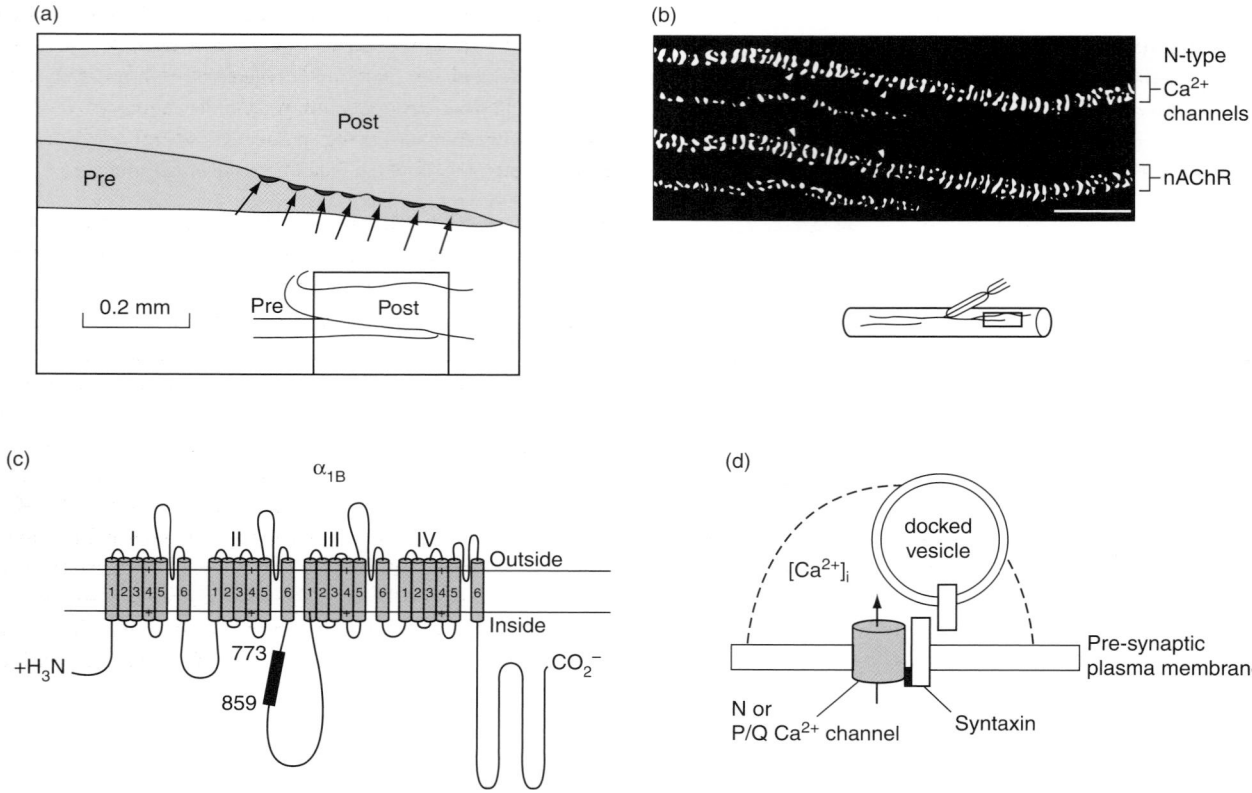

Figure 8.7 Presynaptic N-type Ca^{2+} channels are clustered at active zones.
(a) In the squid giant synapse, presynaptic zones of [Ca^{2+}]$_i$ increase in response to a train of brief presynaptic stimuli (0.5 s at 80 Hz) are visualized with the FURA-2 technique. They are localized at active zones. The diagram below illustrates the synapse and the box indicates the region studied. **(b)** In the frog neuromuscular junction, N-type Ca^{2+} channels and nicotinic acetylcholine receptors (nAChR) are labelled with two different selective toxins coupled to different fluorescent dyes. The preparation is viewed with a confocal laser microscope. The diagram below illustrates the structure of the neuromuscular junction and the box indicates the region scanned by the microscope. The images showing the distribution of presynaptic Ca^{2+} channels (top) and postsynaptic nAChRs (bottom) are separated for clarity but they are in fact superimposed. **(c)** Predicted topological structure of the α$_1$ subunit of class B of N-type Ca^{2+} channel. Rectangle indicates region of interaction with syntaxin. **(d)** Theoretical model of interaction between presynaptic N- or P/Q-type Ca^{2+} channels, syntaxin and docked vesicles at the presynaptic plasma membrane. Part (b) from Robitaille R, Adler EM, Charlton MP (1990) Strategic location of calcium channels at transmitter release sites of frog neuromuscular synapses, *Neuron* **5**, 773–779, with permission. Part (c) from Sheng ZH, Rettig J, Takahashi M, Catterall WA (1994) Identification of a syntaxin-binding site on N-type calcium channels, *Neuron* **13**, 1303–1313, with permission.

The clustering of presynaptic N- and P/Q-type Ca^{2+} channels at active zones has been confirmed by the discovery of a physical link between these Ca^{2+} channels and syntaxin, an integral protein of the presynaptic plasma membrane involved in vesicle docking at the presynaptic active zones (see Section 8.3.2). This was shown (i) by co-precipitation of N and P/Q channels (labelled with their specific toxins) with syntaxin (labelled with a specific antibody), and (ii) by the identification of a syntaxin-binding domain on N- and P/Q-type α$_1$-subunits (pore forming subunit of the class B and A, respectively). For N-type Ca^{2+} channels, the binding involves an 87-amino-acid domain of the α$_{1B}$-sub-

unit, located on the cytoplasmic loop linking homologous domains II and III (**Figure 8.7c**) and the COOH-terminal of syntaxin (amino-acids 181–288) which is thought to be anchored in the presynaptic plasma membrane (see **Figure 8.12**). Such a tight physical coupling ensures the proximity of the trigger for exocytosis (Ca^{2+}) with docked vesicles (**Figure 8.7d**) and makes release as fast as possible.

These results exemplify some general principles of rapid Ca^{2+} signalling in neurotransmitter release:

■ Ca^{2+} entry into the presynaptic element occurs in close proximity to the exocytotic apparatus.

■ Clustering of Ca^{2+} channels close to release sites ensures that a Ca^{2+} signal is rapidly available (in the hundreds of microseconds timescale) to the nearby Ca^{2+}-sensitive proteins which initiate transmitter release.

8.2.4 Ca^{2+} clearance makes presynaptic $[Ca^{2+}]_i$ increase transient: it shapes its amplitude and duration

Ca^{2+} clearance is the removal of Ca^{2+} ions (in excess compared to the resting state) from the presynaptic terminal. The aim of Ca^{2+} clearance mechanisms is to rapidly re-establish the resting level of $[Ca^{2+}]_i$. Ca^{2+} clearance is achieved by proteins that extrude Ca^{2+} ions toward the extracellular space or toward organelles such as the endoplasmic reticulum: these are Ca^{2+} pumps (Ca^{2+}-ATPases) and Ca^{2+}-transporters (Na–Ca exchanger) (see Section 3.4 and **Figure 8.8**). Ca^{2+} ions that enter the presynaptic terminal will also rapidly bind to cytosolic proteins (Ca^{2+}-buffers, Ca-B). Because such binding confiscates Ca^{2+} ions, it can rapidly diminish freely diffusing Ca^{2+} ions.

But such buffering is not a real clearance since Ca^{2+} ions will unbind from these proteins; it is a temporary clearance. Unbound Ca^{2+} ions will have then to be extruded by pumps and transporters. Therefore, the more numerous the number of Ca^{2+} pumps and transporters, the more efficient and rapid is Ca^{2+} clearance.

Extrusion of Ca^{2+} to the extracellular medium by the plasma membrane Ca-ATPase (PMCA) pump and by the Na–Ca exchanger

The former uses the hydrolysis of ATP as a source of energy and is independent of the extracellular Na^+ concentration. The latter is driven by the Na^+ electrochemical gradient across plasma membrane and is thus sensitive to extracellular Na^+ concentration. The Ca-ATPase pump is proposed to be a low-capacity high-affinity system ($K_D = 0.2$–$0.3\ \mu M$) whereas the Na–Ca exchanger would have a high-capacity low-affinity system ($K_D = 0.5$–$1.0\ \mu M$). The Ca-ATPase pump would thus be the most efficient system in the presence of a low presynaptic activity, and the two systems would act in synergy to regulate the intracellular Ca^{2+} concentration after a train of action potentials.

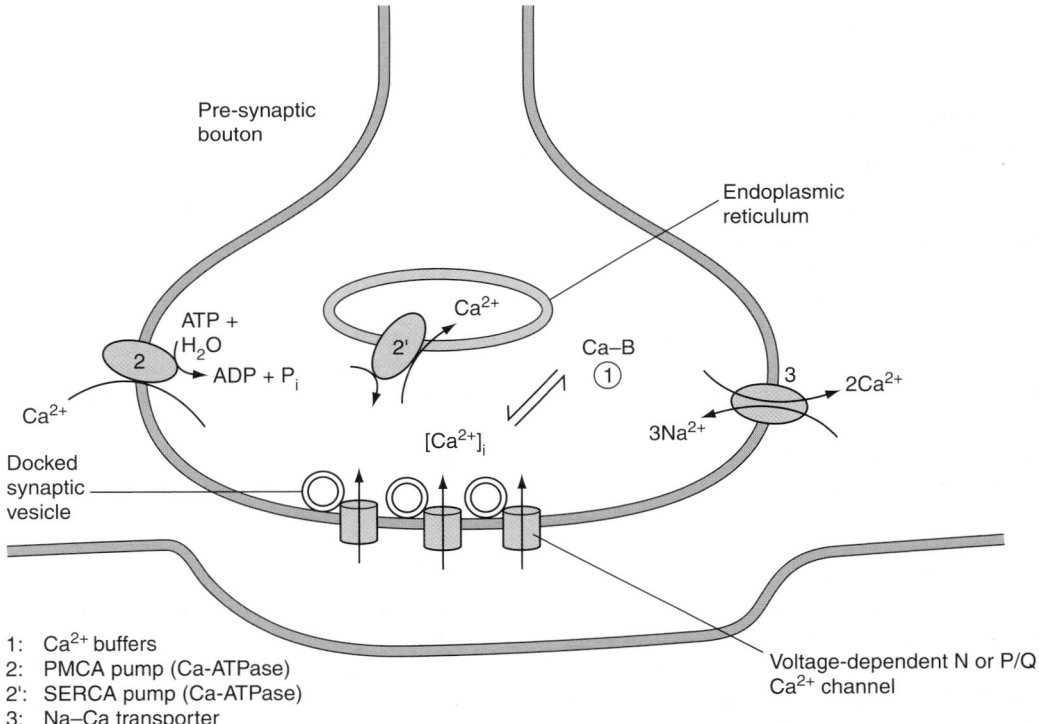

1: Ca^{2+} buffers
2: PMCA pump (Ca-ATPase)
2': SERCA pump (Ca-ATPase)
3: Na–Ca transporter

Figure 8.8 Ca^{2+} clearance mechanisms in a presynaptic terminal.
While Ca^{2+} ions enter at the level of the presynaptic active zone through high-voltage-activated Ca^{2+} channels, they are rapidly buffered by cytoplasmic Ca^{2+}-binding proteins (Ca-B). Ca^{2+} ions are also actively cleared from the intracellular medium towards the extracellular medium via Ca-ATPases of the plasma membrane (PMCA pumps) and the Na–Ca exchangers. They are also cleared by active transport toward endoplasmic reticulum via another type of Ca-ATPase (SERCA pumps). This clearing has a time constant of the order of tens of milliseconds to seconds.

Sequestration of Ca²⁺ ions in smooth endoplasmic reticulum and mitochondria

This is achieved by sarco-endoplasmic Ca-ATPase (SERCA) pumps present in the membrane of these organelles. The smooth endoplasmic reticulum is a Ca^{2+} storage compartment. In the different cell types studied, the smooth endoplasmic reticulum Ca-ATPase pump has a better affinity for Ca^{2+} than that of mitochondrion. This latter would function in very rare situations in cases of massive Ca^{2+} entry. Noteworthy, following an appropriate signal (such as the formation of inositol trisphosphate, IP_3), the Ca^{2+} ions stored in these compartments can be released in the cytoplasm through Ca^{2+}-permeable channels.

Ca²⁺ buffering by cytosolic proteins

Different cytosolic proteins have the ability to bind Ca^{2+} with a high affinity. These proteins have, in general, a low molecular weight and act primarily as Ca^{2+} buffers (such as parvalbumin and calbindin) or subserve messenger functions (calmodulin). Parvalbumin is found in great amount in most GABAergic neurons in the mammalian central nervous system (the co-localization of GABA and parvalbumin has been shown immunohistochemically using highly specific antibodies to GABA and parvalbumin); whereas in other neurons the concentration of parvalbumin is much lower. The high concentration of parvalbumin might have a consequence on a neuron's ability to rapidly buffer Ca^{2+}. This is especially important for neurons that have a high tonic activity since trains of action potentials trigger repetitive $[Ca^{2+}]_i$ increases in their synaptic terminals. Calbindin is a protein that was originally found in the gut, where it binds Ca^{2+} and is vitamin D-dependent. Its presence has been shown in neurons of the mammalian central nervous system, notably the Purkinje cells of the cerebellar cortex and the dopaminergic neurons of the substantia nigra. Calmodulin has a high affinity for Ca^{2+} and a role of intracellular messenger. The buffering of free intracellular Ca^{2+} ions by cytoplasmic calcium binding proteins is a very efficient system responsible for the rapid disappearance of Ca^{2+} ions.

The relative contribution of the clearance systems: example of Purkinje cells

Cerebellar Purkinje cells are GABAergic neurons that have powerful systems to control $[Ca^{2+}]_i$. Immunocytochemical studies demonstrate considerable amounts of cytosolic Ca^{2+}-binding proteins, particularly calbindin D_{28K} and parvalbumin. There are also numerous Ca^{2+} pumps localized in the endoplasmic reticulum (SERCA pumps) or the plasma membrane (PMCA pumps). In order to understand the respective roles of these clear-ance systems, Purkinje cells are loaded with the fluorescent Ca^{2+} dye FURA-2 (see Appendix 6.1), $[Ca^{2+}]_i$ transients are evoked by direct membrane depolarization and measured by microfluorometry, and clearance systems are pharmacologically inhibited one at a time. Since all these experiments are achieved with the use of a whole-cell electrode, the duration of the study is limited to 25 minutes in order to avoid washing out of intracellular constituents that would give an artefactual diminution of $[Ca^{2+}]_i$.

The contribution of SERCA pumps on the amplitude and decay phase of $[Ca^{2+}]_i$ transients is studied by applying cyclopiazonic acid (CPA) or thapsigargin, specific inhibitors of this ATPase. For blocking PMCA pumps, 5,6-succinimidyl carboxyeosin (CE) is applied; and for blocking the Na–Ca exchanger, external Na^+ is replaced with Li^+, choline or N-methyl-D-glucamine, cations that cannot substitute for Na^+ in the exchange reaction. The rate of decay of $[Ca^{2+}]_i$ transients with similar peaks value are compared in control and experimental conditions in order to calculate the rate of clearance. All these inhibitors do not affect resting $[Ca^{2+}]_i$ levels, indicating that the passive leak of Ca^{2+} into the somata is small. For low-intensity $[Ca^{2+}]_i$ transients (0.5 μM at the peak), the proportion of intracellular Ca^{2+} removed by SERCA pumps, PMCA pumps and the Na–Ca exchanger is balanced (**Figure 8.9**). They equally remove 78% of the intracellular Ca^{2+}.

8.3 Presynaptic processes II: From [Ca²⁺]ᵢ increase to synaptic vesicle fusion

In a resting nerve terminal the small synaptic vesicles loaded with the neurotransmitter are either localized in the cytoplasm of the active zone (linked to cytoskeletal elements) or docked to the presynaptic plasma membrane. Depolarization of the presynaptic membrane by an action potential leads to an influx of Ca^{2+} ions that *may* trigger fusion (exocytosis) of a docked vesicle.

8.3.1 Overview of the hypothetical vesicle cycle in presynaptic terminals

From observations and experiments described in the following sections, synaptic vesicle traffic in nerve terminals is considered to involve several hypothetical stages (**Figure 8.10**).

■ *Mobilization.* After they fill with neurotransmitter by active transport, synaptic vesicles translocate to the active zone (translocation of vesicles from the reserve pool to the releasable pool).

■ *Targeting and docking.* Vesicles dock at morphologically defined sites of the presynaptic plasma membrane.

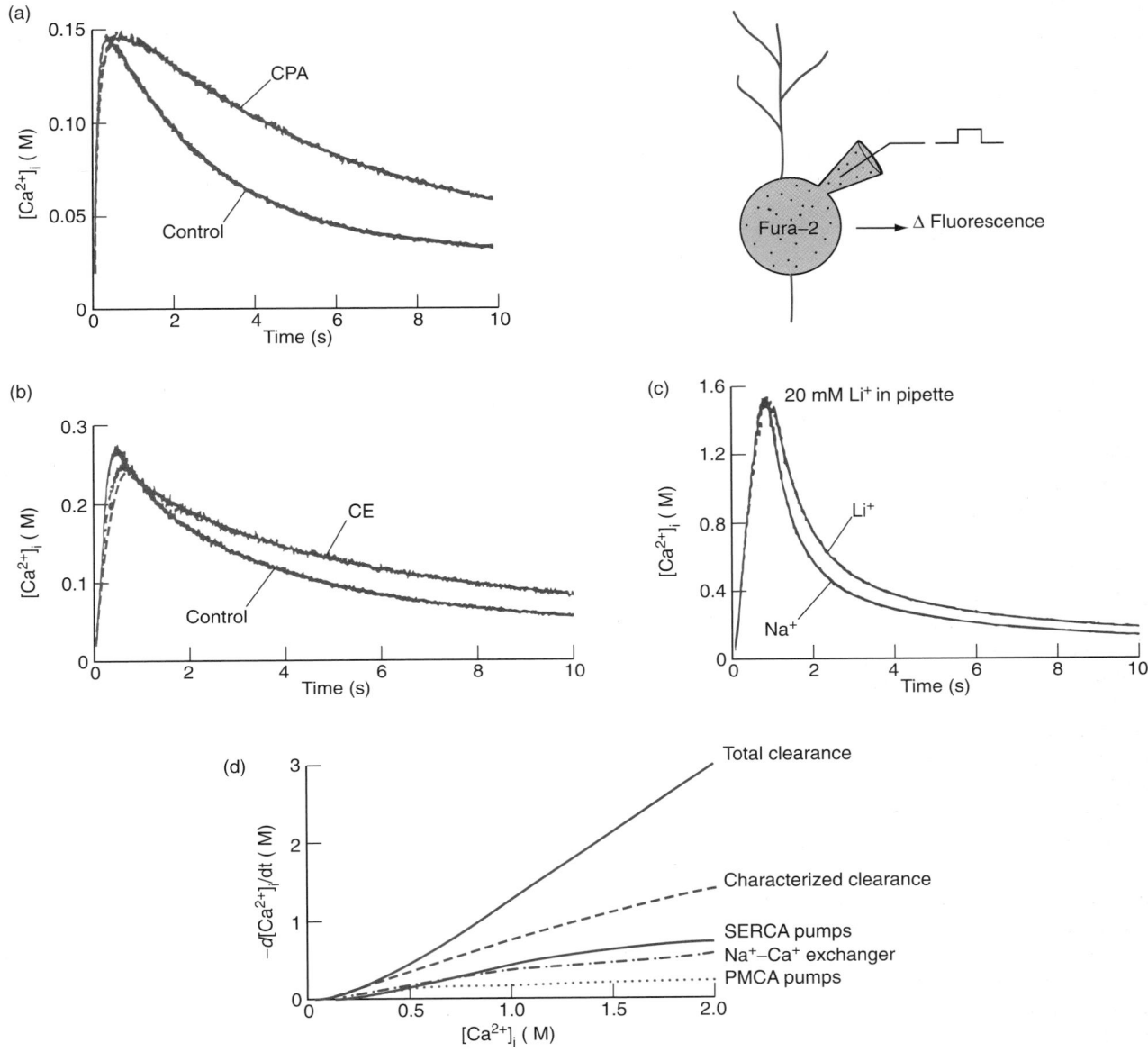

Figure 8.9 Relative contribution of the different mechanisms of Ca²⁺ clearance in Purkinje somata.
[Ca²⁺]$_i$ transients are evoked in FURA-2-loaded Purkinje cells by a depolarizing current pulse of varying duration (60–250 ms). Effects on [Ca²⁺]$_i$ transients of **(a)** cyclopiazonic acid (CPA), a blocker of SERCA pumps, **(b)** 5,6-succinimidyl carboxyeosin (CE), a blocker of PMCA pumps, and **(c)** Li²⁺ saline, a blocker of Na–Ca exchanger. **(d)** Total Ca²⁺ clearance rate is presented in comparison with the rate of the different components characterized in the above experiments. Clearance rate is plotted as a function of the [Ca²⁺]$_i$ in the range between 50 nM and 2 μM. The clearance rate is calculated as follows: (i) The decay phase of each transient is fitted by a single or double exponential function and the derivative function (d[Ca²⁺]$_i$/dt) is calculated from the fit. (ii) $-d$[Ca²⁺]$_i$/dt is then plotted as a function of the [Ca²⁺]$_i$ values obtained from the experimental fit. (iii) The plots from transients with equal peak [Ca²⁺]$_i$ in each condition (control *versus* inhibitor) are pooled and fitted with a polynomial function of fifth to seventh order. Adapted from Fierro L, DiPolo R, Llano I (1998) Intracellular calcium clearance in Purkinje cell somata from rat cerebellar slices, *J. Physiol.* **510**, 499–512, with permission.

■ *Priming*. This includes the ATP-dependent reaction(s) that occur before exocytosis can take place.

■ *Fusion*. The local increase of [Ca²⁺]$_i$ triggers exocytosis of docked vesicles; i.e. fusion of synaptic vesicle membrane with the presynaptic plasma membrane (mixing of protein and lipid bilayers) and release of the full vesicular content.

■ *Retrieval and recycling*. Empty vesicles form coated pits that undergo endocytosis.

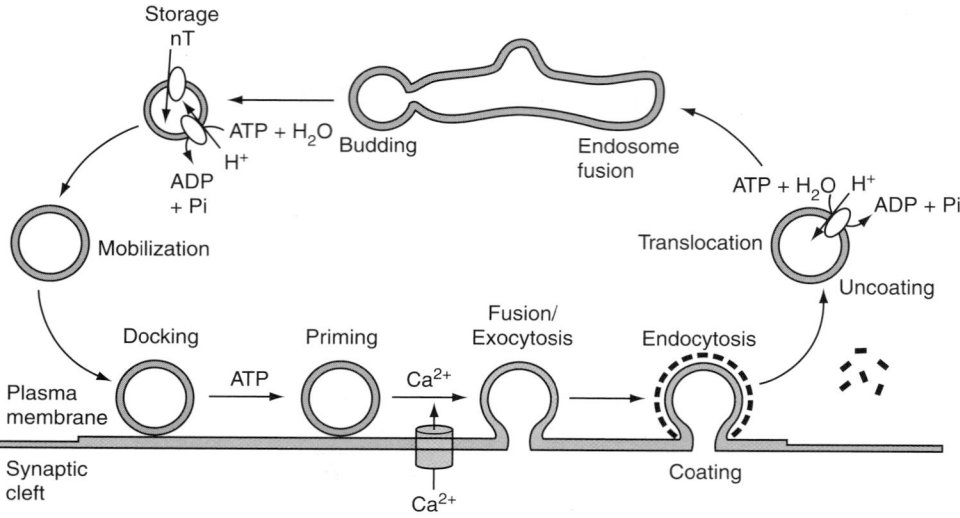

Figure 8.10 Diagram of the hypothetical synaptic vesicle cycle in a presynaptic terminal.
The same synaptic vesicle is shown at different stages. Sites of docking, priming and fusion have been separated for clarity. NT, neurotransmitter. Adapted from Südhof TC (1995) The synaptic vesicle cycle: a cascade of protein–protein interactions, *Nature* **375**, 645–653, with permission.

Comparison of neurotransmitter release with other secretory systems shows that targeting, docking and fusion of vesicles involve common mechanisms. Synaptic transmission makes use of a mechanism that is common to biology. We will look at the docking, priming and fusion steps.

8.3.2 Docking: a subpopulation of synaptic vesicles is docked to the active zone close to Ca²⁺ channels by means of specific pairing of vesicular and plasma membrane proteins

In nerve terminals observed with quick freeze deep-etch electron microscopy, two populations of vesicles are distinguished. A subpopulation of vesicles is suspended in a complex network of filaments – numerous 40 nm long filaments having globular heads that cross each other, thus enabling the filaments to contract, and a few filaments having a larger diameter, extending from the presynaptic membrane to the axoplasm, with length about 50 nm and in contact with the vesicles or the smaller filaments. Another subpopulation of synaptic vesicles is docked to the presynaptic plasma membrane.

How do synaptic vesicles recognize the presynaptic plasma membrane for docking?

Selective targeting of a vesicle to its correct destination has been proposed by G. Palade in 1970 to result from specific recognition sites between vesicle and plasma membranes. Later, the molecular basis of this specific interaction was studied by J. Rothman and colleagues in a cell-free preparation of Golgi membranes that reconstitutes vesicle-mediated transport between Golgi cisternae, a model of constitutive vesicle fusion with a membrane. The experiments described briefly here led to the discovery and purification of several proteins crucial for docking and fusion processes. Proteins essential in the fusion process were identified first, and integral membrane proteins essential for docking were purified later. Though docking occurs before fusion in the synaptic vesicle cycle, the results will be described here as they were obtained, first for the fusion proteins then for the docking proteins.

The experiments were performed in a cell-free preparation of Golgi stacks, a model of constitutive vesicle fusion. Everything began with the discovery that N-ethyl maleimide (NEM), a sulphydryl reagent, blocks the fusion of Golgi vesicles with Golgi stacks: the vesicles still bud off from cisternae but the released vesicles no longer fuse with the next stack membrane; they accumulate docked to the target membrane. This suggested the involvement of a NEM-sensitive fusion protein (NSF) in the fusion step. That protein was purified according to its ability to restore fusion after NEM inactivation. NSF is a 76 kDa protein, a water-soluble ATPase with two distinct ATP-binding sites. To attach to membranes, it requires additional proteins, the 40 kDa soluble NSF-attachment proteins (α, β, γ SNAPs) (**Figures 8.11a** and **8.12b, c**).

(a)

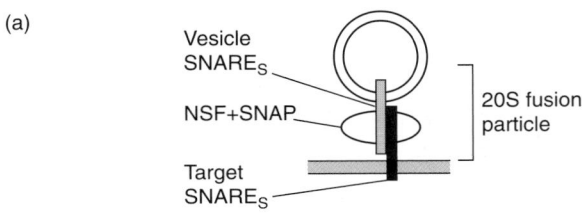

(b)

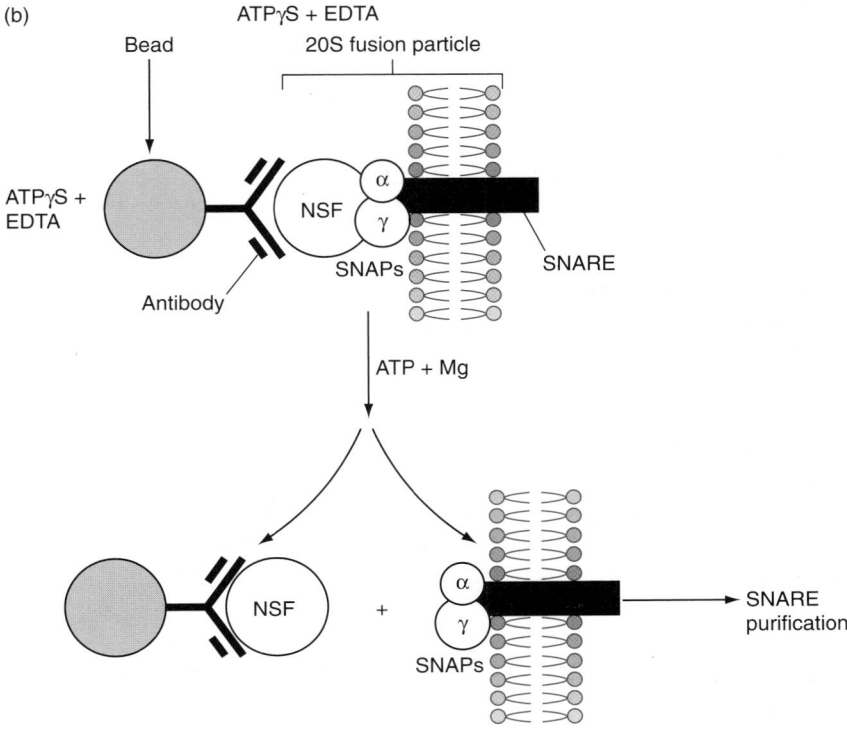

(c)

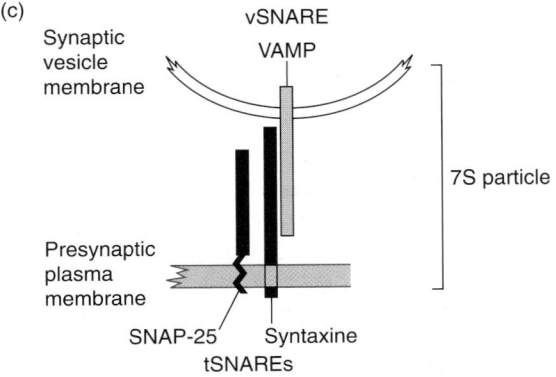

Figure 8.11 The SNARE hypothesis.
(a) Model of the 20S particle that includes SNAPs, membrane receptors to SNAPs (SNAREs) and the fusion protein NSF. (b) Scheme of the experiment that identified the integral membrane proteins (SNAREs) of the vesicle or presynaptic plasma membranes of brain synapses. See text for explanations. Parts (a) and (c) adapted from Söllner T, Rothman JE (1994) Neurotransmission: harnessing fusion machinery at the synapse, *Trend. Neurosci.* **17**, 344–348, with permission. Part (b) adapted from Tixier-Vidal A (1997) *Biologie Cellulaire de la Sécrétion des Protéines*, Paris: Polytechnica editions, with permission.

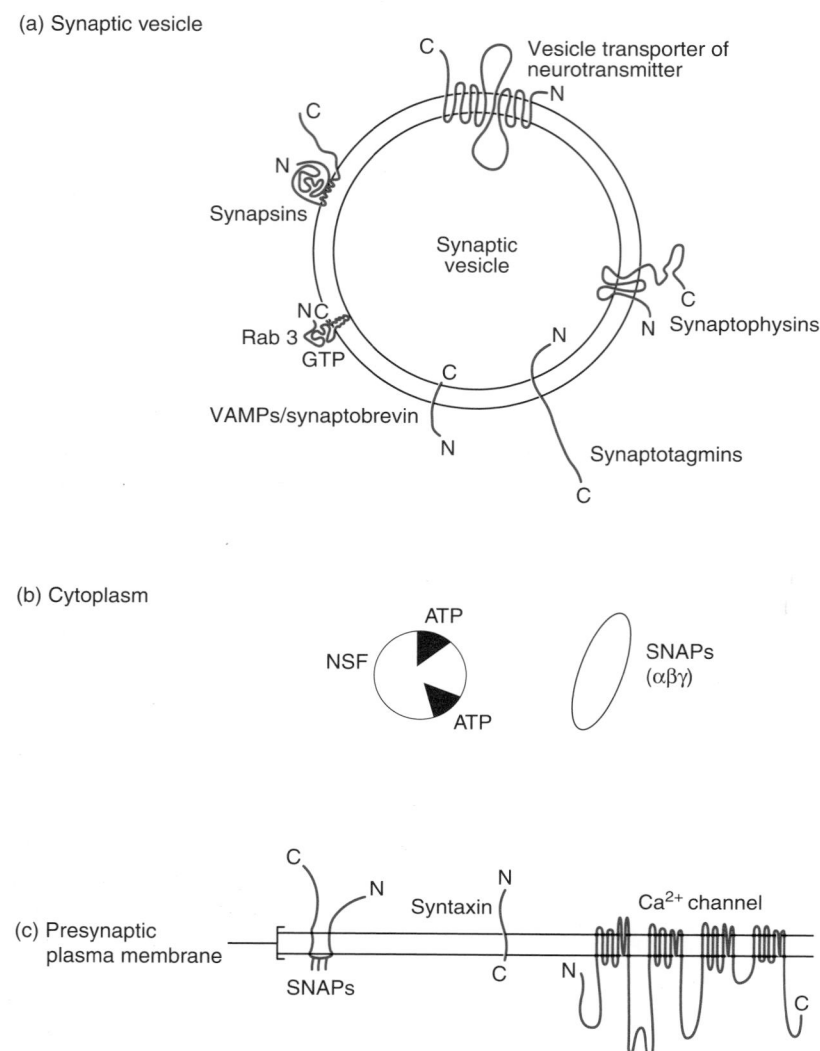

Figure 8.12 Proteins.

Selected proteins present in **(a)** the membrane of synaptic vesicles, **(b)** the presynaptic cytoplasm, and **(c)** the presynaptic plasma membrane. Predicted membrane topology is indicated. Molecules are not necessarily drawn to scale. The proton pump of the synaptic vesicle is omitted. Adapted from Calakos N, Scheller H (1996) Synaptic vesicle biogenesis, docking and fusion: a molecular description, *Physiolog. Rev.* **76**, 1–29, with permission.

This complex (NSF + SNAPs + membrane) migrates in velocity centrifugation with a sedimentation coefficient of 20 Svedberg and is therefore called the 20 S fusion particle. The existence of such a membrane-bound form of NSF + SNAPs suggested that these proteins recognized specific receptors situated in the membrane. These receptors were called SNAREs (for SNAP REceptors).

The membrane-bound form of the NSF protein is released from the membranes to the cytoplasm by ATP hydrolysis (i.e. in the presence of ATP and Mg^{2+}). Inversely, a stable complex between the NSF protein, the SNAPs and the membranes can be isolated in the presence of a non-hydrolysable analogue of ATP (ATPγS).

Since the complex NSF–SNAP is attached to membranes via SNAREs in the absence of hydrolysable ATP, this property was utilized to purify SNAREs of the vesicle membrane (v-SNARE; v for vesicle) and SNAREs of the target presynaptic plasma membrane (t-SNARE; t for target).

Solubilized brain membranes and NSF–SNAPs are immobilized on beads via a specific anti-*myc* antibody (NSF is tagged with the marker *myc*), in the presence of the non-hydrolysable analogue of ATP, ATPγS, and in the absence of Mg^{2+} (**Figure 8.11b**). The stable complex [NSF–SNAP–membrane proteins] is thus captured. It is then dissociated in the presence of ATP and Mg^{2+} in NSF on the one hand and the complex SNAPs-membrane proteins on the other hand. Membranes are collected and SNAREs are characterized. In the vesicle membrane, synaptobrevin (VAMP/synaptobrevin) was thus identified as a v-SNARE. In the presynaptic membrane, syntaxin and SNAP 25 (synaptosome-associated protein 25, a protein of 25 kDa which has no relation to the similarly named SNAPs) were thus identified as t-SNAREs (**Figure 8.11c**). Both v- and t-SNAREs are integral membrane proteins with a short extracellular domain (**Figure 8.12**). These proteins are also the selective target proteins of toxins such as botulinum and tetanus toxins known to block synaptic transmission (see **Figure 8.15b**).

The three SNAREs, syntaxin, SNAP-25 and VAMP/synaptobrevin form a stable ternary (heterotrimeric) complex of 7 S (**Figure 8.11c**). This 7 S complex has been proposed to mediate the docking of synaptic vesicles at the presynaptic plasma membrane. Docking would therefore require that v-SNAREs are tightly associated with t-SNAREs. NSF and SNAPs would be absent at that stage (to avoid fusion to occur). They would act later, for the fusion process.

The SNARE hypothesis has been proposed to generalize this specific model of vesicle docking at the synapse. It postulates that each transport vesicle has its own specific v-SNARE that pairs up in a unique match with a cognate t-SNARE found only at the intended target membrane. The SNAREs differ from one secretion system to the other, while NSF proteins and soluble NSF attachment proteins (SNAPs) are very general cytoplasmic proteins. Syntaxin, SNAP-25 and VAMP/synaptobrevin each have structurally conserved domains predicted to be capable of forming coiled-coil structures, which consist of an interaction between two to four amphipathic helices. Thus pairing of coiled-coil domains would provide a mechanism for the specific matching of v- with t-SNAREs.

In summary, at the docking stage, synaptic vesicles are 'attached' to the target plasma membrane via the tight of v-SNAREs (VAMP/synaptobrevin) and t-SNAREs (syntaxin, SNAP-25) that are respectively vesicular and plasma membrane proteins.

8.3.3 Three to four Ca²⁺ ions must bind to Ca²⁺ receptor(s) to initiate vesicle fusion (exocytosis)

What is the local Ca²⁺ concentration required to trigger vesicle fusion?

The Ca²⁺ sensor, that is also called Ca²⁺ receptor, has an affinity in the order of tens of micromolars as shown recently in the crayfish neuromuscular junction and the calyx of Held (see section on Ca²⁺ sensor affinity in Further reading).

Why is Ca²⁺ entry close to docked vesicles and release sites?

As explained in Section 8.2.3, syntaxin is tightly coupled to both N- or P/Q-type Ca²⁺ channels and docked vesicles. This makes Ca²⁺ entry close to docked vesicles and release sites (see **Figure 8.7**).

What is the identity of the Ca²⁺ receptors that transduce the [Ca²⁺]ᵢ rise in secretory trigger?

In Ca²⁺-regulated exocytosis as in synapses, the docked vesicles do not fuse with a high probability until a significant [Ca²⁺]ᵢ increase occurs. In constitutive exocytosis models (such as between Golgi stacks), once the vesicles are docked to the target membrane they fuse with it and release their content. However, we have seen (Section 8.3.2) that synaptic vesicle exocytosis uses a constitutively operating mechanism similar to that isolated from Golgi membranes (v- and t-SNAREs, NSF + SNAPs). J. E. Rothman proposed that the difference is the existence at synapses of a 'fusion clamp' which prevents a docked vesicle from fusing with the plasma membrane in the absence of an adequate [Ca²⁺]ᵢ increase.

One of the candidate proteins for the role of Ca²⁺ receptor is synaptotagmin, an integral membrane protein of synaptic vesicles (see **Figure 8.12**). Synaptotagmin was identified originally as an antigen for a synapse-specific antibody. This 58 kDa protein contains Ca²⁺-binding domains (the affinity for this binding is in the 2–30 μM range *in vitro*) and forms a stable complex with the three SNAREs: VAMP, syntaxin and SNAP-25. It is displaced from this complex by α-SNAP, suggesting that these two proteins compete for the same binding sites on the SNARE complex. It is therefore an obvious candidate for transducing an elevation of [Ca²⁺]ᵢ into a fusion trigger. In the absence of Ca²⁺, synaptotagmin would operate as a 'fusion clamp' to prevent fusion from proceeding. More precisely, synaptotagmin when bound to SNAREs would keep fusion 'off' by preventing α-SNAP, and therefore NSF, from binding to the SNAREs.

Interestingly, synaptotagmin does not dissociate from SNAREs in the presence of Ca²⁺, in the absence of α-SNAP. This suggests that even though synaptotagmin is a Ca²⁺-binding protein, and may be a Ca²⁺-sensor, its dissociation from the SNARE complex may not be directly triggered by Ca²⁺ ions alone. Other Ca²⁺-binding proteins with a high affinity for Ca²⁺, present in the vesicle membrane or associated with it, may play also a role in triggering vesicle fusion and there would not be a single candidate as a Ca²⁺ sensor in neurosecretion.

How many Ca^{2+} ions must bind to the Ca^{2+} receptor to initiate exocytosis?

In a slice preparation of cerebellar cortex, presynaptic Ca^{2+} channels are partially blocked and the reduction of presynaptic Ca^{2+} entry and EPSC amplitude measured (see **Figure 8.5**). When a saturating dose of ω-conotoxin, an N-type channel blocker, reduces Ca^{2+} influx by around 25% (measured as a fluorescence transient), it reduces the corresponding EPSC by around 55% (**Figure 8.5b**). The P/Q-type channel blocker ω-agatoxin at a dose that reduces Ca^{2+} influx by around 45% nearly abolishes the synaptic current since it reduces the EPSC by around 90% (**Figure 8.5c**). Neither toxin has a direct effect on postsynaptic glutamatergic currents. Therefore, the most likely hypothesis to account for the high-order Ca^{2+} dependence of synaptic strength is that exocytosis is promoted by the cooperative binding of Ca^{2+} ions to one or multiple receptors.

Results obtained by lowering external Ca^{2+} or by adding Cd^{2+} or selective toxins are expressed as peak EPSC as a percentage function of $\Delta F/F$ (**Figure 8.13**). The double logarithmic plot shows that the relationship between $[Ca^{2+}]_i$ and release is well approximated by an expression of the form:

$$Release = k(Ca^{2+}_{influx})^n,$$

where k is a constant and $2 < n < 4$. *In all models studied so far, there has been a nonlinear dependence between presynaptic $[Ca^{2+}]_i$ and transmitter release: several Ca^{2+} ions must bind with positive cooperativity and affinities of 10–100 μM to target protein(s) to trigger secretion.*

8.3.4 Fusion: from Ca^{2+} binding to exocytosis

Fusion between synaptic vesicles and presynaptic plasma membrane is called exocytosis: it is a regulated fusion (as opposed to constitutive fusion which is Ca-independent). In synapses, synaptic vesicle fuses only upon receipt of a signal, the increase of $[Ca^{2+}]_i$.

How does binding of Ca^{2+} to its receptor(s) initiate exocytosis?

Fusion is a lipid–lipid interaction. For fusion to occur, the pairing of v-SNARE with t-SNARE which docks the synaptic vesicle must be broken up at some stage. This

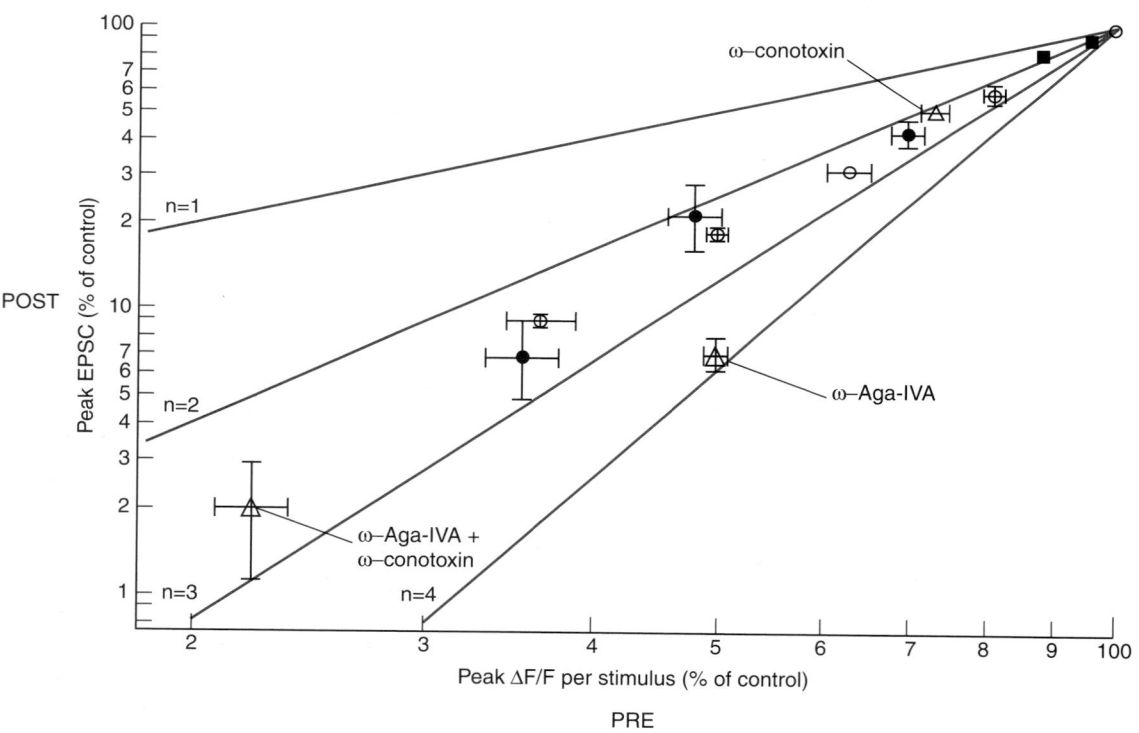

Figure 8.13 Relationship between postsynaptic current amplitude and presynaptic Ca^{2+} influx.
The plot of synaptic strength (peak EPSC) versus Ca^{2+} influx ($\Delta F/F$) summarizes the data obtained from the experiments shown in Figure 8.5. The four lines correspond to the equation Release = $k(Ca^{2+}_{influx})^n$, with n as indicated. All values are normalized to the peak EPSC or the peak $\Delta F/F$ measured in control solution. Adapted from Mintz I, Sabatini BL, Regehr WG (1995) Calcium control of transmitter release at a cerebellar synapse, *Neuron* **15**, 675–688, with permission.

includes of course Ca^{2+} ions but also energy. The SNARE complex being itself a stable entity, an energy input is needed, such as ATP hydrolysis (by NSF). The destabilization of the protein complex between the docked vesicle and the plasma membrane would be triggered by Ca^{2+} binding to specific protein(s) to suppress 'fusion clamp'. One must also keep in mind that even when all the proper conditions come together (a presynaptic spike, opening of Ca^{2+} channels, Ca^{2+} entry, Ca^{2+} binding), the average probability of the exocytosis of a synaptic vesicle still remains below 1 (see Appendix 8.2). In fact, the mean release probability is between 0.05 and 0.5 according to the synapse studied.

The one-site/one-vesicle hypothesis

Ca^{2+}-triggered exocytosis is *inefficient*: only one in every three to ten action potentials leads to exocytosis and only one of many docked vesicles fuses. The 'one-site/one-vesicle' hypothesis states that the number of released vesicles per presynaptic action potential is never larger than, although sometimes equal to, the number of structurally defined release sites. The generally accepted hypothesis is that a presynaptic action potential activates the fusion of a maximum of one synaptic vesicle (one or none) at each release site. This is explained in Appendix 8.2.

Exocytosis involves the formation of a fusion pore

The development of patch-clamp capacitance techniques demonstrated the formation of a fusion pore during exocytosis. There are three basic proposals regarding the nature of the fusion pore: a protein with a structure similar to that of connexin, the protein of gap junctions (see **Figure 3.9**); a protein with a lipid-lined pore or a purely lipidic pore. After formation, the pore would expand in order to allow rapid transmitter release in the cleft. Theoretical models propose that the fusion pore expands at a rate approaching 100 nm ms^{-1} within a few tens of microseconds to achieve the observed transmitter time course.

8.3.5 Pharmacology of neurotransmitter release

Agents blocking K^+ currents potentiate neurotransmitter release

K^+ channels present at the presynaptic membrane are voltage-gated K^+ channels of the Na^+ action potential (see Section 5.3) and Ca^{2+}-activated K^+ channels ($K_{(Ca)}$; Section 6.3). The outflow of K^+ ions through these chan-

nels repolarizes the presynaptic membrane and limits Ca^{2+} entry (in amplitude and duration). At the neuromuscular junction, simultaneous labelling with specific fluorescent toxins of presynaptic $K_{(Ca)}$ and Ca^{2+} channels showed that they are localized close to one another, at presynaptic active zones. This organization ensures a rapid activation of these K^+ channels during Ca^{2+} entry triggered by an action potential.

When these K^+ channels are blocked, Ca^{2+} entry is increased and so is transmitter release. At the neuromuscular junction, potassium channel blockers such as TEA and 3,4-diaminopyridine, when used in conjunction with TTX (to block voltage-dependent Na^+ channels), potentiate the postsynaptic response (**Figure 8.14**). In the presence of K^+ blocking agents, the endplate current has an average time of decline much longer than that of the miniature current. This is due in part to the fact that, in this case, the release of vesicles is asynchronous and there is a temporal spread of quantal release during the entire presynaptic calcium spike. On the other hand, the massive release possibly saturates the enzyme acetylcholinesterase and as a result there is a repeated activation of postsynaptic nicotinic receptors.

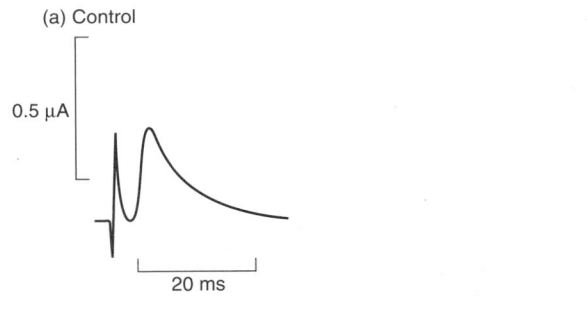

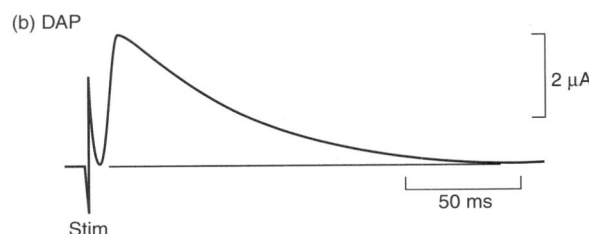

Figure 8.14 Diaminopyridine (DAP) increases the duration and amplitude of motor endplate current.
The postsynaptic endplate current of a frog sartorius muscle cell is evoked by stimulation (2 μA intensity, 5 ms duration) of the motor nerve ($V_H = -90$ mV). **(a)** The average amplitude of the evoked postsynaptic current is 0.5 μA in control Ringer solution. **(b)** The postsynaptic current evoked by the same stimulation in the presence of DAP (1 mM) is always greater than 1 μA and can reach 3.3 μA. These inward currents are represented upwardly, which is unusual. Adapted from Katz B, Miledi R (1979) Estimates of quantal content during chemical potentialization of transmitter release, *Proc. R. Soc. Lond. B* **205**, 369–378, with permission.

In summary, K$^+$ channel blocking agents potentiate acetylcholine release 10–100 times following a presynaptic Ca^{2+} spike. This potentiating effect of TEA and 3,4-diaminopyridine shown at the neuromuscular junction is valid for all chemical synapses.

Example of botulinum toxins

Botulinum toxins derived from the microorganism *Clostridium botulinum* is a powerful neurotoxin made up of seven different toxins (A to G). These proteins have a heavy chain (100 kDa) joined by a single disulphide bond to a light chain (50 kDa). The heavy chain is responsible for the selective binding of the toxin to neuronal cells and for the penetration of the light chain into neurons; the light chain bears the activity. Botulinum toxin blocks synaptic transmission at all peripheral cholinergic synapses. The transmission is blocked for several months. The patient usually dies from asphyxia (paralysis of respiratory muscles) and, in cases where the patient survives, he suffers from muscle atrophy owing to the non-functioning of muscle cells.

Botulinum toxin enters nerve terminals and decreases the number of acetylcholine vesicles released in the synaptic cleft without affecting acetylcholine synthesis or action potential conduction in the motor nerve (it blocks synaptic transmission). In cases where the decrease is not total, the effect of the toxin can be reversed by increasing Ca^{2+} concentration in the extracellular medium or by adding TEA or 3,4-diaminopyridine, agents that potentiate Ca^{2+} influx. Aminopyridines are used to cure patients poisoned by the botulinum toxins contained, for example, in damaged preserves.

Knowing these facts, it was hypothesized that botulinum toxin affected either Ca^{2+} entry or the coupling between intracellular Ca^{2+} concentration increase and exocytosis of synaptic vesicles. To verify the first proposition, Ca^{2+} entry was recorded in terminals 'paralysed' by botulinum toxins. The results showed that presynaptic Ca^{2+} current is not significantly changed (**Figure 8.15a**). The botulinum toxin would therefore act at the presynaptic level to decrease acetylcholine release, after the entry of Ca^{2+} ions.

In order to identify the intracellular target of botulinum toxins, synaptic vesicles from rat cerebral cortex were purified. Of the many proteins detected in these purified synaptic vesicles, one protein band was altered by incubation of the vesicles with botulinum toxin. The electrophoretic mobility of this band corresponds to that of VAMP/synaptobrevins, one of the vesicle proteins thought to play a role in vesicle docking. Syntaxins and SNAP-25 are also targets for botulinum toxin. Botulinum toxins are proteases, each of which cleaves a single target at a single site. The light chain of botulinum toxins contains a consensus sequence of the catalytic site of metallopeptidases. It has a Zn^{2+}- dependent endopeptidase activity. Botulinum toxins B, D, F and G are specific for VAMPs, botulinum toxin C cleaves syntaxins, and botulinum toxins A and E are specific for SNAP-25 (**Figure 8.15b**). The cleavage of one of these SNAREs greatly reduces the probability of neurotransmitter release. The exact mechanism of this inhibition of release is not known.

8.4 Processes in the synaptic cleft: from transmitter release in the cleft to transmitter clearance from the cleft

The time course of transmitter in the cleft depends on the balance between the amount of transmitter released per unit of time and the efficacy of clearance mechanisms that clear transmitter molecules from the cleft.

8.4.1 The amount of neurotransmitter released in the synaptic cleft

The amount of transmitter released per vesicle and per unit of time in the synaptic cleft depends on (i) the concentration of the transmitter in the exocytotic vesicle, (ii) the volume of the vesicle, and (iii) the rate of transmitter release through the vesicle fusion pore into the cleft (i.e. the dimension of the fusion pore).

What is the concentration of neurotransmitter in a synaptic vesicle?

Consider the example of synaptic vesicles that contain glutamate as a neurotransmitter. To isolate synaptic vesicles, antibodies against a vesicular protein (such as synaptophysin) are immobilized on the surface of non-porous methacrylate microbeads. Using these immunobeads, synaptic vesicles are isolated. To avoid the loss of glutamate, the vesicular H$^+$ gradient (responsible for the transport of neurotransmitter molecules into vesicles; see Section 3.4.2) is preserved by adding an ATP-regenerating system. Under these conditions, high levels of glutamate are found in vesicles: 0.8 μmol of glutamate per milligram of synaptophysin. Knowing that synaptophysin represents 7% of total vesicle protein, it gives 60 nmol of glutamate per milligram of protein. This gives an intravesicular concentration of 60 mM, assuming an internal volume of 1 μl mg^{-1} of protein. The concentration of glutamate in synaptic vesicles is estimated at 60–210 mM depending on the preparation studied. The concentrations of other transmitters such as GABA and glycine are not known.

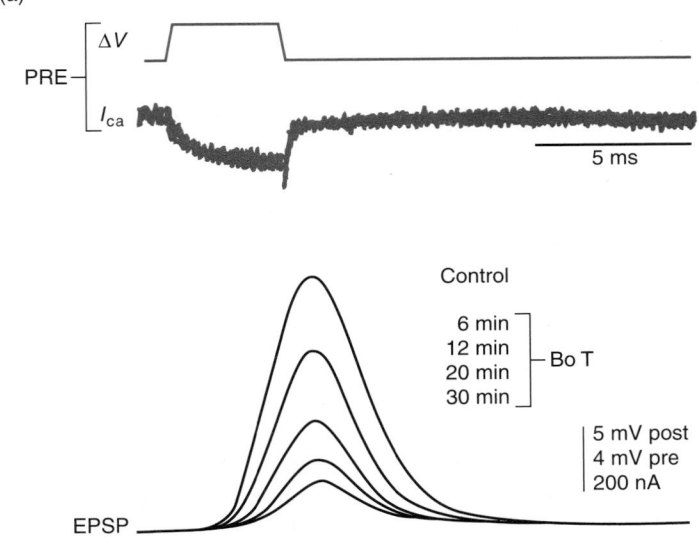

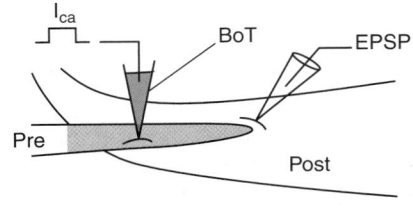

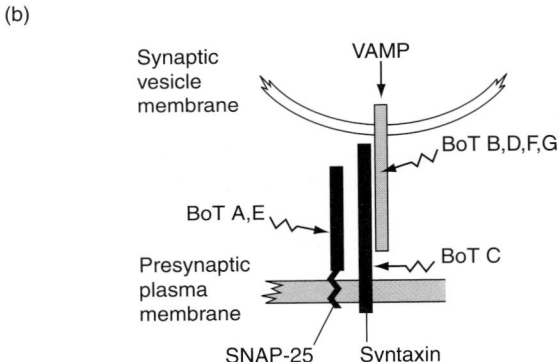

Figure 8.15 Presynaptic injection of botulinum toxin strongly decreases synaptic transmission without affecting presynaptic Ca²⁺ current.

(a) In the squid giant synapse, at the stellate ganglion, presynaptic and postsynaptic intracellular electrodes are implanted to allow simultaneous recording of the presynaptic Ca^{2+} current (voltage-clamp mode) and the postsynaptic response (EPSP, current-clamp mode). A presynaptic voltage step (ΔV) evokes a presynaptic Ca^{2+} current (I_{Ca}) and after a delay, a postsynaptic response (EPSP, control). After injection of botulinum toxin (BoT) through the presynaptic electrode, the EPSP decreases with time. Note that in the same time the presynaptic Ca^{2+} current is unchanged. (b) Target proteins of botulinum toxins (BoT). Part (a) adapted from Marsal J, Ruiz-Montasell B, Blasi J *et al.* (1997) Block of transmitter release by botulinum C1 action on syntaxin at the squid giant synapse, *Proc. Natl Acad. Sci. USA* **94**, 14871–14876, with permission.

Is the vesicle content stable? If yes, how does a vesicle know it is full?

Miniature spontaneous postsynaptic responses that correspond to the exocytosis of a very small number of vesicles (say one, two or three; see Appendix 8.1) have a quite stable amplitude. This suggests that the vesicle content is relatively stable. Therefore, at a given synapse, synaptic vesicles would contain the same amount of transmitter. Such a stable content could be achieved by regulating the number of synaptic transporters in the vesicle membrane. Another hypothesis is that the amount of transmitter in a vesicle is variable but very high so that it saturates postsynaptic receptors; in such a condition, variations in the vesicle content would not be 'seen' by the postsynaptic ligand-gated channels and the size of miniature potentials would show minimal variation.

How does the transmitter diffuse from the vesicle into the cleft?

The detailed nature of the vesicle fusion process remains unclear. In particular, the formation of the fusion pore, its opening rate as well as how molecules diffuse out from the vesicle are not known.

What is the peak concentration of neurotransmitter in the cleft?

The time course of neurotransmitter concentration can be evaluated experimentally. The technique utilizes the non-equilibrium displacement of a competitive antagonist following the synaptic release of transmitter. A specific antagonist of the postsynaptic ionotropic receptors that mediate the transmission is applied. Attenuation of synaptic response amplitude is measured at one or more concentrations of a rapidly dissociating competitive antagonist and a dose–response curve is constructed for the inhibition of synaptic transmission. Transmitter peak concentration in the cleft would be around 1 mM for glutamate and achieved in around 20 μs.

8.4.2 Transmitter time course in the synaptic cleft is brief and depends mainly on transmitter binding to target proteins

The speed of transmitter clearance from the synaptic cleft is a fundamental parameter influencing many aspects of synaptic function. The amount of time the neurotransmitter stays in the cleft depends on (i) the amount of transmitter released, (ii) the transmitter diffusion coefficient, the geometry of the cleft and adjacent extrasynaptic space, (iii) the distribution and affinity of transmitter binding sites, and (iv) the transporter uptake rate and/or degradative enzymes turnover rate. Therefore the transmitter time course varies significantly from synapse to synapse.

Theoretical models predict that within 50 μs the transmitter is evenly distributed throughout the cleft and by 500 μs the cleft is clear of transmitter (**Figure 8.16**). Only transporters, degradative enzymes and diffusion achieve the real removal of neurotransmitter molecules from the cleft. Binding to pre- and postsynaptic receptors is a temporary clearance (buffering) since transmitter molecules will be back in the cleft as soon as they unbind from receptors (as already seen for Ca^{2+} clearance; see Section 8.2.4). The turnover rate for known neurotransmitter transporters is in the range $1–15 s^{-1}$: a single transporter requires at least 60 ms to complete its cycle. This is extremely slow compared with the turnover rate for AChEsterase which is in the order of $10^4 s^{-1}$. It shows how highly efficient is this enzyme to remove acetylcholine from the cleft at nicotinic synapses (for example the neuromuscular junction). Therefore, for glutamate and GABA, which are not enzymatically

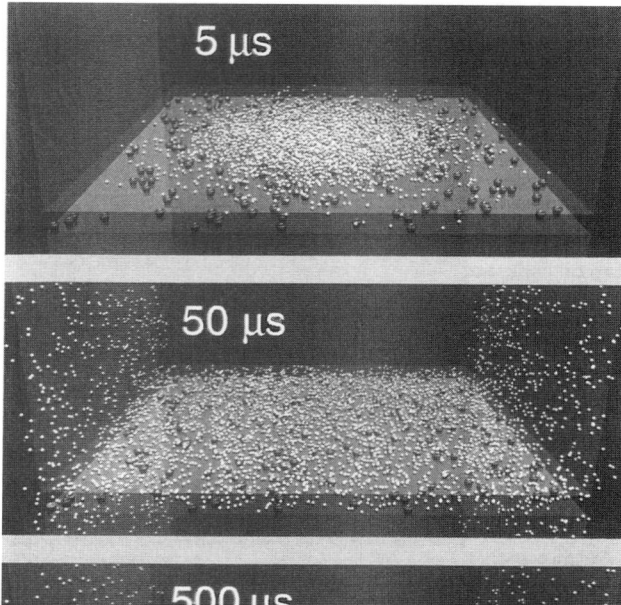

Figure 8.16 The Monte Carlo model of neurotransmitter clearance.

The series of four images describes the distribution and concentration of transmitter molecules (green spheres) in a synaptic cleft (width 20 nm, area 0.5×0.5 μm) at different times after transmitter release. The mathematical model incorporates the geometry of the cleft and adjacent extracellular space, the binding of transmitter to receptors and uptake sites and other details. Postsynaptic receptors are shown as objects embedded in the postsynaptic membrane at a density of 100 μm^{-2}, and their colour indicates the presence or not of bound transmitter molecules (black = 0, white = 1 or 2). At $t = 0$, 5000 transmitter molecules are released instantaneously at the centre of the synaptic cleft. Snapshots of their distribution are taken at 5, 50 and 500 μs. At 50 μs after release, the average concentration of transmitter in the cleft had fallen by 50%. At 500 μs, the cleft is now 90% clear of transmitter and binding to postsynaptic receptors is approaching 50% saturation. From images created by T. Bartol and J. Stiles, in Clements JD (1996) Transmitter time course in the synaptic cleft: its role in central synaptic function, *Trend. Neurosci.* **19**, 163–170, with permission.

degraded in the cleft, uptake transporters are too slow to achieve a rapid disappearance of transmitter molecules from the cleft.

In central synapses, rapid buffering of transmitter molecules from the cleft arises from the binding of these molecules to receptor proteins: postsynaptic receptor-channels (ionotropic receptors), and pre- and post-synaptic G protein-linked receptors (metabotropic receptors). These receptors bind the transmitter molecules tightly enough (i.e. with a high affinity) to prevent release from binding sites for tens of milliseconds, sufficient time for transporters to become less saturated. In other words, each transporter stands ready to bind a transmitter molecule as soon as it is released from a receptor. Otherwise, neurotransmitter molecules would

be released a second time in the cleft and evoke a second postsynaptic response or amplify the duration of the first one.

8.5 Summary

The answers to the questions raised in Section 8.1.3 are as follows (refer to **Figure 8.17**):

■ The opening of presynaptic high-voltage-activated Ca^{2+} channels (N- and P/Q-type Ca^{2+} channels) is triggered by membrane depolarization that occurs during the depolarizing phase of presynaptic action potentials.

■ Presynaptic $[Ca^{2+}]_i$ increase is local in response to a

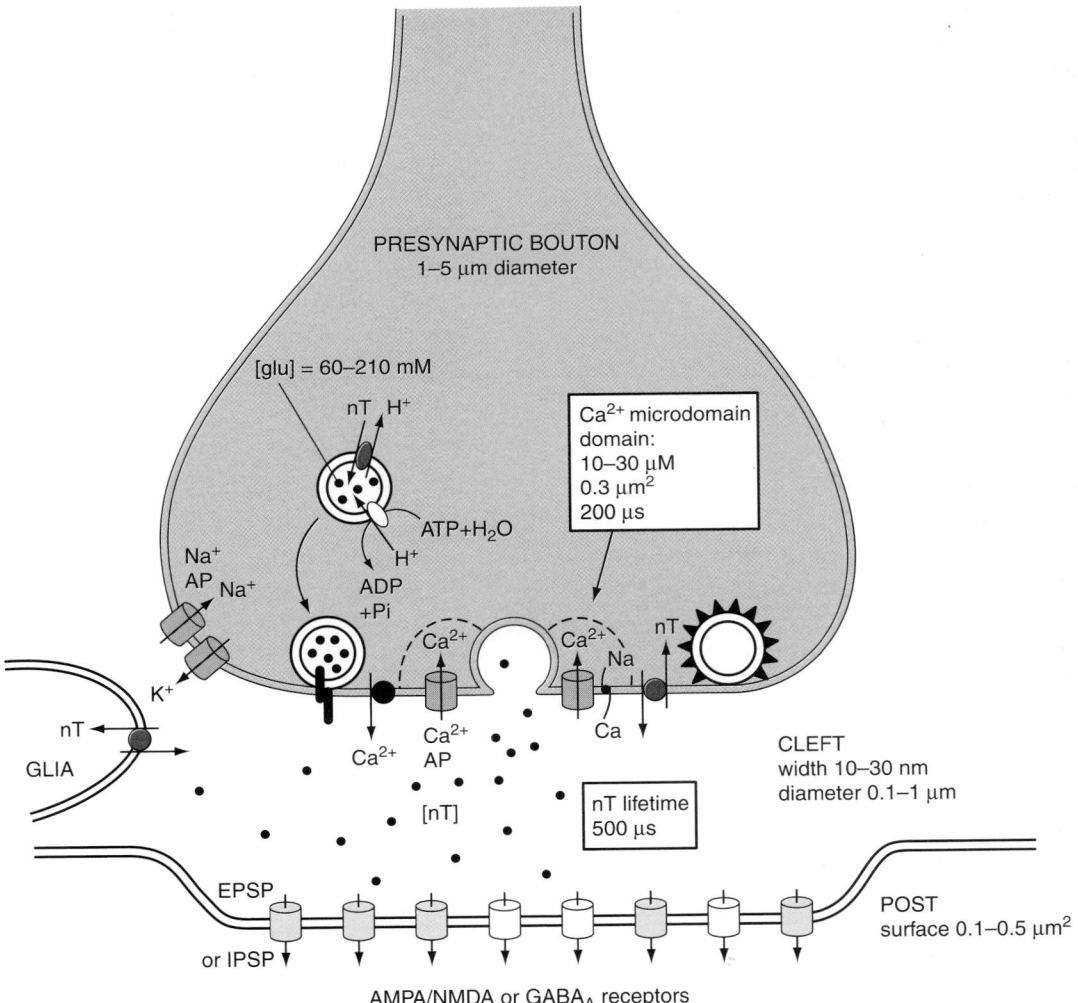

Figure 8.17 Cascade of events leading to neurotransmitter release and its clearance from the synaptic cleft.
Schematic of some steps of synaptic transmission (between the presynaptic action potential and the postsynaptic response, EPSP or IPSP). In the presynaptic and glial plasma membranes only one example of each channel, pump or transporter, is represented owing to the lack of space. In the postsynaptic membrane many examples of ionotropic glutamatergic (AMPA and NMDA) or GABAergic (GABA_A) channels are represented. nT, neurotransmitter.

presynaptic spike due to the clustering of N- and P/Q-type Ca^{2+} channels close to docked vesicles, at release sites. $[Ca^{2+}]_i$ increase is transient since Ca^{2+} channels open and close quickly and Ca^{2+} ions are cleared from the cytoplasm by binding to receptor proteins (cytoplasmic Ca^{2+}-binding proteins and transmembrane proteins such as Ca/ATPase or Na–Ca exchanger).

■ Exocytosis of a docked vesicle is triggered when local $[Ca^{2+}]_i$ increase is around 10–30 µM. The first step includes binding of 3–4 Ca^{2+} ions to Ca^{2+}-binding protein(s) (Ca^{2+}-sensor(s)) but the exact mechanism of vesicle fusion is not yet known. Exocytosis is rapidly triggered since Ca^{2+} entry is close to release sites and each docked vesicle is ready to fuse.

■ The accepted hypothesis is that a maximum of one vesicle fuses at each active zone with the presynaptic plasma membrane in response to a single presynaptic spike.

■ The concentration of transmitter in the cleft resulting from the release of the content of one vesicle is around 1 mM for glutamate. Theoretical models predict that by 500 µs the cleft is clear of neurotransmitter molecules.

■ Buffering of neurotransmitter molecules present in the cleft results from binding to specific receptors such as pre- and postsynaptic ionotropic and metabotropic receptors, but its clearance (total disappearance from the cleft) is achieved by its binding to neuronal and glial transporters and/or to degradative enzymes and by its diffusion out of the cleft.

Neurotransmitter release, from Ca^{2+} entry into the presynaptic terminal to vesicle exocytosis, is achieved by a cascade of chemically gated events (**Table 8.1**). It differs fundamentally from electrical events such as action potentials that are achieved by a cascade of voltage-gated events. Once presynaptic Ca^{2+} channels open, synaptic transmission is determined by the different affinity constants of the reactions between ligands and receptors that underlie synaptic transmission: this includes binding of Ca^{2+} to Ca^{2+} sensor(s), unbinding of v-SNARE to t-SNARE, binding of neurotransmitter molecules to pre- and postsynaptic receptors (receptor channels, G-protein coupled receptors, uptake transporters). Transmitter release from presynaptic elements is a Ca^{2+}-regulated, multiprotein process.

Location of reactions	Type of reaction	Steps of Fig. 7.4a	Reactions			Effect
PRE	Voltage-gated	Step 2	N channels closed P/Q	action potential ⇌	N channels open P/Q	**Ca^{2+} entry**
	Ligand-gated	Step 3a	2–4 Ca^{2+} + sensors	10–30 µM ⇌	$_{2-4}$ Ca-sensor	**Exocytosis**
		Step 3b	Ca^{2+} + pumps Ca^{2+} + transporters	0.2–1.0 µM ⇌	Ca-pumps Ca-transporters	**Ca^{2+} clearance**
CLEFT	Ligand-gated	Step 5a/6	2 Glu + AMPAR	0.25–1.50 mM ⇌	Glu_2-AMPAR	**EPSP**
			2 Glu + NMDAR	1 µM ⇌	Glu_2-NMDAR	
		Step 5a/6	2Gaba + $GABA_A$	8–40 µM ⇌	$Gaba_2$-$GABA_A$	**IPSP**
		Step 5b/5c	nT + transporter	high affinity ⇌	nT + transporter	**nT uptake**

Table 18.1 Some of the reactions (voltage-gated and ligand-gated) from the opening of N- and P/Q-type Ca^{2+} channels to transmitter release into the synaptic cleft and its clearance from the synaptic cleft. The numbers indicate the values of K_D or EC_{50}. All the vesicle steps preceding fusion step have been omitted.

Appendix 8.1
Quantal nature of neurotransmitter release

A8.1.1 Spontaneous release of acetylcholine at the neuromuscular junction evokes miniature endplate potentials: the notion of quanta

At the neuromuscular junction, when an intracellular electrode is implanted in a muscle fibre at the level of the postsynaptic membrane in the presence of TTX and in the absence of extracellular Ca^{2+}, spontaneous postsynaptic potentials of very small amplitude (0.5–1.0 mV on average) are recorded, though presynaptic spikes and synaptic transmission are blocked (**Figure A8.1**). They occur randomly at a low frequency (about 1 s^{-1}). They have been called 'miniature' endplate potentials (mEPP) by Fatt and Katz (1952). As explained by Katz (1966): 'Except for their spontaneous occurrence and their small size, the miniatures are indistinguishable from the EPSPs evoked by presynaptic nerve stimulation; for example curare suppresses them and acetylcholinesterase inhibitors enhance their amplitude and duration with the same doses and to approximately the same extent. Normally, miniature potentials are well below the firing level of the muscle cell and so remain localized and produce no contraction. Since they disappear after the motor nerve has been cut and inthe presence of botulinum toxin, they are evoked by presynaptic release of Ach.' The interpretation is that motor nerve terminals at rest are in a state of intermittent secretory activity: they liberate small quantities of ACh at random intervals at an average rate of about one per second.

Miniature endplate potentials, being the smallest recorded event with a relatively constant amplitude and an all-or-nothing characteristic, were named *quanta* (with reference to quantum physics) by Del Castillo and Katz in 1954. Considering the fast risetime of miniatures, they hypothesized that miniatures arise from the synchronous action of a packet of a large number of ACh molecules at a time: 'At this stage, the characteristic presynaptic vesicles were revealed by electron microscope and the suggestion arose that they could be the subcellular particles in which the transmitter is stored and from which it is released in an all-or-none fashion.' This was confirmed by the observation of exocytosis at active zones of the neuromuscular junction (Couteaux and Pécot-Dechavassine 1970).

However, direct visualization of exocytosis at a neuromuscular junction was achieved only 20 years later by using electron microscopy combined with new methods to rapidly freeze nerve terminals (Heuser *et al.* 1979). The tissue is freeze-fractured during synaptic activity at precise times following nerve stimulation. A metal replica of the presynaptic membrane after fracture is observed under the electron microscope. Images of exocytosis are observed only in the presence of 4-aminopyridine (a blocker of K^+ channels which prolongs depolarization of the presynaptic membrane; see Section 8.3.5), when important ACh release occurs. In the absence of drugs, rearrangement of presynaptic intra-membranous particles is the most common ultrastructural observation. This low probability of observation of exocytosis in the absence of 4-aminopyridine is not surprising, considering the low probability of exocytosis at a synaptic complex at a given time (see Appendix 8.2).

Similar spontaneous miniature potentials are recorded from synapses of the central nervous system. They are called 'miniature postsynaptic potentials' or 'miniature currents' (mEPSPs and mIPSPs).

(a)

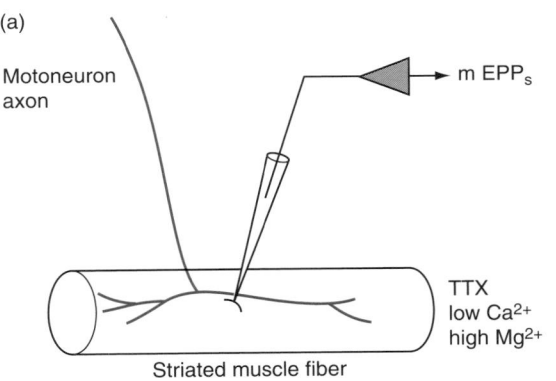

(b)

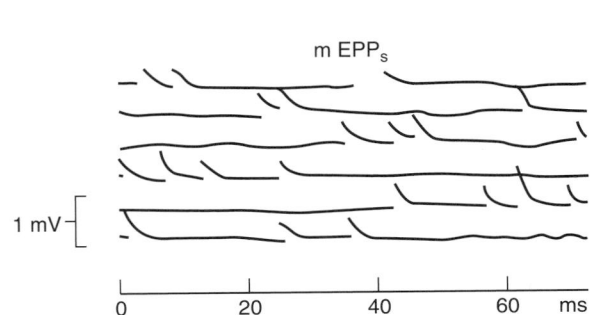

Figure A8.1 Miniature postsynaptic potentials.
Miniature endplate potentials **(b)** recorded at the frog neuromuscular junction **(a)**. Recordings are obtained in the presence of a low external Ca^{2+} concentration. Part (a) adapted from Fatt P, Katz B (1952) Spontaneous subthreshold activity at motor nerve endings, *J. Physiol. (Lond.)* **117**, 109–128, with permission.

The theory of vesicular release of neurotransmitter, or the quantal nature of chemical transmission, states that one quantum equals one vesicle. The size of a quantum is designated by q.

A8.1.2 The quantal composition of EPSPs and IPSPs

At the neuromuscular junction, a quantum produces a 0.5–1 mV miniature potential (mEPP). In response to a presynaptic action potential and in the presence of control concentrations of external Ca^{2+}, an endplate potential (EPP) is recorded: it has a much larger amplitude (50–70 mV) than miniatures. The quantal theory assumes that EPPs are made up of n quanta released simultaneously (200–300 mEPPs). This evidence is obtained by lowering external Ca^{2+} concentration and thus reducing the amplitude of evoked EPPs. If one lowers the normal Ca^{2+} concentration and adds magnesium to the muscle bath, the amount of acetylcholine delivered by an impulse can be reduced to a very low level, and under these experimental conditions, the quantal composition of the endplate potential becomes immediately apparent (see Appendix 8.2). This result has been confirmed in various synapses of vertebrates and invertebrates.

If one admits that only one vesicle fuses at a time at each active zone, a miniature of amplitude q therefore corresponds to the activity of only one active zone at a time (among the hundreds or thousands present).

Appendix 8.2
The probabilistic nature of neurotransmitter release

Neurotransmitter release is probabilistic. In response to a presynaptic action potential, each docked synaptic vesicle has a probability p to fuse with the presynaptic plasma membrane (i.e. to undergo exocytosis). This probability p varies from 0 to 1 ($0 < p < 1$). This means that even when all the proper conditions are fulfilled, the synaptic transmission can fail (see **Figure 8.3a**). What fails exactly is vesicle exocytosis. Of course, when chemical transmission at a single synapse is achieved by only one active zone (mammalian CNS synapses), failures are much more commonly observed than when it is achieved by a large number of active zones (neuromuscular junction).

A8.2.1 The neuromuscular junction as a model

The first studies on the probability of neurotransmitter release were performed on the neuromuscular junction (also called the motor endplate), this preparation offering the possibility of simultaneously recording the activity of pre- and postsynaptic elements and of manipulating the parameters related to neurotransmitter release, here acetylcholine. At the motor endplate level, the number of active zones is estimated at between 300 and 1000. For this reason, the recorded postsynaptic response is global, representing the summation of evoked responses at each active zone.

In the absence of any nerve stimulation, miniature endplate postsynaptic potentials of 0.5–1.0 mV average amplitude are recorded. They occur randomly. These miniature endplate potentials, being the smallest recorded event and having a relatively constant amplitude, were named 'quanta' by Del Castillo and Katz. They proposed that each quantum corresponds to the content of one synaptic vesicle. The size of a quantum is q.

In contrast, in response to nerve stimulation, the probability of synaptic vesicle exocytosis is very high and the size of the endplate potential is in the order of tens of millivolts. In order to test whether EPSPs are made up of quanta, the size of EPSPs is reduced by immersing the preparation in an extracellular medium containing a low Ca^{2+} concentration. In these conditions, following motor nerve stimulation, one can record postsynaptic depolarizations (motor endplate potentials) having a low and variable amplitude and also numerous failures (absence of postsynaptic response) (**Figure A8.2a**). These amplitude variations are in graduated steps, each one corresponding to a quantum of amplitude q (**Figure A8.2b**).

The postsynaptic response is constantly a multiple of 0, 1, 2, ..., x quanta, x always being a whole number. If one admits that a quantum corresponds to the release of a synaptic vesicle, it appears that 0, 1, 2, ..., x synaptic vesicles are released (x being a natural number as each synaptic vesicle is an entity). This produces fluctuations in the amplitude of the postsynaptic response. The distribution of these fluctuations on a graph shows the presence of regularly spaced peaks, the first three peaks clearly corresponding to amplitudes $1q$ (0.4 mV), $2q$ (0.8 mV) and $3q$ (1.2 mV), but the presence of other peaks ($4q$, ..., xq) is less evident (**Figure A8.2c**). The first two amplitudes ($1q$ and $2q$) are more frequent than others. In other words, the probability of recording postsynaptic potentials of amplitude $1q$ or $2q$ is greater than that of recording potentials of amplitude $3q$ or above in the presence of a low external Ca^{2+} concentration.

The demonstration that postsynaptic potentials are composed of discrete units has necessitated the application of statistical tests to the experimental data. Poisson's Law was applied to test that each response is made up of discrete (0, 1, 2, 3, ...) units. As stated earlier,

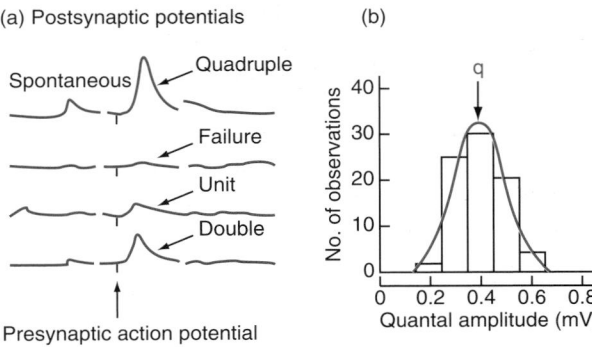

(a) Postsynaptic potentials

(b)

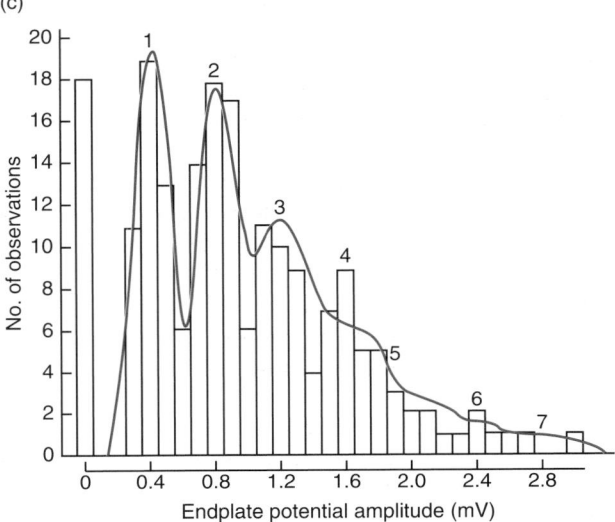

(c)

Figure A8.2 Demonstration of the probabilistic nature of acetylcholine release at the neuromuscular junction.

(a) Recordings of spontaneous miniatures and evoked endplate potentials (mEPP and EPP). The nerve-muscle preparation is bathed in a low-Ca^{2+} high-Mg^{2+} concentration medium. In such condition, spontaneous mEPPs have nearly the same unitary amplitude whereas evoked EPPs have an amplitude that is a multiple of the mEPP amplitude. (b) The distribution of mEPP amplitude is unimodal and their average amplitude is $q = 0.4$ mV. (c) Histogram of evoked EPPs recorded in response to a presynaptic action potential. The cases where no postsynaptic response is recorded (failures) are represented at 0 mV (18 cases). The theoretical distribution calculated from Poisson's Law (represented by the green line) fits the distribution of the amplitude of recorded EPPs (histogram). Part (a) adapted from Liley AW (1956) The quantal component of the mammalian endplate potential, *J. Physiol. (Lond.)* **133**, 571–587, with permission. Parts (b) and (c) from Boyd IA, Martin AR (1956) The endplate potential in mammalian muscle, *J. Physiol. (Lond.)* **132**, 74–91, with permission.

the results shown in **Figure A8.2** were obtained in conditions where p is reduced (reduced extracellular Ca^{2+} concentration). This is a necessary condition for the use of the Poisson distribution. In other words, each time an

action potential invades the axon terminals, it causes the release of a few vesicles out of a very large available population. In the Poisson distribution, the probability of observing a postsynaptic potential composed of x miniature potentials $p(x)$ is:

$$p(x) = e^{-m}m^x/x!,$$

where m is the mean number of quanta (miniature potentials) that compose the postsynaptic response (i.e. the average number of released vesicles in response to a presynaptic spike). N is the total number of observations (the number of recordings of the postsynaptic potential in response to a presynaptic spike) and $n(x)$ is the number of times that the recorded postsynaptic potentials is composed of x miniature potentials (amplitude of the postsynaptic response = xq). The probability that a postsynaptic potential is composed of x miniature potentials, $p(x)$, is equal to the number of times this event is observed, $n(x)$, over the total number of experiments, N:

$$p(x) = n(x)/N. \tag{1}$$

When N is large enough, $Np(x)$ is close to the observed number of responses which contain x quanta (which are made up of a summation of x miniatures).

The difficulty here is to determine the value of m, the mean number of quanta that compose the postsynaptic response (also called the average quantal content). To determine m, two methods can be used.

First, given that the amplitude of miniature potentials is a unit, one can calculate:

$$m = \frac{\text{average amplitude of evoked responses}}{\text{average amplitude of miniature potentials}}$$

This method is used in Chapter 9.

The second option is the so-called failure method. In conditions where p is artificially reduced (reduced external Ca^{2+} concentration), the number of times the synaptic transmission fails is high: numerous presynaptic action potentials are not followed by vesicle release. In these cases of failure, $x = 0$ (the postsynaptic responses of null amplitude composed of 0 miniature potentials). From equation (1), $p(0)$ is the number of failures over the total number of stimulations N; it is large and equal to:

$$p(0) = e^{-m} = \frac{\text{number of failures}}{\text{number of simulations}} = n(0)/N.$$

Therefore $m = \ln (N/n(0))$. The $n(0)/N$ ratio, determined from experimental results (**Figure A8.2c**), leads to an easy deduction of m.

With m known, p can be calculated for each value of x, and a theoretical curve is drawn, showing the distribution of postsynaptic potentials. **Figure A8.2c** shows the correlation between experimental data and the Poisson distribution. Quantal acetylcholine release at the neuromuscular junction is a valid model. The following hypothesis has been proposed.

Acetylcholine release is a discontinuous quantal phenomenon, each quantum corresponding to the total content of one synaptic vesicle. The probability p that the postsynaptic response will be composed of 1, 2, ..., x quanta depends on the experimental conditions (composition of the extracellular medium) and on the frequency of presynaptic activity. Once again, the results in **Figure A8.2** have been obtained in a medium where p is reduced, a condition necessary to the use of the Poisson distribution. We will see in Section A8.2.2 that the binomial distribution allows a more general description of p.

A8.2.2 Inhibitory synapses between interneurons and the Mauthner cell in the teleost fish bulb, as a model

To determine whether the theory on the quantal release of neurotransmitters is applicable to central synapses, and to describe the release probability, the inhibitory synapses between inhibitory afferent neurons and the postsynaptic Mauthner cell (M cell) was the chosen model (**Figure A8.3**). Glycine is the neurotransmitter and it opens receptor channels in the postsynaptic membrane that are selectively permeable to Cl⁻ ions.

In this preparation, one can identify electrophysiologically the presynaptic neurons making inhibitory synapses with the Mauthner cell, perform simultaneous intracellular recordings of the presynaptic axon and the postsynaptic Mauthner cell, and also inject horseradish peroxidase (HRP, a marker) into the presynaptic neurons in order to visualize the terminals and to establish

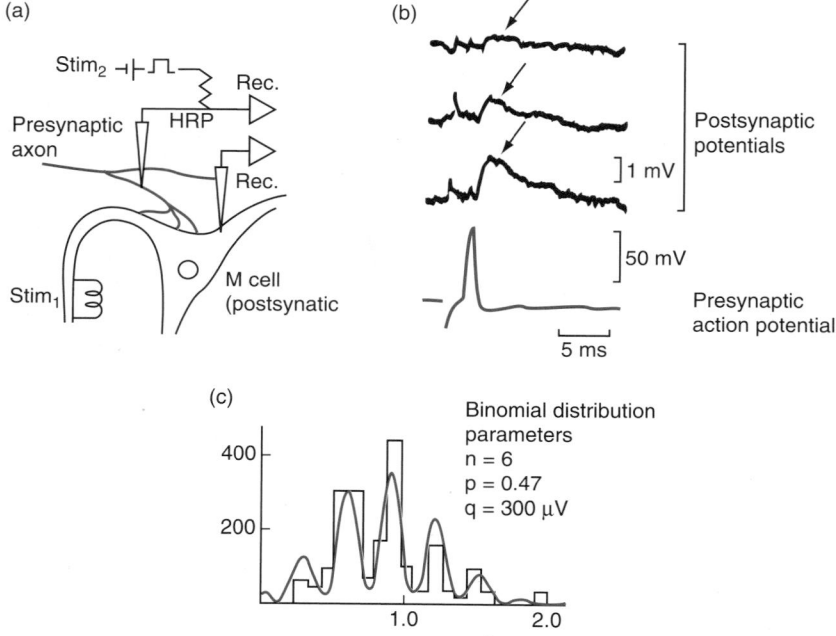

Figure A8.3 Demonstration of quantal release of neurotransmitter in a central synapse.
(a) Experimental design. The Mauthner cell (M cell) in a teleost fish bulb receives afferents from inhibitory glycinergic neurons (PHP cell). Antidromic activation (Stim) allows the identification of cells whose activity is recorded in current clamp. The recording electrodes are filled with a solution of KCl. The Cl⁻ ions diffuse in the intracellular medium, thus changing the reversal potential of Cl⁻ ions and consequently the potential at which the glycine response reverses polarity (glycine opens receptor channels selectively permeable to Cl⁻ ions). For this reason, the recorded postsynaptic response is not a hyperpolarization but a depolarization, called 'inverted IPSP'. At the end of the experiment, HRP is injected into the presynaptic neuron to study its synaptic contacts with the Mauthner cell at the electron microscopic level. **(b)** In response to a presynaptic spike (lower trace), inverted IPSP of variable amplitudes are recorded (arrows, top three traces). The measure of the amplitude of postsynaptic responses necessitates the elimination of thermal noise by mathematical calculations. **(c)** Distribution of amplitudes of evoked postsynaptic potentials. This histogram is adjusted by a binomial distribution with $n = 6$, $p = 0.47$ and $q = 300\,\mu V$ parameters (see text). In this preparation, the number n of synaptic contacts between the presynaptic neuron and the Mauthner cell is also 6 and there is only one active zone per synaptic contact. Adapted from Korn H, Faber DH (1987) Regulation and significance of probabilistic release mechanisms at central synapses. In: Edelman GM, Gall WE, Cowan WM (eds) *Synaptic Function*, New York: John Wiley, with permission.

the number of synaptic contacts (**Figure A8.3a**). Morphological data have shown that the afferent inhibitory neurons make between 3 and 60 synaptic boutons, and that *one and only one* active zone is associated with each bouton.

As in the neuromuscular junction model, the distribution of amplitudes of evoked responses has been confronted by the predictions of a mathematical model to determine whether the response fluctuations are in graduated discrete steps (**Figure A8.3b**) and to determine the fluctuations' parameters. For the analysis of the Mauthner cell synapse, the binomial distribution was used because the Poisson distribution cannot be used when the variable p has a high value; in other words when a large number of synaptic vesicles are released in each assay. The binomial distribution indicates that there are two possible results for each assay: the synaptic vesicle is released or is not released.

The binomial function permits the prediction of the distribution of events; that is, the probability $p(x)$ of having a postsynaptic response of x amplitude (the probability that x quanta are released out of the n quanta available):

$$p(x) = \binom{n}{x}p^x(1-p)^{n-x},$$

where p is the probability of each quantum being released; so $(1-p)$ is the probability of each quantum *not* being released. The quantity $\binom{n}{x}$ represents the number of combinations by which n sites can emit x quanta; it is given by:

$$n!/[(n-x)!x!].$$

The variable m, the average number of released quanta in response to a single presynaptic spike, is np, where n is the maximum number of quanta that can be released and p is the average probability of each quantum being released. The question now becomes: can we give a biological significance to n? When p is not too small, the use of binomial distribution allows the evaluation of both p and n while the Poisson distribution, used when p is very small (low extracellular Ca^{2+} concentration) allows only the calculation of m.

Experimental results have indeed shown that the distribution of amplitudes of postsynaptic responses is best described by the binomial distribution (**Figure A8.3c**). Moreover these results, when set against morphological data on active zones, show that the value of n which best describes the response bar graph corresponds to the number of active zones in all presynaptic terminals. This means that the exocytosis of only a single synaptic vesicle could occur at each active zone. In both the Poisson and binomial distributions, one considers that an event (vesicle exocytosis) may occur at n release sites with a probability p.

Figure A8.4 illustrates the conclusions drawn. The schematized presynaptic axon establishes six contacts (six synaptic boutons) with the postsynaptic M cell (not shown). There is only one active zone per bouton. In response to a presynaptic action potential, a variable number x of boutons release neurotransmitter in the synaptic cleft (success, indicated by a cross, with a probability p) whereas other contacts remain inactivated (failure, with a probability $1-p$). Here, each action

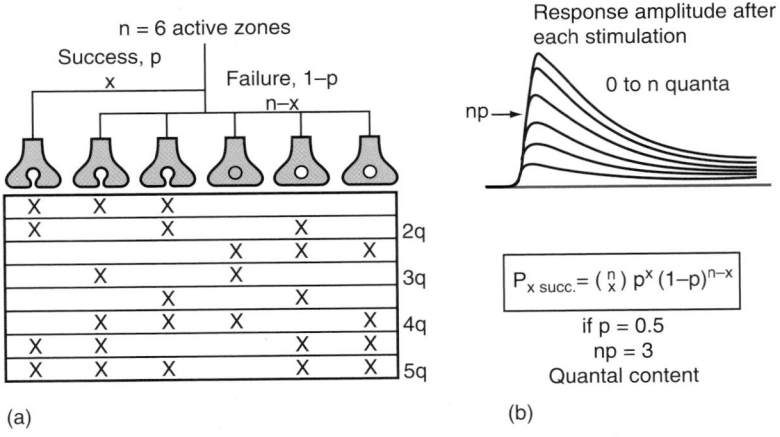

(a)   (b)

Figure A8.4 Diagram explaining the one-vesicle/one-active zone hypothesis.
(a) The presynaptic neuron establishes six synaptic contacts with the postsynaptic Mauthner cell. See text for explanation. (b) Variations of the amplitude of the postsynaptic response. The amplitude depends on the number of released quanta in response to each presynaptic action potential. Responses composed of three quanta are the most frequent (average quantal content $m = np = 3$), whereas responses of amplitude $np = 2$, 4 or 5 are rare. Binomial distribution allows the calculation of the $p(x)$ probability that a response will be composed of x quanta. Adapted from Korn H (1988) Libération des neurotransmetteurs dans le système nerveux central, *Méd. Sci.* **8**, 476–483, with permission.

potential (8 trials) can provoke the release of a synaptic vesicle at 1, 2, ..., 6 boutons. Cases where exocytosis occurs (success) are represented with an opened vesicle and correspond to the first line of the table. Seven other cases are presented in this table. In this experiment the average probability p is equal to 0.5 (1 failure in 2 trials), thus an average of 3 active and 3 inactive contacts with various possible combinations. Electrophysiological data analysed along with morphological data revealed that n, the number of quanta that can be actually released, is equal to the total number of active zones established by a neuron on the Mauthner cell. In other words, a maximum of one synaptic vesicle is released at one active zone in response to a presynaptic spike. The next question that is unresolved is how each release site controls its coterie of docked and fused vesicles.

Thus n is now a physical reality: the number of active zones established by a neuron on a target cell (also corresponding to the number of synaptic contacts). The parameter q, being the size of a quantum or average content of a synaptic vesicle, also has a physical reality: it corresponds to the amount of neurotransmitter released by a presynaptic element at the level of each synaptic complex. This amount is the same for each complex. Only the p parameter has yet to have a physical counterpart. n and q have constant values and thus p is the only variable of synaptic activity.

In summary, when one studies the postsynaptic response to a single presynaptic action potential: m is the mean number of quanta found in the single-spike postsynaptic response or mean quantal content, n is the maximal number of quanta that can be released at each trial, p is the probablility of one quantum being released, and $m = np$. p can be calculated from this equation, but only when n is known. n has been proposed to correspond to the maximal number of active zones that can be activated by a presynaptic spike; i.e. the number of synapses formed by the presynaptic axon multiplied by the number of active zones per synapse. When n is unknown, the Poisson distribution is used (one needs only to know m for calculating p). This needs to be in conditions where p is very small (in the presence of very low concentrations of external Ca^{2+}).

Further reading

Ca²⁺ sensor affinity

Bollmann JH, Sakamnn B, Borst JGG (2000) Calcium sensitivity of glutamate release in a calyx-type terminal. *Science* **289**, 953–957.

Parnas H, Segel L, Dudel J, Parnas I (2000) Autoreceptors, membrane potential and the regulation of transmitter release. *Trends Neurosci.* **23**, 60–68.

Ravin R, Parnas H, Spira ME, Volfovsky N, Parnas I (1999) Simultaneous measurement of evoked release and $[Ca^{2+}]_i$ in a crayfish release bouton reveals high affinity of release to Ca^{2+}. *J. Neurophysiol.* **81**, 634–642.

Schneggenburger R, Neher E (2000) Intracellular calcium dependence of transmitter release rates at a fast central synapse. *Nature* **406**, 889–893.

Bennett MK, Calakos N, Scheller RH (1992) Syntaxin: a synaptic protein implicated in docking of synaptic vesicles at presynaptic active zones. *Science* **257**, 255–259.

Burger PM, Mehl E, Cameron PL, Maycox PR *et al.* (1989) Synaptic vesicles immunoisolated from rat cerebral cortex contain high levels of glutamate. *Neuron* **3**, 715–720.

Calakos N, Scheller RH (1996) Synaptic vesicles, docking and fusion: a molecular description. *Physiological Reviews* **76**, 1–29.

Catterall WA (1999) Interactions of presynaptic Ca^{2+} channels and SNARE proteins in neurotransmitter release. *Ann. NY Acad. Sci.* **868**, 144–159.

Clements JD (1996) Transmitter time course in the synaptic cleft: its role in central synaptic function. *Trends Neurosci.* **19**, 163–171.

Lester HA, Cao Y, Mager S (1996) Listening to neurotransmitter transporters. *Neuron* **17**, 807–810.

Leveque C, el Far O, Martin-Moutot N *et al.* (1994) Purification of the N-type calcium channel associated with syntaxin and synaptotagmin: a complex implicated in synaptic vesicle exocytosis. *J. Biol. Chem.* **269**, 6306–6312.

Mochida S (2000) Protein–protein interactions in neurotransmitter release. *Neurosci. Res.* **36**, 175–182.

Piccolino M, Pignatelli A (1996) Calcium-independent synaptic transmission: artifact or fact? *Trend. Neurosci.* **19**, 120–125.

Rettig J, Heinemann C, Ashery U *et al.* (1997) Alteration of Ca^{2+} dependence of neurotransmitter release by disruption of Ca^{2+} channel/syntaxin interaction. *J. Neurosci.* **17**, 6647–6656.

Sheng ZH, Westenbroek RE, Catterall WA (1998) Physical link and functional coupling of presynaptic calcium channels and the synaptic vesicle docking/fusion machinery. *J. Bioenerg. Biomembr.* **30**, 335–345.

Söllner T, Whiteheart SW, Brunner M *et al.* (1993) SNAP receptors implicated in vesicle targeting and fusion. *Nature* **362**, 318–324.

Song H, Ming G, Fon E *et al.* (1997) Expression of a putative vesicular acetylcholine transporter facilitates quantal transmitter packaging. *Neuron* **18**, 815–826.

Part 2

Ionotropic and Metabotropic Receptors in Synaptic Transmission and Sensory Transduction

The Ionotropic Nicotinic Acetylcholine Receptors

The nicotinic acetylcholine receptor (nAChR) is a glyco-protein present at nicotinic cholinergic synapses. The preparation that has been used most extensively to study the nicotinic receptor is the electric organ of the electric ray, *Torpedo* (Torpedo nAChR; **Figure 9.1a**), or of the electric eel. In part because this preparation is extremely rich in nicotinic receptors, and because snake venom α-toxins had been identified as highly selective markers of nAChRs. In mammals, nAChRs have been mostly studied at the neuromuscular junction (muscle nAChR; **Figure 9.1b**) but also in the peripheral nervous system (synapses between pre- and post-ganglionic neurons of the autonomic nervous system), and more recently in the central nervous system where they are also present (neuronal nAChR; see Appendix 9.1).

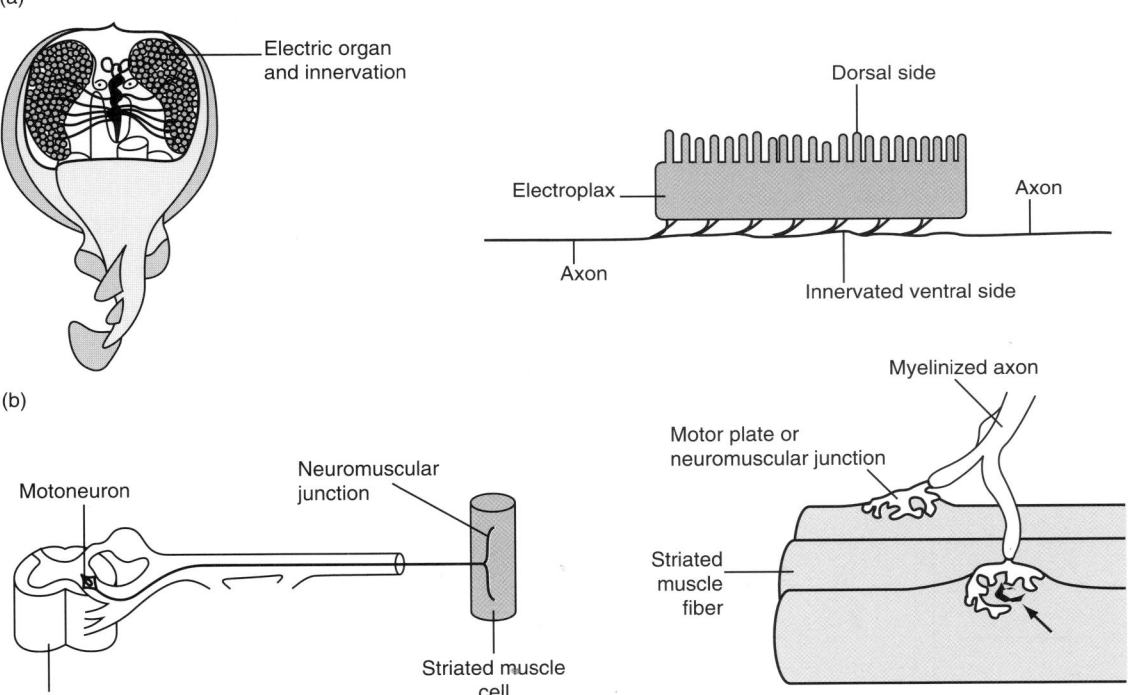

Figure 9.1 Examples of preparations in which nicotinic receptors have been extensively studied.
(a) The electric organ of the electric ray. On a dissected *Torpedo* (left) we can see the electric organs and their innervation. These organs constitute electroplax membranes (right) which are modified muscle cells that do not contract. Nicotinic receptors are present at the command neuron's synapse level, on the ventral side of the postsynaptic membrane of the electroplax. The electroplax are simultaneously activated and the summation of their electric discharges can be of the order of 500 V. **(b)** The neuromuscular junction. Striated muscle cells are innervated by motoneurons whose cell bodies are located in the ventral horn of the spinal cord (horizontal section, left). In mammals, each muscle cell is innervated by one nerve fibre. As the axon makes contact with the muscle cell, it loses its myelin sheath and divides into several branches that are covered by unmyelinated Schwann cells. The thick arrow (right) points to one terminal that has been lifted to show the postsynaptic folds where nicotinic receptors are located.

The nicotinic acetylcholine receptor is a pentamer composed of transmembrane subunits from a repertoire of 16 known different types referred to as α1–α9, β1–β4, γ, δ and ε. Each pentamer presents two acetylcholine receptor sites on its surface, contains the elements to form an ionic channel, and contains all the necessary structural elements for the required interactions between the different functional domains. The acetylcholine receptor sites and the ionic channel controlled by acetylcholine are, therefore, part of the same protein: the nicotinic receptor is a receptor channel (also called an ionotropic receptor).

The nicotinic receptors present in the Torpedo and neuromuscular synapses shown in **Figure 9.1a and b** have comparable structures and functions. For this reason they are presented simultaneously throughout this chapter. Acetylcholine also activates another type of receptor, the muscarinic receptors, also termed metabotropic cholinergic receptors (mAChR) which belong to the family of receptors linked to G-proteins. They will not be studied in this book.

9.1 Observations

The axon of a motoneuron is stimulated in the presence of a low Ca^{2+} concentration (0.5 mM) and a high Mg^{2+} concentration (6 mM) in the extracellular medium to reduce synaptic transmission. In this condition, a postsynaptic depolarizing potential is recorded with the use of an intracellular electrode implanted in the muscle fibre at the level of the neuromuscular junction (current clamp mode) **(Figure 9.2a)**. It is an excitatory postsynaptic potential (EPSP) also called end plate potential (EPP). Its amplitude varies with the intensity of stimulation. In contrast, when the postsynaptic recording electrode is

far from the end plate, no response is recorded **(Figure 9.2b)**.

The low Ca^{2+} and high Mg^{2+} concentrations in the extracellular medium is a necessary condition to avoid muscle fibre contraction during recording. The number of active zones per neuromuscular junction is in fact so high (around 300 to 1000) that a presynaptic axonal spike always triggers a very large EPP that in turn depolarizes the muscle membrane to the threshold potential for voltage-gated Na^+ channels opening and thus evokes a postsynaptic action potential (not shown) and muscle fibre contraction. The elimination of the muscle fibre action potential by lowering the release of acetylcholine from presynaptic terminals allows one to record the EPP in isolation.

Questions

- When released in the synaptic cleft, to which type(s) of postsynaptic receptor do the molecules of acetylcholine bind?
- How is the binding of acetylcholine transduced into a depolarization of the postsynaptic membrane?
- Why is the postsynaptic depolarization recorded only at the level of the neuromuscular junction?

9.2 The torpedo or muscle nicotinic receptor of acetylcholine is a heterologous pentamer $\alpha_2\beta\gamma\delta$

The only type of acetylcholine receptor present in the postsynaptic membrane of neuromuscular junctions or at electrical synapses of *Torpedo* is the nicotinic receptor (nAChR). It is named 'nicotinic' after its sensitivity to

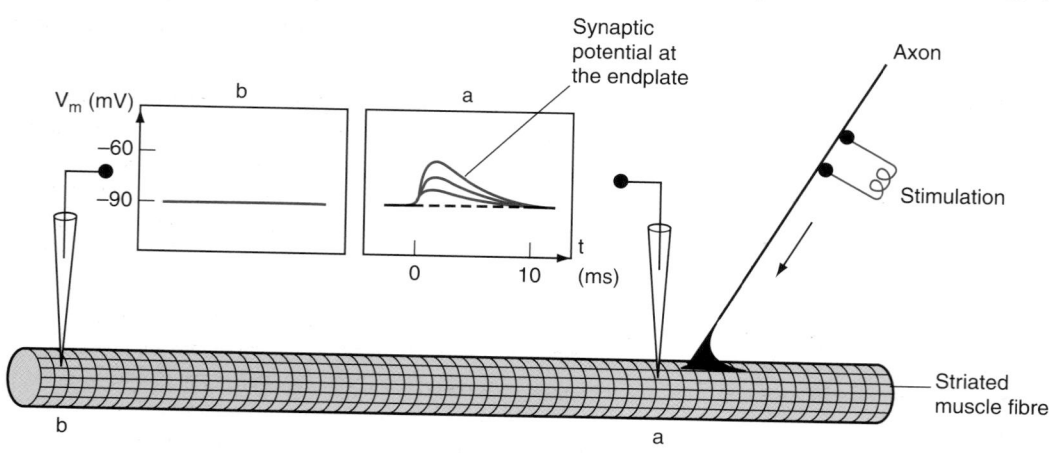

Figure 9.2 The endplate potential.
The axon of a motoneuron is stimulated and the postsynaptic response is recorded in the presence in the bath of a low Ca (0.5 mM) and a high Mg (6 mM) concentration. Two intracellular electrodes are implanted in the muscle fibre, one close to the neuromuscular junction **(a)** and the other more than 5 mm away **(b)**. The evoked response is a transient depolarization called an endplate potential.

nicotine (nicotine is an agonist of nAChR).

9.2.1 Nicotinic receptors have a rosette shape with an aqueous pore in the centre

Under the electron microscope, the nicotinic receptor of the neuromuscular junction, located in the postsynaptic muscular membrane, has a rosette shape with an 8–9 nm diameter and a central depression of diameter 1.5–2.5 nm. This depression corresponds to the channel portion of the protein (**Figure 9.3**). Each rosette is made up of five regions of high electronic density arranged

(a)

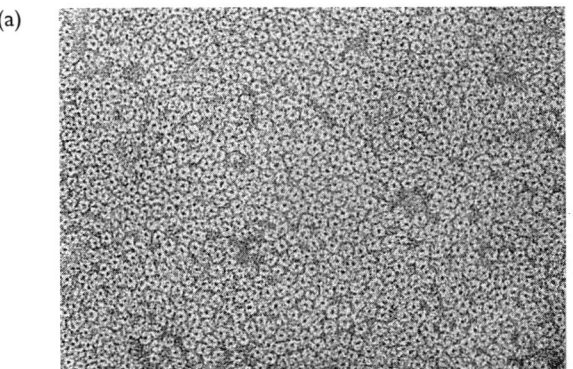

(b)

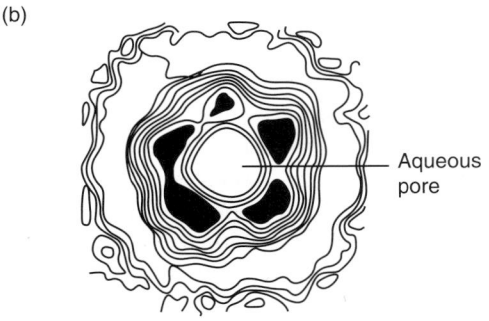

Aqueous pore

(c)

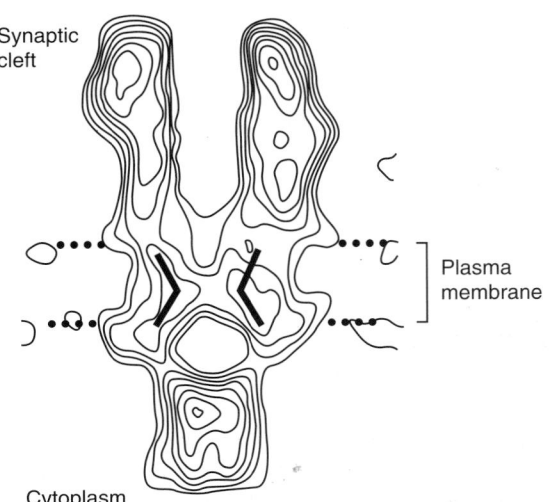

Synaptic cleft

Plasma membrane

Cytoplasm

around an axis perpendicular to the plane of the plasma membrane. In transverse section the rosette appears as a cylinder 11 nm long, extending beyond each side of the membrane (6 nm towards the synaptic cleft and 1.5 nm towards the cytoplasm).

9.2.2 The four subunits of the nicotinic receptor are assembled as a pentamer $\alpha_2\beta\gamma\delta$

The nicotinic receptor is normally purified from the electric organ of *Torpedo* or the electric eel. A 290–300 kD glycoprotein is obtained when this purification is performed on an affinity column using an agarose bound cholinergic ligand (**Figure 9.4**). When this glycoprotein is incorporated into a planar lipid bilayer or into lipid vesicles, it presents the same functional characteristics as the native receptor: if acetylcholine is present in the extracellular side at a concentration of 10^{-5}–10^{-4} mol l^{-1}, it allows the passage of cations across the bilayer.

The nicotinic receptor is composed of four glycopolypeptide subunits $\alpha,\beta,\gamma,\delta$

In the presence of the detergent SDS (sodium dodecyl sulphate), the 290–300 kD protein dissociates into four different subunits, which migrate on a polyacrylamide gel as molecules with apparent molecular weights of 38 kD (α), 49 kD (β), 57 kD (γ) and 64 kD (δ) (**Figure 9.5a**). The same experiment carried out with nicotinic receptors obtained from the neuromuscular junction shows very similar results (**Figure 9.5b**).

Genes coding for each subunit of the nicotinic receptor of the electric ray and of the mammalian receptor have been cloned. When the corresponding mRNAs are

Figure 9.3 The nicotinic receptor has a rosette shape.
(a) Membrane surface of *Torpedo* electric cells (electroplax). Each rosette constitutes one nicotinic receptor. (b) This computer reconstructed image of a single nicotinic receptor provides a more detailed view (superior view). (c) Electron microscopic analysis of tubular crystals of *Torpedo* nAChR viewed from the side. Part (a) from Cartaud J, Benedetti EL, Sobel A, Chargeux JP (1978) A morphological study of the cholinergic receptor protein from Torpedo narmorata in its membrane environment and in its detergent-extracted purified form, *J. Cell Sci.* **29**, 313–337, with permission. Part (b) from Bon F *et al.* (1982) Orientation relative de deux oligomères constituant la forme lourde du récepteur de l'acétylcholine chez la torpille marbrée, *C. R. Acad. Sci.* **295**, 199, with permission. Part (c) from Unwin N (1993) The nicotinic acetylcholine receptor at 9 Å resolution, *J. Mol. Biol.* **229**, 1101–1124, with permission.

(a)

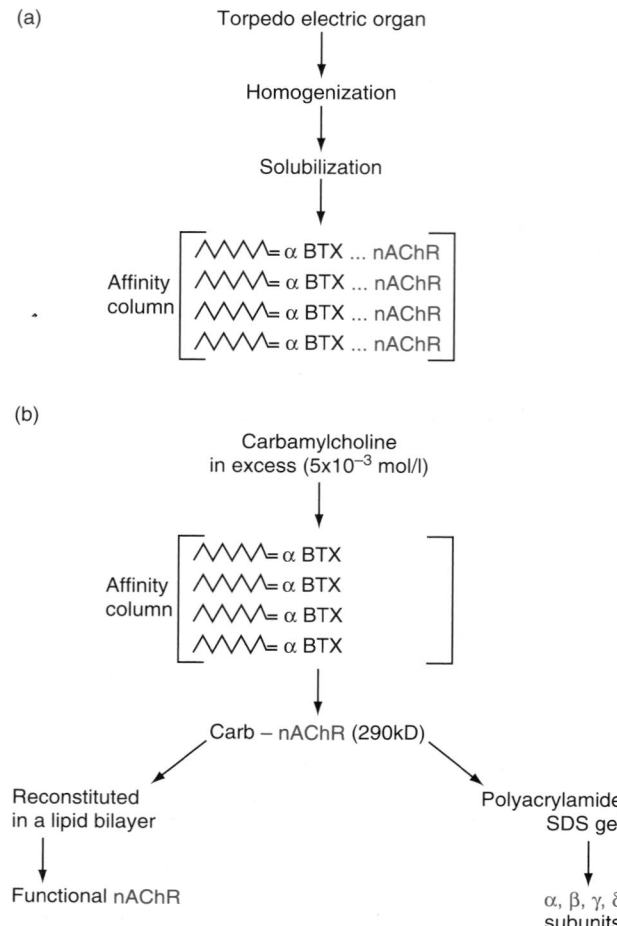

(b)

Figure 9.4 Stages of affinity column purification of the nicotinic receptor.

(a) The electric organ of the electric ray is homogenized and membrane proteins solubilized. The resulting extract is run through an affinity column, on to whose sepharose (^^^=) a nicotinic cholinergic ligand α-bungarotoxin (α-BTX) has been covalently bound. Owing to their affinity to α-BTX, the nicotinic receptors bind to it. (b) In order to recover the nicotinic receptors, another nicotinic ligand, carbamylcholine (Carb), is run in excess through the column to displace the binding of α-BTX to the receptor. Carbamylcholine-bound nicotinic receptor is obtained at the outflow of the column. Carbamylcholine is eliminated by dialysis and the nicotinic receptor is thus obtained in an isolated form. The nicotinic receptor can then be reincorporated into a lipid bilayer to study its functional characteristics. It may also be treated with a detergent (SDS) to dissociate its subunits.

injected into *Xenopus* oocytes, functional nicotinic receptors are synthesized and incorporated into the oocyte membrane. It has, therefore, been confirmed that the subunits α, β, γ and δ are sufficient to obtain a functional nicotinic receptor containing the acetylcholine receptor sites and the elements that form the ionic channel. The

(a)

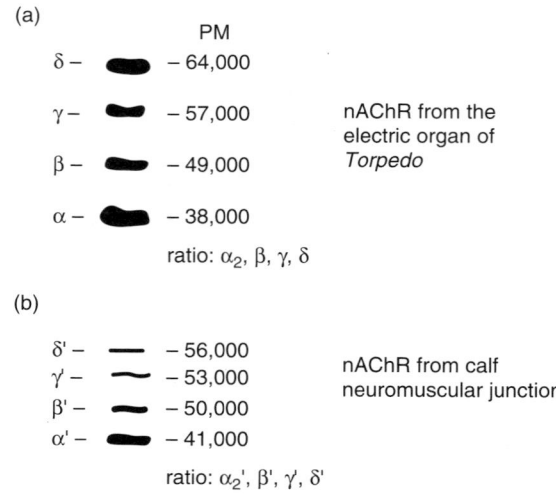

Figure 9.5 Separation of the different nicotinic receptor subunits on a gel.

The subunits of the purified nicotinic receptor have been dissociated with the detergent sodium dodecyl sulphate (SDS) and separated on a polyacrylamide gel: subunits of (a) the nicotinic receptor of electric organ, and of (b) the calf neuromuscular junction. The four subunits obtained, α, β, γ, δ and α', β', γ, δ', have similar molecular weights. From Anholt R, Lindstrom J, Montal M (1984) The molecular basis of neurotransmission: structure and function of the nAChR. In Martinosi A (ed) *The Enzymes of Biological Membranes*, New York: Plenum Press, with permission.

receptor also contains the necessary elements for the interactions between the various functional domains.

Organization of the subunits: the nicotinic receptor model

Images observed under the electron microscope, and results obtained with biochemical techniques, have shown that the nicotinic receptor is made up of five units. However, they did not show in which proportion and in which order the subunits α, β, γ and δ are assembled.

The molecular weight of the isolated and purified nicotinic receptor is consistent with the existence of two α chains for each β, γ or δ-subunit. This stoichiometry has been confirmed by quantitative analyses of the different chains extracted from an electrophoresis gel (**Figure 9.5**). Likewise, when the purified nicotinic receptor is centrifuged in a sucrose gradient in the presence of monoclonal antibodies directed against the α-subunit, it appears that two α chains exist per receptor channel.

Using various procedures to label both α-subunits (notably α-bungarotoxin) it has been possible to show that both subunits subtend an angle of 150°. This means that the two α chains are not adjacent (**Figure 9.6a**).

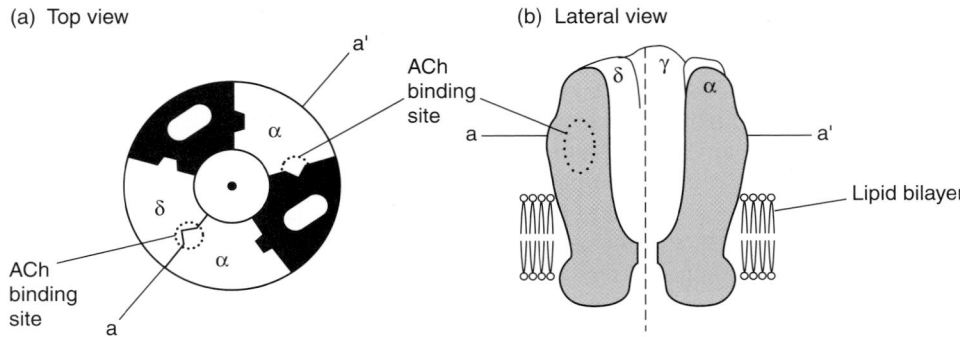

Figure 9.6 Nicotinic receptor (nAChR) model.
(a) Viewed from above, the nAChR has a rosette shape. Both α-subunits carry one acetylcholine (ACh) receptor site each. The subunits are attached to each other by non-covalent interactions. αβαγδ or αγαβδ are the two possible orders of the subunits around the symmetrical axis. **(b)** Profile view of the nAChR *in situ* (cut along the plane aa'). Adapted from Changeux JP, Revah F (1987) The acetylcholine receptor molecule: allosteric sites and the ion channel, *TINS* **10**, 245–250, with permission.

9.2.3 Each subunit presents two main hydrophilic domains and four hydrophobic domains

The amino acid sequence of each subunit α, β, γ and δ has been deduced from the corresponding DNA nucleotide sequence. This has shown that the subunits exhibit among themselves a high percentage of sequence homology and a very similar organization (**Figures 9.7a and b**). For each subunit one finds:

- an NH_2 terminal region which forms a large hydrophilic domain of 210–224 amino acids and carries the glycosylation sites;
- it is followed towards the COOH end by three hydrophobic sequences (M1, M2 and M3) of 20–30 residues each with short connecting hydrophilic loops;
- a second large hydrophilic domain of about 150 residues containing functional phosphorylation sites;
- a fourth hydrophobic sequence and a short carboxy terminal tail.

(a)

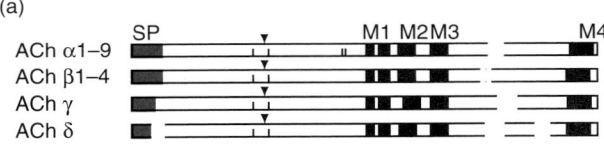

(b)

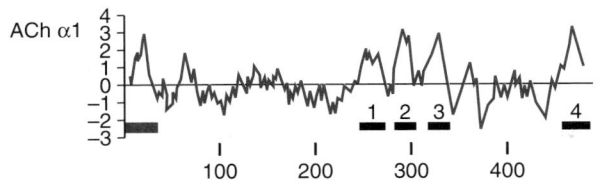

(c)

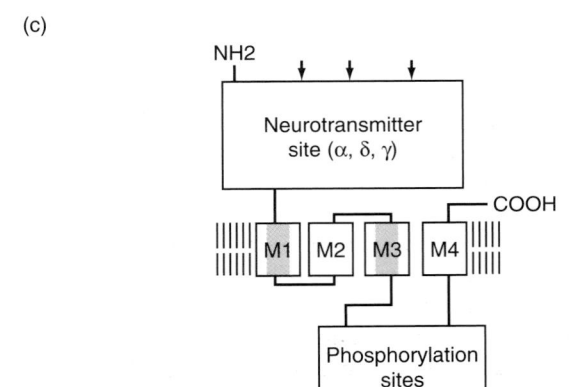

Figure 9.7 Diagrammatic representation of the primary structure of nicotinic acetylcholine receptor subunits from electric organ, muscle cells and neurons.

(a) The sequences are aligned to bring homologous regions into phase; gaps in sequences are indicated by blank spaces (polypeptide lengths are normalized), and cysteinyl residues by vertical bars. SP, signal peptide; α, β, γ and δ chains. One can distinguish two hydrophilic domains, the largest of which is located in the NH_2 terminal, and four hydrophobic segments M1, M2, M3 and M4. This observation has led to the assumption that all four subunits have identical transmembrane organizations. **(b)** Hydropathy plot of the α_1-subunit from *Torpedo* electric organ receptor showing the four hydrophobic segments assumed to span the lipid bilayer, the large hydrophilic amino terminal domain and the hydrophilic domain separating M3 from M4. **(c)** Model of subunit transmembrane organization. The large hydrophilic amino-terminal domain of receptor subunits is exposed to the synaptic cleft and carries the neurotransmitter site and glycosylation sites (arrows). Each subunit spans the membrane four times (M1, M2, M3 and M4). The hydrophilic domain separating M3 from M4 faces the cytoplasm. It contains functional phosphorylation sites. Adapted from Changeux JP (1994) Functional architecture and dynamics of the nicotinic acetylcholine receptor: an allosteric ligand-gated ion channel: *Fidia Research Foundation Neuroscience Award Lecture*, New York: Raven Press, with permission.

A model of the transmembrane organization common to all subunits has been proposed (**Figure 9.7c**): the hydrophilic NH_2 terminal domain is located on the extracellular side of the membrane (in the synaptic cleft), the second hydrophilic domain is located on the cytoplasmic side and the four hydrophobic sequences are membrane-spanning segments. Each subunit therefore crosses the membrane four times and the carboxy terminal tail is oriented towards the synaptic cleft.

9.2.4 Each α-subunit contains one acetylcholine receptor site located in the hydrophilic NH_2 terminal domain

Before the structure of the nicotinic receptor was known, it had been demonstrated that two acetylcholine molecules had to be bound to the receptor in order to initiate an ionic flux (see Section 9.3). It seemed logical that these two sites had to be located on identical subunits; i.e. one on each α-subunit. Additionally, based on the organization of the hydrophilic sequences (**Figure 9.7b**), it was proposed that this site is located in the large hydrophilic NH_2 terminal domain which is exposed to the synaptic cleft.

This proposal has been confirmed by covalent binding studies of cholinergic agonists on α-subunits, isolated either from nicotinic receptor-rich membranes, or expressed in frog oocytes from the corresponding mRNA. Of the four subunit types α, β, γ and δ, the α-subunits have been shown to be the main contributors to cholinergic agonist binding.

The next step was to determine which amino acids are part of the acetylcholine receptor site. To this end, labelled cholinergic ligands are used. These ligands are able to bind covalently to the acetylcholine receptor sites. One of the most used is MBTA (4-(N-maleimido) benzyl trimethylammonium iodide) which binds covalently to α-subunit receptor sites after reduction of disulphide bridges. Once labelled, the α chain is sequenced and the labelled regions identified. In this way a region containing cysteines 192 and 193 was identified and proposed as one of the potential sites of interaction with cholinergic ligands (**Figure 9.8**).

Other data have provided additional evidence of the participation of cysteine residues 192 and 193 in the acetylcholine receptor site. In the first place, these cysteine residues are present only in the α-subunits. Furthermore, when frog oocytes are injected with mRNA coding for α-subunits that have been mutated at the level of cysteines 192 and 193 (serines replaced for cysteines), the α-subunits obtained are unable to bind cholinergic ligands.

However, all these results have the shortcoming of having been obtained from preparations previously treated with disulphide bond-reducing agents (such as dithiothreitol). This treatment is necessary in order to allow the covalent binding of the cholinergic ligand MBTA to the receptor site but it alters the receptor site selectivity for cholinergic ligands.

In order to obtain a more detailed map of the native protein's acetylcholine receptor site, a labelled photoactivated cholinergic ligand has been used: ^{3}H-DDF (para-N,N-dimethylamino benzene diazonium fluoroborate). ^{3}H-DDF is a competitive antagonist of acetylcholine which, once photoactivated, binds covalently (irreversibly) to the acetylcholine receptor sites. This reaction is carried out on the whole nicotinic receptor channel and the α-subunits are then isolated, the segments labelled by ^{3}H-DDF are purified and their sequence analysed. This led to the demonstration that the residues tyr 93, trp 149, tyr 190, cys 192 and cys 193, all labelled by ^{3}H-DDF, are part of the acetylcholine receptor site. This labelling is in fact inhibited by other nicotinic agonists and competitive antagonists (**Figure 9.8b**). This result is valid for the nicotinic receptor of the electric organ as well as for that of the neuromuscular junction.

9.2.5 The pore of the ion channel is lined by the M2 transmembrane segments of each of the five subunits

The ion channel can be considered as functionally equivalent to the active site of allosteric enzymes: its states (open, closed, blocked) are determined by the effectors of the receptor (binding of agonists, competitive antagonists and non-competitive antagonists; see Appendix 7.1). Concerning the channel structure, the question is which of the four hydrophobic membrane-spanning segments M1 to M4 (**Figure 9.7b**) are part of the walls of the ionic channel. On the basis of the hypothesis that non-competitive inhibitors bind to a high-affinity site located inside the open ion channel (channel blockers; see Section 9.6.3), photoactivable non-competitive inhibitors are used to label residues participating in the walls of the ion channel (this is a similar approach to that used for determination of the ACh binding site). Radioactive chlorpromazine activated with ultraviolet light labels serine, leucine and threonine residues from the M2 membrane-spanning segment from all subunits of the *Torpedo* acetylcholine receptor. These results point to a contribution of the M2 membrane-spanning segment to the walls of the ion channel.

In the M2 segments of nAChR subunits there are remarkable amino acids which, in the proposed model, form rings, assuming that the M2 segments of each of the subunits are symmetrically arranged around the central axis of the molecule (**Figure 9.9**): a cytoplasmic ring of negatively charged amino acids that repel negative ions, a hydrophobic ring of leucines, a ring of serines, a ring of threonines and again a ring of negatively charged amino acids that repel negative ions.

Site-directed mutagenesis of some amino acids located in the M2 segment confirmed the contribution of M2 segments to the regulation of ion transport through the nicotinic channel. Chimeric cDNAs are constructed to add or substitute amino acids in the M2 segment. The results obtained will be explained in detail in the section describing the study of ionic selectivity (Section 9.3.2).

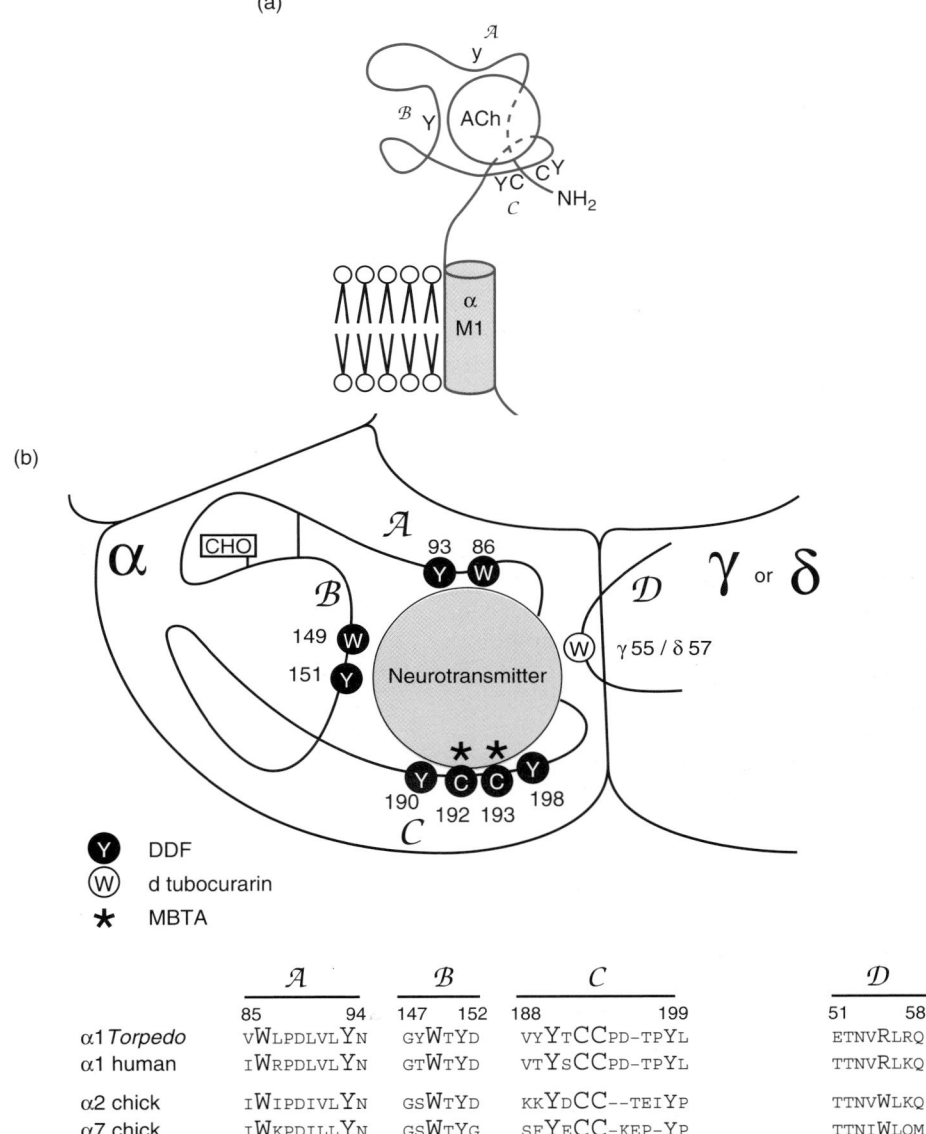

	$\mathcal{A}$		$\mathcal{B}$		$\mathcal{C}$		$\mathcal{D}$	
	85	94	147	152	188	199	51	58
α1 *Torpedo*	vWLPDLVLYn		GYWTYD		vYYtCCPD-TPYL		ETNVRLRQ	
α1 human	IWRPDLVLYn		GTWTYD		vTYsCCPD-TPYL		TTNVRLKQ	
α2 chick	IWIPDIVLYn		GSWTYD		KKYDCC--TEIYP		TTNVWLKQ	
α7 chick	IWKPDILLYn		GSWTYG		sFYeCC-KEP-YP		TTNIWLQM	

Figure 9.8 Model of the acetylcholine binding site.
(a) The amino acids labelled with the nicotinic antagonist ³H-DDF are localized on different regions of the α-chain. In the three-dimensional structure of the protein, these regions fold into positions that are close to each other. (b) More precise view of the labelling of the receptor site. The acetylcholine binding site is located at the interface between α- and γ- or δ-subunits. The amino acids covalently labelled with ³H-DDF are in the α-subunit: W86 and Y93 in loop A, W149 and Y151 in loop B, Y190, C192, C193 and Y198 in loop C. d-Tubocurarine, an antagonist of nAChR, labels one amino acid in loop D of the γ- or δ-subunit. C, cysteine; W, trytophan, Y, tyrosine. Drawing (a) adapted from Dennis M, Giraudat J, Kotzyba-Hibert F *et al.* (1988) Amino acids in the *Torpedo marmorata* acetylcholine receptor α subunit labelled by a photoaffinity ligand for the acetylcholine binding site, *Biochemistry* **27**, 2346–2357, with permission. Drawing (b) adapted from Galzi JL, Changeux JP (1994) Neurotransmitter-gated ion channels as unconventional allosteric proteins, *Curr. Opin. Struct. Biol.* **4**, 554–565, with permission.

9.3 Binding of two acetylcholine molecules favours conformational change of the protein towards the open state of the cationic channel

9.3.1 Demonstration of the binding of two acetylcholine molecules

It has been demonstrated that two acetylcholine molecules must bind to the receptor to trigger the opening of the channel and allow cations to flow through. The proof of this has been obtained from dose–response curves. The response to acetylcholine (i.e. the flux of cations measured at very short intervals after the application of acetylcholine), or the opening probability of the channel (see below), is proportional to the square of the acetylcholine concentration:

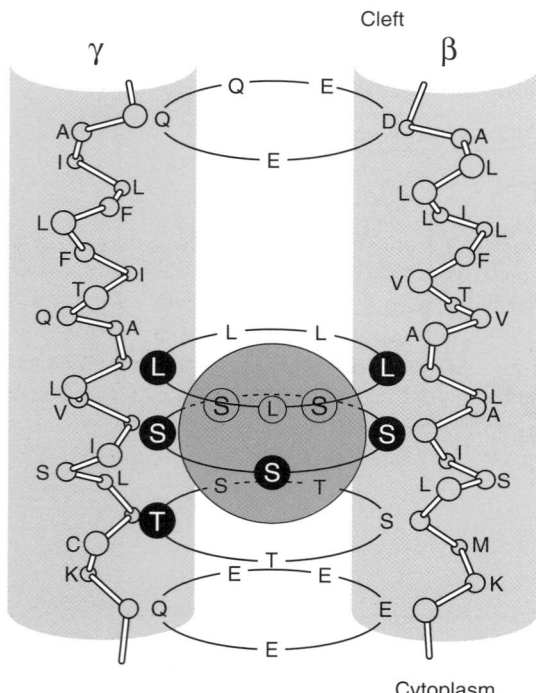

Figure 9.9 Characteristic amino acid residues along the M2 segment of the subunits of the nAChR.
The M2 membrane-spanning segments are symmetrically arranged around the central axis of the molecule (two of them are represented). The relative position of the α-carbons of the amino acids is shown as one-letter code. E, glutamic acid, S, serine, T, threonine, L, leucine, Q, glutamine. Adapted from Revah F, Galzi JL, Giraudat J et al. (1990) The noncompetitive blocker [³H]-chlorpromazine labels three amino acids of the acetylcholine receptor γ subunit: implications for the α-helical organization of the M2 segments and the structure of the ion channel, *Proc. Natl Acad. Sci. USA* **87**, 4675–4679, with permission.

$$\text{Response} = f(\text{ACh})^2.$$

However, this demonstration is obscured by the consequences of receptor desensitization, which have to be eliminated from the recordings (see Section 9.4). For this reason this demonstration will not be presented in detail here. The conformational change of the protein towards the open state is clearly favoured when two acetylcholine molecules bind to the receptor. The following model accounts for these observations (however, as we shall see in Section 9.4, this model is in fact much more complex):

$$R \rightleftharpoons AR \rightleftharpoons A_2R \rightleftharpoons A_2R^* \rightarrow cationic\ current$$

where R is the nicotinic receptor in its closed configuration; R* is the nicotinic receptor in its open configuration; and A is acetylcholine.

The rate of isomerization between R and R* lies in the microsecond to millisecond timescale. The passage of cations through the open channel is the result of the conformational change ($A_2R \rightleftharpoons A_2R^*$). Electrophysiological techniques (patch clamp recordings of the unitary cationic current flowing through a single channel) can be used to study this flow of cations. Based on the results obtained with electrophysiological techniques, we shall look at the properties of the nicotinic channel and of the protein conformational changes.

9.3.2 The nicotinic channel has a selective permeability to cations: its unitary conductance is constant

When the unitary current crossing a nicotinic channel in the presence of acetylcholine is recorded in patch clamp, all the preparations tested show an inward current at negative holding potentials (and under physiological ionic conditions) (**Figure 9.10**).

The nicotinic current reverses at 0 mV

If the imposed membrane potential (V_m) is varied between –100 mV and +80 mV while recording unitary currents with the patch clamp technique (i_{ACh}), one can trace an i_{ACh}/V curve (**Figure 9.10**). This curve is approximately linear between –80 and +80 mV. The measured current is inward for negative voltages and outward for positive voltages.

The i_{ACh}/V curve crosses the voltage axis at a value where the current is zero. This value is called the *reversal potential of the nicotinic response*, or E_{ACh}. The value of this reversal potential is close to 0 mV in the experimental conditions of **Figure 9.11** but may vary slightly towards negative voltages depending on the preparation.

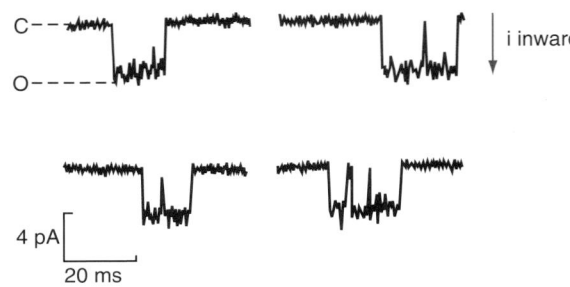

Figure 9.10 Patch-clamp recording of nicotinic receptor activity in rat sympathetic neurons.
Channel activity is recorded in the attached-cell configuration. While the membrane is kept at a negative potential an inward current is recorded in the presence of acetylcholine under physiological conditions. C, closed channel; O, open channel. Adapted from Colquhoun D, Ogden DC, Mathie A (1987) Nicotinic acetylcholine receptors of nerve and muscle: functional aspects, *TIPS* **8**, 465–472, with permission.

The unitary conductance is constant

The linear i_{ACh}/V relationship observed in **Figure 9.11b** (between −80 and +80 mV) is described by the equation $i_{ACh} = \gamma_{ACh}(V_m - E_{ACh})$, where V_m is the membrane potential, E_{ACh} is the reversal potential of the nicotinic response, and γ_{ACh} is the conductance of a single nicotinic channel, or its unitary conductance. The value of γ_{ACh} is given by the slope of the linear i_{ACh}/V curve. It has a constant value at any given membrane potential. This value varies between 35 and 55 pS depending on the preparation and is a fundamental property of a nicotinic channel.

The nicotinic channel is a cationic channel

The reversal potential of the nicotinic response ($E_{Ach} = 0$ mV) does not correspond to the equilibrium potentials of any of the ions in solution (**Figure 9.11**). It is not an Na+ channel because, in the experimental conditions of **Figure 9.11**, $E_{Na} = 58 \log (160/3) = +100$ mV. It is not a K+ channel either, since $E_K = 58 \log (3/160) = -100$ mV. And it is not a Cl− channel because, if the chloride ions are replaced by large anions that cannot cross the channel, such as SO_4^{2-}, no reversal potential change of the nicotinic response is observed.

By performing extracellular ionic substitution experiments, it has been shown that the nicotinic channel is permeable to Na+, K+, Ca2+ and Mg2+ ions. However, Ca2+ and Mg2+ ions contribute only a small fraction to the nicotinic current, which is essentially due to the flux of Na+ and K+ ions through the open channel. If different cations cross the same channel and have similar permeabilities, we define:

$$E_{cations} = 58 \log ([cations]_e/[cations]_i),$$

where $[cations] = [Na^+] + [K^+]$. In our case we obtain $E_{cations} = 0$ mV. In other words, $E_{cations} = E_{Ach} = 0$ mV.

In what direction do Na+ and K+ ions cross the open nicotinic channel at different membrane potentials?

When the membrane is at a voltage of −80 mV, the Na+ ion driving force is inward and equal to −180 mV, while the K+ ion driving force is outward and equal to +20 mV (**Figure 9.12**). If channels open, more Na+ will enter the cell than K+ ions will leave it. The net flux of positively charged ions is, thus, inward: an inward current is recorded (**Figures 9.10** and **9.11a**).

If the same reasoning is followed for different membrane potential values, the same result is obtained as with the i_{ACh}/V curve: the unitary current is inward for negative membrane potentials (net flux of positive charges is inward), and the unitary current is outward for positive membrane potentials (net flux of positive charges is outward) (**Figures 9.11a** and **9.13**).

Effect of a decrease in [Na+]ₑ

When extracellular Na+ ions are partially replaced with a non-permeant substance such as sucrose (without changing the osmotic pressure), the reversal potential of the nicotinic response shifts towards more negative potentials (**Figure 9.14**). This is explained by the fact that, at this point, extracellular Na+ ions contribute less to the nicotinic current, and the nicotinic reversal potential E_{ACh} shifts towards the K+ equilibrium potential (E_K).

Substitution of K+ ions for extracellular Na+ ions

When almost all extracellular Na+ ions are replaced by extracellular K+ ions, the I/V curve obtained superposes on the control I/V curve (**Figure 9.15**). Thus, extracellular K+ ions can replace extracellular Na+ ions; i.e. the nicotinic channel does not distinguish between Na+ and K+ ions. In other words, it presents similar permeabilities for both ions. For this reason the reversal potential of the nicotinic response is independent of the relative concentrations of extracellular Na+ and K+ ions. It depends solely on the sum of these concentrations.

Mutations in the M2 membrane-spanning segment can convert ion selectivity from cationic to anionic

The question was: do substitutions and/or additions of

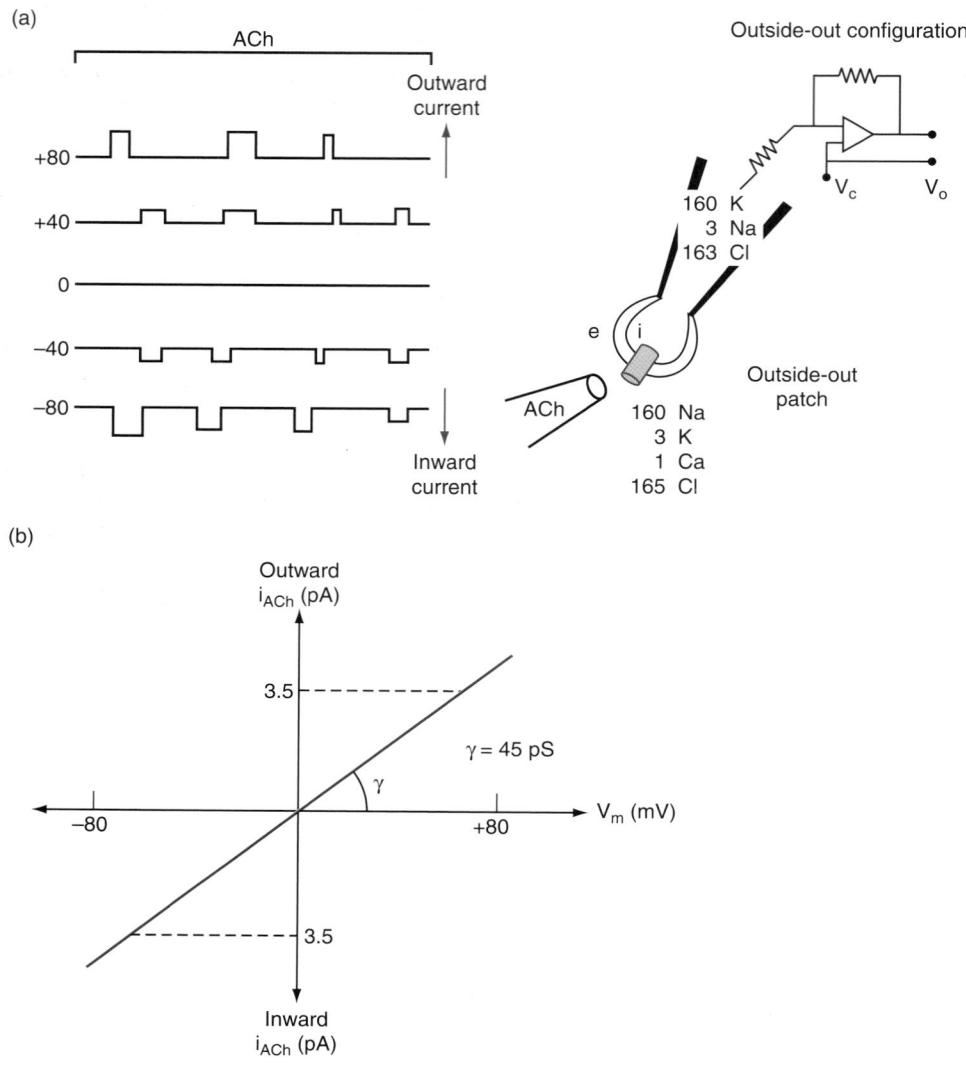

Figure 9.11 Nicotinic unitary current recorded in patch clamp (outside-out configuration) at various membrane potentials (from −80 mV to +80 mV).

(a) Nicotinic unitary current recorded at different membrane potentials in response to the application of acetylcholine (ACh). A downward deflection indicates an inward current and an upward deflection indicates an outward current. (b) i_{ACh}/V curve obtained from the average values of i_{ACh} at each membrane potential V_m. The curve reverses at 0 mV and the slope corresponds to the unitary conductance γ.

amino acids within (or near) the M2 segment from a nicotinic α-subunit (here neuronal α₇-subunit) with homologous amino acids of the glycine receptor suffice to convert α subunit ion-channel selectivity from cationic to anionic? (The glycine receptor is a receptor channel selectively permeable to anions, Cl⁻ ions). The M2 sequences of α-subunits of a cationic channel (nAchR) and anionic channels (GlyR and GABA_AR) show similarities at the level of the threonine (244) and leucine (247) rings and differences at the level of rings of negative amino acids, Glu 237 and Glu 258 (**Figure 9.16a**). A chimeric cDNA encoding the α₇-subunit of neuronal nAChR is constructed in which in the M2 segment, a pro-

line residue, is added at position 236 bis, and amino acids at positions 237, 240, 251, 254, 255 and 258 are exchanged with those found in the M2 segment of the glycine receptor α-subunit (nAChRα₇*; **Figure 9.16a**). Interestingly, glutamates (E) 237 and 258 which form negative rings in the nAChR (repelling negative ions) are exchanged with alanine (A) and asparagine (N) residues, respectively. The chimeric cDNA is injected into oocytes that express homomeric mutated nAChR* (formed by five identical mutated α₇-subunits). The current recorded with double-electrode voltage clamp (see Appendix 5.2) is compared with that recorded in oocytes expressing wild-type (non-mutated) homomeric AChR.

Ionic currents recorded in response to ACh application (100 µM, 2 s duration) from oocytes expressing wild-type homomeric α_7nAChR (in the presence of a Ca²⁺ chelator inside the oocyte) reverses around +3 mV. Substitution of 90% of the external chloride ions did not change the value of the reversal potential. These data thus support the con-clusion that wild-type homomeric αnAChR, like native nAChR, is selective for cations.

Ionic currents recorded in response to ACh application (100 µM, 2 s duration) from oocytes expressing mutated homomeric α*nAChR reverses around –20 mV. Substitution of 90% external chloride ions by isethionate (an impermeant anion) shifts the reversal potential towards positive voltage (around +30 mV) (**Figure 9.16b, left**). This shift is well described by the Goldman–Hodgkin relationship for chloride specific channels (**Figure 9.16b right**). This indicates that ACh-activated currents are almost entirely carried by chloride ions in oocytes expressing mutated homomeric nAChR*. Then, introducing appropriate amino acid residues from the putative channel domain of a chloride-selective GlyR α-subunit into that of a cation selective nAChR α-sub-unit allows the design of an ACh-gated channel now selective for chloride. This confirms that the M2 segment forms the walls of the channel and strongly suggests that the exchanged residues face the lumen of the channel.

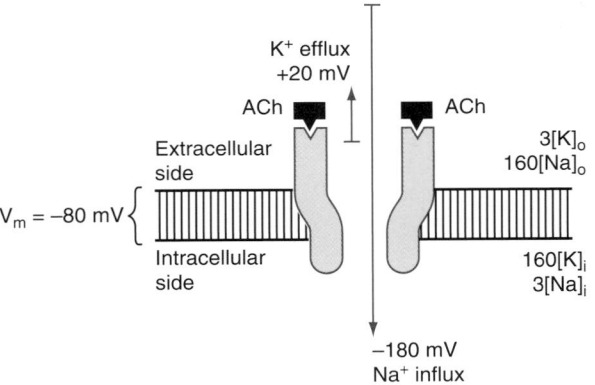

Figure 9.12 Determination and vectorial representation of the Na⁺ ion driving force ($V_m - E_{Na}$) and K⁺ ion driving force ($V_m - E_K$) for a membrane potential of –80 mV.
Observe that 90% of the current is due to Na⁺ ions. The net flux of positive charges is inward. This explains why ACh induces an inward current at $V_m = -80$ mV.

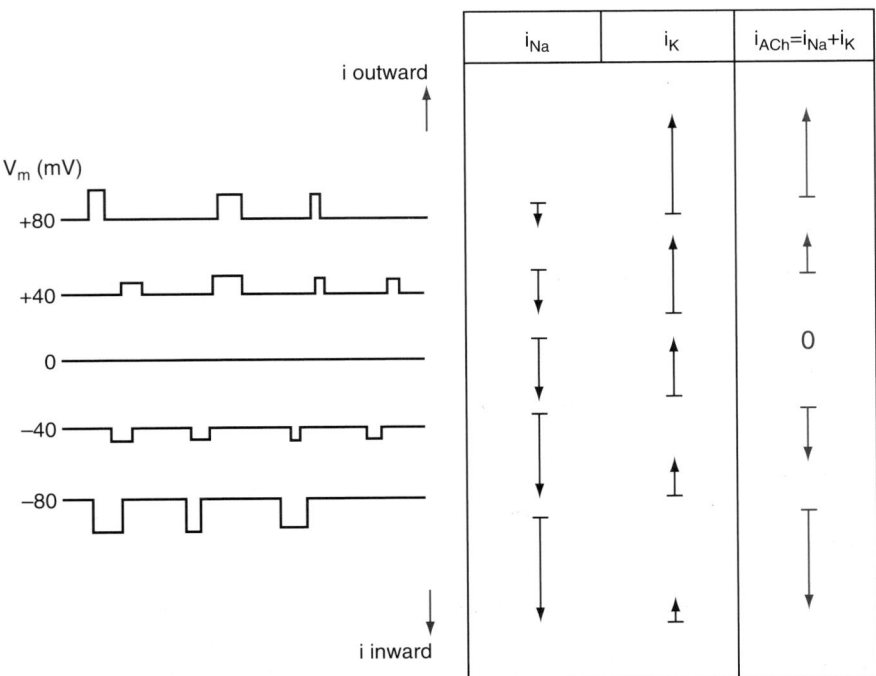

Figure 9.13 Evolution of sodium and potassium currents (i_{Na} and i_K) through the nicotinic channel as a function of membrane potential V_m.
The current induced by acetylcholine i_{ACh} corresponds to the sum of two currents: $i_{ACh} = i_{Na} + i_K$. When $i_{Na} = -i_K$ the current is zero. This occurs at the reversal potential of the nicotinic response ($V_m = E_{ACh}$). A deflection of the traces (left) or an arrow of the chart (right) in the downward direction represents an inward current, and in the upward direction an outward current.

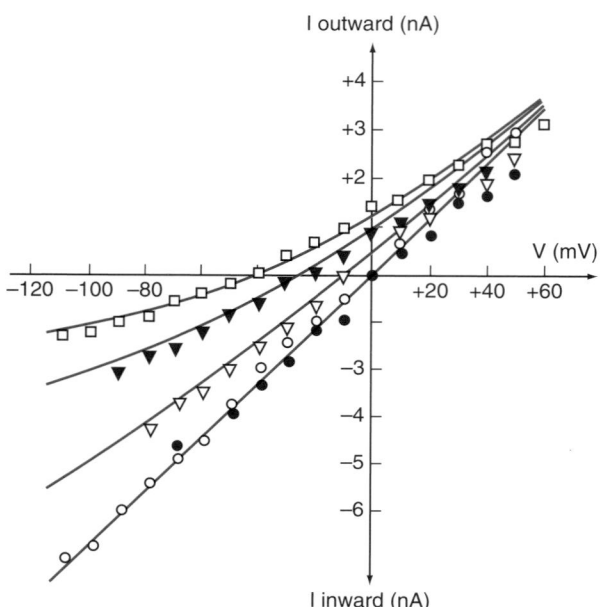

Figure 9.14 Effect of lowering the external Na+ concentration on the I_{ACh}/V curve.
The composition of the external environment is: 5 mM of K+; 0.1 mM of Ca2+; and 21 (□), 46 (▼), 96 (▽) or 146 (● and ○) mM of Na+. Each point represents the average of 25 measurements of I_{ACh}. When [Na+]$_e$ decreases, the reversal potential of the nicotinic response shifts towards the K+ equilibrium potential. Control E_{ACh}: (●, ○) 58 log (146 + 5)/[cations]$_i$; (▽) 58 log (96 + 5)/[cations]$_i$; (▼) 58 log (46 + 5)/[cations]$_i$; (□) 58 log (21 + 5)/[cations]$_i$. Adapted from Linder TM, Quastel DMJ (1978) A voltage clamp study of the permeability change induced by quanta of transmitter at the mouse end plate, *J. Physiol. (Lond.)* **281**, 535–556, with permission.

9.3.3 The time during which the channel stays open varies around an average value τ_o, the mean open time, and is a characteristic of each nicotinic receptor

When recording in patch clamp from myotubes (embryonic muscle cells) or from denervated muscle cells, in the presence of very small doses of acetylcholine, openings of the nicotinic channels separated by periods of silence are observed (**Figure 9.17**). The nicotinic receptor switches between states in which the channel is closed and the unitary current is zero (R, AR, A$_2$R), and a state in which the channel is open and shows a measurable unitary current (A$_2$R*) (**Figure 9.18**). These conformational changes can be modelled as:

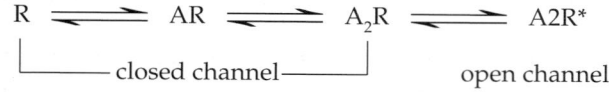

where A is acetylcholine or any nicotinic agonist; R is the

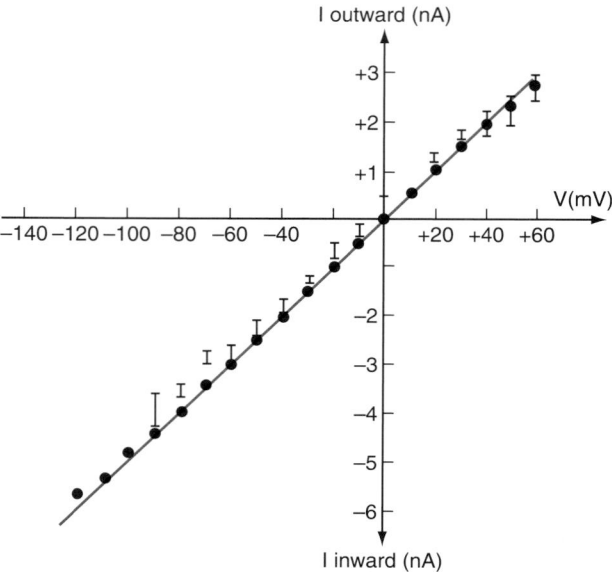

Figure 9.15 Replacing external K+ for Na+ ions has no effect.
Control I/V curve (●) 146 mM of Na+ and 5 mM of K+, and (I) 2 mM of Na+ and 149 mM of K+. Observe that K+ ions can replace Na+ ions without affecting the I/V curve. The nicotinic channel does not distinguish between these two cations. Adapted from Linder TM, Quastel DMJ (1978) A voltage clamp study of the permeability change induced by quanta of transmitter at the mouse endplate, *J. Physiol. (Lond.)* **281**, 535–556, with permission.

receptor in the closed conformation; and R* is the receptor in the open conformation.

In **Figure 9.17a** one observes that the periods during which the channel is open, t_o, are variable. To obtain the mean open time of the channel, τ_o, one can build a frequency histogram of the different t_o. The exponential curve obtained provides the value of τ_o (see **Figure 9.17b** and Appendix 5.3). The functional significance of this value is as follows: during a time equal to τ_o the channel has a high probability of being open.

τ_o is a characteristic of the nicotinic receptor channel type

Nicotinic receptors from the electric organ of *Torpedo* and from the calf neuromuscular junction can be studied in patch clamp after the expression of the corresponding mRNA injected into *Xenopus* oocytes (outside-out configuration). Recording of such channels shows that electric organ and neuromuscular junction channels present very similar conductances (40 and 42 pS) but very different mean open times ($\tau_o = 0.6$ and 7.6 ms, respectively).

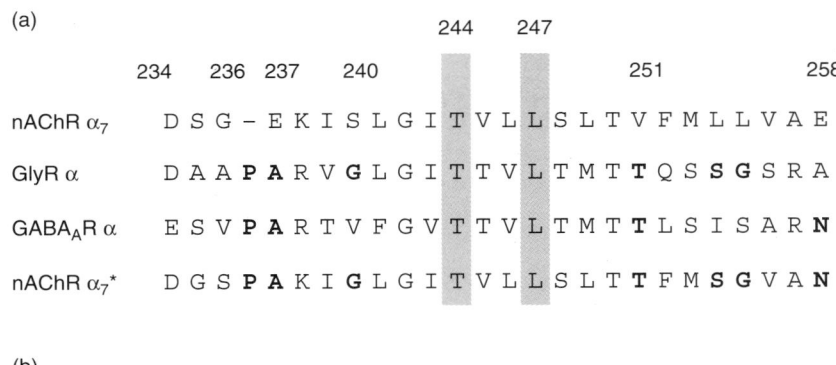

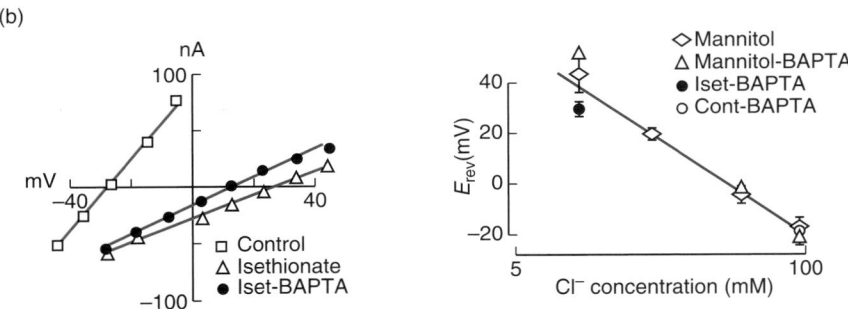

Figure 9.16 Mutations in the M2 segment of an α-subunit of the nAChR convert ion selectivity of the homomeric nAChR from cationic to anionic.

(a) Comparison of M2 sequences from subunits of the cation selective nicotinic α7 receptor subunit with those of the anion-selective glycine α1, GABA$_A$ α1 and β1 and mutated nicotinic α7* receptor subunits. (b, left) I/V relationship of the α7* mutant receptor is first determined in control conditions (control) with 2 s ACh (100 μM) applications (outside-out patch clamp recordings of a patch of membrane containing a large number of nicotinic receptors called macropatch). Then, 90% of chloride ions of the extracellular medium were replaced by the non-permeant anion isethionate and the I/V curve determined (isethionate). This last experiment was also performed in the presence of a chelator of Ca^{2+} ions (BAPTA) injected inside the cell (iset-BAPTA) in order to reduce secondary currents that could be triggered by the entry of Ca^{2+} ions through the nicotinic receptors. (b, right) Reversal potential values as a function of the logarithm of external chloride concentration (92, 50.5, 19.75 and 9.5 μM external chloride after substitution of NaCl by mannitol or isethionate). The solid line corresponds to the theoretical Nernst relation. From Galzi JL, Devillers-Thiéry A, Hussy N (1992) Mutations in the channel domain of a neuronal nicotinic receptor convert ion selectivity from cationic to anionic, *Nature* **359**, 500–505, with permission.

Another example is given by the study of nicotinic receptors from fetal or adult bovine muscle. A study of the subunit structure of the bovine muscle nAChR showed the presence of the α, β, γ and δ-subunits as in the case for *Torpedo* electroplax nAChR. In addition, a novel subunit termed the ε-subunit has been discovered by cloning and sequencing the DNA complementary to the muscle mRNA encoding it. The ε-subunit shows higher sequence homology with the γ-subunit than with any other subunit. In order to study the properties of the γ and ε-subunits, various combinations of the subunit-specific mRNAs are injected in *Xenopus* oocytes and their functional properties are studied in the presence of acetylcholine.

Figure 9.19a shows recordings of ACh-activated single channels from outside-out patches isolated from oocytes injected with the α, β, γ and δ-subunit-specific mRNAs (left) or with the α, β, ε and δ-subunit-specific mRNAs (right). The conductance and mean open time τ_o

(**Figures 9.19c and d**) of the channels formed in a given oocyte differ in relation to the mRNA combination with which it was injected. This suggests that a single subunit can change the conductance and gating properties of the nAChR channel.

To compare the two classes of nAChR channels produced in *Xenopus* oocytes with native bovine nAChR channels, the ACh-activated channels of fetal and adult bovine muscle are recorded. **Figure 9.19b** shows ACh-activated single currents from outside out patches of native fetal (left) and adult (right) bovine muscle. nAChR single-channel current in fetal muscle is similar to that of nAChRγ whereas the nAChR single-channel current in adult muscle is similar to that of nAChRε (compare **Figures 9.19a and b**). This suggests that the nAChR channel in fetal muscle is assembled from α, β, γ and δ-subunits whereas the endplate channel in adult muscle is assembled from the α, β, ε and δ-subunits. To study this developmental

(a)

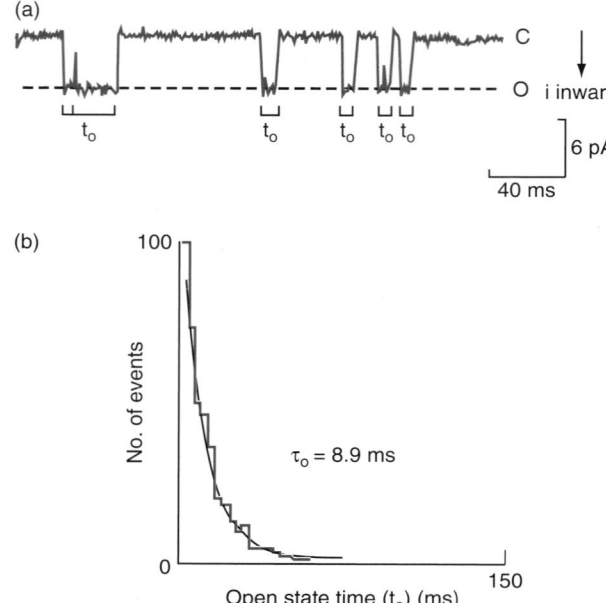

(b)

$\tau_o = 8.9$ ms

Figure 9.17 Patch clamp recording (attached-cell configuration) of myotube nicotinic receptor channel activity (V_m = –170 mV).

(a) Myotubes (embryonic muscle cells) are recorded in the presence of a low concentration of acetylcholine (200 nM). At this concentration, the channels open during periods t_0. This recording does not correspond to a single nAChR because one finds approximately 100 000 nAChR per patch. The repeated openings (downward deflections) correspond, therefore, to the opening of different nAChR. However, all the nAChR being identical, it seems as though the activity of the same nAChR was recorded from. **(b)** The mean open time τ_o can thus be calculated. C, closed channel; unitary current is zero. O, open channel; inward unitary current (downward deflections).

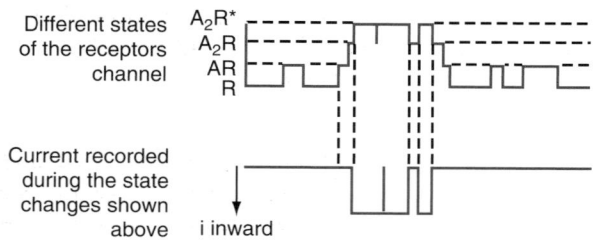

Figure 9.18 Correlation between the nicotinic current and the states of the channel.

The channel opens only (inward current, lower trace) when the protein is in the A_2R^* state. The rapid fluctuations between states A_2R^* and A_2R correspond to short-lived closures. When the receptor channel loses one or two of its acetylcholine molecules, the closures last longer. Adapted from Colquhoun D, Ogden DC, Mathie A (1987) Nicotinic acetylcholine receptors of nerve and muscle: functional aspects, *TIPS* **8**, 465–472, with permission.

change in the contents of the five nAChR-subunit mRNAs in bovine muscle, total RNA is extracted from the diaphragm muscle at various stages of fetal and postnatal development. It is then subjected to blot hybridization analysis using the respective cDNA probes. The results show that the contents of the γ- and ε-subunit mRNAs varies markedly during muscle development showing reciprocal changes: the γ-subunit mRNA is abundant at earlier fetal stages (3–5 months' gestation), but is hardly or not detectable after birth; conversely, considerable amounts of ε-subunit mRNA appear only at postnatal stages and is not detectable at earlier fetal stages (3–4 months' gestation). Therefore, the replacement of the γ-subunit by the ε-subunit in the nAChR complex is responsible for the changes in the properties of the nAChR channel that occur during muscle development. This phenomenon of subunit replacement during development cannot be generalized to all the other mammalian nAChR.

9.4 The nicotinic receptor desensitizes

During the recording of a nicotinic receptor channel with the patch clamp technique (whole-cell configuration) in the presence of a high and constant concentration of acetylcholine, there is a progressive diminution of the total current I_{ACh} (**Figure 9.20a**). This decrease in current corresponds to the progressive desensitization of the nicotinic receptor present in the membrane.

When recording unitary nicotinic currents (outside-out or cell-attached configuration) in the presence of a strong concentration of acetylcholine, there are repeated openings separated by long periods of silence (**Figure 9.20b**). These sequences of openings are known as *unitary current bursts*. Within a burst, the protein rapidly fluctuates between the closed and open states, symbolized as follows:

$$R \rightleftharpoons AR \rightleftharpoons A_2R \rightleftharpoons A_2R^*$$

closed channel states — open channel state

The long silent periods correspond to desensitization of the receptor in the presence of acetylcholine. In the desensitized state, the nicotinic receptor is refractory to activation. Consequently, the channel does not open despite the fact that two molecules of ACh are bound to the receptor.

In summary, desensitization is a phenomenon that renders the nicotinic receptor incapable of being activated by its agonists. The desensitized nicotinic receptor presents two main characteristics: (i) a high affinity for

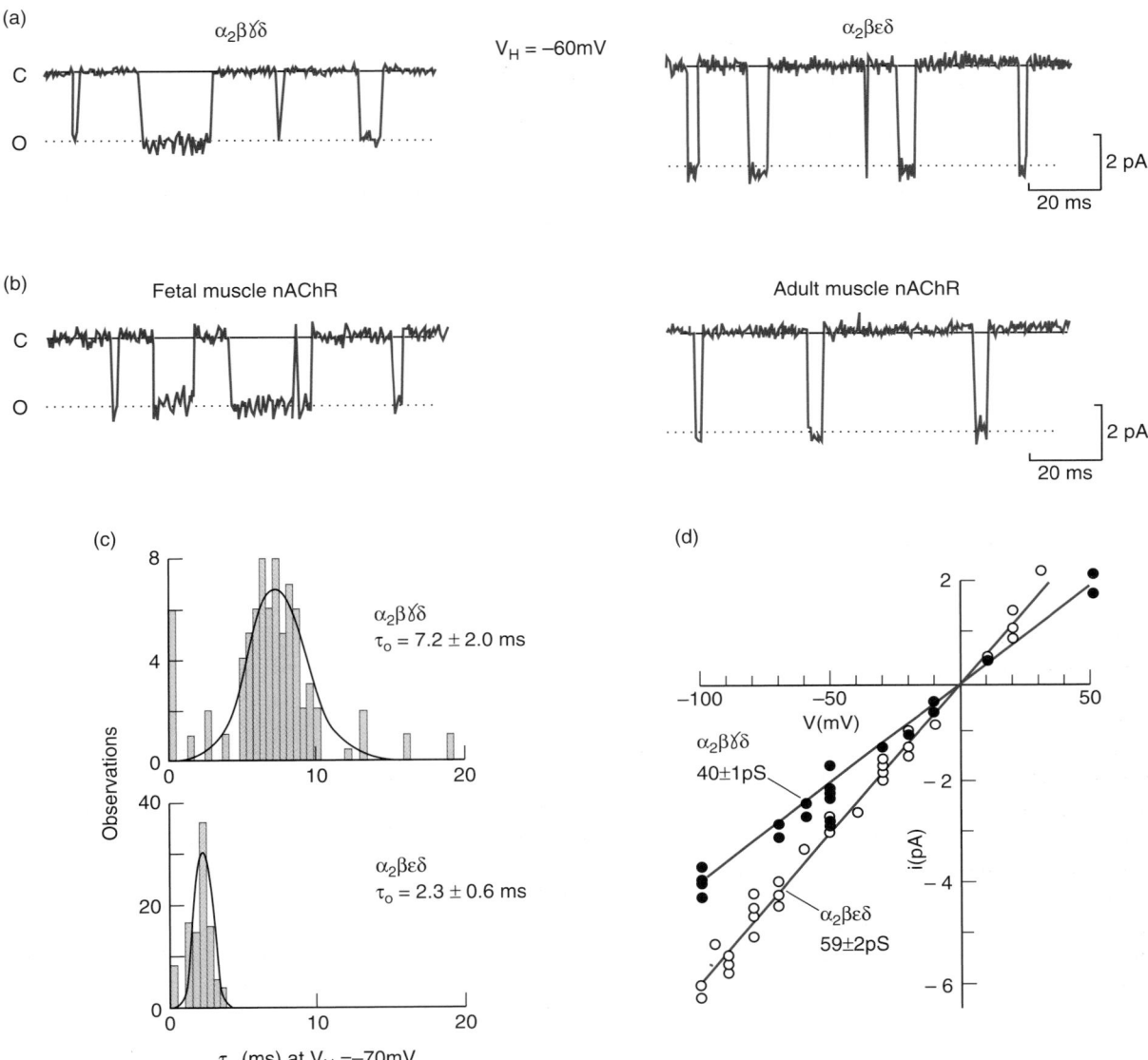

Figure 9.19 The subunit structure participates in determining the nicotinic channel conductance and mean open time.
See text for explanations. C, closed channel; O, open channel. Adapted from Mishina M, Takai T, Imoto K *et al.* (1986) Molecular distinction between fetal and adult forms of muscle acetylcholine receptor, *Nature* **321**, 406–411, with permission.

acetylcholine; and (ii) a closed ionic channel: the unitary current is zero (long silent periods).

At least two desensitized states exist: D_1 and D_2, or according to other authors, I and D, so that:

$$A_2R \rightleftharpoons A_2R^* \underset{k_{-3}}{\overset{k_3}{\rightleftharpoons}} A_2D_1$$

$$k_{-4} \big\updownarrow k_4$$

$$A_2D_2$$

These two states D_1 and D_2, which are closed channel

states, are distinguished from one another other and also from the R state by their affinity constants for acetylcholine (**Table 9.1**) and by the rate constants $k_3 = 0.01$ s^{-1} and $k_4 = 1$ s^{-1}.

Table 9.1 Affinity constants for acetylcholine

State	Affinity constant for ACh K_D
R	10 µM to 1 mM
D_1	1 µM
D_2	3–10 nM

The concept of nicotinic receptor desensitization has been proposed by different authors, notably by Katz and Thesleff, from measurements of the time course of the global synaptic response during an iontophoretic application of acetylcholine.

The process of desensitization appears slowly and is slowly reversible. This is an intrinsic property of the protein. In order to study in patch clamp the states R and R* of the nicotinic receptor channel, it is necessary to choose conditions under which desensitization is negligible. To this end, researchers work with very low doses of acetylcholine (of the order of the nanomoles per litre) because high doses favour the conformational change of the protein into desensitized states (see **Figure** 9.17). An alternative approach is the use of high doses of acetylcholine (of the order of micromoles per litre; see **Figure 9.20b**). In this case, the receptors desensitize (silent periods known as interburst periods) and eventually one or several of the channels open and close repetitively (opening bursts) before re-desensitizing. Desensitization can be minimized by excluding the first and the last opening during the bursting periods, and thus the values calculated for τ_o are then related only to the R* state.

The rate of desensitization of the nicotinic receptor seems to be related to its state of phosphorylation. In fact, studies of the ionic flux through nicotinic receptors incorporated into liposomes have shown that an increase

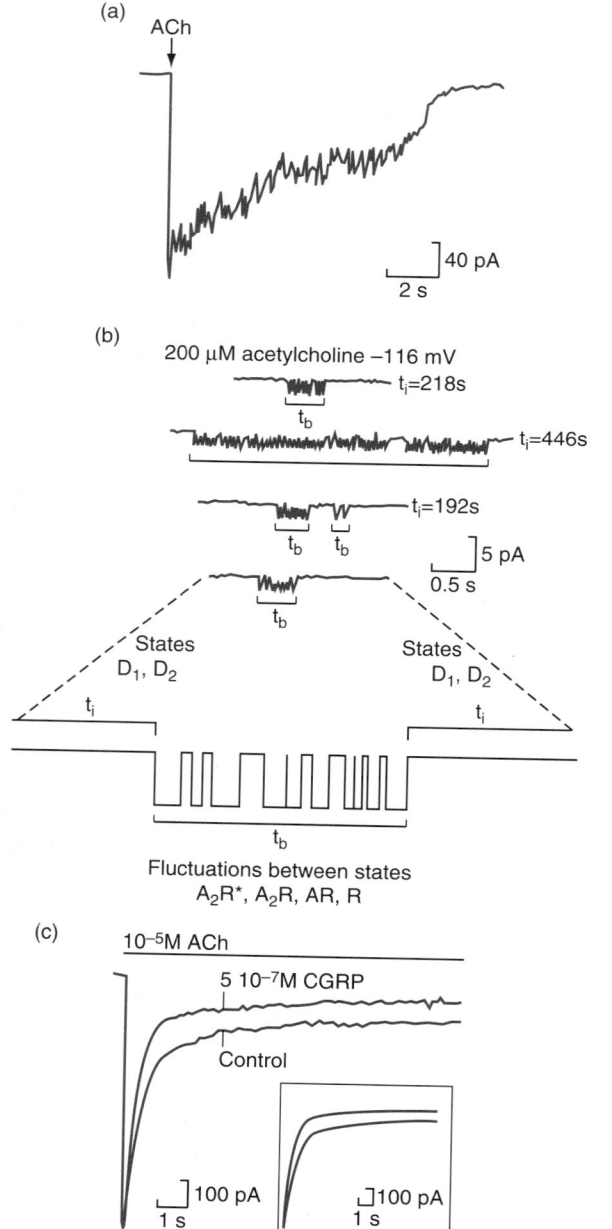

Figure 9.20 Nicotinic receptor desensitization.
(a) Patch clamp recording (whole-cell configuration) of the nicotinic current from adrenal chromaffin cells ($V_m = -70$ mV). In the presence of a high concentration of acetylcholine (20 μM) the inward current reaches a peak of 235 pA, and then decreases despite a constant acetylcholine concentration. This current corresponds to the sum of several unitary currents crossing all the activated nicotinic channels. The decrease in current is due to the desensitization of a large fraction of cellular nicotinic receptors.
(b) Single-channel recordings (cell-attached or outside-out configurations) illustrating another consequence of desensitization. The membrane patch is exposed to a high concentration of acetylcholine (200 μM) for an extended period. Under these conditions, nicotinic receptors present in the patch desensitize. After a certain time, one of the channels reopens and fluctuates between the states A_2R^*, A_2R, AR and R during a time t_b (duration of the burst of openings) before desensitizing again for a duration t_i (interburst duration). The traces shown correspond to segments of a continuous recording. The duration of the desensitized periods t_i between two successive traces is indicated at the end of each trace (218, 446 and 192 s). **(c)** Cultured muscle cell recording (whole-cell configuration). Nicotinic current evoked by the application of 10 μM acetylcholine recorded in the presence of 500 nM CGRP (calcitonin gene related peptide) and in the absence of the peptide (control) ($V_m = -60$ mV). The nicotinic current reaches a peak with a 200 ms delay and then begins to decrease. The sum of two exponentials can describe this decrease in current. CGRP increases the speed of the fast component. Part (a) from Clapham DE, Neher E (1984) Trifluoperazine reduces inward ionic currents and secretion by separate mechanisms in bovine chromaffin cells, *J. Physiol. (Lond.)* **353**, 541–564, with permission. Part (b) from Colquhoun D, Ogden DC, Mathie A (1987) Nicotinic acetylcholine receptors of nerve and muscle: functional aspects, *TIPS* **8**, 465–472, with permission. Part (c) from Mulle C, Benoit P, Pinset C *et al.* (1988) Calcitonin gene-related peptide enhances the rate of desensitization of the nicotinic acetylcholine receptor in cultured mouse muscle cells, *Proc. Natl Acad. Sci. USA* **85**, 5728–5732, with permission.

in the level of phosphorylation of the receptors by cyclic AMP augments the desensitization rate of these receptors. In the neuromuscular junctions a peptide present in the motoneurons is released at the same time as acetylcholine. This peptide, CGRP (calcitonin gene-related peptide), is capable of increasing the level of cyclic AMP in cultured embryonic muscle cells, consequently increasing the number of phosphorylated nicotinic receptors. In patch clamp recordings (whole-cell configuration) of embryonic muscle cells, the simultaneous application of this peptide and acetylcholine accelerates the rapid phase of desensitization of the nicotinic receptors (**Figure 9.20c**). In unitary recordings (cell-attached configuration), CGRP decreases the opening frequency of the nicotinic channels (while at the same time leaving unaffected their mean open time and unitary conductance). These effects are mimicked by the application of substances that augment the intracellular cyclic AMP level (such as forskolin). The following hypothesis has been proposed. CGRP activates a specific membrane receptor. This leads to an increase in the intracellular cyclic AMP concentration and an activation of protein kinase A. Protein kinase A, directly or indirectly, phosphorylates certain subunits of the nicotinic receptor, leading to a rapid desensitization of the receptors.

Generalization

Nicotinic receptors are allosteric receptors as defined by Monod, Wyman and Changeux (MWC model, 1965). The MWC model hypothesizes the following:

■ nAChRs are oligomers made up of a finite number of identical subunits that occupy equivalent positions and as a consequence possess at least one axis of rotational symmetry.
■ nAChRs can exist spontaneously in the four freely interconvertible and discrete conformational states described above (R, R*, D_1, D_2), even in the absence of ligand. The closed states are R, AR and A_2R; the open states are R*, AR* and A_2R*; the desensitized states are D_1, AD_1, A_2D_1 and D_2, AD_2, A_2D_2.
■ The affinity and activity of the stereospecific sites carried by the nAChR differ between these four states.

This gives a tetrahedral model for interactions between the four conformational states instead of the sequential model previously described for simplicity:

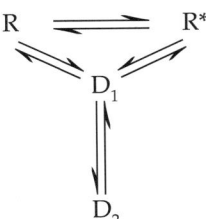

As a result, gating of the nAChR cannot be viewed solely as a ligand-triggered process but as reflecting an intrinsic structural transition of the receptor molecule, which may even occur in the absence of ligand. Moreover, at low agonist concentrations, desensitized states can be stabilized under conditions of negligible channel opening.

9.5 nAChR-mediated synaptic transmission at the neuromuscular junction

A nicotinic synaptic current is evoked by a brief augmentation of the concentration of acetylcholine in the synaptic cleft. This increase, caused by the asynchronous release of synaptic vesicles, is brief because (**Figure 9.21a**): (i) the release is brief; and (ii) acetylcholine rapidly disappears from the synaptic cleft. In fact, when acetylcholine is released into the synaptic cleft, it may either bind to acetylcholine-gated channels, diffuse out of the synaptic cleft, or be rapidly degraded by acetylcholinesterase.

During the analysis of synaptic currents induced by the release of endogenous acetylcholine, the desensitized states of the receptor can be neglected because of the rapid elimination of acetylcholine from the synaptic cleft (in the order of microseconds). The model for this is:

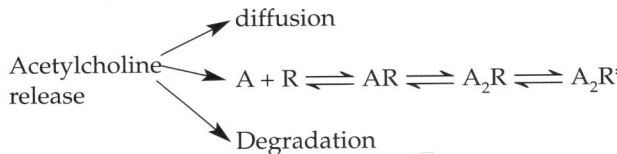

This is very different from what occurs during the recording of the activity of a nicotinic receptor in a patch of membrane in the inside-out configuration, when the acetylcholine is continuously present in the patch pipette, or the recording of the activity of a nicotinic receptor channel in a patch of membrane in the outside-out configuration in response to acetylcholine pressure applied from another pipette. Even the shortest applications in this case are of the order of tens of milliseconds.

9.5.1 Miniature and endplate synaptic currents are recorded at the neuromuscular junction

Two main types of postsynaptic currents can be recorded at any synapse: spontaneous and evoked synaptic currents. The former is recorded in the absence of presynaptic stimulation whereas the latter represents the response to a presynaptic stimulation. Spontaneous

(a)

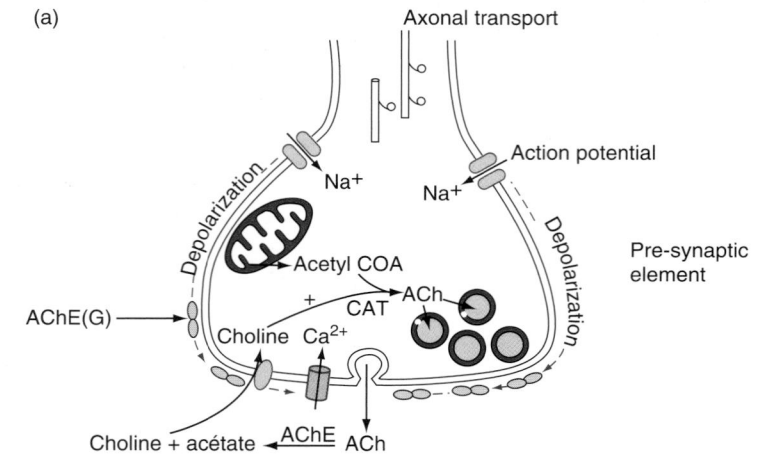

Axonal transport

Action potential

Na+

Pre-synaptic element

Depolarization

Na+

Acetyl COA

ACh

CAT

+

AChE(G)

Choline   Ca2+

Choline + acétate ← AChE ← ACh

(b)

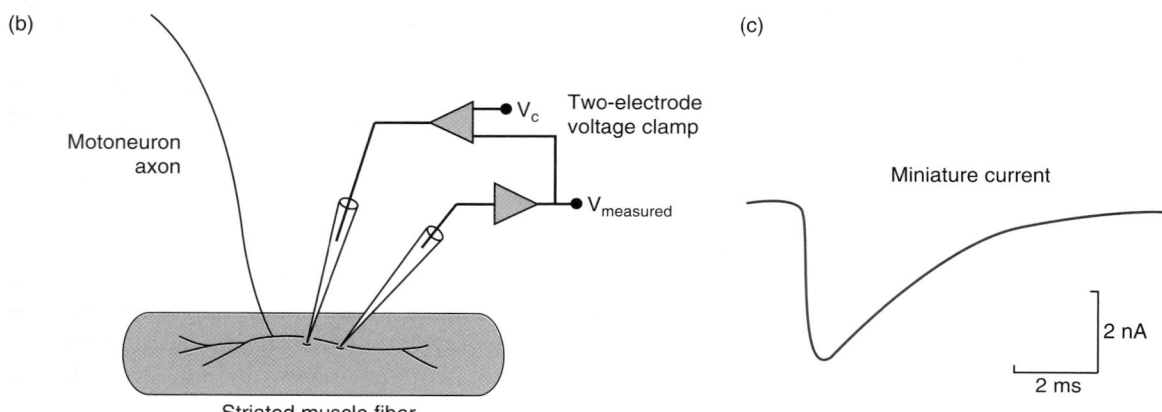

Motoneuron axon

V_c Two-electrode voltage clamp

$V_{measured}$

Striated muscle fiber

(c)

Miniature current

2 nA

2 ms

(d)

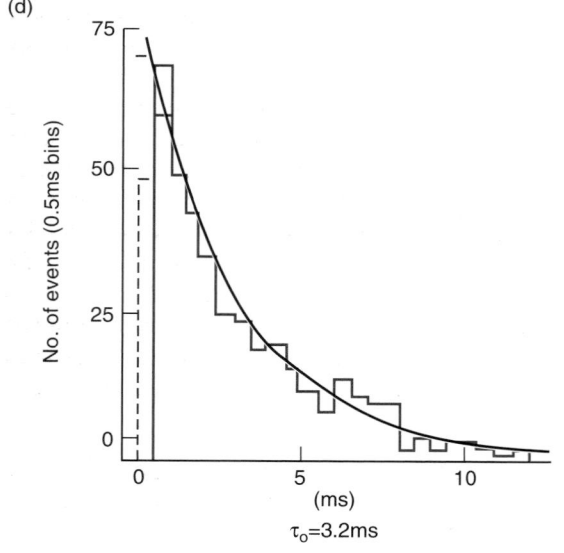

No. of events (0.5ms bins)

75

50

25

0

0   5   10
(ms)
$\tau_o = 3.2$ms

(e)

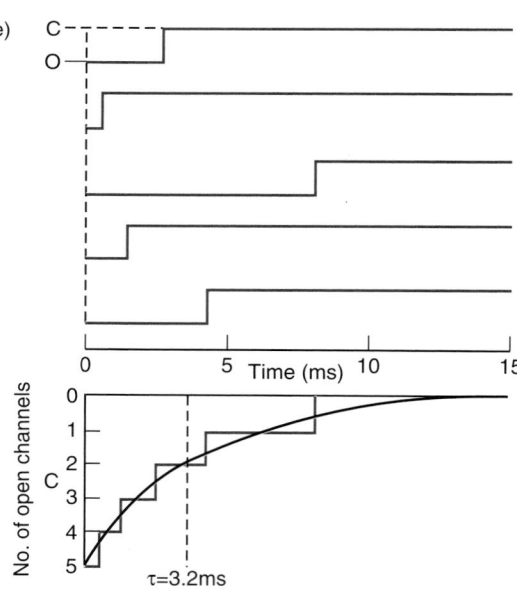

C

O

0   5   Time (ms)   10   15

No. of open channels

0
1
C 2
3
4
5

$\tau = 3.2$ms

Figure 9.21 (left) A cholinergic presynaptic terminal and miniature nicotinic current.
(a) Functional scheme of the presynaptic component of the neuromuscular nicotinic cholinergic synapse. The enzymes choline acetyl transferase (CAT) and acetylcholinesterase (AChE) are synthesized in the cell body of the motoneuron and carried to axon terminals via anterograde axonal transport. Acetylcholine (ACh) is synthesized in axon terminals from choline and acetyl coenzyme A (acetylCOA). About 50% of the released choline is recaptured by the presynaptic terminals. Acetylcholine is actively transported from the cytoplasm into synaptic vesicles via a vesicular ACh carrier using the H^+ gradient as an energy source (antiport). **(b)** Miniature current recorded in two-electrode voltage clamp from a normally innervated muscle fibre in the absence of stimulation and in the presence of TTX. **(c)** The neuromuscular junction miniature current I_{ACh} is the current crossing N nicotinic channels activated by spontaneously released endogenous acetylcholine. The current rising phase is fast owing to the quasi-synchronous activation of the N nicotinic channels. The exponential falling phase of the current is slower ($V_m = -80$ mV). **(d)** Since the opening of the channels is synchronous, their closure appears after a variable time t_o whose distribution is exponential. The mean open time of the N channels is $\tau_o = 3.2$ ms. **(e)** The same value of τ_o is obtained for the time constant of the falling phase (τ) of the total current I_{ACh}. In the example given in (d), $N = 5$, but N is in fact always larger (see text). Parts (c) and (d) adapted from Colquhoun D (1981) How fast do drugs work? *TIPS* **2**, 212–217, with permission.

synaptic currents can be further divided into those evoked by spontaneous presynaptic spikes in a Ca^{2+}-dependent manner, and miniature currents evoked even in the absence of spontaneous spikes (in the presence of TTX). Miniature currents have a very small amplitude and correspond to the release of one or a few synaptic vesicles (see Appendix 8.1).

Miniature currents

Miniature currents are the currents recorded at the neuromuscular junction in the total absence of stimulation of the motor nerve and in the presence of TTX (**Figure 9.21b**). These currents are evoked by the spontaneous liberation of acetylcholine from the presynaptic terminal. Thus, if an innervated muscle fibre in the absence of nerve stimulation is recorded from under voltage clamp (**Figure 9.21b**), from time to time a miniature current will be recorded (**Figure 9.21c**). The recorded current is due to the spontaneous release of a synaptic vesicle or quantum of acetylcholine (1 vesicle = 1 quantum; see Chapter 8). This current is inward at –80 mV and has a maximum amplitude of about 4 nA.

How many receptor channels are opened by acetylcholine at the peak of a miniature current? Knowing the amplitude of the unitary current and the amplitude of a miniature current at the same membrane potential, we can calculate the number of nicotinic receptor channels opened by acetylcholine at the peak of the miniature response. At $V_m = -80$ mV, we have:

$$i = 2.5 \text{ pA, and } I = 4 \text{ nA} = 4 \times 10^3 \text{ pA;}$$

i.e. $4.10^3/2.5 = 1600$ nicotinic receptor channels opened by acetylcholine.

Since two molecules of acetylcholine are needed to open one channel, the average number of acetylcholine molecules released is $1600 \times 2 = 3200$ molecules of ACh per vesicle. In other words, 1 quantum equals about 3000 molecules of ACh.

What is the time course of a miniature current? The time it takes to reach the maximal amplitude of the miniature current is approximately 100 µs while it takes longer to disappear. The decrease of the current has an exponential time course with a time constant of the order of milliseconds (**Figure 9.21e**). This current decrease depends solely on τ_o (**Figures 9.21d and e**).

Motor endplate current

The endplate current is recorded (in voltage clamp) at the neuromuscular junction while the motor nerve is being stimulated (**Figure 9.22**). At $V_m = -80$ mV the current is inward and has an amplitude of approximately 400 nA.

How many channels are opened at the peak of the motor endplate current? The motor endplate current is composed of $400 \text{ nA}/4 \text{ nA} = 100$ miniature currents produced by $1600 \times 100 = 16 \times 10^4$ nicotinic receptors opened by released acetylcholine.

What is the time course of the motor endplate current? Approximately 100 vesicles are released in an asynchronous manner by the stimulated presynaptic terminal. This is the reason why the time it takes to reach the maximal or peak amplitude of this current is relatively longer than the time it takes to reach the peak of a miniature current (300 µs instead of 100 µs).

In current clamp recordings, this endplate inward current depolarizes the postsynaptic membrane thus evoking the endplate potential recorded in **Figure 9.2**.

9.5.2 Synaptic currents are the sum of unitary currents appearing with variable delays and durations

There is a variable delay in the appearance of current flow through each one of the postsynaptic receptor channels. The reason for this is that the synaptic vesicles are released in an asynchronous manner. Furthermore,

(a)

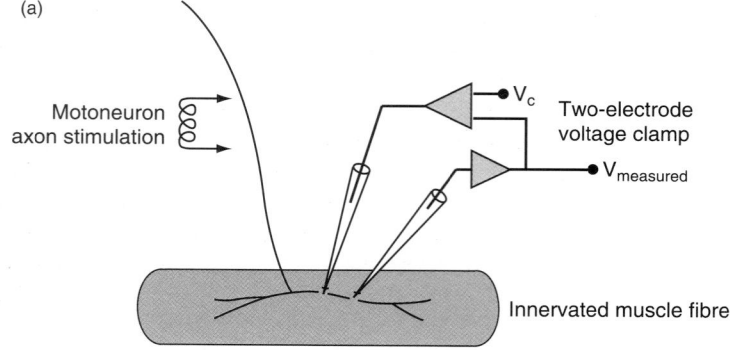

(b)

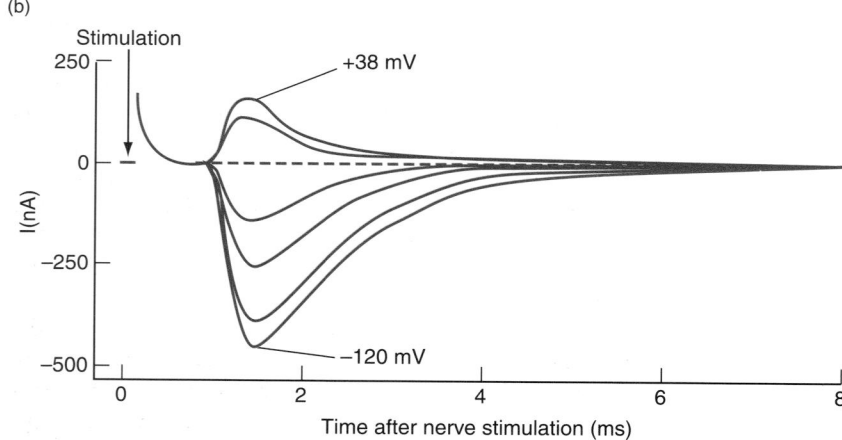

Figure 9.22 Motor endplate current.
(a) Current recorded in response to a stimulation of the nerve fibre under two-electrode voltage clamp. **(b)** This current is inward for negative membrane potentials and outward for positive voltages. As in the case of the unitary current, the motor endplate current reverses around 0 mV (frog's neuromuscular junction). Muscular action potentials are blocked by voltage clamping the corresponding muscle region. The muscle contraction induced by the inward current can be blocked by the destruction of T tubules (with a hyperosmotic shock). Adapted from Magleby KL, Stevens CF (1972) A quantitative description of end plate currents, *J. Physiol. (Lond.)* **223**, 173–197, with permission.

acetylcholine molecules must diffuse for a certain time before they reach a free receptor channel. We have seen that the concentration of acetylcholine in the synaptic cleft decreases so rapidly that a receptor channel has very few chances of being reopened a second time by binding again two acetylcholine molecules.

Determination of the value of the total synaptic current, I_{Ach}, at steady state is:

$$I_{Ach} = N p_o i_{Ach},$$

where N is the number of nicotinic channels in the membrane, i_{ACh} is the unitary current, and p_o is the open-state probability of the channel and depends on the acetylcholine concentration and on the receptor channel open-

ing (β) and closing (α) rate constants.

In the model below we have the following rate constants:

$$\begin{array}{ccccccc} & k_1 & & k_2 & & \beta & \\ R & \rightleftharpoons & AR & \rightleftharpoons & A_2R & \rightleftharpoons & A_2R^* \\ & k_{-1} & & k_{-2} & & \alpha & \end{array}$$

where α and β are the closing and opening rate constants of the channel. The channel's probability of being in the open state at steady state (see Appendix 5.3) is then:

$$p_o = \beta' / (\beta' + \alpha),$$

where β' is the apparent opening rate constant of the channel, which depends on β but also on the rate constants of the preceding stages k_1 and k_2 ($\beta' = f[ACh]$). Thus, if α is short (i.e. the mean open time τ_o is long, because $\tau_o = 1/\alpha$), then p_o is high (it approaches its maximum value), and I_{ACh} is large. The falling phase of the total current is exponential, with a time constant equal to τ_o.

Let us assume that at a time t a certain number of ionic channels are opened more or less synchronously (this is the case of miniature currents). Because acetylcholine disappears very rapidly from the synaptic cleft, a channel has very few chances of reopening. Each one of the open channels has an opening duration t_o. We have seen that the duration t_o during which each channel remains open can be described by an exponential distribution (see **Figure 9.17**). **Figure 9.21e** shows that the total current crossing N channels decreases exponentially with a time constant equal to τ_o.

In conclusion, the falling phase of the total current is not due to the progressive disappearance of acetylcholine from the synaptic cleft (because it disappears with a time constant of the order of microseconds) but depends only on τ_o, an intrinsic property of the channel.

9.6 Nicotinic transmission pharmacology

9.6.1 Nicotinic agonists

Nicotinic receptor agonists (see Appendix 7.1) bind to the same receptor site as acetylcholine and favour the conformational changes of the protein towards the open state. These agonists are, for example, suberyl-dicholine, carbachol and PTMA (phenyl trimethyl ammonium) (**Figure 9.23a**). The application of one of these on a patch of muscle membrane (outside-out configuration) leads to the onset of a current whose amplitude at each membrane potential tested is equal to the current evoked by acetylcholine. However, the duration of the openings of the channel depends on the agonist used (**Figures 9.23b and c**).

9.6.2 Competitive nicotinic antagonists

Competitive antagonists (see Appendix 7.1) bind to the same receptor site as acetylcholine but *do not favour* its conformational change towards the open state. By binding to the acetylcholine receptor sites, competitive antagonists prevent acetylcholine from binding to its receptor sites and activating the nAChR. They decrease the number of sites available to acetylcholine and, therefore, decrease or completely block (depending on the dose used) the nicotinic cholinergic response. A distinc-

tion is made between competitive antagonists whose effect is reversible ((+)tubocurarine) and those whose effect is irreversible (DDF).

The application of (+)tubocurarine on a patch of muscle membrane in the outside-out recording configuration and in the presence of a low dose of acetylcholine causes a drop in the opening frequency of the channels. This occurs because (+)tubocurarine reduces the number of receptor sites available for acetylcholine. It should be noted, however, that the amplitude of the unitary current i_{ACh} evoked in the presence or absence of (+)tubocurarine is identical. The application of (+)tubocurarine on an isolated nerve–muscle preparation induces a reduction in the amplitude of the spontaneous miniature currents (currents evoked by the endogenous and spontaneous liberation of acetylcholine). The effect of (+)tubocurarine can be reversed by elevating the concentration of acetylcholine applied or released. Since the binding of (+)tubocurarine to the nicotinic receptor is reversible, increasing the acetylcholine concentration will increase the probability that the receptor sites are occupied by acetylcholine.

The binding of α-bungarotoxin (venom from the snake *Bungarus multicinctus*) to the nicotinic receptor of the neuromuscular junction is very stable. For this reason, this toxin is used as a marker of acetylcholine receptor sites in this preparation. This labelling permits localizing and counting of these receptors. Labelled α-bungarotoxin also allows identification of the receptor during its purification process (see **Figure 9.4**).

9.6.3 Channel blockers

Channel blockers are substances that bind to the aqueous pore of the open receptor, preventing the passage of cations through it. Among these substances are procaine and its derivatives (QX 222, lidocaine, benzocaine), and also histrionicotoxin and chlorpromazine.

Application of acetylcholine in the presence of benzocaine to a muscle membrane patch in the outside-out recording configuration evokes the onset of opening bursts. These bursts of unitary currents are due to the numerous fluctuations of the receptor between its open and its closed state (**Figure 9.24a**). The following model describes this process:

$$R \rightleftharpoons R^* \rightleftharpoons R^*B,$$

where R represents the nicotinic receptor in its closed state, R* the nicotinic receptor in its open state, and R*B the nicotinic receptor in the open but blocked state. In the R* state, the cations cross the aqueous pore, while in the states R and R*B the ions cannot cross it.

In the presence of benzocaine, a change in the kinetics of the falling phase of the current (**Figure 9.24b**) is

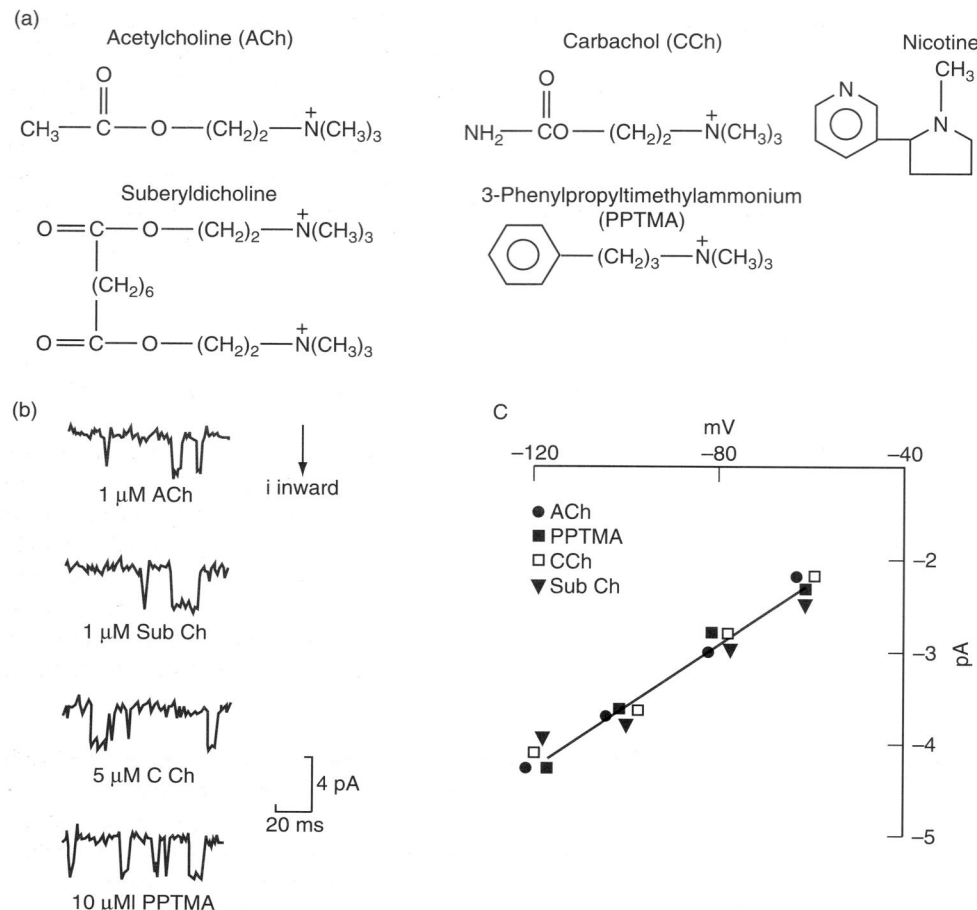

Figure 9.23 Unitary currents evoked by nicotinic agonists.

(a) Structure of the nicotinic agonists tested. (b) Inward unitary currents evoked by different nicotinic agonists ($V_m = -80$ mV) recorded in patch clamp (outside-out configuration) from isolated rat myotubes. Solutions (in mM): intracellular 150 KCl, 5 Na_2EGTA, 0.5 $CaCl_2$; extracellular 135 NaCl, 5.4 KCl. (c) i/V curves built from results similar to those shown in (b), but at different membrane potentials, are completely superimposable. The slope of each curve gives a unitary conductance γ of approximately 34 pS. Adapted from Gardner P, Ogden DC, Colquhoun D (1984) Conductances of single ion channels opened by nicotinic agonists are indistinguishable, *Nature* **289**, 160–163, with permission.

observed during the recording of spontaneous miniature currents of an isolated nerve–muscle preparation ($V_m = -100$ mV). In the absence of benzocaine, the falling phase is described by a single exponential with a time constant of $\tau = 3.8$ ms. In the presence of benzocaine, the falling phase is described by two exponentials with time constants $\tau_1 = 1.0$ ms and $\tau_2 = 7.6$ ms. The explanation of this effect is that the channels opened by acetylcholine are very rapidly blocked by benzocaine, which quickly blocks the unitary current. Thus, one observes a fast initial decrement of the miniature current (with a shorter time constant than in the absence of benzocaine). The channels then reopen and reblock repeatedly. This increases the duration of the miniature current and one observes a second slower decrementing phase (with time constant τ_2).

9.6.4 Acetylcholinesterase inhibitors

These inhibitors have a reversible effect, as in the case of prostigmine, or an irreversible effect, as in the case of DFP (difluorophosphate). The application of prostigmine to an isolated nerve–muscle preparation significantly increases the miniature current duration (**Figure 9.25**). In the presence of prostigmine, acetylcholine molecules degrade much more slowly, and thus are able to bind repeatedly and trigger the reopening of nicotinic receptors. This repeated binding considerably increases the duration of the miniature current falling phase. As we have already seen (see Section 9.5), the miniature-current time constant in the absence of acetylcholinesterase inhibitors reflects the nicotinic receptor average open time. However, the average open time of the nicotinic receptor is clearly not the same in the presence of prostigmine.

9.7 Summary

Upon release of acetylcholine in the synaptic cleft of the neuromuscular junction, two molecules of acetylcholine bind to each postsynaptic nAChRs, at specific sites. Upon ACh binding, each nAChR undergoes fast activation leading to an open-channel state, and a slow desensitization reaction leading to a closed-channel state refractory to activation. nAChR opening occurs in the millisecond range, fast desensitization in the 0.1 s range and slow desensitization in the minute range.

To which type(s) of postsynaptic receptor do the molecules of acetylcholine bind?

At the neuromuscular junction, ACh binds to the muscle-type nAChR. Muscle nAChRs have a fixed composition $[\alpha 1]_2[\beta 1][\delta][\gamma$ or $\varepsilon]$ in vertebrates. Each subunit contains a large N-terminal hydrophilic domain exposed to the synaptic cleft, followed by three transmembrane sgements (M1 to M3), a large intracellular loop and a C-terminal transmembrane segment (M4). Acetylcholine binding sites are located at the interface between α and non-α subunits in the N-terminal regions. The ion channel is lined by the M2 segment from each of the five subunits.

How is the binding of acetylcholine transduced into a depolarization of the postsynaptic membrane?

Upon binding of two molecules of ACh, nAChRs undergo a fast conformational change to a state where the pore is open. The pore is selectively permeable to cations. At −90 to −80 mV, the resting potential of mucle fibres, the electrochemical gradient $(V_m − E_{ion})$ for Na^+ and Ca^{2+} ions is large whereas that for K^+ ions is small. As a result, there is a net inward flux of cations through open nAChRs measured as a transient inward current.

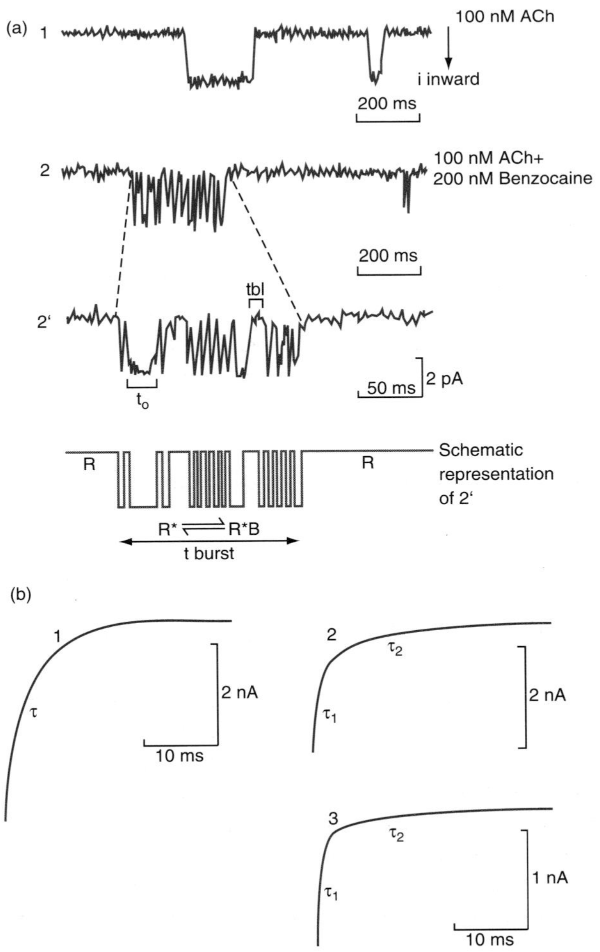

Figure 9.24 Benzocaine effect on the time course of ACh evoked unitary and miniature nicotinic currents.
(a) Patch clamp recording (cell-attached configuration) of nicotinic unitary currents evoked by the application of ACh (i_{ACh}). (1) In the presence of 100 nM of ACh, the channels open for a mean duration of $\tau_o = 19$ ms ($V_m = −110$ mV). (2) In the presence of 100 nM of ACh + 200 μM of benzocaine, bursts of openings ($V_m = −130$ mV) are recorded. (2′) The same recording as (2) but with a different time scale and with an added diagram of the openings and closings of the channel. t_o, time during which the channel stays open; t_{bl}, time during which the channel is blocked by benzocaine; t_{burst}, duration of a burst of openings. The histograms of t_o and of t_{bl} are described by a single exponential with the following average values: $\tau_o = 2.8$ ms, and $\tau_{bl} = 3.5$ ms (extrajunctional muscle membrane of 4- to 6-week-old muscle cells). (b) Two-electrode voltage clamp recording of miniature nicotinic currents. Each curve corresponds to the average of 8 to 14 miniature currents ($V_m = −100$ mV). (1) In the absence of benzocaine, the miniature currents reach their maximum in approximately 1 ms. Their decrement is described by a single exponential with a time constant $\tau = 3.8$ ms. (2) In the presence of extracellular benzocaine (300 μM, 15 min), the peak amplitude of miniature currents decreases, and the falling phase is described by two exponentials with time constants $\tau_1 = 1.0$ ms and $\tau_2 = 7.6$ ms. (3) In the presence of a higher concentration of benzocaine (500 μM, 17 min), the amplitude of the miniature current peak is further diminished and the time constants of the falling phase become $\tau_1 = 0.7$ ms and $\tau_2 = 11.6$ ms (frog cutaneous pectoris muscle). Parts (a) and (b) adapted from Ogden DC, Siegelbaum SA, Colquhoun D (1981) Block of acetylcholine-activated ion channels by an uncharged local anesthetic, *Nature* **289**, 596–598, with permission.

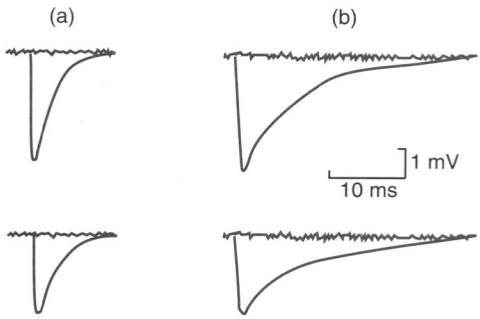

Figure 9.25 Effect of the acetylcholinesterase inhibitor prostigmine on the duration of miniature currents.

Recordings **(a)** in the absence of and **(b)** in the presence of prostigmine (10^{-6} g ml^{-1}), showing that prostigmine augments the duration of the miniature current. Adapted from Katz B, Miledi R (1973) The binding of acetylcholine to receptors and its removal from the synaptic cleft, *J. Physiol. (Lond.)* **231**, 549–574, with permission.

This inward current transiently depolarizes the muscular membrane and thus evokes the endplate potential (EPP). EPP is transient (it lasts several milliseconds) owing to the rapid closing of nAChRs and the rapid elimination of ACh from the synaptic cleft by degradation by acetylcholinesterases. In physiological conditions, desensitization of nAChRs does not play a major role.

Why is the postsynaptic depolarization restricted to the postsynaptic membrane?

nAChRs are restricted to the membrane of the postsynaptic element where they are anchored by cytoskeletal proteins. Therefore, the ACh-evoked postsynaptic inward current is triggered at the level of the postsynaptic element only. It is then passively conducted along the postsynaptic muscular membrane. This conduction is decremental (see **Chapter 16**) such as that at several millimetres from the junction, the EPP amplitude is nearly close to zero.

The function of the nicotinic receptor is to ensure rapid synaptic transmission. This is achieved by converting the binding of two acetylcholine molecules into a rapid and transient increase in cationic permeability. This permeability increase is made possible by conformational changes of the receptor channel: it transiently switches from the state in which the channel is closed into a state in which the channel is open. The nicotinic acetylcholine receptor also presents allosteric binding sites, topographically distinct from the neurotransmitter binding site, to which a variety of pharmacological agents and physiological ligands can bind. In doing so they regulate the transitions between the different states of the nAChR.

Appendix 9.1 The neuronal nicotinic receptors

Nicotinic acetylcholine receptors are a family of ligand-gated cationic channels whose opening is controlled by acetylcholine and other agonists of nicotinic receptors. Each receptor consists of five subunits arranged to delimit the aqueous channel in the centre. The family can be regarded as having three branches:

- muscle nAChR labelled and blocked by α-bungarotoxin;
- neuronal heteromeric nAChRs which do not bind α-bungarotoxin and consist of pairwise combinations of α_2, α_3, α_4, α_6 subunits with β_2, β_4 subunits;
- neuronal homomeric nAChRs which bind α-bungarotoxin and consist of α_7, α_8 or α_9 subunits.

Permeability to Ca^{2+} ions distinguishes neuronal from muscle nAChRs: neuronal nAChRs have a greater Ca^{2+} permeability as determined by using current and fluorescence measurements. Single-channel currents evoked by ACh are recorded in outside-out patches from freshly dissociated neurons of the rat central nervous system (habenula nucleus). In outside-out patches, single-channel inward currents are recorded in response to acetylcholine in pure external Ca^{2+} medium (**Figure A9.1a**). This shows that Ca^{2+} permeates neuronal nAChRs channels. Similarly, in whole-cell recordings, ACh evokes an inward current even when all external cations are replaced with Ca^{2+} (**Figure A9.1b**).

When habenula neurons are loaded with FURA-2 (see **Appendix 6.1**), an increase of [Ca^{2+}]$_i$ up to the micromolar range is observed upon acetylcholine application. This increase is reversibly abolished when Ca^{2+} is removed from the perfusion medium. To exclude a possible involvement of Ca^{2+} entry through voltage-gated Ca^{2+} channels opened by the depolarization subsequent to the activation of nAChRs, the membrane is clamped at −60 mV. In this condition, application of high K$^+$ (140 mM) external medium, which would depolarize a poorly clamped neuronal membrane, yields no detectable increase of [Ca^{2+}]$_i$. In contrast, application of nicotine evokes an inward whole-cell current and a concomitant rapid increase of [Ca^{2+}]$_i$ up to the micromolar range (**Figure A9.1c**).

For native neuronal nAChRs from α_7 gene product, another property is the very rapid desensitization of the whole cell current. For example in neurons of the chick peripheral nervous system (ciliary ganglion), fast perfusion of nicotine allows one to record a large quickly desensitizing current, strongly depressed by α-bungarotoxin (**Figure A9.2**).

In conclusion, neuronal nAChRs allow Ca^{2+} entry in the postsynaptic element at resting membrane potential.

They are in that sense similar to the subtype of AMPA receptors that are permeable to Ca²⁺ ions (glutamate receptors; see Section 11.2). Other Ca²⁺-permeable channels such as voltage-gated Ca²⁺ channels and NMDA receptors (glutamate receptors; see Section 11.4) require prior membrane depolarization to allow Ca²⁺ entry.

Further reading

Abakas MH, Kaufmann C, Archdeacon P, Karlin A (1995) Identification of acetylcholine receptor channel-lining residues in the entire M2 segment of the α subunit. *Neuron* **13**, 919–927.

Changeux JP, Edelstein SJ (1998) Allosteric receptors after 30 years. *Neuron* **21**, 959–980.

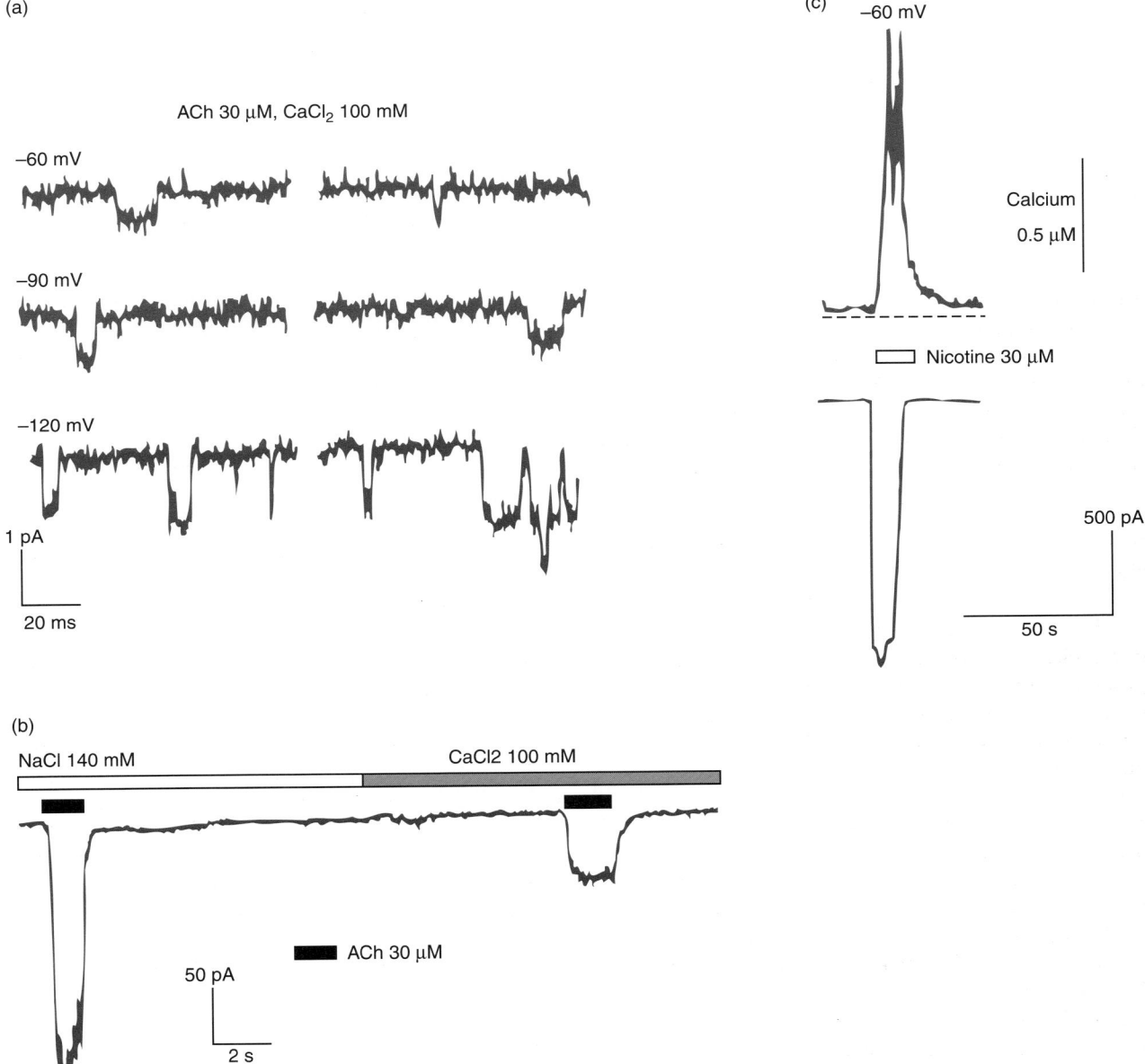

Figure A9.1 Ca²⁺ permeates neuronal nAChR channels.
(a) Single-channel currents evoked by ACh in outside-out patches of habenula neurons at three holding potentials (–60, –90, –120 mV) in the presence of a pure CaCl₂ external medium. (b) Whole-cell currents evoked by ACh in control (140 mM NaCl, 1 mM CaCl₂) and pure CaCl₂ medium. (c) Increase in [Ca²⁺]ᵢ (top trace) and whole-cell current (bottom trace) evoked by a 10 s application of nicotine (30 μM) at V_H = –60 mV. Adapted from Mulle C, Choquet D, Korn H, Changeux JP (1992) Calcium influx through nicotinic receptor in rat central neurons: its relevance to cellular regulation. *Neuron* **8**, 135–143, with permission.

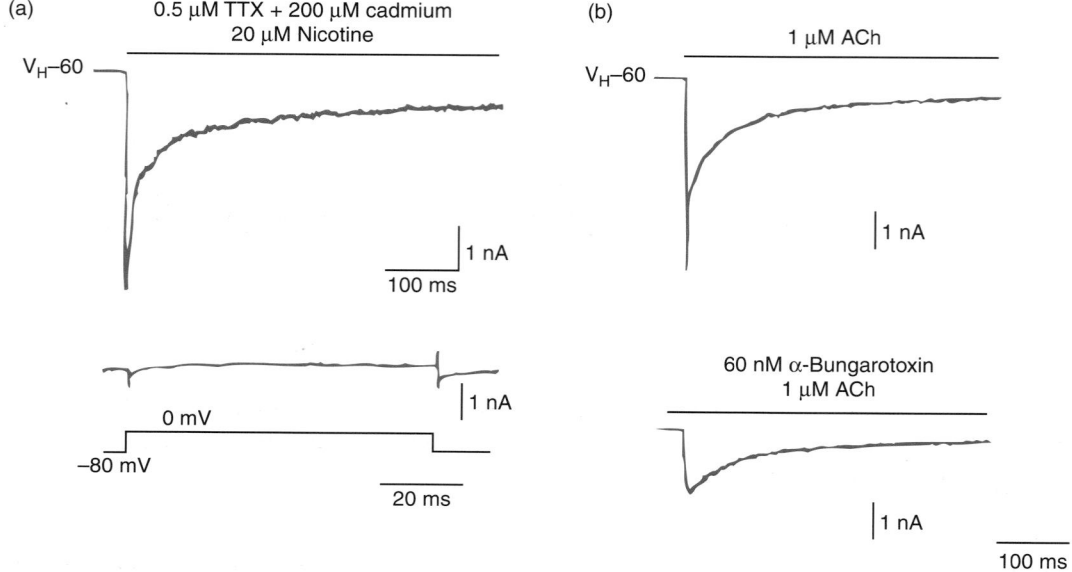

Figure A9.2 The neuronal nAChR-mediated whole-cell current sensitive to α-bungarotoxin rapidly desensitizes.
(a) Rapidly-decaying whole-cell current evoked by nicotine in the presence of blockers of Na⁺ and Ca²⁺ voltage-gated channels (top trace). The bottom traces show the absence of voltage-activated currents in response to a depolarizing pulse to 0 mV in these conditions (TTX + Cd²⁺). (b) The whole-cell current evoked by ACh is sensitive to α-bungarotoxin (incubated for 2 h before recording). Adapted from Zhang ZW, Vijayaraghavan S, Berg DK (1994) Neuronal acetylcholine receptors that bind α-bungarotoxin with high-affinity function as ligand-gated ion channels, *Neuron* **12**, 167–177, with permission.

Corringer PJ, Bertrand S, Bohler S *et al.* (1998) Critical elements determining diversity in agonist binding and desensitization of neuronal nicotinic acetylcholine receptors. *J. Neurosci.* **15**, 648–657.

Couturier S, Bertrand D, Matter JM *et al.* (1990) A neuronal nicotinic acetylcholine receptor subunit (α₇) is developmentally regulated and forms a homo-oligomeric channel blocked by α-BTX. *Neuron* **5**, 847–856.

Czajikowski C, Karlin A (1995) Structure of the nicotinic acetylcholine-binding site: identification of acidic residues in the δ subunit with 0.9 nm of the α subunit-binding site disulfide. *J. Biol. Chem.* **270**, 3160–3164.

Edelstein SJ, Changeux JP (1998) Allosteric transitions of the acetylcholine receptor. *Adv. Protein Chem.* **51**, 121–184.

Katz B, Miledi R (1973) The binding of acetylcholine to receptors and its removal from the synaptic cleft. *J. Physiol. (Lond.)* **231**, 549–574.

Leonard RJ, Labarca CG, Charnet P *et al.* (1988) Evidence that the M2 membrane-spanning region lines the ion channel pore of the nicotinic receptor. *Science* **242**, 1578–1581.

Monod J, Wyman J, Changeux JP (1965) On the nature of allosteric transitions: a plausible model. *J. Mol. Biol.* **12**, 88–118.

Murray N, Zheng YC, Mandel G *et al.* (1995) A single site on the ε subunit is responsible for the change in ACh receptor channel conductance during skeletal muscle development. *Neuron* **14**, 865–870.

The Ionotropic GABA$_A$ Receptor

K. Krnjevic and S. Schwartz observed in 1967 that γ-aminobutyric acid (GABA), applied by micro-iontophoresis on intracellularly recorded cortical neurons, evokes a hyperpolarization of the neuronal membrane which has properties similar to synaptically evoked hyperpolarization. This led to the hypothesis that GABA mediates inhibitory synaptic transmission in the *adult* vertebrate central nervous system.

GABA released by presynaptic terminals activates two main types of receptors: (i) ionotropic receptors called GABA$_A$ and GABA$_C$, which have different pharmacological properties (though GABA$_C$ receptors have been suggested to be a particular class of GABA$_A$, they will not be explained in this chapter); and (ii) metabotropic receptors, i.e. receptors coupled to GTP-binding proteins called GABA$_B$ receptors that are covered in Chapter 13.

The aim of the present chapter is to study how a GABA$_A$ receptor converts the binding of two GABA molecules to a rapid and transient hyperpolarization of the membrane in the *adult* vertebrate central nervous system. In the developing brain, however, GABA$_A$ receptors have a different function (see Chapter 23).

10.1 Observations and questions

In the rat hippocampus, in response to a single spike evoked in a presynaptic GABAergic interneuron, a transient hyperpolarization of the membrane mediated by GABA$_A$ receptors is recorded in the postsynaptic pyramidal cell (in the presence of blockers of GABA$_B$ receptors). This hyperpolarization of synaptic origin is called the 'single-spike inhibitory postsynaptic potential' (single-spike IPSP). A GABA$_A$-mediated IPSP has the following characteristics (**Figure 10.1**). It is:

- totally blocked in the presence of bicuculline thus showing it is mediated by GABA$_A$ receptors;
- potentiated by diazepam (a benzodiazepine, an anxiolytic and anticonvulsant drug);

- potentiated by pentobarbitone sodium (a barbiturate, a sedative and anticonvulsant drug).

These observations raise several questions:

- How does a GABA$_A$ receptor mediate the binding of GABA into a transient hyperpolarization of the membrane; i.e. what are the permeant ions, does GABA induce the entry of negatively charged ions or does it induce the exit of positively charged ions?
- Do benzodiazepines and barbiturates act directly on GABA$_A$ receptors? Are there selective and distinct binding sites on the receptor for each of these drugs? How do they potentiate the hyperpolarizing effect of GABA? Are there other modulators of GABA$_A$ receptors?

10.2 GABA$_A$ receptors are hetero-oligomeric proteins with a structural heterogeneity

10.2.1 The diversity of GABA$_A$ receptor subunits

The first subunits to be identified are α_1 and β_1. A GABA$_A$ receptor purified on affinity columns (see **Figures 9.4 and 9.5**) from calf, pig, rat or chick brain, dissociates in the presence of a detergent into two major subunits which migrate on polyacrylamide gels and have apparent molecular masses of 53 kD (α_1-subunit) and 56 kD (β_1-subunit). Electrophoretic studies based on receptors purified from different regions of the central nervous system show the presence of multiple bands corresponding to apparent molecular masses of 48–53 kD and of 55–57 kD. This strongly suggests the occurrence of several isoforms of α and β subunits.

Demonstration of the structural heterogeneity of the GABA$_A$ receptor came from cloning of cDNAs for different α (α_1–α_6) and β (β_1–β_3) subunits. The diversity of GABA$_A$ receptor subunits (α, β, γ, δ, ε, π, ρ) and the existence of different isoforms for the different subunits

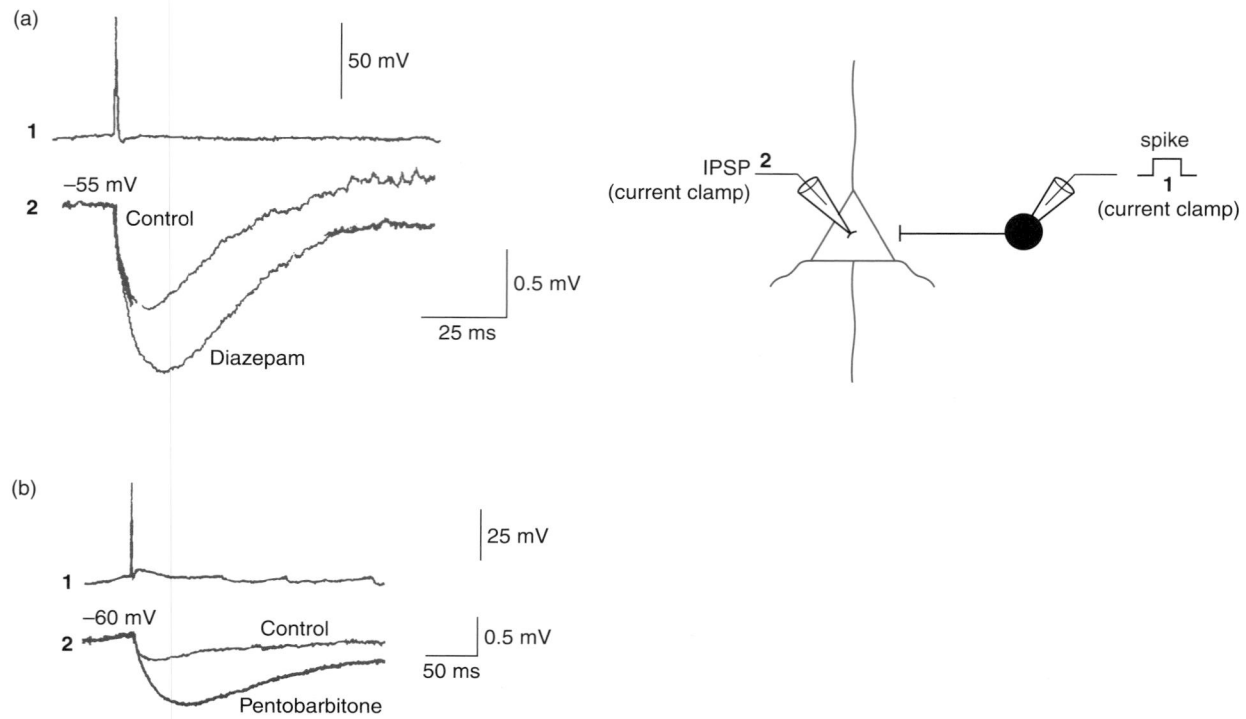

Figure 10.1 GABA$_A$ receptor-mediated IPSPs recorded in pyramidal cells of the hippocampus and two examples of their modulation.

The activity of a pair of connected neurons, a presynaptic GABAergic interneuron and postsynaptic pyramidal cell, is recorded with two intracellular electrodes. **(a)** A single spike is triggered in the presynaptic GABAergic interneuron in response to a current pulse (1). It evokes an IPSP (averaged single-spike IPSP; 2 control) in the postsynaptic pyramidal neuron. This IPSP is increased in amplitude and duration in the presence of a benzodiazepine (2; diazepam 1 μM). **(b)** Similar experiment in a different cell pair with pentobarbitone sodium (250 μM), a barbiturate. Adapted from Pawelzik H, Bannister AP, Deuchars J et al. (1999) Modulation of bistratified cell IPSPs and basket cell IPSP by pentobarbitone sodium, diazepam and Zn²⁺: dual recordings in slices of adult hippocampus, *Eur. J. Neurosci.* **11**, 3552–3564, with permission.

was then revealed (**Figure 10.2a**). All subunits are similar in size, contain about 450–550 amino acids and are strongly conserved among species. A high percentage of sequential identity (70–80%) is found between subunit isoforms (between α and between β isoforms for example). Sequential identity is also found, but to a lesser extent (30–40%), between subunit families.

The common elements of the subunit structure include (**Figures 10.2b and c**):

- a large N-terminal hydrophilic domain exposed to the synaptic cleft (extracellular);
- then four hydrophobic segments named M1 to M4, each composed of approximately 20 amino acids which form four putative membrane-spanning segments (TM1 to TM4).

The segment M2 of each of the subunits composing the GABA$_A$ receptor is thought to line the channel (as for the nAChR) and to contribute to ion selectivity and trans-

port. Apparently, a small number of amino acids within the M2 sequence is responsible for anionic versus cationic permeability (see Section 9.3.2 and Figure 9.16).

There is also a large, poorly conserved hydrophilic domain separating the M3 and M4 segments, located in the cytoplasm, which contains putative phosphorylation sites.

10.2.2 Subunit composition of native GABA$_A$ receptors and their binding characteristics

To form a GABA$_A$ receptor, with the large number of known subunits taken four or five at a time, thousands of combinations are possible. So far a total of six α, three β, three γ, one δ, one ε, one π and three ρ subunits of GABA receptors have been cloned and sequenced from the mammalian central nervous system. Two approaches are currently used to elucidate which subunit combinations exist:

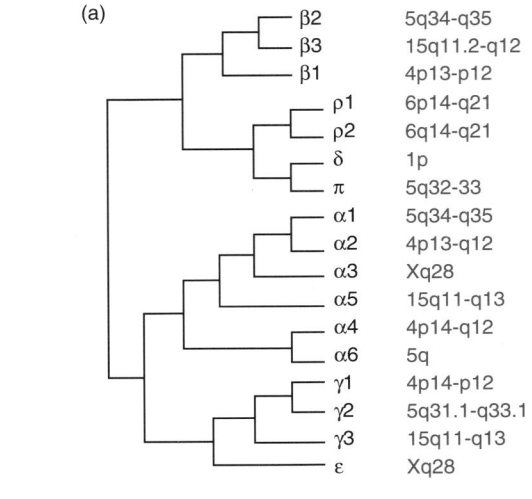

(a)

β2	5q34-q35
β3	15q11.2-q12
β1	4p13-p12
ρ1	6p14-q21
ρ2	6q14-q21
δ	1p
π	5q32-33
α1	5q34-q35
α2	4p13-q12
α3	Xq28
α5	15q11-q13
α4	4p14-q12
α6	5q
γ1	4p14-p12
γ2	5q31.1-q33.1
γ3	15q11-q13
ε	Xq28

(b)

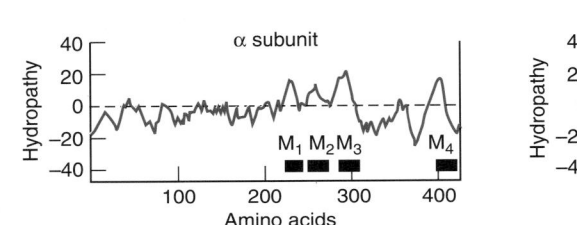
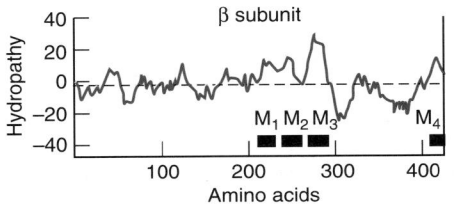

(c)

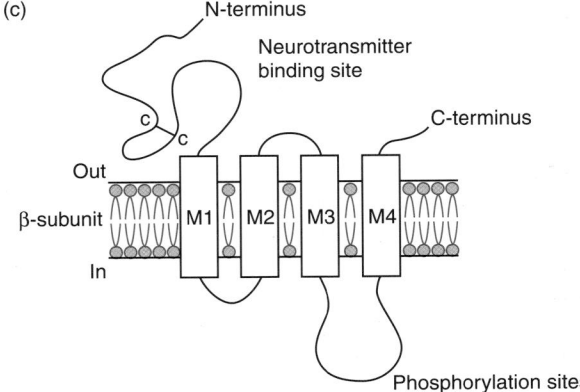

Figure 10.2 GABA$_A$ receptor subunits.
(a) The human GABA$_A$ receptor gene family. The dendrogram indicates the homologies between the deduced amino-acid sequences of the subunits. The human chromosome assigment of each gene is also indicated. (b) Hydropathy plots of an α and a β subunit of the GABA$_A$ receptor. The bars indicate the position of the hydrophobic segments (M1 to M4) assumed to span the lipid bilayer. The other regions are more hydrophilic. Note that the two subunits have similar hydropathic profiles. (c) Model of transmembrane organization of GABA$_A$ receptor subunits. The large hydrophilic N-terminal domain is exposed to the synaptic cleft and carries the neurotransmitter site and glycosylation sites. The four M segments span the membrane. The hydrophilic domain separating M3 and M4 faces the cytoplasm and contains phosphorylation sites. The C-terminus is extracellular. Part (a) adapted from Whiting PJ, Bonnert TP, McKernan RM *et al.* (1999) Molecular and functional diversity of the expanding GABA-A receptor gene family, *Ann. NY Acad. Sci.* **868**, 645–653, with permission. Part (b) from Barnard EA, Darlison MG, Seeburg P (1987) Molecular biology of the GABA$_A$ receptor: the receptor channel superfamily, *TINS* **10**, 502–509, with permission. Part (c) from Lovinger DM (1997) Alcohols and neurotransmitter gated ion channels: past, present and future, *Naunyn-Schmiederberg's Arch Pharmacol* **356**, 267–282, with permission.

- a comparative study of the functional properties of receptors expressed in oocytes or in transfected mammalian cells from known combinations of cloned subunits (with the restriction that *Xenopus* oocyte does not automatically assemble a channel composed of all injected subunits);
- a comparative study of the distribution of the various subunit mRNAs in the brain using the *in situ* hybridization technique (see Appendix 7.2).

Surprisingly, the transient expression in transfected cells of identical α or β subunits gives functional homomeric GABA$_A$ receptors; i.e. receptors which induce a current in the presence of GABA. This current is blocked by GABA$_A$ antagonists and potentiated by barbiturates but is unaffected by benzodiazepines. These properties can be attributed to the conserved structural features of all the subunits. However, these channels resulting from expression of single subunits are assembled inefficiently (are rare and slightly detectable) and it is unlikely that native receptors are formed from identical subunits. Expression of a γ-subunit together with an α- and a β-subunit in transfected cells gives rise to the expression of a GABA$_A$ receptor with all the features of the homomeric receptor with in addition the sensitivity to benzodiazepines. This does not necessarily imply that the receptor site for benzodiazepines is situated on the γ-subunit, but that expression of the latter is required for the action of benzodiazepines. The conclusion of these studies is that the combination αβγ is the minimal requirement for reproducing consensus properties known for the vertebrate GABA$_A$ receptor-channel *in situ*. For example, α$_{1/2}$β$_{2/3}$γ$_2$ coexist in most of the native GABA$_A$ receptors. In contrast, ρ-subunits seem not to combine with other classes of GABA$_A$ receptor subunits. Receptor assemblies derived from various isoforms of the ρ-subunit are suggested to be classified as GABA$_C$ receptors which may be a specialized set of GABA$_A$ receptors.

10.3 Binding of two GABA molecules leads to a conformational change of the GABA$_A$ receptor into an open state; the GABA$_A$ receptor desensitizes

10.3.1 GABA binding site

The amino acids identified by site-directed mutagenesis to affect channel activation by GABA are in the β-subunit: tyrosine (Y) 157, threonine (T) 160, threonine (T) 202 and tyrosine (Y) 206 (**Figure 10.3**). Mutations of the corresponding tyrosines in the α and γ subunits do not play a role in GABA-mediated activation. In the α$_1$-sub-

unit, the mutation of phenylalanine (F) 64 to leucine (L) impairs activation of the GABA channel indicating a role for this α-subunit residue in GABA binding. Therefore, two identified domains (loops B and C) of the β-subunit and at least one domain (loop D) for the neighbouring α-subunit contribute to the GABA-binding site. It is thought that most αβγ receptors are pentameric and have the stoichiometry 2α, 2β and 1γ. This is consistent with data indicating that GABA sites are located at the interface between α and β subunits and that there are two GABA sites per receptor (see below). GABA$_A$ receptors have a relatively low affinity for GABA, of the order of 10–20 μM.

10.3.2 Evidence for the binding of two GABA molecules

Analysis of dose–response curves suggests the binding of two GABA molecules prior to opening of the channel. The response studied, the peak amplitude of the total current I_{GABA} evoked by GABA in whole-cell patch-clamp recording, is proportional to the square of the dose of GABA (but only at low doses of GABA):

$$I_{GABA} = f[GABA]^2.$$

At very low doses of GABA, when receptor desensitization is negligible, it seems that upon binding of two GABA molecules to the receptor, the conformational change of the receptor channel to an open state is favoured. These observations can be accounted for by the following model:

$$2G + R \underset{k_{-1}}{\overset{k_1}{\rightleftharpoons}} G + GR \underset{k_{-2}}{\overset{k_2}{\rightleftharpoons}} G_2R \underset{\alpha}{\overset{\beta}{\rightleftharpoons}} G_2R^*$$

where G is GABA; R is the GABA$_A$ receptor in closed configuration; GR or G$_2$R is the mono- or doubly liganded GABA$_A$ receptor in the closed configuration; and G$_2$R* is the doubly liganded GABA$_A$ receptor in the open configuration.

10.3.3 The GABA$_A$ channel is selectively permeable to Cl$^-$ ions

The reversal potential of the GABA current varies with the Cl$^-$ equilibrium potential, E_{Cl}

The ionic selectivity of the channel is studied in outside-out patch-clamp recording from cultured spinal neurons. This patch-clamp configuration allows control of the membrane potential as well as the composition of

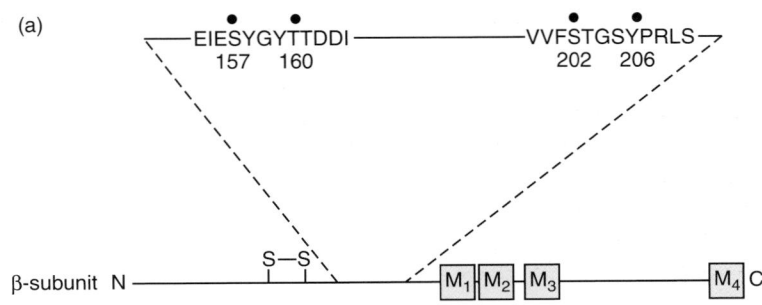

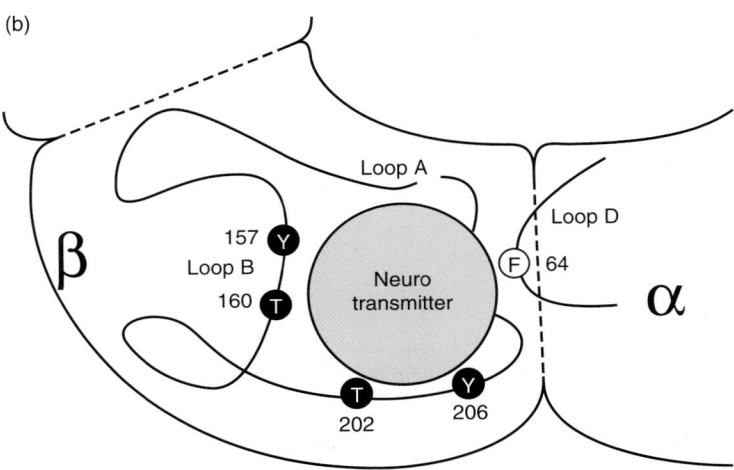

Figure 10.3 GABA binding site on the GABA$_A$ receptor.
(a) Linear representation of the β$_2$-subunit. The amino acids crucial for GABA-dependent gating (black dots) are located in the N-terminal hydrophilic domain between the disulphide bridge and the first membrane spanning segment M1. **(b)** Model of the GABA binding site. The amino acids labelled belong to different regions of the N-terminal extracellular domain of β-subunits and to one domain of α-subunits. Part (a) adapted from Amin J, Weiss DS (1993) GABA$_A$ receptor needs two homologous domains of the β-subunit for activation by GABA but not by pentobarbital, *Nature* **366**, 565–569, with permission. Part (b) from Galzi JL, Changeux JP (1994) Neurotransmitter-gated ion channels as unconventional allosteric proteins, *Curr. Opin. Neurobiol.* **4**, 554–565, with permission.

the intracellular fluid. When the intracellular and extracellular fluids contain the same Cl$^-$ concentration (145 mM), the unitary current evoked by GABA reverses at E_{rev} = 0 mV (**Figures 10.4a–c** and **10.6a**). In this case E_{Cl} is also equal to 0 mV:

$$E_{Cl} = -58 \log (145/145) = 0 \text{ mV}.$$

If part of the intracellular Cl$^-$ is replaced with non-permeant anions such as isethionate (HO-CH$_2$-CH$_2$-SO$_3^-$), for a 10-fold change in intracellular Cl$^-$ concentration a shift in the reversal potential of approximately 56 mV is observed (**Figure 10.4d**). This value approaches very closely that of 58 mV predicted by the Nernst equation for E_{Cl} at 20°C:

$$E_{Cl} = -58 \log (145/14.5) = -58 \text{ mV}.$$

Finally, changes in extracellular Na$^+$ or K$^+$ concentration have very little effect on the reversal potential of the GABA$_A$ response. Taken together, these results demonstrate that the GABA$_A$ channel is selectively permeable to Cl$^-$.

In physiological extracellular and intracellular solutions, the GABA$_A$ current recorded in isolated spinal neurons reverses at –60 mV

Using the technique of patch-clamp recording one can record the unitary currents (i_{GABA}) across the GABA$_A$

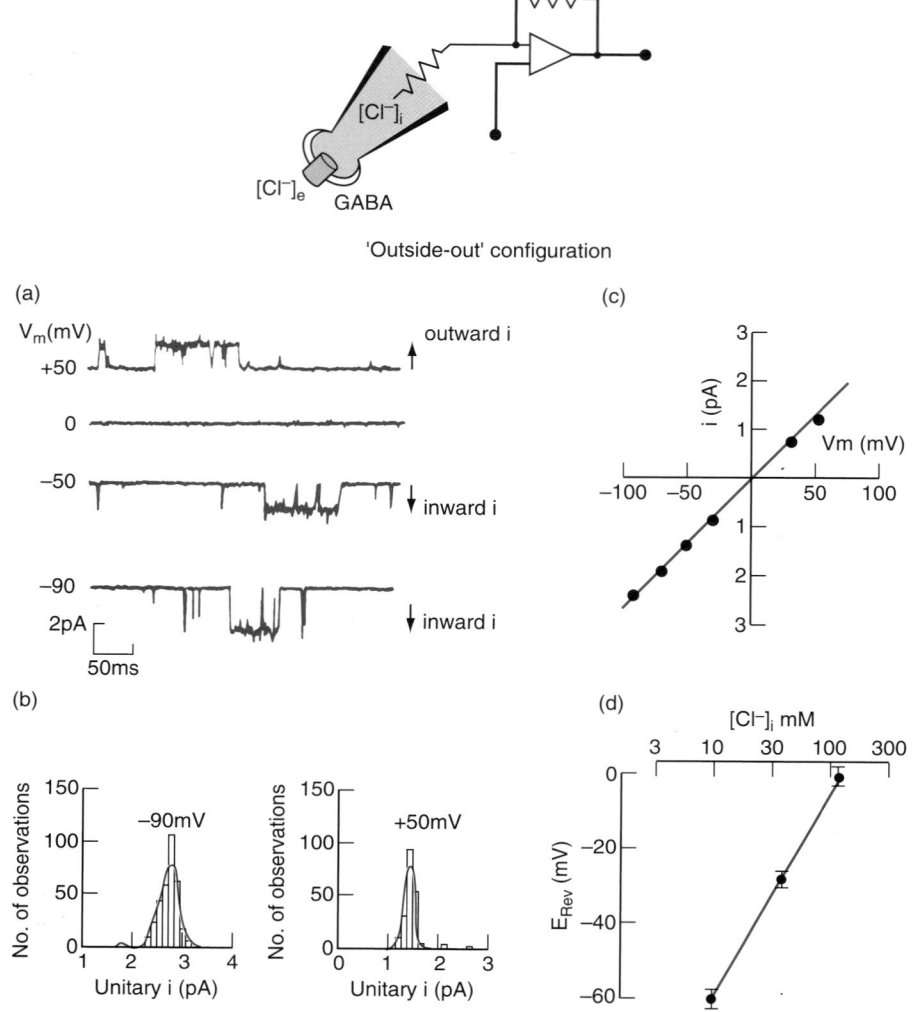

'Outside-out' configuration

Figure 10.4 Variations of the reversal potential of the GABA$_A$ response as a function of the Cl$^-$ equilibrium potential.
The single-channel current i flowing across the GABA$_A$ channel is recorded in cultured mouse spinal neurons (outside-out patch-clamp recording; equal concentrations of Cl$^-$ on both sides of the patch: 145 mM). **(a)** In the presence of GABA (10 mM), the single-channel current i is outward at V_m = +50 mV (upward deflection), null at V_m = 0 mV and inward at V_m = −50 mV or −90 mV (downward deflections). **(b)** The distribution of single channel currents i in different patches of membrane held at V_m = −90 mV (left) and +50 mV (right) shows the existence of a single peak of current of −2.70 ± 0.17 pA and 1.48 ± 0.10 pA, respectively. These two values give a single channel conductance γ equal to 30 pS ($\gamma = i/V_m$ as E_{rev} = 0 mV). **(c)** i/V curve obtained by averaging the most frequently observed single-channel currents. It is a straight line according to the equation $i = \gamma(V_m - E_{rev})$. The relationship is linear between V_m = −90 mV and +50 mV and the slope is γ = 30 pS. **(d)** Reversal potential of the GABA$_A$ response (in mV) as a function of the intracellular Cl$^-$ concentration [Cl$^-$]$_i$ (in mM). Each point represents the mean value of E_{rev} from four different cells. Note that, at the three [Cl$^-$]$_i$ tested, E_{rev} (experimental value) is very close to E_{Cl} (calculated by the Nernst equation):

[Cl$^-$]$_i$ (mM)	E_{Cl} (mV)	E_{rev} (mV)
14.5	−58	−56
45	−29	−28
145	0	0

Parts (a)–(c) adapted from Borman J, Hamill OP, Sakmann B (1987) Mechanism of anion permeation through channels gated by glycine and γ-aminobutyric acid in mouse cultured spinal neurones, *J. Physiol. (Lond.)* **385**, 246–286, with permission. Part (d) from Sakmann B, Borman J, Hamill OP (1983) Ion transport by single receptor channels, *Cold Spring Harbor Symposia in Quantitative Biology* **XLVIII**, 247–257, with permission.

channel (spinal neurones in culture, cell-attached configuration). The GABA present in the solution inside the recording pipette (5 μM) evokes outward single-channel currents at –30, 0 and +20 mV (**Figure 10.5a**). The magnitude of the single-channel current increases with depolarization, suggesting that the reversal potential for the GABA$_A$ response is negative to –30 mV. The i/V curve, obtained by plotting the unitary current i_{GABA} against the membrane potential V, shows in this experiment a reversal potential of the GABA-induced current around –60 mV (**Figure 10.5**). Thus, at a potential close to the resting membrane potential (–60 mV) the current evoked by GABA is not detectable. At potentials more depolarized than rest (for example –30 mV) (**Figure 10.6b**), an outward current is recorded whose magnitude increases with depolarization of the postsynaptic membrane.

As E_{Cl} is close to the resting membrane potential (–60 mV) in physiological intracellular and extracellular solutions, the electrochemical gradient for the Cl$^-$ ions $(V_m - E_{Cl})$ for $V_m = -60$ mV $= E_{Cl}$, is close to 0 mV. The net flux of Cl$^-$ ions at a potential close to rest is therefore null or very small: no current is recorded even though the GABA$_A$ channels are open. On the other hand, as the membrane potential depolarizes, the net flux of Cl$^-$ ions becomes inward. An inward net flux of negative charges corresponds to an outward current. At potentials more depolarized than V_{rest}, an outward current is recorded (**Figure 10.5**). At potentials more hyperpolarized than –60 mV, i_{GABA} is inward (the net flux of Cl$^-$ ions is outward) but of very small amplitude.

10.3.4 The single-channel conductance of GABA$_A$ channels is constant in symmetrical Cl$^-$ solutions, but varies as a function of potential in asymmetrical solutions

Experiments have been performed on mouse spinal neurons in culture, in conditions of equal intra- and extracellular Cl$^-$ concentration (145 mM) to minimize

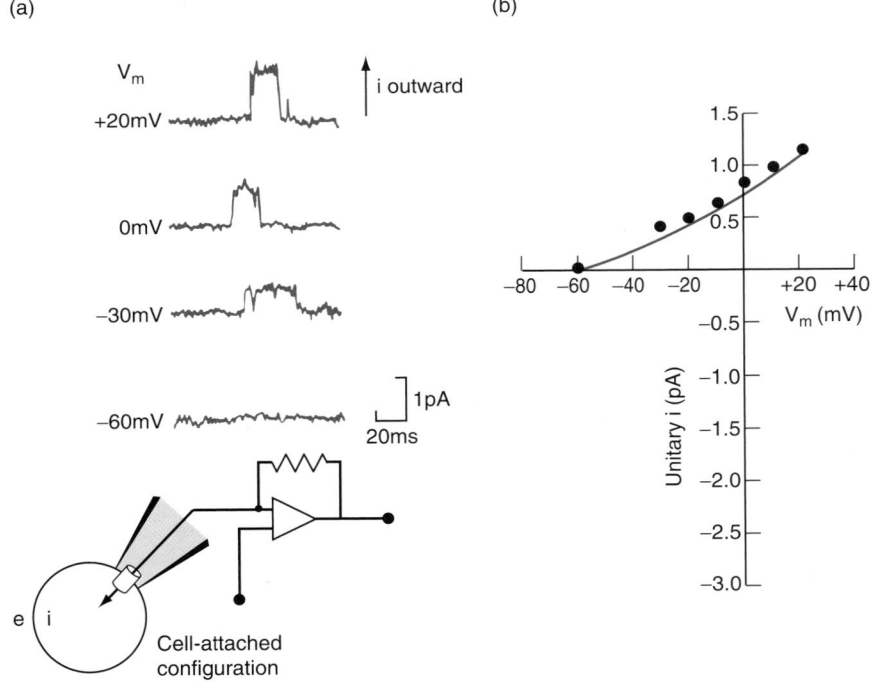

(a)   (b)

Figure 10.5 Activity of a single GABA$_A$ receptor channel in physiological solutions.
The single-channel GABA$_A$ current recorded in cell-attached configuration in rat spinal neurons. **(a)** At $V_m = -30$, 0 and +20 mV respectively, the GABA present in the patch pipette at a concentration of 10 μM elicits an outward current (upward deflection). This current increases with depolarization of the patch. At $V_m = -60$ mV, no current is recorded. **(b)** i/V curve obtained by plotting the amplitude of the recorded unitary current i (pA) against the membrane potential V_m (mV). The intracellular medium is the physiological cytosol and the extracellular or intrapipette solution contains 144.6 mM Cl$^-$. The intracellular Cl$^-$ concentration is estimated at 13 mM, which gives a value of –60 mV for the Cl$^-$ reversal potential: $E_{Cl} = -58 \log (144.6/13) = -60$ mV. As all Na$^+$ ions are replaced by K$^+$ ions in the extracellular solution, the K$^+$ concentration is similar in both solutions, which gives a reversal potential for the K$^+$ current near 0 mV. The membrane potential values indicated in (a) and (b) are evaluated on the basis that the value 0 mV is the potential at which the K$^+$ currents across the K$^+$ channels are zero. From Sakmann B, Bormann J, Hamill OP (1983) Ion transport by single receptor channels, *Cold Spring Harbor Symposia in Quantitative Biology* **XLVIII**, 247–257, with permission.

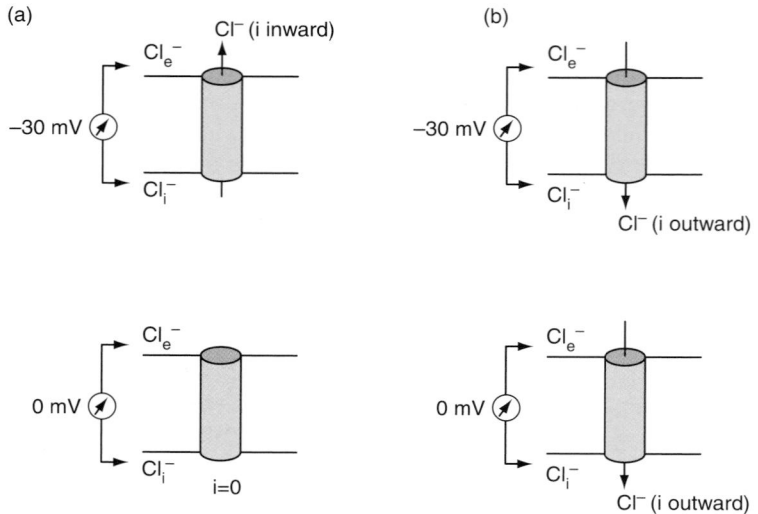

Figure 10.6 Variations of the flux of Cl⁻ ions as a function of membrane potential and intracellular and extracellular Cl⁻ concentrations.

(a) Symmetrical media: $[Cl^-]_e = [Cl^-]_i = 145$ mM; $E_{Cl} = 0$ mV. (b) Physiological media: $[Cl^-]_e = 145$ mM; $[Cl^-]_i = 14.5$ mM; $E_{Cl} = -58$ mV.

rectification (variation of conductance γ as a function of membrane potential). Histograms of single-channel currents evoked by GABA and recorded at $V_m = +50$ mV (outward i_{GABA}) and $V_m = -90$ mV (inward i_{GABA}) show at each potential a single peak of current equal to +1.48 and −2.7 pA respectively (**Figure 10.4b**). From these values of i_{GABA}, the mean single-channel conductance γ can be calculated, as $i_{GABA} = \gamma_{GABA}(V_m - E_{rev})$ and $E_{rev} = 0$ mV in these conditions. A value of 30 pS is obtained for both experimental conditions. This value of γ_{GABA} is also the slope of the i_{GABA}/V curve obtained by averaging the most frequent single-channel current i_{GABA} recorded at each membrane potential studied. This curve, based on the equation $i = \gamma(V_m - E_{rev})$ is linear between −90 mV and +50 mV and has a slope of 30 pS (**Figure 10.4c**).

However, in physiological conditions, when Cl⁻ concentration is approximately 10-fold lower in the intracellular than in the extracellular fluid, the unitary conductance γ_{GABA} varies with the membrane potential. The conductance in fact decreases progressively as the outward Cl⁻ current decreases (**Figure 10.5b**). This phenomenon is called *rectification*. This rectification (nonsymmetrical inward and outward currents) results from the difference in Cl⁻ concentration on either side of the membrane.

10.3.5 Mean open time of the GABA$_A$ channel

With patch-clamp recording of GABA$_A$ channels (in chromaffin cells of the adrenal medulla or cultured hippocampal neurones, in outside-out configuration),

two types of openings are observed in the presence of low concentrations of GABA (**Figure 10.7a**): (i) brief openings, and (ii) longer duration openings interrupted by brief periods of closure: such a group of repeated openings and closures is called a burst of openings.

Brief openings (triangles)

Brief openings have a mean duration, τ_o, of 2.5 ms and contribute little to the total current.

Bursts of openings (open circles)

A burst is defined as a sequence of openings each one having a duration t_o, separated by brief closures of duration t_c. Brief durations are defined as less than 5 ms in the example illustrated in **Figure 10.7**. The duration of each burst t_b is $\Sigma t_o + \Sigma t_c$ and its mean duration τ_b is equal to 20–50 ms depending on the preparation used (**Figure 10.7b**). The openings and the brief closures observed within each burst in the presence of GABA are thought to correspond to fluctuations of the receptor between the double-liganded open state and the double-liganded closed state (before the two molecules of GABA leave the receptor site). Thus, upon a single activation by two molecules of GABA, the double-liganded receptor would open and close several times:

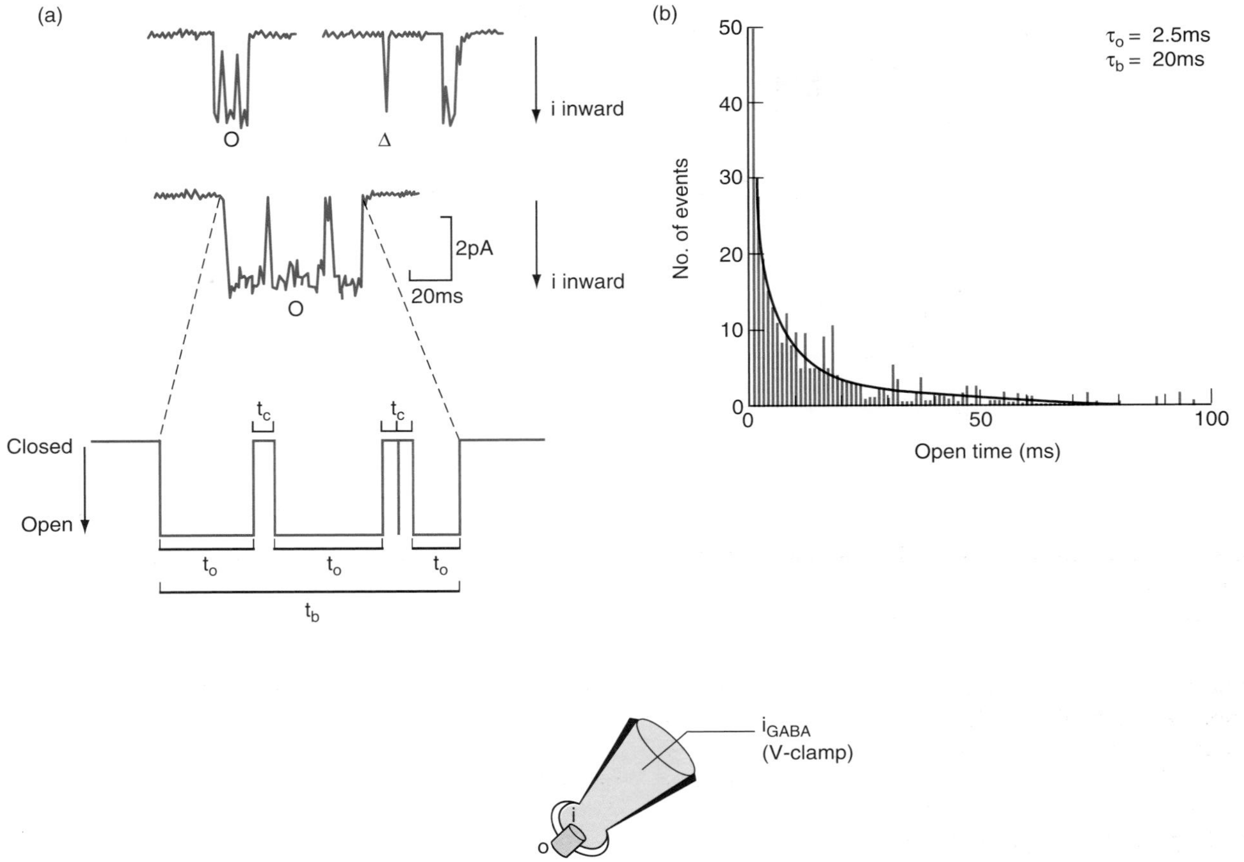

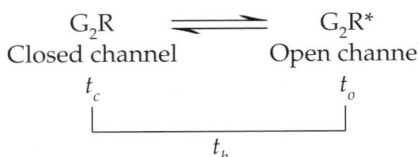

Figure 10.7 Mean open time of GABA$_A$ channels.
Patch-clamp recording of the activity of the GABA$_A$ receptor channels from chromaffin cells of the adrenal medulla (outside-out configuration). The intracellular and extracellular Cl$^-$ concentrations are similar and the membrane potential is maintained at −70 mV. **(a)** Inward unitary currents through a single GABA$_A$ channel evoked by GABA (10 µM). Brief openings (triangle) and bursts of openings (O, long duration openings interrupted by short closures defined in this experiment as less than 5 ms). **(b)** Histogram of open times measured in a homogeneous population of channels (mean value of i = −2.9 pA). The open times plotted on the graph represent the duration of short openings (t_o) and the duration of bursts of openings (t_b). The histogram is described by the sum of two exponentials with decay time constants of τ_o = 2.5 ms and τ_b = 20 ms. τ_o corresponds to the mean open time of short openings and τ_b to the mean open time of bursts of openings. From Borman J, Clapham DE (1985) γ-aminobutyric acid receptor channels in adrenal chromaffin cells: a patch clamp study, *Proc. Natl Acad. Sci. USA* **82**, 2168–2172, with permission.

$$G_2R \rightleftharpoons G_2R^*$$

Closed channel	Open channel
t_c	t_o

$$t_b$$

Silent periods

Silent periods separate single openings or bursts; they are periods during which the channel is closed and the unitary current is zero. In the presence of very low concentrations of GABA (when the receptor has a low probability to desensitize) they correspond to the G$_2$R, GR and R states of the GABA$_A$ receptor.

If one compares the opening characteristics of the GABA$_A$ receptor with those of the nicotinic receptor (see Section 9.3.3), one finds that they are very similar. However, the short openings observed within bursts are approximately twice as abundant in the case of the GABA$_A$ receptor. This implies that opening (β) and closing (α) rate constants have much closer values in the case of the GABA$_A$ receptor (see Appendix 10.1) than in the case of the nicotinic receptor (Appendix 5.3).

10.3.6 The GABA$_A$ receptor desensitizes

Recordings in outside-out configuration show a rundown of the frequency of opening of the GABA$_A$ channels upon prolonged application of GABA (0.5 µM), whereas neither the intensity of the unitary current nor the mean open time of the channels τ_o appears to be affected (**Figure 10.8a**). Considering that $I = Np_oi$, if p_o (open probability of the channel) decreases as a result of a decrease in the frequency of opening events, the current I_{GABA} decreases even though i_{GABA} remains constant. Similarly, G_{GABA}, the total conductance, decreases (since

$G = Np_o\gamma$). As the GABA$_A$ receptors gradually desensitize, p_o becomes progressively smaller with time, and I_{GABA} as well as G_{GABA} gradually decrease to practically zero.

This is confirmed in recordings of the total current I_{GABA} evoked by a prolonged application of GABA: the amplitude of I_{GABA} decreases with time

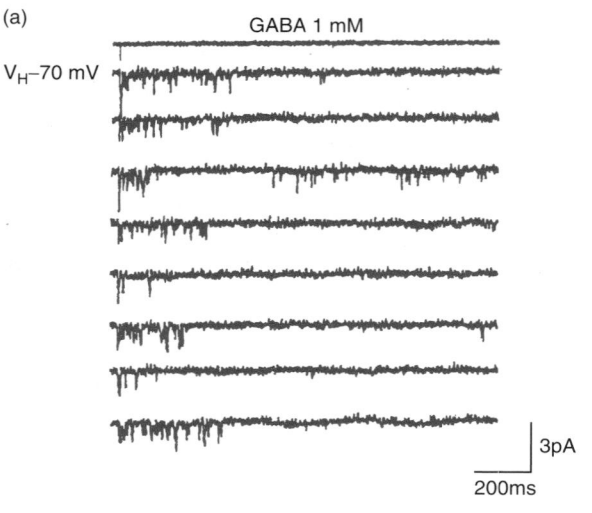

(a)

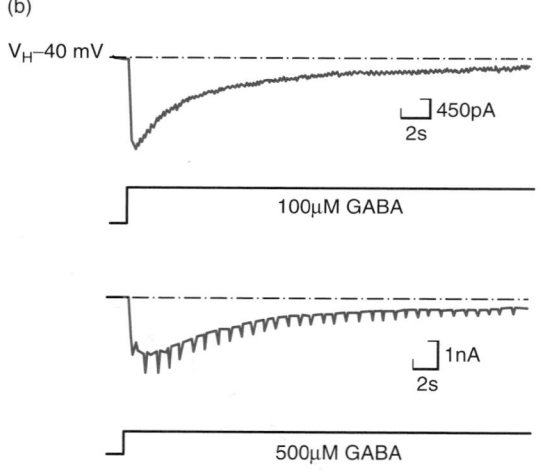

(b)

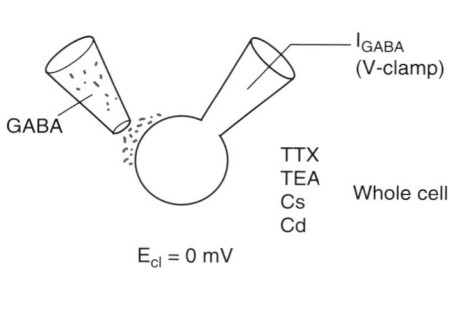

Figure 10.8 Desensitization of the GABA$_A$ receptor.
(a) Outside-out patch excised from a cell transfected with $\alpha_1\beta_2\gamma_2$ cDNAs. A 2 ms pulse of GABA (1 mM) evokes single GABA$_A$ channel activity. (**b**, top) Patch clamp recording (whole-cell configuration, $V_H = -40$ mV) from a chick cerebral neuron. A prolonged application of GABA at high concentration (100 μM) evokes a total current I_{GABA} which decreases with time to almost zero. The total current I_{GABA} corresponds to the sum of the unitary currents i_{GABA}, passing through the open GABA$_A$ channels, while the other currents have been blocked with TTX and TEA as well as with Cs$^+$ and Cd^{2+} ions. (**b**, bottom) The same experiment in the presence of 500 μM of GABA and with hyperpolarizing voltage steps applied at a constant rate. The decrease in amplitude of the step current during the GABA$_A$ response shows that the decrease of I_{GABA} is associated with a decrease in G_m (as $i_{step} = G_mV_{step}$, V_{step} being constant), a decrease of i_{step} implies a decrease of G_m. There are symmetrical Cl$^-$ concentrations in (a) and (b). Part (a) from Zhu WJ, Wang JF, Corsi L, Vicini S (1998) Lanthanum-mediated modification of GABA$_A$ receptor deactivation, desensitization and inhibitory synaptic currents in rat cerebellar neurons, *J. Physiol. (Lond.)* **511**, 647–661, with permission. Part (b) from Weiss DS, Barnes EM, Hablitz JJ (1988) Whole-cell and single-channel recordings of GABA-gated currents in cultured chick cerebral neurons, *J. Neurophysiol.* **59**, 495–513, with permission.

as well as G_{GABA} (**Figure 10.8b**). This rundown of the GABA$_A$ response which increases with increasing concentrations of GABA is largely attributed to the desensitization of the GABA$_A$ receptor. Therefore, upon long-lasting activation by GABA, the doubly liganded receptor goes into at least one desensitization state:

States of the doubly liganded receptor:

$$G_2R \underset{\alpha}{\overset{\beta}{\rightleftharpoons}} G_2R^* \underset{k_{-3}}{\overset{k_3}{\rightleftharpoons}} G_2D$$

State of the channel: closed   open   closed

10.4 Pharmacology of the GABA$_A$ receptor

Benzodiazepines, barbiturates and neurosteroids enhance GABA$_A$ receptor current, whereas bicuculline, picrotoxin and β-carbolines reduce GABA$_A$ current, by binding to specific sites on the GABA$_A$ receptor channels.

10.4.1 Bicuculline and picrotoxin reversibly decrease total GABA$_A$ current; they are respectively competitive and non-competitive antagonists of the GABA$_A$ receptor

Excised outside-out patches are obtained from spinal cord neurons and held at −75 mV to prevent spontaneous openings of voltage-gated channels

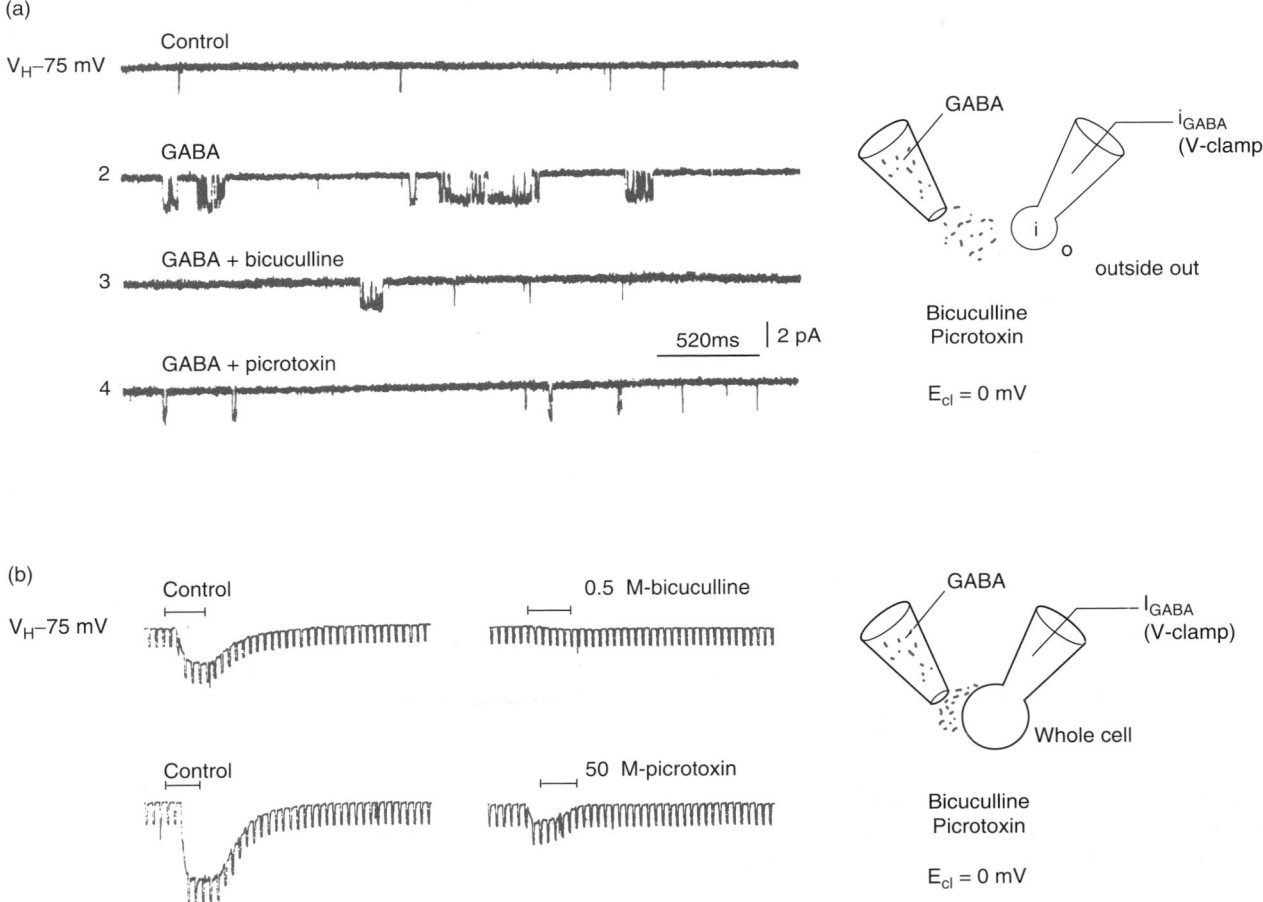

Figure 10.9 Antagonists of the GABA$_A$ receptor.
(a) Activity of an outside-out patch from spinal cord neurons recorded in symmetrical Cl⁻ solutions. GABA (2 μM) is applied in the presence of bicuculline (0.2 μM) or picrotoxin (10 μM). **(b)** The same experiment in the whole-cell configuration. Steps are applied as in Figure 10.8 to evaluate membrane conductance G_m during the response. Adapted from MacDonald RL, Rogers CJ, Twyman RE (1989) Kinetic properties of the GABA$_A$ receptor main conductance state of mouse spinal cord neurones in culture, *J. Physiol. (Lond.)* **410**, 479–499, with permission.

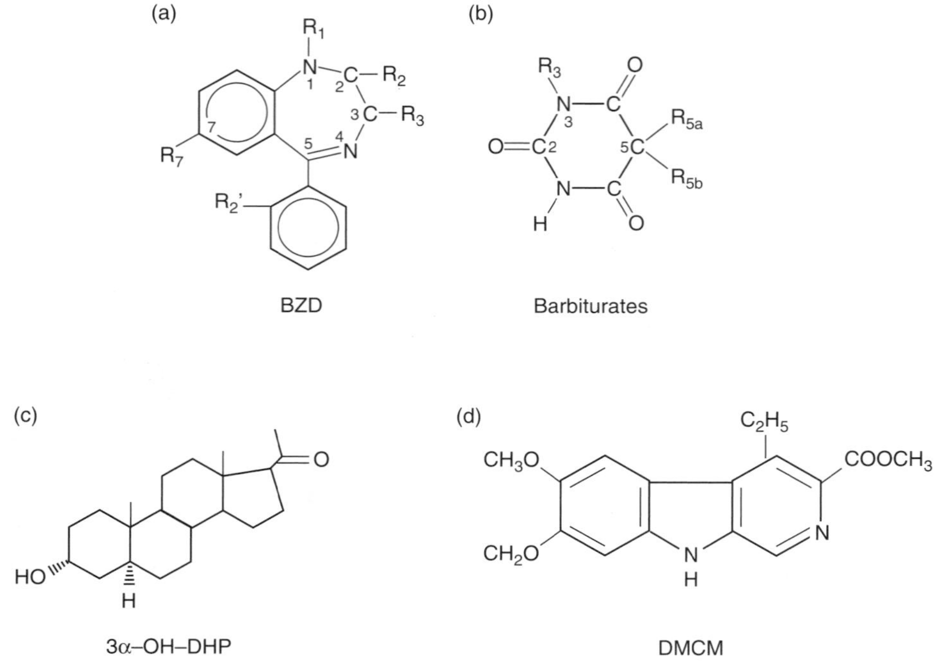

Figure 10.10 Allosteric modulators of the GABA$_A$ receptor.
(a) Structure of benzodiazepines (BZD). For diazepam, the radicals are: R_1 = CH$_3$, R_2 = O, R_3 = H, R_7 = Cl, R_2' = H. **(b)** Structure of barbituric acid derivatives. For phentobarbital, the radicals are: R_{5a} = ethyl, R_{5b} = H and R_3 = phenyl. **(c)** Structure of a neurosteroid, allopregnanolone (3α-OH-DHP). **(d)** Structure of a β-carboline, methyl 6, 7-dimethoxy-4-ethyl β-carboline 3 carboxylate (DMCM).

(Figure 10.9a). Recordings are performed in symmetrical chloride solutions. Prior to GABA application, occasional brief spontaneous currents are recorded (1). Following GABA (2 μM) application, bursting inward chloride currents are evoked (2). These GABA-induced bursting currents are reversibly reduced in frequency by the concomitant application of bicuculline (3; 0.2 μM) or picrotoxin (4; 10 μM). In whole-cell recordings, this effect is recorded as a decrease of the amplitude of the total current I_{GABA}: if p_o decreases, $Np_oi_{GABA} = I_{GABA}$ decreases **(Figure 10.9b)**.

When the dose of GABA is increased and the dose of antagonist is kept constant, the inhibition by bicuculline is reduced whereas that by picrotoxin is unchanged (not shown). This shows that bicuculline is a competitive antagonist whereas picrotoxin is a non-competitive antagonist. Bicuculline binds to the same receptor sites as GABA. It is selective for the GABA$_A$ receptor and therefore serves as a good tool to identify GABA$_A$-mediated responses. Picrotoxin in contrast binds to the ionic channel (it is a channel blocker). Its binding site involves the M2 segment, the region thought to line the chloride ion channel. In insects, resistance to picrotoxin (used as an insecticide) can be conferred to a single amino acid substitution in the M2 segment sequence: alanine 302 replaced by serine. Both bicuculline and picrotoxin are potent convulsants when administered intravenously or intraventricularly.

10.4.2 Benzodiazepines, barbiturates and neurosteroids reversibly potentiate total GABA$_A$ current; they are allosteric agonists at the GABA$_A$ receptor

Benzodiazepines and barbiturates are two classes of clinically active agents **(Figures 10.10a and b)**. Barbiturates are hypnotic and antiepileptic agents and the benzodiazepines are anxiolytic agents, muscle relaxants and anticonvulsants. Various progesterone metabolites that are synthesized in the brain and thus called neurosteroids act directly on the GABA$_A$ receptor. One example is allopregnanolone **(Figure 10.10c)**.

Benzodiazepines, barbiturates and neurosteroids bind to the GABA$_A$ receptor at specific receptor sites

First, it was shown that co-expression of α or β subunits with a γ-subunit is required for the positive modulation of GABA-evoked Cl⁻ currents by benzodiazepines and for photoaffinity labelling of the benzodiazepine receptor site (see Section 10.2.2). With site-directed mutagenesis, His 101 and Gly 200 amino acid residues of the α-subunit and Phe 77, Met 130 and Thr 142 amino acid residues of the γ-subunit are reported to be key determinants of the benzodiazepine site of the rat

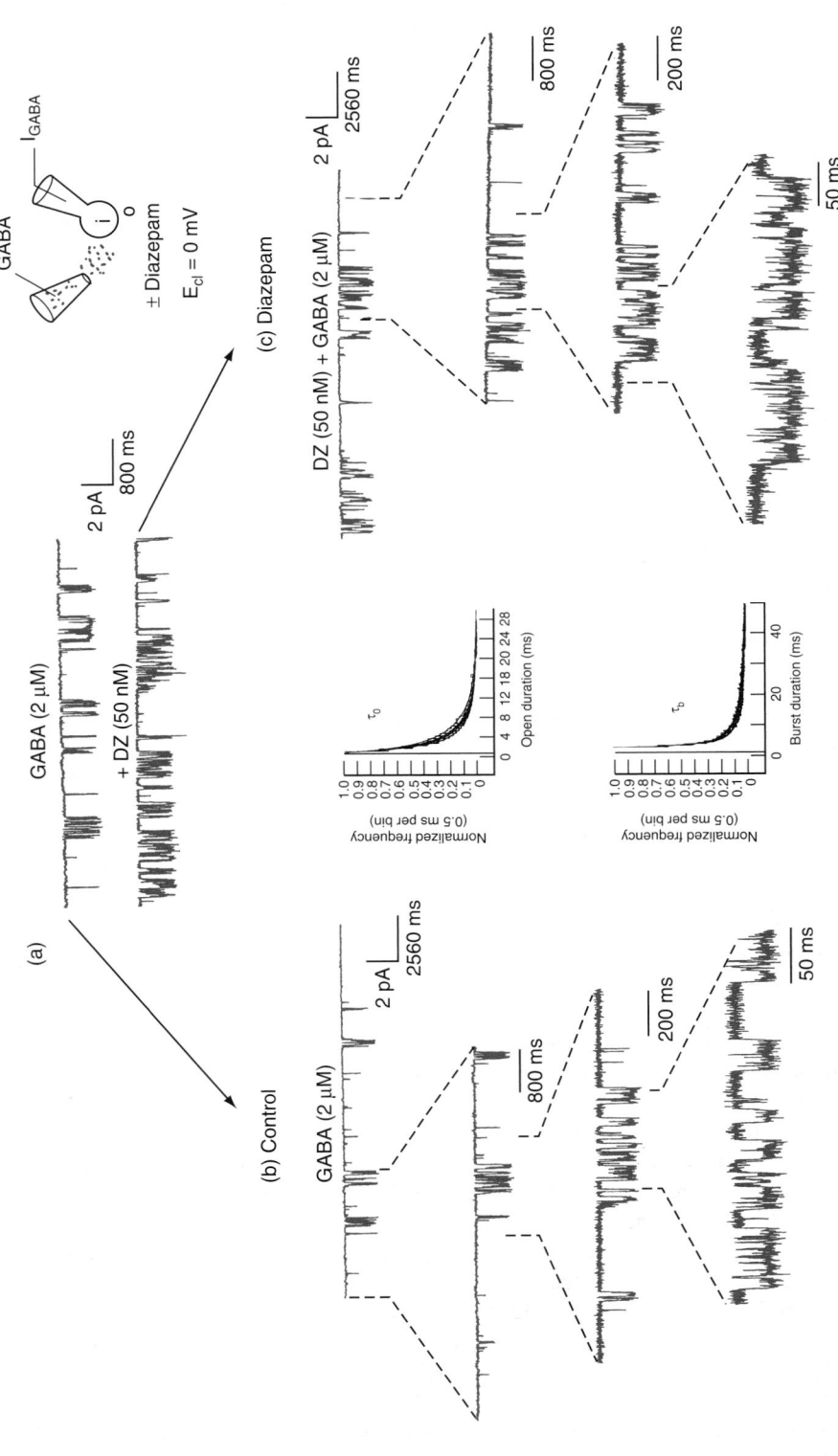

Figure 10.11 GABA_A single-channel current in the presence or absence of diazepam.
(a) Bursting inward currents in outside-out patches from spinal cord neurons evoked by GABA alone or GABA with diazepam (DZ). (b, c) The same experiment at increasing time resolution to demonstrate typical features of the unitary current. Open-duration/frequency and bursts-duration/frequency histograms for GABA are not significantly altered by addition of diazepam from 20 to 1000 nM (middle histograms). From Rogers CJ, Twyman RE, MacDonald RL (1994) Benzodiazepine and β-carboline regulation of single GABA_A receptor channels of mouse spinal neurones in culture, *J. Physiol. (Lond.)* **475**, 69–82, with permission.

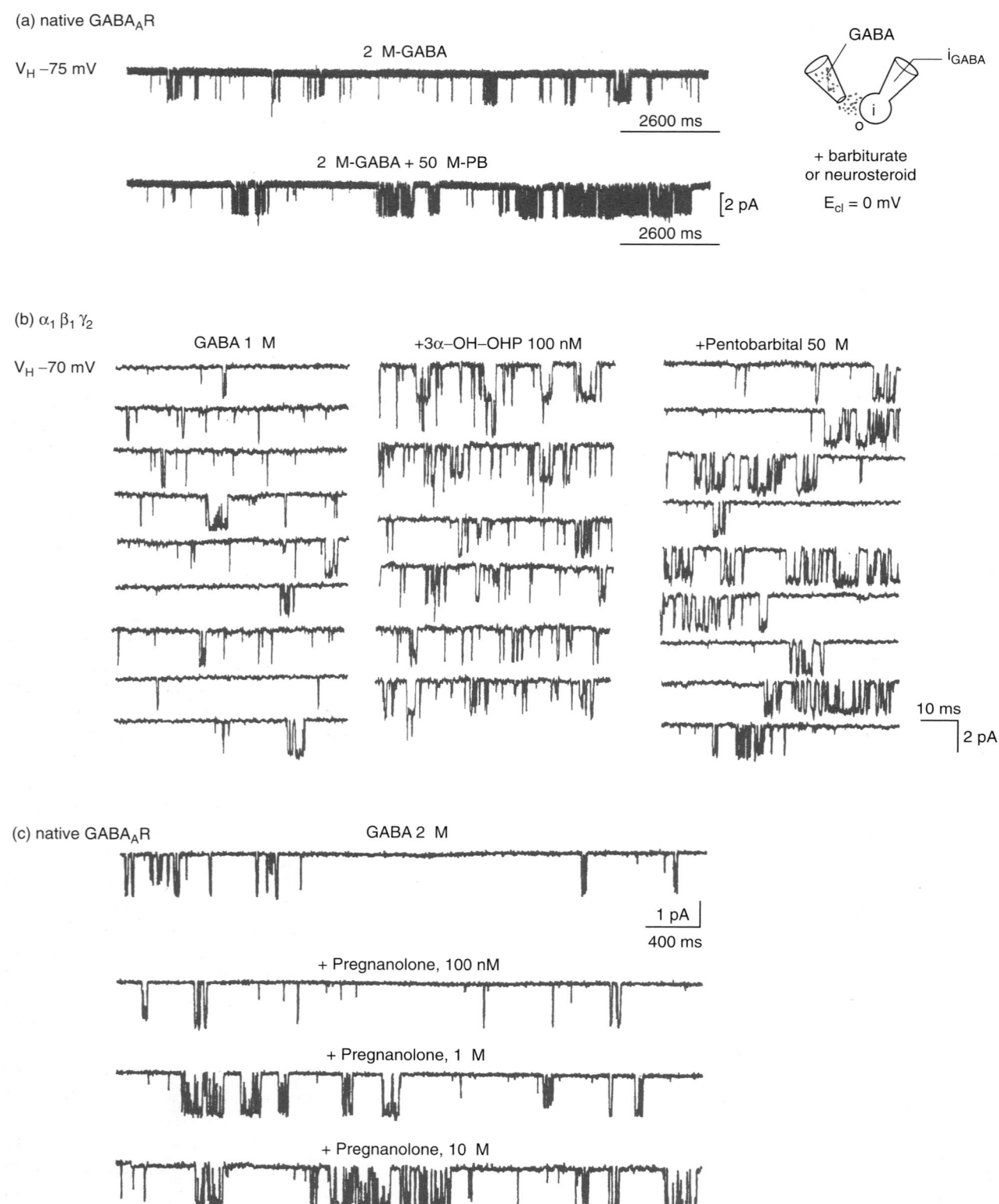

(a) native GABA$_A$R

V_H −75 mV

2 M-GABA

2600 ms

2 M-GABA + 50 M-PB

2 pA

2600 ms

GABA

i$_{GABA}$

+ barbiturate
or neurosteroid

E_{cl} = 0 mV

(b) $\alpha_1 \beta_1 \gamma_2$

V_H −70 mV

GABA 1 M   +3α–OH–OHP 100 nM   +Pentobarbital 50 M

10 ms

2 pA

(c) native GABA$_A$R

GABA 2 M

1 pA

400 ms

+ Pregnanolone, 100 nM

+ Pregnanolone, 1 M

+ Pregnanolone, 10 M

Figure 10.12 (left) GABA$_A$ single-channel current in the presence or absence of barbiturates or neurosteroids.
(a) Unitary GABA$_A$ currents in outside-out patches of spinal cord neurons evoked by GABA alone or GABA with phenobarbitone (PB). (b) Unitary GABA$_A$ currents recorded in outside-out patches excised from $\alpha_1\beta_1\gamma_2$ transfected cells evoked by GABA alone (left) or in combination with the neurosteroid 3α-OH-DHP (centre) or pentobarbital (right). (c) Unitary GABA$_A$ currents in outside-out patches of spinal cord neurons evoked by GABA alone or GABA with pregnanolone at increasing concentration. Part (a) from MacDonald RL, Rogers CJ, Twyman RE (1989) Barbiturate regulation of kinetic properties of the GABA$_A$ receptor channel of mouse spinal neurones in culture, *J. Physiol. (Lond.)* **417**, 483–500, with permission. Part (b) from Twyman RE, MacDonald RL (1992) Neurosteroid regulation of GABA$_A$ receptor single channel kinetic properties of mouse spinal cord neurons in culture, *J. Physiol. (Lond.)* **456**, 215–245, with permission. Part (c) from Puia G *et al.* (1990) Neurosteroids act on recombinant human GABA$_A$ receptors, *Neuron* **4**, 759–765, with permission.

GABA$_A$ receptors. However, GABA$_A$ receptor assemblies derived from the α_4- or α_6- subunits fail to bind conventional benzodiazepines such as diazepam, flunitrazepam and clonazepam. This suggests that the benzodiazepine binding site is localized at the interface of the $\alpha_{1/2/3/5}$ and γ-subunits. Aside from these regions responsible for benzodiazepine binding, there are separated domains required for coupling benzodiazepine binding to potentiation of the GABA$_A$ current that would be localized close to M1 and M2 segments. However, results based on site-directed mutagenesis need to be interpreted in the light of the possibility that amino acids identified may not be directly at the binding site but could be affecting the modulation of the compound at a distant site.

The exact locations of the receptor sites for barbiturates and neurosteroids are presently unknown. The presence of receptor sites on the GABA$_A$ receptor, for benzodiazepines or barbiturates that are not endogenous molecules, suggests the existence of endogenous ligands capable of binding to the barbiturate or benzodiazepine receptor sites and mimicking their effects. At first, research focused on the identification of endogenous ligands at the benzodiazepine receptor site. To this end, monoclonal antibodies were raised that recognize the epitopes of this site so that the secondary antibodies (anti-anti-epitope antibodies; see Appendix 7.2) would recognize endogenous ligands.

Benzodiazepines, barbiturates and neurosteroids potentiate the GABA$_A$ response

To test whether *benzodiazepines* have a direct effect on the GABA$_A$ receptor channel and to identify their effect, the unitary current i_{GABA} is recorded in voltage clamp (V_H = –75 mV) in outside-out patches (cultured spinal cord neurons). In the presence of GABA, the benzodiazepine diazepam (DZ, 50 nM) increases the opening frequency of the channel but does not change i_{GABA} amplitude nor the time spent by the channel in the open configuration at each opening (**Figure 10.11**).

Consistent with this finding, diazepam decreases the mean closed time τ_c; i.e. the time spent by the channel in

the closed configuration (see **Figure 10.13c**). With decreasing or increasing doses, the effect of diazepam was less pronounced (U-shaped concentration dependency). Diazepam (50 nM) also increases the burst frequency without changing the mean burst duration (τ_b) nor the mean number of openings per burst. All the currents evoked by GABA alone or GABA with diazepam are blocked by bicuculline, thus showing that they are mediated by the GABA$_A$ receptor. Since the i_{GABA}/V relationship shows that the unitary conductance is unchanged, it is hypothesized that diazepam alters the gating properties of the GABA$_A$ receptor channel: it increases the probability of the channel being in the open state, p_o.

The equation $I_{GABA} = Np_oi_{GABA}$ tells us that when p_o increases, I_{GABA} increases. Therefore, benzodiazepines should increase the amplitude of the total current I_{GABA} recorded in the whole-cell configuration (see **Figure 10.14**). The I/V curves show that the total currents I_{GABA} evoked in the presence or absence of benzodiazepines reverse at the same potential (not shown). This indicates that the potentiation of I_{GABA} by these drugs is not the result of a change in the ion selectivity of the channel.

Barbiturates also increase the bicuculline-sensitive current I_{GABA} but via a different mechanism: they do not increase the frequency of GABA$_A$ channel openings, instead they increase the duration of single openings and bursts of native GABA$_A$ receptors (**Figure 10.12a**) or transfected $\alpha_1\beta_1\gamma_2$ receptors (**Figure 10.12b**, right). An increase in the time spent in the open configuration at each opening results in an increase of the probability of the channel being in the open state and therefore in an increase of I_{GABA} (see **Figure 10.14**).

Neurosteroids at physiological concentrations increase the total bicuculline-sensitive current I_{GABA}. To study the mechanism of action, the effect of neurosteroids on single GABA$_A$ channel activity is recorded. Transformed human embryonic kidney cells 293 are transfected with the GABA$_A$ subunit combination $\alpha_1\beta_1\gamma_2$. The activity of expressed single GABA$_A$ channels is recorded in the outside-out configuration with symmetrical Cl$^-$ concentrations on both sides of the patch of membrane. Allopregnanolone (3α-OH-DHP) in combination with GABA increases the GABA$_A$ channel activity: it

Table 10.1 Pharmacology of GABA$_A$ receptors

	GABA site	Benzodiazepine site
Selective agonists	Muscimol Isoguvacine THIP	Flunitrazepam
Inverse agonists	–	β-carbolines Ro 15 1788
Competitive antagonist	Bicuculline	–
Channel blocker	Picrotoxin	–

THIP: 4,5,6,7-tetrahydroisoxazolopyridin-3-ol.

increases the number of active channels in the patch and the channel open probability (**Figure 10.12b**). On native GABA$_A$ receptors of spinal cord neurons, pregnanolone in combination with GABA was also seen to increase the duration of single and burst openings. Either one or both these effects on frequency of openings or opening duration result in an increase of p_o and thus an increase of I_{GABA} (see **Figure 10.14**).

In conclusion, benzodiazepines, barbiturates and neurosteroids can be considered as allosteric agonists of the GABA$_A$ receptor: they modulate the efficacy of activation of the receptor by GABA. They act via distinct receptor sites on the GABA$_A$ receptor and via different mechanisms.

10.4.3 β-carbolines reversibly decrease total GABA$_A$ current; they bind at the benzodiazepine site and are inverse agonists of the GABA$_A$ receptor

β-carbolines such as methyl-6,7-dimethoxyl-4-ethyl-β-carboline-3-carboxylate (DMCM) are convulsant and anxiogenic drugs. They bind to the benzodiazepine receptor site but have reverse effects: they are called 'benzodiazepine inverse agonists' (Table 10.1).

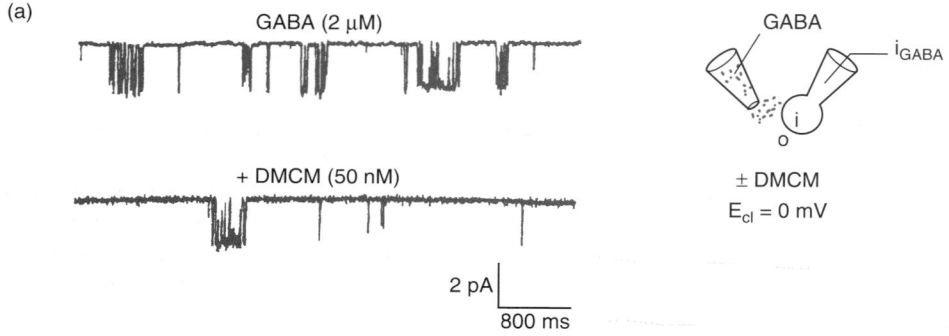

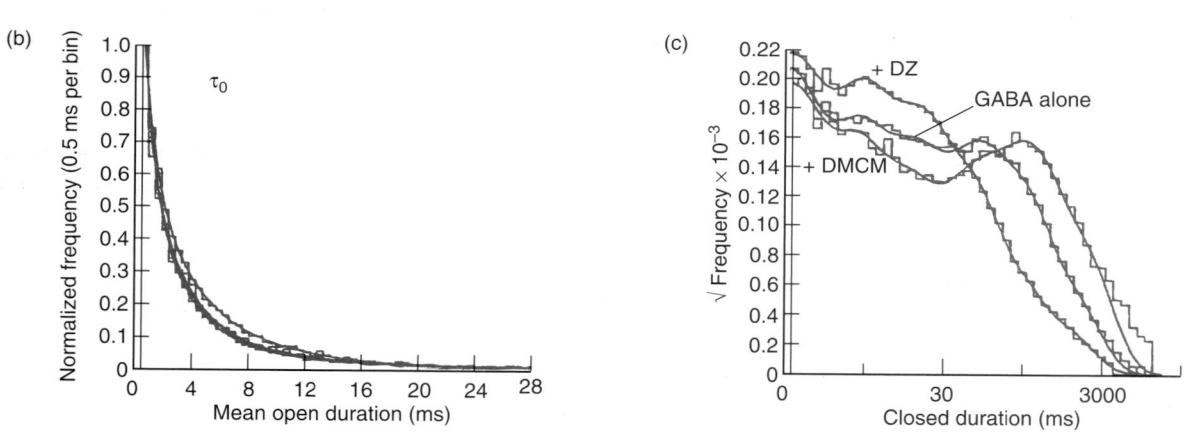

Figure 10.13 GABA$_A$ single-channel current in the presence or absence of a β-carboline.
(a) Unitary GABA$_A$ currents in outside-out patches of spinal cord neurons evoked by GABA alone or GABA with the β-carboline DMCM. (b) Histograms for open durations are plotted for GABA (2 μM, uppermost curve, τ_o = 4.10 ± 0.03 ms) and for GABA and DMCM (20–100 nM, τ_o' = 4.40 ± 0.07 ms). (c) Closed duration-frequency histograms for GABA (2 μM), for GABA with diazepam (DZ, 100 nM) and for GABA with DMCM (100 nM). DZ shifts long closed durations to shorter durations while DMCM shifts long closed durations to longer ones. From Rogers CJ, Twyman RE, MacDonald RL (1994) Benzodiazepine and β-carboline regulation of single GABA$_A$ receptor channels of mouse spinal neurones in culture, *J. Physiol. (Lond.)* **475**, 69–82, with permission.

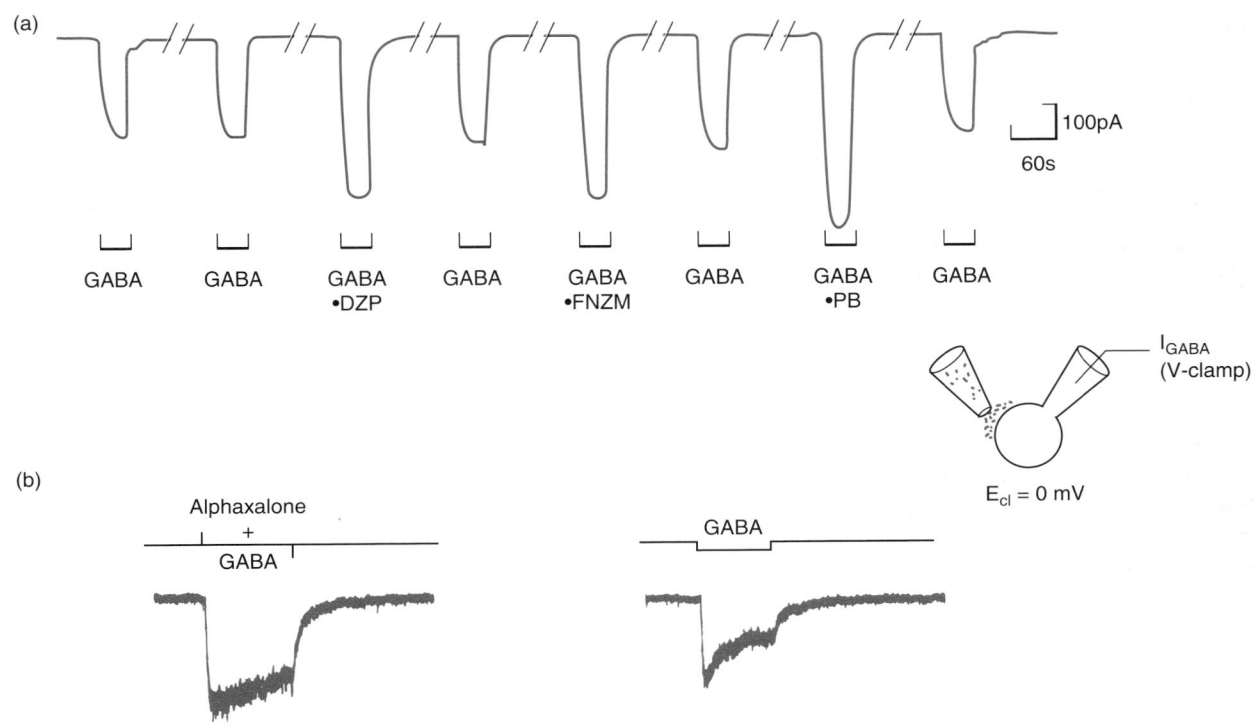

Figure 10.14 Potentiation of the total current I_{GABA} by benzodiazepines, barbiturates and neurosteroids.
(a) GABA_A receptors are expressed in transfected cells with the α, β and γ cDNA subunits. This model is interesting because these cells do not normally express GABA receptors (neither GABA_A nor GABA_B); the GABA applied in the bath activates therefore only the number (N) of GABA_A receptors expressed. On the other hand, it is a model where the presynaptic release of GABA is excluded because of the absence of synapses. The total current I_{GABA} is recorded using the patch-clamp technique (whole-cell configuration). The total current I_{GABA} recorded at $V_m = -60$ mV (GABA, 10 μM) is inward and is significantly potentiated by the simultaneous application of the two benzodiazepines, diazepam (DZP, 1 μM) and flunitrazepam (FNZM, 1 μM) and by pentobarbital (PB, 50 μM). **(b)** Whole-cell GABA_A current evoked by 10 μM of GABA in spinal neurons in culture in the absence (right) or in the presence (left) of the neurosteroid alphaxalone (3α-hydroxy-5α-pregnane-11,20-dione, 1 μM). In (a) and (b), E_{Cl} is estimated to be near 0 mV. Part (a) adapted from Pritchett DB, Southeimer H, Shivers BD, *et al.* (1989) Importance of a novel GABA_A receptor subunit for benzodiazepine pharmacology, *Nature* **338**, 582–585, with permission. Part (b) from Barker JL, Harrison NL, Lange GD, Owen DG (1987) Potentiation of γ-aminobutyric-acid-activated chloride conductance by a steroid anaesthetic in cultured rat spinal neurones, *J. Physiol. (Lond.)* **386**, 485–501, with permission.

The activity of outside-out patches of spinal cord neurons in culture is recorded in voltage clamp. When DMCM is applied with GABA, it decreases the number of GABA_A receptor openings compared with what is observed with GABA alone (**Figure 10.13a**). DMCM (20–100 nM) reduces single openings as well as burst frequency. However, the number of openings per burst is unchanged. The times spent by the GABA_A channel in the open or bursting states are also unchanged but the time spent in the closed state is increased, consistent with a decrease in opening frequency (**Figure 10.13b, c**). Like diazepam, DMCM does not alter GABA_A receptor single-channel conductance nor single-channel open or bursts properties. DMCM decreases p_o and thus decreases I_{GABA}.

Since burst frequency, but not intraburst opening frequency, is altered, it is unlikely that receptor channel opening rates (α and β) are altered by diazepam or DMCM. Several hypotheses have been proposed but the exact mechanism is still unknown.

10.5 GABA_A-mediated synaptic transmission

10.5.1 The GABAergic synapse

To identify a synapse as GABAergic, several techniques can be used such as immunocytochemistry for the GABA synthetic enzyme, glutamate decarboxylase (GAD). Now to identify a synaptic response as mediated by GABA_A receptors, the simplest test is the block by bicuculline. Benzodiazepines significantly potentiate and prolong GABA_A-mediated IPSPs (see **Figure 10.1a**).

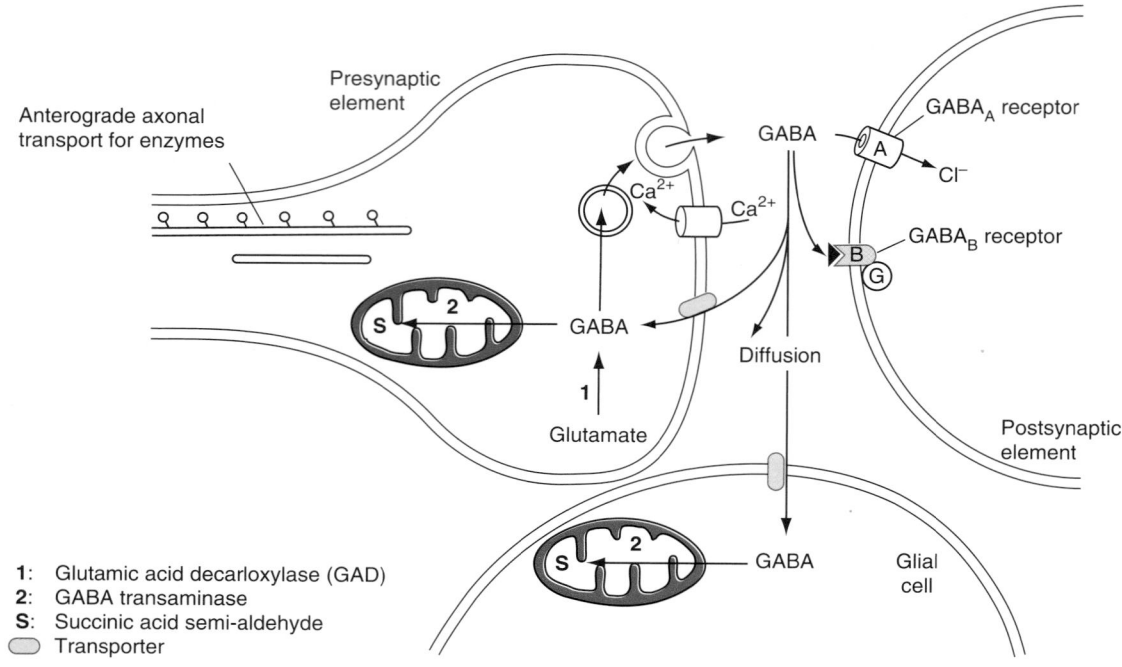

Figure 10.15 The GABAergic synapse.

Functional scheme of a GABAergic synapse where the ionotropic (receptor-channel) GABA$_A$ receptors and the metabotropic (G-protein linked) GABA$_B$ receptors are co-localized. Presynaptic receptors are omitted. In order to study in isolation the GABA$_A$ response, GABA$_B$ receptors are selectively blocked. GABA is formed by the irreversible decarboxylation of glutamate catalysed by the enzyme glutamic acid decarboxylase (GAD) and is metabolized by the mitochondrial enzyme GABA transaminase (GABA-T) into succinic acid semi-aldehyde. Enzymes are synthesized in the soma and carried to axon terminals via fast anterograde axonal transport. GABA is synthesized in the cytoplasm and transported actively into synaptic vesicles by a vesicular carrier. A percentage of the GABA released in the synaptic cleft is uptaken into presynaptic terminals and glial cells by GABA transporters which co-transport Na$^+$ and Cl$^-$. These transports are inhibited by nipecotic acid or β-alanine.

Because of the selective action of benzodiazepines on the GABA$_A$ channel, these substances can be used experimentally together with bicuculline to identify a GABA$_A$ response. They are also widely used clinically.

When GABA is released in the synaptic cleft, it can (see **Figure 10.15**):

- bind to postsynaptic GABA$_A$ receptors;
- bind to postsynaptic or presynaptic GABA$_B$ receptors;
- bind to glial and neuronal transporters and thus be taken up by presynaptic elements or glial cells;
- diffuse away from the synaptic cleft.

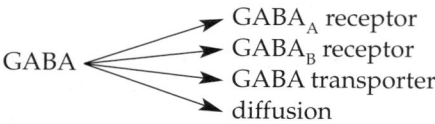

When it binds to postsynaptic GABA$_A$ receptors at resting potential, GABA evokes an inhibitory postsynaptic potential (IPSP).

10.5.2 The synaptic GABA$_A$-mediated current is the sum of unitary currents appearing with variable delays and durations

From single GABA$_A$ current to IPSC

In a slice of hippocampus for example, GABAergic afferents are still spontaneously active and evoke spontaneous synaptic GABA$_A$-mediated postsynaptic currents (called IPSCs) that can be recorded in whole-cell configuration in voltage clamp. Since they are blocked by bicuculline, they are mediated by postsynaptic GABA$_A$ receptors. In symmetrical Cl$^-$ solutions, at a holding potential of -70 mV, GABA$_A$-mediated currents are inward (outward flow of Cl$^-$ ions) (**Figure 10.16a**). When IPSCs are observed at a higher magnification and a faster timebase, unitary current steps can be identified. For example, during a very small IPSC (**Figure 10.16b**), the peak is an integer of 7 unitary currents. During a larger IPSC, steps cannot be identified at the level of the peak but are clear during the decay phase (**Figure 10.16c**). IPSCs result from the activation of N postsynaptic GABA$_A$ receptors.

Single-spike IPSC

When simultaneous intracellular recordings of connected neurons are performed, a presynaptic GABAergic interneuron and a postsynaptic pyramidal cell, one can correlate each presynaptic action potential with the post-synaptic current that it evokes, called *single-spike IPSC*. This postsynaptic current is outward at –30 mV in control intracellular Cl$^-$ concentration. Its amplitude varies at each trial due to the fact that a presynaptic action potential activates, at each trial, a variable number of active zones from the total number of active zones established by the presynaptic axon with the postsynaptic membrane (see Appendix 8.2).

Single-spike IPSP

The same experiment performed in current-clamp mode allows one to record the postsynaptic variation of potential resulting from the postsynaptic GABA$_A$-mediated current (**Figure 10.17**). In response to a single presynaptic action potential (trace 1) an inhibitory postsynaptic potential called *single-spike IPSP* (traces 2; V_m = –62 to –66 mV) is recorded. It is a transient hyperpolarization of the membrane. The amplitude of this single-spike IPSP varies in amplitude at each trial, from 0.6 to 4.2 mV. This is due to the fact that a presynaptic action potential activates, at each trial, a variable number of active zones from the total number of active zones established by the presynaptic axon. The conductance G_{IPSP} can be calculated knowing I_{IPSP}, V_m and E_{Cl}. In this experiment, G_{IPSP} = 6.7 nS ± 2.3 nS at the peak of the IPSP. Knowing that the unitary conductance of the GABA$_A$ channel is estimated in these neurons to be γ_{GABA} = 20–30 pS, it can be deduced that approximately 300 GABA$_A$ channels are

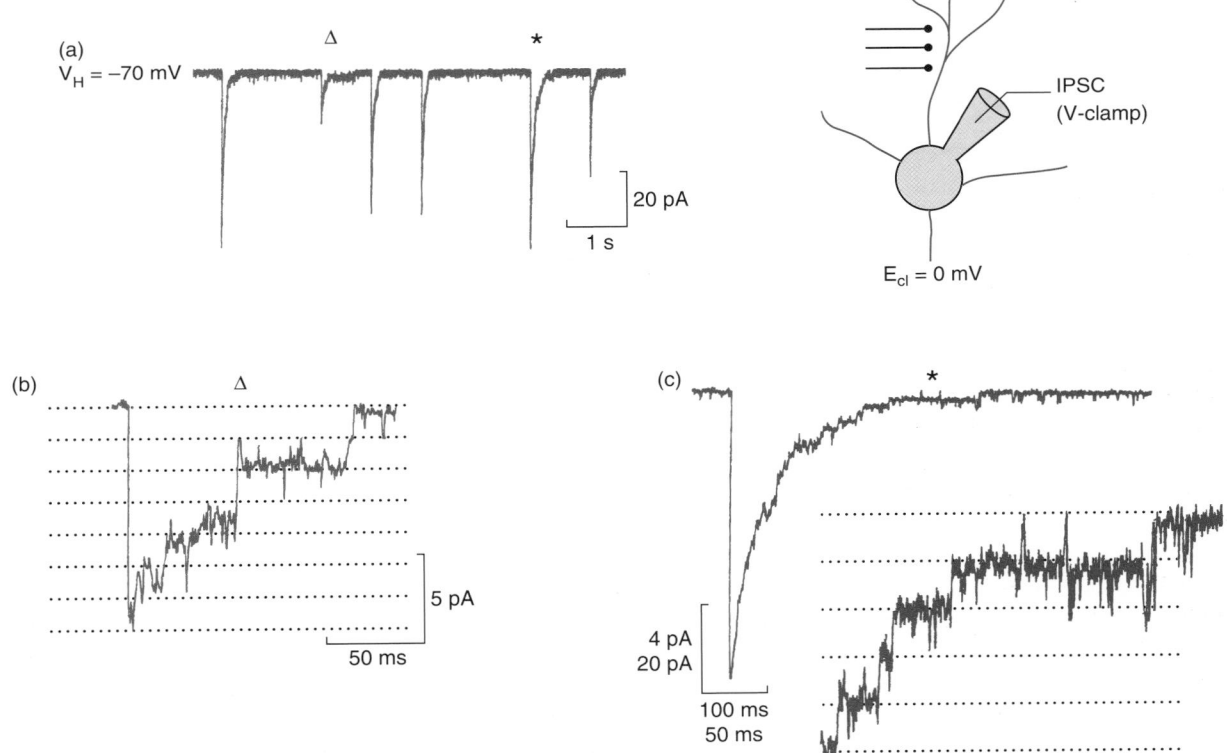

Figure 10.16 Inhibitory postsynaptic currents (IPSCs) result from the summation of unitary GABA$_A$-mediated currents. (a) Spontaneous IPSCs are recorded from a cerebellar granule cell (whole-cell configuration, voltage-clamp mode). IPSCs are inward at –70 mV since E_{Cl} in this experiment is at 0 mV. (b, c) Two IPSCs of different amplitude from trace (a) are enlarged to show that unitary step currents can be resolved in their decay phase. Ionotropic glutamatergic transmission is pharmacologically blocked. From Brickley SG, Cull-Candy SG, Farrant M (1999) Single-channel properties of synaptic and extrasynaptic GABA$_A$ receptors suggest differential targeting of receptor subtypes, *J. Neurosci.* **19**, 2960–2973, with permission.

open at the peak of the single-spike IPSP ($G_{IPSP} = Np_o\gamma_{GABA}$).

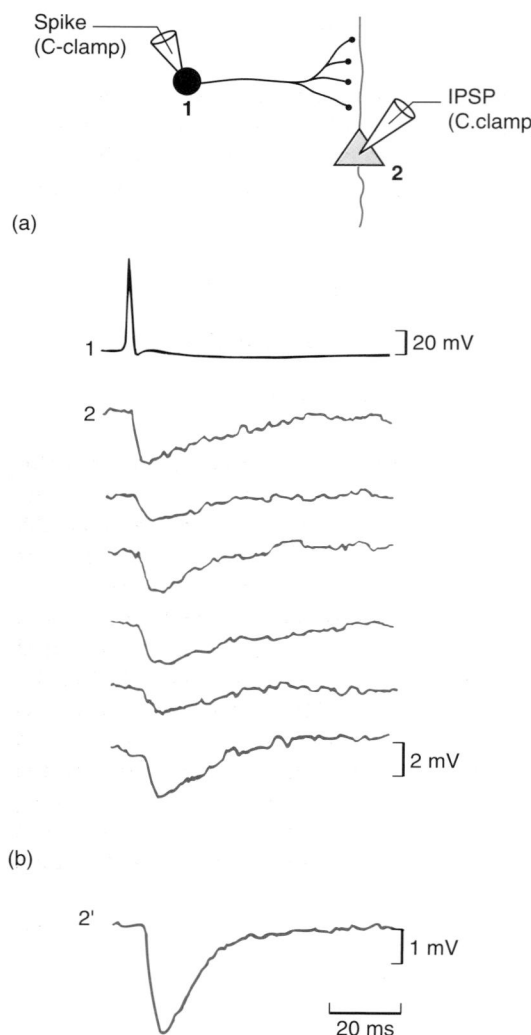

(a)

(b)

Figure 10.17 Characteristics of a single-spike IPSP mediated by GABA$_A$ receptors.
(a) The activity of a pair of connected presynaptic GABAergic interneuron and postsynaptic pyramidal cell of the hippocampus *in vitro* is recorded with two intracellular electrodes. In response to each action potential evoked in neuron 1 (presynaptic GABAergic interneuron), a single-spike IPSP is recorded in neuron 2 (postsynaptic pyramidal neuron) with a mean latency of 0.7 ± 0.2 ms. Each single-spike IPSP results from the activation of several boutons which are not all activated at each trial as shown by their variable amplitude (mean amplitude = -2.1 ± 0.7 mV). They are blocked by picrotoxin (10^{-4} M, not shown), a GABA$_A$ channel blocker. (b) Average of 20 IPSPs obtained by triggering each trace from the peak of the presynaptic action potential. Adapted from Miles R, Wong RKS (1984) Unitary inhibitory synaptic potentials in the guinea-pig hippocampus *in vitro*, J. *Physiol.* **356**, 97–113, with permission.

10.5.3 The consequences of the synaptic activation of GABA$_A$ receptors depend on the relative values of E_{Cl} and V_m

It has just been noted that synaptically released GABA evokes a transient hyperpolarization of the postsynaptic membrane, called IPSP, via the activation of GABA$_A$ receptors. However, this is not always the case.

When E_{Cl} is more negative than V_{rest}, GABA$_A$ receptor activation leads to a hyperpolarizing postsynaptic potential (IPSP) and inhibition of the postsynaptic activity

In recordings with electrodes filled with potassium acetate (instead of potassium chloride, in order not to change the intracellular concentration of Cl$^-$), E_{Cl} is generally more negative than the postsynaptic resting membrane potential (V_{rest}) and a hyperpolarizing postsynaptic potential (IPSP) is recorded in response to the stimulation of GABAergic afferent fibres (**Figures 10.17b and 10.18a**).

When E_{Cl} is close to V_{rest}, activation of GABA$_A$ receptor leads to a 'silent inhibition' of postsynaptic activity

If E_{Cl} is close to V_{rest}, the electrochemical gradient for Cl$^-$ is very weak or null and no IPSP is observed even though GABA$_A$ channels are open. However, GABA still has an inhibitory effect on postsynaptic activity, as any EPSP occurring during the effect of GABA is strongly inhibited (see Section 16.2.3). This inhibitory effect of GABA is called a *shunting effect*. It is due to an increase in the membrane conductance (G_{IPSP}) during the silent inhibition owing to the opening of GABA$_A$ channels. If this effect is large, the membrane resistance decreases and any other synaptic current evoked at this time will produce only a small change in membrane potential (according to Ohm's Law, when I_{EPSP} is constant but R_m diminishes, then V_{EPSP} diminishes). The silent GABA$_A$ inhibition reduces the amplitude of postsynaptic depolarizations and consequently prevents the generation of postsynaptic action potentials (**Figure 10.18b**).

When E_{Cl} is more positive than V_m but below the threshold for action potential generation, GABA$_A$ receptor activation leads to a depolarizing current and an inhibition of postsynaptic activity

If E_{Cl} is more positive than V_m, the activation of GABA$_A$ receptors causes an inward current (outward flow of Cl$^-$

ions) and a depolarization of the membrane. As long as E_{Cl} remains below the threshold for activation of voltage-dependent Na$^+$ channels, postsynaptic activity is inhibited (**Figure 10.18c**).

However, when E_{Cl} is more positive than the threshold for activation of voltage-dependent Na$^+$ channels, GABA$_A$ receptor activation causes a postsynaptic depolarization or EPSP (by analogy with synaptic currents with reversal potentials more depolarized than threshold: nicotinic currents or currents evoked by excitatory amino acids). Note that this depolarizing excitatory effect of GABA has never been described in adult GABA$_A$ synapses but is observed in very young GABAergic synapses (see Chapter 23).

10.5.4 What shapes the decay phase of GABA$_A$-mediated currents?

GABA$_A$ receptor-mediated IPSCs peak rapidly (in 0.5–5 ms) and usually decay with two time constants ranging from a few milliseconds to tens or hundreds of milliseconds. To determine the factors responsible for the duration of IPSC is interesting since IPSC decay determines the time course of the resistive shunt or hyperpolarization that prevents neuronal firing in response to excitatory inputs.

The duration of the synaptic current is determined by the period during which each activated GABA$_A$ receptor remains in the G$_2$R* state. Various factors may determine the duration of the G$_2$R* state and therefore the time course of the postsynaptic GABA$_A$ response:

■ *Case 1:* The GABA$_A$ receptor deactivates due to unbinding of GABA and does not reopen because GABA has disappeared from the cleft:

$$G_2R^* \rightarrow G_2R \rightleftharpoons 2G + R$$

■ *Case 2:* The GABA$_A$ receptor deactivates due to unbinding of GABA but it reactivates several times before closing since removal of GABA from the synaptic cleft by neuronal/glial uptake or diffusion is very slow:

$$G_2R^* \rightleftharpoons G_2R \rightleftharpoons 2G + R$$

■ *Case 3:* The GABA$_A$ receptor desensitizes:

$$G_2R^* \rightleftharpoons G_2D$$

If the decay of the synaptic current is due to rapid closure of the GABA$_A$ channels without any reopenings (case 1), this implies that the concentration of GABA decreases very rapidly in the synaptic cleft after its release (as a consequence, for example, of rapid diffusion or very efficient uptake mechanisms). In this case, the channels have very little chance of being reactivated by the repeated binding of two molecules of GABA: the time constant of the decay of the postsynaptic current is τ_o; i.e. the mean open time of the channels which depends only on the closing time constant of the channels (in the absence of desensitization). GABA$_A$ receptors have a low affinity for GABA (10–20 μM) and display brief openings and bursts (0.2–25 ms).

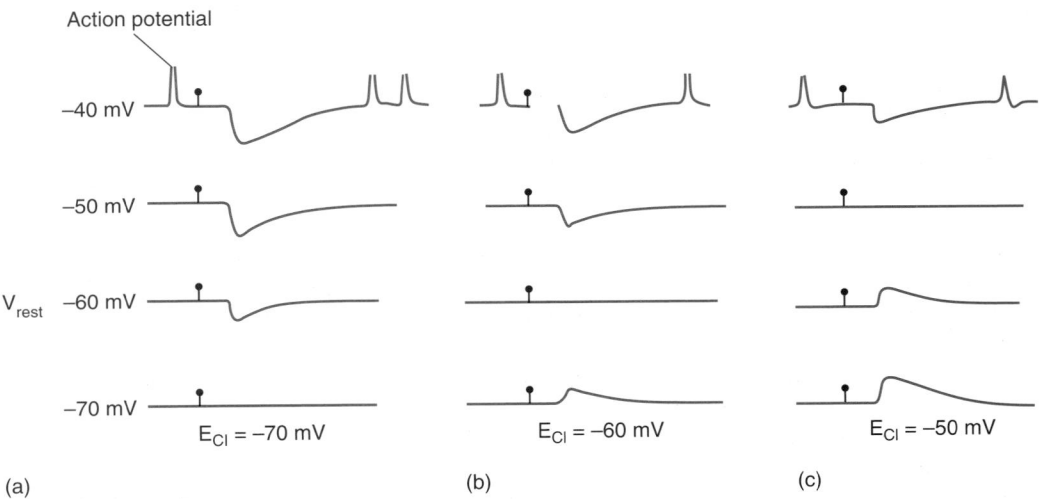

(a)   (b)   (c)

Figure 10.18 Reversal potential of GABA$_A$-mediated IPSPs as a function of membrane potential.
E_{Cl} is **(a)** more negative (–70 mV), **(b)** equal (–60 mV) or **(c)** more positive (–50 mV) than the resting membrane potential of the neuron. A resting membrane potential for the neuron of –60 mV and a threshold for action potential generation at –40 mV are assumed. Action potentials are truncated owing to their large amplitude. In the three cases represented, inhibition of activity is produced during the IPSP (upper trace).

Assuming a brief increase of GABA concentration in the synaptic cleft, these properties predict an IPSC decay of no more than 10–25 ms, much shorter than is frequently observed. This discrepancy could indicate that GABA stays longer in the cleft (case 2) or synaptically activated GABA$_A$ receptors visit desensitized states (case 3).

If the decay of the synaptic current is due to the slow disappearance of GABA from the vicinity of the receptors (removal due to GABA uptake and/or diffusion), this implies, in contrast, a prolonged presence of GABA in the synaptic cleft. The prolonged presence of GABA may result from a slow mechanism of uptake or from a restricted diffusion of GABA away from the synaptic cleft. Hence, GABA may reactivate GABA$_A$ channels which have previously opened and the decay time constant will exceed the value of τ_o. However, uptake inhibitors have very little effect on GABA$_A$ synaptic responses. When applied by micro-iontophoresis in hippocampal slices, nipecotic acid, a neuronal and glial uptake inhibitor, has only a weak effect on the duration of the postsynaptic potential (IPSP) evoked by stimulation of GABAergic afferent fibres: it prolongs the later phase of the IPSP (**Figure 10.19a**). Thus, as mentioned earlier, the uptake process may be too slow to have much influence on the time course of the IPSP.

If the decay of the synaptic current is due to the transition of the channel to a desensitized state, the decay time constant would be related to the kinetics of desensitization. Moreover if there is a prolonged presence of the GABA in the synaptic cleft, and rapid kinetics of desensitization and recovery from desensitization, the channels may reopen once they have recovered from desensitization. To test this hypothesis, GABA is very briefly applied (for 1–10 ms) to outside-out patches of pyramidal neurons. The ensemble average of patch

(a)

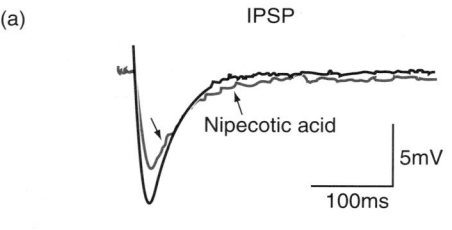

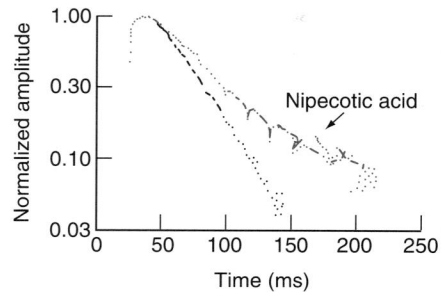

(b)

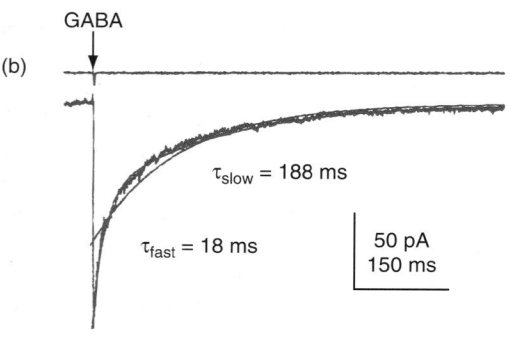

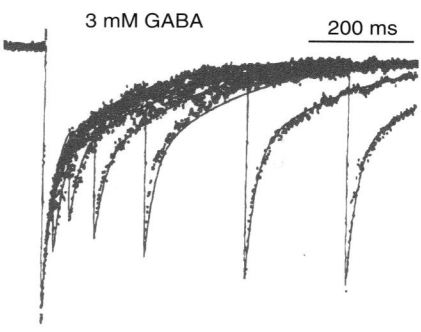

Figure 10.19 Modulation of the decay phase of GABA$_A$-mediated IPSPs and current.
(a) Current clamp recording from hippocampal neurons in rat brain slices. An orthodromic IPSP is recorded in response to stimulation of GABAergic afferents. This IPSP is sensitive to bicuculline (not shown). The IPSP is recorded before and after (arrows) application of nipecotic acid (1 mM for 40 min, left). Each trace represents the average of six responses. Nipecotic acid decreases the amplitude of the IPSP, which obscures the analysis of its effect on the time course of the IPSP. After normalizing the IPSPs to the same peak (right), the analysis of their time course reveals that nipecotic acid prolongs the later phase of the repolarization. **(b)** GABA$_A$ receptor current is evoked in outside-out macropatches of cultured hippocampal neurons by a brief GABA pulse (1 mM for 5 ms). The patch current decay is well fitted by the sum of two exponentials with time constants as indicated (left). Pairs of GABA pulses are given at 25, 50, 100, 200, 400 and 600 ms intervals (right). The second response in each pair is reduced at short interpulse intervals. Part (a) from Dingledine R, Korn SJ (1985) γ-aminobutyric acid uptake and termination of inhibitory synaptic potentials in the rat hippocampal slices, *J. Physiol. (Lond.)* **366**, 387–409, with permission. Part (b) from Jones MV, Westbrook GL (1995) Desensitized states prolong GABA$_A$ channel responses to brief agonist pulses, *Neuron* **15**, 181–191, with permission.

currents decay with bi-exponential kinetics similar to that of the IPSC (**Figure 19.19b**). When pairs of 1–3 ms GABA pulses are given at variable intervals, the second pulse evokes a smaller peak current than the first pulse, demonstrating that channels do not return to the unbound state immediately after closing but rather enter an agonist-insensitive (desensitized) state. This suggests that after a brief pulse, GABA occupies receptors long enough for many channels to accumulate in desensitized state(s). Rapidly-equilibrating desensitized state(s) prolongs the GABA$_A$-mediated IPSC and provides a mechanism for low affinity receptors to support long-lasting currents.

In the case of the nicotinic channel, the removal of acetylcholine is very rapid and desensitization of the nAChR is slow relative to deactivation and does not affect the shape of the endplate current. The kinetic properties of the deactivation of the channel mostly determine the time course of the endplate current (see Section 9.5.2). In the case of the GABA$_A$ receptor, the situation appears to be more complex. For very low-amplitude postsynaptic currents, the mean open time of the GABA$_A$ channel may determine their time course, the released GABA being rapidly removed by diffusion from the cleft. However, for larger postsynaptic currents, evoked by a greater presynaptic release of GABA, the slower removal of GABA from the synaptic cleft together with the desensitization of the channel that recovers over the course of deactivation can prolong synaptic currents.

10.6 Summary

The GABA$_A$ receptor channel is a ligand-gated channel activated by γ-aminobutyric acid, the neurotransmitter at numerous synapses in the mammalian central nervous system. The GABA$_A$ receptor is a glycoprotein composed of several subunits, seven of which have been described to date: α, β, γ, δ, ε, π and ρ. The GABA$_A$ receptor comprises the GABA receptor sites on its surface, the elements that make the ionic channel selectively permeable to chloride ions, as well as all the elements necessary for interactions between different functional domains. Thus, the GABA receptor sites and the chloride channel are part of the same unique protein.

How does GABA$_A$ receptor mediate the binding of GABA into a transient hyperpolarization of the membrane?

The fixation of GABA to the GABA$_A$ receptor induces a conformational change of the receptor and opening of the GABA$_A$ channel. This channel opens in bursts (it rapidly fluctuates between closed and open bi-liganded states). It is permeable to Cl$^-$ ions. Depending on the membrane potential and the concentration of Cl$^-$ in the extracellular and intracellular media, there is an influx or an efflux of Cl$^-$. In adult neurons, there is generally an influx of Cl$^-$; i.e. an outward current which hyperpolarizes the membrane. This hyperpolarization is the inhibitory postsynaptic potential (IPSP) mediated by GABA$_A$ receptors. Even when the membrane is not hyperpolarized by GABA (when $E_{Cl} = V_m$), the opening of GABA$_A$ channels is inhibitory: opening of GABA$_A$ channels reduces membrane resistance and thus reduces the depolarizing effect of concomitant inward currents ($\Delta V_m = R_m \Delta I_{inward}$; when ΔI_{inward} is constant and R_m diminishes, ΔV_m is reduced).

Do benzodiazepines and barbiturates act directly on GABA$_A$ receptors? Are there selective and distinct binding sites on the receptor for each of these drugs? How do they potentiate the hyperpolarizing effect of GABA? Are there other modulators of GABA$_A$ receptors?

Aside from the GABA receptor sites, the GABA$_A$ receptor contains a variety of topographically distinct receptor sites capable of recognizing clinically active substances, such as benzodiazepines (anxiolytics and anticonvulsants), barbiturates (sedatives and anticonvulsants), neurosteroids and ethanol (see **Table 10.1**). There are selective allosteric binding sites on GABA$_A$ receptors such as (i) the benzodiazepine site that recognizes the allosteric agonists benzodiazepines and the inverse agonists β-carbolines, (ii) the barbiturate site, and (iii) the ethanol site. Benzodiazepines increase the opening frequency of the GABA$_A$ receptor whereas barbiturates increase the duration of each opening; they both potentiate GABA$_A$ current. In contrast, inverse agonists depress GABA$_A$ current. GABA$_A$ receptors are probably a pentameric assembly derived from a combination of various subunits. This leads not only to structural heterogeneity but also to pharmacological heterogeneity of the GABA$_A$ receptors, especially regarding the sensitivity to benzodiazepines.

Appendix 10.1
Mean open time and mean burst duration of the GABA$_A$ single-channel current

The conformational changes of the GABA$_A$ channel are modelled as follows:

$$2G + R \underset{k_{-1}}{\overset{k_1}{\rightleftharpoons}} GR \underset{k_{-2}}{\overset{k_2}{\rightleftharpoons}} G_2R \underset{\alpha}{\overset{\beta}{\rightleftharpoons}} G_2R^*$$

Upon application of GABA, the conformational change of the GABA$_A$ receptor towards the G$_2$R* state is favoured (opening of the channel). However, it has been found that the GABA$_A$ receptor closes and opens rapidly several times upon opening: these are bursts of openings (see **Figure 10.7**). The short-duration closures represent the fluctuation of the receptor between the G$_2$R and G$_2$R* states. During these bursts, the receptor returns much less frequently to the GR state, and even less frequently to the R state, before reopening.

The mean open time is $\tau_o = 1/\alpha$. When the receptor is in the G$_2$R* state, it can only transfer to the G$_2$R state with a rate constant of α (this is true when desensitization is negligible). τ_o is calculated experimentally from the different open times t_o within each burst.

The mean closed time within bursts is $\tau_c = 1/(\beta + 2k_{-2})$. When the receptor is in the G$_2$R state, it can either reopen with the rate constant β or transfer to the GR state with a rate constant $2k_{-2}$. The average number of short closures per burst is $nf = \beta/2k_{-2}$ (see Colquhoun and Hawkes 1977).

Once the values of τ_o, τ_c and nf are experimentally defined, the values of α and β can be deduced: $\alpha = 50$ s^{-1}; $\beta = 330$ s^{-1}.

Note that α and β differ by a factor of about 6 (whereas for the acetylcholine nicotinic receptor nAChR, they differ by a factor of 40). This illustrates numerically the fact that fluctuations between the double-liganded open and closed states are more frequent for the GABA$_A$ receptor, the probability that the channel opens in a given time being only six times greater than the probability that the channel closes.

Further reading

Colquhoun D, Hawkes AG (1977) Relaxations and fluctuations of membrane currents that flow through drug-operated channels. *Proc. R. Soc. Lond. B Biol. Sci.* **199**, 231–262.

Krnjevic K, Schwartz S (1967) The action of γ-aminobutyric acid on cortical neurones. *Exp. Brain Res.* **3**, 320–336.

Mehta AK, Ticku MK (1999) An update on GABA$_A$ receptors. *Brain Res. Rev.* **29**, 196–217.

Sieghart W, Fuchs K, Tretter V *et al.* (1999) Structure and subunit composition of GABA(A) receptors. *Neurochem. Int.* **34**, 379–385.

Smart TG (1997) Regulation of excitatory and inhibitory neurotransmitter-gated ion channels by protein phosphorylation. *Curr. Opin. Neurobiol.* **7**, 358–367.

The Ionotropic Glutamate Receptors

From the original observations of Curtis and collaborators (1961) it is known that glutamate has a depolarizing effect on neurons. Glutamate is with GABA the major neurotransmitter in the vertebrate central nervous system. It activates two main types of postsynaptic receptors: (i) ionotropic glutamate receptors (iGluRs) that are ligand-gated channels, and (ii) metabotropic glutamate receptors (mGluRs) that are receptors coupled to GTP-binding proteins. The latter type is covered in Chapter 14.

Ionotropic glutamate receptors are divided into three major subtypes, on the basis of their affinity for glutamate selective structural analogues, notably for N-methyl-D-aspartate (NMDA). A distinction is made between those glutamate receptors activated by NMDA (NMDA receptors) and those not activated by NMDA (non-NMDA receptors) (**Figures 11.1a and b**). Cloning studies have demonstrated that these non-NMDA receptors can be further distinguished in AMPA and kainate receptors, and agonists and antagonists that selectively act on one or the other have been developed in recent years.

11.1 The three different types of ionotropic glutamate receptors have a common structure and participate in fast glutamatergic synaptic transmission

11.1.1 Ionotropic glutamate receptors have the name of their selective or preferential agonist

NMDA, AMPA and kainate receptors are glycoproteins composed of several subunits. To date, molecular cloning has identified 14 cDNAs, four for AMPA receptor subunits (termed GluR1, GluR2, GluR3 and GluR4), five for kainate receptor subunits (termed GluR5, GluR6, GluR7, KA1 and KA2) and five for NMDA receptor subunits (termed NR1, NR2A, NR2B, NR2C and NR2D) (**Figure 11.1c**). iGluR subunits have in common a

large extracellular N-terminus domain and four hydrophobic segments. Immunocytochemical and biochemical studies have indicated that the C-terminus is intracellularly located. This challenged for iGluRs the conventional model of four transmembrane domains. When N-glycosylation consensus sequences were introduced at different sites along the entire length of a GluR1 subunit, to test which part of the protein was extracellularly located (glycosylation at a particular site is taken as a proof of its external location), the hypothesis was put forward that the receptor has only three transmembrane domains, corresponding to TM1, TM3 and TM4. In this model, M2 does not span the membrane but is considered to lie in close proximity to the intracellular surface of the plasma membrane and to have a hairpin structure. Furthermore, the entire region between M3 and M4 is extracellular. This model is applicable to all iGluR subunits (**Figure 11.2**).

11.1.2 The three ionotropic receptors participate in fast glutamatergic synaptic transmission

In the cat neocortex, in response to a single spike in a presynaptic pyramidal neuron, a transient depolarization of the membrane mediated by ionotropic glutamate receptors is recorded in the postsynaptic interneuron. This depolarization of synaptic origin is called a *single-spike excitatory postsynaptic potential* (single-spike EPSP) (**Figure 11.3a**). Note the small amplitude of this EPSP. It is insensitive to APV (the antagonist of NMDA receptors) and totally abolished by CNQX (an antagonist of both AMPA and kainate receptors) (not shown), thus showing that it results from the activation of postsynaptic non-NMDA receptors.

In the rat hippocampus, a large-amplitude EPSP is recorded from an interneuron in response to the stimulation of the presynaptic pyramidal neuron. This EPSP presents two components: an early one abolished by CNQX and a late one abolished by APV. In the presence of APV there is a clear reduction in the EPSP duration

(a)

iGluRs	Non-NMDA receptors		NMDA receptors	
	AMPA R	**Kainate R**	Glu site	Gly site
Selective agonists		ATPA (GluR5)	NMDA	Glycine D-serine
Non-selective agonists	Glutamate AMPA Kainate		Glutamate	–
Selective antagonists	GYKI 53655 NBQX (1 µM)	LY 293558 (GluR5)	D-APV (or AP5)	5,7-dichloro-kynurenate
Selective antagonists	CNQX DNQX NBQX		–	–
Channel blockers	–	–	MK 801 ketamine	–

(b)

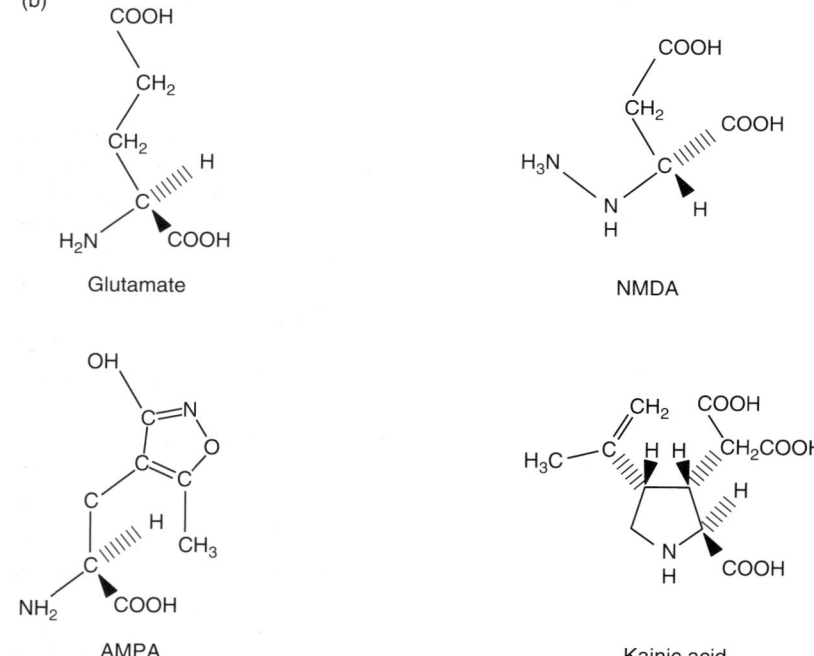

Glutamate

NMDA

AMPA

Kainic acid

(**Figure 11.3b**). The early component of the EPSP which remains is APV-insensitive; i.e. mediated by non-NMDA receptors. It is abolished by CNQX, a non-selective antagonist of AMPA and kainate receptors (not shown).

In the same preparation, the non-NMDA component recorded in the presence of APV can be further sepa- rated in AMPA-mediated and kainate-mediated thanks to GYKI 53655, a selective antagonist of AMPA recep- tors. The kainate component of the EPSP is thus revealed (**Figure 11.3c**). It is a very small-amplitude component that is antagonized by LY 293558, a selective antagonist GluR5-containing kainate receptor.

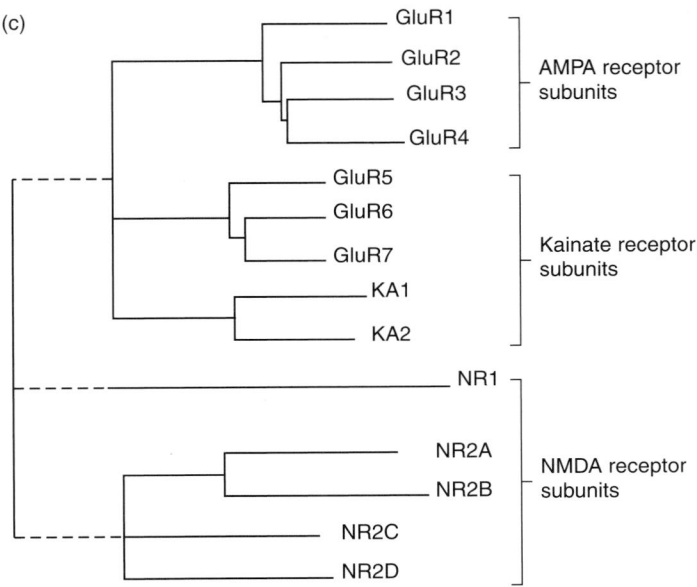

(c)

GluR1
GluR2
GluR3
GluR4
} AMPA receptor subunits

GluR5
GluR6
GluR7
KA1
KA2
} Kainate receptor subunits

NR1
NR2A
NR2B
NR2C
NR2D
} NMDA receptor subunits

Figure 11.1 (left and above) Pharmacology of ionotropic glutamate receptors.
(a) *Key:* AMPA, α amino-3-hydroxy-5-methyl-4-isoxalonepropionate; ATPA, (*RS*)-2-amino-3-(3-hydroxy-5-tert-butylisoxazol-4-yl)propionate; CNQX, 6-cyano-7-nitroquinoxaline-2,3-dione; D-APV, D-2-amino-5-phosphonopentanoate; DNQX, 6,7-dinitroquinoxaline-2,3-dione; GYKI 53655, atypical 2,3-benzodiazepines; MK 801, 5-methyl-10,11-dihydro-5H-dibenzocyclohepten-5,10-imine maleate; NBQX, 2,3-dihydroxy-6-nitro-7-sulphamoyl-benzo(F) quinoxaline; NMDA, *N*-methyl-D-aspartate. **(b)** Agonists of iGluRs: L-glutamate, NMDA, AMPA and kainate. **(c)** Dendrogram of the members of the ionotropic glutamate receptor family. Part (c) from Ozawa S, Kamiya H, Tsuzuki K (1998) Glutamate receptors in the mammalian central nervous system, *Prog. Neurobiol.* **54**, 581–618, with permission.

These observations raise several questions:

- Do all ionotropic glutamate receptors have the same properties, for example the same sensitivity to glutamate, the same ionic permeability?
- Do they have the same conditions of activation?
- Are all three always present in postsynaptic elements of glutamatergic synapses?

11.2 AMPA receptors are an ensemble of cationic receptor-channels with different permeabilities to Ca²⁺ ions

11.2.1 The diversity of AMPA receptors results from subunit combination, alternative splicing and post-transcriptional nuclear editing

Cloning studies have demonstrated that AMPA selective ionotropic glutamate receptors are built from the four closely related subunits GluR1, GluR2, GluR3 and GluR4. The four predicted polypeptide sequences, each approximately 900 amino acids in length, revealed similarities between 70% (GluR1 and 2) and 73% (GluR2 and 3). These subunits when expressed *in vitro* constitute a high-affinity ³H AMPA and low-affinity kainate receptor type of glutamate-gated ion channel. These different subunits are abundantly and differentially expressed in the brain, as revealed by *in situ* hybridization studies (see Appendix 7.2). Although these different GluR subunits exhibit some ability to form homomeric channels when expressed by themselves in *Xenopus* oocytes or cultured mammalian cells, it is considered likely that channels are formed *in vivo* by different combinations of subunits. Thus, with four receptor subunits there are already a very large number of potential combinations.

The diversity of GluR receptors results not only from subunit combinations but also from two genetic processes: *alternative splicing* and *editing* of the pre-messenger RNA (or primary transcript). Alternative splicing concerns the 38-amino-acid sequence preceding the most C-terminal putative transmembrane domain TM4 of each of the four receptor subunits (**Figure 11.2**). This small segment has been shown to exist in two versions (with different amino acid sequences), designated 'flip' and 'flop', and encoded by adjacent exons of the receptor genes. As a consequence, each of the four subunits exists in two molecular forms (GluR1 flip and GluR1 flop, GluR2 flip and Glu R2 flop...). When these splicing derivatives are expressed in oocytes, the proteins exhibit different properties (see Section 11.2.4). Native GluRs

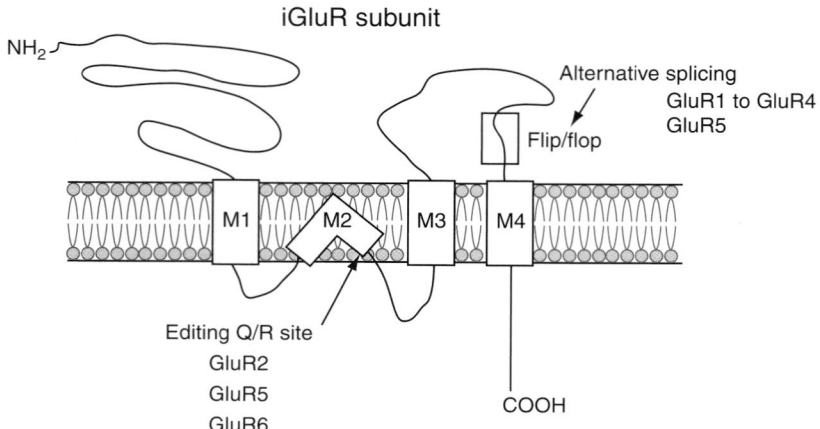

Figure 11.2 iGluR subunit topology.
See text. From Hollmann M, Maron C, Heinemann S (1994) N-glycosylation site tagging suggests a three transmembrane domain topology for the glutamate receptor GluR1, *Neuron* **13**, 1331–1343, with permission.

may be composed of heteromeric assemblies of different subunits which contain either flip or flop sequences.

Editing is a post-transcriptional change of one or more bases in the pre-mRNA such that the codon(s) encoded by the gene and the codon(s) present in the mRNA differ. It has been established that the sequences necessary for editing lie in the introns. Thus, only primary transcript can be edited. Therefore, editing is not a regulatory mechanism for mature mRNA, but results from post-transcriptional nuclear editing. In AMPA receptors, editing concerns only the GluR2 subunit. GluR2 subunit possesses an arginine (R) in the M2 putative membrane spanning segment at position 586; whereas in GluR1, 3 and 4 subunits, glutamine (Q) lies in the homologous position. This functional critical position is referred to as the Q/R site (see **Figure 11.2**). The arginine codon (CGG) is not found in the GluR2 gene. It is introduced into the GluR2 mRNA by an adenosine to inosine conversion in the respective glutamine codon (CAG) of the GluR2 transcript by a double-stranded RNA adenosine deaminase. The inosine is subsequently read as a guanosine, resulting in the change of codon identity (CGG). Editing is developmentally regulated such that 99% of the GluR2 subunit in postnatal stages is in the edited (R) form. The consequences of the GluR2 editing at the Q/R site are analysed in Section 11.2.3.

11.2.2 The native AMPA receptor is permeable to cations and has a unitary conductance of 8 pS

When quisqualate (1–10 μM) is applied in the extracellular milieu of cultured central neurons recorded in the outside-out patch clamp configuration, an inward unitary current, i_q, is observed at $V_m = -60$ mV (**Figure 11.4a**). If the application of quisqualate is repeated on different membrane patches recorded at the same membrane potential, one observes that the recorded inward unitary currents are not a homogeneous population. The unitary conductance values corresponding to the four peaks of **Figure 11.4b** are calculated from the different i_q recorded with the equation $i_q = \gamma_q(V_m - E_{rev})$ given that $E_{rev} = 0$ mV. One set of similar unitary currents appears with a higher frequency than the others, the one of $\gamma_q = 8$ pS. Plotting the mean unitary current amplitude of this population as a function of the membrane potential, we obtain an i_q/V_m relation (**Figure 11.4c**) that follows the equation $i_q = \gamma_q(V_m - E_{rev})$. Between −80 mV and +80 mV this curve is linear (i.e. voltage-independent), has a slope of 8 pS, and shows a quisqualate current reversal potential of approximately 0 mV.

These results show that the majority of the channels activated by quisqualate have a unitary conductance of 8 pS, and that this conductance is only slightly or not at all sensitive to membrane potential variations. Additionally, the unitary current i_q reverses at a value close to 0 mV if the extracellular and intracellular environments contain similar concentrations of monovalent cations (**Figure 11.4c**). This suggests that the quisqualate-activated channel is permeable to cations.

To test this hypothesis, the reversal potential of the current is recorded at different intracellular and extracellular concentrations of Na⁺ and K⁺ ions. When the extracellular Na⁺ concentration is lowered from 140 to 50 mM by replacing Na⁺ ions with choline ions, the reversal potential becomes negative (it shifts from 0 mV to about −20 mV). When Cs⁺ ions substitute for intracellular K⁺ ions, the reversal potential is not affected. These results suggest that the quisqualate-activated channel is

(a) Non-NMDA-mediated EPSP

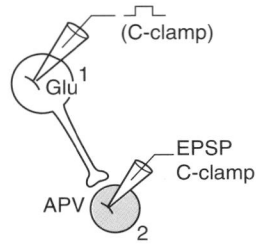
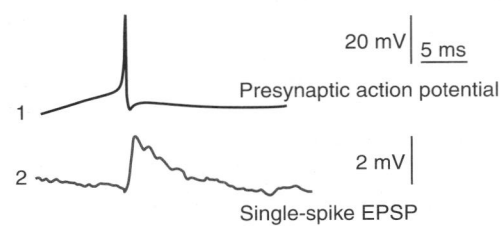

Presynaptic action potential

Single-spike EPSP

(b) NMDA and non-NMDA-mediated EPSP

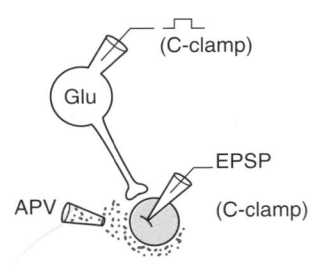
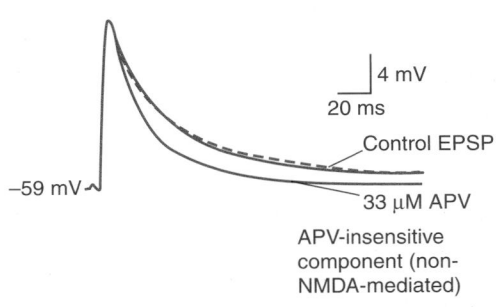

Control EPSP

33 µM APV

APV-insensitive component (non-NMDA-mediated)

(c) Kainate-mediated EPSP

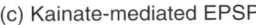
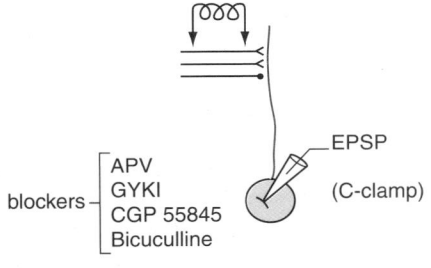
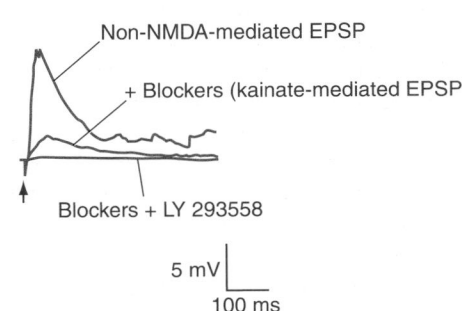

Non-NMDA-mediated EPSP

+ Blockers (kainate-mediated EPSP

Blockers + LY 293558

Figure 11.3 iGluR-mediated EPSPs and their components.
(a) Current clamp recordings of a presynaptic glutamatergic pyramidal neuron and a postsynaptic interneuron in the cat neocortex *in vitro*. A spike triggered by a current pulse in the presynaptic neuron evokes a single-spike EPSP in the postsynaptic interneuron (intracellular recordings). (b) The same experiment in the hippocampus *in vitro*. In response to a stronger stimulation of the presynaptic pyramidal neuron and in the absence of external Mg^{2+}, a postsynaptic EPSP of larger amplitude (control) with a fast rising phase and a long duration (sometimes up to 500 ms) is recorded. The same experiment in the presence of APV (APV, 33 µM). Picrotoxin is added to the extracellular solution in order to block $GABA_A$ synaptic receptors. (c) In response to the stimulation of afferent fibres, a control EPSP is recorded from a hippocampal interneuron. In the presence of blockers of NMDA (APV), AMPA (GYKI 53655), $GABA_B$ (CGP 55845) and $GABA_A$ (bicuculline) receptors, a low-amplitude component is still present. It is mediated by kainate receptors since it is totally blocked by LY 293558. Part (a) from Buhl EH, Tamas G, Szilagyi T *et al.* (1997) Effect, number and location of synapses made by single pyramidal cells onto aspiny interneurons of cat visual cortex, *J. Physiol. (Lond.)* **500**, 689–713, with permission. Part (b) from Forsythe ID, Westbrook GL (1988) Slow excitatory postsynaptic currents mediated by *N*-methyl-D-aspartate receptors on cultured mouse central neurons, *J. Physiol. (Lond.)* **396**, 515–533, with permission. Part (c) from Cossart R, Esclapez M, Hirsch J *et al.* (1998) GluR5 kainate receptor activation in interneurons increases tonic inhibition of pyramidal cells, *Nature Neurosci.* **1**, 470–478, with permission.

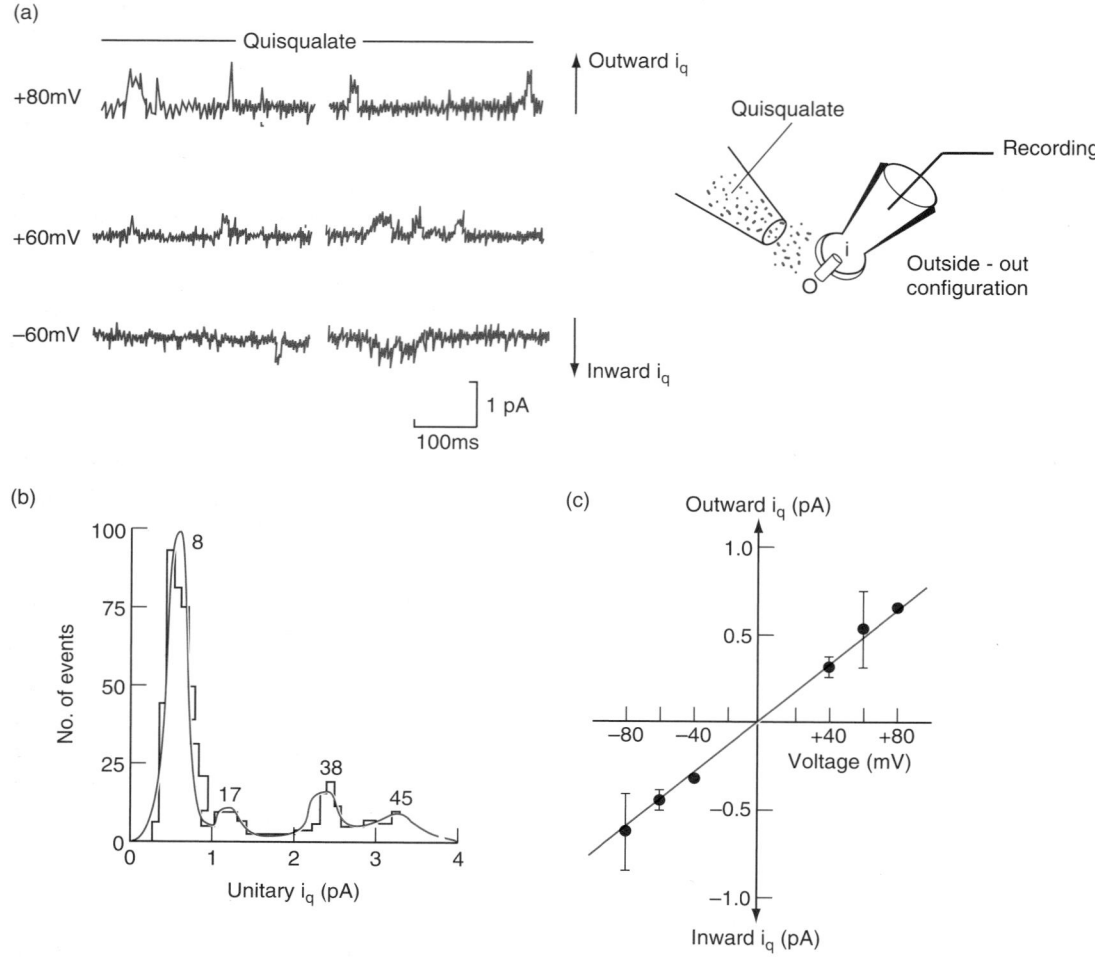

Figure 11.4 Electrophysiological properties of native AMPA receptor-channel.
(a) Patch clamp recording (outside-out configuration) of the activity of a quisqualate-activated channel. When the membrane is held at −60 mV, the unitary current i_q is inward (downward deflection). At +60 mV or +80 mV, i_q is outward (upward deflection). **(b)** Unitary current amplitude histogram (in pA). Currents recorded at the same voltage but from different membrane patches. **(c)** i_q/V curve obtained from the averages of unitary currents recorded from a homogeneous population of channels (8 pS population). Intrapipette solution (in mM): 140 CsCl, 5 K-EGTA, 0.5 $CaCl_2$; extracellular solution: 140 NaCl, 2.8 KCl, 1 $CaCl_2$. Parts (a) and (c) from Ascher P, Nowak L (1988) Quisqualate and kainate-activated channels in mouse central neurons in culture, *J. Physiol. (Lond.)* **399**, 227–245, with permission. Part (b) from Cull-Candy SG, Usowicz MM (1987) Patch clamp recording from single glutamate-receptor channels, *TIPS* **8**, 218–224, with permission.

permeable to Na^+, K^+ and Cs^+ ions, and impermeable to choline ions.

This quisqualate-activated channel shows a low permeability to divalent cations, especially to Ca^{2+}. Thus, variations by a factor of 20 of the extracellular Ca^{2+} concentration have no effect on the reversal potential of the quisqualate current recorded from neurons in the whole-cell configuration. Likewise, only small changes of the photometrically recorded intracellular Ca^{2+} concentration (see Appendix 6.1) can be measured during a quisqualate-evoked response at a constant voltage of −60 mV. It should be noted that it is essential to carry out these recordings in cells maintained at membrane

potentials lower than the activation threshold of the voltage-sensitive Ca^{2+} channel in order to prevent Ca^{2+} inflow through these channels.

In conclusion, this native quisqualate-activated channel, recorded in spinal neurons in culture, is permeable to monovalent cations: the application of quisqualate at a membrane potential of $V_m = -60$ mV evokes a unitary inward current that results from the inflow of Na^+ ions and an outflow of K^+ ions through the same channel (the Na^+ inflow is stronger than the K^+ outflow). This AMPA receptor is a classic cationic channel receptor: it has a negligible permeability to Ca^{2+} ions ($P_{Ca}/P_{Na} = 0.1$) and its conductance is only weakly voltage-dependent.

However, studies performed in other preparations show that some AMPA receptors are permeable to Ca^{2+} ions. The above pioneering electrophysiological experiments which characterized the properties of native AMPA receptor-channels were carried out before molecular cloning of glutamate receptor subunits had been achieved, which showed that the Ca^{2+} permeability of AMPA receptor channels varies with their subunit composition. In the example of Figure 11.4, the native AMPA receptors studied probably contained in their structure the edited form of GluR2 (GluR2(R)) as explained below.

11.2.3 AMPA receptors are permeable to Na^+, K^+ and Ca^{2+} ions unless the edited form of GluR2 is present; in the latter case, AMPA receptors are impermeable to Ca^{2+} ions

The mRNA editing at the Q/R site for AMPA receptors concerns only the GluR2 subunit. This change from glutamine (Q) to arginine (R) (**Figure 11.5a**) has a major consequence on the channel permeability: those channels with a GluR2(R) edited subunit are Ca^{2+}-impermeable while those with a GluR2(Q) non-edited subunit or with no GluR2 subunit are Ca^{2+}-permeable.

To show this, the current response to glutamate of homomeric GluR channels expressed in transfected cells is studied in extracellular solutions containing Na^+ or Ca^{2+} as the only cations. In cells expressing the GluR2(R) subunit only, the glutamate-evoked current is present in high Na^+ solution and nearly absent in high Ca^{2+} solution, indicating that this homomeric channel has a low divalent/monovalent permeability ratio. Moreover, heteromeric GluR2(R) + GluR1 subunit association forms Ca^{2+}-impermeable oligomeric channels in oocytes (**Figure 11.5b**). The situation is different in the absence of the GluR2(R) subunit since homomeric GluR1, GluR3 or heteromeric GluR1 + GluR3 channels allow the influx of Ca^{2+}. Therefore, the presence of a positively charged side-chain of one amino acid (R) would determine the divalent/monovalent permeability ratio and thus GluR2(R) would dominate the properties of ion flow through the heteromeric GluR channel. The positive charge of arginine at the Q/R site hinders the permeation of divalent cations in AMPA channels.

11.2.4 The presence of flip or flop isoforms plays a role on the amplitude of the total AMPA current

Each of the GluR1–GluR4 subunits exists in two different forms, flip and flop, created by alternative splicing of a 115-base-pair region immediately preceding TM4 (**Figures 11.2 and 11.5a**). Nine amino acids in this region are different between flip and flop versions. When these splicing derivatives are expressed in oocytes, the AMPA receptors exhibit different properties: AMPA receptors incorporating the flip sequence allow more current entry into the cell in response to glutamate than receptors containing solely flop modules (**Figure 11.5c**). Native AMPA receptors may be composed of heteromeric assemblies of different subunits which contain either flip or flop sequences. For example, native AMPA receptors expressed in rat cerebellar granule cells are known to be composed of both flip and flop forms of GluR2 and GluR4, with the flop isoform increasing with age.

11.3 Kainate receptors are an ensemble of cationic receptor channels with different permeabilities to Ca^{2+} ions

Kainic acid is a powerful neurotoxin, which kills neurons by means of overexcitation. It is isolated from a seaweed known for its potency at killing intestinal worms. The word 'kainic' is derived from the Japanese *kaininso* which means the 'ghost of the sea'. At nanomolar concentrations, kainate is a preferential agonist of kainate receptors but at higher concentrations it also activates AMPA receptors (see **Figure 1.1a**).

11.3.1 The diversity of kainate receptors

A family of kainate receptors has been cloned and five subunits termed GluR5, GluR6, GluR7, KA1 and KA2 have been identified (see **Figure 11.1c**). GluR5 to GluR7 may represent the low-affinity kainate-binding site with K_D around 50 nM, whereas KA1 and KA2 correspond to the high-affinity kainate-binding site (K_D around 5 nM) in neuronal membranes. GluR5 to GluR7 are of similar size and share 75–80% amino acid sequence identity with each other and around 40% with AMPA receptors. KA1 and KA2 share 70% amino acid sequence identity with each other and around 40% with either GluR1–GluR4 or GluR5–GluR7. Homomeric GluR7, KA1 and KA2 expression does not generate agonist-sensitive channels. Kainate-evoked currents are observed only in homomeric receptors of GluR5 or GluR6 subunits and when KA2 is co-expressed with GluR5 or GluR6 subunits.

For GluR5 and GluR6, mRNA editing occurs at the Q/R site in the M2 segment (but not in GluR7) (see **Figure 11.2**). For GluR6 there are two additional sites of editing in the first transmembrane segment (TM1) (see **Figure 11.7a**). In contrast to GluR2, the Q/R site editing is incomplete during development and significant amounts of both edited and non-edited versions of

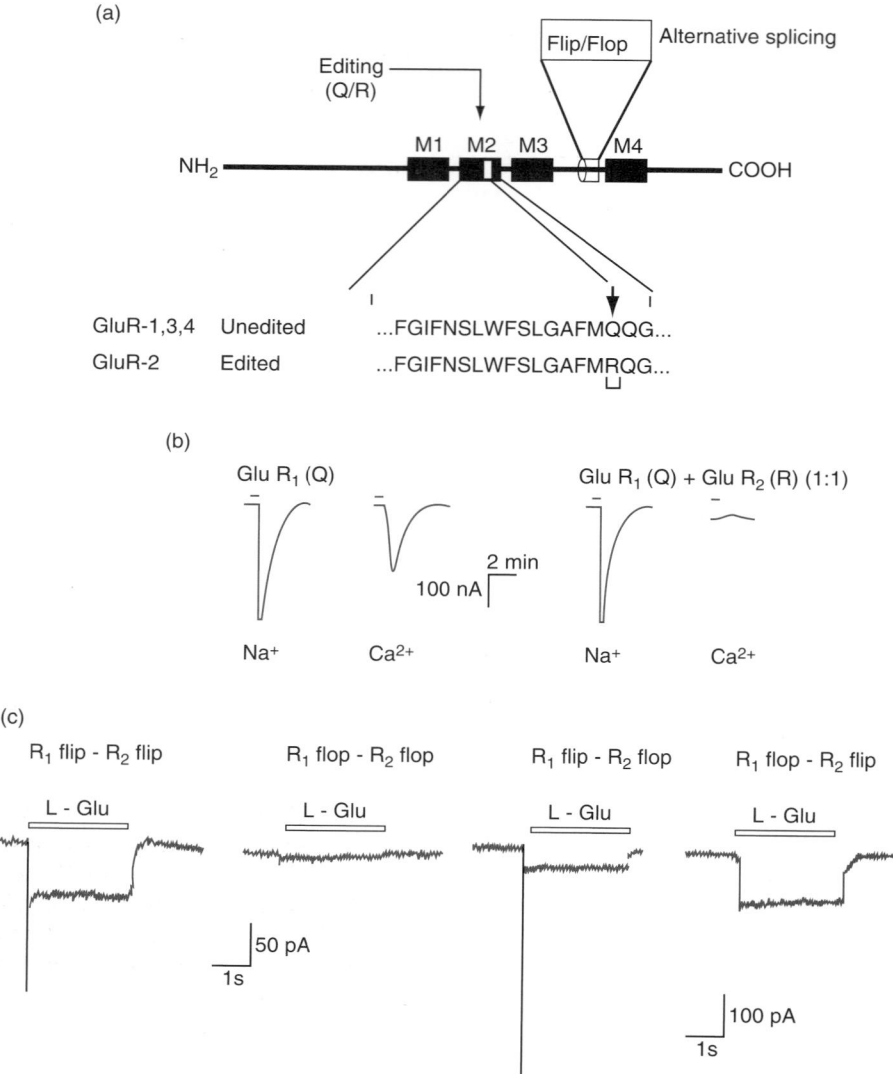

(a)

Editing (Q/R)

Flip/Flop   Alternative splicing

M1 M2 M3   M4

NH₂ —————————————————— COOH

GluR-1,3,4   Unedited   ...FGIFNSLWFSLGAFMQQG...
GluR-2   Edited   ...FGIFNSLWFSLGAFMRQG...

(b)

Glu R₁ (Q)   Glu R₁ (Q) + Glu R₂ (R) (1:1)

2 min
100 nA

Na⁺   Ca²⁺   Na⁺   Ca²⁺

(c)

R₁ flip - R₂ flip   R₁ flop - R₂ flop   R₁ flip - R₂ flop   R₁ flop - R₂ flip

L - Glu   L - Glu   L - Glu   L - Glu

50 pA
1s

100 pA
1s

Figure 11.5 Functional properties of AMPA receptors.
(a) Linear representation of the predicted structure of AMPA receptors. The regions where alternative splicing and Q/R occur are indicated. **(b)** Comparison of whole-cell currents evoked by pulse application (25 s, bars) of a glutamate agonist to homomeric GluR1(Q) (left) or heteromeric GluR1(Q) + GluR2(R) (right) channels expressed in oocytes and recorded in normal Ringer (Na⁺) and Ca²⁺-Ringer (Ca²⁺) solutions. Oocytes were injected with a single GluR subunit cRNA (2 ng) or a combination of two types of GluR subunit cRNA (2 ng + 2 ng for 1:1 combination). Intrapipette solution (in mM): 250 CsCl, 250 CsF, 100 EGTA. Na-external solution (in mM): 115 NaCl, 2.5 KCl, 1.8 CaCl₂, 10 Hepes; Ca²⁺-external solution (in mM): 10 CaCl₂, 10 Hepes. **(c)** Whole-cell recordings of the inward current evoked by rapid application of an L-glutamate agonist (300 μM) at a holding potential of –60 mV in cultured mammalian cells engineered for the transient expression of the flip forms or the flop forms of GluR1 and GluR2. Part (a) from Sommer B, Keinänen K, Verdoorn TA *et al.* (1990) Flip and flop: a cell-specific functional switch in glutamate-operated channels of the CNS, *Science* **249**, 1580–1585, with permission. Part (c) from Hollmann M, Hartley M, Heinemann S (1991) Ca²⁺ permeability of KA-AMPA-gated glutamate receptor channels depends on subunit composition, *Science* **252**, 851–853, with permission.

GluR5 and GluR6 coexist in adult brain. RNA editing at these sites are critical determinants of the Ca²⁺ permeability and rectification properties of kainate receptors. Alternative splicing of GluR5 further adds to receptor diversity.

11.3.2 Native kainate receptors are permeable to cations

In comparison with AMPA and NMDA channels, relatively little is known about the properties of kainate

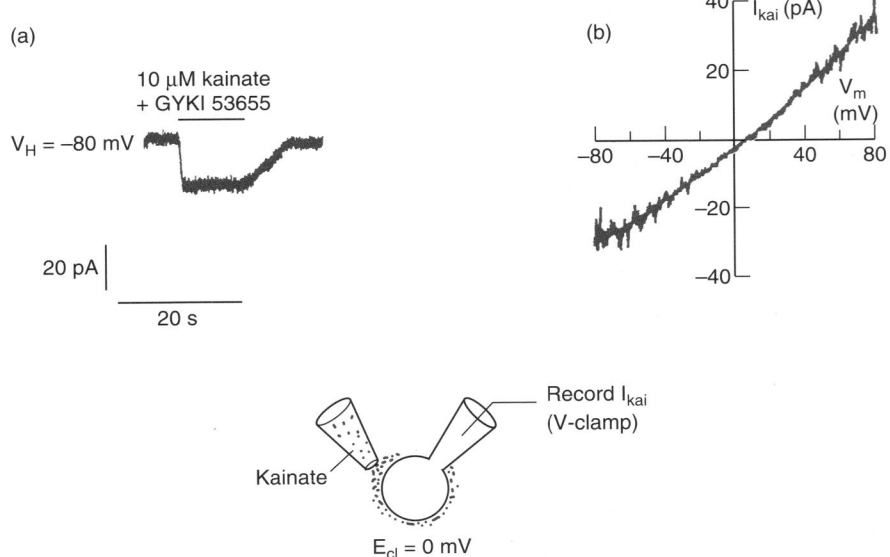

Figure 11.6 Whole-cell kainate current in cerebellar granule cells.

(a) Whole-cell current (I_{kai}) evoked by the application of 10 μm of kainate in the presence of GYKI 53655 (100 μM) in a concanavalin A-treated granule cell. **(b)** I_{kai}/V relationship. I_{kai} is measured during 500 ms voltage ramps from −80 to +80 mV. From Pemberton KE, Belcher SM, Ripellino JA, Howe JR (1998) High affinity kainate-type ion channels in rat cerebellar granule cells, *J. Physiol. (Lond.)* **510**, 401–420, with permission.

channels in central neurons despite their widespread expression in the brain. One way to study kainate channels in isolation is to apply kainate (or the agonist SYM 2081) in the presence of the selective antagonist GYKI 53655 to block AMPA responses.

Granule cells of the rat cerebellar cortex are dissociated and plated in culture dishes. Whole-cell recordings are performed in voltage clamp mode in order to record the total kainate current (I_{kai}). Concanavalin A is added in the extracellular solution to reduce kainate receptor desensitization. Kainate 10 μM in the presence of GYKI 53655 evokes an inward current when the membrane is held at −80 mV (**Figure 11.6a**). The current/voltage curve obtained by varying the holding potential is shown in **Figure 11.6b**. I_{kai} reverses around 0 mV, suggesting that it is carried by cations (in the presence of control extra- and intracellular solutions). Experiments in high Na⁺ or Cs⁺ solutions have confirmed the cationic permeability of kainate channels. Changes in Ca^{2+} permeability due to editing of either TM1 or TM2 sites of GluR6 subunits (**Figure 11.7a**) have been shown but the exact correlation between editing of the specific sites and permeability to Ca^{2+} ions is still under study.

Editing at the Q/R site affects the I_{kai}/V relationship in hippocampal neurons. In cells expressing GluR6(Q), the non-edited form of GluR6 at the TM2 site, as shown by single-cell RT-PCR, the current/voltage relationship shows a strong inward rectification (**Figure 11.7b**); whereas in a cell expressing the edited form, GluR6(R),

the curve is almost linear (**Figure 11.7c**). This shows a clear relationship between the rectification properties of native kainate receptors and RNA editing of Q/R site in the GluR6 subunit mRNA. One of the possible physiological consequences for the presence of rectification is that in a membrane depolarized to around −20 mV, the GluR6(Q)-mediated current is extremely small.

11.4 NMDA receptors are cationic-receptor-channels highly permeable to Ca^{2+} ions; they are blocked by Mg^{2+} ions at voltages close to the resting potential, which confers strong voltage-dependence

11.4.1 Molecular biology of NMDA receptors

Molecular cloning has identified to date cDNAs encoding NR1 and NR2A, B, C, D subunits of the NMDA receptor (see **Figure 11.1c**), the deduced amino acid sequences of which are 18% (NR1 and NR2), 55% (NR2A and NR2C) or 70% (NR2A and NR2B) identical. When the *Xenopus* oocyte system and transfected mammalian cells are employed to study the functional properties of these subunits, large currents are measured only in oocytes co-expressing NR1 and NR2 subunits.

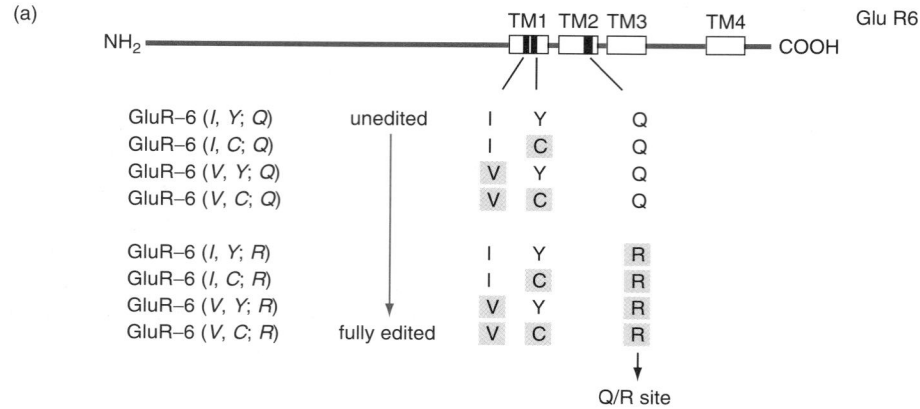

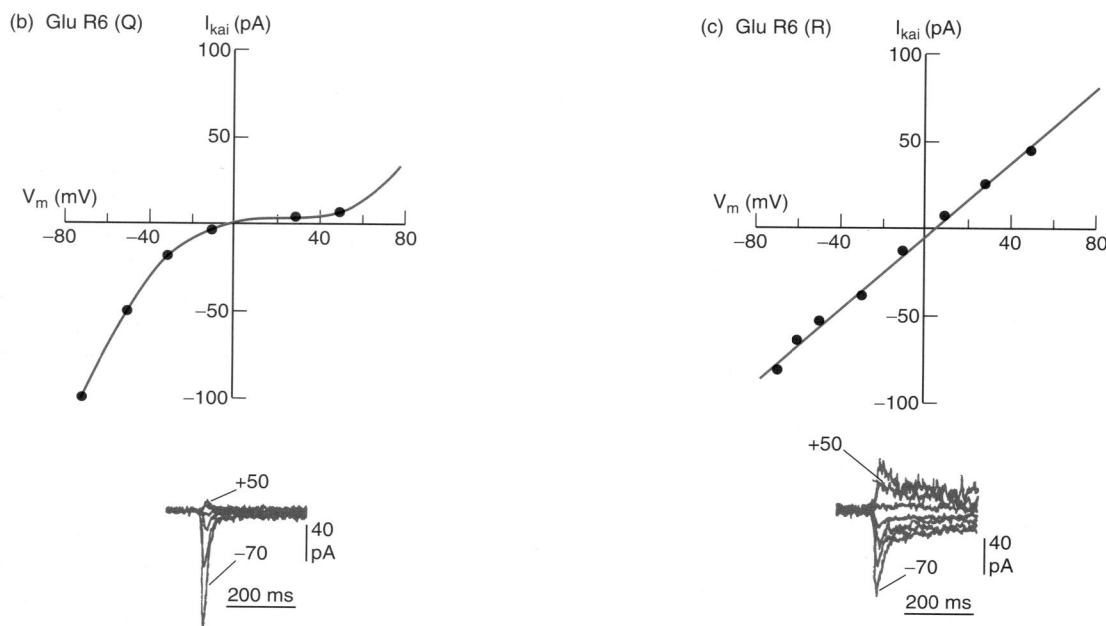

Figure 11.7 Correlation of functional properties of native kainate receptors and RNA editing of the Q/R site of the GluR6 subunit.

(a) Eight GluR6 variants generated by editing codons in the TM1 and TM2 segments. An approximate relative frequency for each variant is indicated on the right. **(b, c)** Current/voltage relationships of the kainate-induced current in two different hippocampal neurons, (b) expressing homomeric GluR6(Q) and (c) expressing homomeric GluR6(R). Kainate (300 μM) is rapidly applied while holding the membrane potential at different voltages, from −70 to +50 mV. Insets show the current traces at these different voltages. Part (a) from Köhler M, Burnashev N, Sakmann B, Seeburg PH (1993) Determinants of Ca^{2+} permeability in both TM1 and TM2 of high affinity kainate receptor channels: diversity by RNA editing, *Neuron* **10**, 491–500, with permission. Part (b) from Ruano D, Lambolez B, Rossier J *et al.* (1995) Kainate receptor subunits expressed in single cultured hippocampal neurons: molecular and functional variants by RNA editing, *Neuron* **14**, 1009–1017, with permission.

This result tends to predict that natural NMDA receptors would occur as hetero-oligomers like other ligand-gated channels. Since recombinant heteromeric NMDA receptors display different properties depending on which of the four NR2 subunits are assembled with NR1, the NR2 subunits can be regarded as modulatory subunits whereas the NR1 serves as a fundamental subunit.

Site-directed mutagenesis has revealed that the NR2 subunit carries the binding site for glutamate within the N-terminal domain and the extracellular loop between membrane segments M3 and M4; whereas the homologous domains of the NR1 subunit carries the binding site for the co-agonist glycine. NR1 and NR2 subunits carry in the M2 segment (which forms a re-entrant loop) an asparagine residue in a position homologous to the Q/R site of AMPA receptors (see **Figure 11.11a**). Expression of modified subunits in *Xenopus* oocytes showed that these asparagines are crucial for the particular properties of divalent ion permeation of NMDA channels.

11.4.2 Native NMDA receptors have a high unitary conductance of 40–50 pS

The experiments related in this section allowed the characterization of the electrophysiological properties of native NMDA channels. They were carried out before molecular cloning of NMDA receptor subunits had been achieved. As has already been pointed out, the NMDA channel has the property of being blocked by extracellular Mg^{2+} ions at voltages close to the resting potential of the cell, Mg^{2+} ions blocking the channel in the open state thus preventing the passage of other ions. The concentrations of Mg^{2+} that produce a significant block are similar to the concentrations of Mg^{2+} normally present in the extracellular milieu. For the sake of clarity, we shall first look at the conductance and permeability properties of the NMDA channel in the absence of extracellular Mg^{2+}. Subsequently we shall consider the nature of the changes that occur in a medium containing Mg^{2+} ions.

Let us look at patch clamp recordings (outside-out configuration) of cultured central neurons in the absence of Mg^{2+} ions. The application of NMDA (10 nM) in the extracellular milieu at $V_m = -60$ mV induces an inward unitary current, i_N (**Figure 11.8a**). The i_N/V relation obtained under these conditions is linear (between -80 mV and $+60$ mV) and is described by the equation $i_N = \gamma_N(V_m - E_{rev})$ (**Figure 11.8b**). The slope of this curve corresponds to the unitary conductance of the NMDA channel, γ_N. The average value of γ_N is in the range 40–50 pS. The unitary conductance of NMDA channels is only slightly voltage-dependent in the absence of Mg^{2+} ions.

11.4.3 The NMDA channel is highly permeable to monovalent cations and to Ca^{2+}

The i_N/V relation shows that i_N reverses at a membrane potential value close to 0 mV when the extracellular and intracellular ion concentrations are similar. This value suggests that the NMDA channel is permeable to cations. If one replaces any of the monovalent cations (Na^+, K^+ or Cs^+) by another, one observes only minor changes in the reversal potential; i.e. the channel discriminates only slightly between the different monovalent cations.

In order to establish whether the NMDA channel is permeable to Ca^{2+} or not, two types of experiments have been performed.

The first type of experiment consisted of photometric measurements (see Appendix 6.1) of the variations of intracellular Ca^{2+} in response to NMDA. To carry out these experiments and to prevent the activation of voltage-dependent Ca^{2+} channels, spinal neuron activity is recorded in patch clamp (whole-cell configuration) at a holding potential of -60 mV (**Figure 11.9a**). Under these conditions one observes a strong increase of the intracellular Ca^{2+} concentration during an NMDA-evoked response. This augmentation is selectively blocked by the antagonist APV and by the NMDA channel blocker MK 801. It clearly results from an influx of Ca^{2+} through the NMDA channels and is not due to a release of these ions from intracellular storage pools of Ca^{2+}, since it disappears in Ca^{2+}-free external solution.

A second type of experiment has shown that changes in the extracellular Ca^{2+} concentration is accompanied by changes in the reversal potential of the macroscopic NMDA current (**Figure 11.9b**). This indicates that Ca^{2+} ions actually carry part of the NMDA current. Furthermore, if the activity of a NMDA channel is recorded under conditions where Ca^{2+} is the only cation present in the extracellular milieu, at -60 mV one can observe an inward current. Ca^{2+} ions are the only ions that can carry this current under these conditions.

What does molecular biology tell us about Ca^{2+} permeability?

The molecular substrate for Ca^{2+} permeability of NMDA channels is analysed by exchanging (by site-directed mutagenesis) either glutamine (Q) or arginine (R) for asparagine (N) in the TM2 domain of NR1 or NR2A subunits (see **Figure 11.11a**). Wildtype and mutant NR subunits are co-expressed by cells transfected with cDNAs. Whole-cell currents are activated by application of L-glutamate to transfected cells expressing heteromeric wild type or mutant NMDA receptors and differences in Ca^{2+} permeability are analysed. Replacing the asparagine (N) by arginine (R) in the NR1 subunit generates 'mutant NR1-wildtype NR2A' channels that do not exhibit a measurable Ca^{2+} permeability (see **Figure 11.11b**). In high Ca^{2+} solution, glutamate evokes a small outward current at $V_H = -60$ mV, indicating a low Ca^{2+} permeability of the mutant channel. Thus, when the positively charged arginine (R) occupies the critical position in TM2 of the NR1 subunit, Ca^{2+} ions appear to be prevented from entering the channel, suggesting that the size and the charge of the amino acid present at this critical position in the M2 segment are important for Ca^{2+} permeability.

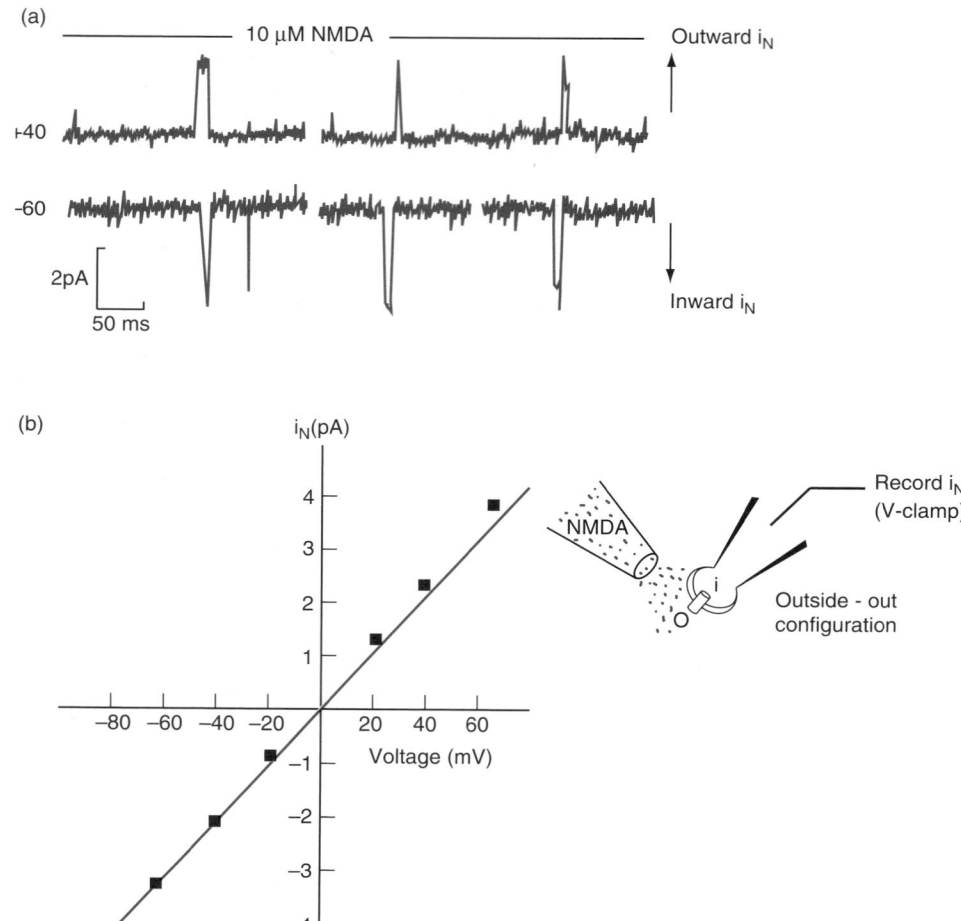

Figure 11.8 Unitary NMDA current in the absence of extracellular Mg^{2+}.
(a) Outside-out patch clamp recordings of the activity of a NMDA (10 μM) activated channel at two holding potentials, −60 and +40 mV.
(b) i_N/V relation obtained from the averages of unitary currents i_N recorded from a homogeneous population of channels (a population that shows a 40–50 pS unitary conductance). Intrapipette solution (in mM): 140 CsCl, 5K-EGTA, 0.5 CaCl$_2$; extracellular solution: 140 NaCl, 2.8 KCl, 1 CaCl$_2$. Part (a) from Ascher P, Bregestovski P, Nowak L (1988) N-methyl-D-aspartate-activated channels of mouse central neurons in magnesium free solutions, *J. Physiol. (Lond.)* **399**, 207–226, with permission. Part (b) from Cull-Candy SG, Usowicz MM (1987) Patch clamp recording from single glutamate-receptor channels, *TIPS* **8**, 218–224, with permission.

11.4.4 NMDA channels are blocked by physiological concentrations of extracellular Mg^{2+} ions; this block is voltage-dependent

Single NMDA channel current evoked by NMDA (10 nM) is recorded in the presence of increasing concentrations of extracellular Mg^{2+} ions (in nM: 0, 10, 50, 100) **(Figure 11.10a)**. At V_H = −60 mV, NMDA (10 nM) evokes an inward unitary current whose amplitude remains constant at all the Mg^{2+} concentrations tested (i_N = 2.7 pA). However, while in the absence of Mg^{2+} the NMDA channel opens for periods of several milliseconds (0), in the presence of Mg^{2+} (10, 50, 100 nM) the

recordings show bursts of short openings during which the channel fluctuates between open (t_o) and blocked (t_{bl}) periods. For a Mg^{2+} concentration of 100 nM, the unitary current appears to have a lower amplitude. This is actually due to its higher closing frequency which the recording system is unable to follow. The repeated closures of the channel (which actually correspond to fluctuations between the open and the blocked states) strongly diminish the average time during which the channel is open. Note that when the recorded unitary current is outward at V_H = +40 mV, the presence of Mg^{2+}, even at a concentration of 100 nM, has no effect on the channel open time. The most interesting aspect of

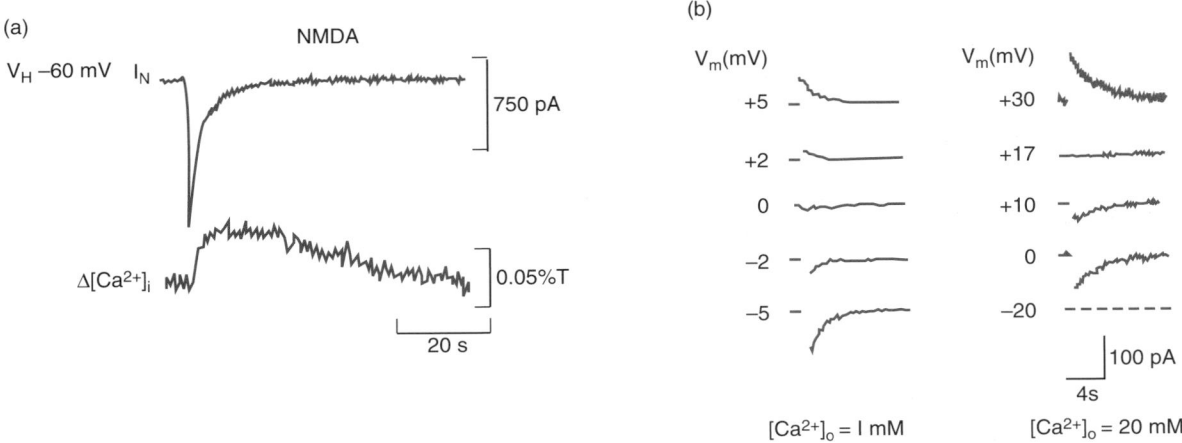

Figure 11.9 Optical measurements of intracellular Ca²⁺ concentration changes during a NMDA-evoked response.
The Ca^{2+}-sensitive dye Arsenazo III is used. The absorption coefficient of this dye varies at certain wavelengths when it complexes Ca^{2+} ions. The activity of cultured spinal neurons is recorded in the whole-cell patch clamp configuration in the absence of external Mg^{2+}. **(a)** Pressure application of 1 μM of NMDA (20 ms) in the presence of 2.5 mM of Ca^{2+} in the extracellular milieu evokes an inward current I_N (top trace). During this response there is an increase of $[Ca^{2+}]_i$ (bottom trace). **(b)** Reversal potential of the whole-cell NMDA current (I_N) as a function of extracellular $[Ca^{2+}]_o$. Currents activated by the application of 1 mM of NMDA are recorded at different membrane potentials in the presence of 1 mM (left) or 20 mM (right) of $[Ca^{2+}]_o$. Part (a) from Mayer ML, MacDermott AB, Westbrook GL et al. (1987) Agonist- and voltage-gated calcium entry in cultured mouse spinal chord neurons under voltage clamp using Arsenazo III, J. Neurosci. **7**, 3230–3244, with permission. Part (b) from MacDermott AB, Mayer ML, Westbrook GL et al. (1986) NMDA-receptor activation increases cytoplasmic calcium concentration in cultured spinal neurons, Nature **321**, 519–522, with permission.

this block is its voltage dependence. Mg^{2+} ions block the channel atnegative potentials while at positive voltages (wherethe current i_N is outward) they have almost no effect at all.

The same properties as those of the unitary current are observed in macroscopic recordings (whole-cell configuration). Recall that $I_N = Np_o i_N$. We know that i_N is approximately constant at a given membrane potential irrespective of the Mg^{2+} concentration, and that the mean open time of each channel (and therefore, the open state probability p_o of the channel as well) decreases as a function of the Mg^{2+} concentration. From the recordings in **Figure 11.10a** we can predict that at negative potentials, in the presence of Mg^{2+}, the macroscopic current I_N will be small.

As a matter of fact, the I_N/V curve described by the equation $I_N = G_N(V_m - E_{rev})$ in the presence of extracellular Mg^{2+} ions (500 nM) is not linear. This nonlinearity appears at negative voltages; i.e. when the current is inward (**Figure 11.10b**). Furthermore, we observe that for V_H between –35 and –80 mV, the current amplitude diminishes instead of increasing (region of negative conductance), as would be expected from the increasing electrochemical gradients for Na^+ and Ca^{2+} and the decreasing electrochemical gradient for K^+. This peculiar property of the I_N/V curve in this region of voltage

is due to the block of the channel by Mg^{2+}. Since Mg^{2+} ions are normally found in the extracellular milieu at concentrations of approximately 1 mM, at membrane potentials close to the resting potential a majority of NMDA channels are blocked.

Mechanism of action of Mg²⁺ ion block: a hypothesis

Mg^{2+} ions block open NMDA channels, thus preventing the passage of Na^+, Ca^{2+} and K^+ ions. The probability that a Mg^{2+} ion will enter the NMDA channel increases with the level of membrane hyperpolarization: the greater the electrical gradient, the stronger are the Mg^{2+} ions attracted into the channel. For this reason, the block of NMDA channels by Mg^{2+} is voltage-sensitive. This block can be symbolized as follows:

$$R + NMDA \rightleftharpoons NMDA - R^* \overset{Mg^{2+}}{\underset{\perp}{\rightleftharpoons}} NMDA - R^*\text{-}Mg$$

where R is the NMDA channel in the closed state, R* is the NMDA channel in the open state, and R*-Mg is the open NMDA channel blocked by Mg^{2+} ions. The reaction $R^* + Mg^{2+} \rightleftharpoons R^*\text{-}Mg$ is strongly favoured to the right when $[Mg^{2+}]$ is increased and when $V_m < 0$ mV.

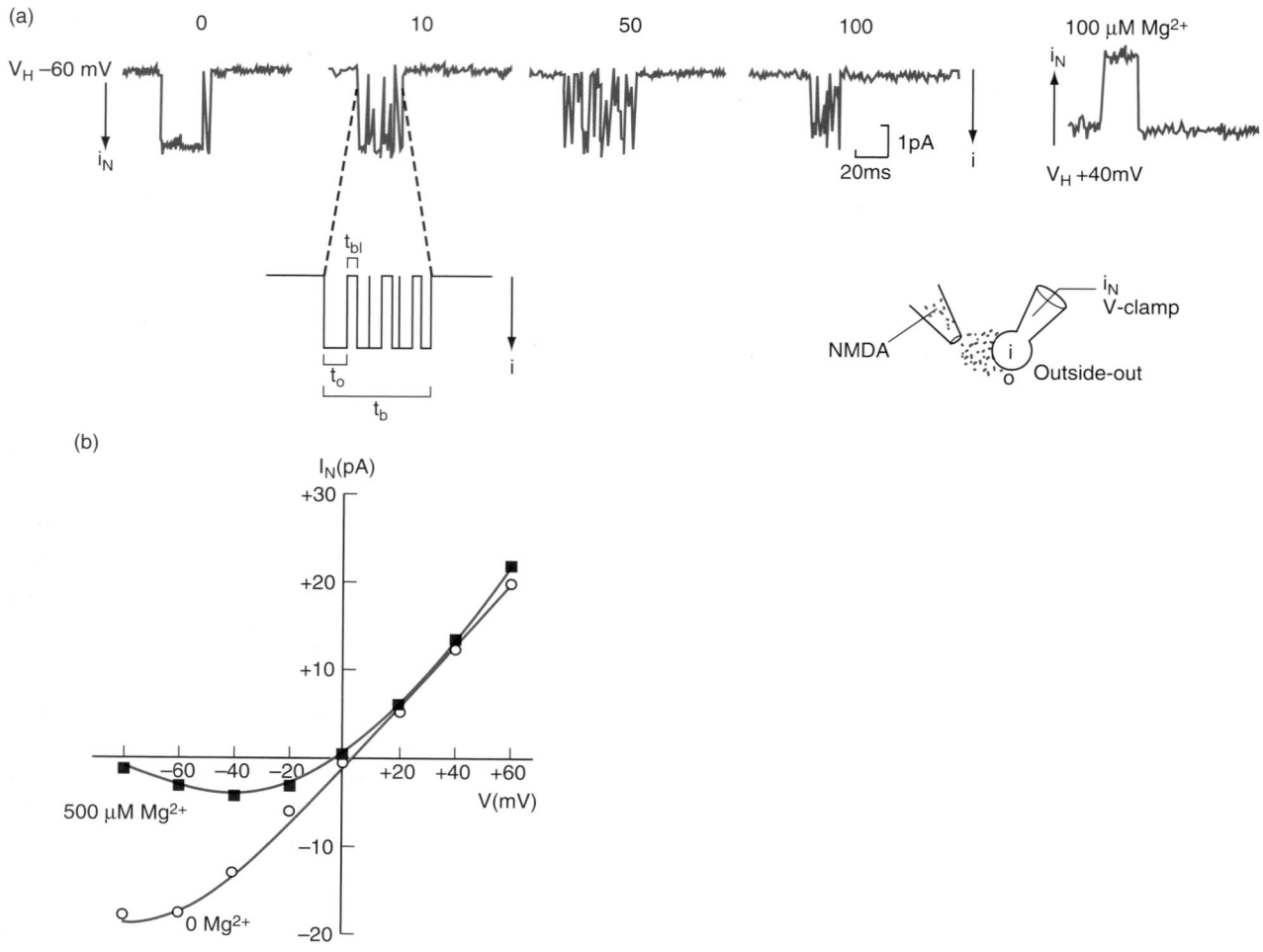

Figure 11.10 NMDA channel block by extracellular Mg^{2+} ions.
(a) Outside-out patch clamp recording of the activity of cultured central neurons. Application of NMDA (10 μM) in the absence of external Mg^{2+} ions (0) and in the presence of Mg^{2+} 10, 50, 100 μM at $V_H = -60$ mV. At $V_H = +40$ mV, i_N is outward. (b) Voltage sensitivity of the NMDA response in the presence of extracellular Mg^{2+} ions. The total current I_N is recorded in the whole-cell patch clamp configuration in the absence (o), and in the presence (■) of 500 μM of Mg^{2+}. Part (a) from Ascher P, Nowak L (1988) The role of divalent cations in the N-methyl-D-aspartate responses of the mouse central neurons in culture, *J. Physiol. (Lond.)* **399**, 247–266, with permission. Part (b) from Nowak L, Bregestovski P, Ascher P *et al.* (1984) Magnesium free glutamate-activated channels in mouse central neurones, *Nature* **307**, 463–465, with permission.

Why is the NMDA channel permeable to Ca^{2+} ions and blocked by Mg^{2+} ions?

One can separate the effects of cations into two groups:

■ those, like Ca^{2+}, which pass through the NMDA channel (e.g. Ba^{2+}, Cd^{2+});
■ those which mimic the Mg^{2+} effect, i.e. block the NMDA channel (e.g. Co^{2+}, Ni^{2+}, Mn^{2+}).

The difference between the ions that pass through the channel and those that block it coincides with the difference in the speed with which the water molecules surrounding these ions can exchange with other water molecules of the aqueous solution. In fact, this exchange is a thousand times faster for the group of permeable (Ca^{2+}-like) ions than for the group of blocking (Mg^{2+}-like) ions.

These differences have led to the suggestion that both ions can cross the channel but only in their dehydrated forms. The following model of the channel has been proposed. The channel has a large extracellular entrance and presents a narrow constriction towards the intracellular side through which the ions can cross only in their dehydrated form. Because of the slow rate of dehydration of the cations from the Mg^{2+} group these ions are trapped in the interior of the channel, thus blocking it.

Another hypothesis for the blockade by Mg^{2+} ions is the following: a high affinity binding site for Mg^{2+} ions could exist inside the channel so that Mg^{2+} ions would cross the channel slowly and thus block it for the time of passage (see Chapter 3).

What does molecular biology tell us about Mg^{2+} block?

The molecular substrate for the hypothesis of a high-affinity site in the NMDA channel for Mg^{2+} ion binding is analysed by exchanging (by site-directed mutagenesis) either glutamine (Q) or arginine (R) for asparagine (N) in the TM2 domain of NR1 or NR2A. Wildtype and mutant NR subunits are co-expressed by cells transfected with cDNAs. Whole-cell currents are activated by application of L-glutamate to transfected cells expressing heteromeric wildtype or mutant NMDA receptors, and differences in Ca^{2+} or Mg^{2+} permeability and channel block by extracellular Mg^{2+} are analysed. Replacing the asparagine (N) by arginine (R) in the NR1 subunit generates 'mutant NR1-wildtype NR2A' channels that do not exhibit a measurable Ca^{2+} permeability (**Figure 11.11b**), as already pointed out. Whole-cell I_N/V curves in (1) divalent ion-free external solution and (2) after adding 0.5 mM of Mg^{2+} to the external solution superimpose almost completely, showing that the mutant channel is not blocked by external Mg^{2+} ions (**Figure 11.11c**). Conversely, the presence of glutamine (Q) instead of asparagine (N) in the NR2A subunit generated 'wildtype NR1-mutant NR2A' channels with increased Mg^{2+} permeability and thus reduced sensitivity to block by extracellular Mg^{2+}. The whole-cell current evoked by glutamate is recorded in (1) divalent ion-free Ringer and (2) after addition of 0.1 mM of Mg^{2+} as a function of membrane potential. The I_N/V relations show that the wildtype channel consisting of NR1 and NR2A subunits (**Figure 11.11d**) is blocked by external Mg^{2+}, while the mutant channel comprising wildtype NR1 and mutant NR2A (N595Q) subunits is permeable to Mg^{2+} since it is only slightly blocked by external Mg^{2+} (**Figure 11.11e**). The effect observed suggests that the M2 segment forms part of the channel of NMDA receptors.

11.4.5 Glycine is a co-agonist of NMDA receptors

Glycine is an amino acid that acts as an inhibitory neurotransmitter at certain central nervous system synapses in vertebrates. However, this amino acid also plays a role in modulating the NMDA response. The effect of glycine on the NMDA receptor-channel has been demonstrated in cultured central neurons recorded in the whole-cell patch clamp configuration. When NMDA was applied by slow perfusion the response is much larger than when NMDA was rapidly perfused into the bath. The following hypothesis was proposed. The cultured cells (neurons and glia) tonically release a substance that accumulates in the bath due to the slow perfusion and thus potentiates the NMDA response. In order to characterize the active substance present in the medium, a variety of treatments were applied. It was established that its activity was still present after heating the medium to 90°C, and that its molecular weight is below 700 D. After testing the most common amino acids, glycine proved to be the most effective in reproducing the effects of the conditioning medium on the NMDA response (**Figure 11.12a**).

Patch clamp outside-out recordings showed that glycine potentiates the NMDA response by augmenting the NMDA receptor-channel opening frequency (thus increasing the open state probability of the channel, p_o). The molecular mechanisms of this potentiating effect remained to be determined. Nevertheless, the fact that glycine has an effect on excised outside-out patch clamp recorded NMDA receptor-channels rules out the mediation of its effect by a diffusible second messenger. It was then suggested that glycine would in fact be indispensable for the activation of the NMDA receptor channel by its agonists. When the activity of NMDA receptor channels expressed in oocytes is recorded in the whole-cell patch clamp configuration, a current in response to NMDA application is observed only when glycine is also present in the bath (**Figure 11.12b**).

How can these results be interpreted from a physiological perspective? This question still remains unanswered. Glycine is in fact present at relatively high concentrations in the cerebrospinal fluid (several μM). This level is close to the concentration required to produce its maximum effect. However, a high-affinity glycine pump may lower extracellular glycine concentration at the level of glutamatergic synapses. These transporters, via the modulation of extracellular glycine concentration, could play a significant role in determining the NMDA response. The discovery of selective antagonists for the glycine receptor site should bring some insight as to the role of glycine in vivo.

Site-directed mutagenesis has identified determinants of the glycine binding site in distinct regions of the NR1 subunit. A glycine binding domain is composed of residues from both the N-terminal extracellular domain and the extracellular loop that joins M3 to M4. Recall that glutamate binds to homologous regions on the NR2 subunit.

11.4.6 Conclusions on NMDA receptors

The NMDA receptor-channel is unusual in that there are at least two conditions required for its activation: the

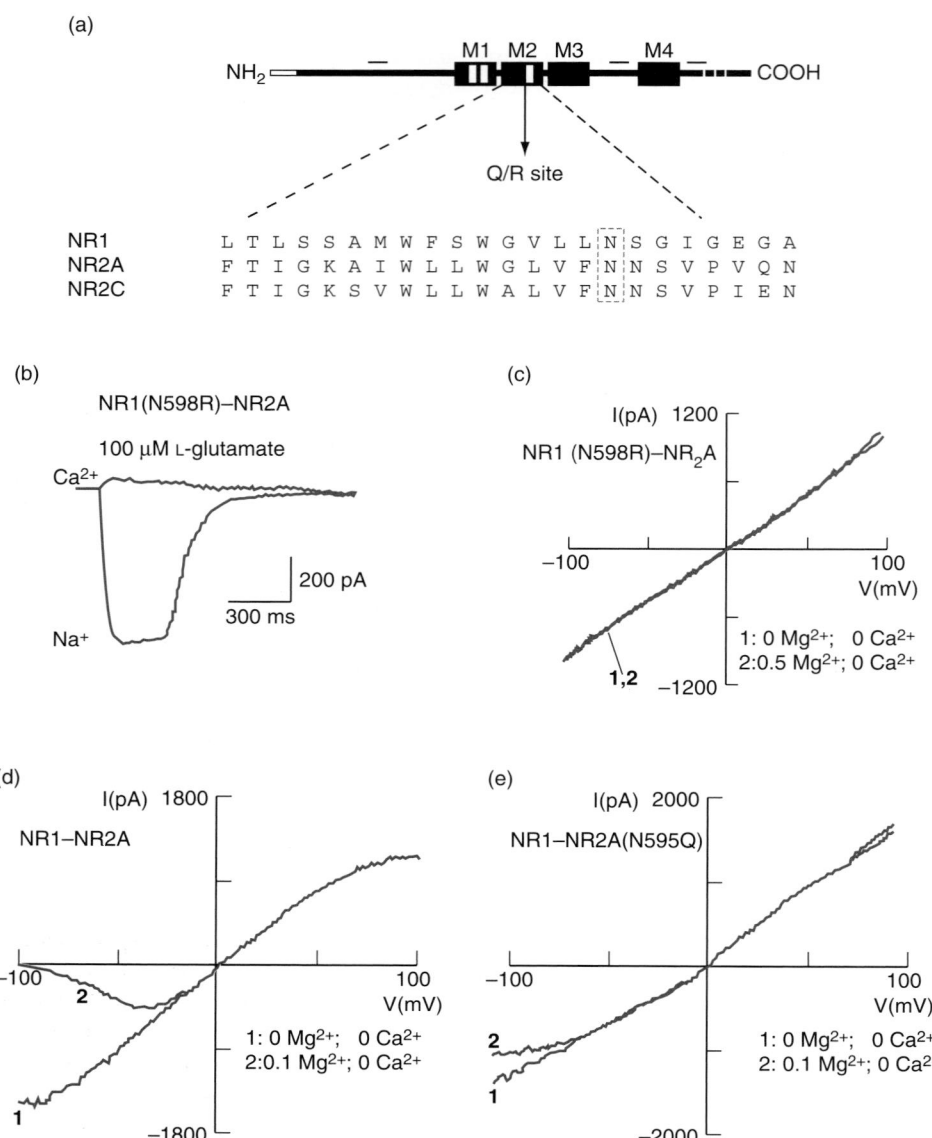

Figure 11.11 Permeability of NMDA channels to divalent cations.
(a) Linear representation of a NMDA receptor subunit. Hydrophobic regions (M1 to M4) are boxed. The M2 segment is expanded to list sequences of subunits belonging to NMDA receptors: NR1, NR2A, NR2C. They carry an asparagine residue (N) in a position homologous to the Q/R site of AMPA and kainate receptor-subunits. (b, c) Reduction of Ca^{2+} permeability and channel block by extracellular Mg^{2+} in a mutant channel where asparagine (N) in the M2 segment of the NR1 subunit is replaced by arginine (R). (b) Whole-cell current elicited by 100 µM of glutamate (bar) at $V_H = -60$ mV in high Na^+ (inward current) or high Ca^{2+} (small outward current) extracellular solution. (c) Whole cell I_N/V relations in (1) divalent ion-free external solution and (2) after adding 0.5 mM of Mg^{2+} to the external solution. (d, e) Difference in channel block by extracellular Mg^{2+} between wildtype and mutant NMDA receptor-channels. In the NR2A (N595Q) subunit, one asparagine (N) in the M2 segment is replaced by glutamine (Q) by site-directed mutagenesis. The whole-cell current evoked by glutamate is recorded in (1) divalent ion-free Ringer and (2) after addition of 0.1 mM of Mg^{2+} as a function of membrane potential from (d) wildtype channels and (e) a mutant channel. Extracellular high Na^+ solution (in mM): 140 NaCl, 5 HEPES; high Ca^{2+} solution: 110 $CaCl_2$, 5 HEPES. Divalent ion-free Ringer's solution: 135 NaCl, 5.4 KCl, 5 HEPES. Part (a) from Wisden W, Seeburg PH (1993) Mammalian ionotropic glutamate receptors, *Curr. Opin. Neurobiol.* **3**, 291–298, with permission. Parts (b)–(e) from Burnashev N, Schoepfer R, Monyer H *et al.* (1992) Control of calcium permeability and magnesium blockade in the NMDA receptor, *Science* **257**, 1415–1419, with permission.

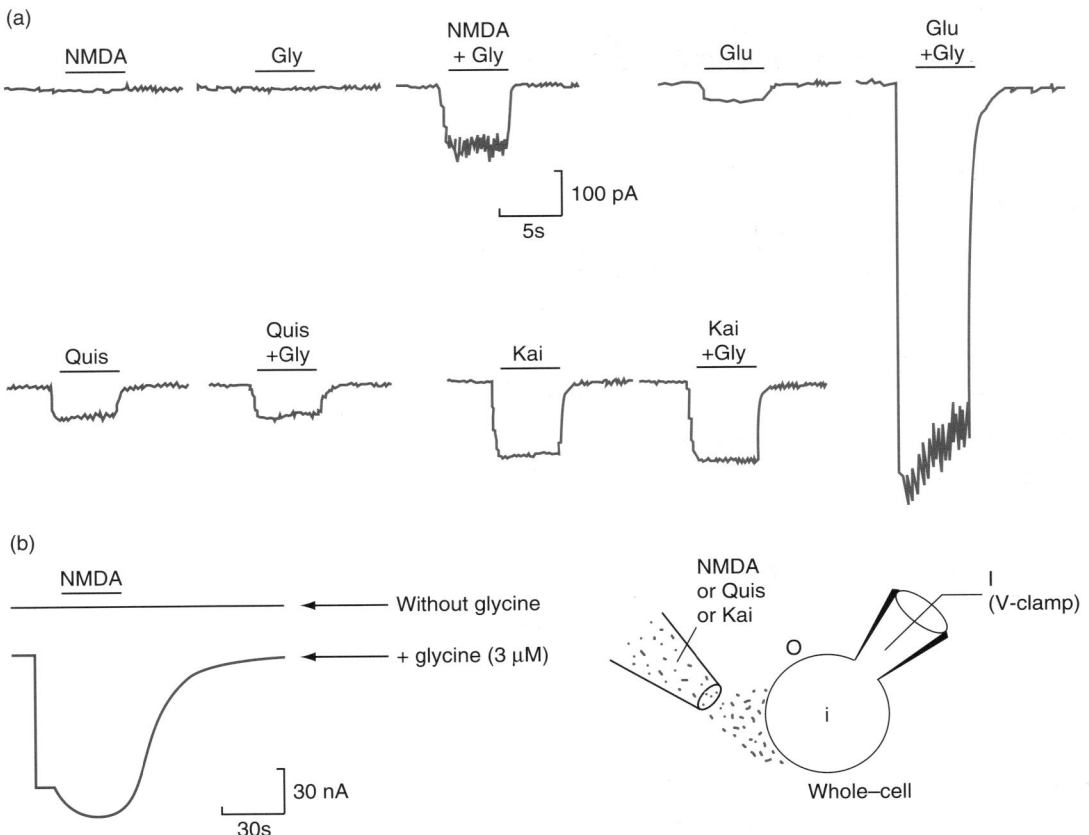

Figure 11.12 Potentiation of the NMDA response by glycine.
(**a**, top) Whole-cell currents evoked in cultured central neurons in response to 10 μM of NMDA or 10 μM of glutamate at $V_H = -50$ mV in the absence or presence of 1 μM of glycine (Gly). (**a**, bottom) The same experiment with quisqualate (Quis) or kainate (Kai) applications. Glycine by itself does not trigger an inward current at any concentration, through either NMDA or non-NMDA channels. (**b**) Whole-cell inward current (66 ± 13 nA) evoked in *Xenopus* oocytes which express NMDA receptors, in response to 300 μM of NMDA at $V_H = -60$ mV in the absence or presence of 3 μM of glycine. In (a) and (b) the extracellular solution is devoid of Mg^{2+} ions. Part (a) from Johnson JW, Ascher P (1987) Glycine potentiates the NMDA response in cultured mouse brain neurons, *Nature* **325**, 529–531, with permission. Part (b) from Kleckner N, Dingledine R (1988) Requirements for glycine in activation of NMDA receptors expressed in *Xenopus* ovocytes, *Science* **241**, 835–837, with permission.

presence of a ligand (glutamate and perhaps also glycine) and the depolarization of the membrane. It is a doubly gated channel. It should be noted that the voltage sensitivity of the NMDA channels (a sensitivity due to an extrinsic ion, namely Mg^{2+}) differs radically from that of voltage-dependent Na^+ and Ca^{2+} channels. In the two latter cases, the voltage sensitivity is an intrinsic property of the protein which does not require extracellular or intracellular blocking ions.

The voltage sensitivity of the NMDA channel has important physiological implications. Since these channels are blocked by Mg^{2+} ions at voltages close to the resting potential of the cell, does the presence of the neurotransmitter in the synaptic cleft suffice to evoke a postsynaptic NMDA response? Knowing that the non-NMDA and the NMDA receptors coexist in the postsy-

naptic membrane, what is the fraction of the synaptic current that is due to the activation of NMDA receptors? These questions are analysed in the following section.

11.5 Synaptic responses to glutamate are mediated by NMDA and non-NMDA receptors

11.5.1 Glutamate receptors are co-localized in the postsynaptic membrane of glutamatergic synapses

The glutamatergic synapses typically exhibit an electron-dense postsynaptic density where ionotropic glutamate receptors are concentrated as shown by immunogold labelling. To date, among iGluRs, only NMDA and AMPA receptors can be labelled for electron microscopy observation. In contrast to iGluRs, metabotropic glutamate receptors (mGluRs) appear to occur at highest concentrations in the perisynaptic annulus; i.e. the narrow zone surrounding the postsynaptic specialization (**Figure 11.13**).

The receptors localized in the postsynaptic specialization are directly apposed to the presynaptic active zone. The enrichment of iGluRs at the site of the postsynaptic specialization reflects their roles in mediating fast glutamatergic transmission. Such enrichment depends on anchoring synaptic proteins (see Chapter 8).

Glutamate released into the synaptic cleft diffuses to the postsynaptic membrane and binds to postsynaptic NMDA as well as non-NMDA receptors (**Figure 11.13**) and evokes a synaptic response which is a postsynaptic excitatory current (EPSC). In turn this EPSC depolarizes the membrane; i.e. it evokes an excitatory postsynaptic potential (EPSP; see **Figure 11.3**). *In vivo*, when the membrane potential is near the resting potential of the cell, a large fraction of the NMDA receptors are blocked by Mg^{2+} ions present in the synaptic cleft. Therefore, glutamate first activates non-NMDA receptors.

■ Is the synaptic response to glutamate mediated by non-NMDA receptors only?
■ If not, under which conditions are NMDA receptors activated by synaptically released glutamate and how do they contribute to the synaptic response?

To answer these questions it is necessary to differentiate, in the postsynaptic current, between the component due to the activation of non-NMDA and that due to NMDA receptors (**Figure 11.13**, inset).

11.5.2 The glutamatergic postsynaptic current is inward and can have at least two components in the absence of extracellular Mg^{2+} ions

A global postsynaptic inward current (excitatory postsynaptic current; EPSC), evoked by the stimulation of a

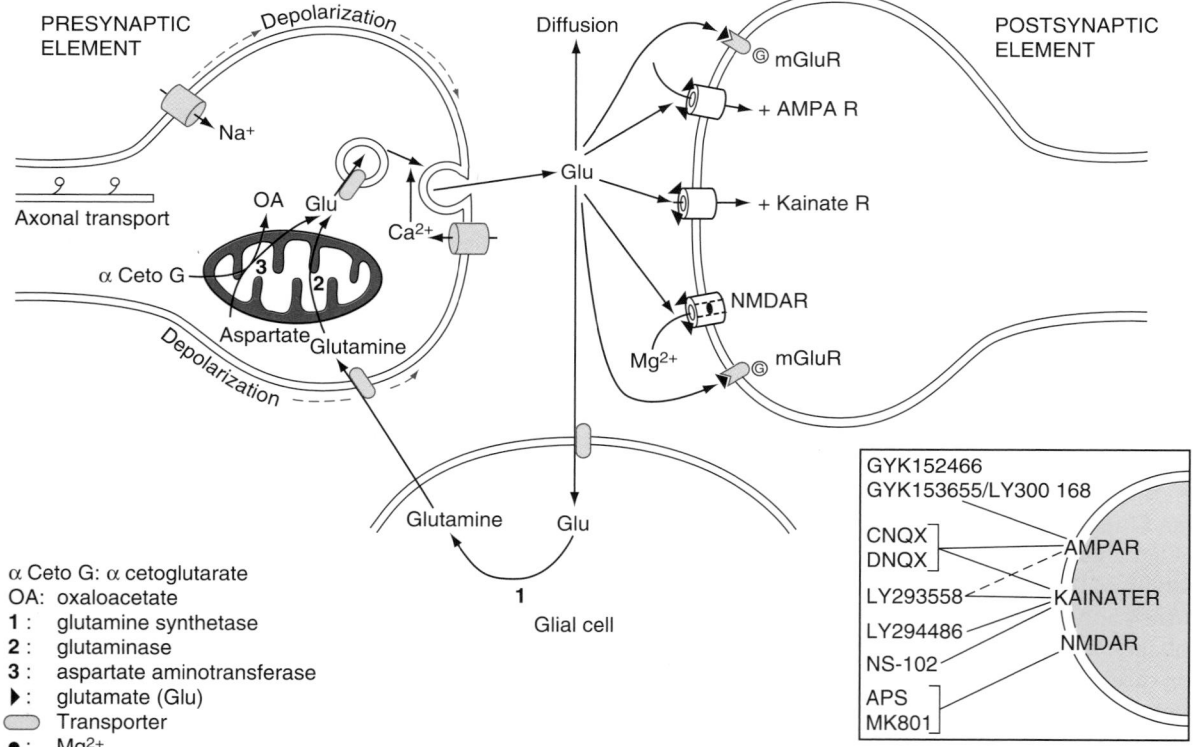

α Ceto G: α cetoglutarate
OA: oxaloacetate
1 : glutamine synthetase
2 : glutaminase
3 : aspartate aminotransferase
▶ : glutamate (Glu)
⬭ Transporter
● : Mg^{2+}

Figure 11.13 The glutamatergic synapse.
Functional scheme of a glutamatergic synapse where ionotropic and metabotropic glutamate receptors are co-localized. Presynaptic receptors are omitted. The enzymes (1 to 3) and mitochondria are carried to axon terminals via anterograde axonal transports. Glutamate synthesized in mitochondria of the presynaptic element is transported actively into synaptic vesicles by a vesicular carrier. A percentage of the glutamate released in the synaptic cleft is uptaken into presynaptic terminals and glial cells by transporters. Inset shows iGluRs antagonists. Inset from Mody I (1998) Interneurons and the ghost of the sea, *Nature Neurosci.* **1**, 434–436, with permission.

presynaptic glutamatergic neuron, is recorded in the whole-cell configuration (voltage clamp mode). When the presynaptic neuron is stimulated in the absence of extracellular Mg^{2+} ions and the postsynaptic membrane is held at –46 mV, an inward current showing two components is recorded (**Figure 11.14a**):

- an early component: an initial peak of current of great amplitude and rapid inactivation;
- a late component: a current of smaller amplitude that inactivates slowly.

To identify the NMDA and non-NMDA components of the postsynaptic current we can make use of the different properties of the non-NMDA and the NMDA channels summarized in **Figure 11.1a**. The non-NMDA component is not affected by different concentrations of extracellular Mg^{2+} ions, nor by the presence of APV, but disappears in the presence of CNQX, an antagonist of non-NMDA receptors. On the other hand, the NMDA component is present in a medium devoid of Mg^{2+} ions but disappears in the presence of APV, the competitive antagonist of NMDA receptors.

In the presence of Mg^{2+} ions the late component is largely attenuated at negative potentials but is present at all positive voltages (**Figure 11.14b**, black square). In the absence of Mg^{2+} ions and the presence of APV in the extracellular environment (**Figure 11.14c**), the late component disappears at all voltages tested. These results strongly suggest that the late component of the synaptic current results from the activation of NMDA receptors (APV-sensitive and blocked by Mg^{2+} at negative voltages). The reverse experiment in the presence of CNQX is not shown.

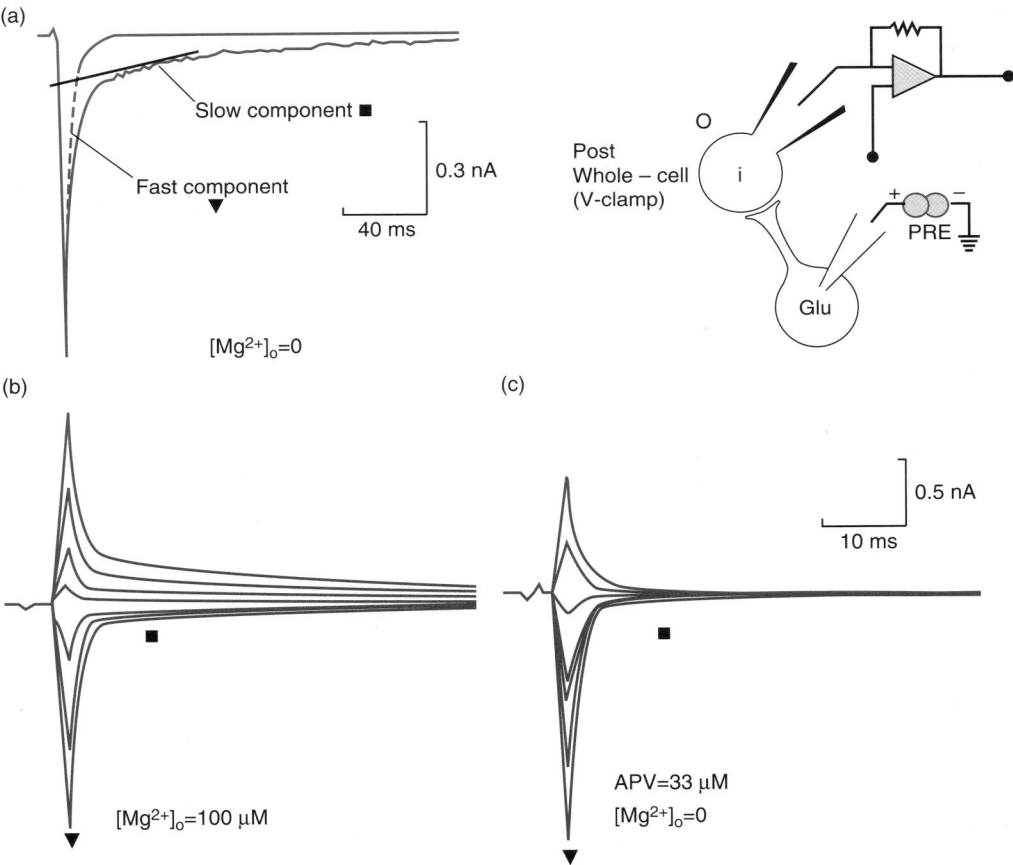

Figure 11.14 Postsynaptic inward current evoked by the stimulation of a glutamatergic presynaptic neuron.
(a) Whole-cell postsynaptic inward current (EPSC) recorded at V_H = –46 mV in the absence of Mg^{2+}, in response to the activation of a presynaptic glutamatergic neuron. The peak current decays with a time constant τ_1 = 4.2 ms and the slow components decays with a time constant τ_2 = 81.8 ms. **(b)** The EPSC is recorded at different V_H in the presence of Mg^{2+} (100 μM). **(c)** The EPSC is recorded at different V_H in the presence of 33 μM of D-APV and in the absence of extracellular Mg^{2+}. Picrotoxin (10–100 μM) is added to the extracellular solution to block GABAergic inhibitory synaptic activity. From Forsythe ID, Westbrook GL (1988) Slow excitatory postsynaptic currents mediated by N-methyl-D-aspartate receptors on cultured mouse central neurons, *J. Physiol. (Lond.)* **396**, 515–533, with permission.

*Which receptor channels contribute to the
non-NMDA component of the synaptic current?*

Until recently, there was little evidence for which of the
AMPA and kainate receptors participate in the non-
NMDA component of the synaptic glutamatergic current, since antagonists such as CNQX are not selective of
either one of these receptors. Only after the fortuitous
discovery that the 2,3-benzodiazepine muscle relaxant
GYKI 53655 is a specific AMPA antagonist (see **Figure
11.1a**) could physiologists begin to distinguish between
the separate activation of AMPA and kainate receptors
at synapses. In many glutamatergic synapses, the non-
NMDA postsynaptic current results solely from AMPA
receptors. But there are few places where synaptically
activated kainate receptors were identified. One of them
is the CA3 region of the hippocampus where pyramidal
neurons and interneurons receive excitatory input from
glutamatergic mossy fibres (see **Figure 7.3**).

EPSCs evoked by the stimulation of afferents are
recorded from interneurons in the whole-cell configuration (voltage clamp mode) in the continuous presence of
D-APV to block NMDA receptors. A large, rapidly
decaying control EPSC with a small, long-lasting tail is
recorded (**Figure 11.15a**). Application of GYKI, the
AMPA antagonist, blocks the rapid component but the
slow component is mostly unaffected. The subsequent
addition of the AMPA/kainate antagonist CNQX blocks
the GYKI-resistant slow component. When the synapse
between afferent glutamatergic fibres and pyramidal
CA1 neurons is now studied, no GYKI-resistant
(kainate-mediated) component can be shown, although
the EPSC in pyramidal cells is more than twice as large
as the EPSC in interneurons (**Figure 11.15b**). This indicates that, at this synapse, kainate receptors are absent
and that the non-NMDA component of the EPSC is
mediated only by AMPA receptors.

11.5.3 The glutamatergic postsynaptic depolarization (EPSP) has at least two components in the absence of extracellular Mg^{2+} ions

The postsynaptic potential variations in response to the
stimulation of the presynaptic neurons (same preparation as above) is recorded in the whole-cell configuration (current clamp mode to leave the voltage free to
vary) in the absence of Mg^{2+} ions. Such stimulation
evokes a postsynaptic depolarization (EPSP), which
results from the evoked synaptic inward current
through postsynaptic ionotropic glutamate receptors.
As in the case of the synaptic current, the EPSP shows
two identifiable components (see **Figure 11.3b**). In the
presence of APV the early component is only slightly

affected or not at all. This APV-insensitive early component is a result of the early synaptic inward current; i.e.
the inward current through non-NMDA receptors.

In these conditions (absence of Mg^{2+} ions, presence of
APV), the duration of the EPSP is reduced. The difference between the APV-insensitive component of the
EPSP and the total EPSP corresponds to the APV-sensitive component; i.e. the component resulting from the
inward current through NMDA receptors.

In summary, the component resulting from the activation of the NMDA receptors has a slower rising phase
and lasts longer than the component mediated by the
non-NMDA receptors. Thus, when the NMDA receptors
are activated, the peak of the EPSP is not always affected
but the duration of the EPSP is much longer. As for
EPSCs, the non-NMDA component of glutamatergic
EPSPs is mediated either by AMPA receptors alone or by
both AMPA and kainate receptors (see **Figure 11.3c**).

11.5.4 Synaptic depolarization recorded in physiological conditions: factors controlling NMDA receptor activation

The recordings of **Figure 11.14** have shown the presence
of two components in the synaptic current and depolarization, when the extracellular medium is Mg^{2+}-free.
What is the situation in physiological conditions, when
the extracellular physiological milieu has a Mg^{2+} concentration of approximately 1 mM. Since at this Mg^{2+}
concentration and at membrane potentials close to the
resting potential of the cell, most of the NMDA channels
are closed, under which conditions will NMDA receptors participate to synaptic transmission?

It seems unlikely that the extracellular Mg^{2+} concentration *in vivo* will vary sufficiently to allow the 'unblocking' of NMDA receptors. However, depolarizations
reduce the level of Mg^{2+} block of the NMDA channel.
Thus, one can imagine that a depolarization of the membrane is precisely what allows the NMDA channels to
become 'unblocked'. A depolarization can be the consequence of the activation of other receptors present in the
postsynaptic membrane, such as non-NMDA receptors.
It can also result from the activation of a subpopulation
of NMDA receptors that are not blocked at the resting
potential. This hypothesis can be summarized as follows.

*When NMDA and non-NMDA receptors coexist in
the postsynaptic membrane*

When the glutamate concentration is sufficiently high to
activate non-NMDA receptor channels, a current is generated through these channels and an APV-insensitive
depolarization is recorded:

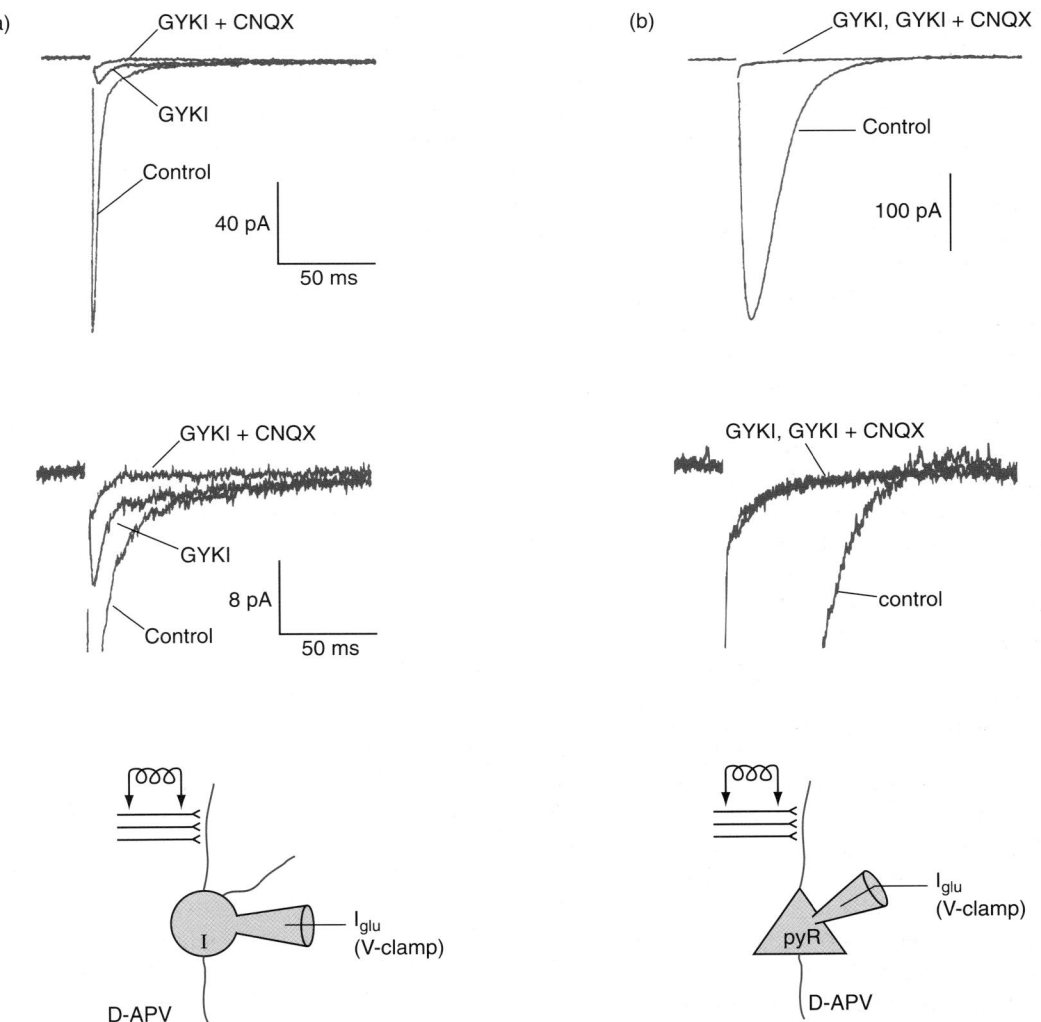

Figure 11.15 The AMPA- and kainate-mediated component of EPSCs.
Experiments performed in slices of the rat hippocampus (CA1 region). **(a)** Averaged EPSCs recorded from an interneuron (I) in control conditions (continuous presence of 100 μM of D-APV), after bath application of 70 μM of GYKI 53655 and after addition of 100 μM of CNQX. Middle traces are the same EPSCs at high gain. **(b)** The same experiment performed in pyramidal cells (pyR). V_H in (a) and (b) is −80 mV. From Frerking M, Malenka RC, Nicoll RA (1998) Synaptic activation of kainate receptors on hippocampal interneurons, *Nature Neurosci.* **1**, 479–486, with permission.

- If this non-NMDA mediated depolarization is not strong enough to allow 'unblocking' of the NMDA receptors, only the early component of the depolarization (non-NMDA component) is recorded (**Figure 11.3a**).
- If this non-NMDA mediated depolarization is sufficiently strong to 'unblock' NMDA receptors, it triggers the activation of an inward NMDA current through these channels and an additional depolarization of the membrane. This depolarization allows the 'unblocking' of additional NMDA receptors which, activated by glutamate, evoke an enhanced depolarization. The more depolarized the membrane, the higher the number

of NMDA receptors activated by glutamate. This regenerative phenomenon, due to the voltage sensitivity of the NMDA receptors (associated with the negative-slope region of the I_N/V curve), reminds us of a similar phenomenon observed with the action potential generating Na^+ channels. In the present case, an important postsynaptic depolarization made up of the non-NMDA early component and the NMDA late component is recorded. However, the NMDA component not only prolongs the EPSP but also allows a significant influx of Ca^{2+} ions. These ions have numerous roles: one of them is the activation of channels sensitive to intracellular Ca^{2+} ions. Another role of intracellular

Ca^{2+} is as a second messenger. Consequently it participates in the regulation of a number of intracellular Ca^{2+}-sensitive processes.

NMDA receptors are the only receptors present in the postsynaptic membrane

In certain preparations the postsynaptic depolarization recorded in response to the endogenous release of glutamate shows only one component, the NMDA component. This has led to the assumption that not all the NMDA receptors are blocked by Mg^{2+} ions at resting membrane potential. The mechanism of NMDA receptor activation in this case would be the following. When the glutamate concentration in the synaptic cleft is high enough to activate the few NMDA receptors that are not blocked by Mg^{2+} at the resting potential, a small inward current is activated. This current produces a small depolarization of the membrane which allows the 'unblocking' of additional NMDA receptors and, as in the previous example, this triggers a regenerative phenomenon. The resulting Ca^{2+} influx through the NMDA channels further triggers Ca^{2+}-dependent processes.

11.6 Summary

The function of postsynaptic iGluRs is to mediate fast excitatory synaptic transmission by converting the binding of glutamate to a rapid and transient increase in cationic permeability. Glutamate receptors comprise the glutamate receptor sites on their surface, the elements that make the ionic channel selectively permeable to cations, as well as all the elements necessary for interactions between different functional domains. Thus, the glutamate receptor sites and the cationic channel are part of the same unique protein. NMDA, AMPA and kainate receptors are co-expressed in many neurons. Therefore, to study them separately, patch clamp techniques and the use of selective agonists for each receptor type have proven to be particularly useful.

Do all ionotropic glutamate receptors have the same properties; for example the same sensitivity to glutamate, the same ionic permeability?

NMDA and kainate receptors have a higher affinity (around 1 μM) for glutamate than do AMPA receptors (250–1500 μM). All iGluRs are cationic channels permeable to Na$^+$ and K$^+$. Some AMPA receptors and all NMDA receptors are also permeable to Ca^{2+}.

Do all these receptors have co-agonists acting at modulatory sites?

No – to date, only NMDA receptors have been shown to contain a co-agonist binding site (for glycine).

What are the exact conditions of the activation of the different iGluRs?

AMPA receptors open rapidly and briefly, once glutamate is released in the cleft, allowing a transient Na$^+$ influx (inward current) and sometimes a Ca^{2+} influx, through the postsynaptic membrane. This AMPA-receptor-mediated EPSC generates a fast-rising (time to peak in the order of 1 ms) EPSP (or EPSP component).

When kainate receptors are present in the postsynaptic element, they are activated once glutamate is released in the cleft. They allow a transient Na$^+$ influx (inward current) and sometimes a Ca^{2+} influx, through the postsynaptic membrane (inward current). This kainate receptor-mediated EPSC is smaller and slower (time to peak of the order of 5–10 ms) than the AMPA-mediated one, thus giving a slow-rising, low-amplitude EPSP component.

NMDA-type receptors have a more complex role based on three characteristic properties. They open more slowly (they require more than 2 ms to open) and remain open longer than AMPA receptors; this slow time course allows the summation of responses to events tens of milliseconds apart. They are also regulated by voltage-dependent block by Mg^{2+}. As a result they can be activated only when the membrane is sufficiently depolarized to remove this block. NMDA receptors function as a coincidence detector that admits current only when agonist binding and cell depolarization take place simultaneously. When they open, they allow a large Na$^+$ and Ca^{2+} influx through the postsynaptic membrane. The resulting EPSC triggers a slow-rising, long-duration EPSP (or EPSP component) and the resulting increase of intracellular Ca^{2+} concentration triggers a cascade of molecular events in the postsynaptic cell.

The risetime of EPSPs depends on the agonist binding rate and on the opening rate of postsynaptic receptors. The amplitude of EPSPs depends on the number of open channels in the postsynaptic element; i.e. on the number N of receptors present in the membrane, on the open probability (p_o) of the channel, and on the concentration of neurotransmitter in the synaptic cleft.

Further reading

Bigge CF (1999) Ionotropic glutamate receptors. *Curr. Opin. Chem. Biol.* **3**, 441–447.

Burnashev N, Monyer H, Seeburg PH, Sakmann B (1992) Divalent ion permeability of AMPA receptor channels is dominated by the edited form of a single subunit. *Neuron* **8**, 189–198.

Conti F, Weinberg RJ (1999) Shaping excitation at glutamatergic synapses. *Trend. Neurosci.* **22**, 451–458.

Gregor P, Mano I, Maoz I *et al.* (1989) Molecular structure of the chick cerebellar kainate-binding subunit of a putative glutamate receptor. *Nature* **342**, 689–692.

Hirai H, Kirsch J, Laube B *et al.* (1996) The glycine binding site of the *N*-methyl-D-aspartate receptor subunit NR1: identification of novel determinants of co-agonist potentiation in the extracellular M3–M4 loop region. *Proc. Natl Acad. Sci.* **93**, 6031–6036.

Hume RI, Dingledine R, Heinemann SF (1991) Identification of a site in glutamate receptor subunits that controls calcium permeability. *Science* **253**, 1028–1031.

Laube B, Hirai H, Sturgess M *et al.* (1997) Molecular determinants of agonist discrimination by NMDA receptor subunits: analysis of the glutamate binding site on the NR2B subunit. *Neuron* **18**, 493–503.

Sheng M, Pak DT (1999) Glutamate receptor anchoring proteins and the molecular organization of excitatory synapses. *Ann. NY Acad. Sci. USA* **868**, 483–493.

Sommer B, Kohler M, Sprengel R, Seeburg PH (1991) RNA editing in brain controls a determinant of ion flow in glutamate-gated channels. *Cell* **67**, 11–19.

Takumi Y, Matsubara A, Rinvik E, Ottersen OP (1999) The arrangement of glutamate receptors in excitatory synapses. *Ann. NY Acad. Sci. USA* **868**, 474–482.

Wada K, Dechesne CJ, Shimasaki S *et al.* (1989) Sequence and expression of a frog complementary DNA encoding a kainate binding protein. *Nature* **342**, 684–689.

Ionotropic Mechanoreceptors: the Mechanosensitive Channels

Detection of changes in local physical force by mechanosensitive cells plays many important roles in sensory physiology. Our ability to feel the external world via the sense of touch represents the most obvious case. Other familiar examples include: the sense of hearing, which is generated upon perception of vibrations in the tympanic membrane; the sense of position, which depends on proprioceptors in the body's muscles and joints; and the sense of balance, which arises from detection of head movements by vestibular hair cells.

In addition to having multiple roles in sensory perception, the detection of mechanical stimuli is also important for a number of involuntary physiological events. Thus, direct physical stress can modulate local processes such as structural plasticity in bone and the secretion of renin by renal glomerular mesangeal cells. Peripheral mechanosensors can also modulate homeostatic responses via connections with the central nervous system. For example, information concerning changes in vascular distension, detected at baroreceptors and volume receptors, is relayed to the brain from where it can modulate sympathetic outflow, and the secretion of various hormones involved in the regulation of blood pressure and body fluid balance.

In all of these examples the perception of a sensation or the production of a homeostatic response becomes possible only once a physical stimulus has been detected and transduced into a signal that can be recognized by the mechanosensory cell itself, or by its extrinsic cellular targets. This chapter focuses on the possible involvement of mechanosensitive ion channels as 'ionotropic mechanoreceptors' responsible for the transduction of mechanical stimuli into electrical signals.

12.1 Mechanoreception in sensory neurons is associated with the production of a receptor potential

Some of the cells specialized for the production of mechanically regulated effector responses are intrinsically sensitive to mechanical perturbation. Elongation of some muscle cells, for example, can provoke self-contraction. In such cases, local electrical or biochemical events resulting from the mechanical stimulus are sufficient to trigger an appropriate cellular response. In other instances, however, information concerning the stimulus must be relayed to distinct effector cells. This is particularly important in the nervous system, where the information must be processed by higher order neurons in order to be perceived, or to produce a coordinated homeostatic response. In these cases mechanical stimuli first modify the frequency or pattern of action potential discharge in a mechanosensory neuron, which subsequently relays these signals to the brain.

Patterns of neuronal spike discharge are strongly influenced by the density and subtypes of ion channels present in the region of the cell responsible for the initiation of action potentials. In mechanosensory neurons, however, the principal factors governing stimulus-evoked changes in firing are the magnitude and time course of the receptor potential (see **Figure 12.7**), the primary change in membrane voltage provoked by the physical stimulus itself. The process by which a physical stimulus is converted into an ionic current and receptor potential is termed *mechanotransduction*. While the molecular basis for this process remains largely undefined, introduction of the patch clamp technique has led to the discovery of a category of ion channels that are uniquely suited to perform such a task: *the mechanosensitive channels*.

12.2 Discovery of mechanosensitive ion channels provided a potential molecular mechanism for mechanotransduction

In 1984, Guharay and Sachs reported that during patch clamp experiments on embryonic muscle cells they frequently encountered a cation-permeable channel whose probability of opening could be increased by applying suction to the inside of the recording pipette. The discovery of channels whose activity could be directly controlled by physical stimulation was exciting because it provided a potential molecular mechanism for mechanotransduction. Unfortunately, while mechanosensitive ion channels remain the most likely candidates, direct evidence of their involvement in mechanically regulated physiological processes has been difficult to obtain using single-channel recording. This problem stems primarily from the fact that membranes responsible for mechanotransduction are usually embedded within complex cellular structures specialized for the capture and transfer of physical energy. Structural elements required for the channels to operate as mechanotransducers, therefore, are often destroyed by procedures related to cell isolation or patch clamp recording.

12.3 Structural basis for the mechanical gating of ion channels

Regulation of mechanosensitive channels does not result from physically evoked changes in the size of the ionic pore. Indeed, during single-channel recordings changes in activity are observed as variations in the rate of transitions between discrete closed and open states (see **Figures 12.11** and **12.12**). Thus, as for other types of channels, ion flux through mechanosensitive channels appears to be regulated as if controlled by an all-or-none gate. In ligand- and voltage-sensitive channels the energy required to control the gate is delivered via allosteric and electrostatic forces generated by ligand binding or changes in transmembrane potential, respectively. In mechanosensitive channels, energy delivered to the gating apparatus appears to be derived from mechanical force via direct physical links with the local environment.

12.3.1 Intrinsic and extrinsic forms of mechanical gating

Interestingly, some channels appear to be intrinsically capable of sensing changes in shape or tension within the lipid bilayer itself. For example, in 1990 Martinac and colleagues reported that the activity of mechanosensitive channels in liposomes reconstituted from *E. coli* could be modulated by the addition of amphipathic molecules causing differential expansion of the inner or outer leaflets of the lipid bilayer. This observation suggests that interactions with local lipid structure may play a key role in the regulation of some mechanosensitive channels. In most other mechanosensitive channels, however, mechanical gating is modified or abolished by disrupting interactions with extracellular or intracellular elements. The nature of the molecular complex required for this extrinsic regulation of

mechanosensitive channels is not yet known. Possible structure/function relations, however, can be inferred by considering the ways by which such channels might be coupled to their physical environment.

12.3.2 Channels regulated by coupling molecules oriented orthogonally to the membrane

Figure 12.1 illustrates hypothetical situations in which force is delivered to the channel gate via extracellular or cytoplasmic coupling molecules whose axes lie normal to the plasma membrane. In both cases, therefore, channel gating would be strongly influenced by orthogonal displacements of the plasma membrane relative to the site of anchoring.

During cell-attached single-channel recordings, axial tension within an orthogonal coupling molecule anchored intracellularly should increase in response to the application of negative pipette pressure and decrease in response to positive pressure (**Figure 12.2**). Theoretically, axial tension in a coupling molecule anchored extracellularly would increase in response to positive pipette pressure and decrease in response to suction. Consequently, if an orthogonal coupling molecule regulates channel activity, the latter should vary as a monotonic function of pipette pressure, where the polarity of the response is determined by the site of anchoring. Ion channels with coupling molecules anchored in a quasi-orthogonal orientation may be present in vertebrate hair cells, where extracellular filamentous 'tip-links' attached to adjacent stereocilia appear to serve as gating springs for the mechanosensitive transduction channels involved in hearing and vestibular function.

12.3.3 Channels regulated by coupling molecules parallel to the membrane

Figure 12.3 shows a different hypothetical architecture for mechanotransduction. In this case the long axes of the coupling molecules are oriented in a plane lying parallel to the plasma membrane. Regardless of how their coupling molecules are anchored (to each other or to other proteins or channels within or near the membrane), channels of this type would be most sensitive to changes in physical force applied in a plane tangential to the cell membrane. Under cell-attached patch-clamp recording conditions, increases in patch curvature evoked by applying either positive or negative pressure to a recording pipette would cause similar increases in tangential force or 'membrane tension' (**Figure 12.4**). Consequently, the activity of such channels should vary as approximately symmetric functions of positive and negative pipette pressures. Mechanosensitive channels

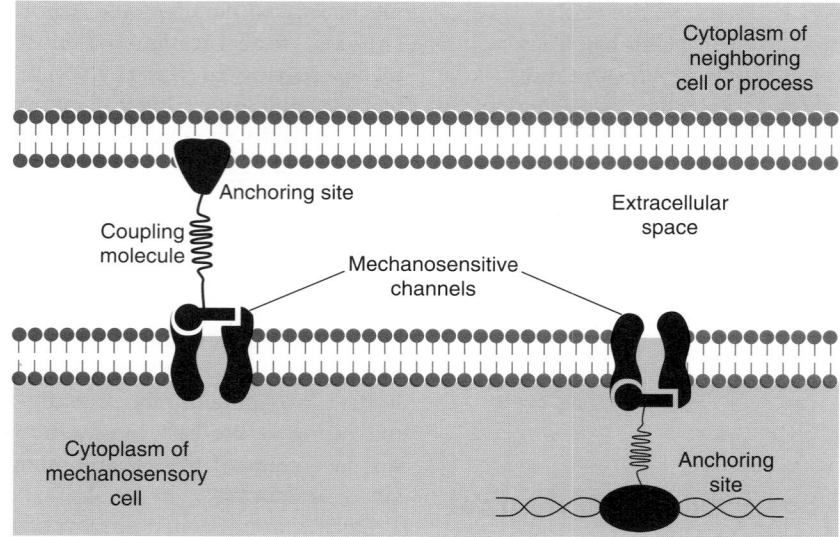

Figure 12.1 Channels with orthogonally anchored gating springs.
The channel on the left features a gating mechanism regulated via a coupling molecule attached to an extracellular anchoring site, in this case a membrane-bound protein in an adjacent cell. An arrangement of this type is believed to regulate the mechanoreceptor channels of vertebrate hair cells – see Gillespie PG (1995) Molecular machinery of auditory and vestibular transduction, *Curr. Opin. Neurobiol.* **5**, 449–455. The gating apparatus of the channel shown on the right is anchored to a cytoplasmic support site, such as a component of the cytoskeleton. Note that in reality the gates are not directly 'pulled' open or shut by the coupling molecule. Rather, the application of force supplies the energy that biases the frequency at which the gate is opened and closed.

of this type appear to be the ones most frequently encountered during single-channel recordings in a variety of preparations. The apparent preponderance of such channels, however, may simply indicate that channels with a functional parallel coupling architecture are easier to isolate by patch clamp methods.

12.3.4 Other gating configurations

The simplified orthogonal and parallel coupling architectures hypothesized in **Figures 12.1** and **12.3** predict distinct functional properties for extrinsically regulated mechanosensitive channels during patch clamp experiments (see **Figures 12.2** and **12.4**). While it is possible that these structural configurations may resemble those found in real channels, it must be emphasized that the molecular organization of mechanosensitive channels is presently unknown, and may be much more elaborate. Moreover, the presence of angled, or non-elastic, coupling molecules would introduce complicated vectorial bias to channel stretch-sensitivity. Indeed, it is likely that the evolution of multiple varieties of specialized mechanoreceptors has been paralleled by the appearance of varied architectural designs. The recent cloning of a variety of putative mechanosensitive ion channels may lead to a more detailed understanding of the molecular scaffold responsible for mechanical gating.

12.4 Classification of stretch-sensitive ion channels

In the absence of definitive structural information, the classification of mechanosensitive channels identified during patch clamp experiments has been organized according to their ionic permeability and functional responses to modifications of pipette pressure.

12.4.1 Patch clamp experiments reveal the existence of stretch-activated and stretch-inactivated channels

As indicated above, the activity of many of the mechanosensitive channels characterized to date has been found to vary symmetrically in response to increases or decreases in pipette pressure. Such channels, therefore, appear to be regulated by tangential membrane forces, as might result from the intrinsic monitoring of lateral tension within the bilayer or from an extrinsic parallel coupling architecture (**Figure 12.4**). Functionally, two classes of symmetrically stretch-sensitive channels are recognized during patch clamp recordings: those whose probability of opening increases with stretch, or stretch-activated channels; and those whose probability of opening decreases with stretch, or

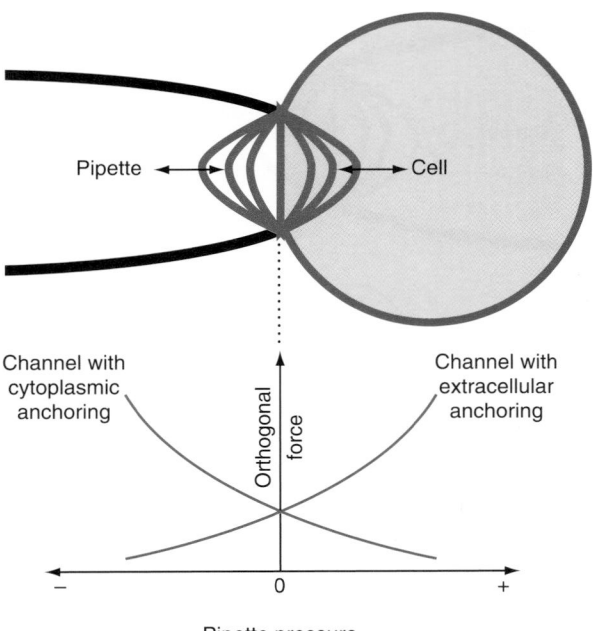

Figure 12.2 Relationship between orthogonal force and pipette pressure during cell-attached patch clamp recordings. The patch of membrane isolated during a cell-attached recording is pulled away from the cell as pressure inside the pipette is made negative and pushed toward the cell interior as pipette pressure is made positive. Since the tension within an orthogonally directed coupling spring increases with length, orthogonal forces vary as monotonic functions of pipette pressure. However, as shown on the graph, the polarity of the force/pressure relationship depends on the site of anchoring of the coupling spring. The force/pressure relationship of a channel with extracellular anchoring is illustrated for completeness, but could not be measured in the recording configuration illustrated.

stretch-inactivated channels. Because tangential forces increase symmetrically as a function of positive and negative pressures (**Figure 12.4**), stretch-activated channels recorded during patch clamp experiments display a U-shaped activation curve, whereas stretch-inactivated channels exhibit a characteristic bell-shaped activity profile (**Figure 12.5**).

12.4.2 Ionic permeability of stretch-sensitive channels

Stretch-sensitive ion channels have also been characterized according to their various relative permeabilities to different ions. Among the forms most commonly observed are the stretch-activated K^+ channels, which are K^+-selective, and the stretch-activated cationic channels, which are permeable to Ca^{2+}, Na^+ and K^+. Channels selective for either anions (including Cl^-), Ca^{2+} or Na^+ have also been reported. Through its effect on the equilibrium potential for transmembrane current flux, ionic permeability plays a key role in determining the functional role of mechanosensitive channels.

A wide diversity of mechanically gated channels are therefore recognized during patch clamp experiments. In the absence of definitive information concerning the molecular biology of defined subtypes of mechanosensitive ion channels, however, it is difficult to predict whether differences in mechanical gating and ionic permeability result from small differences in a common structural motif, or whether completely distinct structural units explain the large diversity of mechanosensitive channel types.

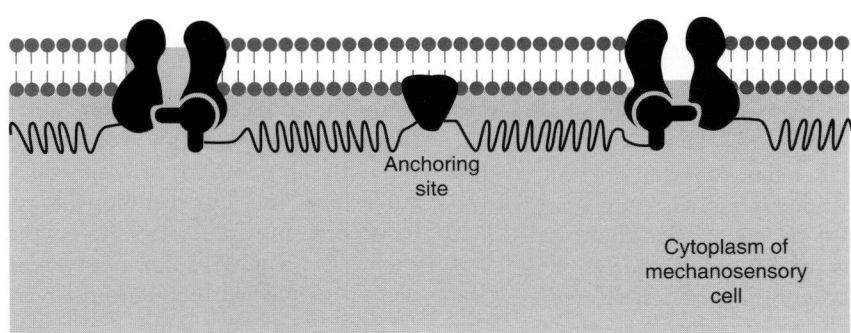

Figure 12.3 Channels with gating springs oriented parallel to the cell membrane. In this sketch, the gating mechanisms of two channels are coupled to a common anchoring site. The anchoring site is illustrated as a membrane-bound protein but could have been replaced by another channel, or by a fixed cytoplasmic molecule located just beneath the plasma membrane. An important functional aspect is that for the channel's gating spring to impart changes in tangential force, the channel must move relative to the site anchoring the coupling molecule. The channels illustrated, therefore, are also attached via springs extending in opposite directions. The latter, which could be anchored to other proteins or channels, are simply placed to emphasize that for relative movements to occur, the channels must be stabilized to a component that is physically isolated from the anchoring point of the gating spring.

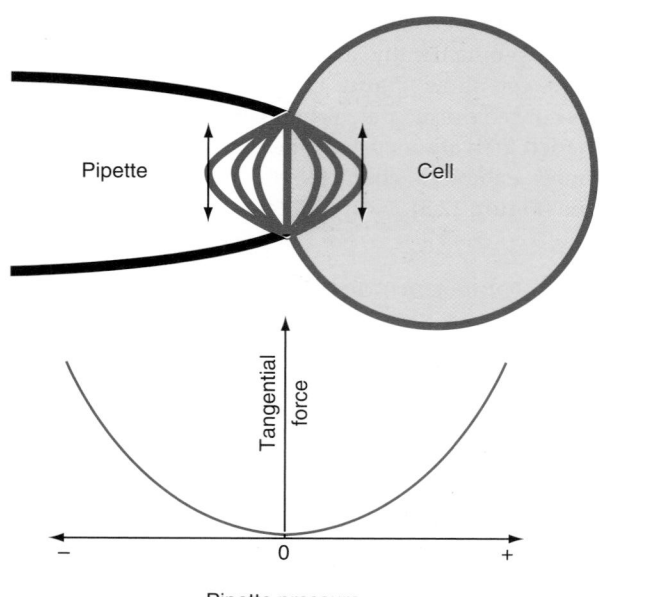

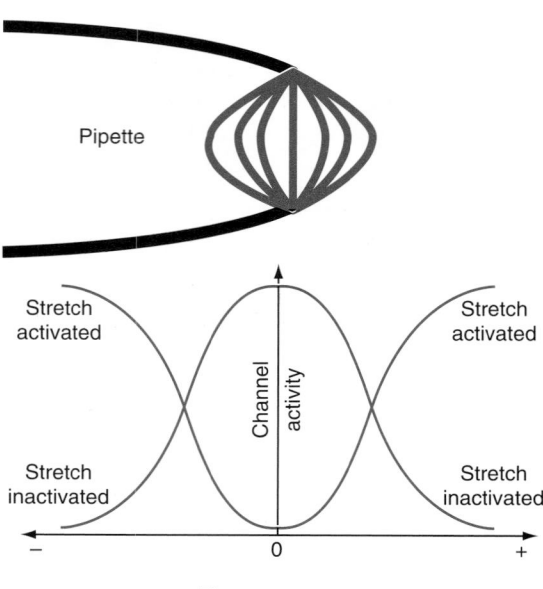

Figure 12.4 Relationship between tangential force and pipette pressure during cell-attached patch clamp recordings. Relative to the cell interior, increases in pipette pressure cause the membrane patch to become concave, whereas suction provokes patch convexity. In both situations, however, the patch of membrane is effectively stretched, such that increased tangential forces are experienced by coupling molecules lying parallel to the plasma membrane.

Figure 12.5 Activity/pressure profiles of symmetrical stretch-activated and stretch-inactivated channels during patch clamp experiments. Since tangential forces within a membrane patch increase symmetrically as a function of absolute pipette pressure (see Figure 12.4), the activity of mechanosensitive channels having a parallel coupling architecture should also vary in a similar manner. During patch clamp experiments, stretch-activated channels are distinguishable from stretch-inactivated channels by the opposite profiles of activity they show in response to changes in pipette pressure. The demonstration of U-shaped (stretch-activated) and bell-shaped (stretch-inactivated) response profiles under experimental conditions provides strong support for the existence of a parallel coupling architecture in some mechanosensitive channels.

12.5 Mechanosensitive ion channels and mechanotransduction

As indicated earlier, many stretch-sensitive channels appear to require extrinsic molecules in order to display normal mechanosensitive gating. Since mechanosensory membranes are frequently embedded within cellular structures specialized for the detection of a particular type of stimulus, it has been difficult to obtain direct evidence that mechanosensitive channels function as physiological mechanotransducers using single-channel recording.

One exception has been the demonstration that stretch-inactivated cationic channels may serve as the molecular mechanoreceptors responsible for signal detection and transduction in osmoreceptors. The remainder of this chapter briefly reviews the physiological role of these unique receptors and examines the biophysical basis for their operation in specialized neurons.

12.6 Osmoreceptors in the central nervous system

The existence of specific osmoreceptors in the central nervous system has been recognized for more than 50 years. In mammals, osmoreceptors are important for the coordination of behavioural, autonomic and neuroendocrine responses to perturbations in the volume and osmolality of the extracellular fluid. Thus, receptors of this type have been shown to control sensations such as thirst and appetite for salt, as well as sympathetic vascular tone and the secretion of hormones regulating blood pressure and body fluid balance. Perhaps the best example of osmoreceptor involvement concerns the regulation of the hypothalamo-neurohypophyseal system (**Figure 12.6a**). In mammals, circulating concentrations of the neurohypophyseal hormone vasopressin increase during hyperosmolality and decrease during hypoosmolality (**Figure 12.6b**). Because it is the body's chief antidiuretic hormone, increases in vasopressin secretion promote water reabsorption from the kidney and reduce the osmolality of extracellular fluids. Osmotically evoked changes in vasopressin release, therefore, play a fundamental role in systemic osmoregulation.

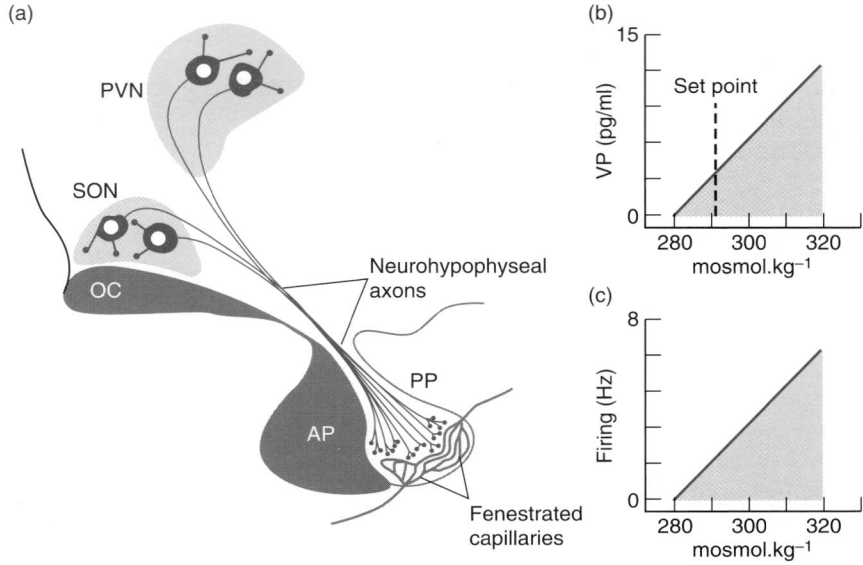

Figure 12.6 A classic example of osmoreceptor involvement: the osmotic regulation of the hypothalamo-neurohypophyseal system.

(a) Sketch of a sagittal view of the hypothalamo-neurohypophyseal system which comprises the somata of magnocellular neurosecretory cells (MNCs) in the supraoptic (SON) and paraventricular (PVN) nuclei of the hypothalamus, and their axon terminals in the posterior pituitary (PP). The axon terminals abut fenestrated capillaries which carry the secreted peptides into the systemic circulation. Individual cells secrete either oxytocin or vasopressin, and both types of MNCs are present in the PVN and SON. Anatomical landmarks illustrated include the optic chiasma (OC) and the anterior pituitary (AP). (b) Summary of results of radioimmunoassay experiments in rats, which have characterized how the concentration of vasopressin (VP) varies as a function of plasma osmolality. Note that physiologically significant hormone concentrations are present at the osmotic set point. Threshold and slope values correspond to regression fits of data obtained in control rats – see Robertson GL (1985) Osmoregulation of thirst and vasopressin secretion: functional properties and their relationship to water balance, in: Schrier RW (ed) *Vasopressin*, New York: Raven Press, 203–212. Comparable data have been obtained for oxytocin release in rats – see Verbalis JG, Dohanics J (1991) Vasopressin and oxytocin secretion in chronically hyposmolar rats, *Am. J. Physiol.* **261**, R1028–1038. (c) Summary of results of electrophysiological experiments in anaesthetized rats, which have shown that the basal firing rate of MNCs is increased by hyperosmolality and decreased by hypo-osmolality. Threshold and slope values represent averages of data obtained from control rats – see Walters JK, Hatton GI (1974) Supraoptic neuronal activity in rats during five days of water deprivation, *Physiol. Behav.* **13**, 661–667; and Wakerley JB, Poulain DA, Brown D (1978) Comparison of firing patterns in oxytocin and vasopressin-releasing neurones during progressive dehydration, *Brain Res.* **148**, 425–440, with permission.

As illustrated in **Figure 12.6a**, the somata of the neurons that secrete the neurohypophyseal hormones vasopressin and oxytocin are located in the supraoptic and paraventricular nuclei of the hypothalamus, from where each cell sends an axon to the posterior pituitary. Collectively, these cells are referred to as *magnocellular neurosecretory cells* (MNCs) in order to distinguish them from the smaller 'parvocellular' hypothalamic neurons that do not project to the posterior pituitary. Hormone release from nerve terminals in the posterior pituitary has been shown to increase as a steep function of the frequency of action potential firing in the neurohypophyseal axons. Thus, hormone secretion into blood is primarily determined by the rate at which the somata of MNCs generate action potentials. The basis for the osmotic regulation of MNCs has been extensively studied in rats, where the release of both oxytocin and vaso-

pressin is regulated in a similar manner by changes in plasma osmolality.

12.6.1 Electrical activity and neurohypophyseal hormone secretion

Electrophysiological recordings in rats have confirmed that the mean rate at which action potentials are discharged by MNCs *in vivo* varies as a positive function of plasma osmolality. Moreover, as shown in **Figures 12.6b and c**, the apparent osmotic threshold for neurohypophyseal hormone secretion corresponds to the osmolality at which MNCs become electrically active. Osmoreceptor-mediated control of the hypothalamo-neurohypophyseal system, therefore, primarily reflects the mechanisms by which changes in osmolality modify the rate at which action potentials are discharged by the somata of MNCs.

12.6.2 Magnocellular neurosecretory cells in the hypothalamus are intrinsic osmoreceptors

Osmoreceptor neurons located in a number of brain regions contribute to the osmotic control of vasopressin secretion via synaptic mechanisms. For example, osmosensitive neurons in the organum vasculosum lamina terminalis, a midline circumventricular organ, have been found to regulate the firing rate of MNCs via the release of glutamate from axon terminals in the supraoptic nucleus. Osmotically evoked changes in firing rate, however, can also be recorded from MNCs in the absence of synaptic transmission, indicating that these cells behave as intrinsic osmoreceptors. Since they can be easily identified during physiological experiments, rat MNCs have been the focus of recent experiments examining the biophysical basis of osmoreception.

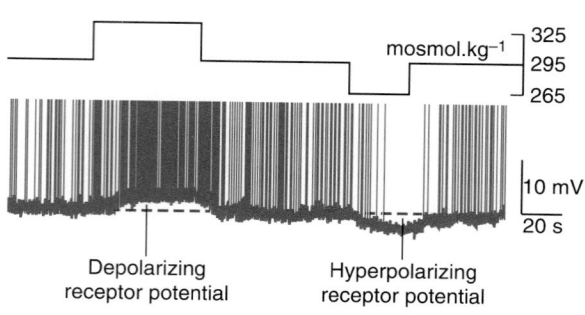

Figure 12.7 Hypothalamic magnocellular neurosecretory cells (MNCs) are intrinsic osmoreceptors.
Effects of osmotic stimulation on whole-cell membrane potential recorded from an MNC acutely dissociated from the rat supraoptic nucleus. Spike hyperpolarizing afterpotentials have been erased to highlight changes in membrane potential. Note that an individual cell responds to increased osmolality with membrane depolarization and to hypo-osmolality with hyperpolarization. Adapted from Oliet SHR, Bourque CW (1993) Steady-state osmotic modulation of cationic conductance in neurons of the rat supraoptic nucleus, *Am. J. Physiol.* **265**, R1475–1479, with permission.

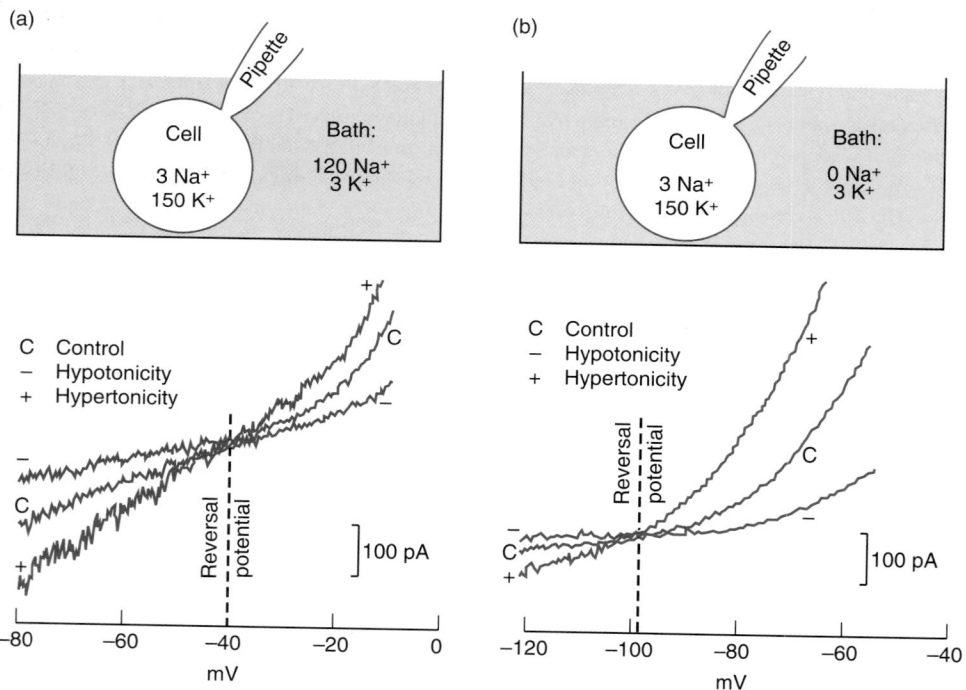

Figure 12.8 Osmotic stimuli modulate a non-selective cationic conductance in osmoreceptor neurons.
Current/voltage relations from isolated MNCs exposed to various osmotic conditions were recorded using the whole-cell configuration of the patch clamp technique. The osmolality of the extracellular fluid was modified by addition or removal of mannitol in order to maintain constant concentrations of Na^+ and K^+ (upper panels). **(a)** Traces show that in normal extracellular solution hypertonic stimuli increase membrane conductance (slope) whereas hypotonic stimuli reduce it. The reversal potential for both responses is approximately −40 mV. **(b)** Removing Na^+ ions from the external solution does not prevent osmotically evoked changes in slope conductance, but causes a shift of the reversal potential toward the equilibrium potential for K^+ ions (about −98 mV in these recording conditions). Adapted from Oliet SHR, Bourque CW (1993) Steady-state osmotic modulation of cationic conductance in neurons of the rat supraoptic nucleus, *Am. J. Physiol.* **265**, R1475–1479, with permission.

12.7 Osmoreception in magnocellular neurosecretory cells

12.7.1 Osmoreceptor potentials reflect the modulation of a non-selective cationic conductance

Increases in firing rate recorded from MNCs during hypertonic stimulation are accompanied by membrane depolarization, whereas decreases in firing frequency associated with hypotonicity result from hyperpolarization (**Figure 12.7**).

Current/voltage analysis of MNCs under voltage clamp has revealed that the inward and outward currents generating these osmotic receptor potentials are associated with increases and decreases in membrane conductance, respectively (**Figure 12.8**). Under physiological conditions, the membrane currents evoked by both stimuli display a common reversal potential (−40 mV), suggesting that they may be mediated by the modulation of a single population of ionic channels. The reversal potential of these currents is not affected by changing the concentration of chloride ions in the external solution. In contrast, lowering the concentration of external Na^+ shifts the reversal potential of the response towards E_K, whereas increasing the concentration of external K^+ shifts the reversal potential towards E_{Na}. These findings indicate that the receptor potentials asso-

ciated with osmoreception in vasopressin-releasing neurons result from the osmotic regulation of a macroscopic conductance permeable to both Na^+ and K^+.

12.7.2 Changes in cell volume directly regulate the macroscopic cationic conductance in magnocellular neurosecretory cells

Changes in fluid osmolality provoke inversely proportional changes in cell volume due to the flux of water across the semi-permeable cell membrane. Changes in cell volume, therefore, have long been assumed to be involved in the transduction mechanism responsible for osmoreception. In agreement with this hypothesis, osmotically evoked changes in cell volume have been found to mirror changes in macroscopic conductance in MNCs, but not in non-osmosensitive neurons (**Figure 12.9**). The tight temporal coupling between changes in cell volume and membrane conductance suggests that the two events are intimately coupled, and may not require the generation of long-lived second messengers.

However, transmembrane water fluxes associated with osmotic stimulation produce immediate and proportional changes in the concentration of cytoplasmic solutes (**Figure 12.10a**). It is possible, therefore, that the cationic membrane conductance of MNCs is regulated by changes in the concentration of one or more cytosolic

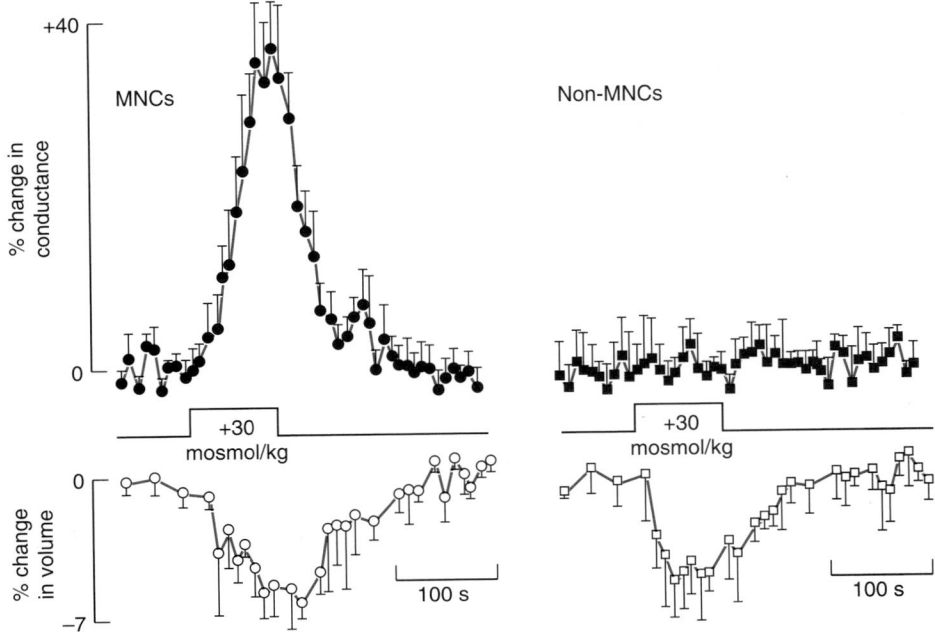

Figure 12.9 Osmotically evoked changes in cationic conductance parallel changes in cell volume in osmoreceptor neurons.
In response to the application of a hypertonic stimulus both MNCs (left) and control neurons (right) undergo a decrease in somatic volume (bottom panels). Only MNCs, however, display an accompanying change in membrane conductance (top panels). Adapted from Oliet SHR, Bourque CW (1993) Mechanosensitive channels transduce osmosensitivity in supraoptic neurons, *Nature* **364**, 341–343, with permission.

constituents. This hypothesis was tested directly by examining the effects of eliciting changes in cell volume under constant osmotic conditions. As shown in **Figure 12.10b**, decreases in cell volume provoked by applying negative pressure to the recording pipette cause increases in cationic conductance similar to those evoked by hypertonic stimulation (**Figure 12.10a**).

Conversely, decreases in membrane conductance are evoked by increasing cell size either by blowing into the recording pipette, or by exposing the cell to a hypotonic solution. Interestingly, upon changing the concentration of external Na^+ or K^+, identical shifts in reversal potentials are observed for the responses evoked by osmotic stimuli (e.g. **Figure 12.8**) and those produced by changes in pipette pressure (not illustrated). The membrane conductance regulated by changes in pipette pressure, therefore, appears to be the same as that modulated by osmotic stimuli. Since the pressure-evoked changes in volume are not associated with changes in solute concentration, the cationic conductance of MNCs appears to be specifically regulated by variations in cell volume, rather than by the concentration, or dilution, of an internal solute.

12.7.3 Magnocellular neurosecretory cells express stretch-inactivated cationic channels

The existence of a cationic conductance directly regulated by cell volume suggests that volume-regulated ion channels might transduce the effects of osmotic stimuli in MNCs. Cell-attached patch-clamp recordings (**Figure 12.11a**) were therefore performed on these cells using pipettes containing various blockers of known voltage- and ligand-gated channels. These experiments revealed the presence of single channels exhibiting a reversal potential of –40 mV and an open channel conductance of about 30 pS (**Figures 12.11b and c**). In individual membrane patches, comparable changes in channel activity could be evoked either by changing the osmolality of the extracellular fluid, or by modifying the pressure inside the recording pipette (**Figure 12.11d**).

These findings suggest that mechanosensitive channels may be responsible for osmoreception in MNCs. Since an unknown amount of residual pipette pressure remains following the formation of a seal

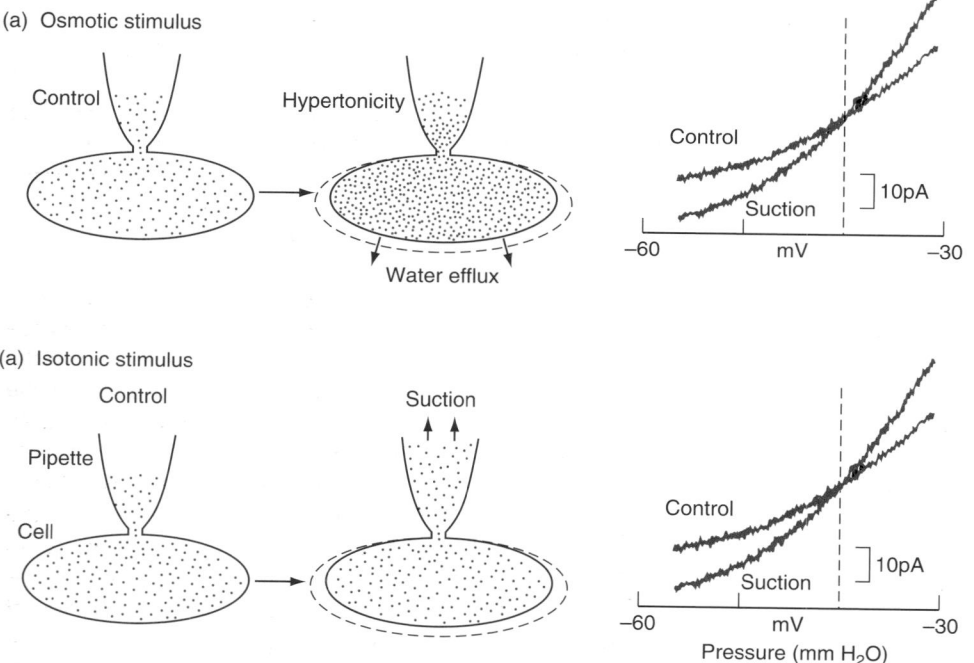

(a) Osmotic stimulus

Control   Hypertonicity

Water efflux

Control

Suction

10pA

−60   mV   −30

(a) Isotonic stimulus

Control   Suction

Pipette

Cell

Control

Suction

10pA

−60   mV   −30

Pressure (mm H₂O)

Figure 12.10 Volume changes directly regulate the cationic conductance in magnocellular neurosecretory cells.
(a) Decreases in volume evoked by hypertonicity are associated with increases in cytoplasmic solute concentration. (b) An isotonic decrease in cell volume can be caused by applying suction to the inside of a recording pipette. Corresponding whole-cell current-voltage relations, recorded from a single acutely isolated MNC, reveal that decreases in cell volume evoked either by hypertonicity (a), or by the application of pipette suction (b), cause similar changes in cationic conductance. Note that the reversal potentials of both responses are similar (vertical dashed line drawn through –40 mV). Adapted from Bourque CW, Oliet SHR (1995) Mechanosensitive ion channels and osmoreception in magnocellular neurosecretory neurons, in: Saito T, Kurokawa K, Yoshida S (eds) *Neurohypophysis: Recent Progress of Vasopressin and Oxytocin Research*, Amsterdam: Elsevier Science, 205–213, with permission.

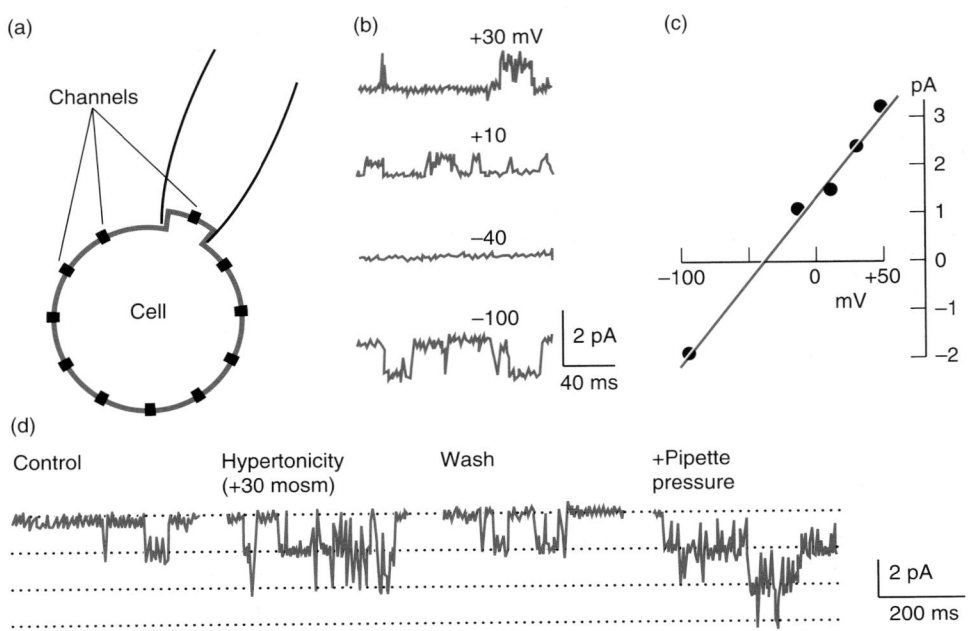

Figure 12.11 Osmoreceptor neurons express cationic channels modulated by osmotic stimuli and changes in pipette pressure.
(a) Single-channel recordings were obtained from isolated MNCs using the cell-attached configuration of the patch clamp technique. **(b)** Single-channel currents observed at the membrane potentials indicated. **(c)** This plot reveals that the single channel has a slope conductance of about 30 pS and a reversal potential near –40 mV. **(d)** Recordings from a membrane patch containing at least three channels. Note that channel activity was increased either by applying a hypertonic stimulus (addition of mannitol to the bath), or by raising the pressure inside the recording pipette. Changes in pipette pressure were achieved by blowing or sucking into a tube connected to the patch pipette and were monitored using a manometer. Adapted from Bourque CW, Oliet SHR (1995) Mechanosensitive ion channels and osmoreception in magnocellular neurosecretory neurons, in: Saito T, Kurokawa K, Yoshida S (eds) *Neurohypophysis: Recent Progress of Vasopressin and Oxytocin Research*, Amsterdam: Elsevier Science, 205–213; and from Oliet SHR, Bourque CW (1993) Mechanosensitive channels transduce osmosensitivity in supraoptic neurons, *Nature* **364**, 341–343, with permission.

between the tip of the pipette and the cell membrane, the functional nature of mechanosensitive channels cannot be determined by examining their response to a single pulse of pressure (see **Figure 12.5**). As shown in **Figure 12.12**, the activity of the channels recorded on MNCs varied as a bell-shaped function of pipette pressure, indicating that they are of the stretch-inactivated variety.

12.7.4 The inhibitory effects of Gd^{3+} provide pharmacological evidence for the involvement of the stretch-inactivated cation channels in osmoreception

Cation-permeable mechanosensitive channels recorded in many preparations are blocked by micromolar concentrations of the trivalent lanthanide gadolinium (Gd^{3+}). In agreement with such observations, addition of Gd^{3+} to the recording pipette was found to cause a profound reduction in the mean open time of stretch-inactivated cation channels in MNCs (**Figure 12.13a**). As

shown by the graph in **Figure 12.13b**, the mean open time of the channels was reduced by 50% when a concentration of Gd^{3+} of about 30–35 μM was present in the recording pipette. Thus if these channels underlie the generation of osmoreceptor potentials (see **Figure 12.7**), responses to osmotic stimuli recorded from the whole cell should also be reduced by approximately 50% in the presence of an equivalent concentration of Gd^{3+} in the bath. As shown in **Figure 12.13c**, excitatory responses to hypertonic perturbations were potently inhibited in the presence of Gd^{3+}, with a half-maximal concentration of the order of 30 μM (**Figure 12.13d**). These findings provide strong support for the involvement of the stretch-inactivated cation channels in the generation of osmoreceptor responses.

12.7.5 Molecular basis for mechanotransduction in osmoreceptors

Under hypotonic conditions, cell swelling would increase tangential force, reducing the activity of the

(a)

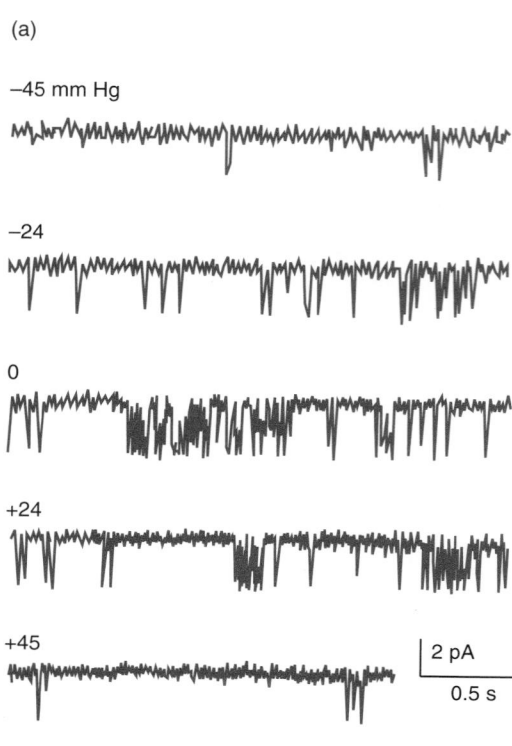

−45 mm Hg

−24

0

+24

+45

2 pA

0.5 s

(b)

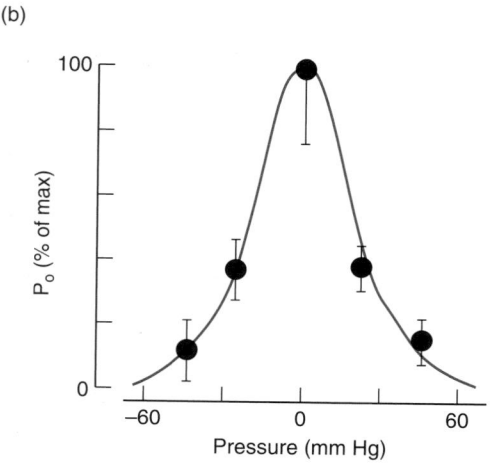

P_o (% of max)

Pressure (mm Hg)

Figure 12.12 (left) Mechanosensitive channels in magno-cellular neurosecretory cells are stretch-inactivated. The effects of exposing a single mechanosensitive channel to a wide range of pipette pressures were examined during cell-attached patch-clamp recording from an acutely isolated MNC. **(a)** Representative excerpts of channel activity recorded at the pressures indicated. **(b)** Mean changes in probability of opening (p_o) observed during recordings from many patches, expressed as a percentage of the maximal activity recorded in individual patches. The bell-shaped relation between channel p_o and pipette pressure suggests that mechanosensitive channels in MNCs are inactivated by stretch. Part (b) from Bourque CW, Oliet SHR (1995) Mechanosensitive ion channels and osmoreception in magnocellular neurosecretory neurons, *Excerpta Medica International Congress Series* 1098; and adapted from Oliet SHR, Bourque CW (1993) Mechanosensitive channels transduce osmosensitivity in supraoptic neurons, *Nature* **364**, 341–343, with permission.

in **Figure 12.15** confirm this prediction by revealing that the inhibition of macroscopic conductance observed during progressive hypo-osmolality saturates near 275 mOsmol kg^{-1}. Thus the osmolality at which the stretch-inactivated channels become active is strikingly similar to the osmotic pressure at which the electrical activity of MNCs and systemic neurohypophyseal hormone secretion become detectable *in vivo* (**Figure 12.6**). This observation provides strong support for the functional involvement of stretch-inactivated cation channels in osmoreception.

12.8 Conclusions

Mechanosensitive ion channels represent obvious candidates as molecular mediators of mechanotransduction, the process by which local physical force is transformed into an electric current. Given the broad range of functions apparently regulated by mechanoreceptors, it is not surprising that a large and diverse group of functionally distinct stretch-sensitive channels has been characterized during patch-clamp recording experiments. The observation of channels displaying symmetric or asymmetric forms of mechanosensitive gating further implies the existence of a variety of different structural mechanisms by which the gating apparatus may receive physical force from the local environment. Thus, in addition to cloning the subunits comprising the pore region of mechanosensitive channels, it will be important to identify the structure of extrinsic molecules comprising the transduction apparatus regulating their function in specialized types of mechanoreceptors.

Mechanosensitive channels have been observed in a wide variety of cell types, suggesting that they may also

cationic channels and hyperpolarizing the cell (**Figure 12.14**). Conversely, hypertonic cell shrinking would reduce tangential force, increasing the opening probability of cationic channels and depolarizing the cell. The presence of stretch-inactivated cation channels in rat MNCs, therefore, is consistent with their role as intrinsic osmoreceptors.

The involvement of these channels has functional implications concerning the osmotic regulation of the hypothalamo-neurohypophyseal system. Indeed, since channel activity can be virtually abolished by pressure-evoked membrane stretch (see **Figure 12.12**), one should observe complete suppression of the macroscopic conductance under strong hypotonic conditions. The plots

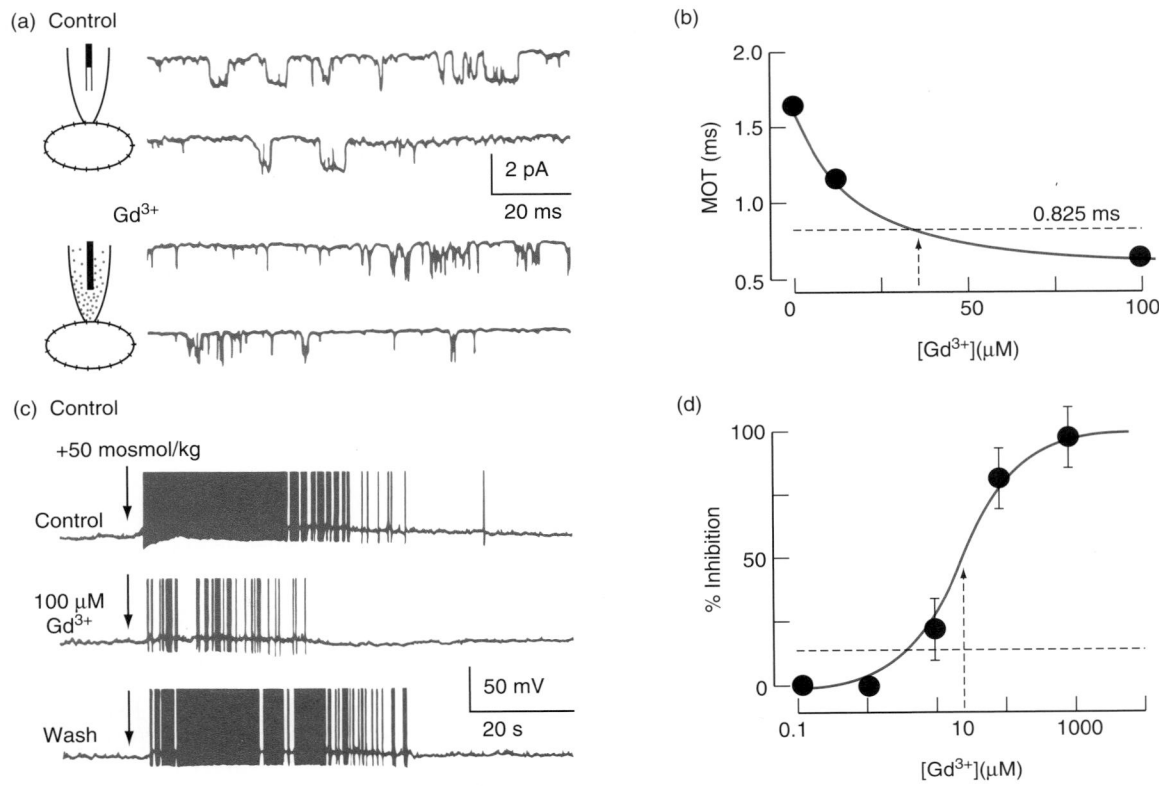

Figure 12.13 Effects of gadolinium (Gd³⁺) on stretch-inactivated cation channels and osmoreception in magnocellular neurosecretory cells.

(a) The top two traces show typical openings recorded from a stretch-inactivated cation channel under control, cell-attached recording conditions (see inset). The lower traces show openings recorded from the same ion channel after a small bolus (1 mM) of GdCl$_3$ was infused into the recording pipette (inset). Note that the duration of individual openings was dramatically reduced in the presence of Gd³⁺. (b) The channel mean open time (MOT; the average duration of all openings recorded under a particular condition) decreased as a function of the concentration of Gd³⁺ present in the recording pipette. Note that at a concentration of approximately 32 μM (vertical arrow) the MOT is reduced by 50%. (c) Whole-cell current clamp responses to the application of brief hypertonic stimuli consisting of saline plus 50 mM of mannitol (vertical arrow). The amplitude of the depolarization and the number of spikes evoked by the stimulus were dramatically inhibited in the presence of 100 μM of Gd³⁺ in the bath (middle trace). (d) Quantification of the inhibitory effects of different concentrations of Gd³⁺ on macroscopic responses to hypertonic stimuli revealed an IC$_{50}$ value near 30 μM, a value which corresponds to the effects of Gd³⁺ on channel MOT. Adapted from Oliet SHR, Bourque CW (1996) Gadolinium uncouples mechanical detection and osmoreceptor potential in supraoptic neurons, *Neuron* **16**, 175–181, with permission.

perform functions unrelated to mechanosensory transduction. Moreover, recent experiments have revealed that ligand- or voltage-gated channels can display mechanosensitive gating under certain experimental conditions. Whether the mechanosensitivity of such channels is an artifact, or is physiologically relevant, remains to be established. As indicated by Morris (1992), observations of this kind highlight the need for caution when considering the possible role of a mechanosensitive channel in a physiological process.

The biophysical characteristics of stretch-inactivated cation channels in magnocellular neurosecretory cells correspond well with the osmotic regulation of macroscopic conductance, membrane potential and action potential firing. The role of stretch-inactivated channels in osmoreception, therefore, provides one of the clearest demonstrations of the involvement of mechanosensitive channels in a mechanically regulated physiological process. Interestingly, very recent studies have shown that the activity of the mechanosensitive channels mediating osmoreception in magnocellular neurosecretory cells can in fact be modulated by neuropeptides known to be present in synaptic pathways targeting these hypothalamic neurons. It is likely, therefore, that neuromodulatory effects can contribute to the regulation of gain and dynamic range in these and other mechanotransducers.

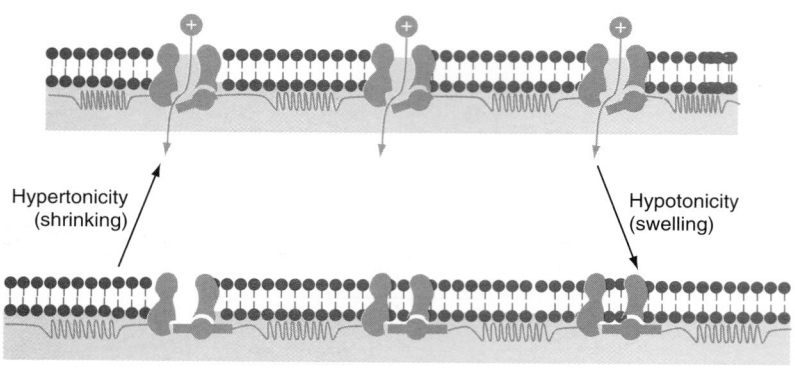

Hypertonicity (shrinking)

Hypotonicity (swelling)

Figure 12.14 (left) Osmotic modulation of stretch-inactivated channels.
The diagram illustrates how cell swelling evoked by hypotonic stimuli may increase tangential force in parallel coupling molecules regulating the gating mechanism of mechanosensitive channels in magnocellular neurosecretory cells. Because channel activity is reduced by stretch, the associated decrease in macroscopic cationic conductance generates a hyperpolarizing receptor potential. Reversing the mechanism explains how a depolarizing receptor potential is generated in response to a hypertonic stimulus.

Further reading

Bourque CW (1998) Osmoregulation of vasopressin neurons: a synergy of intrinsic and synaptic processes. *Prog. Brain Res.* **119**, 59–76.

Bourque CW, Oliet SHR (1997) Osmoreceptors in the central nervous system. *Ann. Rev. Physiol.* **59**, 601–619.

Chakfe Y, Bourque CW (2000) Excitatory peptides and osmotic pressure modulate mechanosensitive cation channels in concert. *Nature Neurosci.* **3**, 572–579.

Guharay F, Sachs F (1984) Stretch-activated single ion channel currents in tissue-cultured embryonic chick skeletal muscle. *J. Physiol.* **352**, 685–701.

Martinac B, Adler J, Kung C (1990) Mechanosensitive ion channels of *E. coli* activated by amphipaths. *Nature* **348**, 261–263.

Morris CE (1992) Are stretch-sensitive channels in molluscan cells and elsewhere physiological mechanotransducers? *Experentia* **48**, 852–858.

Voisin DL, Chakfe Y, Bourque CW (1999) Coincident detection of CSF Na⁺ and osmotic pressure in osmoregulatory neurons of the supraoptic nucleus. *Neuron* **24**, 453–460.

Walker RG, Willingham AT, Zuker CS (2000) A *Drosophila* mechanosensory transduction channel. *Science* **287**, 2229–2234.

(a)

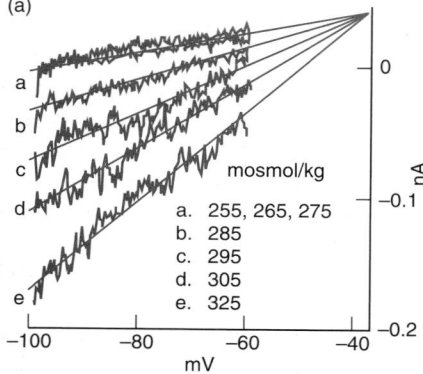

mosmol/kg

a. 255, 265, 275
b. 285
c. 295
d. 305
e. 325

(b)

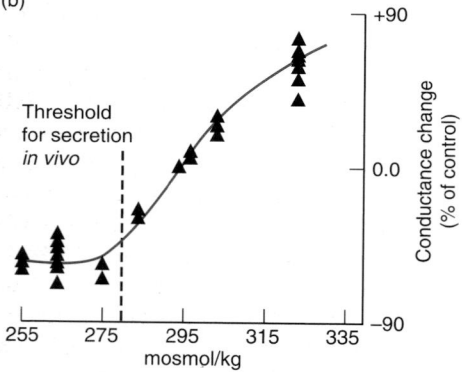

Threshold for secretion *in vivo*

Figure 12.15 Osmotic modulation of macroscopic conductance shows saturation during strong hypotonicity.
(a) Currents recorded in response to voltage ramps applied between –100 and –60 mV during exposure of a single cell to solutions of varying osmolalities. The solid lines extrapolate current–voltage relations to the reversal potential of the cationic conductance (–40 mV). (b) Changes in membrane conductance observed in 22 cells during osmotic stimulation from 295 mOsmol kg⁻¹. Note that decreases in conductance saturate under hypotonic conditions and that the resulting apparent threshold for the osmotically evoked conductance is similar to the threshold for hormone secretion observed *in vivo* (see Figure 12.6). Adapted from: Oliet SHR, Bourque CW (1993) Steady-state osmotic modulation of cationic conductance in neurons of the rat supraoptic nucleus, *Am. J. Physiol.* **265**, R1475–1479, with permission.

The Metabotropic GABA$_B$ Receptors

Gamma-aminobutyric acid (GABA) is the primary inhibitory neurotransmitter in the mammalian central nervous system. It is found in virtually every area of the brain. It exerts fast and powerful synaptic inhibition by acting on GABA$_A$ receptors. These receptors are directly coupled to an integral chloride channel and produce inhibition by increasing the membrane chloride conductance. This form of synaptic inhibition is critical for maintaining and shaping neuronal communication.

However, like other neurotransmitters that activate fast, ionotropic responses lasting for milliseconds, GABA can also activate a second class of receptors which produce slow synaptic responses capable of lasting for seconds. The receptors producing these slow, metabotropic responses are called GABA$_B$ receptors. They play a major role in regulating neurotransmission, which makes them potentially important therapeutic targets in the treatment of a variety of neurological conditions including epilepsy, spasticity, pain and psychiatric illness. GABA$_B$ receptors are G-protein coupled to a number of cellular effector mechanisms. These different effectors enable GABA$_B$ receptors to produce, not only inhibition, but a diversity of other effects on neuronal function as well. Thus, GABA$_B$ receptors enable GABA to modulate neuronal activity in a fashion that is not possible through GABA$_A$ receptors alone.

This chapter focuses on GABA$_B$ receptors and the effects these receptors can have on cellular function.

13.1 GABA$_B$ receptors were originally discovered because of their insensitivity to bicuculline and their sensitivity to baclofen

The discovery of GABA$_B$ receptors was made possible by the development in the early 1970s of the compound β-parachlorophenyl GABA (baclofen). Baclofen is a GABA analogue which can be administered orally and will penetrate the blood–brain barrier. It was hoped that after gaining access to the brain this compound would act on GABA receptors and be an effective anticonvulsant. Indeed, baclofen did mimic many of the actions of GABA and was found to reduce skeletal muscle tone and inhibit spinal reflex activity, making it a successful agent in treating spinal cord spasticity. Yet, despite these similarities with GABA, several important differences between the actions of GABA and baclofen were reported, the most notable of which was that the actions of baclofen were insensitive to the classical GABA antagonist, bicuculline.

It was at this time that Norman Bowery and his colleagues found that application of GABA decreased the release of norepinephrine from a preparation of the rat isolated atrium. Interestingly, this effect of GABA was insensitive to bicuculline as well as another GABA antagonist, picrotoxin, and was not mimicked by classical GABA agonists, such as isoguvacine and THIP. Bowery *et al.* found similar results when they measured the effect of GABA on the release of norepinephrine in another peripheral preparation, the rat isolated anococcygeus muscle. In both of these preparations the GABA analogue, baclofen, mimicked the action of GABA by depressing the release of norepinephrine in a dose-dependent manner (**Figure 13.1**). Furthermore, neither the effect of GABA nor that of baclofen appeared to be mediated by an increase in chloride conductance, suggesting that a receptor other than the classical GABA receptor was responsible for the presynaptic inhibition of norepinephrine release.

To determine whether this bicuculline-insensitive action of GABA was confined to the periphery, Bowery and coworkers tested the effect of GABA and baclofen on potassium-evoked norepinephrine release from brain slices. They found that, as in the periphery, GABA suppressed norepinephrine release by acting on a bicuculline-insensitive receptor that was separate from the classical bicuculline-sensitive GABA receptor. This action of GABA was mimicked by the GABA analogue baclofen, but not by other known GABA agonists. Radioligand receptor binding in brain using ^{3}H-GABA demonstrated two distinct binding sites for GABA with different distributions. These results led Bowery and his

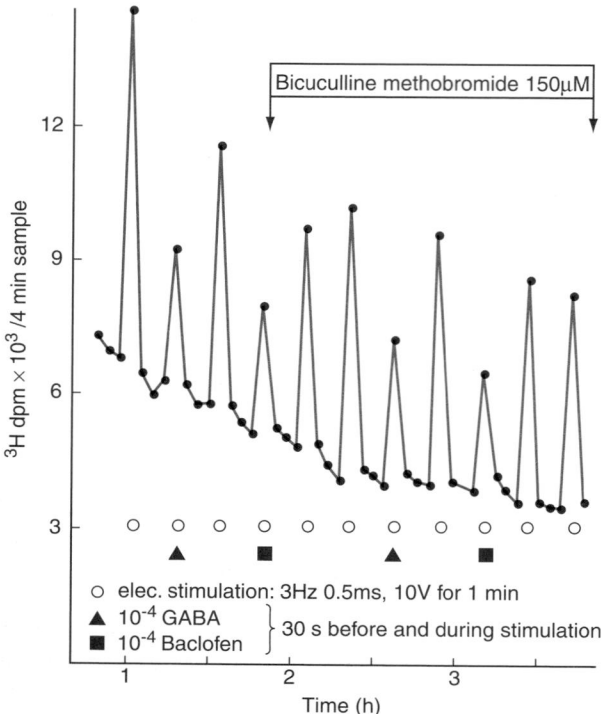

Figure 13.1 GABA and baclofen suppress ³H-norepineph-rine release from the rat atrium.

The release of ³H-norepinephrine was assessed by taking samples of the superfusate every 4 minutes and measuring the tritium content (in dpm) by liquid scintillation spectrometry. Electrical stimuli were delivered to the tissue at times indicated by the open circles. These stimuli caused the release of ³H-norepinephrine and so increased the tritium content of the sample. GABA (filled triangles) and baclofen (filled squares) reduced the release of ³H-norepinephrine by the stimulus. The effect of these drugs was insensitive to co-application of bicuculline methobromide. From Bowery NG, Doble A, Hill DR *et al.* (1981) Structure/activity studies at a baclofen-sensitive, bicuculline-insensitive GABA receptor. In: DeFeudis FV, Mandel P (eds) *Amino Acid Neurotransmitters*, New York: Raven Press, with permission.

coworkers in 1981 to propose the existence of a new class of GABA receptor, which they termed the GABA$_B$ receptor, while designating the classical GABA receptor as the GABA$_A$ receptor.

13.2 Structure of the GABA$_B$ receptor

Using a high-affinity antagonist, the structural properties of the GABA$_B$ receptor were recently characterized by expression cloning. Expression of a fully functional GABA$_B$ receptor requires coupling between two separate and distinct gene products, GABA$_B$ R1 and R2. GABA$_B$ receptors are thus the first example of a functional heterodimeric metabotropic receptor.

13.2.1 GABA$_B$ receptors belong to family-3 G-protein-coupled receptors

Cloning of the GABA$_B$ receptor

In 1997, Bettler and colleagues successfully cloned the first GABA$_B$ receptor, GABA$_B$R1, by expression cloning in mammalian COS-1 cells, using the high-affinity GABA$_B$ antagonist [¹²⁵I]CGP 64213. The derived sequence of GABA$_B$R1 indicated that it shares no significant sequence similarity to GABA$_A$ or GABA$_C$ receptors, but that it is distantly related to family-3 G-protein-coupled receptors (GPCRs). This family of receptors includes metabotropic glutamate receptors (mGluRs), the Ca^{2+}-sensing receptor, a family of pheromone receptors and certain mammalian taste receptors. Family-3 GPCRs have several characteristic features, including a large extracellular N-terminus which plays a critical role in ligand binding, followed by seven closely spaced putative transmembrane domains, indicative of GPCRs. In family-3 GPCRs the third intracellular loop, which is short and highly conserved, is critical for G-protein activation, whereas the second intracellular loop is important for G-protein coupling selectivity. The carboxy-terminal intracellular tail is the most variable region of these receptors and is subject to major changes by alternative splicing of the mRNA. This region is likely the target of multiple interacting proteins, such as the Homer proteins, which have been shown to interact with certain mGluR receptors. When compared with mGluRs, GABA$_B$R1 shares only 18–23% sequence homology, but hydrophobicity profiles indicate clear conservation of structural architecture between these receptors. The N-terminal extracellular domain of both mGluRs and GABA$_B$R1 shares limited, but significant similarity with bacterial periplasmic amino acid-binding proteins (PBPs) such as the leucine-binding protein (LBP) and the leucine/isoleucine/valine-binding protein (LIVBP). However, the intracellular loops of the GABA$_B$ receptor are not as well conserved as in other family-3 receptors. In particular, most cysteine residues, which are highly conserved in other family-3 receptors, are not conserved in GABA$_B$R1.

GABA$_B$R1 exists in at least four isoforms

Four isoforms of GABA$_B$R1 have been identified to date. These isoforms are generated by alternative splicing of a single GABA$_B$R1 gene.

The first two GABA$_B$ receptor isoforms to be discovered were termed GABA$_B$R1a and GABA$_B$R1b and possess molecular weights of 130 and 100 kDa, respectively. These isoforms are pharmacologically identical with similar ligand binding affinities and differ only in the length of their N-terminal sequences. The N-terminus of each contains the LBP-like sequence thought to be important for ligand binding; however, unlike GABA$_B$R1b, the N-terminus of GABA$_B$R1a also contains a tandem pair of consensus sequences for the complement protein module.

The third isoform of the GABA$_B$ receptor, designated GABA$_B$R1c, is generated by an in-frame insertion of 31 amino acids between the second extracellular loop and the fifth transmembrane region of either GABA$_B$R1a or GABA$_B$R1b.

The final identified isoform, designated GABA$_B$R1d, is identical to GABA$_B$R1b but has an insertion of 566 base pairs which generates a divergent amino acid sequence in the carboxy-terminal end.

Whereas the specific function of these different isoforms is unclear, they may provide a mechanism for differential targeting of GABA$_B$ receptors within the cell or the coupling of these receptors to different effector systems. Current studies are under way to identify additional GABA$_B$R1 isoforms. Significantly, no pharmacological differences between these splice variants have been reported to date.

GABA$_B$ receptor pharmacology

GABA is the endogenous agonist at both GABA$_A$ and GABA$_B$ receptors. GABA$_B$ receptors are pharmacologically distinguished from GABA$_A$ receptors by their insensitivity to the GABA$_A$ antagonist bicuculline and their selective activation by the prototypic agonist baclofen (**Figure 13.2**). Baclofen activates GABA$_B$ receptors in a stereospecific manner with the (−)isomer being about 100 times more potent than the (+)isomer. In contrast, GABA$_B$ receptors are not sensitive to classical agonists at the GABA$_A$ receptor, such as muscimol and isoguvacine, or to modulators of GABA$_A$ receptors such as benzodiazepines, barbiturates and neurosteroids.

The discovery of selective GABA$_B$ receptor antagonists with increased receptor affinity and improved pharmacokinetic profile has been an important element in establishing the significance and structure of GABA$_B$ receptors. The first GABA$_B$ receptor antagonists, phaclofen and 2-hydroxysaclofen (**Figure 13.2**), represented a major breakthrough in the study of GABA$_B$ receptors even though they possessed relatively low potencies. Subsequently, Froestl and coworkers introduced CGP 35348, the first GABA$_B$ receptor antagonist capable of crossing the blood–brain barrier. This was soon followed by CGP 36742, the first orally active GABA$_B$ receptor antagonist. Whereas both of these compounds displayed rather low potency, Wolfgang Froestl and coworkers found that the substitution of a dichloroben-

zene moiety into these antagonist molecules resulted in the production of antagonists with affinities about 10 000-fold higher than previously described. This breakthrough resulted in the production of a host of compounds, such as CGP 52432, CGP 55845, CGP 64213 and CGP 71872 which had affinities in the nanomolar and even subnanomolar range. This series of compounds eventually led to the development of the radio-iodinated, high-affinity antagonist [^{125}I]-CGP 64213, which was used to clone GABA$_B$R1.

The agonist binding site on GABA$_B$R1 is in the extracellular amino-terminal domain

The ligand-binding domain for family-3 GPCRs has been shown to be located in the extracellular N-terminus of the receptor in a region with significant homology to bacterial periplasmic amino-acid-binding proteins (PBP). Recent experiments with truncated versions of mGluR1 confirmed the importance of this domain for agonist binding. The binding of mGluR1 ligands to the PBP-like domain requires the cysteine-rich region, a hallmark of family-3 GPCRs, which is absent in GABA$_B$Rs. These structural differences, as well as the low sequence similarity between GABA$_B$ receptors and other family-3 receptors, suggest that their N-terminal domains may not necessarily function in the same manner during agonist binding.

To address this issue, Bettler and colleagues have recently constructed chimeric receptors which contain the N-terminus of GABA$_B$R1 on the body of the mGluR1 receptor. They found that these chimeric receptors and wildtype GABA$_B$ receptors possessed similar binding affinities for GABA$_B$ receptor ligands. Furthermore, radio-iodinated antagonist binding affinities were also unaltered in GABA$_B$ truncation mutants in which the entire carboxy-terminus after the first transmembrane domain was deleted. Finally, when the N-terminus of the GABA$_B$ receptor was produced as a soluble miniprotein it bound radiolabelled GABA$_B$ receptor antagonist with a similar affinity to control wildtype receptor. These studies indicate that, like the N-terminal domain of other family-3 GPCRs, the N-terminal domain of GABA$_B$R1 is both necessary and sufficient for ligand binding.

Mutagenesis studies support the LBP-like domain in the N-terminus of GABA$_B$R1 as a critical region for ligand binding. Mutation of several key residues in this area markedly alters the affinity of the GABA$_B$ receptor for antagonist, suggesting that the architecture of this region bears structural homology to that of the PBPs. Three-dimensional modelling of the GABA$_B$-binding domain based on the known structure of LBP supports a Venus flytrap model for receptor activation. According

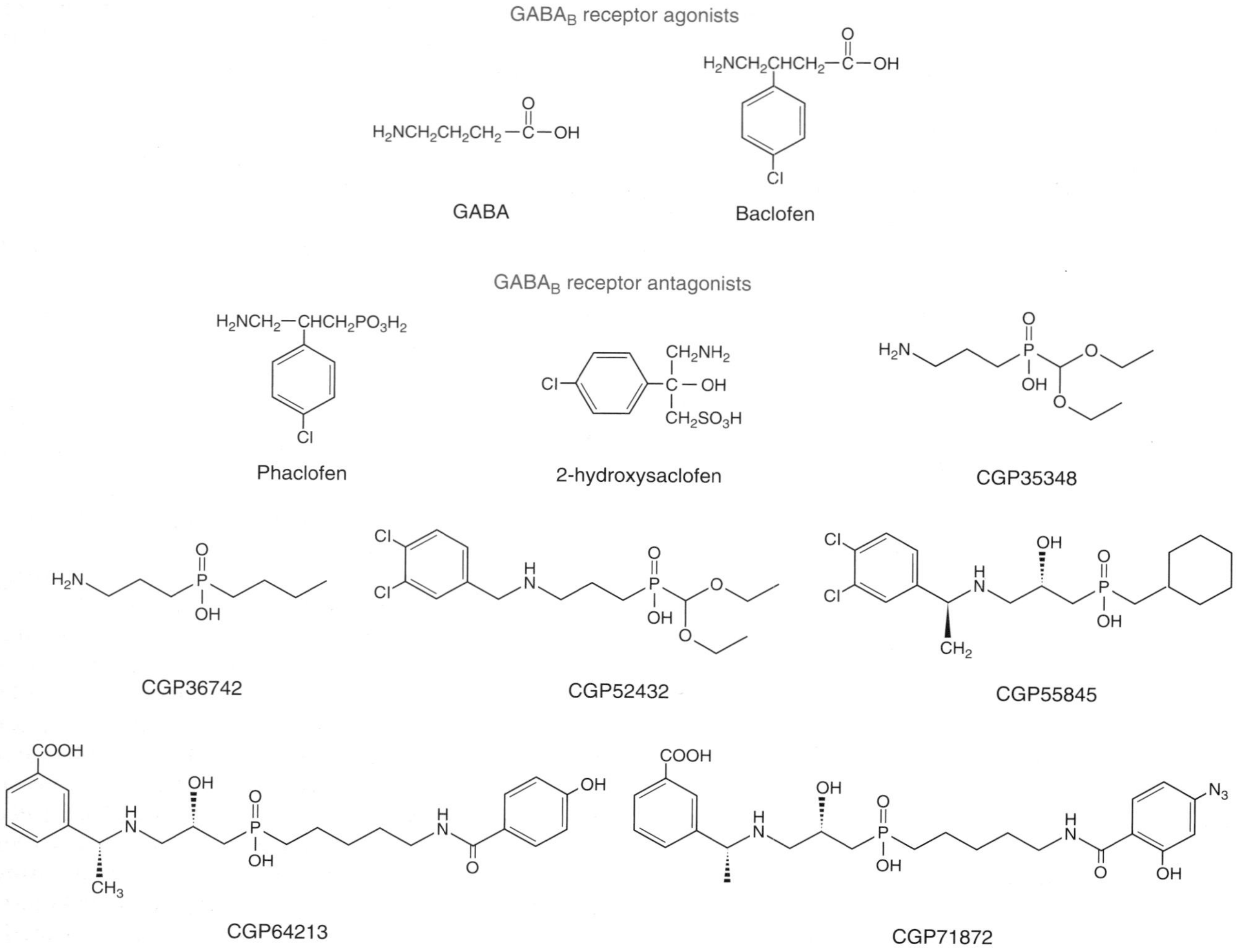

Figure 13.2 Structures of selected GABA$_B$ receptor agonists and antagonists.
Adapted from Mott DD, Lewis DV (1994) The pharmacology and function of central GABA$_B$ receptors, *Int. Rev. Neurobiol.* **39**, 97–223, with permission.

to this model, the ligand-binding site is formed in a groove between two large globular domains in the N-terminus. Activation of the receptor results from the closure of these two lobes upon agonist binding. This model is similar to that proposed for other members of family-3 GPCRs.

Ligand binding to GABA$_B$ receptors requires the presence of divalent cations

GABA$_B$ receptor-binding assays using ^{3}H-GABA reveal that divalent cations are required for binding. This differs from GABA$_A$ receptors which have no such requirement. A number of different divalent cations were tested for their ability to increase GABA$_B$ binding and were found to have the following order of potency $Mn^{2+} = Ni^{2+} > Mg^{2+} > Ca^{2+} > Sr^{2+} > Ba^{2+}$. The effect of divalent cations is concentration dependent with physiological concentrations of calcium or magnesium being near optimal to promote GABA$_B$ receptor binding. Calcium increases the affinity of GABA, but not of baclofen, on GABA$_B$R1. Mutational analysis has revealed that a specific highly conserved residue in the GABA$_B$ ligand-binding site (Ser269) is critical for this effect of calcium. The calcium-sensing properties of the GABA$_B$ receptor are similar to those of other family-3 GPCRs, such as the Ca^{2+}-sensing receptor and metabotropic glutamate receptor, both of which have been shown to respond to extracellular calcium. Interestingly, other divalent cations, including Hg^{2+}, Pb^{2+}, Cd^{2+} and Zn^{2+}, were found to inhibit GABA$_B$ receptor binding. The ability of some divalent cations to enhance binding while others inhibit it suggests that the GABA$_B$ receptor is modulated by distinct excitatory and inhibitory cation binding sites.

13.2.2 GABA_B receptors are heterodimers

GABA_BR1 receptors are nonfunctional

Whereas GABA_BR1 displays binding and biochemical characteristics similar to those of native GABA_B receptors, several important discrepancies were noted between these cloned receptors and native GABA_B receptors. For example, the affinity of agonists, but not antagonists, was 100–150 fold lower for GABA_BR1 than for native receptors. Most importantly, when expressed in cell lines GABA_BR1 coupled only weakly to adenylyl cyclase and did not couple to other effector systems, such as Ca^{2+} or K^+ channels. The reason for the failure of GABA_BR1 to produce functional receptors was examined using epitope tagged versions of GABA_BR1a to study the cellular distribution of the receptor protein in a variety of cell types. It was found that GABA_BR1 was retained in the endoplasmic reticulum and therefore failed to reach the cell surface. Thus, it appeared as though GABA_BR1 required additional information for functional targeting to the plasma membrane.

GABA_BR2 receptors are structurally similar to GABA_BR1 but exhibit functional and pharmacological differences from native GABA_B receptors

The failure of GABA_BR1 to produce functional GABA_B receptors inspired database searches for other related genes, ultimately resulting in the discovery of a second GABA_B receptor gene, termed GABA_BR2. This receptor subtype was 35% homologous with GABA_BR1 and exhibited many of the structural features of GABA_BR1, including a large molecular weight (110 kDa), an extended extracellular N-terminus and seven transmembrane spanning domains. In contrast, the intracellular carboxy-terminus of GABA_BR2 was longer than that of GABA_BR1.

Increasing evidence supports the ability of GABA_BR2 to act as a functional GABA_B receptor. Unlike GABA_BR1, GABA_BR2 is expressed predominantly at the cell surface in heterologous systems. GABA_BR2 can also bind GABA in many, but not all, expression systems. The inability of GABA_BR2 to bind GABA in some expression systems may reflect different levels of GABA_BR2 expression, different G proteins or the presence of an accessory protein for GABA_BR2.

Whereas GABA_BR2 displays similar agonist pharmacology to GABA_BR1, its antagonist pharmacology profile exhibits some important differences. In particular, GABA_BR2 binds 2-hydroxysaclofen, but none of the more potent GABA_B receptor antagonists. This inability to bind antagonists most likely results because of a single amino acid difference in the binding pocket of GABA_BR2; the substitution of a proline in GABA_BR2 for a critical serine (Ser246) in GABA_BR1a.

Fully functional GABA_B receptors require coupling between GABA_BR1 and GABA_BR2

Differences in the pharmacology between GABA_BR2 and native GABA_B receptors as well as the difficulty in expressing functional GABA_B responses prompted the continued search for a recombinant GABA_B receptor which would mimic the properties of the native receptor. Two lines of evidence suggested that the functional form of the GABA_B receptor might be formed from co-expression of GABA_BR1 and GABA_BR2. First, GABA_BR1 and GABA_BR2 share a similar distribution in the brain and are expressed in the same neuronal cells. Second, co-expression of GABA_BR1 and GABA_BR2 markedly increases the agonist affinity of the expressed GABA_B receptor to a level similar to that of native receptors.

Two series of experiments were used to determine whether GABA_BR1 and GABA_BR2 interact to form a functional GABA_B receptor. First, a yeast two hybrid system was used to identify proteins which interact with the carboxy terminal of GABA_BR1. Screening of a human brain cDNA library revealed GABA_BR2 as the major hit. GABA_BR1 and GABA_BR2 formed a tightly coupled heterodimer via an interaction of coiled-coil domains in the carboxy-termini. Coiled-coil domains are present in a wide variety of proteins and are known to mediate protein–protein interactions. Further experiments demonstrated that the interaction between GABA_BR1 and GABA_BR2 was specific and that neither receptor formed homodimers. The existence of GABA_B heterodimers in neurons was confirmed in immunoprecipitation experiments. In these experiments antibodies raised against GABA_BR2 efficiently co-precipitated the GABA_BR1 proteins from cortical membranes. Conversely, antibodies which recognize GABA_BR1 co-precipitated the GABA_BR2 receptor. Thus, native GABA_B receptors appear to be heterodimers composed of GABA_BR1 and GABA_BR2 which interact at their carboxy termini in a stoichiometry of 1 : 1.

The ability of GABA_BR2 to couple to GABA_BR1 fulfils several functions which allows the heterodimeric receptor to exhibit properties similar to those of the native receptor, further confirming the heteromeric nature of the GABA_B receptor. First, as with native GABA_B receptors, the heterodimer is functional and displays robust coupling to a variety of effector systems, including inhibition of adenylyl cyclase, inhibition of calcium current and activation of a potassium conductance. Second, GABA_BR2 acts as a translocator for GABA_BR1 by shepherding the receptor to the cell membrane. Finally, the agonist affinity of the heterodimer is similar to that of native GABA$_B$ receptors. In contrast, antagonist affinity of the heterodimer is unchanged compared with that of GABA$_B$R1. Interestingly, since GABA$_B$ receptor antagonists do not bind to GABA$_B$R2, their ability to inhibit the heterodimer suggests that the ligand-binding site on GABA$_B$R1 is critical for activation of the heterodimer.

GABA$_B$ receptors are the first functional heterodimers to be identified within the metabotropic class. Only among the ionotropic receptors have heterodimers been previously recognized (i.e. GABA$_A$ receptors). Other members of the family-3 GPCRs, including mGluR1–5 and the Ca^{2+}-sensing receptor have previously been reported to form homodimers. As opposed to the GABA$_B$ receptor, dimer formation for these receptors has been shown to be caused by the disulphide interaction of cysteine residues in the extracellular N-terminal domain. These cysteine residues are absent in the GABA$_B$ receptor, which dimerizes through an interaction at the carboxy-terminus. That such closely related receptors have evolved different mechanisms of dimerization suggests that dimerization is important for this class of receptors.

13.2.3 GABA$_B$ receptors are located throughout the brain at both presynaptic and postsynaptic sites

GABA$_B$ receptors can be found in most regions of the brain. In the majority of these areas the number of GABA$_B$ receptors is either less than or equal to the number of GABA$_A$ receptors. However, there are a few brain regions, such as the brainstem and certain thalamic nuclei, where GABA$_B$ receptors can account for up to 90% of the total GABA-binding sites. Autoradiography or antibody labelling of GABA$_B$R1 and GABA$_B$R2 suggests that these subunits are similarly distributed; however there are some brain regions, such as the caudate putamen, where GABA$_B$R1 is present but GABA$_B$R2 appears to be absent. The brain regions possessing the highest density of GABA$_B$ receptors are the thalamic nuclei, the molecular layer of the cerebellum, the cerebral cortex and the interpeduncular nucleus. GABA$_B$ receptors are also found in high density in laminae II and III of the spinal cord.

Electrophysiological studies have suggested for many years that GABA$_B$ receptors are located extrasynaptically. However, this may not always be the case. For example, immunogold electron microscopic studies have revealed that in the cerebellum GABA$_B$ receptors are enriched in synapses, whereas in thalamic nuclei GABA$_B$ receptors are found in extrasynaptic membrane, having no enrichment in synapses.

Both electrophysiological recordings and immunogold electron microscopic techniques have been used to demonstrate that at a subcellular level GABA$_B$ receptors are located on both presynaptic terminals, where they modulate the release of a variety of different neurotransmitters, as well as on postsynaptic membrane, where they produce postsynaptic inhibition. *In situ* hybridization techniques have suggested a differential localization of GABA$_B$R1 splice variants to pre- and postsynaptic sites. These studies have suggested that GABA$_B$R1a is more closely associated with presynaptic receptors, whereas GABA$_B$R1b may participate in the formation of postsynaptic GABA$_B$ receptors. The role of presynaptic and postsynaptic GABA$_B$ receptors is discussed in greater detail in Section 13.4.

13.2.4 Summary

The GABA$_B$ receptor was characterized pharmacologically almost 20 years ago, but it was not until recently that the first GABA$_B$ receptor subunit, GABA$_B$R1, was cloned. Whereas GABA$_B$R1 showed some of the expected properties of native GABA$_B$ receptors, it was not transported to the cell membrane surface and therefore was largely nonfunctional. The inability of GABA$_B$R1 to faithfully reproduce the properties of the native receptor led to the continued search for GABA$_B$ receptors. This search ended with the discovery of a second GABA$_B$ receptor gene, GABA$_B$R2. It was found that GABA$_B$R2 must heterodimerize with GABA$_B$R1 to form a functional receptor. Although receptor homodimers have previously been described for GPCRs, the GABA$_B$ receptor represents the first example of a heterodimeric GPCR. The functional importance of this heterodimerization process is under study.

13.3 GABA$_B$ receptors are G-protein-coupled to a variety of different effector mechanisms

GABA$_B$ receptors have the potential to produce a variety of different neuronal responses because they are coupled to several intracellular effectors (**Figure 13.3**). These different effectors enable GABA, acting through GABA$_B$ receptors, to have a broader range of effects than it could by acting on GABA$_A$ receptors alone. The primary actions of GABA$_B$ receptor activation include modulation of adenylyl cyclase activity, inhibition of voltage-dependent calcium channels, and activation of inwardly rectifying potassium channels. GABA$_B$ receptors have also been reported to alter both inositol triphosphate synthesis and phospholipase A$_2$ activity. However, few studies have addressed these latter two effects and so they will not be discussed in this chapter. Instead, we will focus on the effector systems through which GABA$_B$ receptors mediate the majority of their known actions. GABA$_B$ receptors are coupled to each of these effectors through inhibitory G proteins. Therefore, the evidence linking GABA$_B$ receptors to G proteins is looked at first, and then the different cellular actions mediated by GABA$_B$ receptors.

13.3.1 GABA$_B$ receptors are coupled to inhibitory G proteins

Guanyl nucleotide-binding proteins (G proteins) carry signals from activated membrane receptors to effector enzymes and channels. These molecules enable a single receptor to be functionally connected to a variety of different effector mechanisms in a single cell or to different effectors in different cells. A number of different G proteins have been identified and these can be divided into several subfamilies, including G_s, G_i, G_q and G_{12}/G_{13}. The G_i protein subfamily contains at least nine members, including G_{i1}, G_{i2}, G_{i3}, G_{oA}, G_{oB}, G_{oC} and G_z. Members of the G_i and G_o protein class contain sites susceptible to modification by pertussis toxin (PTX) and are therefore expected to mediate PTX-sensitive processes. G_s, G_i and G_o proteins have opposing effects on adenylyl cyclase, with G_s protein stimulating and G_i and G_o protein inhibiting the accumulation of cAMP.

All G proteins are composed of three subunits, termed α, β and γ. Whereas it was thought for many years that the α-subunit alone was able to stimulate effector systems, it has now become apparent that under many circumstances it is the βγ-subunit which carries the signal. The pathway by which G proteins carry a signal to an effector begins when agonist, in this case GABA or baclofen, binds to the low-affinity conformation of the GABA$_B$ receptor. This causes the receptor to undergo a conformational change which enhances the binding of the G protein. G protein binding, in turn, increases the affinity of the receptor for agonist. Binding of G protein to the receptor catalyses the exchange of GDP for GTP on the α-subunit of the G protein. This promotes the dissociation of the G protein from the receptor, causing the receptor to convert back to its low-affinity conformation. The G protein further dissociates into its α- and βγ-subunits which are now free to act independently on a variety of effector systems. The signal ends when endogenous GTPase in the α-subunit converts the GTP back to GDP. This promotes dissociation of the α-subunit from the effector and reassociation with the βγ-subunit. Binding of the α-subunit inhibits the interaction of the βγ-subunit with its effectors.

Coupling of GABA$_B$ receptors and G proteins was originally deduced from binding studies of ^{3}H-GABA and ^{3}H-baclofen to crude synaptic membranes prepared using whole rat brain. In these experiments the addition of guanyl nucleotides, such as GTP, did not effect the binding of ^{3}H-GABA to GABA$_A$ receptors, but potently inhibited GABA$_B$ receptor binding (**Figure 13.4**). This effect was concentration-dependent and was not mimicked by adenosine 5′-triphosphate (ATP), indicating that

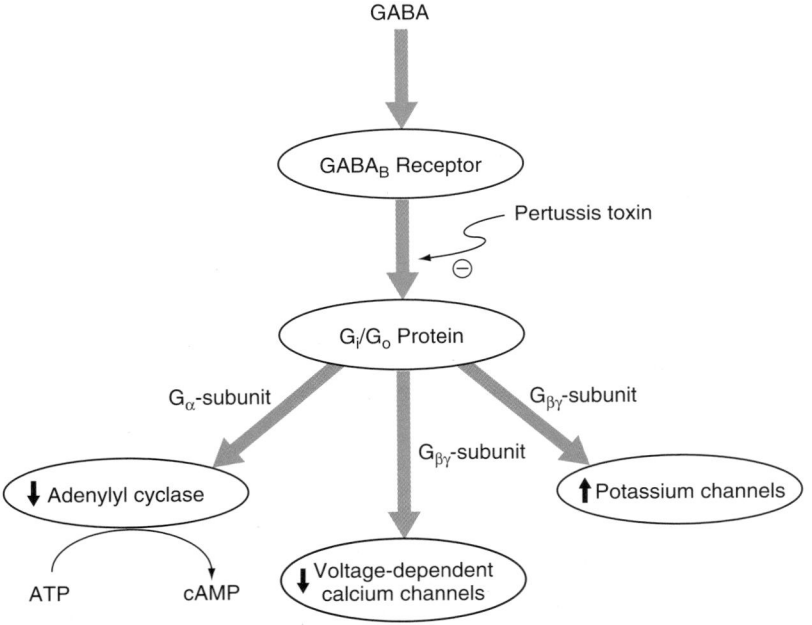

Figure 13.3 Schematic depicting the major effector systems to which GABA$_B$ receptors are coupled.

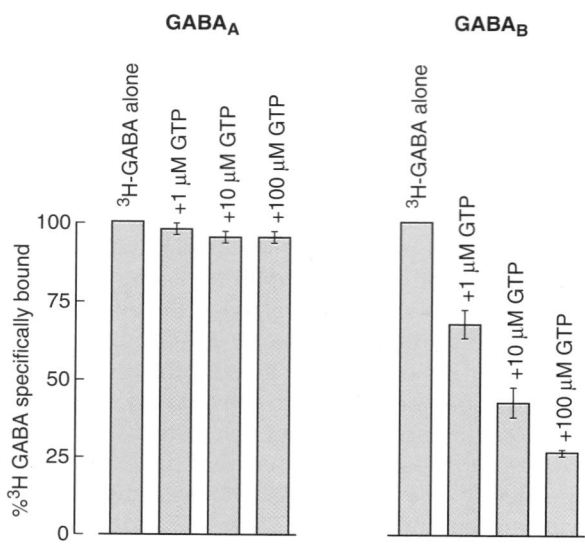

Figure 13.4 The effect of GTP on ³H-GABA binding to GABA_A and GABA_B receptors.

³H-GABA binding to crude synaptic membranes from whole rat brain was measured in the presence of either isoguvacine or baclofen to saturate GABA_A and GABA_B receptors, respectively. The addition of increasing concentration of GTP had no effect on GABA_A receptor binding but produced a concentration dependent inhibition of GABA_B receptor binding. From Hill DR, Bowery NG, Hudson AL (1984) Inhibition of GABA_B receptor binding by guanyl nucleotides, *J. Neurochem.* **42**, 652–657, with permission.

it was specific for guanyl nucleotides. The inhibition of ligand binding produced by GTP was caused by a decrease in GABA_B receptor affinity and not a decrease in the number of available GABA_B receptors. It was concluded that the addition of GTP promoted the dissociation of the G protein from the receptor, causing the receptor to revert to its low-affinity conformation. Thus, GABA_B receptors appeared to couple to G proteins.

A large number of studies have examined the molecular determinants of receptor-G protein coupling selectivity. For most GPCRs the third intracellular loop of the receptor plays a critical role in the selectivity of the interaction with G proteins. However, for family-3 GPCRs, such as the mGluRs, this function appears to be served by the second intracellular loop. Structural homology between mGluR and GABA_B receptors suggests that the second intracellular loop plays a similar role for GABA_B receptors as well. Interestingly, models of GPCR coupling to G proteins have been based on the assumption of a monomeric form of the GPCR. The ability of GABA_B receptors to heterodimerize raises a number of important questions about how this dimeric receptor interacts with G proteins and whether the receptor can interact with more than one G protein or more than one type of G protein simultaneously. These questions are currently under study.

The identity of the G proteins coupled to GABA_B receptors was established through two different experiments. First, it was observed that inhibition of GABA_B receptor binding by GTP was blocked by pertussis toxin. This demonstrated that GABA_B receptors are functionally coupled to the inhibitory G proteins, G_i and/or G_o. This finding was further confirmed using cloned heteromeric GABA_B receptors (GABA_BR1/GABA_BR2) expressed with chimeric G_q proteins in human embryonic kidney cells (HEK 293). Wildtype G_q protein activates phospholipase C (PLC). Ordinarily GABA_B receptors do not stimulate PLC activity, indicating that they do not couple to G_q protein. PLC activity produced by GABA_B receptor activation was then measured following the addition of chimeric G_q proteins in which the five carboxy-terminal residues of the α-subunit had been exchanged for those of either G_i, G_o or G_z protein. The five carboxy-terminal residues of the G protein α-subunit are critical for coupling of G proteins to receptors. Only those chimeric G_q proteins containing the coupling sites of G_i or G_o protein were able to activate PLC, indicating that only G_i and G_o proteins interact with the GABA_B receptor.

13.3.2 GABA_B receptors regulate the activity of adenylyl cyclase

Adenylyl cyclase converts ATP to cyclic AMP. Cyclic AMP, in turn, activates several different target molecules, such as cyclic AMP-dependent protein kinase, to regulate cellular functions including gene transcription, cellular metabolism and synaptic plasticity. Nine isoforms of adenylyl cyclase (types I to IX) have so far been identified. This multiplicity of isoforms enables cells to show a range of responses to regulatory factors, such as calcium, protein kinase C (PKC), and the α- and βγ-subunits of G proteins.

GABA_B receptors are negatively coupled to adenylyl cyclase through inhibitory G proteins

The ability of GABA_B receptors to couple to inhibitory G_i/G_o proteins suggested that GABA_B receptor activation would inhibit adenylyl cyclase activity. To test this hypothesis the effect of GABA_B receptor activation on adenylyl cyclase activity was measured by the enzymatic conversion of [α-³²P]ATP to cyclic [³²P]AMP in crude synaptosomal preparations from a variety of regions of the rat brain. Application of baclofen or GABA caused a decrease in cAMP levels, reflecting a reduction in basal adenylyl cyclase activity (**Figure 13.5a**). This effect was blocked by the GABA_B receptor antagonist CGP 35348, indicating that it was mediated

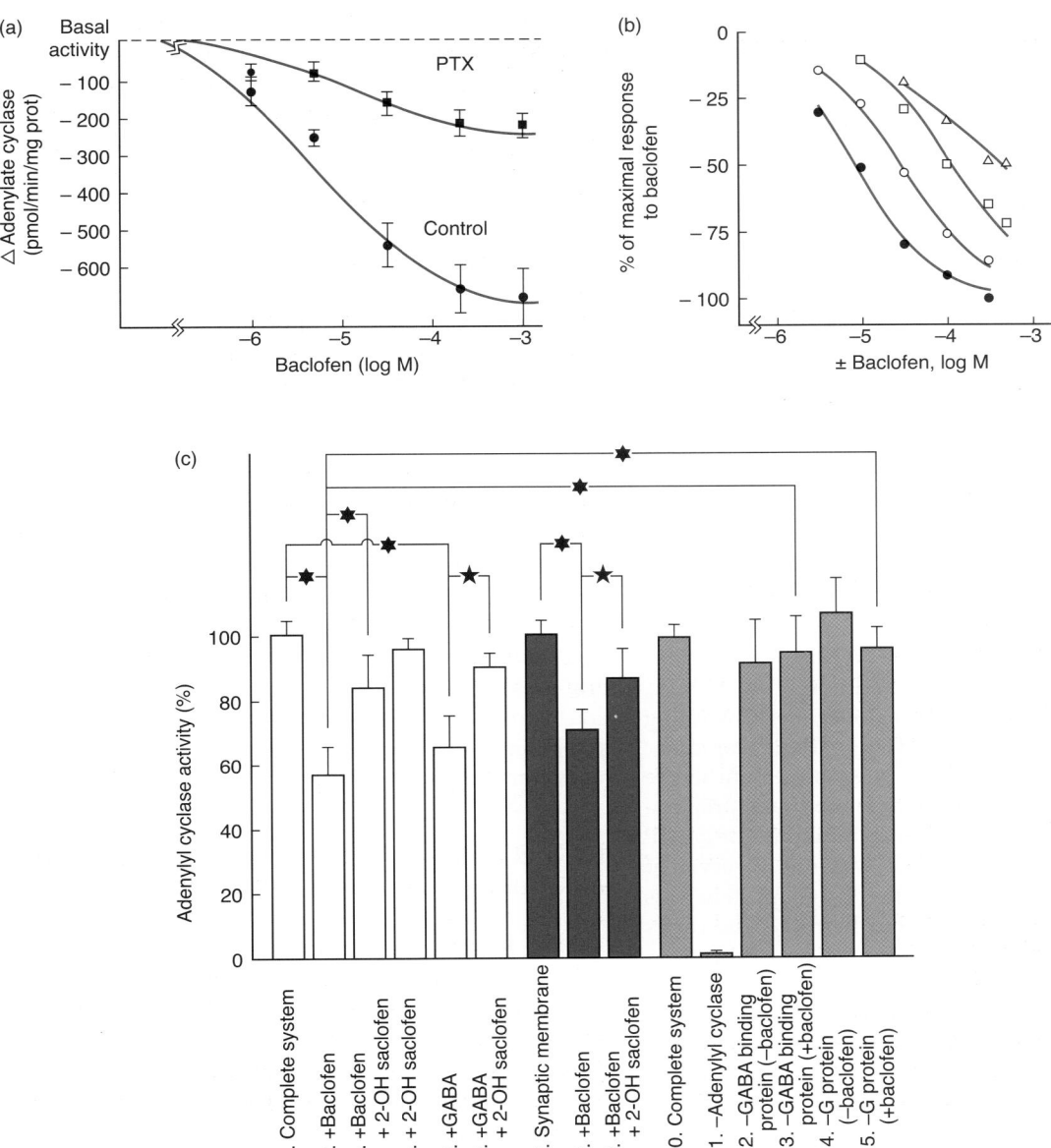

Figure 13.5 GABA$_B$ receptors couple to adenylyl cyclase through inhibitory G proteins.
(a) Adenylyl cyclase activity in membranes of cerebellar granule cells was measured by the conversion of [α-^{32}P]ATP to [^{32}P]AMP. In control preparations baclofen decreased the activity of adenylyl cyclase in a concentration-dependent manner (filled circles). Treatment of the membranes with pertussis toxin (PTX) antagonized the effect of baclofen on adenylyl cyclase activity (filled squares). **(b)** The inhibition of adenylyl cyclase activity by baclofen was antagonized in a concentration-specific manner by the GABA$_B$ receptor antagonist, CGP 35348. The inhibition produced by increasing concentrations of baclofen alone (filled circles) was compared with that observed in the presence of baclofen plus either 0.6 mm (open circles), 1.5 mm (open squares) or 5 mm (open triangles) of CGP 35348. **(c)** The effect of baclofen and GABA on adenylyl cyclase activity measured in reconstituted membranes (open bars), synaptic membranes (dark bars) and partially reconstituted membranes (light bars). Note that the removal of the G protein from the reconstituted system (no. 15) blocked the inhibitory effect of baclofen (no. 2). See text for details. Significant differences are indicated by an asterisk (∗) signifying $P < 0.05$ or a star (★) signifying $P < 0.01$. Part (a) from Xu J, Wojcik WJ (1986) Gamma aminobutyric acid B receptor-mediated inhibition of adenylate cyclase in cultured cerebellar granule cells: blockade by islet-activating protein, *J. Pharmacol. Exp. Ther.* **239**, 568–573, with permission. Part (b) adapted from Holopainen I, Rau C, Wojcik WJ (1992) Proposed antagonists at GABA$_B$ receptors that inhibit adenylyl cyclase in cerebellar granule cell cultures of rat, *Eur. J. Pharmacol. Mol. Pharmacol.* **227**, 225–228, with permission. Part (c) from Nakayasu H, Nishikawa M, Mizutani H *et al.* (1993) Immunoaffinity purification and characterization of γ-aminobutyric acid receptor from bovine cerebral cortex, *J. Biol. Chem.* **268**, 8658–8664, with permission.

by GABA$_B$ receptors (**Figure 13.5b**). Application of PTX dramatically reduced the effect of baclofen on adenylyl cyclase. Since PTX selectively inactivates G$_i$/G$_o$ proteins, these results demonstrate that GABA$_B$ receptors are negatively coupled to adenylyl cyclase through one or both of these inhibitory G proteins.

Reconstitution experiments have also been used to demonstrate that GABA$_B$ receptors are negatively coupled to adenylyl cyclase through inhibitory G proteins. Purified phospholipids were combined with purified GABA$_B$ receptor, partially purified G$_i$/G$_o$ protein, partially purified adenylyl cyclase and GTP to form a reconstituted membrane preparation. This preparation was then incubated with forskolin, to activate the adenylyl cyclase, and either baclofen or GABA, to activate the GABA$_B$ receptors. In theory, during this incubation, the baclofen or GABA should bind to the GABA$_B$ receptor, causing a decrease in the formation of cAMP by adenylyl cyclase as compared with the level of cAMP formation in the absence of baclofen or GABA. This was exactly what happened (**Figure 13.5c**). Furthermore, the inhibitory effect of baclofen and GABA on adenylyl cyclase was antagonized by the addition of the GABA$_B$ receptor antagonist, 2-hydroxysaclofen, demonstrating that the inhibition was mediated by GABA$_B$ receptors.

To demonstrate the necessity of each element in the preparation, partially reconstituted membrane preparations were prepared. As predicted, inhibition of cAMP formation by baclofen or GABA was not observed if either the GABA$_B$ receptor or the G$_i$/G$_o$ protein was omitted from the preparation. Furthermore, the omission of adenylyl cyclase resulted in the almost complete absence of cAMP formation. The inability of GABA$_B$ receptors to inhibit cAMP formation in the absence of G$_i$/G$_o$ protein further confirms that GABA$_B$ receptors can negatively couple to adenylyl cyclase through either or both of these G proteins.

GABA$_B$ receptors facilitate neurotransmitter-mediated activation of adenylyl cyclase

In contrast to its direct inhibition of adenylyl cyclase through G$_i$/G$_o$ proteins, GABA$_B$ receptor activation can also have another seemingly opposite effect on cAMP accumulation. When adenylyl cyclase is stimulated to produce cAMP by a G$_s$ protein-coupled receptor, GABA$_B$ receptor activation will enhance this increase in cAMP accumulation. For example, addition of baclofen enhances by two to three fold the increase in cAMP accumulation produced by norepinephrine (β receptors), adenosine (A2 receptors) or vasoactive intestinal peptide (VIP) receptors (**Figure 13.6**). This effect is contrary to the inhibition of adenylyl cyclase discussed above.

The mechanism of this effect lies in the ability of the βγ-subunit from the G$_i$/G$_o$ protein, liberated by the activation of GABA$_B$ receptors, to synergize the interaction of the α$_s$-subunit of the G$_s$ protein with certain types of adenylyl cyclase. For example, the activation of adenylyl cyclase type II by the α$_s$-subunit is markedly potentiated by the subsequent binding of βγ-subunits. These βγ-subunits can come from either G$_s$ or G$_i$/G$_o$ proteins. In this way adenylyl cyclase type II can act as a molecular 'coincidence detector' by responding only minimally to activation by a single signal but synergistically to the coincident arrival of dual signals through separate pathways.

According to this mechanism, G protein α- and βγ-subunits liberated by the activation of GABA$_B$ receptors could produce opposing effects. The α$_i$/α$_o$ subunits could directly inhibit one type of adenylyl cyclase while the βγ-subunits could synergize the stimulation of adenylyl cyclase type II by α$_s$-subunit. This α$_s$-subunit was generated by the interaction of another neurotransmitter with a G$_s$-coupled receptor. Depending upon the overall balance between the inhibitory and stimulatory effect of these two processes on adenylyl cyclase activity, this could result in a net increase in cAMP accumulation. Thus, GABA$_B$ receptor activation has the potential to regulate the activity of a variety of G$_s$ protein-coupled neurotransmitters.

13.3.3 GABA$_B$ receptor activation inhibits voltage-dependent calcium channels

GABA$_B$ receptors are negatively coupled to voltage-dependent calcium channels. Voltage-dependent calcium channels are one of the major elements controlling the entry of calcium into neurons. These channels are activated by depolarization of the neuronal membrane. Electrophysiological and pharmacological studies distinguish at least six classes of calcium channels, designated types L, N, P, Q, R and T. Based on the level of depolarization required for activation, these channels have been divided into two groups, low-voltage activated (LVA; T-type) and high-voltage activated (HVA; L, N, P, Q and R-type). These different classes of calcium channels play a variety of roles in neuronal function. For example, HVA N-type and P/Q-type channels have been implicated in the control of neurotransmitter release, whereas HVA L-type channels participate in action potential generation and signal transduction. LVA T-type channels are thought to control neuronal oscillatory activity, including spontaneous and repetitive burst firing. By inhibiting calcium entry through these channels, GABA$_B$ receptors have the potential to modulate a variety of neuronal functions, perhaps the most significant of which is the ability to regulate neurotransmitter release.

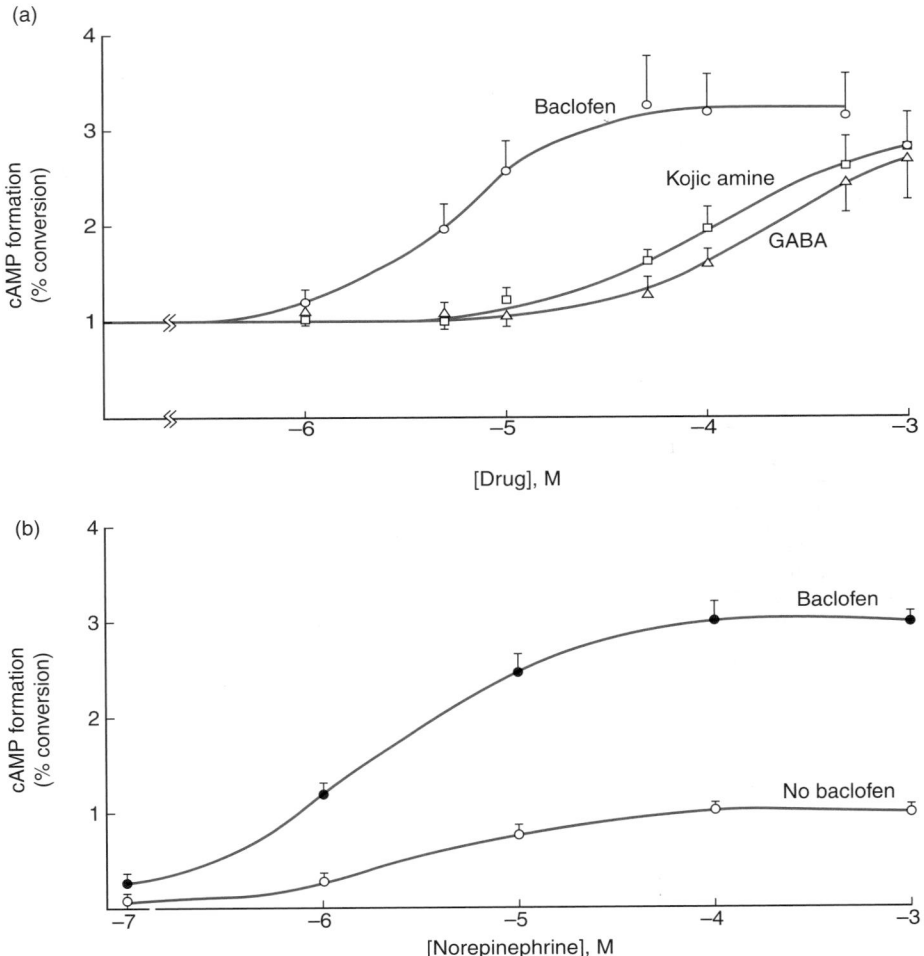

Figure 13.6 The effect of GABA_B receptor activation on norepinephrine stimulated cAMP accumulation.
(a) The effect of different GABA_B receptor agonists on the cAMP accumulation produced by 100 μM of norepinephrine in rat brain cerebellar slices. The GABA_B agonists, baclofen (open circles), kojic amine (open squares) and GABA (open triangles) were applied at increasing concentrations in the presence of norepinephrine. All these GABA_B agonists enhanced cAMP formation produced by the norepinephrine. (b) Baclofen (100 μM) potentiates the cAMP formation induced by increasing concentrations of norepinephrine. The effect of norepinephrine alone (open circles) and norepinephrine plus baclofen (filled circles) is shown. From Karbon EW, Duman RS, Enna SJ (1984) GABA_B receptors and norepinephrine-stimulated cAMP production in rat brain cortex, *Brain Res.* **306**, 327–332, with permission.

Pioneering experiments

Inhibition of calcium currents by GABA_B receptor activation was first observed in electrophysiological recordings made from neurons in the dorsal root ganglion (DRG). In this preparation both GABA and baclofen were found to decrease the calcium-dependent plateau phase of the action potential (**Figure 13.7**). The effect of baclofen was stereospecific with (–)baclofen being the active isomer, and was blocked by the GABA_B antagonist, phaclofen, indicating that the effect was mediated by GABA_B receptors.

To confirm that GABA_B receptor activation directly inhibited calcium currents, the effect of baclofen on phar-

macologically isolated calcium currents in voltage-clamped DRG neurons was examined. The calcium current was pharmacologically isolated by application of blockers of sodium (tetrodotoxin) and potassium (cesium, tetraethylammonium) currents. Under these conditions a depolarizing voltage step from a holding potential of –80 mV evokes a sustained inward calcium current. Baclofen reversibly reduces the amplitude of this current (**Figures 13.7b and c**). In contrast, in the same preparation baclofen had no effect on the pharmacologically isolated voltage-activated potassium current nor did it affect the holding current, suggesting no effect on the resting potassium conductance. This finding indicates that GABA_B receptor activation depresses voltage-dependent calcium

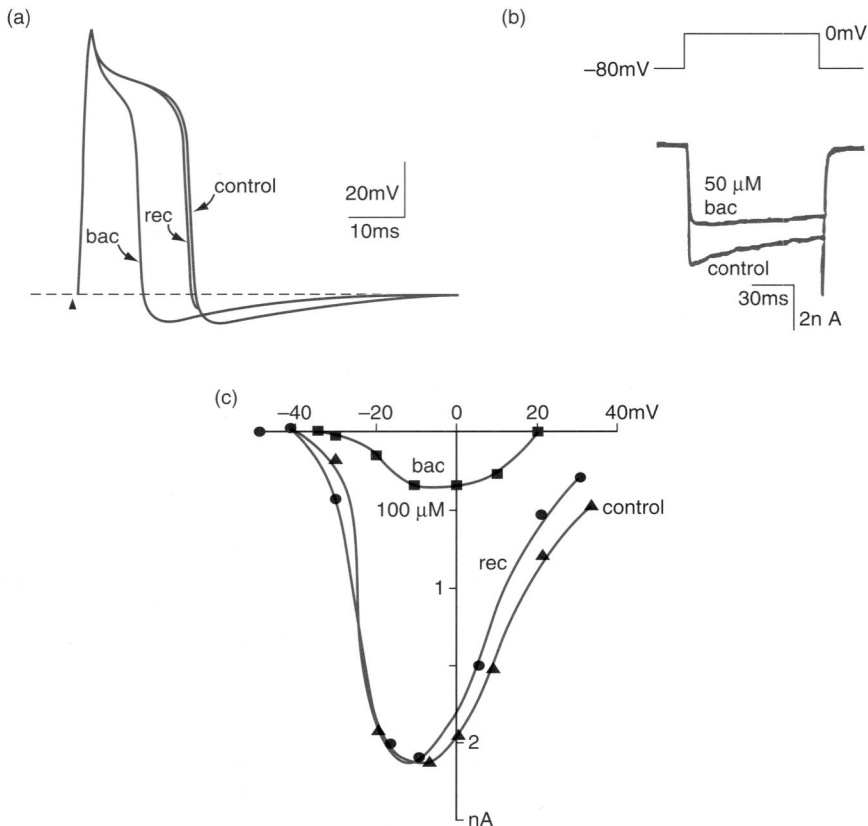

Figure 13.7 Baclofen suppresses voltage-dependent calcium currents in DRG neurons.
(a) The effect of baclofen on the action potential in a DRG neuron. Baclofen (100 µM; bac) reversibly depressed the calcium-dependent plateau phase of the action potential compared to control or wash (rec). **(b)** In the same preparation, 50 µM of baclofen depressed the pharmacologically isolated calcium current (bottom). This current was evoked by a depolarizing voltage step from –80 mV to 0 mV (top). See text for details. **(c)** The current–voltage relationship for the voltage-dependent calcium current in a DRG neurons is shown in control, in 100 µM of baclofen (bac) and after 5 minutes of wash (rec). The current–voltage curve represents the amplitude of the calcium current evoked by a voltage step from the holding potential of –80 mV to a variety of test potentials. Baclofen markedly inhibited the calcium current. From Dolphin AC, Huston E, Scott RH (1990) GABA$_B$-mediated inhibition of calcium currents: a possible role in presynaptic inhibition. In: Bowery NG, Bittiger H, Olpe H-R (eds) *GABA$_B$ Receptors in Mammalian Function*, Chichester: John Wiley, with permission.

currents in DRG neurons. Similar studies have subsequently confirmed that GABA$_B$ receptor activation can inhibit voltage-dependent calcium currents in many different types of both peripheral and central neurons.

A recent study has addressed the question of whether heterodimerization of GABA$_B$ receptors is required for the coupling of these receptors to calcium channels in neurons. In this study GABA$_B$ expression constructs were injected into the nuclei of superior cervical ganglion (SCG) neurons, resulting in the expression of GABA$_B$ receptor protein. Baclofen had no effect on calcium currents in uninjected SCG neurons. However, the expression of heterodimeric GABA$_B$ receptors composed of GABA$_B$R1a or GABA$_B$R1b plus GABA$_B$R2 resulted in a marked baclofen-mediated inhibition of calcium-channel currents in these cells. The actions of baclofen

were blocked by the selective GABA$_B$ receptor antagonist CGP 62349, indicating that the effect was mediated by GABA$_B$ receptors. Injection of an antisense construct to block GABA$_B$R1 expression markedly decreased GABA$_B$R1 protein levels as well as the inhibitory effects of baclofen on calcium currents. These results suggest that heterodimeric assemblies of GABA$_B$R1 and GABA$_B$R2 are necessary for GABA$_B$ receptor-mediated inhibition of calcium-channel currents.

GABA$_B$ receptors inhibit a variety of voltage-gated calcium channels

The voltage-dependent calcium current evoked in a given cell is typically produced by the activation of several different calcium-channel types. Thus, partial suppression of this current by GABA$_B$ receptor activation could be produced by a partial inhibition of several different channel types or the complete inhibition of only a single type. Because of the different physiological functions of the various voltage-dependent calcium channels, it is important to determine the type(s) of calcium channel inhibited by GABA$_B$ receptors. This can be accomplished through the use of calcium-channel antagonists that are specific for different calcium channels. The ability of a selective antagonist to occlude further inhibition of a calcium current by baclofen indicates that the antagonist and baclofen are acting on the same subset of channels. Alternately, specific calcium-channel antagonists can be used to pharmacologically isolate a single type of calcium current and the effect of GABA$_B$ receptor activation assessed. Finally, kinetic analysis of the calcium current inhibited by GABA$_B$ receptors can be used to determine the electrophysiological characteristics of the inhibited current, which can then be compared with the known properties of identified calcium channels.

Using these techniques, GABA$_B$ receptors have been shown to inhibit all types of calcium channels (**Figure 13.8**). Inhibition of N-type and P/Q-type calcium channels by GABA$_B$ receptors is the most common and has been seen in many different cell types. In comparison, GABA$_B$ receptor-mediated inhibition of L-type channels is dependent upon the cell type. For example, it is observed in cerebellar granule neurons and hippocampal pyramidal neurons, but not in cerebellar Purkinje neurons, spinal cord neurons or thalamocortical neurons. Similarly, GABA$_B$ receptor-mediated inhibition of T-type calcium channels is also neuron-dependent. Baclofen suppresses current through these channels in DRG neurons and interneurons in the *stratum lacunosum moleculare* of the hippocampus, but not in thalamocortical neurons or pyramidal neurons of the hippocampus. Thus, GABA$_B$ receptor activation has the potential to inhibit a variety of different voltage-dependent calcium channels, suggesting that through this pathway GABA$_B$ receptors could have profound effects on neuronal function.

Inhibition of calcium channels is dependent upon G$_o$ proteins

Several lines of evidence have been used to demonstrate the involvement of G proteins in the inhibition of calcium channels by GABA$_B$ receptors (**Figure 13.9**).

First, simply omitting GTP from the internal pipette solution during whole-cell recording gradually blocked the effect of baclofen on the calcium current. This occurs because, in the absence of a replacement supply, GTP

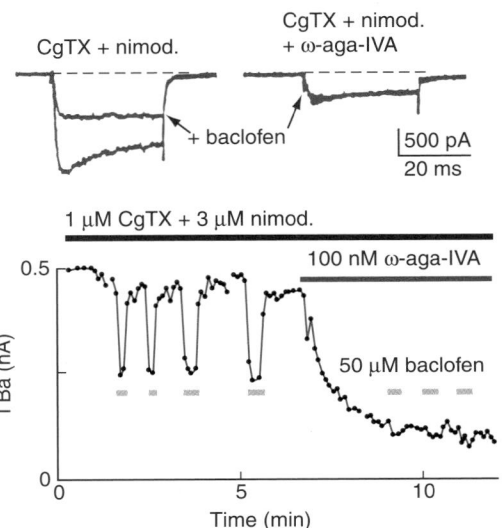

Figure 13.8 Baclofen suppresses the P-type calcium current in cerebellar Purkinje neurons.

In the presence of 1 μM of ω-conotoxin (CgTX) and 3 μM of nimodipine (nimod.) to block N-type and L-type calcium channels, a voltage step from –80 mV to +10 mV elicits an inward calcium current (top left). This current is partially inhibited by 50 μM of baclofen. Application of the P-type calcium-channel antagonist ω-agatoxin-IVA (ω-aga-IVA; 100 μM) partially blocks the current and occludes any further inhibition by baclofen (top right). The time course of the peak calcium-channel current amplitude throughout the experiment is shown below. CgTX and nimod are applied throughout the experiment (black bar), ω-aga-IVA is applied for the period of time indicated by the green bar. Note that ω-aga-IVA suppressed the calcium current and completely occluded any further inhibition by baclofen, demonstrating that baclofen was acting on the P-type calcium current. In this experiment barium was exchanged for calcium so the currents that were measured represent barium flux through calcium channels. From Mintz IM, Bean BP (1993) GABA$_B$ receptor inhibition of P-type Ca^{2+} channels in central neurons, *Neuron* **10**, 889–898, with permission.

slowly washes out of the cell during the experiment, thereby inactivating G proteins. Alternately, loading the cell with guanosine 5′-O-(2-thiodiphosphate) (GDP-β-S), a GDP analogue that inhibits the binding of GTP to G proteins, antagonized the effect of baclofen on calcium currents. Conversely, the effect of baclofen was enhanced when cells were loaded with guanosine 5′-O-(3-thiotriphosphate) (GTP-γ-S), a non-hydrolysable GTP analogue that irreversibly activates G proteins. These findings support a role for G proteins in the coupling of GABA$_B$ receptors to calcium channels.

That GABA$_B$ receptors negatively couple to calcium channels through G proteins was confirmed by the observation that PTX blocks the inhibitory effect of baclofen on calcium channels. Furthermore, this result

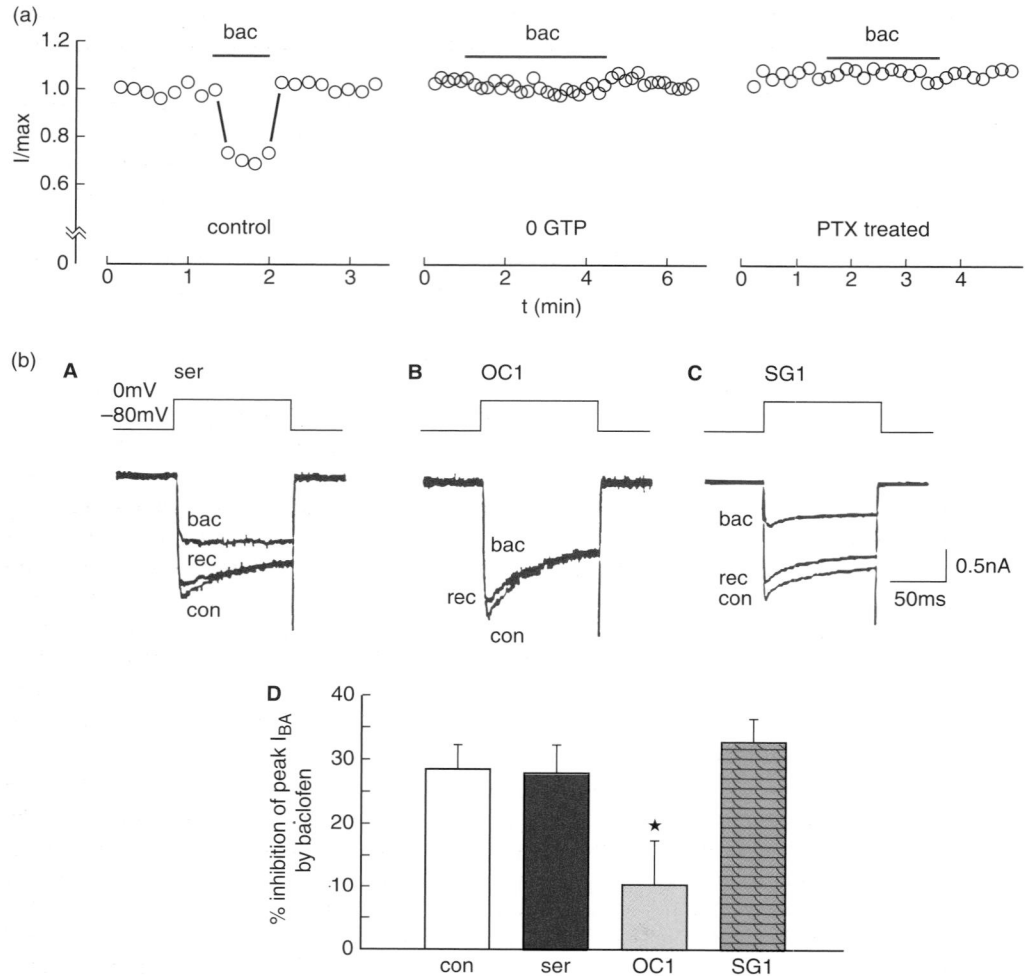

Figure 13.9 GABA$_B$ receptors are coupled to calcium channels through G$_o$ protein.
(a) Calcium currents in cerebellar granule cells are evoked by stepping from a holding voltage of –80 mV to a test voltage of +10 mV. Current was expressed as a percentage of the maximal current in the cell at the beginning of the experiment. Bath application of baclofen (100 μM; baclo) for the time indicated by the bar reduced the size of the calcium current (left). This inhibition was antagonized by removal of GTP from the internal pipette solution (centre) or by pretreatment of the neurons 12–16 h earlier with pertussis toxin (PTX; right). These observations indicate that GABA$_B$ receptors mediate inhibition of calcium channels through inhibitory G proteins. **(b)** The effect of anti-G protein antibodies on the inhibition of the calcium current by baclofen in dorsal root ganglion neurons. Calcium currents were evoked by a voltage step from –80 mV to 0 mV as shown (top records in (a)–(c)). A: In the presence of non-immune serum (ser), 50 μM of baclofen (bac) markedly inhibited the calcium current from its control (con) level. This effect was reversible upon wash-out (rec) of the baclofen. B: In the presence of a 1:50 dilution of anti-G$_o$ antibodies (OC1) targeted to the C-terminal peptide of α$_o$ protein, the effect of baclofen on the calcium current was antagonized. C: At the same dilution, the anti-G$_i$ protein antibodies (SG1) had no effect on the inhibition of the calcium current produced by baclofen. D: Bar chart showing the average maximal inhibition of the calcium current produced by baclofen in cells treated with either no serum (con; $n = 18$), serum with no antibodies (ser; $n = 15$), serum with anti-G$_o$ antibodies (OC1; $n = 4$) or serum with anti-G$_i$ antibodies (SG1; $n = 20$). Part (a) from Amico C, Marchetti C, Nobile M, Usai C (1995) Pharmacological types of calcium channels and their modulation by baclofen in cerebellar granules, *J. Neurosci.* **15**, 2839–2848, with permission. Part (b) from Menon-Johansson AS, Berrow N, Dolphin AC (1993) G$_o$ transduces GABA$_B$-receptor modulation of N-type calcium channels in cultured dorsal root ganglion neurons, *Pflügers Arch.* **425**, 335–343, with permission.

indicates that GABA$_B$ receptors couple to calcium channels through inhibitory G$_i$/G$_o$ proteins. The specific identity of the inhibitory G protein was established through several lines of investigation.

First, cultured DRG neurons, which express N-type calcium channels, were treated with anti-G$_o$ or anti-G$_i$ antibodies, raised against the C-terminal decapeptide of the α$_o$ and α$_i$-subunit of the G$_o$ and G$_i$ protein, respectively (**Figure 13.9b**). The hypothesis was that by binding to the G protein in the DRG neuron one or both of these antibodies would prevent the association of that G protein with the GABA$_B$ receptor and thereby prevent inhibition of N-type calcium channels by baclofen. The amount of inhibition of the N-type calcium current produced by baclofen was evaluated for each group of antibody-treated cells and compared with the level of baclofen-induced inhibition in untreated cells. Inhibition of the N-type calcium current produced by baclofen was reduced only in the group of neurons treated with the anti-G$_o$ antibodies, indicating that baclofen couples to N-type calcium channels through a G$_o$ protein.

Second, the ability of baclofen to inhibit calcium currents in cultured DRG neurons was evaluated after antisense oligonucleotides had been used to knock down the expression of either G$_o$ or G$_i$ proteins. DRG neurons were injected with antisense oligonucleotides complementary to a unique sequence in either the α$_o$-subunit of the G$_o$ protein, the α$_i$-subunit of the G$_i$ protein or a nonsense sequence. Inhibition of calcium current by baclofen was unaffected in neurons injected with the nonsense oligonucleotide and with the oligonucleotide complementary to the α$_i$-subunit. However, baclofen-induced inhibition of the calcium current was reduced in neurons injected with the α$_o$ antisense oligonucleotide. Immunocytochemical localization of the α$_o$-subunit using a confocal microscope demonstrated the presence of this subunit in the plasma membrane of control cells as well as in cells treated with nonsense oligonucleotide and α$_i$ oligonucleotide. However, the level of this subunit was markedly reduced in neurons treated with the α$_o$ oligonucleotide, indicating that this oligonucleotide specifically reduced the expression of G$_o$ protein. Similarly, the G$_i$ protein was present in the membrane of control cells as well as in cells treated with nonsense oligonucleotide and α$_o$ oligonucleotide, but substantially reduced in cells treated with α$_i$ oligonucleotide. These findings indicate that both oligonucleotides were capable of specifically reducing the expression of the G protein for which they were targeted, but that only the reduction in G$_o$ protein resulted in a suppression of the effects of baclofen. Thus, GABA$_B$ receptors appear to couple to calcium channels through G$_o$ protein.

G$_o$ proteins inhibit calcium currents through a direct interaction of the βγ-subunit with the calcium channel

The mechanism by which GABA$_B$ receptor-activated G$_o$ proteins couple to calcium channels is also of importance. In theory, G$_o$ proteins could inhibit calcium channels by physically interacting with the channel itself or by resulting in the production of a second messenger molecule which would diffuse to and inhibit the channel. For L-type calcium channels regulation by G proteins is thought to depend upon the intermediary action of a protein phosphatase. However, the experimental evidence indicates that for N-type and P/Q-type channels a direct interaction between the G$_o$ protein and the calcium channel is most likely. In these experiments, cell-attached patches in DRG neurons were used to determine whether the inhibition of calcium currents produced by baclofen involved a diffusable second messenger. It was found that baclofen, applied outside the patch pipette, did not affect the amplitude of calcium currents in cell-attached patches. However, in the same cell baclofen applied inside the patch pipette produced clear inhibition of the calcium current, demonstrating that baclofen was able to inhibit calcium currents in these cells. The inability of baclofen, applied outside the patch pipette, to inhibit calcium channels under the patch indicates that a diffusable second messenger was not involved in the inhibition. Thus, GABA$_B$ receptor-activated G$_o$ protein appears to inhibit N and P/Q-type calcium channels through a direct interaction with the channel.

G$_o$ proteins inhibit N and P/Q-type calcium channels through a direct interaction of their βγ-subunits with the channels. This idea was originally proposed following experiments which demonstrated that in cells the overexpression or injection of βγ-subunits, but not α$_o$-subunits, mimicked the inhibition of calcium channels produced by activation of GPCRs. Whereas these studies indicated a role for βγ-subunits in the inhibition of calcium channels, they did not demonstrate that these subunits acted directly on the channel. Recently, binding studies using purified βγ dimers and recombinant Q-type calcium-channel subunits have demonstrated a direct interaction between these two proteins. Furthermore, mutational analysis has identified a region on the carboxy-terminus of the α-subunit of the Q-type calcium channel as a critical region for this interaction.

GABA$_B$ receptors inhibit calcium channels by altering their voltage dependence

It was originally proposed that GPCRs, such as GABA$_B$ receptors, which inhibit calcium channels do so by reducing the number of functional channels. However, subsequent experiments demonstrated that strong depolarization of the neuronal membrane could overcome the transmitter-mediated inhibition of the calcium current. This result cannot be explained by a mechanism which involves a reduction in the number of functional channels. Instead, it appears that receptor activation

(a)

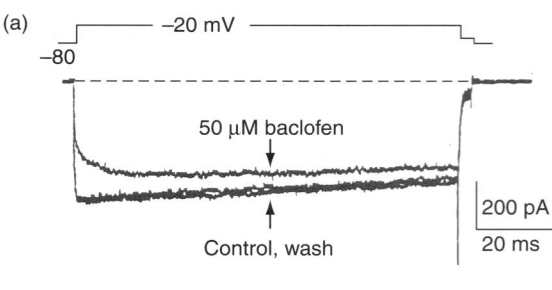

(b)

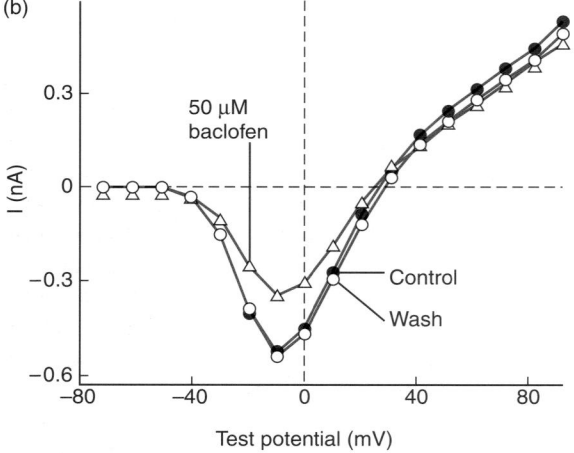

Figure 13.10 Inhibition of the calcium current by baclofen is voltage dependent.

(a) In cerebellar Purkinje neurons a voltage step from –80 mV to –20 mV (top) in the presence of 1 μM of ω-conotoxin and 3 μM of nimodipine evokes a P-type calcium current (bottom). This current is suppressed by the subsequent application of baclofen (50 μM) and recovers following wash-out of the baclofen. (b) Inhibition of P-type calcium currents by baclofen is voltage-dependent. This graph shows the amplitude of the calcium current evoked by depolarizing steps to a variety of different test potentials in control (filled circles), 50 μM of baclofen (open triangles) and after wash-out of the baclofen (open circles). The holding potential was –80 mV. Baclofen inhibited the current most effectively when it was evoked with voltage steps to potentials below +20 mV. Strong depolarizations were able to overcome the inhibition produced by baclofen. Adapted from Mintz IM, Bean BP (1993) GABA$_B$ receptor inhibition of P-type Ca^{2+} channels in central neurons, *Neuron* **10**, 889–898, with permission.

induces a large shift in the voltage dependence of channel activation. Thus, following exposure to the transmitter, almost all of the channels are still fully functional and can be opened by a strong depolarization. However, a percentage of the channels undergo a shift in voltage dependence so that they are no longer opened by small to moderate depolarizations. In practice this means that a transmitter, such as GABA, is able to inhibit the calcium current during activation by low to moderate depolarization, but the inhibitory effect of the transmitter is lost during strong depolarizations (**Figure 13.10**). In light of this, calcium channels have been proposed to exist in two states termed 'willing' and 'reluctant', to describe their ease of activation. These two states exist in equilibrium and according to the following model where $C_{willing}$ is the closed channel in the absence of transmitter, $C_{reluctant}$ is the closed channel in the presence of transmitter, and O is the open channel:

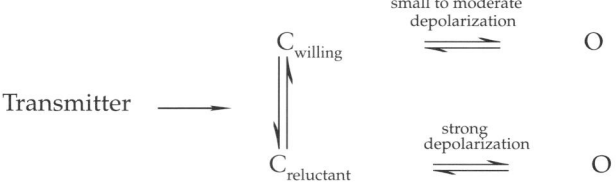

Calcium channels predominantly exist in the willing mode in the absence of transmitter and can be activated by small to moderate depolarizations. In contrast, activation of G$_o$ coupled receptors, like GABA$_B$ receptors, shifts the balance of equilibrium to favour the 'reluctant' state in which large depolarizations are required to open the channels.

13.3.4 GABA$_B$ receptors activate potassium channels

GABA$_B$ receptors activate a potassium current mediated by G protein-activated inwardly rectifying potassium (Kir) channels (previously termed GIRK channels). Through these potassium channels, GABA$_B$ receptors play a critical role in regulating neuronal excitability. Recent molecular biological dissection has shown that the DNAs encoding G-protein-coupled Kir channels constitute a family of potassium channels whose subunits contain two putative transmembrane domains and a pore-forming region. Members of this family include Kir3.1 (GIRK1), Kir3.2 (GIRK2), Kir3.3 (GIRK3), Kir3.4 (GIRK4) and Kir3.5 (GIRK5). In addition, three splice variants of Kir3.2 have been identified (Kir3.2a–c, GIRK2A–C). Kir3.1–3.3 are abundantly expressed throughout the brain with an overall similar distribution. Kir3.4 is expressed in the brain although to a much lesser extent than other Kir3.x transcripts. Kir3.5 was cloned from *Xenopus* oocytes and its mammalian homologue has not yet been reported. Expression of Kir3.x subunits revealed that Kir3.2 and Kir3.4, but not Kir3.1, can form functional homomeric channels. However, when Kir3.x subunits are co-expressed they form heteromultimers. These heteromultimers can form between any pair of Kir3.x subunits and exhibit electrophysiological properties similar to those of native channels.

Further biochemical analysis revealed that in neurons Kir3.x channels have a tetrameric structure, most likely comprised of two pairs of subunits. The identity of the Kir3.x subunits that comprise the tetramer in different brain regions has been the subject of intensive investigation. Co-immunoprecipitation studies have revealed a tight association between Kir3.1 and Kir3.2 in cerebral cortex and hippocampus. Furthermore, in mice whose Kir3.2 genes were genetically deleted, both Kir3.1 and Kir3.2 proteins disappear from the cerebral cortex. These studies indicate that in these brain regions virtually all Kir3.1 proteins are assembled with Kir3.2 subunits. However, in other brain regions, such as cerebellum, Kir3.1 appears to partner with other Kir3.x subunits in addition to Kir3.2.

Thus, neuronal G-protein-coupled Kir channels exhibit a great deal of complexity. The ability of GABA$_B$ receptors to regulate the function of these channels enables these receptors to fine-tune neuronal excitability.

Pioneering experiments

The interaction of GABA$_B$ receptors with potassium channels was initially suggested in a series of pioneering experiments. In these experiments it was found that the application of baclofen to voltage-clamped hippocampal pyramidal neurons produced a strong outward current and an increase in membrane conductance (**Figures 13.11a and b**). Subsequent application of the GABA$_B$ receptor antagonist 2-hydroxysaclofen blocked both the outward current and conductance increase produced by baclofen, confirming that these effects were mediated by GABA$_B$ receptors. The I/V curve for the baclofen-mediated current in these pyramidal neurons displays inward rectification and reverses at a membrane potential of about –80 mV. This reversal potential corresponds well with the calculated equilibrium potential for potassium ions using the ionic conditions in these experiments. The agreement between the equilibrium potential for potassium and the reversal potential of the GABA$_B$ receptor-mediated current suggests that this current was caused by an increase in the potassium conductance of the membrane.

This was further confirmed by measuring the shift in the reversal potential of the GABA$_B$ receptor-mediated current produced by an increase in the extracellular potassium concentration from 5.8 mM to 17.4 mM (**Figure 13.11c**). The reversal potential of the current depolarized 26 mV, an amount close to that predicted by the Nernst equation (29 mV). This close agreement indicated that the GABA$_B$ current was carried by potassium ions. This conclusion was further confirmed when it was observed that compounds that are known to block potassium channels, such as extracellular barium or intracellular caesium, also blocked the response to baclofen and GABA.

Further studies support these early findings and have further demonstrated that GABA$_B$ receptors couple to the Kir3.x family of inwardly rectifying potassium channels. Specifically, heteromeric potassium channels composed of Kir3.1/Kir3.2 (GIRK1/GIRK2) or Kir3.1/Kir3.4 (GIRK1/GIRK4) were found to couple with high efficiency to GABA$_B$ receptors in a variety of heterologous systems. Whereas these studies demonstrate that GABA$_B$ receptors are capable of coupling to Kir3.x channels in recombinant systems, other studies have examined the subunit composition of potassium channels to which GABA$_B$ receptors couple in neurons. One study, using mice whose Kir3.2 genes were genetically deleted, reported that GABA$_B$ receptor-mediated potassium currents were absent in CA3 hippocampal neurons. Analysis of Kir3.x protein levels in these mice revealed a lack of Kir3.2 protein and a substantial reduction in Kir3.1 protein, indicating a critical role for both Kir3.2 and Kir3.1 proteins in mediating the effect of GABA$_B$ receptor activation. Alternately, examination of the electrophysiological and pharmacological properties of the GABA$_B$ receptor-mediated potassium current in hippocampal CA3 pyramidal neurons revealed that this current shared similar properties to that mediated by Kir3.1/Kir3.2 or Kir3.1/Kir3.4 potassium channels. However, several significant differences were apparent. In particular, the neuronal potassium current exhibited less voltage dependence and greater sensitivity to blockade by barium than did the potassium current mediated by multimeric cloned channels. These observations suggest that native channels may contain additional subunits which have yet to be identified.

GABA$_B$ receptors are coupled to potassium channels via inhibitory G proteins

Just as they are linked to their other effector systems, GABA$_B$ receptors are coupled to potassium channels through inhibitory G proteins. This conclusion is based on the observation that GDP-β-S reduced the potassium current produced by baclofen. In contrast, GTP-γ-S mimicked the effect of baclofen. Exposure to PTX blocked the activation of potassium channels by both baclofen and GABA, indicating that the effect of GABA$_B$ receptors on potassium channels is achieved through either one or both of the inhibitory G proteins, G$_i$ and/or G$_o$.

The identity of the G protein through which GABA$_B$ receptors couple to potassium channels was further examined using heteromeric GABA$_B$ receptors (GABA$_B$R1a/GABA$_B$R2 or GABA$_B$R1b/GABA$_B$R2) expressed in HEK 293 cells which stably expressed

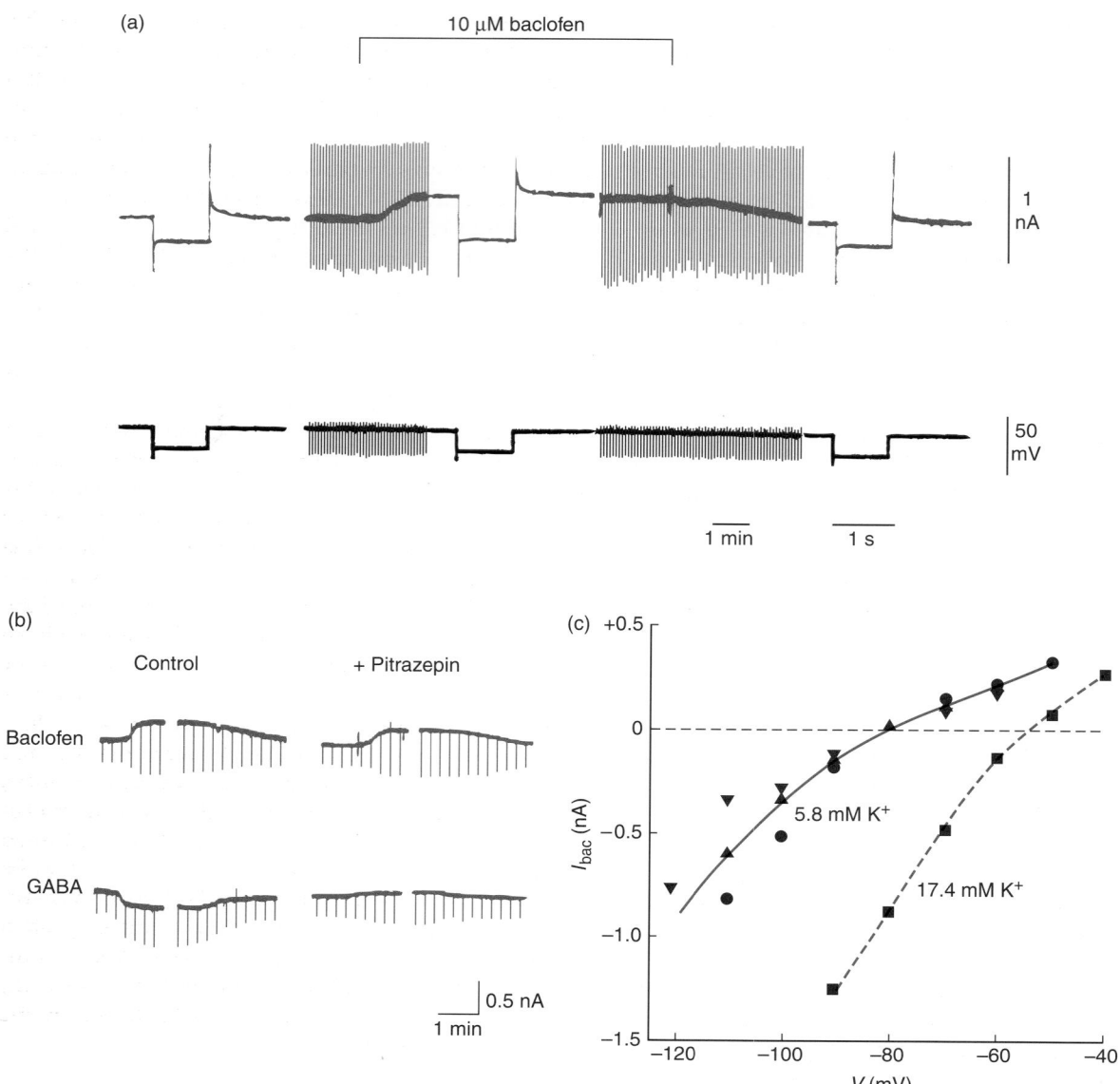

Figure 13.11 GABA$_B$ receptor activation produces an outward current that is mediated by potassium ions.
(a) In a hippocampal pyramidal neuron held in voltage clamp at a membrane potential of –61 mV, baclofen (10 μM) produces an outward current. Both the current (top) and voltage (bottom) recordings are shown. Voltage steps lasting 1 s were delivered repetitively during the experiment to assess the membrane conductance. At three points in the experiment the recording was expanded to better show the response to the voltage step. Note that in the presence of baclofen the current response to the voltage step is larger, indicating an increase in membrane conductance. (b) Another voltage clamped pyramidal cell shows a similar outward current in response to baclofen (top left). Baclofen increased the membrane conductance of this neuron as indicated by an increase in the amplitude of the current deflection in response to repetitive voltage steps (downward deflections). In this cell GABA evoked an inward current and conductance increase (bottom left), suggesting that it was primarily acting on GABA$_A$ receptors. Blockade of the GABA$_A$-linked chloride conductance with pitrazepin (10 μM) had no effect on the baclofen-evoked current (top right), but caused the GABA response to become an outward current (bottom right). This occurred because blockade of the GABA$_A$ receptor-mediated inward chloride current enabled the underlying GABA$_B$ receptor-mediated outward current to become visible. (c) Current–voltage relationship for the baclofen-evoked current in a pyramidal cell when the extracellular concentration of potassium ions was 5.8 mM (circles, triangles) and 17.4 mM (squares). Altering the extracellular potassium concentration depolarized the reversal potential of the baclofen-evoked current by an amount predicted by the Nernst equation, indicating that this current was mediated by potassium ions. Adapted from Gähwiler BH, Brown DA (1985) GABA$_B$-receptor-activated K$^+$ current in voltage-clamped CA3 pyramidal cells in hippocampal cultures, *Proc. Natl Acad. Sci. USA* **82**, 1558–1562, with permission.

Kir3.1+Kir3.2A potassium channels. In these cells all endogenous G$_i$/G$_o$ protein activity was eliminated by PTX treatment, preventing the GABA$_B$ receptors from activating a potassium current. The introduction of mutant PTX-resistant G$_i$/G$_o$ proteins in these cells then allowed determination of those G proteins which would rescue coupling between GABA$_B$ receptors and potassium channels. Interestingly, G protein coupling by the two splice variants of the GABA$_B$ receptor was different. Receptors containing GABA$_B$R1a preferentially coupled to potassium channels via G$_{oA}$ proteins. Receptors containing GABA$_B$R1b coupled to potassium channels via both G$_{oA}$ and G$_{i2}$ proteins with equal efficiency. For both GABA$_B$ receptor splice variants, signalling through other G protein subtypes was not as pronounced. Whereas both GABA$_B$R1 splice variants appear to preferentially signal through G$_{oA}$ protein, the ability of GABA$_B$R1b to also signal through G$_{i2}$ protein suggests differences in effector coupling. Interestingly, in a separate experiment, using CA3 neurons from mice genetically engineered to lack the α_o-subunit of the G$_o$ protein, GABA$_B$ receptors coupled to potassium channels with equal efficiency to that in wildtype littermates.

These results show that modulation of potassium channels by GABA$_B$ receptors does not have an absolute requirement for G$_o$ protein. Thus, it appears that G$_o$ protein is preferentially used but, when absent, can readily be replaced by G proteins with different properties.

GABA$_B$ receptors are directly coupled to potassium channels by $\beta\gamma$-subunits of G proteins

Several lines of evidence indicate that G proteins couple to potassium channels via their $\beta\gamma$-subunits. Initially, it was observed that the application of purified G protein $\beta\gamma$-subunits, but not α-subunits, to the intracellular surface of excised patches of chick embryonic atrial cells activated G-protein-gated potassium channels, suggesting that $\beta\gamma$-subunits carried the functional signal. This suggestion was confirmed by subsequent binding studies which demonstrated a direct interaction between G protein $\beta\gamma$-subunits and Kir3.1, Kir3.2 and Kir3.4. Similarly, it was found, using the yeast two hybrid system, that the G protein β-subunit bound directly with the amino-terminus of Kir3.1. Mutational analysis was then used to determine the binding site for G protein $\beta\gamma$-subunits on the Kir3.x proteins and revealed that $\beta\gamma$-subunits bound to sites on both the amino- and carboxy-terminus of the Kir3.x protein. The role of each of these $\beta\gamma$-binding domains on the Kir3.x channel is currently under study.

Whereas $\beta\gamma$-subunits are necessary for activation of Kir3.x channels by GPCRs, the mechanism by which $\beta\gamma$-subunits activated these potassium channels was not

known. However, recent studies have shed light on this issue. Huang et al. found that the membrane phospholipid, phosphatidylinositol 4,5-bisphosphate (PIP$_2$) binds directly to the carboxy-terminus of Kir3.x subunits and activates Kir3.x channels. Furthermore, the direct association of PIP$_2$ with the carboxy-terminus of the Kir3.x subunit is a prerequisite for channel activity. The binding of G protein $\beta\gamma$-subunits to the channel enhances the sensitivity of the channel for PIP$_2$. In the absence of G protein $\beta\gamma$-subunits the channel has a significantly lower sensitivity for PIP$_2$ and is therefore less likely to be activated. Thus, G protein $\beta\gamma$-subunits activate Kir3.x channels by stabilizing interactions between PIP$_2$ and the potassium channel.

Whereas Kir3.x channels are activated by G protein $\beta\gamma$-subunits, the mechanism by which receptor specificity is achieved is unclear. For example, in native tissues only G$_i$/G$_o$, and not G$_s$ proteins activate Kir3.x channels and yet all of these G proteins release free $\beta\gamma$-subunits upon receptor stimulation. It is known that receptor specificity does not lie at the level of the $\beta\gamma$-subunit since a variety of different $\beta\gamma$-subunits have been shown to be equally effective at stimulating Kir3.x channels. A recent study has shown that in a mammalian expression system (HEK 293 cells) G$_i$/G$_o$-coupled receptors, such as GABA$_B$ receptors, but not G$_s$-coupled receptors, activate Kir3.1/Kir3.2a channels, suggesting that the receptor specificity lies at the level of the G protein α-subunit. This possibility was confirmed by the observation that G$_s$-coupled receptors could be made to stimulate potassium channels by swapping critical residues on the carboxy-terminus of the G$_s$ protein α_s-subunit with those of the G$_i$ protein α_i-subunit. Thus, G protein $\beta\gamma$-subunit directly controls Kir3.x channels, but the G protein α-subunit appears to determine the specificity of receptor action.

GABA$_B$ receptor-activated potassium channels display flickering behaviour

Single-channel potassium currents, activated by baclofen or GABA, can be recorded from cell-attached patches of cultured hippocampal neurons. They are blocked by the GABA$_B$ receptor antagonist, 2-hydroxysaclofen, but are not affected by the GABA$_A$ antagonist bicuculline, indicating that they are GABA$_B$ receptor-dependent. As with the whole-cell current discussed above, GABA$_B$ receptor-mediated single-channel currents are potassium selective. Thus, alterations in the concentration of potassium ions in the pipette cause a corresponding shift in the reversal potential of the single-channel current. The single-channel current amplitude that occurs with highest probability is about 4 pA (**Figure 13.12**). This corresponds to a conductance of 67 pS.

(a)

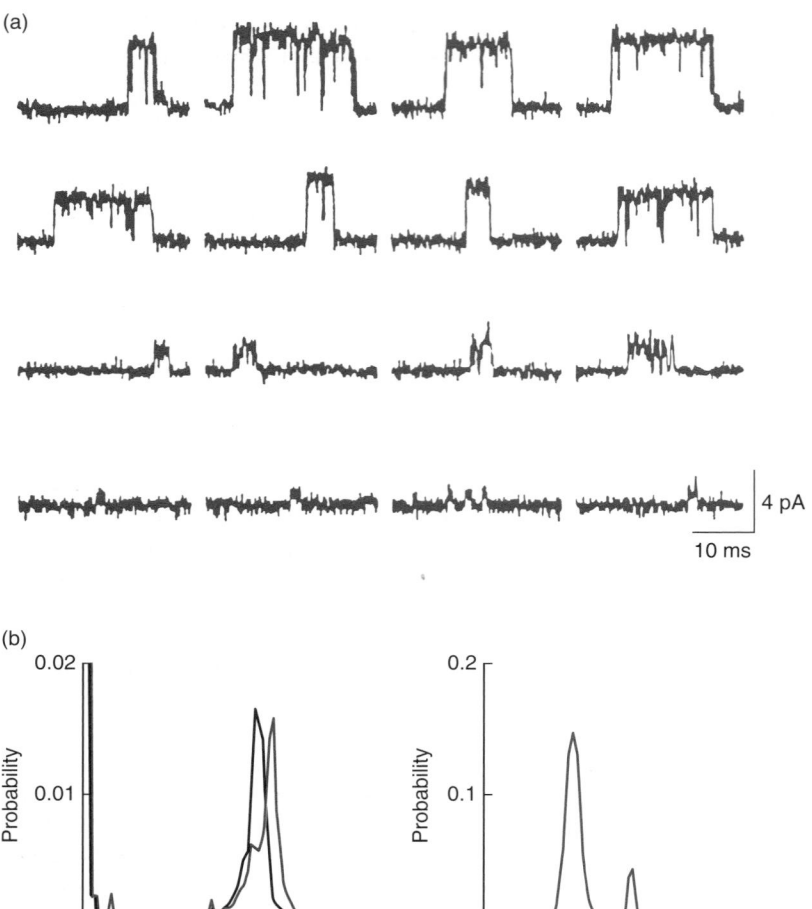

Figure 13.12 Baclofen activates single channel currents with a mean amplitude of 4 pA.
(a) Examples of single-channel currents evoked by GABA in cultured hippocampal neurons. Currents were recorded in the cell-attached patch configuration and GABA was applied through the bath to the membrane outside of the patch. Currents in the lower two rows were selected for this figure because of their small amplitudes. (b) Current-amplitude probability histograms of the GABA$_B$ receptor-mediated single-channel current. These histograms were constructed from data collected from the same patch as in (a). The graph on the left shows two histograms (black and green lines) representing the current amplitudes taken from two unbroken segments of data in this patch. Note that in both cases a channel with an amplitude of about 4 pA occurred with the greatest probability. The histogram on the right was taken from sections of the data which had the smallest currents. The smaller peak corresponds to elementary channel current with an amplitude of 0.36 pA. From Premkumar LS, Chung S-H, Gage PW (1990) GABA-induced potassium channels in cultured neurons, *Proc. R. Soc. Lond.* **B241**, 153–158, with permission.

A prominent characteristic of these single-channel currents is a rapid flickering between open and closed states. In addition to channel closings, this flickering appears to show a variety of different subconductance levels (**Figure 13.13a**). These different conductance levels are particularly prominent during wash-on and wash-out of the baclofen (**Figure 13.13b**). Indeed, histograms of the current amplitudes reveal many peaks which appear to occur at multiples of the smallest peak. This smallest peak represents an elementary current amplitude of 0.36 pA (**Figure 13.12**), corresponding to a conductance of 5–6 pS. Whereas this measurement reflects the conductance coupled to somatic GABA$_B$ receptors, a recent study has used non-stationary variance analysis to estimate the conductance linked to synaptically activated GABA$_B$ receptors. This study reported a small unitary conductance in the range of 5–12 pS, in agreement with the elementary conductance observed at the single-channel level. Taken together, these studies suggest that this small subconductance state predominates during synaptic GABA$_B$ currents.

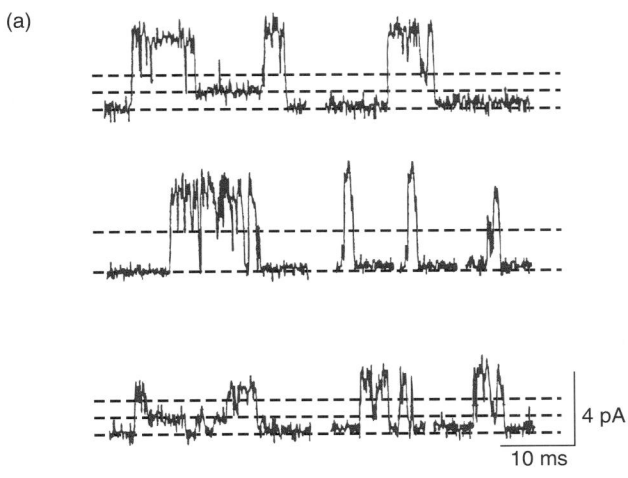

(a)

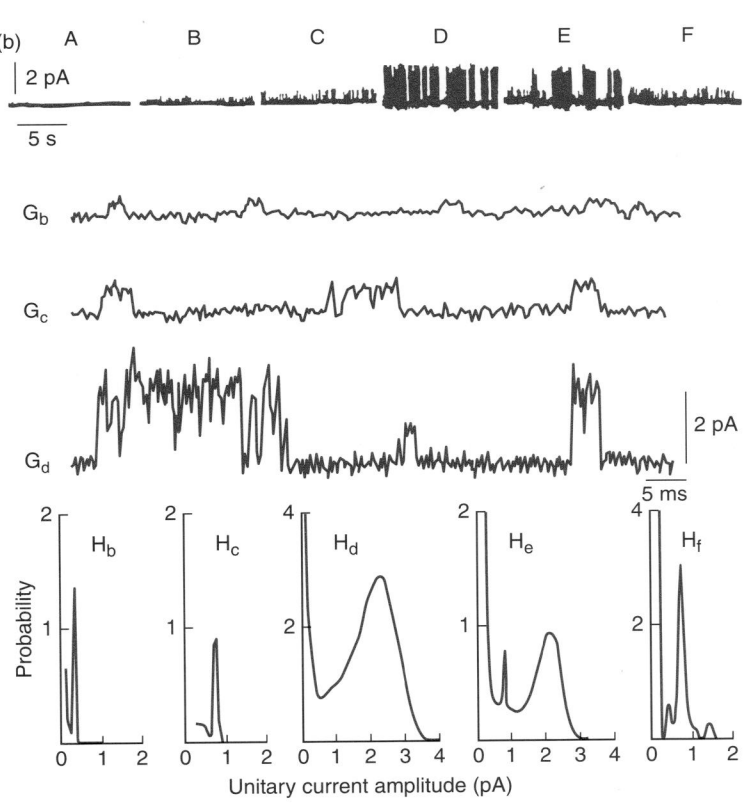

(b)

Figure 13.13 GABA_B single-channel currents have multiple subconductance states.

(a) Examples of single-channel currents recorded from cell-attached patches of cultured hippocampal neurons. These currents were selected to emphasize different subconductance states of the channels. All currents were evoked by application of GABA except for the current in the panel on the upper right which was evoked by baclofen. Dotted lines indicated different conductance levels. (b) Exposure of a cell to GABA (100 μM) and bicuculline (100 μM) causes the slow development of single-channel currents in a cell attached patch. These currents appear to go through several different conductance states until finally reaching their maximal amplitude. The panel in A represents the baseline response of the patch before the addition of agonist. The panels in B–D show activity in the patch at 25 s (B), 1.5 min (C) and 4 min (D) after the addition of agonist. Panels E and F show patch activity after 5 and 10 minutes of wash, respectively. The records in the middle three rows represent an expansion of a portion of the panels shown in B (G_b), C (G_c), and D (G_d). Finally, the current amplitude probability histograms (H_b–H_f) were produced from data collected at the same times as panels B–F. Note the progressive increase in the current amplitude following the application of GABA. From Premkumar LS, Chung S-H, Gage PW (1990) GABA-induced potassium channels in cultured neurons, *Proc. R. Soc. Lond.* **B241**, 153–158, with permission.

In single-channel studies the kinetics of the current activation and deactivation, even during large events (>4 pA), are extremely rapid. Since the elementary current amplitude is only 0.36 pA, many of these elementary channels would need to open or close synchronously to cause these rapid transitions. However, it is extremely unlikely that these channels would behave independently in such a synchronized fashion. Therefore, it has been suggested that these elementary channels function cooperatively. According to this hypothesis, these elementary co-channels would form oligomers of varying size which would function as a single unit. Activation of the oligomer would cause many of the channels to open simultaneously. The flickering behaviour of the current would then represent the transient opening and closing of the elementary channels within the oligomer. However, this hypothesis remains to be conclusively demonstrated.

13.3.5 Summary

$GABA_B$ receptors are coupled through inhibitory G_i/G_o proteins to multiple effector systems. The primary effects of $GABA_B$ receptor activation include inhibition of adenylyl cyclase, inhibition of voltage-dependent calcium channels and activation of inwardly rectifying potassium channels. Future studies may reveal other effector systems to which $GABA_B$ receptors are also coupled. By coupling to these different effector systems, $GABA_B$ receptors enable GABA to have a broader range of effects on neurons than it could by acting only on $GABA_A$ receptors. The discussion so far has focused on the intrinsic properties of the $GABA_B$ receptor and the effector systems to which they are coupled. We now turn attention to the role that these receptors play in synaptic activity.

13.4 The functional role of $GABA_B$ receptors in synaptic activity

GABAergic synapses in the central nervous system contain both $GABA_A$ and $GABA_B$ receptors capable of responding to the synaptic release of GABA. Once released, the lifetime of GABA in the synaptic cleft is very brief (milliseconds) both because the duration of the release is very short and the GABA that is released quickly diffuses away. In addition, there exists an avid uptake system to actively remove GABA from the synaptic cleft. These systems combine to tightly regulate GABA concentration in the synaptic cleft.

Synaptic activation of $GABA_A$ receptors produces a rapid, synchronous opening of chloride channels, resulting in a fast inhibitory postsynaptic current. In contrast, synaptic activation of $GABA_B$ receptors initiates a second-messenger-mediated process which is considerably slower. Because of the delay inherent in the second messenger system, GABA has disappeared from the synaptic cleft before the $GABA_B$ receptor-mediated response even begins. Thus, the kinetics of this response are determined not by the binding/unbinding of GABA from the $GABA_B$ receptor but rather by the kinetics of the second messenger system involved. The functional effects of $GABA_B$ receptors are exerted by both postsynaptic and presynaptic receptors, which play very different roles in neuronal function. The primary functional effect of postsynaptic $GABA_B$ receptors is to hyperpolarize the postsynaptic membrane. In contrast, the primary functional effect of presynaptic receptors is to inhibit the release of neurotransmitter.

13.4.1 Postsynaptic $GABA_B$ receptors produce an inhibitory postsynaptic current

When stimulated by synaptically released GABA, postsynaptic $GABA_B$ receptors increase the potassium conduc-
tance of the neuronal membrane. For a neuron near its resting potential, this increase in potassium conductance produces a large hyperpolarization of the membrane which is seen in a whole-cell voltage clamp recording as an outward current. This outward current, termed an *inhibitory postsynaptic current* (IPSC), is produced by the summation of the elementary current flowing through each of the $GABA_B$ receptor-activated potassium channels (**Figure 13.14a**). The small elementary conductance of the $GABA_B$-coupled potassium channel suggests that a large number of these channels open during an average-sized $GABA_B$ IPSC. In the example shown in **Figure 13.14a**, the conductance of the $GABA_B$ IPSC is 1.25 nS. Therefore, based on an elementary conductance for $GABA_B$-coupled potassium channels of 5–12 pS, it can be calculated that approximately 150 channels opened at the peak of the $GABA_B$ IPSC.

The kinetics of the $GABA_B$ receptor-mediated response are slow

Because it is coupled through a second messenger system, the $GABA_B$ receptor-mediated hyperpolarization has a time course that is very different from that produced by an ionotropic receptor-channel, such as $GABA_A$ (**Figure 13.14b**). Measurements of the time required from stimulation of the presynaptic terminals to the initiation of the postsynaptic hyperpolarization have ranged from 20 to 50 ms. This onset latency is considerably longer than that of the $GABA_A$ receptor-mediated response (<3 ms). Once the $GABA_B$ response begins, its risetime is also slow and it does not reach a peak for 130–300 ms. This compares with the $GABA_A$ response which reaches a typical peak in 1–15 ms. The slower risetime of the $GABA_B$ response is thought to occur because of the asynchronous activation of potassium channels by the diffusing second messenger. Finally, the $GABA_B$ response decays back to baseline over the next 400–1300 ms. This slow rate of decay may reflect the rate of GTP hydrolysis, suggesting that it is the decline of activated G protein that ultimately terminates the response. In contrast, the $GABA_A$ response decays to baseline much more rapidly (80–220 ms). The prolonged duration of the $GABA_B$ response (500–1500 ms) enables GABA to produce inhibition over a much longer period of time than it could acting on $GABA_A$ receptors alone (90–250 ms).

$GABA_B$ receptors are more sensitive than $GABA_A$ receptors to GABA

Dose–response curves can be used to compare the sensitivity of $GABA_A$ and $GABA_B$ receptors to GABA. These dose–response curves reveal that GABA is much more potent in activating $GABA_B$ receptors (EC_{50} 1.6 μM) than

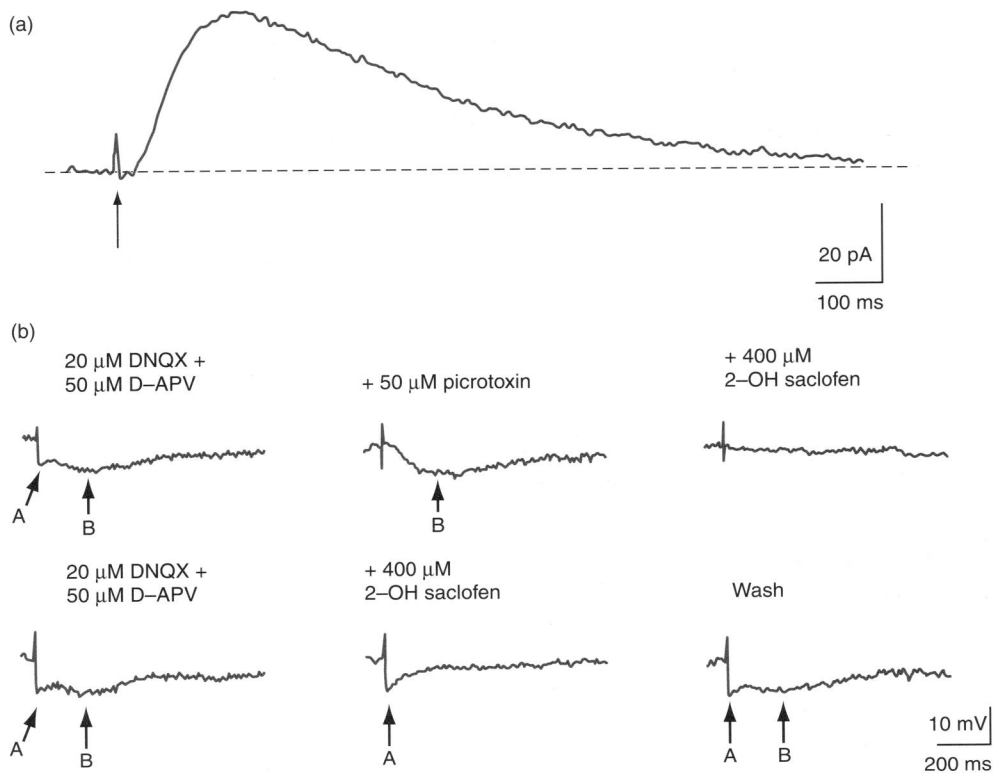

Figure 13.14 Synaptically released GABA activates postsynaptic GABA$_B$ receptors to produce a slow IPSC.

(a) Stimulation of inhibitory fibres evokes a stimulus artifact (arrow) followed by a GABA$_B$ receptor-mediated IPSC in a hippocampal neuron held at a potential of –60 mV in whole-cell voltage clamp. The GABA$_B$ IPSC was pharmacologically isolated from the excitatory synaptic current using DNQX, which blocks AMPA receptors and APV, which blocks NMDA receptors. It was also isolated from the GABA$_A$ inhibitory current using bicuculline which blocks GABA$_A$ receptors. Note the slow onset of the IPSC and its long latency. **(b)** GABA$_A$ and GABA$_B$ inhibitory postsynaptic potentials (IPSPs) were recorded in current clamp from a dentate gyrus granule cell. These hyperpolarizing potentials were evoked by stimulating inhibitory fibres. They were isolated from glutamatergic excitatory potentials by application of DNQX and APV. GABA$_A$ and GABA$_B$ IPSPs are indicated by arrows labelled 'A' and 'B', respectively. In control (top left) a stimulus evoked a stimulus artifact (upward deflection) followed by both a GABA$_A$ and a GABA$_B$ IPSP which can be seen as the fast and slow components of the hyperpolarizing response, respectively. Application of picrotoxin blocks the GABA$_A$ IPSP leaving only the slow GABA$_B$ IPSP (top centre). The subsequent addition of 2-hydroxysaclofen blocks this GABA$_B$ IPSP. Similarly, in another cell, application of 2-hydroxysaclofen to the control response (bottom left) blocks the GABA$_B$ IPSP, leaving an isolated GABA$_A$ IPSP (bottom centre). The effect of this antagonist is reversible (bottom right). Note the difference in the time course of the isolated GABA$_B$ IPSP (top centre) and the isolated GABA$_A$ IPSP (bottom centre). Part (a) from Mott DD, Lewis DV, unpublished observations. Part (b) from Mott DD, Lewis DV (1992) GABA$_B$ receptors mediate disinhibition and facilitate long-term potentiation in the dentate gyrus, *Epilepsy Res.* **Suppl. 7**, 119–134, with permission.

GABA$_A$ receptors (EC$_{50}$ 25 μM). In physiological ionic conditions the current generated by GABA$_A$ receptors in response to a maximal concentration of GABA is far larger than that generated by GABA$_B$ receptors. However, the higher sensitivity of GABA$_B$ receptors to GABA suggests that at low GABA concentrations GABA$_B$ receptors will produce more current.

Despite their higher sensitivity to GABA, numerous electrophysiological studies have reported that activation of GABA$_B$ receptors requires high intensity or repetitive stimulation of the neuronal network. This situation most likely arises because GABA$_B$ receptors are located extrasynaptically and are not activated until

sufficient GABA is released to overcome local uptake systems and spill over on to these receptors. However, the higher sensitivity of GABA$_B$ receptors to GABA enables these receptors to respond to the low concentrations of GABA that are able to reach these extrasynaptic spaces.

The GABA$_B$ IPSC produces inhibition by hyperpolarizing the neuronal membrane

Whole-cell voltage clamp recordings reveal that the maximal peak conductance increase produced by activation of GABA$_A$ receptors is much greater (5 to 10-fold) than that produced by activation of GABA$_B$ receptors. For example, in hippocampal pyramidal neurons the maximal conductance of the GABA$_A$ IPSC ranges from 90 to 140 nS. This compares with a range of 13–19 nS for the maximal conductance of the GABA$_B$ IPSC in these same cells. Similar differences between the maximal conductance values of GABA$_A$ and GABA$_B$ receptor-mediated currents have been reported in other brain regions.

Despite its relatively small conductance, the GABA$_B$ current produces a large hyperpolarization from rest in most neurons. This strong hyperpolarization occurs because activation of GABA$_B$ receptors drives the membrane potential toward the reversal potential for potassium ions. In physiological ionic conditions the equilibrium potential for potassium ions (–80 to –98 mV) is quite negative relative to the resting membrane potential (–50 to –75 mV) of most cells. Therefore, even though the conductance of the GABA$_B$ IPSC is small, the driving force for potassium can be quite large. In fact, because of this large driving force for potassium ions and the long duration of the GABA$_B$ response, the GABA$_B$ IPSC can move an amount of charge that is close to that carried by the GABA$_A$ IPSC. For example, in granule cells of the dentate gyrus about 8 pC of charge leaves the cell during the GABA$_B$ IPSC. This compares favourably with the 9–35 pC that are carried by the GABA$_A$ response in these same cells.

The GABA$_A$ IPSC powerfully inhibits neuronal excitability both by hyperpolarizing the postsynaptic membrane and increasing its conductance. Hyperpolarization moves the postsynaptic membrane away from action potential threshold, whereas the conductance increase produced by the GABA$_A$ IPSC shunts the postsynaptic membrane thereby short-circuiting excitatory responses. This inhibition powerfully suppresses both voltage-dependent and voltage-independent excitatory currents and cannot be overcome by depolarization. In contrast, the GABA$_B$ IPSC produces a large hyperpolarization with a fairly small conductance increase. Thus, it inhibits neurons primarily through hyperpolarization. This hyperpolarizing inhibition is effective in suppressing voltage-dependent currents, such as NMDA receptor-mediated responses. However, since it can be overcome by neuronal depolarization, it does not effectively inhibit voltage-independent currents. Inhibition produced by GABA$_B$ receptors has been suggested to be a more modulatory form of inhibition than that produced by GABA$_A$ receptors, enabling a fine-tuning of neuronal function. Thus, GABA$_B$ receptor-mediated inhibition differs in both kinetics and function from inhibition produced by GABA$_A$ receptors.

13.4.2 Presynaptic GABA$_B$ receptors inhibit the release of many different transmitters

In addition to their presence postsynaptically, GABA$_B$ receptors are also located on presynaptic terminals where they inhibit the release of a variety of neurotransmitters, including GABA, glutamate, dopamine, serotonin and norepinephrine. The majority of evidence suggesting a role for GABA$_B$ receptors in the regulation of neurotransmitter release has been obtained using applied agonists, such as baclofen. However, recent studies have shown that during repetitive stimulation, synaptically released GABA can also activate these presynaptic GABA$_B$ receptors to inhibit neurotransmitter release. Inhibition of transmitter release by synaptically released GABA is dramatically enhanced following pharmacological blockade of GABA uptake, indicating that GABA has to overcome uptake in order to reach these presynaptic GABA$_B$ receptors. By activating presynaptic GABA$_B$ receptors, synaptically released GABA can inhibit transmitter release at the inhibitory terminal from which the GABA was originally released (homosynaptic depression) as well as at neighbouring inhibitory and/or excitatory terminals (heterosynaptic depression).

Presynaptic GABA$_B$ receptors inhibit the release of GABA

Inhibition of GABA release by presynaptic GABA$_B$ receptors has been especially well examined. It has been demonstrated conclusively that synaptically released GABA can feedback onto presynaptic GABA$_B$ receptors located on the activated GABAergic terminal as well as on other neighbouring GABAergic terminals. These presynaptic GABA$_B$ receptors can then suppress the subsequent release of GABA, causing both the GABA$_A$ IPSC and GABA$_B$ IPSC to be smaller.

This effect can be clearly observed if paired electrical stimuli are used to activate GABAergic axons which synapse onto GABA$_A$ receptors on a cortical neuron which is recorded in whole-cell voltage clamp (**Figure 13.15**). The first stimulus evokes the release of GABA, resulting in the production of a GABA$_A$ IPSC. However, a second identical stimulus delivered 300 ms later, during the peak of the GABA$_B$ suppression of GABA release, evokes a GABA$_A$ IPSC that is greatly reduced. Application of the GABA$_B$ antagonist, 2-hydroxysaclofen, blocks the reduction in the second IPSC, indicating that the suppression is mediated through GABA acting on GABA$_B$ receptors. The ability of presynaptic GABA$_B$ receptors to suppress GABA$_A$ IPSCs endows the GABAergic system with a powerful feedback mechanism capable of suppressing GABAergic inhibition in an activity-dependent manner.

The time course of the depression of GABA release is similar to the time course of the postsynaptic GABA_B IPSC

Just like the postsynaptic effect of GABA_B receptors, the time course of the inhibition of GABA release by GABA_B receptors reflects a second-messenger-coupled mechanism. Following the stimulation of an inhibitory pathway, the onset of the presynaptic inhibition is slow, reaching a peak about 200 ms after the initial stimulus

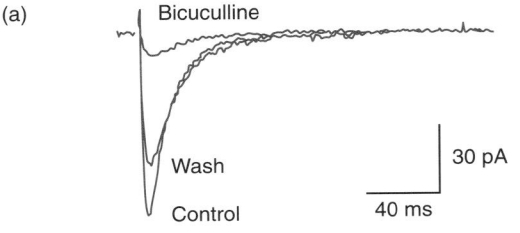

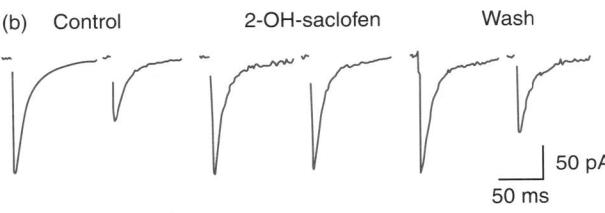

Figure 13.15 Presynaptic GABA_B receptors mediate paired pulse depression of IPSCs.

(a) The pharmacologically isolated GABA_A IPSC in a neuron in the somatosensory cortex is reversibly blocked by bicuculline. This GABA_A IPSC was evoked by electrical stimulation of inhibitory fibres and recorded in whole-cell voltage clamp. It was isolated from the excitatory synaptic current by application of CNQX and APV, antagonists of AMPA and NMDA receptors, respectively. The neuron was held at a membrane potential of −70 mV, causing the GABA_A IPSC to be an inward current. **(b)** Under these same conditions if paired stimuli are delivered 300 ms apart, the GABA_A IPSC evoked by the second stimulus of the pair is reduced (left). This reduction of the second IPSC is blocked by the GABA_B antagonist, 2-hydroxysaclofen (centre). This effect is reversible after wash-out of the antagonist (right). The cell recorded in this experiment was from a very young (postnatal day 10) rat. In animals of this young age the postsynaptic GABA_B response is developmentally immature, whereas the presynaptic GABA_B response is fully developed. This difference in development explains why no GABA_B IPSC is evident in these recordings and gives further confirmation that postsynaptic GABA_B receptors are not necessary for paired pulse depression of IPSCs. In older animals postsynaptic GABA_B IPSCs are fully developed and both GABA_A and GABA_B IPSCs are depressed by presynaptic GABA_B receptors (see Figure 13.16). Adapted from Fukuda A, Mody I, Prince DA (1993) Differential ontogenesis of presynaptic and postsynaptic GABA_B inhibition in rat somatosensory cortex, *J. Neurophysiol.* **70**, 448–452, with permission.

(Figure 13.16). The duration of the effect is also quite prolonged and can extend for up to several seconds. Thus, although GABA has a brief lifetime in the synaptic cleft, the activation of presynaptic GABA_B receptors by this GABA enables it to modulate the subsequent release of transmitter for up to several seconds.

GABA_B receptors suppress transmitter release by inhibiting voltage-dependent calcium channels

There exist several possible mechanisms by which presynaptic GABA_B receptors could suppress neurotransmitter release. For example, GABA_B receptors inhibit currents mediated by N- and P/Q-type calcium channels. These calcium channels have been implicated in the control of neurotransmitter release. Thus, presynaptic GABA_B receptors could inhibit transmitter release by suppressing current flux through these channels. However, activation of presynaptic potassium conductances is also thought to be important in the regulation of transmitter release. The ability of postsynaptic GABA_B receptors to couple to Kir3.x potassium channels suggests that presynaptic GABA_B receptors may inhibit transmitter release by coupling to similar channels in nerve terminals. Finally, it has been suggested that presynaptic GABA_B receptors directly inhibit the transmitter release machinery downstream of calcium influx. Recent studies have begun to distinguish between these alternatives.

It was reported that GABA_B receptors did not activate a postsynaptic potassium conductance in hippocampal neurons from transgenic mice lacking the Kir3.2 gene. Thus, the potassium channel coupled to GABA_B receptors was absent in these mice. However, in these same mice GABA_B receptor-mediated presynaptic inhibition of both glutamate and GABA release was unchanged. Taken together, these findings suggested that potassium channels played no role in the inhibition mediated by presynaptic GABA_B receptors. However, without direct recordings from presynaptic terminals, the possibility could not be ruled out that GABA_B receptors mediated inhibition of transmitter release by coupling to potassium channels which were unique to the presynaptic terminal.

Therefore, to investigate the mechanism of action of presynaptic GABA_B receptors it would be desirable to record directly from presynaptic terminals. Unfortunately, the small size of most synaptic structures in the brain has made direct electrophysiological study of presynaptic terminals and their modulation impossible. However, it is possible to record directly from the giant nerve terminals (calyces of Held) in the medial nucleus of the trapezoid body. Two recent studies have made use of this preparation in order to address the

Figure 13.16 Paired pulse depression of IPSCs is maximal when stimuli are delivered 200 ms apart.

(a) Isolated GABA$_A$ and GABA$_B$ IPSCs recorded in whole-cell voltage clamp from a dentate gyrus granule cell. Since the cell was held at a membrane potential of –80 mV, the GABA$_A$ IPSC is an inward current whereas the GABA$_B$ IPSC is an outward current. Inhibitory fibres were electrically stimulated to evoke IPSCs. Paired stimuli were delivered at increasing intervals to determine the time course of the inhibition of GABA release produced by presynaptic GABA$_B$ receptors. Responses to paired stimuli at four different intervals are shown. In this cell suppression of the second IPSC was greatest when the stimuli were delivered 200 ms apart. GABA$_A$ and GABA$_B$ IPSCs are indicated by arrows labelled 'A' and 'B', respectively. (b) Graph of the averaged data obtained from six cells showing the time course of the suppression of the second IPSC. For both the GABA$_A$ and GABA$_B$ IPSC the second response of the pair was maximally depressed when the stimuli were delivered about 200 ms apart. Asterisks indicate a significant depression of the IPSC ($*P < 0.05$, $**P < 0.01$). The cross (+) indicates that the GABA$_B$ IPSC was significantly more depressed than the GABA$_A$ IPSC. From Mott DD, Xie CW, Wilson WA *et al.* (1993) GABA$_B$ autoreceptors mediate activity-dependent disinhibition and enhance signal transmission in the dentate gyrus, *J. Neurophysiol.* **69**, 674–691, with permission.

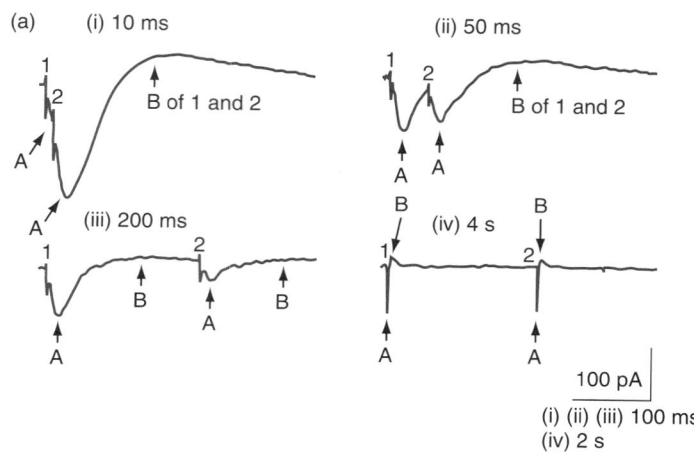

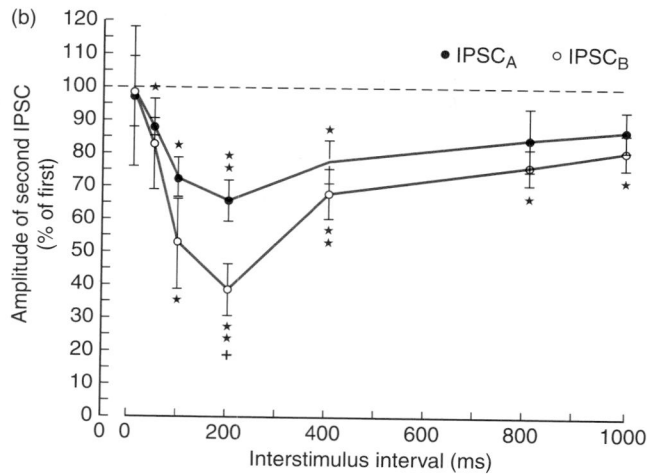

mechanism of action of presynaptic GABA$_B$ receptors. In these studies baclofen suppressed both synaptic transmission recorded postsynaptically as well as the presynaptic calcium current recorded in the nerve terminal. The suppression of synaptic transmission by baclofen was similar to that observed when the external calcium concentration was lowered. This similarity suggested that the presynaptic inhibition produced by baclofen was caused by the suppression of presynaptic calcium influx and not a direct effect on the transmitter release machinery. Furthermore, baclofen did not activate a potassium conductance in the presynaptic terminal, indicating that potassium conductances are not involved in the effect of baclofen at this synapse. Thus, presynaptic GABA$_B$ receptors appeared to suppress transmitter release by directly inhibiting calcium channels. Several observations suggested that these presynaptic GABA$_B$ receptors were coupled to calcium channels via G$_i$/G$_o$ proteins. First, loading of the presynaptic terminal with GDP-β-S blocked the effect of baclofen on calcium currents. In contrast, GTP-γ-S suppressed presynaptic calcium currents and occluded the

effect of baclofen. Finally, inhibition of calcium channels by baclofen was blocked by *N*-ethylmaleimide, a sulphydryl alkylating agent which uncouples G$_i$/G$_o$ proteins from their receptors. These results directly indicate that at this giant synapse GABA$_B$ receptors suppress synaptic transmission by inhibiting presynaptic calcium channels and that GABA$_B$ receptors couple to these calcium channels via G$_i$/G$_o$ proteins. It remains to be demonstrated whether this result generalizes to other synapses in the brain.

13.5 Summary

GABA$_B$ receptors enable GABA to produce a variety of effects on neuronal function. These receptors are located both pre- and postsynaptically where they can be activated by synaptically released GABA. Postsynaptic GABA$_B$ receptors generate a slow inhibitory current which is carried by potassium ions. This current produces a hyperpolarizing inhibition which effectively inhibits voltage-dependent conductances, such as the

NMDA receptor-mediated current. Presynaptic GABA$_B$ receptors inhibit the release of a variety of different neurotransmitters, including glutamate and GABA. The ability of GABA$_B$ receptors to regulate GABA release provides an important mechanism for the feedback control of both GABA$_A$ and GABA$_B$ inhibition. Thus, by acting at both pre- and postsynaptic sites, GABA$_B$ receptors have the potential to produce profound changes in neuronal function.

Further reading

Bowery NG, Enna SJ (2000) γ-Aminobutyric acid$_B$ receptors: first of the functional metabotropic heterodimers. *J. Pharmacol. Exp. Ther.* **292**, 2–7.

De Koninck Y, Mody I (1997) Endogenous GABA activates small-conductance K$^+$ channels underlying slow IPSCs in rat hippocampal neurons. *J. Neurophysiol.* **77**, 2202–2208.

Filippov AK, Couve A, Pangalos MN *et al.* (2000) Heteromeric assembly of GABA$_B$R1 and GABA$_B$R2 receptor subunits inhibits Ca^{2+} current in sympathetic neurons. *J. Neurosci.* **20**, 2867–2874.

Galvez T, Parmentier M-L, Joly C *et al.* (1999) Mutagenesis and modeling of the GABA$_B$ receptor extracellular domain support a Venus flytrap mechanism for ligand binding. *J. Biol. Chem.* **274**, 13362–13369.

Ikeda SR (1996) Voltage-dependent modulation of N-type calcium channels by G-protein beta gamma subunits. *Nature* **380**, 255–258.

Isomoto S, Kaibara M, Sakurai-Yamashita Y *et al.* (1998) Cloning and tissue distribution of novel splice variants of the rat GABA$_B$ receptor. *Biochem. Biophys. Res. Comm.* **253**, 10–15.

Kaupmann K, Huggel K, Heid J *et al.* (1997) Expression cloning of GABA$_B$ receptors uncovers similarity to metabotropic glutamate receptors. *Nature* **386**, 239–246.

Kaupmann K, Malitschek B, Schuler V *et al.* (1998) GABA$_B$-receptor subtypes assemble into functional heteromeric complexes. *Nature* **396**, 683–687.

Leaney JL, Tinker A (2000) The role of members of the pertussis toxin-sensitive family of G proteins in coupling receptors to the activation of the G protein-gated inwardly rectifying potassium channel. *Proc. Natl Acad. Sci. USA* **97**, 5651–5656.

Lüscher C, Jan LY, Stoffel M *et al.* (1997) G protein-coupled inwardly rectifying K$^+$ channels (GIRKs) mediate postsynaptic but not presynaptic transmitter actions in hippocampal neurons. *Neuron* **19**, 687–695.

Malitschek B, Schweizer C, Keir M *et al.* (1999) The N-terminal domain of γ-aminobutyic acid$_B$ receptors is sufficient to specify agonist and antagonist binding. *Mol. Pharmacol.* **56**, 448–454.

Sodickson D, Bean BP (1996) GABA$_B$ receptor-activated inwardly rectifying potassium current in dissociated hippocampal CA3 neurons. *J. Neurosci.* **16**, 6374–6385.

Takahashi T, Kajikawa Y, Tsujimoto T (1998) G-protein-coupled modulation of presynaptic calcium currents and transmitter release by a GABA$_B$ receptor. *J. Neurosci.* **18**, 3138–3146.

Uezono Y, Ueda Y, Ueno S *et al.* (1997) Enhancement by baclofen of the G$_s$-coupled receptor-mediated cAMP production in *Xenopus* oocytes expressing rat brain cortex poly (A)$^+$ RNA: a role of G-protein beta gamma subunits. *Biochem. Biophys. Res. Comm.* **241**, 476–480.

White JH, Wise A, Main MJ *et al.* (1998) Heterodimerization is required for the formation of a functional GABA$_B$ receptor. *Nature* **396**, 679–682.

Yamada M, Inanobe A, Kurachi Y (1998) G protein regulation of potassium ion channels. *Pharmacol. Rev.* **50**, 723–757.

The Metabotropic Glutamate Receptors

Earlier chapters have described how glutamate is the primary excitatory neurotransmitter in the CNS, and that many of the effects of glutamate are mediated through glutamate-gated ion channels, or ionotropic glutamate receptors (iGluRs). However, many effects of glutamate in the brain are mediated by G-protein-coupled or metabotropic glutamate receptors (mGluRs). This chapter discusses structural features of mGluRs and well-defined physiological roles for these receptors in the nervous system.

Initially, the actions of glutamate in the nervous system were thought to be solely mediated by iGluRs. However, in the mid-1980s several groups reported that glutamate can stimulate phosphoinositide (PI) turnover in brain tissue. Several lines of evidence indicated that glutamate stimulation of PI hydrolysis did not occur via iGluRs. First, the pharmacological profile did not match any known profile for iGluRs. Glutamate-stimulated PI hydrolysis was mimicked by quisqualate and *trans*-ACPD (1S,3R-1-amino-1,3-cyclopentanedicarboxylic acid) and was not inhibited by any known antagonist of iGluRs. Second, the stimulation was prevented by inhibitors of G proteins and mimicked by activators of G proteins. Therefore, the existence of a G-protein coupled or 'metabotropic' glutamate receptor was hypothesized.

14.1 What is the receptor underlying glutamate-stimulated PI hydrolysis? – The cloning of metabotropic glutamate receptor genes

A common way to clone a gene with a putative function is to utilize the known function of the protein to screen a library of genes expressed in a heterologous system, such as *Xenopus laevis* oocytes or various cell lines. A metabotropic glutamate receptor coupled to PI hydrolysis was cloned by injecting progressively smaller pools of cDNA into oocytes and then using PI hydrolysis assays to determine which gene confers glutamate-stimulated PI hydrolysis. Using this approach, two groups

cloned the first metabotropic glutamate receptor gene, mGluR1. Hydrophobicity analysis of the deduced amino acid sequence suggested seven transmembrane domains similar to other G-protein coupled receptors. However, mGluR1 shares no sequence homology to other G-protein coupled receptors, indicating that mGluRs form a distinct gene family.

Cloning of other members of the mGluR family was accomplished using low-stringency hybridization of DNA probes derived from mGluR1 looking for mGluRs presumably containing similar sequences. Hybridization approaches uncovered the remainder of mGluRs cloned thus far, mGluR2 to mGluR8. Alternative splicing of many of these mGluR genes results in further diversity among mGluR proteins.

The cloning of eight mGluR subtypes immensely expanded the study of mGluRs as these clones were expressed in heterologous systems to determine coupling to second-messenger systems, establish pharmacological profiles with glutamate analogues, and screen for novel subtype-specific pharmacological agents. Based on sequence homology, pharmacological profile and second-messenger coupling, mGluR subtypes can be classified into three different groups (**Figure 14.1**).

The mGluRs in group I include mGluR1 and mGluR5. These receptors share approximately 60% sequence identity, and appear to couple primarily to PI hydrolysis in heterologous expression systems. The group-I mGluRs are most potently activated by quisqualate, and are selectively activated by 3,5-dihydroxyphenylglycine (DHPG). The group-II mGluRs, which include mGluR2 and mGluR3, inhibit adenylyl cyclase in expression systems. These receptors have about 70% sequence identity with each other, but less than 50% homology with the six other mGluR clones. The group-II mGluRs are potently and selectively activated by (2S,2′R,3′R)-2-(2′,3′-dicarboxycyclopropyl)glycine (DCG-IV) and (2R,4R)-4-aminopyrrolidine-2,4-dicarboxylate (2R,4R-APDC). The group-III mGluRs (mGluR4, mGluR6, mGluR7 and mGluR8) also couple to inhibition of adenylyl cyclase in cell lines. The group-III mGluRs share approximately

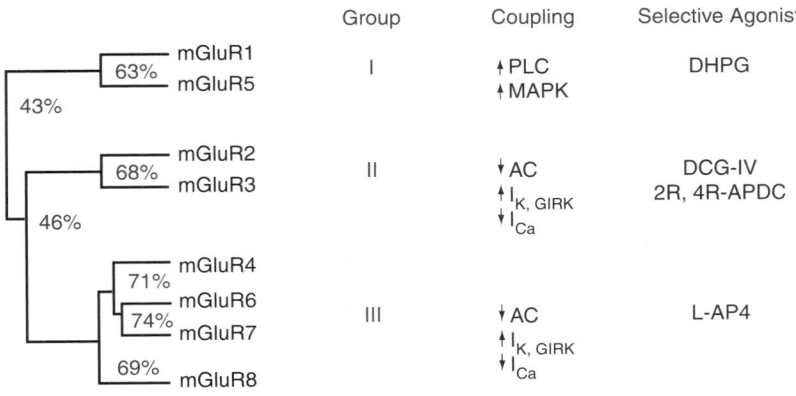

Figure 14.1 Classification of mGluRs.

mGluRs can be divided into three groups based on amino acid identity (left), second-messenger coupling (centre) and pharmacology (right). The dendrogram on the left indicates the percentage identity between various clones at the amino acid level. Coupling mechanisms in the centre indicate the biochemical actions of different mGluR groups as determined in expression systems.

70% sequence identity within the group, and less than 50% identity with the other four mGluRs. L-2-amino-4-phosphonobutyric acid (L-AP4) is the most potent and selective agonist of group-III mGluRs. In addition to inhibition of adenylyl cyclase function, the mGluRs in groups II and III potently activate G-protein coupled potassium channels, known as GIRKs (*G*-protein coupled *I*nwardly *R*ectifying K^+ channels). Pharmacological evidence obtained from brain slice studies indicates that additional mGluR subtypes exist that have not yet been cloned.

14.2 How do metabotropic glutamate receptors carry out their function? – Structure–function studies of metabotropic glutamate receptors

The main function of mGluRs is to activate G proteins upon glutamate binding. Therefore, a logical first step in understanding mGluR function is to determine regions responsible for agonist binding versus regions responsible for G protein coupling. Hydrophobicity analysis of various mGluRs suggests a large extracellular N-terminus with a signal peptide, followed by seven transmembrane domains, and terminating with a cytoplasmic C-terminal tail. While seven transmembrane domains are found in other G-protein coupled receptors, the large N-terminal domain of mGluRs is a divergent structural feature. A simple early hypothesis postulated that the N-terminal domain is responsible for agonist binding, while the transmembrane domains and cytoplasmic loops are responsible for G protein coupling and other functions. Given this hypothesis, a chimera containing a group-II mGluR N-terminal domain followed by the remainder of a group-I mGluR would have the agonist profile of group-II mGluRs (activation by DCG-IV), but the second-messenger coupling of group-I mGluRs (stimulation of PI hydrolysis). As shown in **Figure 14.2**, the predicted result occurred as DCG-IV led to increased PI hydrolysis in the chimera, while having little effect on PI hydrolysis with a group-I or group-II mGluR. Conversely, quisqualate, a group-I agonist, was ineffective at stimulating PI hydrolysis with the chimera or group-II mGluR, but stimulated PI turnover with a group-I mGluR.

Further support for the idea that the N-terminal domain mediates agonist binding is the finding that this domain shares weak sequence homology with bacterial periplasmic amino acid binding proteins. Based on the known crystal structures of these bacterial proteins, the N-terminal domain of mGluRs was modelled as a 'Venus flytrap'-like structure, which clamps together upon ligand binding. Consistent with this model, point mutations of residues modelled to be critical for ligand binding dramatically reduced agonist binding. Finally, the most convincing evidence for a N-terminal agonist binding domain is that expression of this domain alone results in a protein which binds agonist similar to the corresponding full-length mGluR.

Metabotropic glutamate receptors must somehow convert the binding of glutamate by the N-terminal domain into G protein activation. Regions responsible for activating G proteins by other G-protein coupled receptors, such as β-adrenergic receptors and rhodopsin, have been extensively studied. As mentioned earlier, other G-protein coupled receptors contain seven transmembrane domains with three intracellular loops and a cytoplasmic C-terminal tail. Certain regions in other G-protein coupled receptors determine the efficacy of transducing ligand binding to G protein

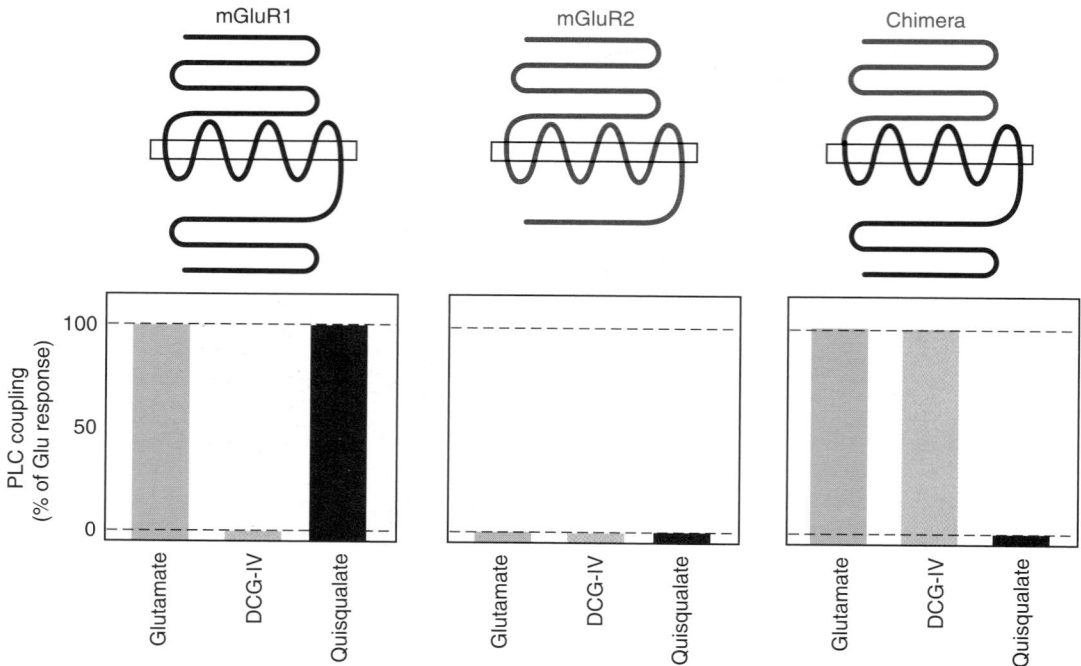

Figure 14.2 Determination of the ligand-binding domain of mGluRs.
In these experiments, the PLC-coupled receptor, mGluR1 and the AC-coupled receptor, mGluR2, were expressed in cells and their coupling to PLC was measured. It was found that the group-I agonist quisqualate, but not the group-II agonist DCG-IV, stimulated PI hydrolysis in the mGluR1-expressing cells, but neither stimulated PI hydrolysis in mGluR2-expressing cells, since mGluR2 does not normally couple to PLC. When the large N-terminal domain of mGluR1 is replaced with the comparable domain from mGluR2, the mGluR2 agonist DCG-IV now stimulated PI hydrolysis in cells expressing this chimeric receptor, whereas the group-I agonist quisqualate now has no effect. Adapted from Takahashi K, Tsuchida K, Taneba Y *et al.* (1993) Role of the large extracellular domain of metabotropic glutamate receptors in agonist selectivity determination, *J. Biol. Chem.* **268**, 19341–19345, with permission.

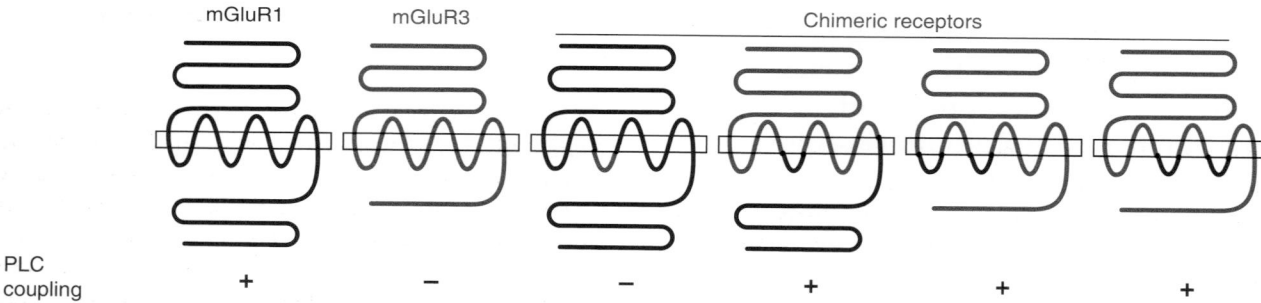

Figure 14.3 Determining regions responsible for the G-protein coupling specificity of mGluRs.
In these experiments, the G_o/G_q-coupled receptor mGluR1 and the G_i-coupled receptor mGluR3 were expressed in cells and their coupling to PLC was measured. It was found that if the second intracellular loop from mGluR1 was replaced with that of mGluR3, all PLC coupling was lost. However, if the second intracellular loop of mGluR3 was replaced with that of mGluR1 along with any of the other intracellular domains from mGluR1, this mGluR3/mGluR1 chimera now couples efficiently to PLC. Adapted from Gomeza J, Joly C, Kuhn R *et al.* (1996) The second intracellular loop of metabotropic glutamate receptor 1 cooperates with other intracellular domains to control coupling to G-proteins, *J. Biol. Chem.* **271**, 2199–2205, with permission.

activation, while other regions determine the specificity or which G proteins are activated after ligand binding. In these G-protein coupled receptors, the second and third intracellular loops play critical roles in coupling efficacy and specificity, respectively. Conversely, chimera studies have identified the second intracellular loop in metabotropic glutamate receptors as the major determinant of coupling specificity with all of the other

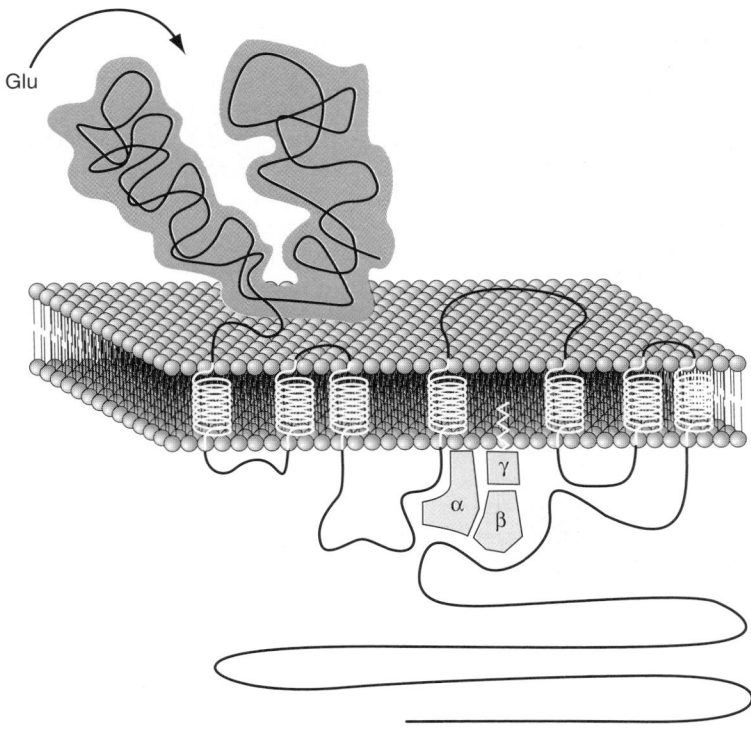

Figure 14.4 Structural model of the metabotropic glutamate receptor family.

intracellular loops contributing to efficacy. For example, a chimera of mGluR3 with the second intracellular loop and cytoplasmic tail of mGluR1 couples to phospholipase C, thus exhibiting the G protein specificity of mGluR1 (**Figure 14.3**).

At first glance, the difference in regions involved in G-protein coupling specificity and the lack of sequence homology between mGluRs and other G-protein coupled receptors may suggest a different structure for the mGluRs. However, the second intracellular loop of mGluRs is predicted to form amphipathic alpha-helices similar to the third intracellular loop of other G-protein coupled receptors. Furthermore, the same amino acid residues on G-protein α-subunits are critical for coupling to both mGluRs and other G-protein coupled receptors. Therefore, while the specific regions involved may differ, the general structural strategy utilized to activate G-proteins is probably shared among all G-protein coupled receptors.

As a result of numerous structure–function studies on mGluRs, a general model of mGluR structure has been developed (**Figure 14.4**). This model includes the large amino-terminal 'Venus flytrap'-like ligand-binding domain attached to a seven transmembrane spanning region reminiscent of other G-protein coupled receptors, with the second intracellular loop being primarily responsible for determining G-protein coupling specificity.

14.3 What biochemical means do metabotropic glutamate receptors utilize to elicit physiological changes in the nervous system? – Signal transduction studies of metabotropic glutamate receptors

Once activated by glutamate, mGluRs initiate a host of intracellular biochemical cascades, which eventually change the physiological behaviour of those cells. As G-protein coupled receptors, they activate heterotrimeric G-proteins, which consist of the GTP hydrolysing α-subunit and a membrane-bound complex of β- and γ-subunits. When G proteins are activated, the α-subunit exchanges GDP with GTP and dissociates from the βγ complex. Both the activated, GTP-bound α-subunit and the freed βγ complex now initiate various downstream processes. βγ-subunits are known to directly modulate the activity of various ion channels, including potassium and calcium channels. For example, group-II and group-III mGluRs activate potassium channels and inhibit calcium channels probably through direct coupling of βγ-subunits. βγ-subunits can also modulate cAMP formation by altering adenylyl cyclase activity. While βγ-subunits execute important functions, historically, the classification and study of G proteins has concentrated on α-subunit function. Two major avenues of α-subunit signalling are the modulation of adenylyl cyclases and phospholipases.

As mentioned earlier, the discovery of metabotropic glutamate receptors was initiated by the finding that glutamate stimulates PI hydrolysis. Phospholipids are major constituents of cell membranes and in addition play a variety of important roles in intracellular signalling. One important phospholipid in intracellular signalling is phosphotidylinositol (PI) and its derivative phosphotidylinositol 4,5-bisphosphate (PIP2). Phospholipases hydrolyse phospholipids including phosphotidylinositols and are classified based on the phospholipid substrate and location of hydrolysis. Phospholipase C hydrolyses PIP2 releasing the inositol moiety as inositol triphosphate (IP3) and forming the membrane-bound, lipid moiety diacylglycerol (DAG). Therefore, a simple way to follow phospholipase C activity is to load cells with radioactively labelled inositol and then determine the release of inositol from the membrane or organic fraction to the cytoplasmic or aqueous fraction. When neuronal cultures or slices from various regions in the brain are loaded with ^{3}H-inositol (which is then incorporated into membrane phospholipids), glutamate stimulation increases the fraction of inositol found in the aqueous fraction, indicating phospholipase C hydrolysis of PIP2.

Based on pharmacological studies of glutamate-stimulated PI hydrolysis in the brain and studies of cloned mGluRs, it is now known that group-I mGluRs (subtypes 1 and 5) stimulate PI hydrolysis. These mGluRs couple to G proteins (mainly G_q), whose α-subunits activate phospholipase C. Phospholipase C hydrolyses PIP2 and causes a rise in intracellular levels of DAG and IP3. IP3 is a potent stimulator of Ca^{2+} release from internal stores, and DAG along with Ca^{2+} activates protein kinase C. DAG may also be further processed to yield various lipid messengers, including arachidonic acid. Therefore, group-I mGluRs exert many of their physiological effects through changes in lipid messengers, intracellular Ca^{2+}, and protein kinase C activation.

Group-II and group-III mGluRs couple to G proteins whose α-subunits modulate adenylyl cyclase activity. The main G proteins coupled to adenylyl cyclase are G_s and G_i, whose α-subunits stimulate and inhibit adenylyl cyclase activity, respectively. Similar to determining phospholipase C activity, adenylyl cyclase activity and stimulation of cAMP formation are measured by loading cultures or slices with radioactively labelled adenine (which is incorporated into intracellular ATP pools) and following its incorporation into cAMP. Activity of both group-II and group-III mGluRs inhibits forskolin-stimulated cAMP accumulation in expression systems and neuronal cultures or

slices. However, a more relevant issue is the effect of group-II and group-III mGluRs on neurotransmitter-induced increases in cAMP accumulation in native systems. Interestingly, group-II mGluR agonists potentiate cAMP accumulation induced by stimulation of β-adrenergic receptors and other G_s coupled receptors. In this case, released G-protein βγ-subunits may actually potentiate type II adenylyl cyclase activation by G_s α-subunits. Conversely, group-III mGluRs inhibit neurotransmitter-induced increases in cAMP, probably through G_i α-subunit activation. Therefore, group-II and group-III mGluRs may exert physiological effects by altering intracellular cAMP levels. However, repeated attempts to find physiological roles for group-II and group-III mGluRs involving changes in intracellular cAMP levels have been unsuccessful, with one exception. In hippocampus, a form of glial–neuron signalling occurs in which group-II mGluRs potentiate cAMP formation induced by β-adrenergic receptors in glial cells. Cyclic AMP metabolites from glia are then released and activate adenosine receptors on nearby neurons, thereby modulating synaptic transmission.

While most studies have concentrated on the roles of PI hydrolysis and cAMP formation in mGluR signalling, other avenues are also becoming increasingly apparent. mGluRs in groups II and III can activate GIRK channels through G-protein βγ subunits. The relative dearth of evidence for group-II and group-III mGluR modulation of cAMP levels leading to physiological effects may indicate that activation of GIRK channels plays an equal or even greater role in the physiology of mGluRs in groups II and III. Indeed, mGluRs in groups II and III seem to couple to these channels more efficiently than to inhibition of cAMP formation in expression systems.

In hippocampus, an mGluR with novel pharmacology has been found to increase the activity of phospholipase D, which metabolizes phosphatidylcholine (PC) into phosphatidic acid (PA) and choline. Subsequent degradation of PA results in the formation of DAG, which stimulates PKC. Interestingly, this mGluR activity seems to be more potently activated by L-cysteine sulphinic acid (L-CSA) over glutamate. In addition to this phospholipase D-coupled receptor, other lines of evidence indicate that L-CSA may be an endogenous neurotransmitter.

Finally, in cultured glial cells and expression systems, group-I mGluRs activate mitogen-activated protein kinase (MAPK), possibly through phosphoinositide 3-kinase (PI3K). Given that MAPK signalling has been implicated in nervous system development and synaptic plasticity, mGluR-mediated activation of MAPK may add great diversity to the roles mGluRs play in the nervous system.

14.4 What are the functions of metabotropic glutamate receptors in the nervous system? – Physiological and genetic studies of mGluRs

mGluRs modulate two major neuronal functions: excitability and synaptic transmission. Altered excitability is mainly exhibited by changes in the threshold for action potential firing or firing pattern after reaching threshold. A powerful mechanism for altering neuronal excitability is to modulate potassium channels. Potentiation of potassium channel function leads to reduced excitability, while inhibition of potassium channel function results in enhanced excitability.

An early experiment involving mGluR-mediated effects on neuronal excitability showed that application of glutamate and related agonists onto hippocampal pyramidal neurons inhibits spike accommodation, a reduction in spike frequency during a suprathreshold depolarizing stimulus (**Figure 14.5**). While many fast-activating potassium currents are involved in spike repolarization, slower activating currents are involved in spike frequency maintenance and accommodation. One of these currents is $I_{K,AHP}$ (potassium *after*hyperpolarization current), a potassium current activated by rises in intracellular Ca^{2+} which occur during repetitive firing. Inhibition of $I_{K,AHP}$ leads to reduced potassium efflux during repetitive firing and therefore firing fails to accommodate. Since $I_{K,AHP}$ is dependent on intracellular Ca^{2+} levels, inhibition of $I_{K,AHP}$ by mGluRs may be due to reduced Ca^{2+} influx with repetitive firing or a direct inhibition of Ca^{2+}-activated potassium channels. In hippocampal neurons, glutamate did not affect calcium currents with depolarizing stimuli (**Figure 14.5**). Therefore, the inhibition of $I_{K,AHP}$ must be mediated by a direct inhibition of potassium channels. $I_{K,AHP}$ inhibition by glutamate was concluded to be mGluR-mediated, since ionotropic antagonists failed to block the inhibition. Furthermore, group-I mGluR agonists replicated $I_{K,AHP}$ inhibition, while agonists in groups II or III had little effect. Interestingly, mice genetically engineered to lack mGluR1 still exhibited $I_{K,AHP}$ inhibition induced by a group-I mGluR agonist, suggesting that this inhibition is likely to be mediated by mGluR5.

Several groups using different preparations have shown that mGluR agonists depolarize neurons. This depolarization is associated with an increase in membrane resistance, thereby suggesting inhibition of a hyperpolarizing current rather than activation of a depolarizing current. Two conductances underlie this hyperpolarizing current, a voltage-independent potassium conductance termed $I_{K,leak}$ and a voltage-dependent current activated near rest termed $I_{K,M}$. Inhibition of $I_{K,leak}$ leads to depolarization, which can either modulate suprathreshold cell firing or result in a subthreshold depolarization. The pharmacological profile in hippocampal neurons suggests that group-I mGluRs mediate the inhibition of $I_{K,leak}$. While G-protein inhibitors block the effect of group-I mGluR agonists, general protein kinase inhibitors had little effect, suggesting a direct inhibition of $I_{K,leak}$ by G-proteins rather than via kinases.

mGluRs can also excite neurons by activating non-selective cation currents. These conductances are often ill-defined, but can include activation of Na^+/Ca^{2+} exchangers, Ca^{2+}-activated non-selective cation conductances (I_{CAN}), and Ca^{2+} independent non-selective cation conductances. In CA3 pyramidal neurons and in dorsal root ganglion neurons, mGluR agonists induce cation conductances. In CA3 neurons, these conductances seem to be mysteriously activated independent of G proteins, while in dorsal root ganglion neurons, these conductances are activated by rises in intracellular Ca^{2+} as a result of IP3 production.

Although the discussion thus far has centred around mGluR-mediated increases in neuronal excitability through inhibition of potassium conductances or activation of non-selective cation currents, in certain preparations, mGluR activation can reduce excitability and induce hyperpolarization. For example, a group-II mGluR agonist induces a potassium conductance based hyperpolarization in basolateral amygdala neurons. In cerebellar Golgi cells, group-II mGluR agonists activate GIRK currents. Given these examples of reduction in neuronal excitability mediated by a group-II mGluR, and the previously mentioned illustrations of increase in excitability mediated by a group-I mGluR, an emerging hypothesis may be that group-I mGluRs generally increase excitability, while mGluRs in groups II and III generally reduce excitability.

mGluR modulation of calcium channels bridges changes in neuronal excitability and synaptic transmission. Calcium channels help generate the action potential upstroke in certain neurons and also mediate the calcium influx required for synaptic transmission. Furthermore, calcium influx at various locations within neurons results in the activation of multiple signal-transduction pathways. In general, mGluRs inhibit calcium currents, and the specific subtype of calcium current varies depending on the preparation. For example, mGluR agonists inhibit L-type, but not N-type, currents in acutely isolated neocortical neurons. However, in cultured cortical and cerebellar granule cells, mGluR activation inhibits both N- and L-type calcium currents. Finally, in hippocampal CA3 pyramidal neurons, mGluR agonists inhibit N-type currents, but not L-type currents. In pyramidal neurons, the agonist profile seems to match the profile for group-I mGluRs. This modulation of N-type currents seems to involve a

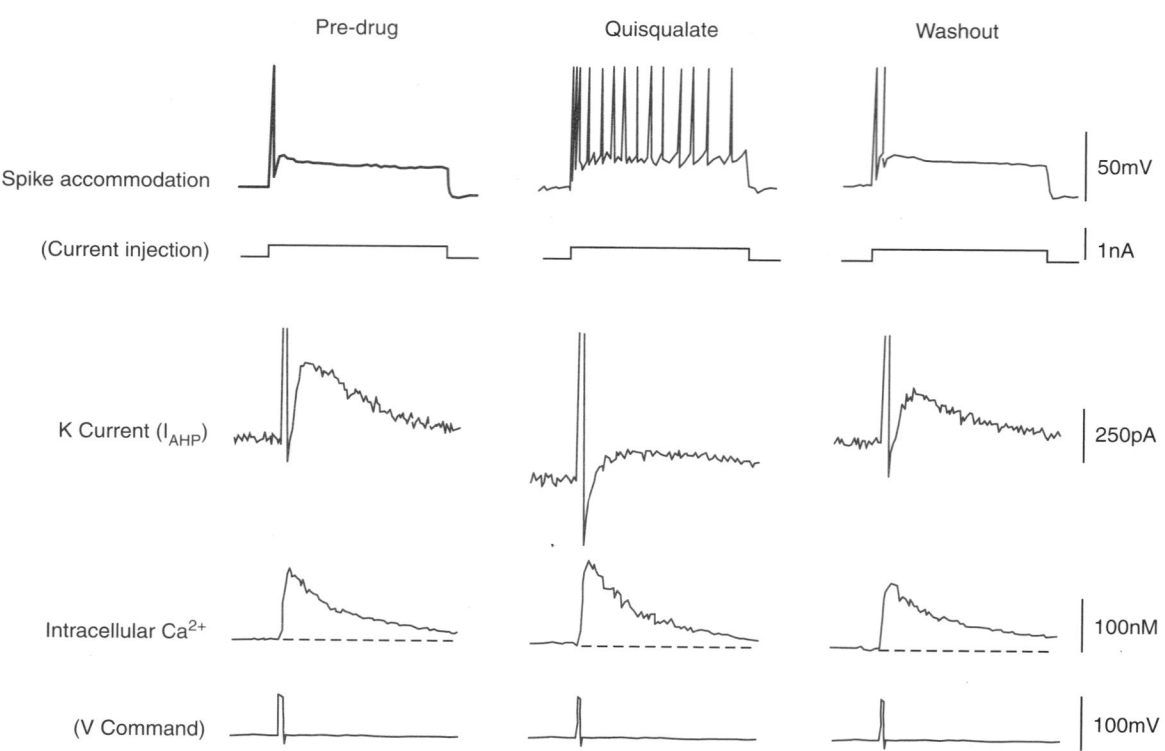

	Pre-drug	Quisqualate	Washout	

Figure 14.5 Modulation of action potential accomodation by inhibition of a calcium-dependent potassium current, rather than calcium influx.

The top row shows the action potential firing pattern in response to a prolonged depolarizing current injection in hippocampal neurons. Only one to two action potentials normally fire even in the presence of a suprathreshold stimulus, since depolarization-induced calcium influx activates $I_{K,AHP}$. The middle row shows the late outward potassium current, $I_{K,AHP}$ under voltage clamp conditions, while the bottom row shows the calcium influx as measured by fluorescence-based techniques. The spike accommodation is reversibly blocked by the group-I mGluR agonist, quisqualate, as is the $I_{K,AHP}$ current. However, the magnitude of the intracellular calcium response is not altered by quisqualate, indicating that group-I mGluRs directly modulate the $I_{K,AHP}$ channel, rather than the calcium influx that activates the channel. Adapted from Charpak S, Gahwiler BH, Do KQ, Knopfel T (1990) Potassium conductances in hippocampal neurons blocked by excitatory amino acid transmitters, *Nature* **347**, 765–767, with permission.

membrane delimited mechanism, such as direct coupling of calcium channels with G-protein βγ-subunits. When a group-I mGluR agonist is applied outside of a cell-attached patch, it has no effect on N-type calcium currents within the patch, indicating that a freely diffusible second messenger is not responsible for the modulation. However, when a group-I mGluR agonist is applied to an outside-out patch, N-type calcium currents are inhibited, indicating that factors responsible for modulation reside in the membrane (**Figure 14.6**).

Besides altering neuronal excitability, mGluRs modulate synaptic transmission. In general, mGluR effects on synaptic transmission can be divided simply into presynaptic and postsynaptic. Presynaptically, mGluRs typically act as glutamate autoreceptors, decreasing glutamate release from presynaptic nerve terminals. mGluRs can also act as heteroreceptors on GABAergic nerve terminals, where they reduce GABA release. The presynaptic mGluR action of reducing transmitter

release is quite ubiquitous, occurring in various brain regions and is not restricted to any single group of mGluRs. As an example, in adult hippocampal CA1, both group-I and group-III mGluRs seem to serve as autoreceptors depressing evoked synaptic transmission (**Figure 14.7**). Pharmacological and immunocytochemical studies mainly point to mGluR5 as the group-I autoreceptor and mGluR7 as the group-III autoreceptor, although other receptor subtypes may also be involved.

The mechanisms for depression of synaptic transmission mediated by mGluRs in groups I and III are partially understood. A presynaptic origin, as opposed to a postsynaptic one, must first be determined. In general, two main presynaptic mechanisms can be envisioned for reduced synaptic transmission: (i) a decrease in presynaptic calcium influx, or (ii) a decrease in release probability downstream of calcium influx. A first step in deciphering these mechanisms is to examine miniature excitatory postsynaptic potentials or currents

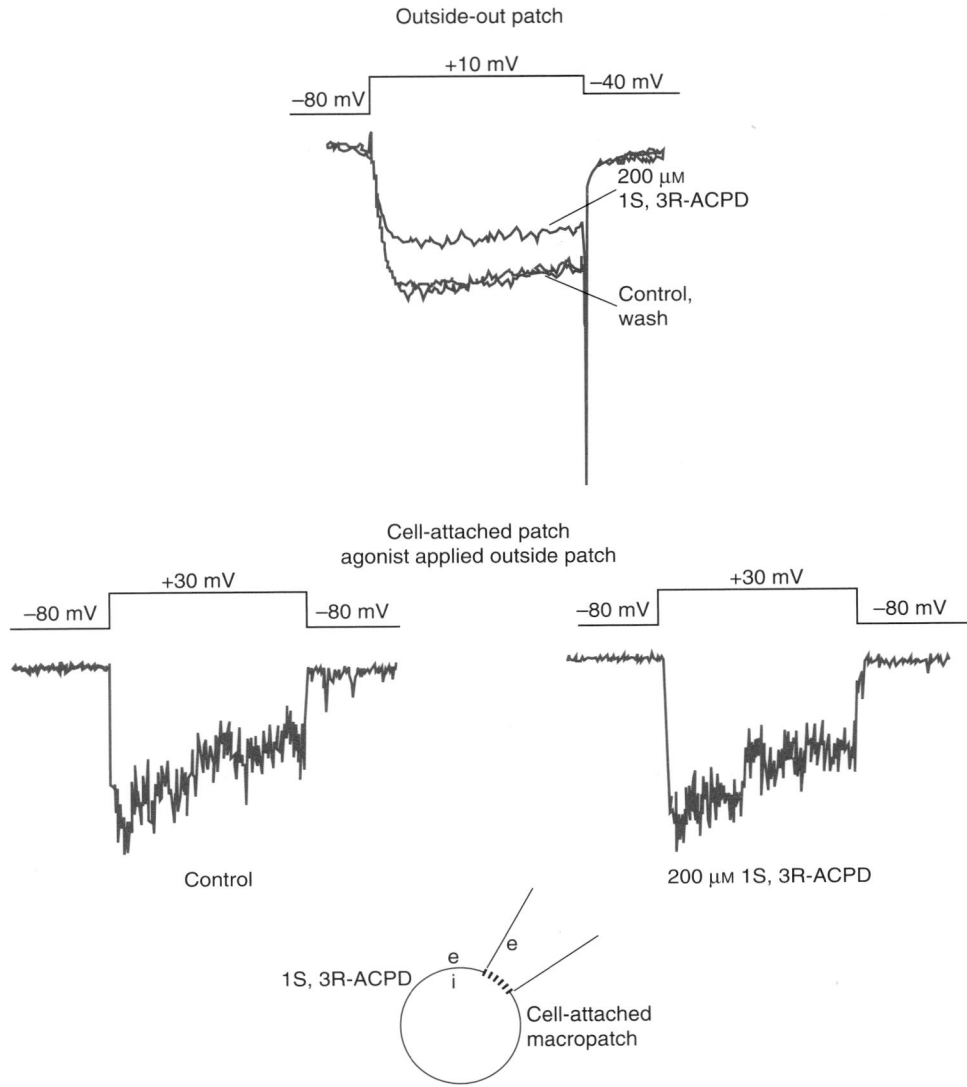

Figure 14.6 mGluR-mediated inhibition of voltage-activated calcium currents in hippocampal pyramidal cells by a membrane delimited mechanism.

The left panel shows a recording of macroscopic calcium currents from a rat CA3 pyramidal cell outside-out patch. The membrane was held at −80 mV and stepped to +10 mV, resulting in activation of voltage-sensitive calcium channels. When 200 μM of *t*-ACPD was applied to the surface of the patch, a reversible reduction of the calcium current resulted. However, when macroscopic calcium currents were recorded in the cell-attached mode and the agonist was applied outside the patch, *t*-ACPD had no effect. These findings suggest that the mGluR-mediated reduction in calcium currents is not mediated by a readily diffusible second messenger in these cells. Adapted from Swartz KJ, Bean BP (1992) Inhibition of calcium channels in rat CA3 pyramidal neurons by a metabotropic glutamate receptor, *J. Neurosci.* **12**, 4358–4371, with permission.

('miniatures' or 'minis'). Miniatures are spontaneous events occurring in the absence of action potentials. Operationally, they are often defined as events occurring in the presence of TTX, which blocks voltage-dependent sodium channels and therefore action potential firing. In classic quantal analysis, miniature frequency is usually determined by the presynaptic release probability, while miniature amplitude is deter-

mined by postsynaptic sensitivity to transmitter. Often, but not always, miniature frequency is independent of action-potential-driven presynaptic calcium influx. A simple verification of this hypothesis is to demonstrate that miniature frequency is unaffected by general calcium-channel blockers; a prediction that seems to hold in adult hippocampal area CA1. When a group-I mGluR agonist is applied, miniature frequency and amplitude are unaffected, thereby indicating that the most likely mechanism for inhibiting evoked release is calcium-channel inhibition (**Figure 14.7**). Earlier it was mentioned that group-I mGluRs were found to inhibit N-type calcium currents. Since N-type calcium channels, but not L-type channels, are commonly found at nerve terminals, it seems plausible that group-I mGluRs inhibit synaptic transmission by reducing calcium influx at synaptic terminals. Conversely, when a group-III mGluR agonist is applied, a significant reduction in miniature frequency is observed, with no effect on miniature amplitude, indicating a reduction in presynaptic release probability (**Figure 14.7**).

While mGluRs ubiquitously act presynaptically as auto- and heteroreceptors, they execute subtype- and location-specific postsynaptic roles. In cerebellar Purkinje cells, postsynaptic mGluR1 plays a pivotal role in synaptic plasticity. Purkinje cells receive excitatory inputs from climbing fibres and parallel fibres. When these inputs are conjunctively stimulated, it results in a long-term depression (LTD) of the parallel-fibre/Purkinje-cell synaptic response. Based on a large body of evidence, it has been established that LTD of the parallel-fibre/Purkinje-cell synapse requires voltage-gated calcium-channel activation in Purkinje cells, presumably due to climbing fibre input and ionotropic and metabotropic glutamate receptor activation secondary to parallel fibre stimulation. When various mGluR agonists are paired with Ca^{2+} spike firing in Purkinje cells, only group-I mGluR agonists are effective in inducing LTD. Furthermore, when Purkinje cell depolarization is paired with glutamate application to induce LTD, the presence of specific mGluR1 blocking antibodies prevents LTD. Finally, Purkinje cell LTD cannot be induced in mice with a targeted disruption of the mGluR1 gene (see **Figure 21.19**). At the behavioural level, LTD is thought to play a role in motor learning. Mice lacking mGluR1 exhibit ataxia and deficient eye-blink

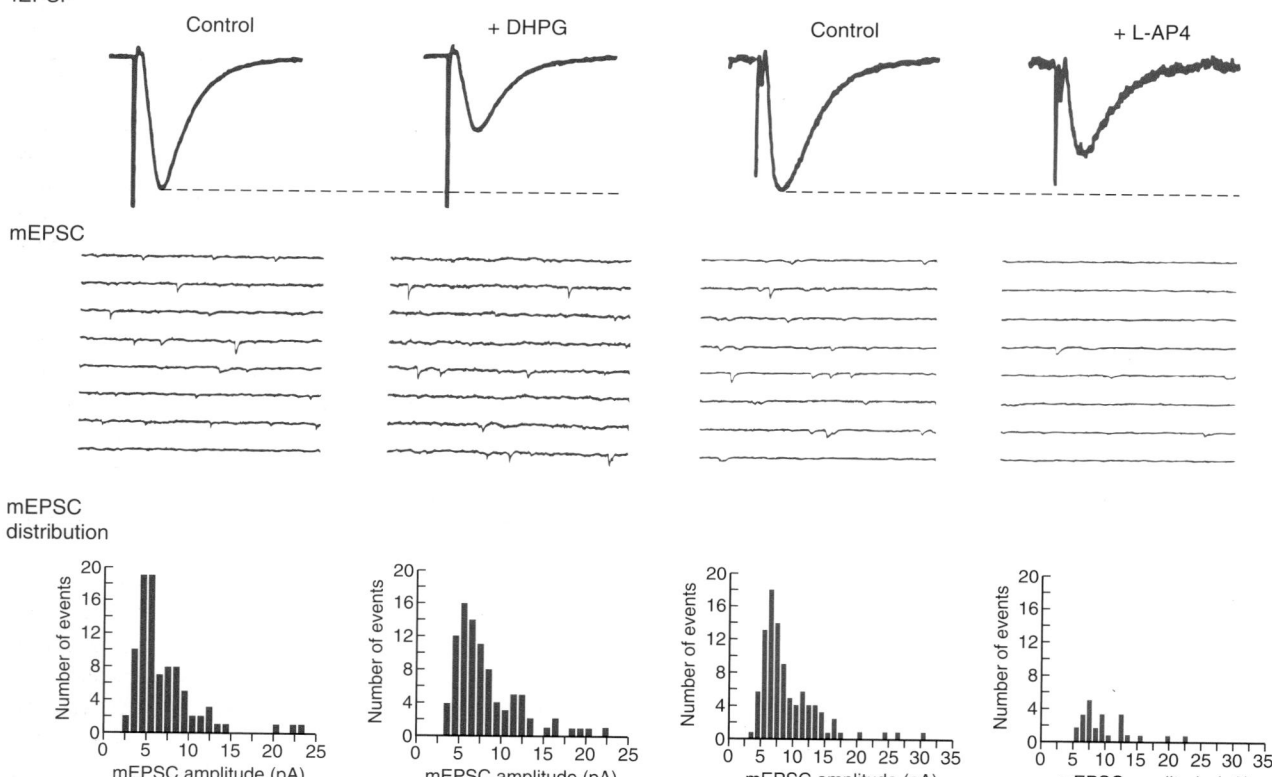

Figure 14.7 Different mechanisms involved in group-I and group-III mGluR modulation of synaptic transmission in hippocampal area CA1.

The top panel shows that the group-I agonist DHPG, and the group III agonist L-AP4, both reduce synaptic transmission at the CA3–CA1 synapse. The bottom panel histograms show that DHPG does not affect mini amplitude or frequency and L-AP4 does not affect mini amplitude, but does reduce mini frequency. The lack of effect on mini amplitude by either drug indicates a presynaptic origin. L-AP4 seems to modulate transmission at this synapse by reducing release probability, whereas DHPG likely reduces voltage-activated calcium influx. Adapted from Gereau RW, Conn PJ (1995) Multiple presynpatic metabotropic glutamate receptors modulate excitatory and inhibitory synaptic transmission in hippocampal area CA1, *J. Neurosci.* **15**, 6879–6889, with permission.

conditioning. Interestingly, some human patients with paraneoplastic syndromes involving ataxia have high serum titres of anti-mGluR1 antibodies. These antibodies have been shown to be effective at blocking mGluR1 function, and the titre of these antibodies correlates well with the degree of ataxia. Finally, injection of serum from these patients into rodents causes ataxia. The mechanism for the role of mGluR1 in LTD is not well understood; but a rise in intracellular Ca^{2+}, activation of PKC, and activation of protein kinase G through nitric oxide (NO) production and guanylyl cyclase activation, are all involved in LTD. Given the previous discussion, all of these events could potentially lie downstream of mGluR1 activation.

In hippocampal CA1 neurons, mGluRs modulate postsynaptic ligand-gated ion channels. Specifically, group-I mGluR agonists potentiate NMDA receptor currents, while having little effect on AMPA receptor currents (see **Figure 21.8**). Such modification of postsynaptic currents may play a role in synaptic plasticity, such as long-term potentiation (LTP) of CA1 pyramidal neurons. In hippocampal CA1 LTP, repetitive stimulation of the input Schaffer collateral pathway results in persistently increased excitatory synaptic responses. Induction of CA1 LTP is NMDA-dependent, while the expression of CA1 LTP may occur through potentiation of both the non-NMDA and NMDA components of glutamatergic synpatic responses. Since group-I mGluRs potentiate NMDA currents, group-I mGluRs may ease LTP induction and play a role in the expression of potentiated NMDA responses. Consistent with this idea, mGluR activation facilitates induction of CA1 LTP (see **Figure 21.8**). Furthermore, mice lacking mGluR5 are specifically deficient in the NMDA component of LTP, while having normal non-NMDA LTP. Against this hypothesis, several groups have reported conflicting evidence on the effect of mGluR antagonists on LTP, which may be due to different stimulation paradigms and experimental conditions. However, the ability of group-I mGluRs to modulate NMDA receptors has been repeatedly confirmed in many preparations, including hippocampal neurons, spinal cord neurons, and expression systems.

mGluRs modulate both neuronal excitability and synaptic transmission. In general, with possible exceptions, group-I mGluRs increase neuronal excitability by inhibiting potassium channels and activating non-selective cationic currents, while mGluRs in groups II and III reduce neuronal excitability by activating potassium channels such as GIRKs. Members of all three mGluR groups can act to depress synaptic transmission as autoreceptors and heteroreceptors throughout various brain regions. Finally, specific mGluR groups at certain locations modify synaptic transmission postsynaptically by various mechanisms.

14.5 How are metabotropic glutamate receptors specifically localized in neurons to execute their functions? – Studies of mGluR postsynaptic localization

In order for mGluRs to carry out their functions, they must be properly localized within neurons. For instance, mGluRs must be located postsynaptically at or near synaptic contact sites in order to 'see' glutamate and modify synaptic transmission. Ultrastructurally, synapses contain electron-dense synaptic densities postsynaptically. Recent studies have begun to uncover the biochemical nature of postsynaptic densities (PSDs) with the identification of PSD proteins. The main breakthrough involved the use of yeast two-hybrid techniques to identify proteins interacting with postsynaptic potassium channels and ionotropic glutamate receptors. These proteins were then utilized to identify other interacting proteins. With the identification of PSD proteins, it has becoming increasingly evident that the PSD is a large multimeric complex, consisting of postsynaptic receptors coupled to scaffold proteins and downstream signalling molecules.

Group-I mGluRs have now been identified as players in the PSD complex. Yeast two-hybrid studies identified the Homer family of proteins, which always contain an N-terminal EVH domain and sometimes contain a C-terminal coiled-coil domain that mediates multimerization of these proteins. The EVH domain was found to bind both mGluR1 and mGluR5 at a consensus sequence consisting of PPXXF. Interestingly, Homer can also bind the IP3 receptor through the EVH domain. Because Homer can multimerize via the coiled-coil domain and interact with both group-I mGluRs and IP3 receptors via the EVH domains, this interaction can place group-I mGluRs in close physical proximity to their downstream effectors. This association may be functionally important, as disruption of these interactions reduces the coupling efficacy of group-I mGluRs to Ca^{2+} release from intracellular stores. Recently, Homer was also found to bind the Shank family of PSD proteins, whose members also contain the PPXXF motif. Furthermore, Shank binds to GKAP (*guanylate kinase-associated protein*), thereby crosslinking the Homer-group-I mGluR complex with the GKAP/PSD-95/NMDA receptor complex. One can now envision the beginnings of a PSD complex consisting of group-I mGluRs, IP3 receptors, Homer, Shank, GKAP, PSD-95 and NMDA receptors (**Figure 14.8**).

Recall that in several preparations, group-I mGluRs are found to modulate NMDA responses, but not AMPA responses. Part of the biochemical answer for this physiological phenomenon probably rests in the physical coupling of group-I mGluRs to NMDA receptors, but not to AMPA receptors in the PSD.

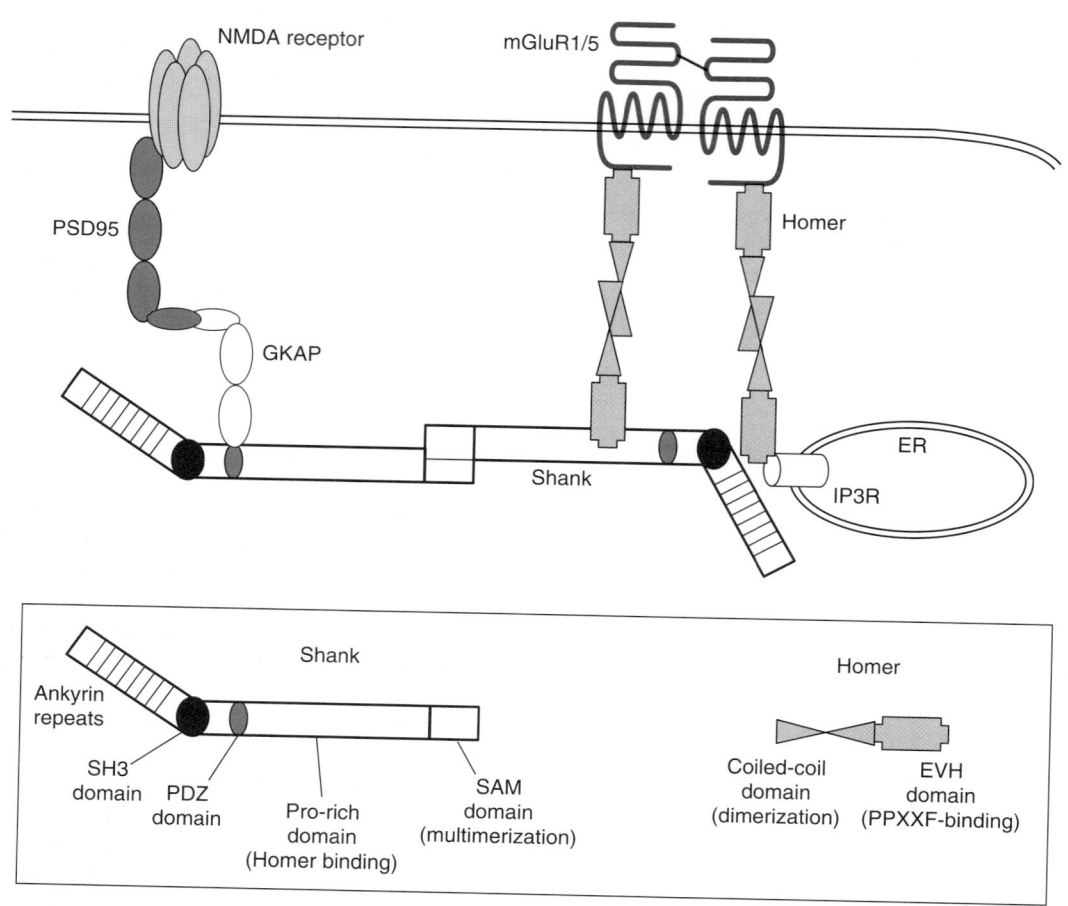

Figure 14.8 Current model for a portion of the glutamatergic postsynaptic density involving NMDA receptors and mGluRs.

14.6 How is the activity of metabotropic glutamate receptors modulated? – Studies of mGluR desensitization

Soon after the discovery that group-I mGluRs underlie glutamate-stimulated PI hydrolysis, it was discovered that preincubation of neuronal cultures or slices with group-I agonists decreases the PI hydrolysis response to subsequent exposures of agonist. This phenomenon commonly occurs with many G-protein coupled receptors and is referred to as *desensitization*. This basically involves a reduced response in the presence of a continuous stimulus. In the case of PI hydrolysis desensitization induced by a group-I mGluR agonist, the reduced response may be due to diminished receptor, G protein, or PLC function. However, studies from β-adrenergic receptors and other G-protein coupled receptors have suggested a major mechanism may be reduced coupling between receptor and G-protein or receptor desensitization. Receptor desensitization is often classified into homologous and heterologous desensitization. The homologous type refers to receptor desensitization that occurs only when the receptor is in a ligand-bound state. Conversely, heterologous desensitization can occur independently of receptor activation. The most common mechanism for reduced receptor to G-protein coupling is phosphorylation of the G-protein coupled receptor. For example, β-adrenergic receptors become desensitized when phosphorylated by β-adrenergic receptor kinase (BARK) or by PKA. BARK phosphorylation occurs only when the β-adrenergic receptor is in a ligand-bound state and therefore is a mechanism for homologous desensitization. In contrast, PKA phosphorylation and β-adrenergic receptor desensitization does not require β-adrenergic receptor activation. Moreover, another receptor, such as a G_s coupled dopamine receptor, may activate PKA leading to β-adrenergic receptor phosphorylation and desensitization to subsequent applications of β-adrenergic agonist. Thus, this PKA-mediated desensitization is classified as heterologous desensitization.

Analogous to β-adrenergic and other G-protein coupled receptors, numerous studies found that protein kinase inhibitors greatly reduced desensitization of PI hydrolysis stimulated by a group-I mGluR.

Subsequently, PKC was determined to be a major determinant of group-I mGluR desensitization, as PKC inhibitors reduced desensitization, while PKC activators enhanced desensitization. Finally, removing PKC phosphorylation consensus sites in mGluR5 produces a receptor highly resistant to desensitization. Since PKC activation does not necessarily require group-I mGluR activation and can occur by other routes, this mechanism fits under the rubric of heterologous desensitization. Therefore, PKC-mediated desensitization of group-I mGluRs represents not only a mechanism for negative feedback, but also a mechanism for crosstalk between different neurotransmitter pathways, as activation of other PKC-coupled neurotransmitter receptors can modulate mGluR activity and signalling.

14.7 Summary

- 'Metabotropic' glutamate receptors were first hypothesized based on glutamate-stimulated, G-protein-dependent PI hydrolysis in various neuronal preparations.
- mGluR1 was cloned using expression cloning. Subsequently, mGluR2 to mGluR8 were cloned using homology-based techniques.
- The mGluRs comprise a novel family of G-protein coupled receptors, which are characterized by a large ligand-binding N-terminal domain and seven transmembrane domains responsible for G-protein coupling.
- The second intracellular loop of mGluRs determines G-protein coupling specificity, while other intracellular loops contribute to coupling efficiency. This differs somewhat from other G-protein coupled receptor families.
- mGluRs can be divided into three groups based on pharmacology, second messenger coupling, and sequence homology:
  Group I – mGluR1 and 5 couple to PLC;
  Group II – mGluR2 and 3 couple to inhibition of AC and activation of GIRK channels;
  Group III – mGluR4, 6, 7 and 8 couple to inhibition of AC and activation of GIRK channels.
- In general, group-I mGluRs tend to increase neuronal excitability by inhibiting potassium conductances and activating non-selective cation currents. Conversely, mGluRs in groups II and III reduce neuronal excitability by activating potassium currents.
- mGluRs act as presynaptic auto- and hetero-receptors, reducing the release of many neurotransmitters. The main mechanisms for presynaptic reduction of transmitter release are inhibiting calcium channels and reducing release probability.

- Postsynaptically, mGluRs mediate location-specific functions in a subtype-specific manner. For example, mGluR1 plays a role in cerebellar LTD, while mGluR5 enhances NMDA currents in hippocampal area CA1.
- mGluRs are specifically localized near postsynaptic contact sites through interactions with PSD proteins, such as Homer and Shank.
- Group I mGluR function is downregulated by PKC-mediated heterologous desensitization. This allows for negative feedback as well as for crosstalk with other transmitter systems.

Further reading

Aiba A, Kano M, Chen C *et al.* (1994) Deficient cerebellar long-term depression and impaired motor learning in mGluR1 mutant mice. *Cell* **79**, 377–388.

Charpak S, Gahwiler BH, Do KQ, Knopfel T (1990) Potassium conductances in hippocampal neurons blocked by excitatory amino acid transmitters. *Nature* **347**, 765–767.

Conn PJ, Pin J-P (1997) Pharmacology and functions of metabotropic glutamate receptors. *Ann. Rev. Pharmacol. Toxicol.* **37**, 205–237.

Gereau RW, Conn PJ (1995) Multiple presynaptic metabotropic glutamate receptors modulate excitatory and inhibitory synaptic transmission in hippocampal area CA1. *J. Neurosci.* **15**, 6879–6889.

Gereau RW, Heinemann SF (1998) Role of protein kinase C phosphorylation in rapid desensitization of metabotropic glutamate receptor 5. *Neuron* **20**, 143–151.

Gomeza J, Joly C, Kuhn R *et al.* (1996) The second intracellular loop of metabotropic glutamate receptor 1 cooperates with other intracellular domains to control coupling to G-proteins. *J. Biol. Chem.* **271**, 2199–2205.

Jia Z, Lu Y, Henderson J *et al.* (1998) Selective abolition of the NMDA component of long-term potentiation in mice lacking mGluR5. *Learn. Mem.* **5**, 331–343.

Pin J-P, Joly C, Heinemann SF, Bockaert J (1994) Domains involved in the specificity of G-protein activation in phospholipase C-coupled metabotropic glutamate receptors. *EMBO J.* **13**, 342–348.

Sladeczek F, Pin J-P, Recasens M *et al.* (1985) Glutamate stimulates inositol phosphate formation in striatal neurons. *Nature* **317**, 717–719.

Smitt PS, Kinoshita A, Leeuw BD *et al.* (2000) Paraneoplastic cerebellar ataxia due to autoantibodies against a glutamate receptor. *New Engl. J. Med.* **342**, 21–27.

Swartz KJ, Bean BP (1992) Inhibition of calcium channels in rat CA3 pyramidal neurons by a metabotropic glutamate receptor. *J. Neurosci.* **12**, 4358–4371.

Takahashi K, Tsuchida K, Taneba Y *et al.* (1993) Role of the large extracellular domain of metabotropic glutamate receptors in agonist selectivity determination. *J. Biol. Chem.* **258**, 19341–19345.

Tu JC, Xiao B, Yuan JP *et al.* (1998) Homer binds a novel proline-rich motif and links group 1 metabotropic glutamate receptors with IP3 receptors. *Neuron* **21**, 717–726.

Tu JC, Xiao B, Naisbitt S *et al.* (1999) Coupling of mGluR/Homer and PSD-95 complexes by the Shank family of postsynaptic density proteins. *Neuron* **23**, 583–592.

The Metabotropic Olfactory Receptors

The olfactory systems of all organisms have the capacity to discriminate between different odorant stimuli. Humans, for example, are capable of distinguishing between thousands of distinct odours. A subtle alteration in the molecular structure of an odorant can lead to a change in the perceived odour. Perception of an odour by the brain can be divided into odorant recognition and neural processing. The first events include the transductory processes, which code the odour stimulation in the generation of propagated action potentials. The second events, the processing of sensory information, occur in the neuronal networks of the olfactory bulb and higher cortical centres.

This chapter focuses on odorant recognition, the initial events that take place in the olfactory neuro-epithelium and more precisely in the olfactory receptor neurons.

15.1 The olfactory receptor cells are sensory neurons located in the olfactory neuroepithelium

15.1.1 The olfactory neurons are bipolar cells that project to the olfactory bulb

The vertebrate olfactory mucosa contains several million sensory neurons that reside in a pseudostratified columnar epithelium 200 μm thick (**Figure 15.1**). Three cell types dominate this epithelium: the olfactory sensory neuron, the sustentacular or supporting cell and the basal cell. The supporting cell is a glia-like cell which secretes part of the mucus components and the basal cell is a stem cell that divides and differentiates throughout life to become functional olfactory sensory neurons.

The olfactory receptor cell is a sensory bipolar neuron that projects a single non-branching dendrite to the epithelial surface and a single unmyelinated axon to the olfactory bulb. Each dendrite terminates in a dendritic knob, which gives rise to 5–20 thin cilia into the nasal lumen. These cilia (0.1–0.2 μm diameter and up to 200 μm long) lie in the thin layer of mucus bathing the epithelial surface. They provide an extensive, receptive surface for the interaction of odours with the cell since they increase the receptive area of an olfactory knob (5 μm^2) up to 100-fold. A small unmyelinated axon projects from the opposite pole of the cell, penetrates through the basement membrane and after making a 90° angle joins between 10 and 100 others to form a bundle of axons ensheathed with Schwann cells. These bundles

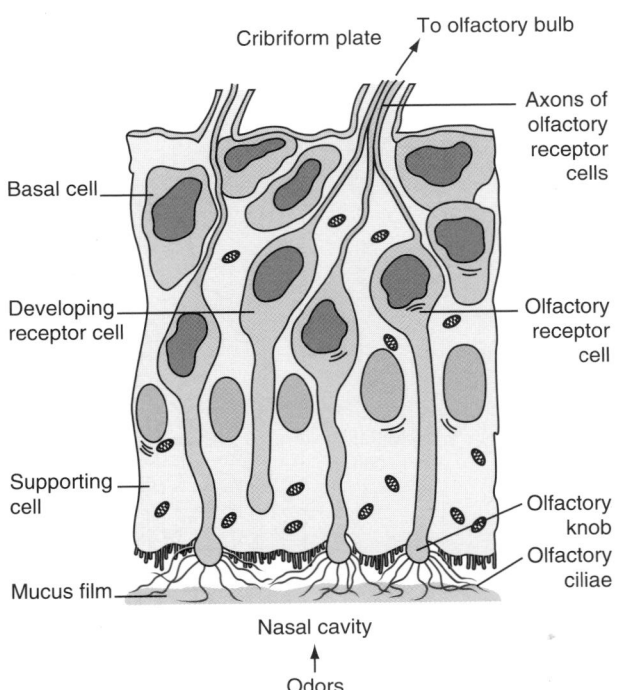

Figure 15.1 Olfactory receptors lie in the olfactory epithelium.

The vertebrate olfactory epithelium is located in the dorsal recess of the nasal cavity, the nasopharynx. It contains olfactory receptor cells, supporting cells and basal cells. Ventilatory air currents bring the odorant molecules to the olfactory mucosa. From Kandel ER, Schwartz JH, Jessel TM (1991) *Principles of Neural Science*, 3rd edn, New York: Elsevier, with permission.

penetrate across the cribriform plate (a porous region of the ethnoid bone), join to form the olfactory nerve (the first cranial nerve) and project to the ipsilateral olfactory bulb. Every axon synapses on to secondary neurons, the mitral cells located in the olfactory bulb where decoding of the odour message is initiated (**Figure 15.2**). This synapse is a complex structure known as a *glomerule* (see

Figure 2.2e) which consists of 100–1000 afferent olfactory axons converging upon the dendritic arbor of a single mitral cell. This allows mitral cells to sample chemosensory information from a wide area of the olfactory epithelium, increasing the chance of detecting small concentrations of odorants that may reach the chemosensory surface in a non-uniform manner.

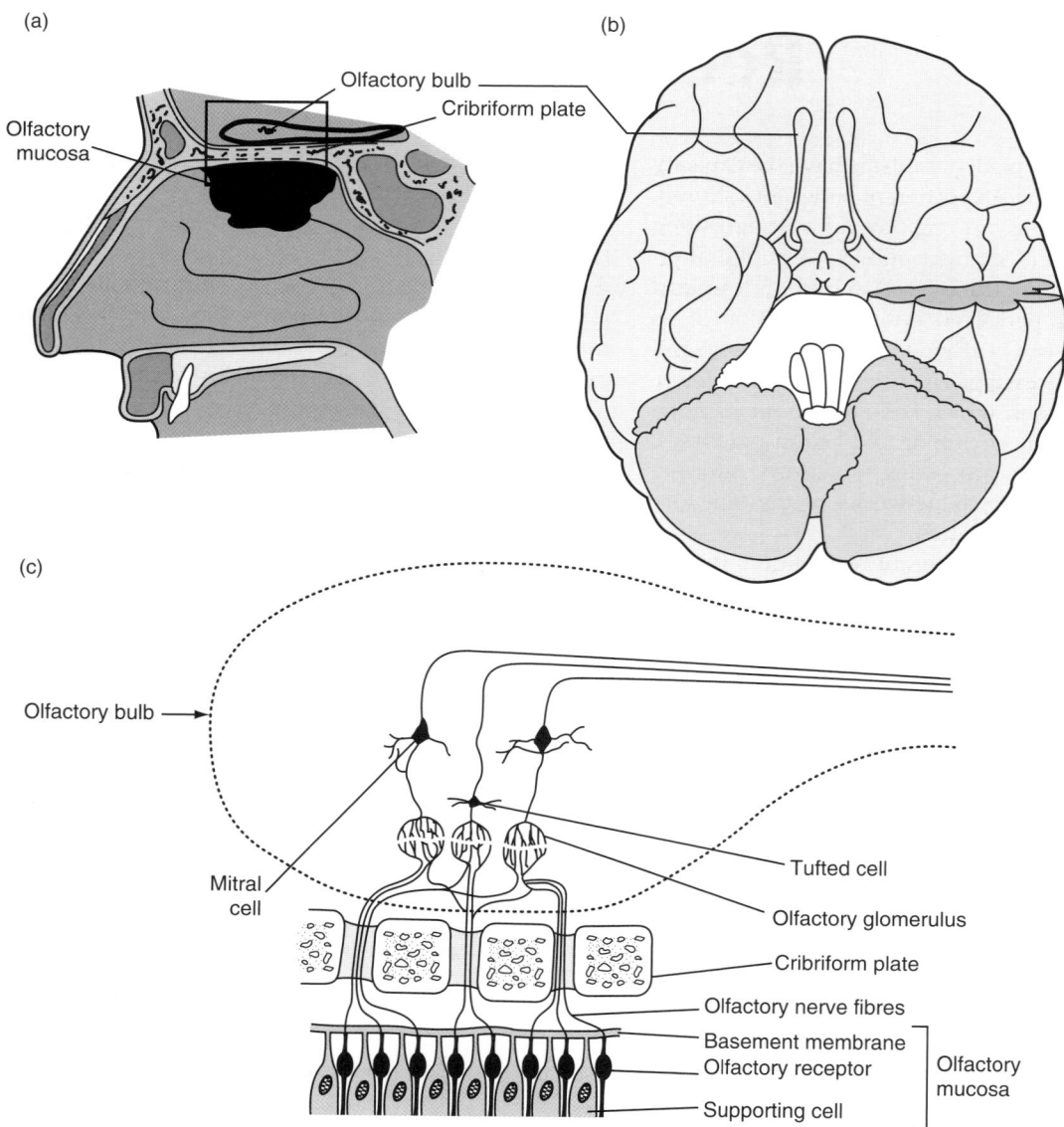

Figure 15.2 The olfactory receptor cells project to mitral cells in the olfactory bulb.
(a) Lateral view of the nasopharynx. The cribriform plate of the ethnoid bone lies over the olfactory mucosa. (b) View from the bottom side of the encephalon to show the olfactory bulbs. (c) Drawing of the neuroepithelium and of a sagittal section through an olfactory bulb (enlargement of the section in (a)). The olfactory epithelium is separated by a basement membrane from the lamina propria, a highly vascular and glandular tissue that lies adjacent to the nasal cartilage. The single axon of each olfactory receptor cell courses through the holes of the ethnoid bone, ramifies and synapses on the dendrites of the neurons of the olfactory bulb to form the olfactory glomeruli. As many as 1000 afferent fibres synapse on the dendrites of a single mitral cell. Local circuit neurons in the olfactory bulb are omitted. Parts (a) and (c) from Berne RM, Levy MN (1993) *Physiology*, 3rd edn, St Louis: YearBook; and House EL, Pansky B (1967) *A Functional Approach to Neuroanatomy*, 2nd edn, New York: McGraw Hill, with permission. Part (b) drawing: Jérôme Yelnik.

15.1.2 Odorants diffuse through the extracellular mucous matrix before interacting with the chemosensory membrane of olfactory receptor neurons

The cilia and dendritic knob are the only parts of the sensory neuron exposed to the external environment. They were therefore candidates for the site of odour recognition and transmembrane signalling. The sense of smell is based on molecular recognition. The molecules of odorants are recognized by specialized receptors located in the cilia of olfactory cells which lie in a 30 µm thick viscous liquid medium, the mucus, which covers the olfactory epithelium (**Figure 15.1**). It is a structured extracellular matrix which contains glycoproteins, mucopeptides, detoxification enzymes and immunoglobulins secreted by supporting cells and Bowman's glands. It protects the epithelium against microorganisms and biological toxins.

The mucus layer represents an aqueous environment into which primarily hydrophobic odorants must partition and gain access to odorant receptors in the cilia membrane. Using radioactively labelled odorants, odorant-binding proteins have been identified in the mucus. They belong to a family of hydrophobic ligand carrier proteins. They may trap odorants entering the nasal cavity and carry them to the nasal area. Alternatively, they may provide a reservoir of binding sites for odorants, protecting olfactory neurons from exposure to high concentrations of odorants.

15.2 The response of olfactory receptor neurons to odours is a membrane depolarization which elicits action potential generation

Pioneering experiments

In order to define the membrane potential changes of olfactory receptor cells in response to an odour, cell activity is recorded with intracellular recording techniques in the salamander (*Ambystoma tigrinum*). The olfactory epithelium is exposed after surgery and cells are penetrated with an electrode filled with a dye. At the end of the recording session, the dye is injected into the cell, allowing the determination of recordings as being from a receptor cell or not on the basis of morphological examination of histological sections.

An example of recordings is shown in **Figure 15.3**. The odour stimulus, ethyl *n*-butyrate, is delivered at the epithelial surface. It evokes a slow membrane depolarization, about 8 mV in amplitude, upon which are superimposed nine action potentials or spikes. A log

dilution of the odorant evokes a smaller depolarization, 6 mV, upon which are superimposed four spikes. In the same cell, a different odorant, anisole, does not evoke a response. These observations suggest that both the amplitude of the membrane depolarization and the number of spikes code for the stimulus strength. However, only the action potentials will propagate to the olfactory bulb along the single axon of the olfactory neuron (see **Figure 15.2**).

Questions

■ How is an odour recognized by the olfactory receptor neurons? (Section 15.3)
■ How does an odour give rise to a membrane depolarization? What underlies membrane depolarization: the generation of an inward current or the inhibition of an outward current? What are the

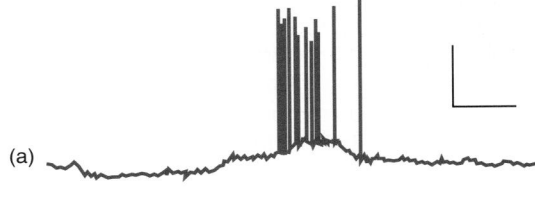
(a)

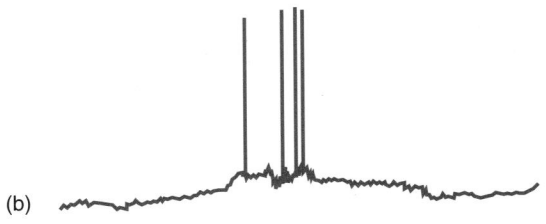
(b)

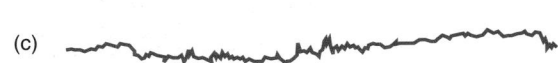
(c)

Figure 15.3 The response of olfactory neurons to an odorant stimulation is a slow membrane depolarization which can evoke action potentials.
Intracellular recordings from an olfactory receptor neuron in response to **(a)** ethyl *n*-butyrate and **(b)** a log step dilution. **(c)** In contrast, in the same cell, anisole does not evoke a response. $V_m = -60$ mV. Calibrations: 20 mV, 500 ms. Adapted from Getchell TV (1977) Analysis of intracellular recordings from salamander olfactory epithelium, *Brain Res.* **123**, 275–286, with permission.

channels opened or closed and responsible for this current? Why do these channels open or close in response to odorant stimulation? All these questions concern the transduction mechanisms and will be explained from the single-channel properties to the membrane depolarization. (Section 15.4)

■ How does the response of the olfactory neuron code for the characteristics of the odorant stimulation (nature of the odorant, its concentration, and the duration of the stimulus)? (Section 15.5)

15.3 Odorants bind to a family of G-protein-linked receptors which activate adenylate cyclase

The different results presented in this section were not obtained in this order. The study of the mechanisms of olfactory transduction began with the development of a cilia-enriched, cell-free preparation of the olfactory epithelium. In this preparation, Doron Lancet and coworkers (1985) obtained evidence that cAMP and G proteins are involved in olfactory transduction since exposure of isolated cilia from rat olfactory epithelium to numerous odorants led to the rapid activation of adenylate cyclase and an elevation of intracellular cAMP concentration. Both effects being dependent on the presence of GTP, this suggested the involvement of a G protein. Then came the characterization of the olfactory receptors and the identification of the G protein linked to these receptors. For clarity, the results are presented in the order of the molecular events that take place from odorant recognition to cAMP formation.

15.3.1 Odorant receptors are a family of G-protein-linked receptors

When the cilia of olfactory neurons are enzymatically removed by application of Triton X-100 to the olfactory mucosa in the frog, the response to odorants is lost and restored upon regeneration of the cilia. This observation that the selective removal of the cilia of olfactory cells results in the loss of olfactory responses led to the suggestion that the olfactory receptors are densely expressed in olfactory cilia. The other observation that the activation of adenylate cyclase by odorants is dependent on the presence of GTP led to the hypothesis that odorant receptors are G-protein linked. Based on this assumption, the authors tried to identify molecules in the olfactory epithelium that resemble members of the seven transmembrane domain superfamily (see Chapter 3).

The expected properties of the odorant receptors deduced from the responses of olfactory cells to odorants *in vivo* are:

■ their diversity, making them capable of interacting with extremely diverse molecular structures since a high diversity of olfactory molecules are recognized;

■ their ability to transduce odorant binding into intracellular signals that generate the membrane response;

■ their specific expression in the olfactory epithelium, the tissue in which odorants are recognized.

Different members of a large multigene family that encodes seven transmembrane domain proteins (a characteristic of the superfamily of G-protein-linked receptors) have been cloned and characterized. Important differences between the olfactory protein family and the other G-protein-linked receptors are present within the third, fourth and fifth transmembrane domains. The olfactory receptors also exhibit between themselves considerable sequence diversity in these transmembrane domains (**Figure 15.4**). These domains are thought to contribute to the formation of the ligand-binding site in group Ia of G-protein-linked receptors. Group Ia contains the receptors for small ligands such as photons (rhodopsin), for catecholamines (α- and β-adrenergic receptors and dopamine receptors), opiates and enkephalins (opioid receptors). *In vitro* mutagenesis experiments showed that adrenergic ligands interact with β-adrenergic receptors by binding within the plane of the membrane such that the ligand contacts many, if not all, of the transmembrane domains. This divergence within transmembrane domains may explain the specific recognition of a large number of odorants of diverse molecular structures (benzene, phenols, camphor, isoamyl acetate, menthol, terpenes, etc.).

Receptors that belong to the superfamily of seven transmembrane domain proteins interact with G proteins to generate intracellular signals. *In vitro* mutagenesis experiments indicate that one site of association between the receptor of the group Ia and G proteins resides between the third cytoplasmic loop. As shown in **Figure 15.4**, this loop is relatively short and shows sequence diversity.

To examine the hypothesis that the cloned cDNA, if they express olfactory receptors, must hybridize preferentially with mRNA from olfactory epithelium, a Northern blot analysis is performed. Poly (A)+ RNA isolated from different tissues are hybridized with a ^{32}P-labelled mixture of segments of the cDNA cloned. No hybridizing RNA can be detected in brain or retina and in non-neural tissues including lung, liver, spleen and kidney. In contrast, hybridization is detected in olfactory epithelium, demonstrating that the expression of the family of olfactory proteins cloned is restricted to the olfactory epithelium.

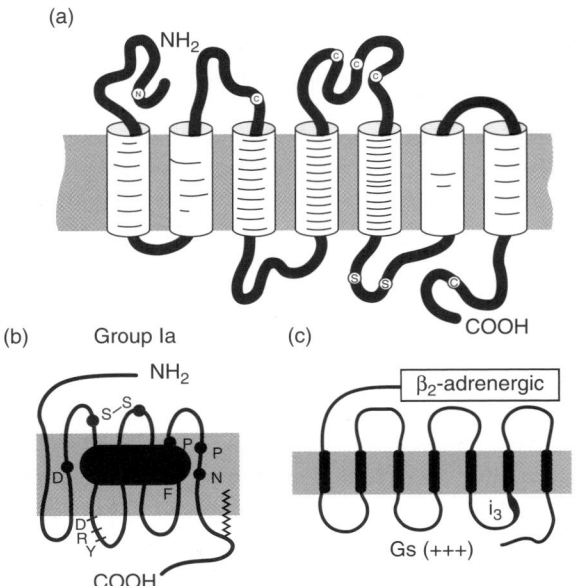

Figure 15.4 Putative transmembrane organization of the olfactory receptor family and transmembrane organization of G-protein-coupled receptors of group I.

(a) Schematic of a putative odorant receptor. The vertical cylinders delineate the seven putative membrane-spanning domains. The degree of shading of the transmembrane domains in the diagram is proportional to the degree of sequence variability found in these domains among different members of the putative odorant receptor family. The high degree of variability encountered in transmembrane domains III, IV and V is apparent. **(b)** Transmembrane organization of group-I G-protein-coupled receptors. This group is characterized by the presence of a sequence DRY (aspartate–arginine–tryptophan) and a disulphide bond (S–S) between the extracellular loops 1 and 2. **(c)** The third intracellular loop i3 in most G-protein-coupled receptors participates in the coupling with G proteins (e.g. the β_2-adrenergic receptor). Part (a) adapted from Buck L, Axel R (1991) A novel multigene family may encode odorant receptors: a molecular basis for odour recognition, *Cell* **65**, 175–187; and Anholt RRH (1993) Molecular biology of olfaction, *Crit. Rev. Neurobiol.* **7**, 1–22, with permission. Parts (b) and (c) from Bockaert J (1995) Les récepteurs à sept domaines transmembranaires: physiologie et pathologie de la transduction, *Méd Sci.* **11**, 382–394, with permission.

15.3.2 The activation of odorant receptors leads to the activation of adenylate cyclase and the rapid formation of cAMP via the activation of a Gs-like protein

Preparations of frog olfactory cilia contain a high concentration of substrate for ADP ribosylation by cholera toxin. This toxin specifically labels the α-subunit of the G_s protein in other tissues. In the olfactory tissue it labels a G-type protein of slightly different motility. To characterize the candidate G-protein mediating odorant

transduction, cDNA clones homologous to a highly conserved region of the G_α subunit were isolated from a rat olfactory library.

The activation of odorant receptors leads to the activation of a $G_{olf\alpha}$ protein

By screening the rat olfactory cDNA library, a $G_{olf\alpha}$ subunit that is expressed abundantly and exclusively by olfactory neurons has been identified. This $G_{olf\alpha}$ subunit shares 88% amino acid identity with $G_{s\alpha}$ present in neurons. In order to play a role in olfaction, this G protein must be expressed preferentially in the olfactory neurons, be coupled to odorant receptors and be able to stimulate the formation of cAMP.

Immunocytochemical experiments demonstrate that $G_{olf\alpha}$ is abundant in crude olfactory cilia preparations where olfactory receptors are also densely expressed (see above), a localization appropriate for a G protein involved in odorant signal transduction. In order to test that $G_{olf\alpha}$ is able to stimulate adenylate cyclase, a murine lymphoma cell line, which is deficient in endogenous stimulatory G proteins, is infected with a recombinant retrovirus encoding $G_{olf\alpha}$. The expressed G proteins are activated by aluminium fluoride ions (AlF_4^-) known to activate G proteins in the absence of receptor activation (the olfactory receptors are of course absent in the cell line). In such conditions, membranes prepared from $G_{olf\alpha}$-expressing cells show an increase in adenylate cyclase activity in response to AlF_4^- though membranes prepared from non-$G_{olf\alpha}$-expressing cells do not. The coupling of $G_{olf\alpha}$ to olfactory receptors could not be tested in these experiments since they were performed before the molecular cloning of olfactory receptors.

An odorant-sensitive adenylate cyclase is present in membranes of olfactory cells

The enzyme adenylate cyclase is present in extraordinarily high amounts in crude olfactory cilia preparations (a cell-free preparation). Activation of adenylate cyclase in this preparation by non-hydrolysable GTP analogues or the diterpene forskolin reveals a specific activity 10-fold higher than in brain membranes. The application of a mixture of odorants enhances the adenylate cyclase activity in a dose-dependent manner. This is observed only in the presence of GTP (**Figure 15.5**) or GTP-γ-S. The concentration of odorants required to activate adenylate cyclase *in vitro* correlates well with that known to give responses *in vivo*. Moreover, non-odorant compounds known to stimulate adenylate cyclase in other membranes such as isoprenaline, prostaglandins and histamine are ineffective. These results suggest that odour reception involves the binding of odour molecules to a family of receptors linked to a G_{olf} protein and the subsequent activation of adenylate cyclase by the α-subunits of activated G_{olf}.

The adenylate cyclase activated by $G_{olf\alpha}$ is type-III adenylate cyclase. Calmodulin is abundant in olfactory cilia, and on isolated dendritic cilia from frog olfactory tissue, the activity of the odorant-sensitive adenylate cyclase (type III) is stimulated by calmodulin. This effect is dose-dependent and strictly Ca^{2+}-dependent. Adenylate cyclase type III is a Ca^{2+}-calmodulin sensitive isoenzyme. Activation by calmodulin can generate concentrations of cAMP three to six times higher than those elicited by maximal concentrations of a mixture of odorants. Thus, enhanced production of cAMP can be evoked by the coincidence of two distinct activation signals, $G_{olf\alpha}$ and Ca^{2+} bound to calmodulin.

The formation of cAMP precedes the onset of the current

One important criterion for a candidate second messenger of chemo-electrical transduction is that its formation must precede the onset of the odorant-induced membrane permeability changes which proceed on a subsecond timescale (see **Figure 15.11**). In order to study the kinetics of cAMP formation in response to odorant stimulation, the basal level of cAMP is first estimated in a preparation of isolated olfactory cilia from rat. The

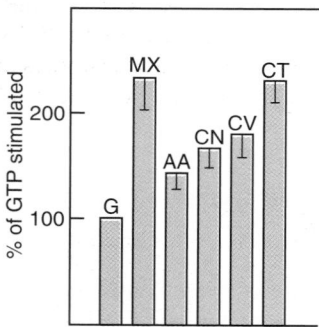

Figure 15.5 Effects of odorants on olfactory cilia adenylate cyclase.

The adenylate cyclase activity of frog olfactory cilia membranes is assayed in the presence of 0.5 mM of IBMX. The experiment is performed in the presence of 10 μM of GTP. The results are normalized with respect to the activity elicited by GTP alone (G), which is about twice the basal activity level. AA: n-amyl acetate; CN: 1,8-cineole; CV: L-carvone; CT: citral (each at 1 mM); MX: a mixture of the preceding four components at a concentration of 0.25 mM each. From Pace U, Hanski E, Salomon Y, Lancet D (1985) Odorant-sensitive adenylate cyclase may mediate olfactory reception, *Nature* **316**, 255–258, with permission.

application of the odorant isomenthone in the presence of GTP (to allow G protein activation) evokes a rapid increase of cAMP, reaching a maximal level between 25 and 50 ms and declining thereafter to the basal level in 250–500 ms (**Figure 15.6a**). This cAMP increase clearly precedes the electrical response and is dependent on the dose of odorant (**Figure 15.6b**). In contrast, no variations in inositol trisphosphate (IP_3) concentration are seen. These observations favour the role of cAMP as a second messenger in rat olfactory transduction.

In antennal preparations from the cockroach, the application of an odorant induces the rapid (250–500 ms) formation of IP_3 and stimulates adenylate cyclase to a lesser extent. IP_3 seems to have a role in olfactory transduction in this preparation. In cells where IP_3 formation is observed in response to odorants, it could have the following role. IP_3 would bind to receptors linked to Ca^{2+} channels located in the ciliary plasma membrane and evoke Ca^{2+} influx; Ca^{2+} would bind to calmodulin and activate adenylate cyclase type III (see above); this pathway would greatly enhance cAMP production when adenylate cyclase type III is at the same time activated by $G_{olf\alpha}$. The involvement of IP_3 or other second-messenger pathways in olfactory transduction is still a matter of debate. This chapter focuses on the olfactory transduction pathway via cAMP.

15.4 cAMP opens a cyclic nucleotide-gated channel and generates an inward current

15.4.1 The olfactory cyclic nucleotide-gated channel is a ligand-gated channel composed of at least two different subunits

A protein similar to the cyclic nucleotide-gated channel from rods (visual cells) was looked for in olfactory epithelium. At present, cDNAs encoding two olfactory cyclic nucleotide-gated channel subunits have been cloned and characterized. Their expression is restricted to olfactory epithelium. The hydropathy plot of the sequence of the channel from rods and cone receptors (cGMP-gated channel) and olfactory receptor neurons led to a model of the secondary structure of the channel (**Figure 15.7**). This model presents six putative membrane-spanning regions. A region located on the C-terminal side of the sixth domain shows significant sequence similarity with cyclic nucleotide binding sites such as, for example, the cGMP-dependent protein kinase.

The first subunit cloned (named $rOCNC_1$) contains sequence motifs reminiscent of voltage-gated channels, in particular K^+ and Ca^{2+} channels. The two classes of

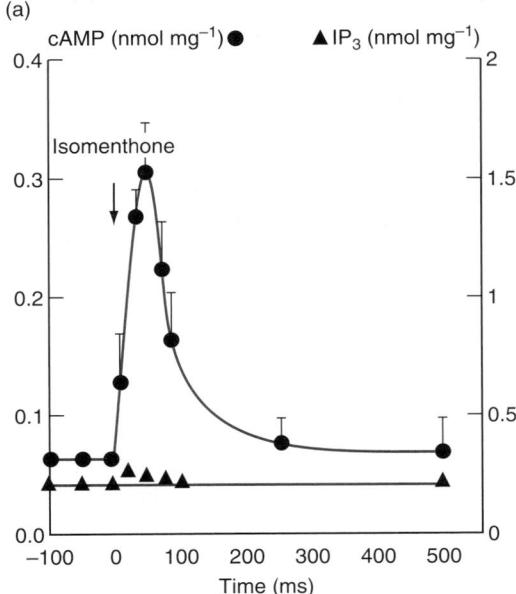

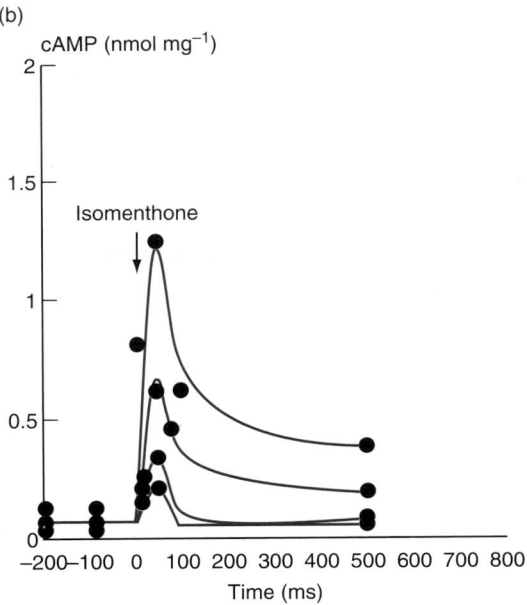

Figure 15.6 Rapid kinetics of odorant-induced accumulation of cAMP in rat olfactory cilia.

(a) In a preparation of isolated olfactory cilia, the application of 1 μM of isomenthone evokes a rapid increase of cAMP concentration which declines thereafter to the baseline. The inositol trisphosphate concentration (IP_3) is not affected. **(b)** Odorant dose-dependence of the cAMP accumulation. Various doses of isomenthone, 0.1 μM, 1 μM, 10 μM and 100 μM (from bottom to top), induce a rise in cAMP accumulation with different onset and decay times. From Breer H, Boekhoff I, Tareilus E (1990) Rapid kinetics of second messenger formation in olfactory transduction, *Nature* **345**, 65–68, with permission.

channels share in fact a common putative transmembrane topology. The subunit $rCOCN_1$ can form functional homo-oligomeric channels activated by cAMP when expressed in *Xenopus laevis* oocytes and mammalian cell lines. It presents a cyclic nucleotide-binding domain, comprising 80–100 amino acids located near the carboxyl terminus.

The second subunit cloned ($rCOCN_2$) cannot form functional channels by itself when expressed alone. However, when co-expressed with the first subunit, the channel activity detected resembles more closely that of the native channel and particularly concerning its low sensitivity to cAMP (see Section 15.4.3). This suggests that the native channel is a hetero-oligomer composed of at least the first and second cloned subunits in an unknown ratio.

15.4.2 cAMP directly opens a cyclic nucleotide-gated channel

The olfactory receptor cells are dissociated from the olfactory epithelium of the toad (*Bufo marinus*) by the action of proteolytic enzymes. A gigaohm seal is formed between the patch pipette and the membrane of a cilium. Because of the small diameter (0.1–0.25 μm) of the cilia, small patch pipette tips are used. The membrane patch is then excised, exposing the cytoplasmic surface of the cilium membrane to the bath solution (inside-out configuration). Nakamura and Gold (1987) were the first to show that in the presence of cAMP in the bath, single-channel events are recorded from inside-out patches. However, they could not resolve single-channel activity because of high densities of the cAMP-gated channels in the cilia membrane and therefore in the patch of membrane.

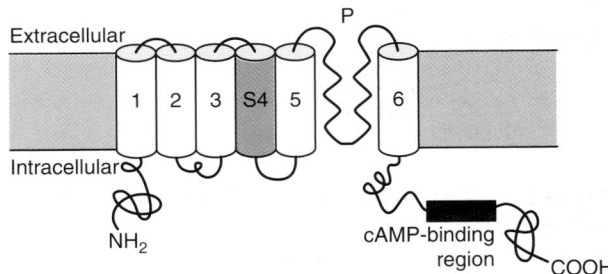

Figure 15.7 Hypothetical model of the two-dimensional architecture of cyclic nucleotide-gated channels.
From Bönigk W, Altenhofen W, Muller F *et al.* (1993) Rod and cone photoreceptor cells express distinct genes for cGMP-gated channels, *Neuron* **10**, 865–877; and Zufall F, Firestein S, Shepherd GM (1995) Cyclic nucleotide-gated channels and sensory transduction in olfactory receptor neurons, *Ann. Rev. Biophys. Biomol. Struct.* **23**, 577–607, with permission.

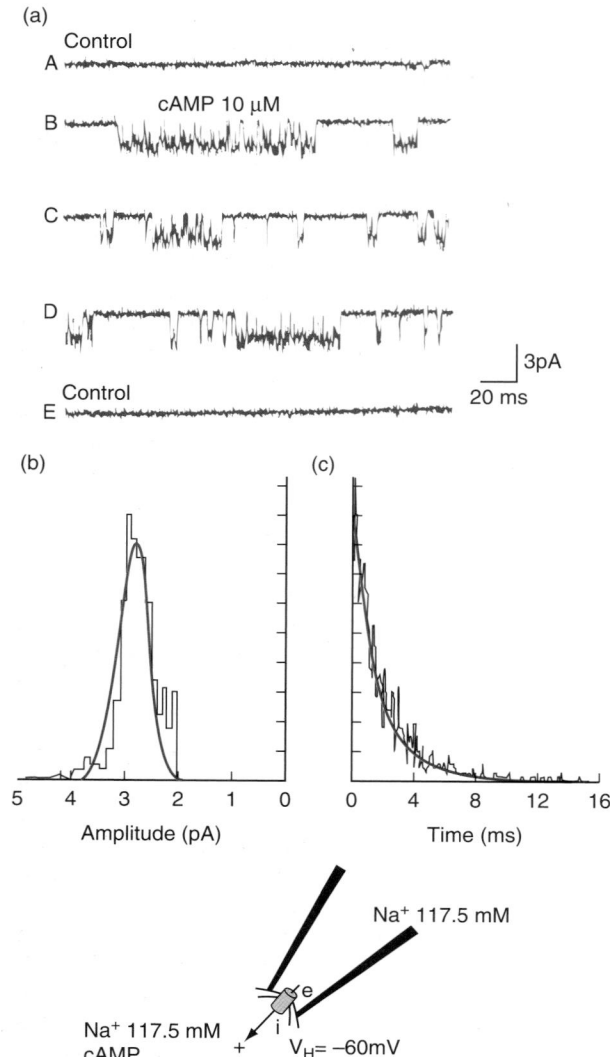

An alternative strategy was offered by the finding that cyclic nucleotide-gated channels also occur at low density in the membrane of the olfactory knob, dendrite and soma of olfactory receptor neurons. In such preparations, the activity of a single channel activated by cAMP can be recorded. Olfactory receptor neurons are isolated from the nasal epithelium of tiger salamanders (*Ambystoma tigrinum*). The activity of the channel is recorded in patch clamp in the inside-out configuration, in the absence of divalent cations (see below). When the holding potential is –60 mV, the control recordings show no channel openings. In the presence of a continuous application of cAMP in the bath, single channel openings occur (**Figure 15.8a**). These effects are fully reversible upon returning to cAMP-free solution.

The inward current steps have a mean amplitude of –3 pA when the driving force is –60 mV (**Figure 15.8b**). This gives a unitary conductance of around 30–45 pS. The activity of the channel consists of single openings and bursts of openings (mean open time 1.9 ms; **Figure 15.8c**). As these results were obtained in inside-out configuration (the cytoplasmic surface of the cilium membrane faces the bath solution), where intracellular components are absent and particularly protein kinases, it is possible to conclude that cAMP directly gates the channel.

$$R + {}_n(cAMP) \rightleftharpoons R - {}_n(cAMP) \rightleftharpoons R^* - {}_n(cAMP) \rightarrow current$$

where R is the cyclic nucleotide-gated channel in the closed state; R* is the cyclic nucleotide-gated channel in the open state; cAMP is the ligand that gates the channel; and *n* is the number of cAMP molecules that bind to the channel.

Figure 15.8 Single-channel recordings of a cyclic AMP-gated channel.
(a) The activity of a single cAMP-gated channel is recorded from inside-out patches of dendritic membrane of an isolated olfactory receptor neuron. Recordings without (A, E) and in the presence (B–D) of a continuous application of cAMP (10 μM) in the medium bathing the intracellular side of the membrane. V_H = –60 mV. (b) Amplitude histogram for the cAMP-induced unitary current. Each division on the ordinate scale is 20 counts, total of 2000 events. Peak = 2.9 pA, V_H = –60 mV. (c) Open time distribution for the cAMP-evoked channel activity. The single exponential fit has a time constant of τ^o = 1.89 ms (bin width 0.2 ms, total of 2000 events). From Zufall F, Firestein S, Shepherd GM (1991) Analysis of single nucleotide-gated channels in olfactory receptor cells, *J. Neurosci.* **11**, 3573–3580, with permission.

cGMP also opens the olfactory cyclic nucleotide-gated channel

The results obtained with the application of cGMP are very similar. On the same patch of membrane cGMP evokes the same single-channel openings as cAMP. Since the patches tested are always sensitive to both nucleotides, it is concluded that cAMP and cGMP act upon the same channel. The role of cGMP *in vivo*, is unclear since there is a very active odour-sensitive adenylate cyclase present in olfactory neurons and no detectable odour-sensitive guanylate cyclase activity.

The unitary cAMP-induced current reverses around 0 mV

The voltage sensitivity of the channel is analysed by exposing inside-out patches to saturating concentrations of cAMP while holding the membrane at different potentials. When measuring the unitary current amplitude, we obtain an i_{cAMP}/V plot (**Figure 15.9b**). This relation is approximately linear between −100 and +80 mV. The unitary current is inward for potentials more negative than +5 mV, reverses polarity at +5 mV and is outward for potentials more positive than +5 mV (**Figures 15.9a and b**). The reversal potential of i_{cAMP} varies slightly according to the experiment or the preparation studied.

The unitary conductance is constant in the absence of divalent cations

The i/V relation of **Figure 15.9b** is described by the equation: $i_{cAMP} = \gamma_{cAMP}(V_m - E_{cAMP})$, where V_m is the membrane potential, E_{cAMP} is the reversal potential of the cAMP-induced current, and γ_{cAMP} is the conductance of the cAMP-gated channel or unitary conductance. The value of γ_{cAMP} is the slope of the i/V plot. In the present experimental conditions (absence of divalent cations), it is equal to 45 pS and does not vary according to the membrane potential.

The cyclic nucleotide-gated channel is a non-specific cationic channel

The recorded value of the reversal potential of i_{cAMP} suggests that i_{cAMP} is either a cationic current or a current carried by Cl⁻ ions. A study of the ionic selectivity of the cAMP-gated channel was performed on macropatches of olfactory cell membrane from which only the macroscopic current is recorded. The results will therefore be explained in the next section.

The cyclic nucleotide-gated channel recorded in inside-out patches does not desensitize

Long exposures of single channels to even saturating concentrations of cAMP does not result in any detectable desensitization (see **Figure 15.9a**). In contrast, as we will see in the next section, recordings of the macroscopic cyclic nucleotide-gated current from intact olfactory neurons show strong desensitization to elevated intracellular cAMP concentration (see **Figure 15.11**). This suggests that the mechanisms of desensitization require intracellular factors.

In the presence of increasing concentrations of external divalent cations the channel displays a flickering behaviour

The effects of external divalent cations on cAMP-activated single-channel currents are studied in inside-out membrane patches taken from the dendritic region of isolated olfactory receptor neurons of the tiger salamander (*Ambystoma tigrinum*). Since the effect of divalent cations was tested on the external side (i.e. in the pipette solution), each experiment with a different concentration of divalent cation corresponds to a new patch of membrane. A comparison of these experiments is reliable since single-channel parameters such as amplitude, kinetics and open probability do not differ considerably among different patches. With increasing concentrations of Ca^{2+}, from 10 nM (control) to 1 mM, in the pipette solution (extracellular solution), in the presence of cAMP in the medium bathing the intracellular side of the membrane, a reduction of the apparent unitary current is observed (**Figure 15.10a**). At higher concentrations of Ca^{2+} ions, the transitions are in fact too rapid to be fully resolved and appear as a reduction of the mean unitary current.

The effect of Ca^{2+} ions also shows a strong voltage-dependence. The i_{cAMP}/V relation (**Figure 15.10b**) is S-shaped in the presence of external Ca^{2+} ions. The same effect is observed in the presence of external Mg^{2+} ions (600 μM). These effects are explained by an open channel block by divalent cations. Therefore, at normal resting membrane potential, about −50 mV, and at physiological extracellular Ca^{2+} concentration (the Ca^{2+} concentration in the mucus is between 2 and 5 mM), single-channel events are no longer resolvable. The block is partially relieved by depolarization. The physiological consequences are analysed in Sections 15.4.3 and 15.5.

In the presence of increasing concentrations of cytoplasmic Ca^{2+} ions the mean open time of the channel is decreased

In inside-out patches of dendritic membrane of an isolated olfactory receptor, the activity of a single cyclic nucleotide-gated channel is first recorded in the continuous presence of a saturating intracellular concentration of cAMP (100 μM) and a control intracellular Ca^{2+} concentration (0.1 μM) (**Figure 15.10c**, upper traces). Single-channel currents are recorded and the mean open probability is 0.6. Even during several second-long exposures to a saturating concentration of cAMP, the channel displays no obvious signs of desensitization. When the intracellular Ca^{2+} concentration is increased 30 times (to 3 μM, middle traces), the amplitude and

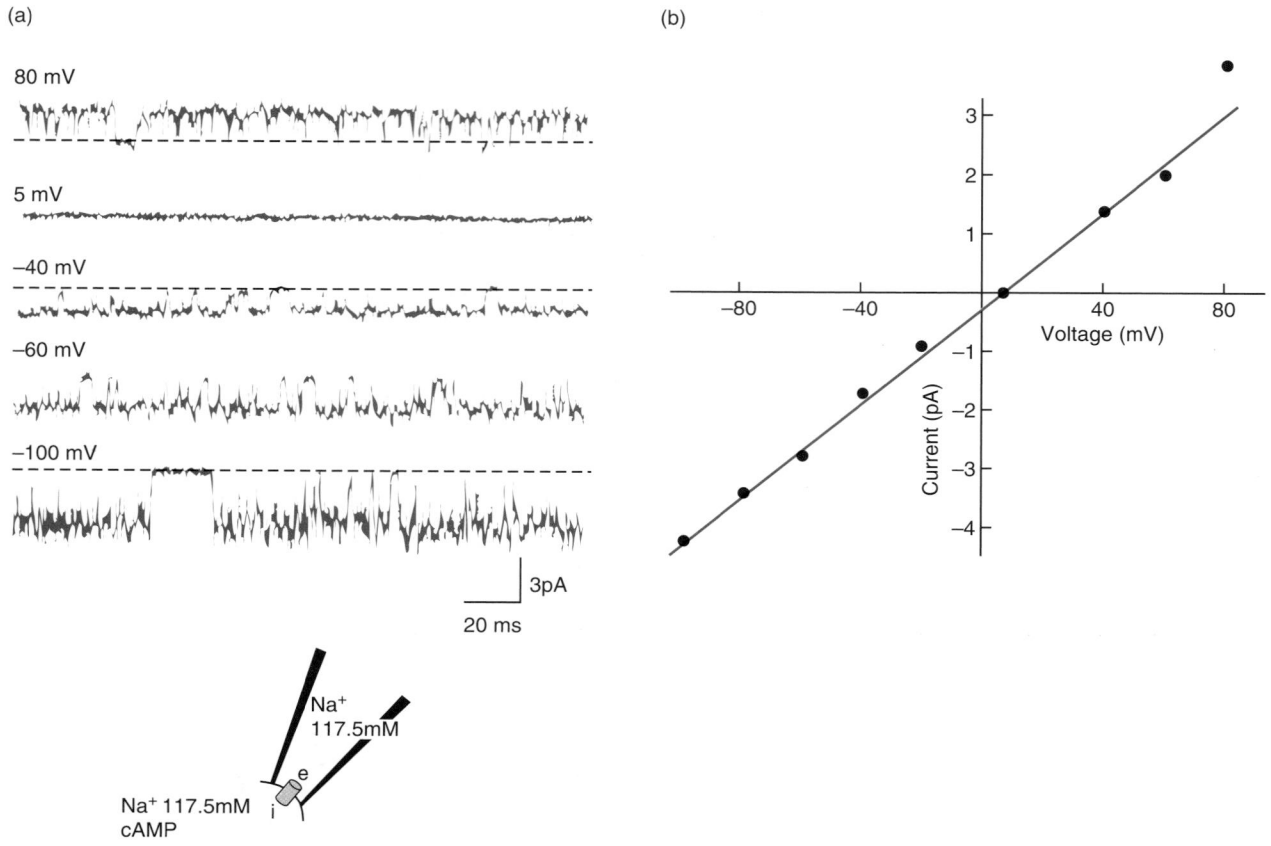

Figure 15.9 Voltage-dependence of the cAMP-induced unitary current.
The activity of a single channel is recorded in inside-out patches of dendritic membrane of an isolated olfactory receptor. A saturating concentration of cAMP (0.1 mM) is continuously present in the medium bathing the intracellular side of the membrane. **(a)** Examples of single-channel openings at different holding potentials as indicated for each trace. The closed state is marked by a broken line. **(b)** i_{cAMP}/V relation. Each point represents 3000 events from the recording shown in (a). From Zufall F, Firestein S, Shepherd GM (1991) Analysis of single nucleotide-gated channels in olfactory receptor cells, *J. Neurosci.* **11**, 3573–3580, with permission.

kinetics of channel openings are unaffected but the recording contains longer intervals between bursts of openings. The channel mean open probability is strongly reduced (to 0.09). Returning to the control solution restores normal channel activity (lower traces). This effect suggests that intracellular Ca^{2+} ions act directly on an intracellular site of the channel and stabilize the channel in the closed state. It is very different from the open channel block by external divalent cations described above.

15.4.3 The activation of N cyclic nucleotide-gated channels evokes an inward depolarizing current carried by cations

In a preparation containing N channels, cAMP induces a macroscopic current I such that $I_{cAMP} = Np_o i_{cAMP}$. To record this macroscopic current in isolation, the activity of an isolated olfactory receptor cell (from the newt olfactory epithelium, *Cynops pyrrhogaster*) in response to a rise of intracellular cAMP is recorded in whole-cell patch clamp in the presence of blockers of all the voltage-gated currents. First a gigaohm seal is formed between the patch pipette and the membrane of the terminal swelling (cell-attached configuration; **Figure 15.11a**). The extracellular solution contains TEACl to block voltage-gated K^+ conductances and $CoCl_2$ to block voltage-gated Ca^{2+} conductances. The pipette solution contains Cs^+ and EGTA to block voltage- and Ca^{2+}-activated K^+ currents. cAMP (or cGMP) is added to the pipette solution. At time zero the patch of membrane is ruptured to allow the pipette solution to diffuse into the olfactory cell from the tip of the opening of the recording pipette through the ruptured hole of the plasma membrane. When the intrapipette solution con-

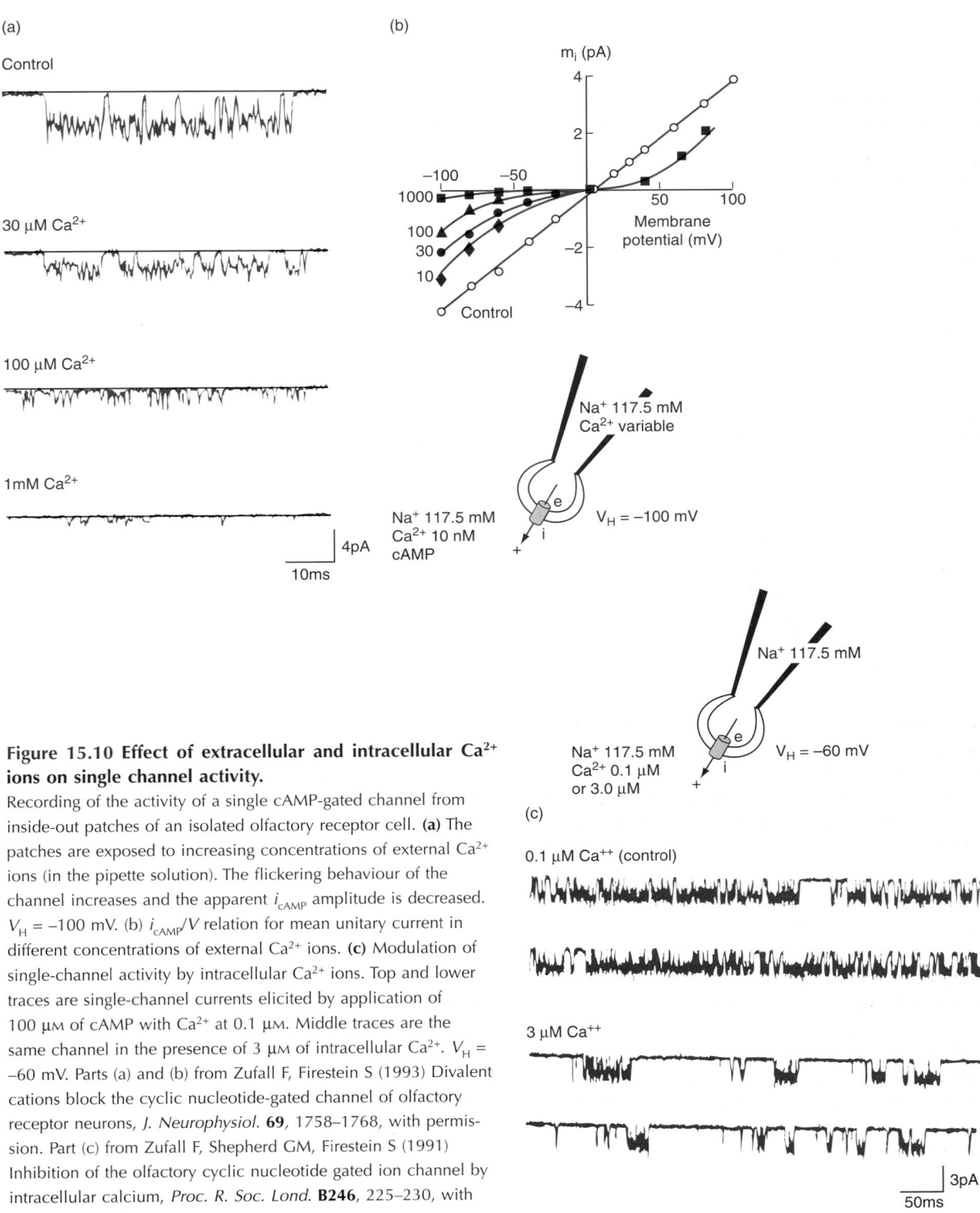

Figure 15.10 Effect of extracellular and intracellular Ca²⁺ ions on single channel activity.
Recording of the activity of a single cAMP-gated channel from inside-out patches of an isolated olfactory receptor cell. **(a)** The patches are exposed to increasing concentrations of external Ca²⁺ ions (in the pipette solution). The flickering behaviour of the channel increases and the apparent i_{cAMP} amplitude is decreased. $V_H = -100$ mV. (b) i_{cAMP}/V relation for mean unitary current in different concentrations of external Ca²⁺ ions. **(c)** Modulation of single-channel activity by intracellular Ca²⁺ ions. Top and lower traces are single-channel currents elicited by application of 100 μM of cAMP with Ca²⁺ at 0.1 μM. Middle traces are the same channel in the presence of 3 μM of intracellular Ca²⁺. $V_H = -60$ mV. Parts (a) and (b) from Zufall F, Firestein S (1993) Divalent cations block the cyclic nucleotide-gated channel of olfactory receptor neurons, *J. Neurophysiol.* **69**, 1758–1768, with permission. Part (c) from Zufall F, Shepherd GM, Firestein S (1991) Inhibition of the olfactory cyclic nucleotide gated ion channel by intracellular calcium, *Proc. R. Soc. Lond.* **B246**, 225–230, with permission.

tains cAMP, an inward current is recorded approximately 100 ms after rupture of the patch membrane (V_H = –50 mV; **Figure 15.11b**). Since in the absence of cyclic nucleotide in the patch pipette, no current is recorded (**Figure 15.11c**), it is concluded that the inward current is induced by the intracellularly introduced cAMP. The amplitude of the cAMP-induced current is dose-dependent (**Figure 15.11d**). The least effective dose is estimated to be in the order of 100 μM and the maximal reponse is observed for 1 mM intracellular cAMP.

The second subunit of the cyclic nucleotide-gated channel confers high sensitivity to cAMP

The olfactory cyclic nucleotide-gated channel subunit cloned first (named rOCNC₁), when functionally expressed in *Xenopus laevis* oocytes and mammalian cell lines, forms functional, presumably homo-oligomeric, channels. Although these channels share some characteristics with the native channels (they are selectively permeable to cations and activated by cAMP), their sensitivity to cAMP is 30-fold less than

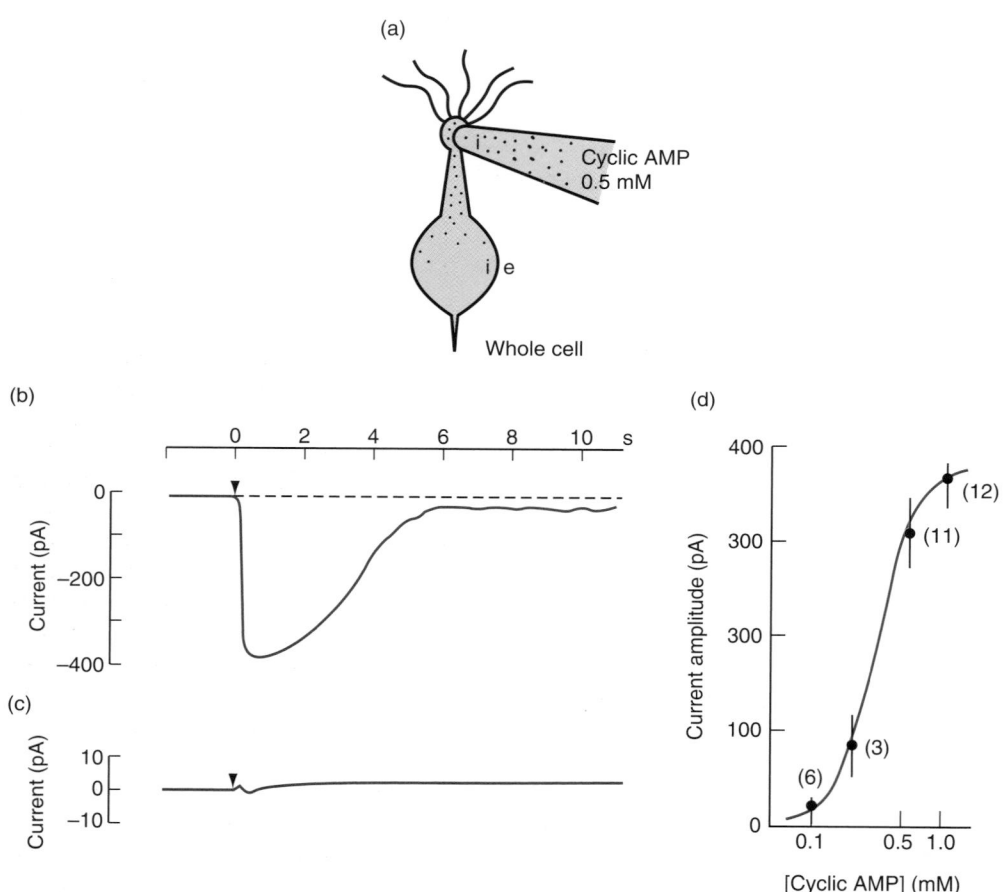

Figure 15.11 A transient macroscopic inward current is induced in an olfactory neuron by the introduction of cAMP from the patch pipette.

(a) First a gigaohm seal is formed on the dendritic knob. **(b)** A brief application of negative pressure ruptures the membrane at the pipette tip (arrowhead) and 0.5 mM cAMP is allowed to diffuse into the terminal knob. It induces a transient inward current. V_H = –50 mV. **(c)** When the pipette solution does not contain a cyclic nucleotide, no inward current is induced after the membrane rupture (arrowhead). **(d)** The dose-dependence is studied by measuring the inward current amplitude (pA) induced by different doses of cAMP (in mM). For each experiment, only one dose can be tested since cAMP is in the patch pipette solution (the number of cells tested for each point are in parentheses). From Kurahashi T (1990) The response induced by intracellular cyclic AMP in isolated olfactory receptor cells of the newt, *J. Physiol.* **430**, 355–371, with permission.

the native channels. The activity of the expressed channels is recorded in patch clamp in the inside-out configuration. These are macropatches which contain a high density of channels and the current recorded is therefore a macroscopic current. Bath application of low doses of cAMP (or cGMP) have no effect but high doses evoke a large inward current (like a whole-cell inward current) (**Figure 15.12a**). One hypothesis could be that additional subunits are missing from the expression system.

A new cDNA cloned from the rat olfactory epithelium that encodes a second subunit of the olfactory cyclic nucleotide-gated channel, $rOCNC_2$, has been found (both these subunits present a structural homology with the voltage-gated K^+ channel subunits). *Xenopus* oocytes are injected with *in vitro* transcribed $rOCNC_2$ RNA. Excised inside-out patches from these oocytes failed to respond to bath application of cAMP or cGMP, suggesting a failure of the protein to incorporate into the oocyte membrane or to form homo-oligomeric channels. When the oocytes are injected with equal amounts of $rOCNC_1$

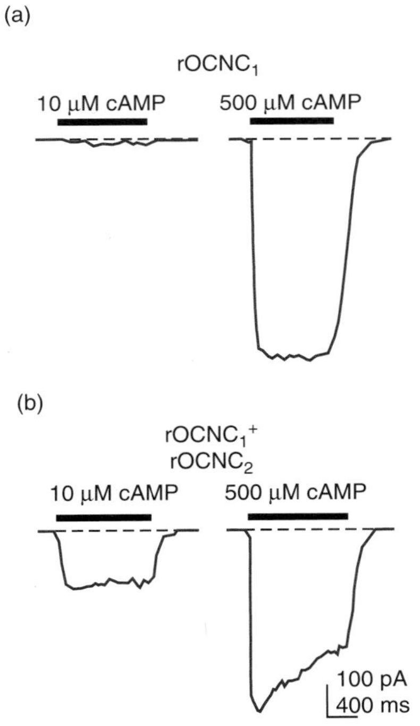

Figure 15.12 cAMP-induced currents in excised macropatches from oocytes injected with cloned rat olfactory cyclic nucleotide-gated channel RNA.

(a) Inward currents recorded from inside-out macropatches from an oocyte injected with $rOCNC_1$ RNA in response to bath application of 10 μM or 500 μM of cAMP. (b) Same experiment as in (a) for a patch excised from an oocyte injected with $rOCNC_1$ and $rOCNC_2$ RNA. From Liman ER, Buck LB (1994) A second subunit of the olfactory cyclic nucleotide-gated channel confers high sensitivity to cAMP, *Neuron* **13**, 611–621, with permission.

and $rOCNC_2$ RNA, the excised inside-out patches now respond with a large current to bath application of low doses of cAMP (**Figure 15.12b**) and cGMP.

The cAMP-induced current is generated in olfactory cilia

The response amplitude and the time course differ markedly depending on the site of the seal; i.e. the site of cAMP introduction. The most effective site is the nearest to olfactory cilia. When cAMP is introduced to the terminal swelling (close to the cilia), it evokes a response of large amplitude, short latency and rapid risetime (**Figure 15.13a**). When cAMP is introduced to the cell body, the amplitude of the response is smaller, the latency longer and the risetime slower (**Figure 15.13b**). This agrees with the finding that excised patches from the ciliary membrane show a high sensitivity to cAMP. The density of cAMP-gated channels in the ciliary membrane is estimated to be about 2500–10 000 μm^{-2} (from a single channel conductance $\gamma = 30$ pS).

The cAMP-gated current is carried by cations

The whole-cell current evoked by intracellular cAMP is recorded in the presence of blockers of voltage-gated channels. The cAMP-induced current–voltage relation is measured by rapidly changing the holding potential. A ramp voltage command varying from −50 to +46 mV is applied at a rate of 195 mV s^{-1} during the evoked current and after the end of the current (**Figure 15.14a**). The curve obtained after the end of the current is subtracted from the one obtained at the peak of the current in order to eliminate the leak current. The I/V relation (**Figure 15.14b**) is almost linear between −50 and +50 mV, and the reversal potential of the cAMP-induced current is around −5 mV. This observed value can be accounted for by either a current carried by cations or by Cl^- ions.

To differentiate between these two possibilities, the I/V relations of the cAMP-induced current are measured under different ionic conditions. When K^+ ions replace all the Na^+ ions present in the extracellular medium, the I/V curve and the reversal potential are unchanged, suggesting that the channel is equally permeable to Na^+ and K^+. Changing the Na^+ extracellular concentration alone induced changes of the reversal potential of the response according to the Nernst equation for a cationic channel. In conclusion, the channel permeates all alkali metal ions such as Li^+, Rb^+ or Cs^+ ions but not Cl^- or choline ions.

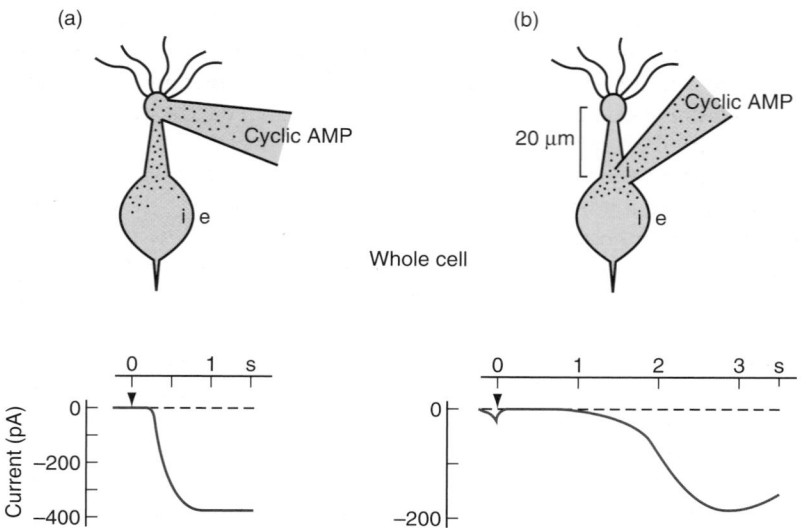

Figure 15.13 Relation between the site of cAMP introduction and the response time course.
(a) When 0.5 mM cAMP is introduced into the terminal knob, it evokes a response of large amplitude, short latency (0.20 ± 0.02 s) and rapid rising time (time from the onset to the peak is 0.9 ± 0.2s). (b) When 0.5 mM of cAMP is introduced into the proximal part of the dendrite, which is about 20 μM long, it evokes a response of small amplitude (approximately half of that in (a)), long latency (1.4 ± 0.4 s) and slow rising time (2.8 ± 0.5 s). Arrowheads indicate the time when the patch membrane is ruptured. V_H = –50 mV. From Kurahashi T (1990) The response induced by intracellular cyclic AMP in isolated olfactory receptor cells of the newt, *J. Physiol.* **430**, 355–371, with permission.

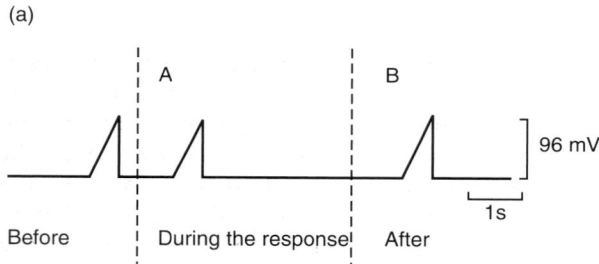

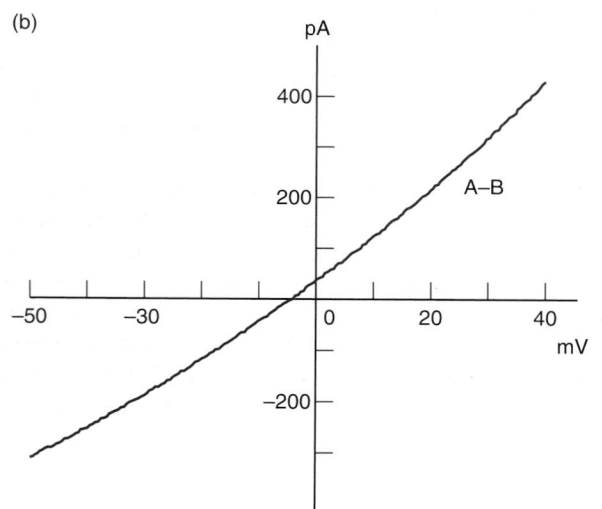

The characteristics of I_{cAMP} are dependent on Ca^{2+} ions

In some olfactory receptor cells recorded in physiological solutions, the I/V relation shows significant outward rectification at potentials more negative than –50 mV, in contrast to the linear behaviour of the I/V relation in the absence of divalent cations. Based on the observations of open channel block in single-channel recordings (see

Figure 15.14 Current–voltage relation of the cAMP-induced response.
(a) Experimental design. Same experiment as in Figure 15.11b but a voltage ramp command from –50 to +46 mV at a rate of 195 mV s⁻¹ is applied to the voltage clamped membrane before, at the peak of the response (A) and after the end of the response (B). Voltage-dependent K⁺ currents are blocked by 35 mM of TEACl and voltage-dependent Ca²⁺ currents by 3 mM of CoCl₂ in the external solution. (b) I/V relation of the cAMP-induced response. This relation is obtained by subtracting the I/V curve recorded after the response (B) to the I/V curve recorded at the peak of the response (A) in order to subtract leak current. The current reverses at –5 mV. The external solution contains (in mM): 85 NaCl, 3 CaCl², 35 TEACl, 3 CoCl², 2 NaOH. The intrapipette solution contains (in mM): 122 K⁺, 120 Cl⁻, 0.5 cAMP. From Kurahashi T (1990) The response induced by intracellular cyclic AMP in isolated olfactory receptor cells of the newt, *J. Physiol.* **430**, 355–371, with permission.

Figures 15.10a and b), it is proposed that extracellular Ca^{2+} ions bind to a site within the pore of the open cAMP-gated channel and block it. A membrane depolarization removes the block (as observed for Mg^{2+} ions and NMDA channels). The physiological consequence of such a block is that the generator current in these olfactory cells induced by odours depends simultaneously on cAMP concentration and membrane voltage.

Moreover, intracellular Ca^{2+} ions play a role. In control conditions we have seen that the macroscopic inward current evoked by a continuous application of cAMP is transient despite the fact that cAMP is continuously supplied from the pipette to the intracellular medium (see **Figure 15.10c**). When the extracellular solution is replaced by a Ca^{2+}-free solution, the cAMP-induced current is sustained during the recording (**Figure 15.15a**). Re-application of a standard extracellular medium containing 3 mM of Ca^{2+} suppresses the maintained current. Conversely, after the end of the cAMP-induced current evoked in control external conditions, the application of a medium containing a low Ca^{2+} concentration (1 μM) re-induces an inward current after the response was once suppressed

(**Figure 15.15b**). Finally, in the presence of control external Ca^{2+} concentration, the intracellular injection of the Ca^{2+} chelator EGTA prior to cAMP application slows down the decay time course of the cAMP-induced current.

In single-channel recordings in the absence of a control intracellular Ca^{2+} concentration, the channel does not desensitize, but in the presence of a high intracellular Ca^{2+} concentration the channel mean open probability is strongly reduced (see **Figure 15.10c**). We know that the cAMP-gated channel is permeable to Ca^{2+} ions since Ca^{2+} influx during the odour response is observed in experiments using the Ca^{2+} indicator FURA-2 (see Appendix 11.1) in conditions where other pathways of Ca^{2+} entry are blocked. It is proposed that the main source of cytoplasmic Ca^{2+} ions is the Ca^{2+} influx as a constituent of the inward current. Cytoplasmic Ca^{2+} ions would act directly on an intracellular site on the channel and reduce the apparent affinity of the channel for cAMP. This would constitute a rapid and effective negative feedback loop, which could account for the short-term adaptation of the response to sustained cAMP or odour exposure recorded in intact neurons.

15.4.4 The cyclic nucleotide-gated conductance and the odour-gated conductance are identical

The unitary activity of a patch of olfactory dendritic membrane is recorded in patch clamp in the cell-attached configuration. A pulse of odour activates a channel present in the patch (**Figure 15.16a**). The external solution is then replaced by a solution containing IBMX (isobutylmethylxanthine), an inhibitor of phosphodiesterase, the enzyme that hydrolyses cAMP in 5′AMP (IBMX enhances the basal and evoked intracellular concentration of cAMP). In the presence of IBMX in the bath the same channel activity is recorded from the same patch of membrane (**Figure 15.16b**). This suggests that the ion channels underlying the odour-induced unitary current and the cyclic nucleotide-induced unitary current are the same.

In whole-cell patch clamp recordings, the odorant-induced current has the same properties as the cAMP-induced current. Cilia are the most sensitive site both to intracellularly applied cAMP and to extracellularly applied odorants. Both responses reverse polarity near 0 mV and are carried by cations. To either stimulation of a long duration, responses show a rapid decay to a very low level, and the decay is strongly dependent on the influx of Ca^{2+} ions.

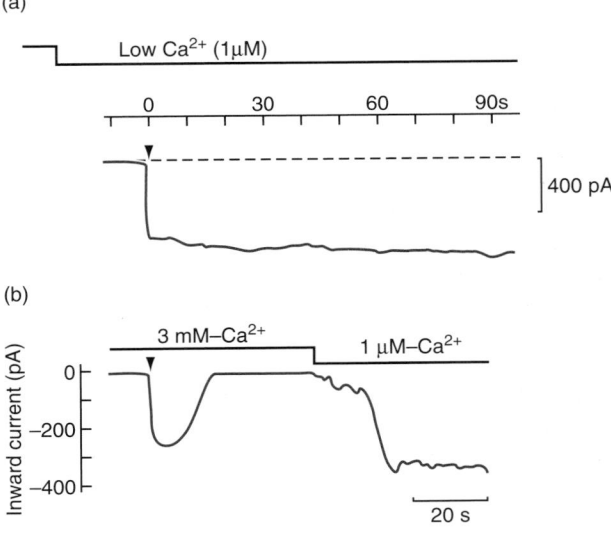

Figure 15.15 In the presence of a low external Ca^{2+} concentration, the cAMP-induced current is sustained.
(a) Same experiment as in Figure 15.11a but in the presence of a Ca^{2+}-free external solution and 1 mM of cAMP in the pipette. (b) The transient response induced by 1 mM of cAMP is first recorded in the presence of 3 mM of external Ca^{2+}. The subsequent application of a low external Ca^{2+} concentration after the end of the first response re-induces an inward current (cAMP is still present inside the patch pipette and freely diffuses inside the cell). V_H = −90 mV. From Kurahashi T (1990) The response induced by intracellular cyclic AMP in isolated olfactory receptor cells of the newt, *J. Physiol.* **430**, 355–371, with permission.

15.4.5 Conclusions (Figure 15.17)

These results, together with the preceding ones, demonstrate that the first event that initiates excitation of olfactory neurons is the binding of odorant to one or more receptors. These receptors are members of a diverse subfamily that itself belongs to the large superfamily of G-protein-linked receptors. Binding of the odorant on its receptor activates G_{olf}, a heterotrimeric protein closely related to the G_s protein. Binding of GTP to the activated α-subunit of the G_{olf} protein triggers stimulation of adenylate cyclase type III. This leads to the formation of cAMP. When the intraciliary concentration of cAMP reaches a threshold level, cAMP opens directly cyclic nucleotide-gated channels present in the ciliary membrane. The cations Na⁺ and

Ca^{2+} flow into the cilia through the open channels and generate an inward depolarizing current. The cAMP concentration returns to its basal levels by the rapid degradation of cAMP by phosphodiesterase, which hydrolyses cAMP in 5′AMP. The increase of cytoplasmic Ca^{2+} concentration caused by Ca^{2+} entry through cyclic nucleotide-gated channels, together with the action of the enzyme phosphodiesterase, contribute to stop the effect of cAMP and to make the cAMP-induced response transient. Such a system allows amplification of the signal: even a few molecules of the odorant that activates a few receptors induce the activation of many G proteins, the formation of many molecules of cAMP and the activation of many cationic channels.

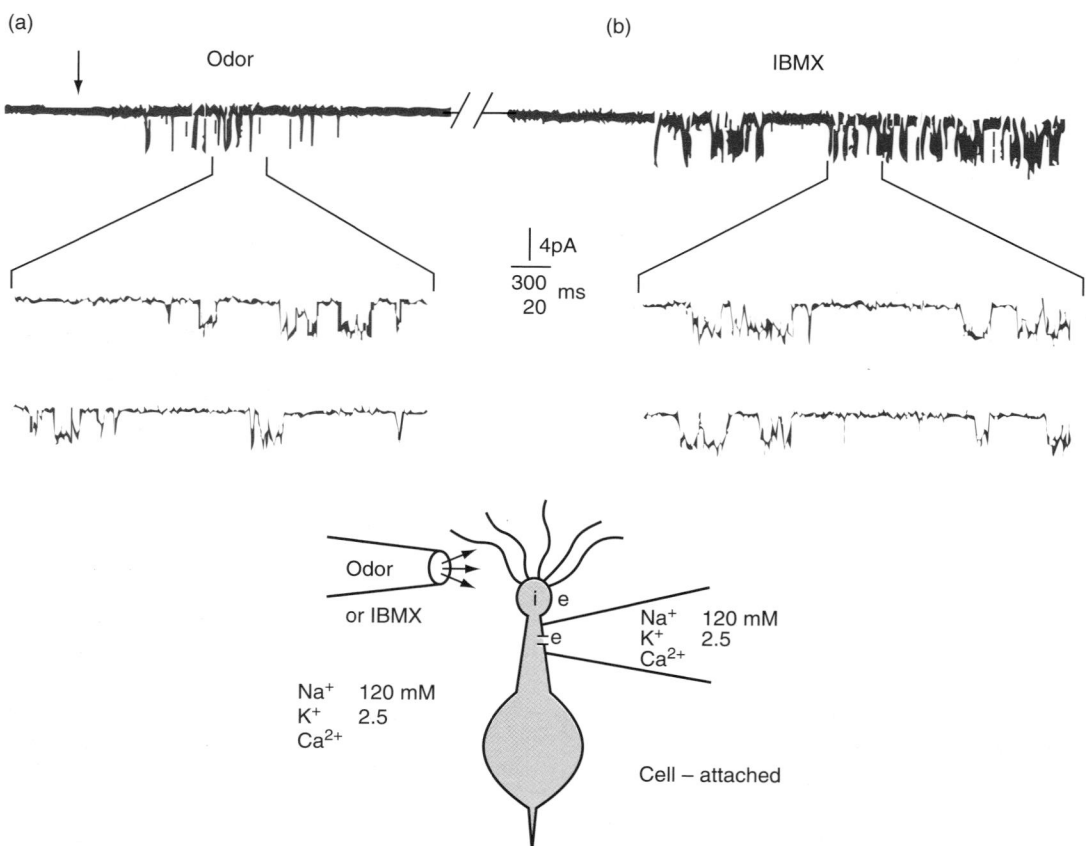

Figure 15.16 Odour and cyclic nucleotide-induced single-channel activity in the same membrane patch.
The activity of a single cyclic nucleotide-gated channel is recorded in cell-attached configuration from an isolated olfactory receptor neuron. **(a)** A 150 ms pulse of odour stimulus is delivered at the arrow. It elicits a burst of single-channel openings. **(b)** A solution with 100 μM of IBMX is then perfused into the bath. It elicits a similar activity in the same patch of membrane. Sample recordings at higher sweep speeds are shown below. Pipette potential: +40 mV. From Firestein S, Zufall F, Shepherd GM (1991) Single odour-sensitive channels in olfactory receptor neurons are also gated by cyclic nucleotides, *J. Neurosci.* **11**, 3565–3572, with permission.

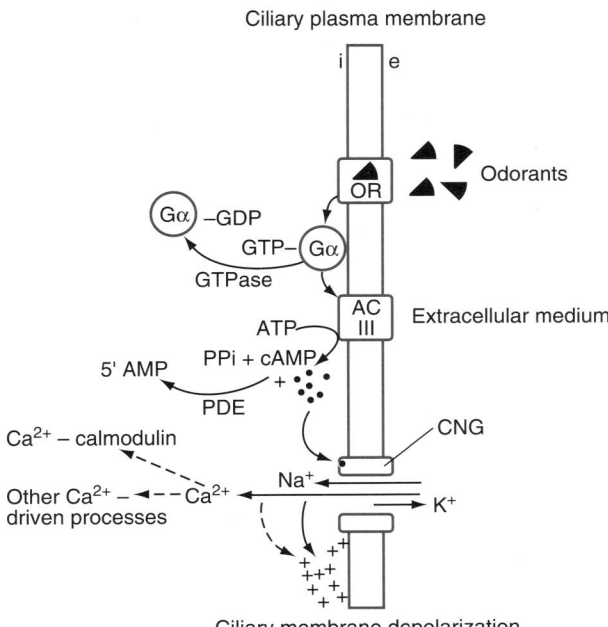

Ciliary plasma membrane

Ciliary membrane depolarization

Figure 15.17 The molecular cascade from odorant stimulation to activation of the cyclic nucleotide-gated channels. See text for explanations. OR, odorant receptor; ACIII, adenylate cyclase type III; CNG, cyclic-nucleotide-gated channel; PDE, phosphodiesterase. The open channel block by Ca^{2+} ions is not represented.

15.5 The odorant-evoked inward current evokes a membrane depolarization that spreads electronically to the axon hillock where it can elicit action potentials

15.5.1 The odorant-induced inward current depolarizes the membrane of olfactory receptors: the generator potential

It was shown in Section 15.2 that an odorant induces a depolarization of the membrane of olfactory receptor cells recorded *in vivo*. The same response is recorded *in vitro*. The *in vitro* preparation allows the analysis of the correspondence between the inward current and its consequence on membrane potential. Receptor cells are dissociated enzymatically from the olfactory epithelium of the newt, *Cynops pyrrhogaster*. Isolated olfactory cells are voltage-clamped by a patch pipette and their activity recorded in the whole-cell configuration. The odorant, *m*-amyl acetate, is dissolved in the external solution, placed in a pipette and ejected by pressure to the surface of the recorded cell. The cell interior is dialysed with the pipette solution. In such conditions, the resting membrane potential recorded is around −45 mV. When the

membrane is clamped at resting level ($I_H = 0$ pA), a brief application of the odorant evokes an inward current of 300 pA (**Figure 15.18a**). Ejection of the vehicle solution alone does not induce any response, ruling out the possibility of a response to mechanical stimulation (pressure). If the recording is now switched to current clamp mode in order to record potential changes, the same

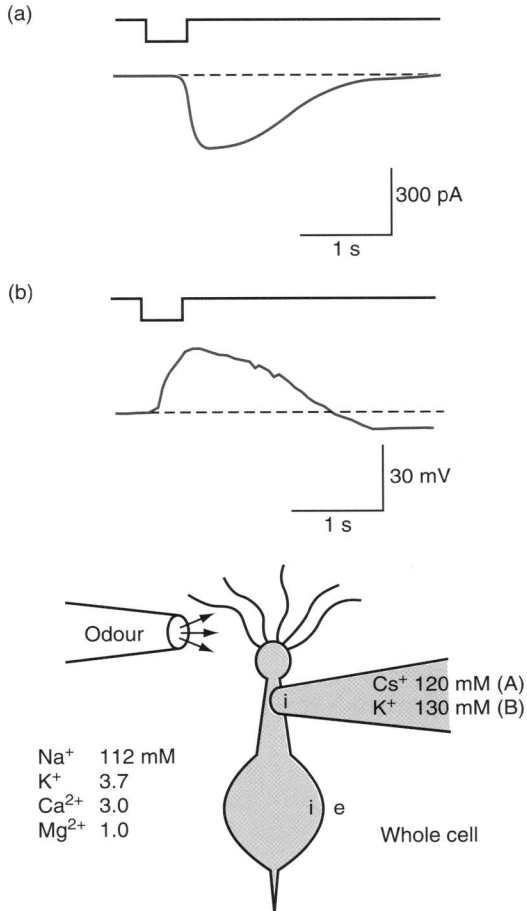

Figure 15.18 Response to odorant in control conditions. The activity of an isolated receptor cell is recorded in patch clamp in the whole-cell configuration. Cells are bathed in a standard solution and pipettes are filled with a pseudo-intracellular medium. Upper traces indicate the timing of ejection of the odorant, *n*-amyl acetate (10 mM). **(a)** In voltage clamp mode, the odorant application induces an inward current ($V_H = -54$ mV). **(b)** In current clamp mode, the odorant application induces a depolarization. The (a) and (b) recordings are obtained from two different olfactory receptor cells and the differences in the latency of the responses are due to a different position of the pipette ejecting the odorant. Adapted from Kurahashi T (1989) Activation of a cation-selective conductance in the olfactory receptor cell isolated from the newt, *J. Physiol. (Lond.)* **419**, 177–192, with permission.

brief application of the same odorant evokes at resting membrane potential a depolarization of 25–30 mV (**Figure 15.18b**). This depolarization is called the *generator potential*.

The membrane of the olfactory cells has a high input resistance in the order of 2–5 GΩ when measured in the isolated preparation with a patch pipette (this is estimated from the amplitude of the passive hyperpolarization evoked by a negative current pulse of known amplitude through the recording electrode). Thus the current required to depolarize the membrane by 10 mV from the resting potential can be as small as 10 pA. The synchronous opening of a few 45 pS channels at −50 mV would in theory be sufficient to drive the membrane potential to the threshold for spike initiation. At physiological Ca^{2+} concentrations, however, the unitary conductance is so reduced that simultaneous activation of at least 100 channels could be required to generate a response.

The divalent cation block is relieved by depolarization. So, we can hypothesize that once a sufficient number of channels are activated, the membrane begins to depolarize. This relieves partly the cation block. Then more current flows through the open channels and the membrane further depolarizes. This hypothesis is based on the model of the glutamatergic NMDA receptor channel studied in Chapter 11. Consequently, the generator potential depends not only on the presence of cAMP but also on the membrane potential of the olfactory receptor neuron.

15.5.2 The odorant-induced depolarization takes place in the cilia; spikes are initiated in the soma–initial axon segment, and the pattern of spike discharge propagated codes for the concentration and duration of the odorant stimulus

The generator potential (the depolarization) is electrotonically conducted from the cilia to the axon initial segment where the voltage-gated Na^+ channels are located and spikes are initiated in response to a membrane depolarization above threshold. In very few isolated olfactory cells (*in vitro* preparation), the depolarization evokes repetitive firing. Usually, depolarization causes only small spike-like events. Amputation of axons by the dissociation procedure may be responsible for the lack of spike initiation. In order to study the coupling between odorant-induced depolarization and the initiation of spikes and the coding of odorant concentration, the *in vivo* preparation is chosen.

Most olfactory neurons increase their firing rate with increasing odorant concentration. When the activity of an olfactory neuron is intracellularly recorded *in vivo*

(see Section 15.2 and **Figure 15.3**), a slow (50 mV s⁻¹) depolarization and evoked action potentials are recorded in response to an odorant application (**Figure 15.19**). The depolarization amplitude increases with the stimulus intensity as well as the instantaneous frequency of firing. For the largest depolarizations, the maximal instantaneous frequency is about 25 s⁻¹. These observations suggest that the stimulus concentration is transduced by the cell into an increased frequency of firing.

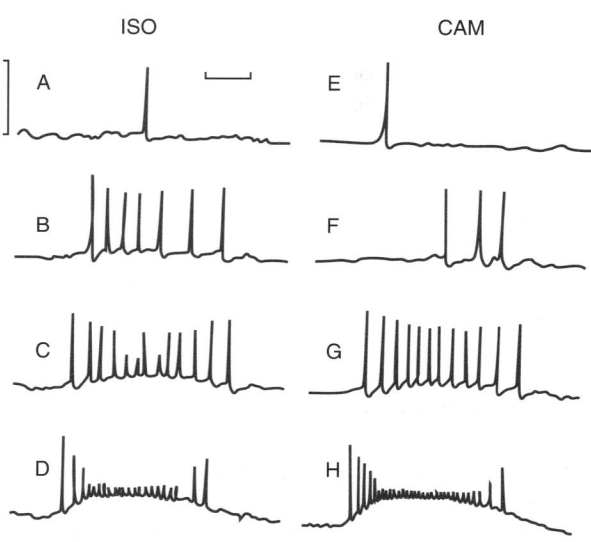

Figure 15.19 Dose–response relation recorded from an olfactory neuron stimulated with increasing concentrations of odorants.

Olfactory stimuli consist of short puffs (200–300 ms) of isoamylacetate (ISO) or camphor (CAM). From *A* to *D* and from *E* to *H* the concentrations of isoamylacetate or camphor are increased. The activity of the neuron is recorded with an intracellular electrode, in current clamp mode (V_m = −62 mV). *A*: The lowest concentration of isoamylacetate evokes a succession of small depolarizations and an action potential is evoked when the membrane reaches −52 mV. *B–D*: A slow and graded depolarization appears when the concentration of isoamylacetate is increased. As the amplitude of the depolarization increases, the number of spikes generated also increases. Note the small amplitude of the spikes when the interval interspike is short. *E–H*: With camphor, the general features of the cell responses were the same. Calibrations: 60 mV, 500 ms. Adapted from Trotier D, MacLeod P (1983) Intracellular recordings from salamander olfactory receptor cells, *Brain Res.* **268**, 225–237, with permission.

15.5.3 The nature of the odorant would be coded by the nature of the olfactory neuron stimulated and the synaptic arrangements in the olfactory bulb

It is hypothesized that each olfactory receptor cell expresses a single type of olfactory receptor. Thus, two odorants that are well discriminated would activate two different populations of olfactory neurons. This would hold true for all the odorants recognized. Now, how can the brain determine which type of neurons has been activated?

Specific recognition is conserved by the characteristic arrangements of the synaptic connections between the axons of olfactory cells and the second-order neurons in the olfactory bulb. There is a high convergence ratio 100–1000 : 1 of olfactory neurons to secondary neurons. It has been shown that the olfactory neurons expressing the same olfactory receptor project to the same region in the olfactory bulb on a small number of glomeruli, or even one. This was studied with *in situ* hybridization techniques. Taking advantage of the fact that copies of mRNA are transported in olfactory neurons to axon terminals, sections of the olfactory bulb are treated with a labelled probe which recognizes a known olfactory receptor mRNA: a single spot of labelled axons is observed in each olfactory bulb (left and right).

15.6 Conclusions

Olfactory receptor neurons amplify the odorant stimulus by a second-messenger cascade that produces hundreds or more of effector molecules (G proteins, cAMP) in response to the capture of one odorant molecule. This mechanism of transduction of sensory information is slow. The delay between a threshold stimulus and the response is up to hundreds of milliseconds. The same type of mechanism underlies visual and gustatory transductions. If we compare with photo-transduction, for example, the activation of rhodopsin by a single photon triggers a G protein (G_T) cascade which activates phosphodiesterase which hydrolyses cyclic GMP. In doing so, light causes closure of cGMP-gated cationic channels located in the plasma membrane of retinal rods and hyperpolarizes the membrane. The processes differ in that chemoreception involves an increase of cAMP concentration with a subsequent depolarization of the membrane whereas photoreception involves a decrease of cGMP concentration with a subsequent hyperpolarization of the membrane. It is striking that receptor cells use conventional G-protein-mediated mechanisms for transduction of the sensory stimulus, mechanisms also encountered in the transduction of neurotransmitter or hormone recognition.

Further reading

Broillet MC, Firestein S (1999) Cyclic nucleotide-gated channels: molecular mechanisms of activation. *Ann. NY Acad. Sci.* **868**, 730–740.

Dudai Y (1999) The smell of representations. *Neuron* **23**, 633–635.

Frings S, Lynch JW, Lindenman B (1992) Properties of cyclic nucleotide-gated channels mediating olfactory transduction. *J. Gen. Physiol.* **100**, 45–67.

Lancet D (1986) Vertebrate olfactory reception. *Ann. Rev. Neurosci.* **9**, 329–355.

Mombaerts P (1999) Seven-transmembrane proteins as odorant and chemosensory receptors. *Science* **286**, 707–711.

Nakamura T, Gold GH (1987) A cyclic-nucleotide gated conductance in olfactory receptor cilia. *Nature* **325**, 442–444.

Reed RR (1990) How does the nose know? *Cell* **60**, 1–2.

Shepherd GM (1994) Discrimination of molecular signals by the olfactory receptor neuron. *Neuron* **13**, 771–790.

Strausfeld NJ, Hildebrand JG (1999) Olfactory systems: common design, uncommon origins? *Curr. Opin. Neurobiol.* **9**, 634–639.

Part 3

Somato-Dendritic Processing and Plasticity of Postsynaptic Potentials

Somato-Dendritic Processing of Postsynaptic Potentials I: Passive Properties of Dendrites

Neurons of the mammalian central nervous system receive many afferents which contact different parts of their somato-dendritic arborization. When these afferents are activated, if their combined effect is depolarizing enough, they trigger the firing of sodium action potentials in the postsynaptic neuron. Classically, it is accepted that these action potentials are generated at a central point in the neuron, at the level of the initial segment of the axon (action potential generating zone; see Section 5.4.3 and **Figure 16.1**).

Action potentials are the response of the postsynaptic neuron. This response may be simple, consisting of a single action potential. In this case it can be described by a single characteristic: its latency. However, the postsynaptic response is generally more complex, consisting of several action potentials. It can then be described by several parameters: the latency of the first action potential, the duration of the response, the frequency of the action potentials that compose the response and the overall form – the pattern, or configuration – of the response (see **Figure 11.1**).

The events that lead to a postsynaptic response can be separated into several stages. When the afferent synapses are activated, an excitatory or inhibitory current is generated at the subsynaptic membrane, as a result of activation of receptor channels by the neurotransmitter(s). These postsynaptic currents propagate through the dendrites to the soma and to the initial segment of the postsynaptic neuron. In the course of their propagation, the postsynaptic currents summate. If the sum of the postsynaptic currents is sufficient to depolarize the membrane of the initial segment as far as the threshold potential for activation of the voltage-sensitive sodium channels, a response is triggered in the postsynaptic neuron (**Figure 16.1**).

However, we will see in the following chapters that the presence of a postsynaptic response and the characteristics of this response are not the result only of the integration of different currents of synaptic origin over

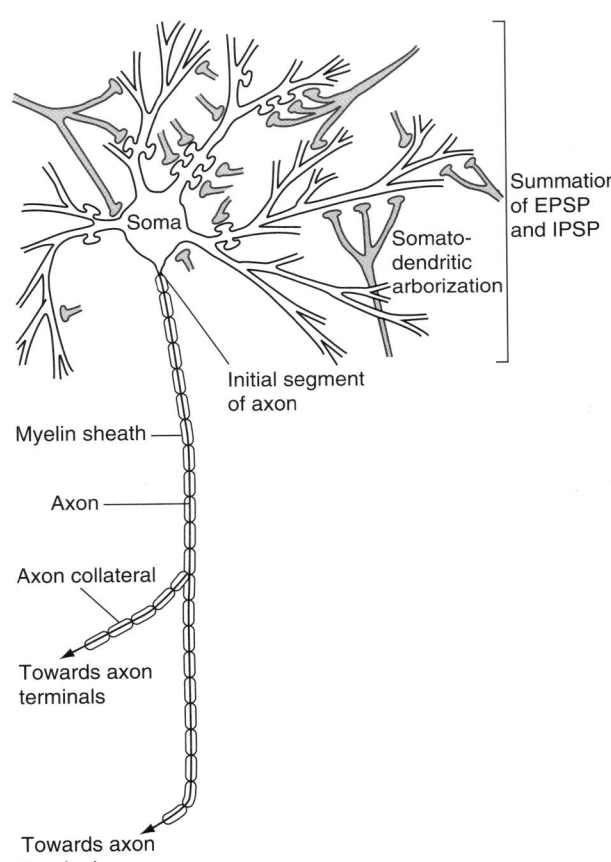

Figure 16.1 Schematic of a neuron and some of its afferents.

Afferent fibres establish synaptic contacts on spines and dendritic branches which are situated at different distances from the soma of the postsynaptic neuron. When these afferents are activated, the depolarizing or hyperpolarizing postsynaptic currents are conducted towards the soma and initial segment of the axon. It is at this level that the response of the postsynaptic neuron is generated. The response is then conducted along the axon and its collateral branches.

the somato-dendritic tree. In fact the response of the postsynaptic neuron is the result of two types of currents: currents across receptor channels in the postsynaptic membrane evoked by neurotransmitters and currents across voltage-sensitive channels present in the non-synaptic membrane. Currents of the first type are generated strictly at the postsynaptic membrane and their presence and duration is determined essentially by the interaction between the transmitter and the receptor channel and the intrinsic properties of the receptor channel. Currents of the second type are generated at the non-synaptic membrane (dendritic, somatic or at the initial segment) by voltage changes resulting from currents of synaptic origin, or from currents generated during the first action potential that is fired. The voltage-gated channels responsible for this second type of current are different from those of the sodium action potential and are generally activated in the sub-threshold range of membrane potentials. The duration of these subliminal voltage-gated currents is determined by the gating properties of the corresponding channels.

This chapter looks at the conduction and the summation of synaptic currents (first type of currents) over the dendritic tree. The characteristics of the diverse non-synaptic, subliminal currents (second type of currents) together with their role in the pattern of the postsynaptic discharge will be studied in the following chapters.

16.1 Propagation of excitatory and inhibitory postsynaptic potentials through the dendritic arborization

Excitatory and inhibitory postsynaptic potentials result, respectively, from depolarizing or hyperpolarizing currents through channels opened by neurotransmitters (receptor channels) in the postsynaptic membrane. These currents are generated over the somato-dendritic tree, at sites more or less distant from the soma (distal dendritic sites or proximal dendritic sites). Once generated, the postsynaptic currents propagate the length of the dendrites to the soma. For a long time it was thought that postsynaptic currents propagated passively and decrementally along the dendrites: passively because dendrites do not generate action potentials, the propagation of the signal depending only on the cable properties of the dendrite; and decrementally because the signal attenuates as it propagates, owing to the leakage properties of the membrane. From this it would be expected that depolarizations evoked by distal excitatory synapses would be smaller in amplitude at the soma and would have a longer risetime than depolarizations evoked by proximal synapses.

In fact, it seems that propagation is not always passive and not always decremental. There may be at least two types of propagation of postsynaptic currents through dendrites:

■ a passive and decremental propagation, which implies an attenuation of distal postsynaptic currents;
■ a passive but only slightly decremental propagation, which occurs where the cable properties of the dendrite are very good and involve no attenuation, or a weak attenuation, of distal postsynaptic currents.

These two alternatives are treated in Sections 16.1.2 and 16.1.3.

16.1.1 The complexity of synaptic organization (Figure 16.1)

Presynaptic complexity

A presynaptic afferent axon gives off many axon terminals (terminal boutons or 'en passant' terminals). In this way, it generally establishes several synaptic contacts with the postsynaptic neuron. In addition, the postsynaptic neuron receives synapses coming from many other presynaptic axons. It is thus possible to distinguish several levels of complexity in postsynaptic potentials:

■ the postsynaptic potential resulting from the activity of a single synaptic bouton: miniature potential;
■ the postsynaptic potential representing the sum of postsynaptic potentials generated by synaptic boutons coming from the same presynaptic axon: unitary postsynaptic potential;
■ the postsynaptic potential representing the sum of all the postsynaptic potentials generated at all the active synaptic boutons: composite postsynaptic potential.

Postsynaptic complexity

Different dendritic postsynaptic regions (spines, branches and main trunks) are not equivalent. The diameter of dendritic trunks is greater than that of branches, particularly distal branches. Thus different dendritic compartments have different resistances (note that $R = \rho l / s$, ρ being the resistivity, l the length and s the cross-section of the dendrite). This means that spines with a neck, or a very small diameter pedicle, have a high resistance. Consequently, synaptic currents generated at different points do not give the same potential change: for the same inward current I, the amplitude of the resulting postsynaptic depolarization (V_{EPSP}) will be greater for the dendritic regions where the resistance $r_m = 1/g_m$ is large ($V_{EPSP} = I_{EPSP}/g_m$).

Complexities of the propagation of postsynaptic action potentials

Postsynaptic potentials (EPSPs and IPSPs) propagate along the dendrites to the action potential initiation zone, which is generally situated in the initial region of the axon (initial segment). Depending on the cable properties of the dendrites, the postsynaptic potentials can change their characteristics (amplitude, risetime) during their propagation.

16.1.2 Passive decremental propagation of postsynaptic potentials

'Decremental' means that the postsynaptic potentials attenuate as they propagate. This implies that the postsynaptic potentials are not regenerated at each point along the dendrites, as is the action potential as it travels along the axon. This passive propagation depends on the cable properties of the dendrite. In order to estimate quantitatively the modifications of postsynaptic potentials in the course of their conduction, a theoretical model of the passive properties of membrane potential changes was first established by Wilfred Rall from data obtained on the squid giant axon. Thus a postsynaptic potential conducted with decrement (i) reduces in amplitude, and (ii) has a risetime (rt) which gets longer as it is propagated along the dendrites (**Figure 16.2a**).

The reduction in amplitude of the postsynaptic current as it gets further from the generation site is due to the fact that the current flows not only longitudinally along the dendrite but also transversely across the channels that are open in the dendritic membrane potential. This 'leak' of ions towards the extracellular medium results in a reduction in the postsynaptic current and a consequent reduction in the amplitude of the postsynaptic potential. Thus, the fewer the number of channels open in the dendritic membrane, the higher will be the value of r_m, the better will be the cable properties of the dendrite and the less will be the reduction in amplitude of postsynaptic potentials of distal origin.

The increase in the risetime of the postsynaptic potentials is due to the fact that part of the postsynaptic current serves to charge the capacity of each unit of membrane along the dendrite. The consequence of this is a change in the time course of the postsynaptic current: as it gets further from its point of generation, its risetime becomes longer (it can also be said that the speed of rising becomes slower).

16.1.3 Passive and non-decremental propagation of postsynaptic potentials

This type of propagation means that postsynaptic potentials are conducted passively along the dendrites but, because of the good cable properties of the dendritic arborization, they are almost unattenuated as they propagate. Thus, in the model of the synapse of Ia afferent fibres with spinal motoneurons, it has been shown that the unitary EPSPs evoked by the activity of afferent fibres and recorded in the soma have very similar amplitudes even though their risetimes may be different; i.e. when they are generated at different distances from the soma. This implies that, in this model, there must be local dendritic mechanisms that allow an almost non-attenuating conduction of the distal postsynaptic potentials.

16.2 Summation of excitatory and inhibitory postsynaptic potentials

16.2.1 Linear and nonlinear summation of excitatory postsynaptic potentials

In general many excitatory synaptic afferents converge on a single neuron. At each excitatory synapse that is activated, there is an inward current of positive charges. When the membrane potential is not held at a fixed value, this inward current of positive charges depolarizes the postsynaptic membrane: this is the postsynaptic potential, or EPSP (see, for example, the current clamp recordings of the synaptic response to glutamate in Chapter 11).

A unitary EPSP (meaning one caused by the activation of a single afferent fibre; Section 16.1.1) cannot trigger action potentials. EPSPs generated in isolation are too small in amplitude to depolarize the membrane of the initial segment to the threshold potential for the opening of voltage-sensitive Na^+ channels. However, if many EPSPs generated at different sites in the dendritic arborization arrive more or less simultaneously at the level of the initial segment, the probability that they will generate action potentials becomes much greater. This is due to the fact that the EPSPs summate.

Linear summation of excitatory postsynaptic potentials

The term 'linear summation' means that the composite EPSP (see Section 16.1.1) resulting from the activity of several excitatory synapses has an amplitude that is equal to the geometric sum of the different EPSPs contributing to it. This is true when the EPSPs are generated

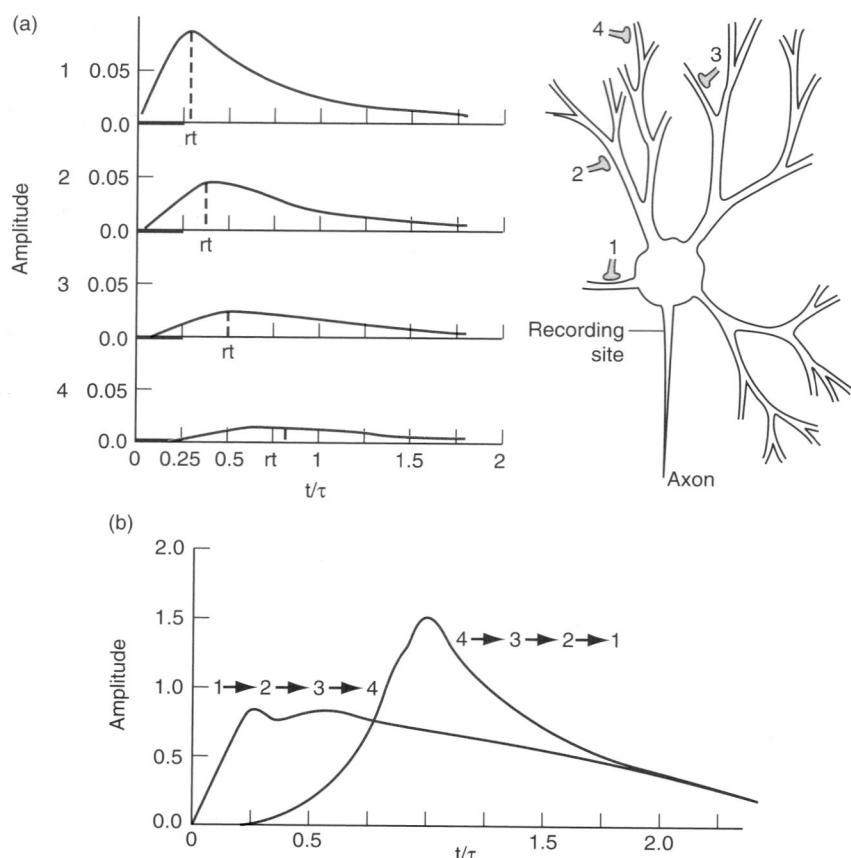

Figure 16.2 Theoretical model of decremental conduction of excitatory postsynaptic potentials (EPSP) along dendrites.
(a) Four EPSPs numbered 1 to 4 are generated at the instant t between $t = 0$ and $t = 0.25$ ms (black bar in simulation diagram on left), at different sites within the dendritic tree (schematic drawing on right). At the site of generation, these EPSPs are identical in amplitude and duration. After conduction along the dendrites, their shapes are different (theoretical recordings at the level of the soma, simulation diagram on left). It can be observed that the further away the site of generation of the EPSP (case 4), the smaller is its amplitude and the longer is its rise-time (rt) when it arrives at the level of the soma (compare the theoretical recordings 1 to 4).
(b) Theoretical model of the linear summation of EPSP (see text for explanation). From Rall W (1977) *Handbook of Physiology*, vol. 1, part 1, Bethesda, MA: American Physiological Society, with permission.)

at sites that are sufficiently far or isolated from one another to avoid interactions between them (on different dendritic branches, or on different dendritic spines, for instance).

A postsynaptic neuron generally receives many excitatory synapses at different points on its somato-dendritic arborization (see **Figures 16.1** and **16.2a**). These EPSPs summate as they propagate, in a temporo-spatial manner. To grasp this phenomenon, it must be understood that the EPSPs generated at different sites in the dendritic arborization and conducted to the initial segment of the axon can arrive spread out in time. The offset between the EPSPs will depend on the distances between the generation sites and on the respective times at which they were generated. The examples demonstrated here are based on theoretical calculations of

the cable properties of dendrites. These data give a qualitative understanding of the phenomena of summation but do not constitute a real experimental demonstration.

Let us consider the example of four EPSPs of the same amplitude, generated at different sites in the dendritic arborization, at times such that their arrivals at the initial segment are offset in time. **Figure 16.2b** shows the 'composite EPSP' obtained in two cases of arrival sequences. In the case $1 \rightarrow 2 \rightarrow 3 \rightarrow 4$, the four EPSPs are generated at the same time t; but since some are generated at more distal sites, their arrivals at the initial segment are staggered, the most proximal arriving first and the most distal arriving last. In the case $4 \rightarrow 3 \rightarrow 2 \rightarrow 1$, the most distal EPSPs are generated well before the proximal EPSPs, so that the distal EPSPs arrive before the proximal EPSPs. The theoretical results show that in the first case in which the proximal EPSPs occur first and are followed by the more distal EPSPs, the 'composite EPSP' has a short latency, a long duration and a small amplitude; while in the second case, in which the distal EPSPs arrive before the proximal EPSPs, the 'composite EPSP' has a long latency and a large amplitude (**Figure 16.2b**).

Nonlinear summation of excitatory postsynaptic potentials

The term 'nonlinear summation' means that the 'composite EPSP' has an amplitude that is not equal to the geometric sum of the different EPSPs contributing to it. This occurs, for instance, when two EPSPs are generated at the same site or at sites that are close.

Let us take the example of two excitatory synapses whose neurotransmitter is glutamate and which are situated close together on the same dendritic segment (**Figure 16.3**), supposing that the membrane potential of the dendritic segment is V_m. When synapse 1 is active alone, EPSP$_1$ is recorded, due to the excitatory postsy-

naptic current I_1, such that $I_1 = g_{cations}(V_m - E_{cations})$, whose amplitude is $V_{EPSP1} = I_1/g_m$, where g_m is the membrane conductance (**Figure 16.3a**). When synapse 2 is active alone, EPSP$_2$ is recorded at level 2, due to the postsynaptic current I_2, such that $I_2 = g_{cations}(V_m - E_{cations})$, whose amplitude is $V_{EPSP2} = I_2/g_m$ (**Figure 16.3b**). If we suppose that when the two EPSPs are generated separately, $V_{EPSP1} = V_{EPSP2}$, what is the amplitude of the 'composite EPSP' when the two synapses are active at the same time?

When synapse 1 is activated first, EPSP$_1$ is recorded in the postsynaptic element and will be conducted passively to neighbouring regions (**Figure 16.3a**). At time $t + \Delta t$, EPSP$_1$ arrives at the postsynaptic element 2. The membrane of the postsynaptic element 2 is then at a potential $V_m{}'$ which is more positive than V_m (**Figure 16.3c**). If at this moment ($t + \Delta t$) synapse 2 is active, the postsynaptic current $I_2{}'$ will be smaller than if it had taken place independently from I_1 because the electrochemical gradient of Na$^+$ and Ca^{2+} ions is reduced. $I_2{}' = g_{cations}(V_m{}' - E_{cations})$ and $I_2{}' < I_2$ because $(V_m{}' - E_{cations}) < (V_m - E_{cations})$. The 'composite EPSP' will have an amplitude less than the geometric sum EPSP$_1$ + EPSP$_2$ (**Figure 16.3c**).

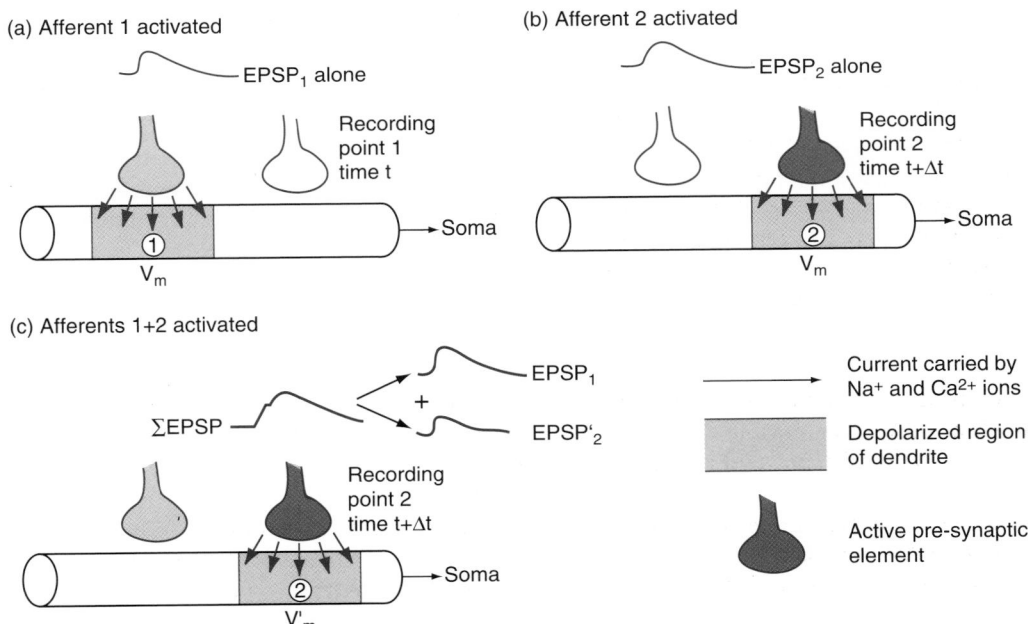

Figure 16.3 Nonlinear summation of excitatory postsynaptic potentials.
Suppose that there are two excitatory synapses situated close together on the same dendritic segment. **(a)** When afferent 1 is activated at time t, a depolarization of the postsynaptic membrane 1 is recorded at time t (EPSP$_1$ alone). This depolarization propagates in the two directions away from 1. **(b)** When afferent 2 is activated, at time $t + \Delta t$, a depolarization of the postsynaptic membrane 2 is recorded (EPSP$_2$ alone). **(c)** When the two afferents 1 and 2 are activated as before, but together, one at time t and the other at time $t + \Delta t$, a depolarization of the postsynaptic membrane 2 (ΣEPSP) is recorded at time $t + \Delta t$, which does not correspond to the geometric sum EPSP$_1$ alone + EPSP$_2$ alone, since EPSP$_2{}'$ has an amplitude which is smaller than EPSP$_2$ (see text for explanation).

This is also the case when a single excitatory synapse is activated repetitively by the arrival of high-frequency presynaptic action potentials. When an excitatory postsynaptic current is generated before the preceding current has ended, it has a smaller amplitude because the postsynaptic membrane is depolarized. Thus, during high-frequency activation, successive excitatory postsynaptic potentials have amplitudes that are smaller and smaller.

16.2.2 Linear and nonlinear summation of inhibitory postsynaptic potentials

When inhibitory synapses are active they cause, in the postsynaptic membrane, an outward postsynaptic current of positive charges (carried by K^+ ions) or an inward current of negative charges (carried by Cl^- ions) which hyperpolarizes the membrane: this is the inhibitory postsynaptic potential, or IPSP.

Linear summation of IPSPs is symmetrically the same as linear summation of EPSPs. Nonlinear summation of IPSPs is symmetrically the same as nonlinear summation of EPSPs.

16.2.3 The integration of excitatory and inhibitory postsynaptic potentials partly determines the configuration of the postsynaptic discharge

In order for an action potential to be triggered at the initial segment, the membrane of the initial segment must be depolarized to the threshold potential for the opening of voltage-sensitive Na^+ channels. It is also necessary for this depolarization to have a relatively rapid risetime so that the Na^+ channels do not inactivate during the depolarization. The characteristics of depolarization of the initial segment (amplitude, duration, risetime) result partly from the summation of excitatory and inhibitory postsynaptic potentials.

Integration of depolarizing (excitatory) postsynaptic potential with hyperpolarizing (inhibitory) postsynaptic potential

A hyperpolarizing postsynaptic potential is due to a current whose reversal potential is more negative than the resting membrane potential of the cell. This type of inhibition is generally due to the opening of K^+ channels ($GABA_B$-type inhibition). Since the equilibrium potential of K^+ ions is more negative than the resting membrane potential, the opening of K^+ channels gives rise to an outward current (an exit of positive charges) and to a

hyperpolarization of the membrane; i.e. an IPSP. If this IPSP is concomitant with an EPSP, it will reduce the amplitude of the EPSP. This type of summation of EPSP and IPSP is summarized in **Figure 16.4**.

Integration of depolarizing (excitatory) postsynaptic potential and silent (inhibitory) postsynaptic potential

A silent postsynaptic potential is due to a current whose reversal potential is close to the resting potential of the cell. Generally, this is caused by a current of Cl^- ions through $GABA_A$ channels (see Chapter 10). When the equilibrium potential of Cl^- ions is close to the membrane resting potential, the opening of Cl^- channels does not reveal a hyperpolarizing current at the resting potential (from which comes the term 'silent' for this inhibition). However, when the membrane is depolarized by an EPSP, the inhibition is no longer silent, but becomes hyperpolarizing and results in a reduction or even a complete suppression of the EPSP (**Figure 16.5**).

Integration of depolarizing (excitatory) postsynaptic potential and depolarizing inhibitory postsynaptic potential

A depolarizing inhibitory postsynaptic potential is due to a synaptic current whose reversal potential is more positive than the resting potential of the membrane but more negative than the threshold for the opening of the Na^+ channels of the action potential. This is generally due to the opening of Cl^- channels in cells in which the reversal potential for Cl^- ions is situated between the resting potential and the threshold potential for the opening of the Na^+ channels of the action potential. Thus, when the membrane is at its resting potential, this Cl^- current causes a slight depolarization of the membrane, but does not trigger action potentials. When the membrane is depolarized (by an EPSP) above the inversion potential of Cl^+ ions, this current causes a hyperpolarization of the membrane and an inhibition of the EPSP.

16.3 Summary

Several types of inhibition appear over the length of the somato-dendritic arborization and these limit the effect of excitatory synapses. The opening or non-opening of the Na^+ channels of the action potential, and in consequence the generation of action potentials which will constitute the response of the postsynaptic neuron, are the result of this summation of excitatory and inhibitory postsynaptic potentials. However, the characteristics of

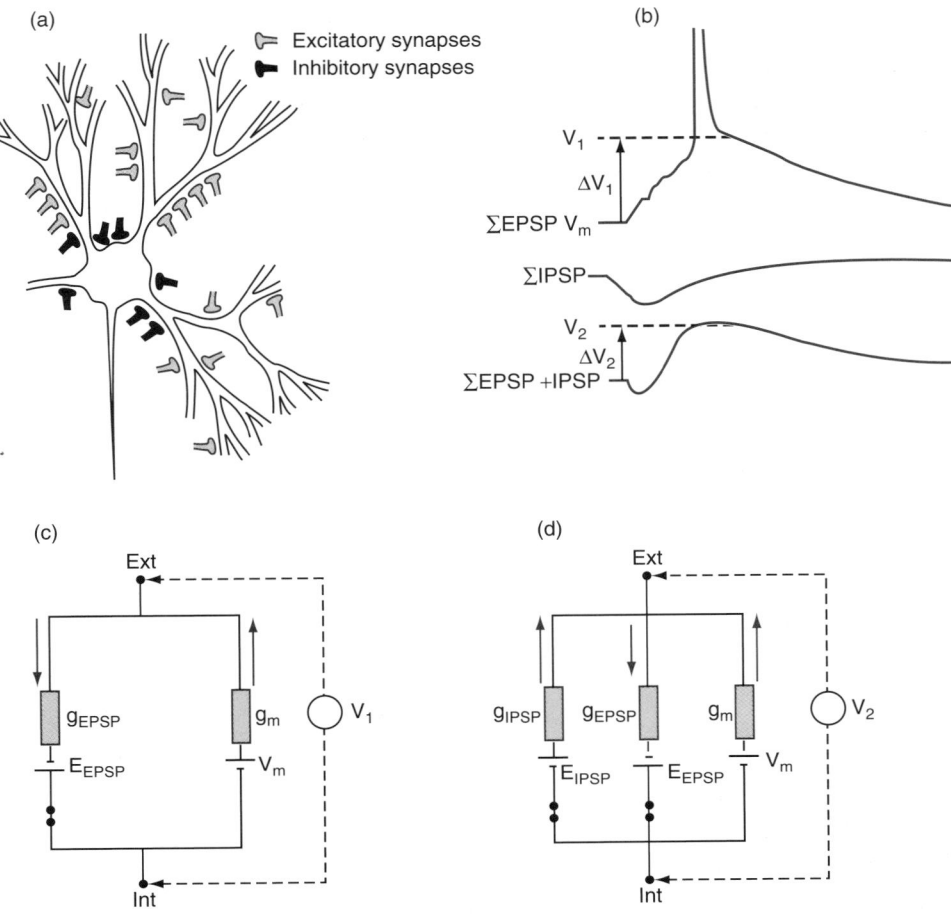

Figure 16.4 Integration of excitatory (EPSP) and inhibitory (IPSP) postsynaptic potentials.
(a) Suppose that on a dendritic tree, there are glutaminergic excitatory synapses which are situated distally, and $GABA_B$-type inhibitory synapses which are situated proximally, and that all of these are active at the same instant t. (b) If only the excitatory synapses are active, a depolarization, a composite EPSP ($\Sigma EPSP$) will be recorded at the soma which corresponds to the linear and nonlinear summation of all the different EPSPs (top trace). We will suppose that the $\Sigma EPSP$ has an amplitude that is sufficient to trigger an action potential (upper trace). If only the inhibitory synapses are active, a hyperpolarization, a composite IPSP ($\Sigma IPSP$) will be recorded at the soma which corresponds to the linear and nonlinear summation of all the different IPSPs (middle trace). When all these different synapses are activated at the same time t, a depolarization preceded by a hyperpolarization, a composite PSP, will be recorded at the soma, corresponding to the sum of the different synaptic potentials ($\Sigma EPSP + \Sigma IPSP$) (bottom trace). In this case the amplitude of the depolarization is no longer sufficient to trigger an action potential. (c) Electrical equivalent of the membrane at the level of the initial segment, for an EPSP alone. (d) Electrical equivalent for the membrane when an EPSP and an IPSP summate. The currents I_{EPSP} and I_{IPSP} are opposite and subtract from one another. By comparing with (c), it is observed that I_{EPSP} in (c) is greater than $I_{EPSP} + I_{IPSP}$ in (d), and $\Delta V_1 > \Delta V_2$.

the response of the postsynaptic neuron are determined not only by the amplitude and duration of the depolarization of synaptic origin but also by the characteristics of the membrane of the initial segment, also known as 'input–output' characteristics.

Further reading

Buhl EH, Halasy K, Somogyi P (1994) Diverse sources of hippocampal unitary inhibitory postsynaptic potentials and the number of release sites. *Nature* **368**, 823–828.

Cauller LJ, Connors BW (1992) Functions of very distal dendrites. In: McKenna TM, Davis J, Zornetzer SE (eds) *Single Neuron Computation*, New York: Academic Press.

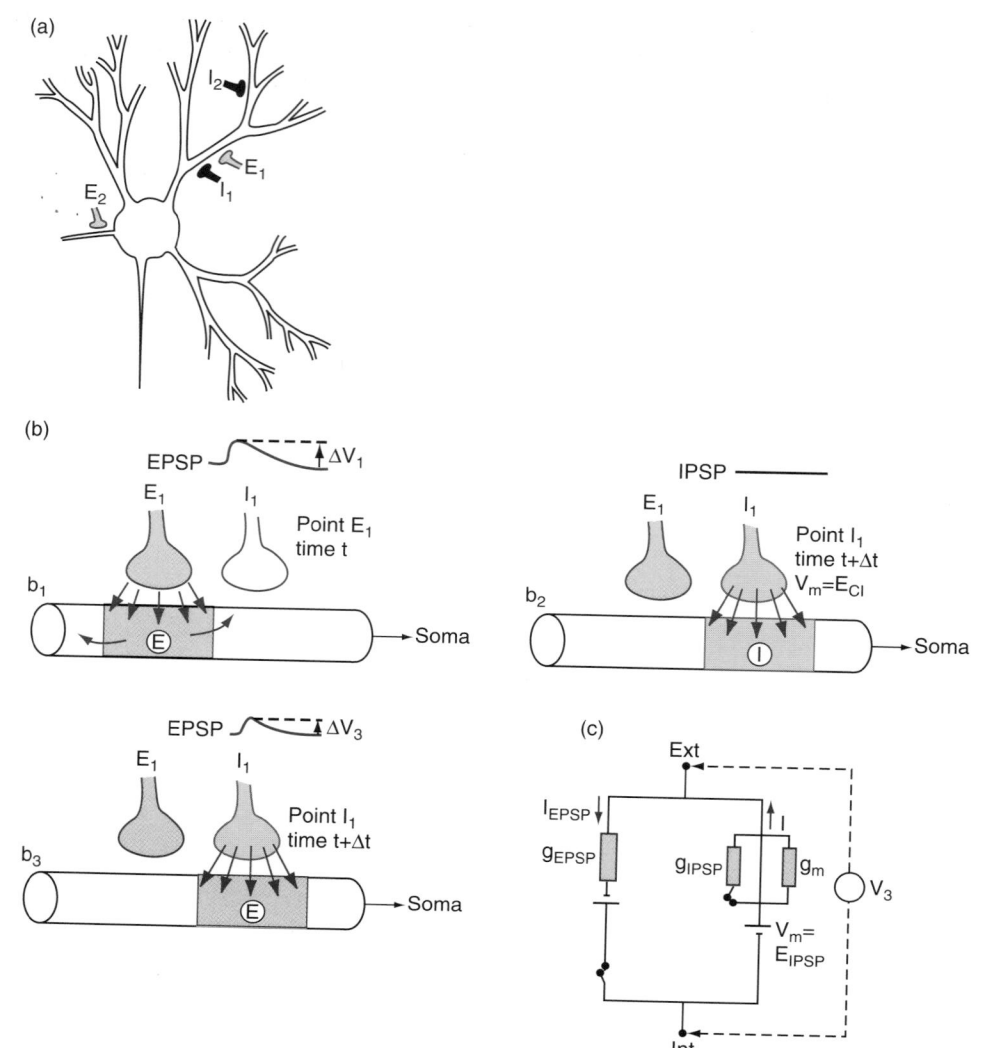

Figure 16.5 Role of silent inhibition.

(a) This diagram shows two synapses, one glutamatergic with postsynaptic AMPA receptors (E_1) and the other GABAergic with GABA$_A$ postsynaptic receptors (I_1), situated close to one another on the same dendritic segment, such that the inhibitory synapse is closer to the soma than the excitatory synapse. (b) When the excitatory synapse is excited alone, an EPSP of ΔV_1 in amplitude is recorded (b_1). When the inhibitory synapse is activated alone, no change in potential is recorded because $V_m = E_{Cl}$ (b_2). When both synapses are activated, the EPSP which propagates towards the soma is reduced in amplitude (amplitude ΔV_3), or even cancelled out. This type of inhibition is selective because it only acts on excitatory synapses that are situated distally. (c) Electrical equivalent of the membrane at the dendritic segment. If this is compared with Figure 16.4c, it can be seen that $\Delta V_3 < \Delta V_1$ because $g_m + g_{IPSP} > g_m$.

Larkum ME, Launey T, Dityatev A, Lüscher HR (1998) Integration of excitatory postsynaptic potentials in dendrites of motoneurons of rat spinal cord slice cultures. *J. Neurophysiol.* **80**, 924–935.

Miles R, Toth K, Gulyas AI, Hajos N, Freund TF (1996) Differences between somatic and dendritic inhibition in the hippocampus. *Neuron* **16**, 815–823.

Rall W (1977) Core conductor theory and cable properties of neurons. In: Brookhart JM, Mountcastle VB, Kandel ER, Geiger SR (eds) *Handbook of Physiology*, vol. 1, part 1, Bethesda, MD: American Physiological Society.

Redman SJ (1973) The attenuation of passively propagating dendritic potentials in a motoneuron cable model. *J. Physiol.* **234**, 637–664.

Shepherd GM (1994) The significance of real neuro-architectures for neural network simulations. In: Schwartz EL (ed.) *Computational Neuroscience*, New York: Oxford University Press.

Spruston N, Johnston D (1992) Perforated patch clamp analysis of the passive membrane properties of three classes of hippocampal neurons. *J. Neurophysiol.* **67**, 508–528.

Spruston N, Jaffe DB, Johnston D (1994) Dendritic attenuation of synaptic potentials and currents: the role of passive membrane properties. *Trends Neurosci.* **17**, 161–166.

Subliminal Voltage-Gated Currents of the Somato-Dendritic Membrane

Not all neurons respond in the same way when they are activated by a depolarizing current pulse or when they are hyperpolarized: it can be said that they do not have the same pattern of firing (**Figure 17.1**). When depolarized, spinal motoneurons may respond with a low-frequency regular discharge, certain pyramidal neurons of the hippocampus with a burst of action potentials followed by a long silence, neurons of the inferior olive nucleus with an irregular sustained activity of bursts of action potentials. Conversely, when hyperpolarized, hippocampal neurons become silent whereas thalamic and subthalamic neurons discharge bursts of action potentials. It should be noted that the term 'firing pattern' is not equivalent to the term 'discharge frequency', except in cases where the response consists of action potentials generated at a regular frequency. In this case only, the mean value of the discharge frequency is sufficient to describe the response of the neuron. In other cases, the mean frequency value has no significance.

Neurons, as pointed out by Llinas (1988), are not interchangeable; i.e. a neuron cannot be functionally replaced by one of another type even if their synaptic connectivity, type of afferent neurotransmitters and receptors to these neurotransmitters are identical. The activity of a neuronal network is related not only to the *excitatory and inhibitory interactions* among neurons but also to their *intrinsic electrical properties* as well. The 'personality' of a neuron is defined by its input–output characteristics; i.e. its firing pattern (output) in response to a depolarization or a hyperpolarization (input).

Input–output characteristics are the result of a rich repertoire of ionic currents other than those of the action potentials. These currents, inward or outward, are called *subliminal voltage-gated currents* because they are activated at voltages subthreshold to that of action potentials. They are located either in the dendritic or the somatic membrane or both. In many experiments, recordings are performed at the level of the soma and the question may remain as to where these currents are generated: at the level of the dendrites, the soma, the initial segment?

17.1 Observations and questions

Figure 17.1 shows the different responses of central neurons recorded in current clamp mode, in response to a depolarizing current pulse and at different membrane potentials.

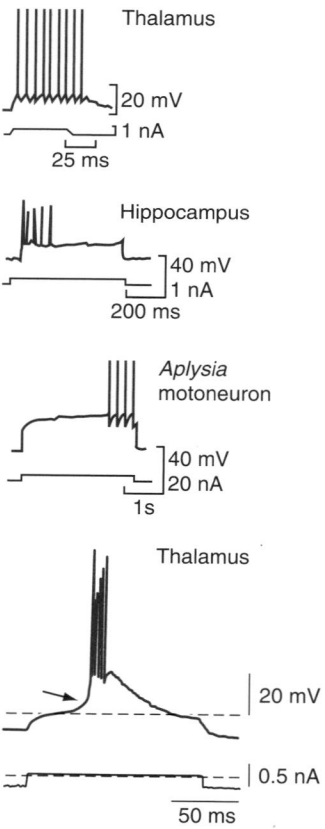

Figure 17.1 Different neuronal responses to a depolarizing current pulse.

From top to bottom: thalamo-cortical neuron, pyramidal neuron of the hippocampus, motoneuron innervating the ink gland of *Aplysia*, and again a thalamo-cortical neuron but from a more hyperpolarized membrane potential.

- What are the currents activated during the depolarizing current pulse that stop the firing of hippocampal neurons after 100–200 ms? Are these currents activated by action potentials?
- What are the currents activated by the depolarizing current pulse that delay the firing of motoneurons innervating the ink gland of *Aplysia*?
- What are the currents that make a thalamic neuron fire in the bursting mode? Why are they activated at a hyperpolarized membrane potential?

To answer these questions, the main subliminal currents must be first explained individually (this chapter). Their influence on postsynaptic potentials and firing patterns are explained in Chapters 18–20.

17.2 The subliminal voltage-gated currents that depolarize the membrane

The common characteristic of these currents is to be inward and turned on at potentials more negative than the threshold for the opening of voltage-gated Na^+ channels of the action potential. Three types of inward subliminal currents will be explained: the persistent Na^+ current (I_{NaP}), the transient Ca^{2+} current (I_{CaT}) and the hyperpolarization-activated cationic current (I_h).

17.2.1 The persistent inward Na^+ current, I_{NaP}

I_{NaP} is a slowly inactivating current. It is thus called 'P' for persistent in comparison with the fast-inactivating Na^+ current of the action potential (I_{Na}). I_{NaP} is activated at potentials of about 10 mV negative to I_{Na}; i.e. at subthreshold potentials. I_{NaP} is present in many vertebrate central neurons, and in particular in Purkinje cells.

I_{NaP} was first described by Prince and coworkers in hippocampal (1979) and neocortical (1982) neurons in slices, as an increase in slope resistance at potentials 10–15 mV positive to resting potential (the I_{NaP}/V relation showed an inward rectification). In the presence of TTX in the extracellular medium or when external Na^+ is replaced by the impermeant ion choline, this inward rectification disappears.

Structure of the main channel subunit

To determine whether the I_{NaP} channel is a non-inactivating subtype of the classical fast-inactivating Na^+ channel, or is a different channel, the Na^+ channel α-subunit transcripts expressed in Purkinje cells are studied using single-cell reverse transcription-PCR

(RT-PCR). Purkinje cells have been chosen because the two different voltage-gated Na^+ currents are recorded from them: one responsible for the fast depolarization phase of action potentials and a second responsible for the TTX-sensitive prolonged potential plateau. mRNA transcripts for two α-subunits have been found. On the basis of mutant studies, the one called CerIII (cerebellum III) is suggested to be responsible for I_{NaP}; the other, called RBI (rat brain I), is suggested to be responsible for I_{Na}. This result tends to favour the hypothesis that I_{NaP} does not result from a Na^+ channel with multiple gating states but corresponds to a different channel.

Gating properties and ionic nature

In whole-cell recordings, in the presence of Cd^{2+} (200 μM) and K^+ channel blockers (20 mM TEA, 2 mM Cs^+), a slowly inactivating Na^+ current is recorded in response to incremental depolarizing steps between −60 and −50 mV from a holding potential of −90 mV (**Figure 17.2a**). Note that at more depolarized levels, the fast-inactivating Na^+ current superimposes on the slow one. I_{NaP} has a fast activation time of 2–4 ms, and once it is evoked it is present for several hundreds of milliseconds and is totally and reversibly blocked by TTX (1 μM) (**Figure 17.2b**). This observation, together with the lack of effect of extracellular Co^{2+} on this current, suggest that it is an inward current which uses Na^+ as the charge carrier.

The I/V relation gives an estimated reversal potential of +49.1 ± 1.3 mV (**Figure 17.2c**). The voltage dependence of activation is determined by applying different voltage steps from a holding potential $V_H = -90$ mV. The normalized peak current amplitude is plotted against the test potential to give the activation curve. In suprachiasmatic neurons, I_{NaP} is half-activated at $V_{1/2} = -43$ mV, at least 10 mV more negative than $V_{1/2}$ of I_{Na} (**Figure 17.2d**). To study the inactivation properties of I_{NaP}, the membrane is clamped at different holding potentials and the current in response to a depolarizing step to −50 mV is recorded. A plot of peak current amplitude against holding potential gives a measure of the voltage dependence of inactivation. In these neurons, I_{NaP} is half inactivated at $V_{1/2} = -68$ mV (**Figure 17.3**).

Pharmacology

I_{NaP} is sensitive to TTX at micromolar doses in the extracellular solution and to internal QX-314 (a derivative of lidocaine) injected into the intracellular medium. These toxins also block I_{Na}, which is a problem when studying the role of I_{NaP} on the pattern of discharge of a neuron. There is no selective blocker of I_{NaP}. To study I_{NaP} in

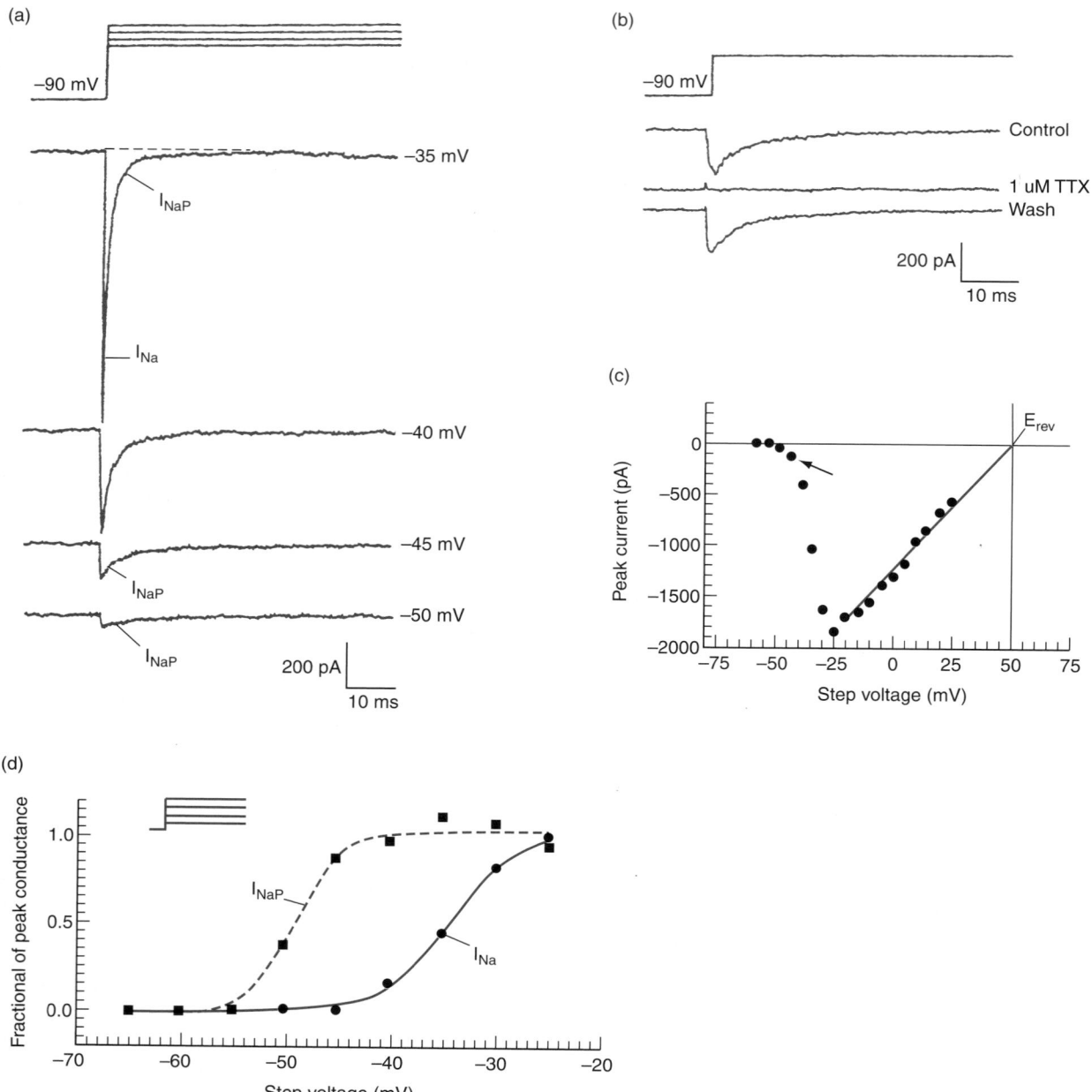

Figure 17.2 Activation properties of the slowly inactivating Na⁺ current, I_{NaP}.
The activity of neurons of the suprachiasmatic nucleus is recorded in slices (whole-cell configuration, voltage clamp mode). **(a)** Incremental steps from a holding potential of –90 mV. **(b)** Reversible block by TTX. **(c)** I/V plot for the peak I_{NaP} measured from records in (a). **(d)** Activation curve ($V_{1/2}$ = –43 mV). Adapted from Pennartz CMA, Bierlaagh MA, Geurtsen AMS (1997) Cellular mechanisms underlying spontaneous firing in rat suprachiasmatic nucleus: involvement of a slowly inactivating component of sodium current. *J. Neurophysiol.* **78**, 1811–1825, with permission.

isolation, Ca^{2+} and K^+ channels must be blocked by Cd^{2+} or Co^{2+} or Ni^{2+} (200 μM to 1 mM), 4-AP (1 mM), TEA (10 mM), Ba^{2+} (1 mM). In these conditions I_{Na} will be also recorded at some voltage steps but is easily recognized by its high amplitude and fast inactivation.

In summary, I_{NaP} is a TTX-sensitive Na⁺ current that activates at around –60 to –50 mV. I_{NaP} can be distinguished from the Na⁺ current of action potential, I_{Na}, by its low threshold of activation and its slow inactivation.

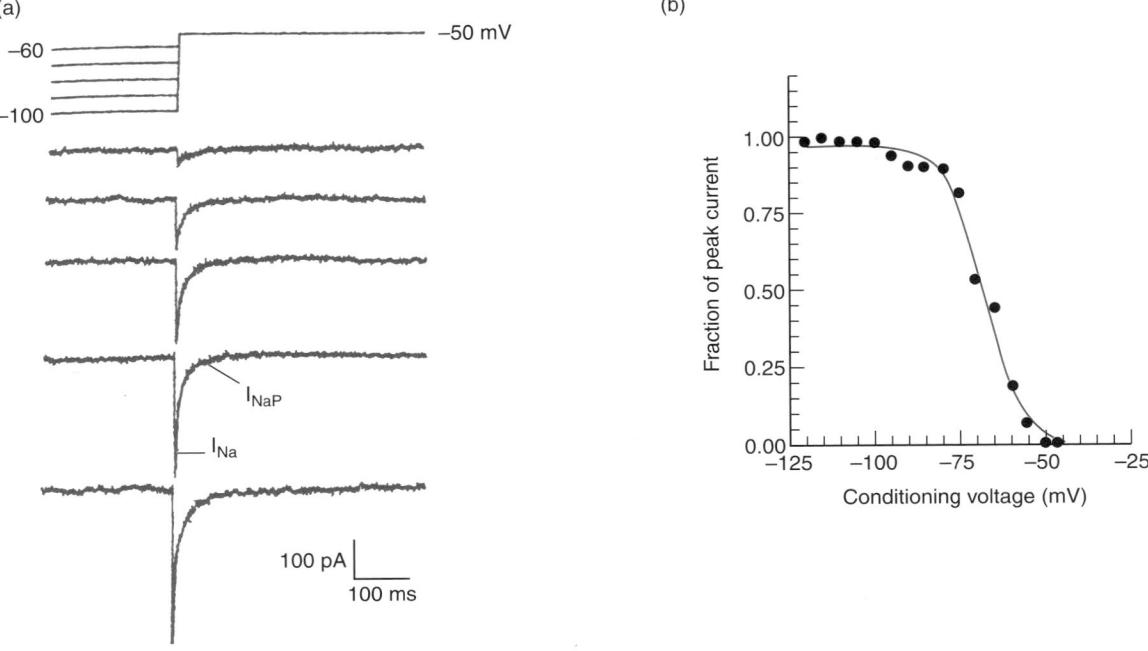

Figure 17.3 Inactivation properties of the slowly inactivating Na+ current, I_{NaP}.
The activity of neurons of the suprachiasmatic nucleus is recorded in slices (whole-cell configuration, voltage clamp mode). **(a)** Currents recorded in response to a fixed step to –50 mV from incremental holding potentials. **(b)** Inactivation curve ($V_{1/2}$ = –68 mV). Adapted from Pennartz CMA, Bierlaagh MA, Geurtsen AMS (1997) Cellular mechanisms underlying spontaneous firing in rat suprachiasmatic nucleus: involvement of a slowly inactivating component of sodium current. *J. Neurophysiol.* **78**, 1811–1825, with permission.

17.2.2 The low-threshold transient Ca²⁺ current, I_{CaT}

I_{CaT} is called 'T' for transient since once activated it rapidly inactivates. It was originally described by Carbone and Lux in 1984 but its existence had first been suggested by Eccles and coworkers in 1964 to explain their observation of a period of enhanced excitability following membrane hyperpolarization in some central neurons.

Structure of the main channel subunit

Three different α-subunits which encode a T-type Ca²⁺ channel have been described: α_{1G}, α_{1H} and α_{1I}. Their primary structure shows the presence of four homologous domains, each containing six putative transmembrane segments (S1 to S6) and a P loop between segments 5 and 6 (**Figure 17.4a**). In contrast to the α-subunits of high-voltage-activated channels (L, N, P), T channel α-subunits contain a large extracellular loop located between S5 and the P loop.

Single-channel conductance

The activity of chick dorsal root ganglion cells in culture is recorded in patch clamp (cell-attached patch). The patch pipette contains 110 mM of BaCl₂ instead of 2 mM of CaCl₂ for the following reasons: Ca²⁺ channels are permeable to Ba²⁺, Ba²⁺ does not inactivate Ca²⁺ channels, Ba²⁺ does not activate Ca²⁺-dependent channels such as Ca²⁺-activated K⁺ channels, and Ba²⁺ current (at such high concentration of charge carrier, 110 mM) through Ca²⁺ channels has in general a large amplitude and is more easy to study. Moreover, when Ba²⁺ is the only external cation, Na⁺ currents are not recorded.

The membrane is held at a hyperpolarized potential (V_H = –80 mV) to keep T channels non-inactivated. When depolarizing voltage steps of small amplitude (30–60 mV) are applied to the patch, unitary inward Ba²⁺ currents are recorded. These unitary inward currents have a small amplitude (**Figure 17.4b**) and the unitary conductance γ_T is very low compared with that of high-threshold activated Ca²⁺ channels: it varies between 5 and 9 pS in 110 mM of Ba²⁺. At physiological concentrations of external Ca²⁺ (2 mM) the expected conductance would be around 1 pS. Single-channel T currents are present at the beginning of the depolarizing step and

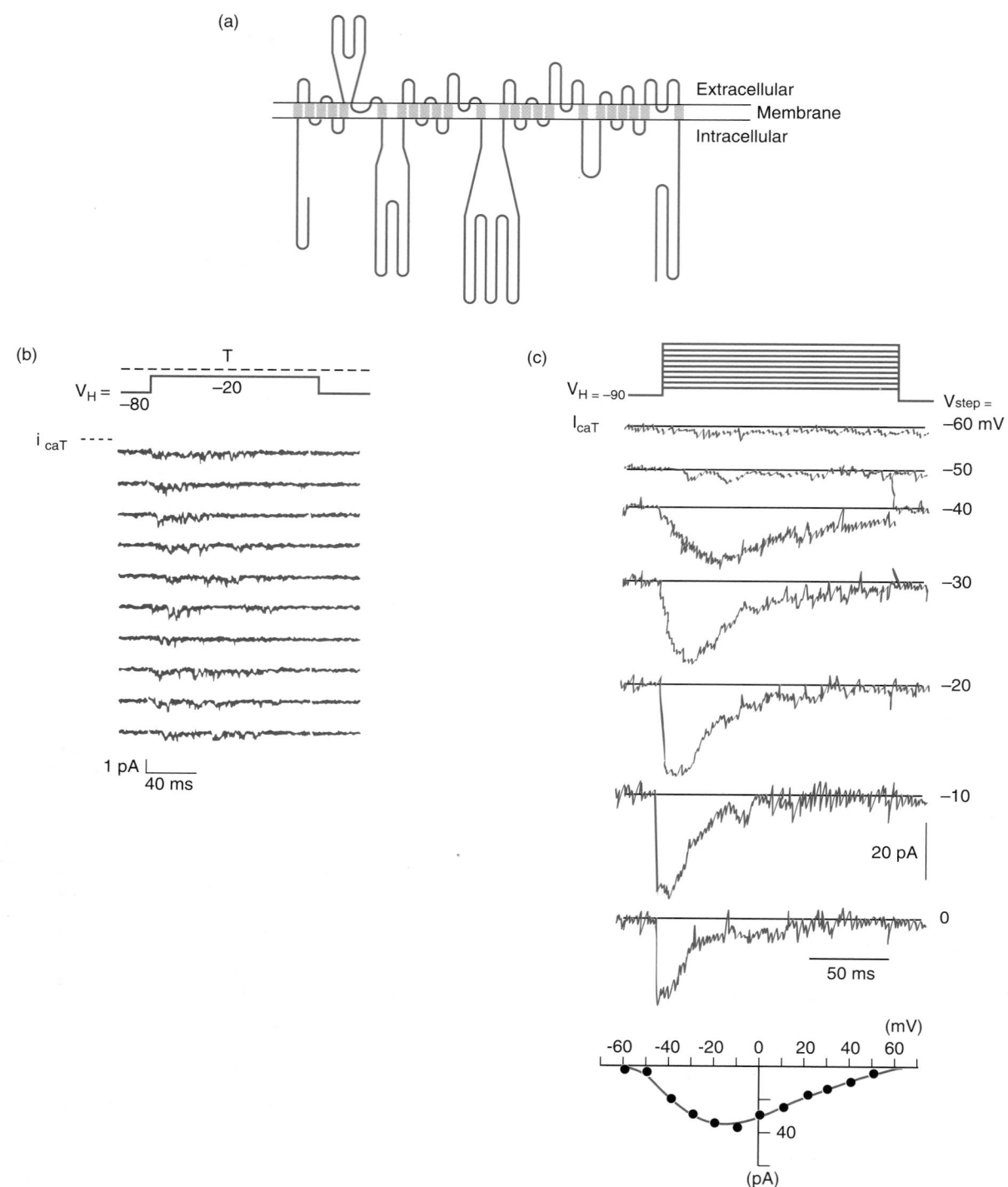

Figure 17.4 T-type Ca²⁺ channel and current, I_T.

(a) Predicted topology of the rat α_{1I} subunit. (b) Activity of a single T channel recorded from dorsal root ganglion cell bodies in patch clamp (cell-attached patch). Mean i_{CaT} amplitude at –20 mV is –0.62 ± 0.03 pA. (c) I/V relation of the whole-cell T current from a freshly plated (5 h) dissociated rat hippocampal neuron recorded in 10 mM of external Ca²⁺. Part (a) adapted from Lee JH, Daud AN, Cribbs LL et al. (1999) Cloning and expression of a novel member of the low voltage-activated T-type calcium channel family, *J. Neurosci.* **19**, 1912–1921, with permission. Part (b) adapted from Nowycky MC, Fox AP, Tsien RW (1985) Three types of neuronal calcium channels with different calcium agonist sensitivity, *Nature* **316**, 440–443, with permission. Part (c) adapted from Yaari Y, Hamon B, Lux HD (1987) Development of two types of calcium channels in cultured mammalian hippocampal neurons, *Science* **235**, 680–682, with permission.

then disappear though the membrane is still depolarized consistent with a rapid inactivation of T channels. T channels are more resistant to rundown of activity following patch excision or whole-cell recording than are L-type Ca^{2+} channels.

Gating properties and ionic nature

The voltage-dependence of the T current is studied in whole-cell recordings. In order to study the I/V relation of the T current in isolation, the other Ca^{2+} currents present in the cell, such as the high-threshold L-, N- and P-type Ca^{2+} currents (see Chapter 6) are pharmacologically blocked. However, in some preparations, T channels predominate and can be studied in the absence of blockers. For example, during development, embryonic hippocampal neurons in culture first express T-type Ca^{2+} channels and then, with neurite extension, also express high-threshold Ca^{2+} channels.

To study the activation properties of I_{CaT}, the membrane potential is held at –90 mV. The I/V relation shows that I_{CaT} activates in response to depolarizations positive to –55 mV and is maximal around –10 mV when recorded in the presence of 10 mM of external Ca^{2+} (**Figure 17.4c**). The voltage-dependence of activation is determined by applying different voltage steps from a holding potential $V_H = –105$ mV (**Figure 17.5b**). The normalized peak current amplitude is plotted against the test potential (**Figure 17.5c**). In chick sensory neurons, I_{CaT} is half-activated at –51 mV (in 10 mM of external Ca^{2+}). Note that the rate of activation is highly voltage-dependent.

During a 150 ms depolarizing pulse to –10 mV, I_{CaT} rapidly inactivates (in 50 ms): it is transient (**Figure 17.4c**). To study the inactivation properties of I_{CaT}, the membrane is clamped at different holding potentials and the current in response to a depolarizing step to –35 mV is recorded (**Figure 17.5a**). A plot of peak current amplitude against holding potential (**Figure 17.5c**) gives a measure of the voltage-dependence of inactivation. In chick sensory neurons, I_{CaT} is half inactivated at –78 mV (in 10 mM of external Ca^{2+}).

The removal of inactivation (de-inactivation) of the T current is time-dependent. This is studied in lateral geniculate cells *in vitro* (in single-electrode voltage clamp) with the following protocol. The membrane is held at –55 mV to inactivate completely the T current. A voltage step to –95 mV of variable duration is then applied. On stepping back to –55 mV, the peak amplitude of the T current is measured (I) and compared with its maximum amplitude (I_{max}). At 35°C, 500–600 ms at –95 mV are needed to totally remove inactivation. The removal of inactivation of the T current is also voltage-dependent: at potentials close to –55 mV the

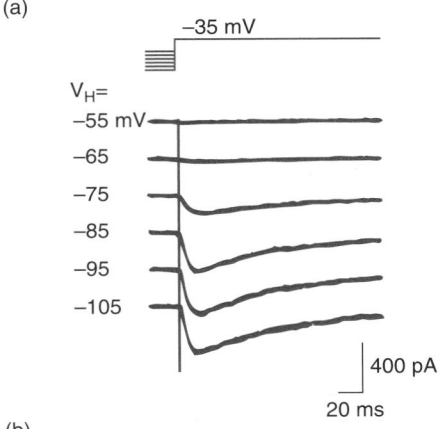

(a)

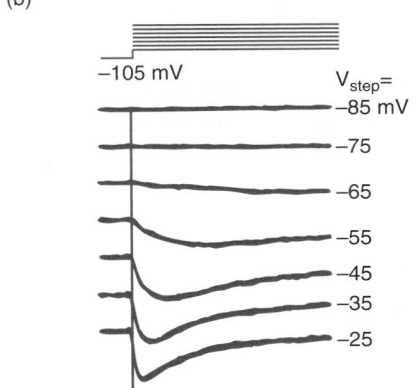

(b)

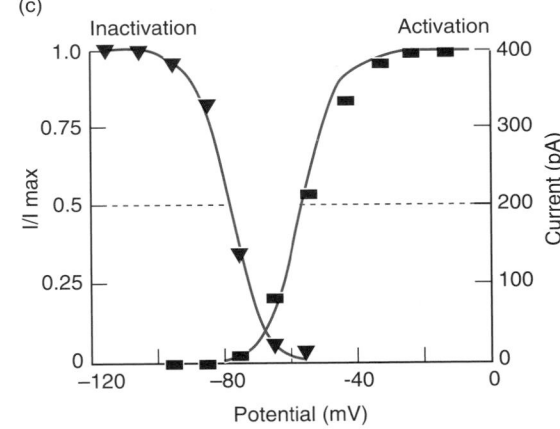

(c)

Figure 17.5 Voltage dependence of activation and inactivation of the T current.

Recorded in 5–10 mM of external Ca^{2+}: **(a)** inactivation; **(b)** activation. See text for explanation. **(c**, left) I_{max} is the maximal peak current amplitude obtained at $V_H = –105$ mV. **(c**, right) I_{max} is the maximal peak current amplitude obtained at $V_{step} = –35$ to –20 mV. Adapted from Fox AP, Nowycky MC, Tsien RW (1987) Kinetic and pharmacological properties distinguishing three types of calcium currents in chick sensory neurones, *J. Physiol.* **394**, 149–172, with permission.

de-inactivation is less complete than at more hyperpolarized potentials.

Pharmacology

There are no highly specific antagonists or toxins for the T-type Ca^{2+} channels. Low concentrations of the inorganic cation Ni^{2+} (20–50 μM) strongly depress I_{CaT}. Ethosuximide and amiloride have been also reported to reduce I_{CaT} in some preparations. Specific toxins acting at HVA channels are inefficient in T channels. To study I_{CaT} in isolation, Na^+ and K^+ channels must be blocked by TTX (1 μM), 4-AP (1 mM), TEA (10 mM), Ba^{2+} (1 mM) and HVA Ca^{2+} channels by their specific blockers (nifedipin, ω-conotoxin GVIA, ω-agatoxin).

In summary, T-type Ca^{2+} current is an inward current carried by Ca^{2+} ions; the activation threshold is around resting membrane potential (−50 to −60 mV), 10–20 mV negative to spike threshold. It is named 'T' for transient (owing to fast inactivation) and also for tiny (owing to small single-channel conductance). T-type current is a low-threshold-activated (LVA) Ca^{2+} current that can be distinguished from the high-threshold-activated (HVA) L-, N- and P-type Ca^{2+} currents by the following criteria: low-voltage activation, tiny single-channel conductance, and slow deactivation (tail current). It is totally inactivated at potentials close to the resting potential and is slowly de-inactivated during a transient hyperpolarization of the membrane. Therefore, it is fully activated by a depolarization only when the membrane potential has been previously maintained at a potential more hyperpolarized than resting membrane potential.

17.2.3 The hyperpolarization-activated cationic current, I_h, I_f, I_Q

I_h has an unusual voltage-dependence since it is activated upon hyperpolarization of the membrane beyond resting membrane potential. For this reason it has several names: 'h' for hyperpolarization, 'f' for funny (in the sinoatrial node of the heart) and 'Q' for queer, in some early studies in view of its odd electrophysiological behaviour and its undefined functional significance. It was originally observed by Ito and coworkers in 1962 in cat motoneurons as a non-ohmic behaviour of the I/V relation in the hyperpolarizing direction.

Structure of the main channel subunit

The I_h channel is a family of channels whose correct name should be HCN: *h*yperpolarization-activated, *c*yclic *n*ucleotide-gated channels; they are at present called BCNG (*b*rain *c*yclic *n*ucleotide-*g*ated channels) or HAC (*h*yperpolarization-*a*ctivated *c*hannels). These channels contain the conserved motifs of K^+ voltage-gated channels including the S1–S6 segments, a charged S4 voltage sensor and a pore-lining P loop (**Figure 17.6a**). In addition, all family members contain a conserved cyclic nucleotide-binding (CNB) domain in their carboxy terminus. This domain is homologous to the CNB domain of protein kinases and of cyclic nucleotide-gated channels (see **Figure 3.8**), suggesting that the gating of I_h channels is directly regulated by cyclic nucleotides such as cAMP or cGMP.

Gating properties and ionic nature

The type of voltage clamp experiment that allows one to record I_h is called a *relaxation experiment*. The activity of dorsal ganglion neurons (sensory neurons) in culture is recorded under two-electrode voltage clamp (**Figure 17.6b**). A 1.5 s hyperpolarizing voltage step to −90 mV while the membrane potential is held at $V_H = -60$ mV evokes an instantaneous inward current (I_{leak}) followed by a slowly developing inward current which shows no inactivation with time (on I_h). I_{leak} reflects the leak current through channels open at $V_H = -60$ mV (mostly K^+ channels). The following slow inward current reflects the slow opening of I_h channels. When the membrane is then repolarized to −60 mV at the end of the voltage step, an instantaneous current (I'_{leak}) is recorded followed by an inward tail current (tail I_h). The instantaneous current reflects the leak current through channels open at −90 mV. The tail current reflects the kinetics of closure (deactivation) of I_h channels. I'_{leak} is larger than I_{leak} because at −90 mV not only the leak channels are open but also the I_h channels that have been opened by the hyperpolarization.

By varying the amplitude of voltage steps, I_h is shown to activate at between −45 and −60 mV and to be half activated at around −75 and −85 mV (**Figure 17.6c**). I_h reverses at around −50 to −30 mV depending on the neuronal type. Decreasing the external Na^+ concentration from 153 to 26 mM reduces the amplitude of I_h (**Figure 17.7a**). When Na^+ ions are totally replaced by the non-permeant cation choline, I_h disappears almost completely (since $E_K = -90$ mV). Similarly, raising the external K^+ concentration from 2.5 mM to 12.5 mM enhances I_h (not shown). These results indicate that I_h is carried by both Na^+ and K^+ ions, which is consistent with the

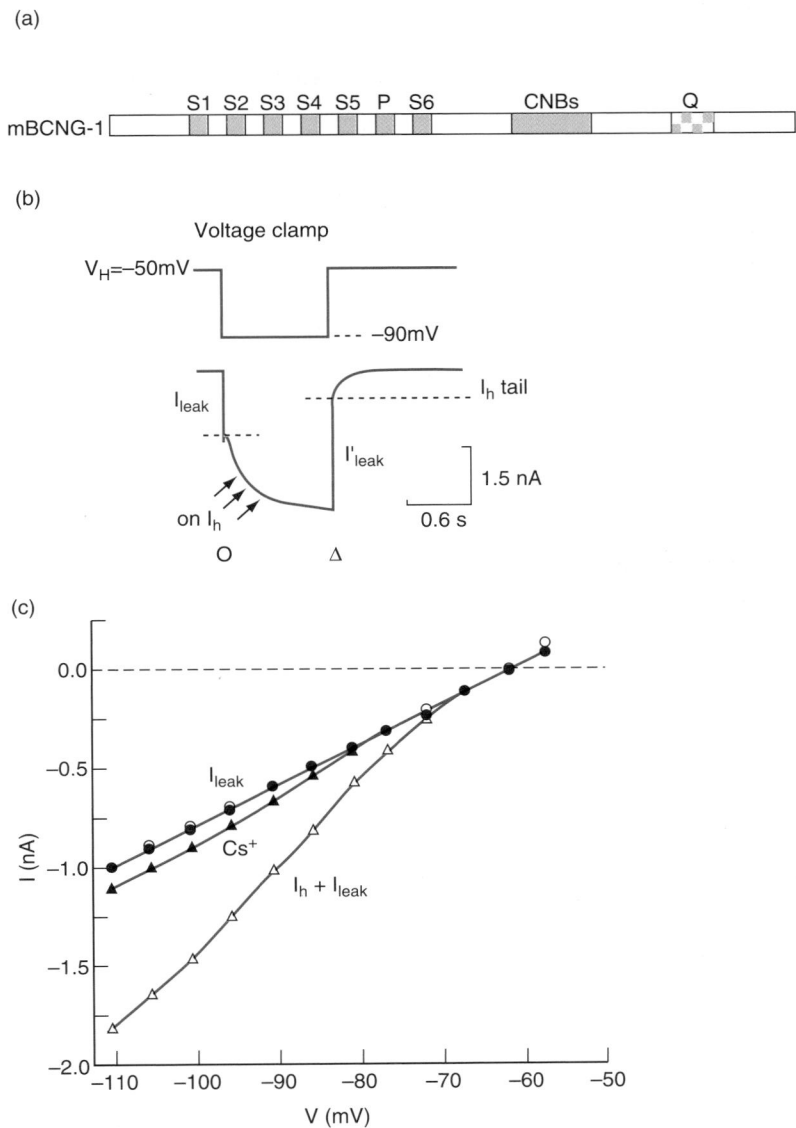

Figure 17.6 The hyperpolarization-activated H channel and current, I_h.
(a) Predicted structure of the mBCNG-1 channel subunit. (b) The activity of a thalamic neuron recorded in slices (intracellular recording, voltage-clamp mode). Relaxation experiment. The extracellular medium contains 14.5 mM of K^+ and 116 mM of Na^+. (c) I/V relation obtained from experiment in Figure 17.7c: instantaneous leak current is plotted as circles, steady-state current ($I_{leak} + I_h$) measured at the end of the voltage steps, is plotted as triangles. Open symbols represent currents under control conditions and filled symbols are currents after application of Cs^+. Part (a) adapted from Santoro B, Liu DT, Yao H *et al.* (1998) Identification of a gene encoding a hyperpolarization-activated pacemaker channel of brain, *Cell* **93**, 717–729, with permission. Part (c) adapted from McCormick DA, Pape HC (1990) Properties of a hyperpolarization-activated cation current and its role in rhythmic oscillation in thalamic relay neurones, *J. Physiol.* **431**, 291–318, with permission.

extrapolated reversal potential. I_h channels are in fact 4-fold selective for K^+ versus Na^+.

The opposite voltage-dependent polarity of I_h channels occurs despite the presence of a highly charged, basic S4 voltage-sensing domain. A similar reversed polarity of voltage-dependent activation has been reported for the Shaker K^+ channel after S4 point mutations. This K^+ channel which normally opens upon depolarization is transformed in a hyperpolarization-activated channel due to the fact that at voltages near the resting potential, mutated Shaker K^+ channels are now in an inactivated state. They are opened by a

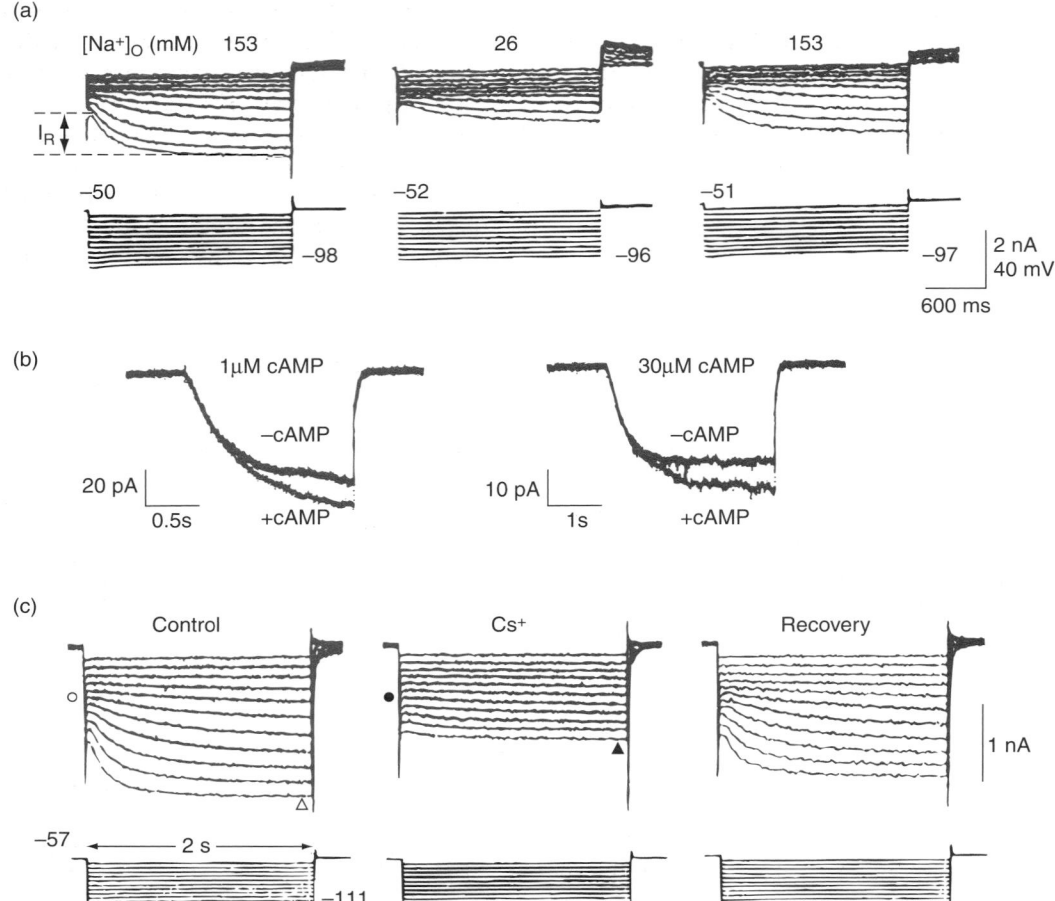

Figure 17.7 Ionic selectivity and pharmacology of I_h.
The activity of thalamic neurons is recorded in slices (intracellular recording, voltage-clamp mode). **(a)** Effect on I_h of changing the extracellular concentration of Na^+ ions. A family of I_h currents (upper traces) are evoked by stepping membrane potential to hyperpolarized potentials from $V_H = -50$ mV (bottom traces), in control condition (153 mM, left and right) and during reduced Na^+ concentration (26 mM, centre). It should be noted that there is no change in the baseline current. **(b)** The mBCNG-1 channel is expressed in *Xenopus* oocytes. The I_h current is evoked in inside-out macropatches by a hyperpolarizing step to –100 mV in the absence or presence of cAMP in the bath. **(c)** Similar experiment as in (a), in control conditions and in the presence of Cs^+. Parts (a) and (c) adapted from McCormick DA, Pape HC (1990) Properties of a hyperpolarization-activated cation current and its role in rhythmic oscillation in thalamic relay neurones, *J. Physiol.* **431**, 291–318, with permission. Part (b) adapted from Santoro B, Liu DT, Yao H *et al.* (1998) Identification of a gene encoding a hyperpolarization-activated pacemaker channel of brain, *Cell* **93**, 717–729, with permission.

hyperpolarization since this procedure removes inactivation. The opening of I_h channels upon hyperpolarization could reflect a similar removal of inactivation. This suggests that at resting potentials, I_h channels are, at least partly, inactivated.

Pharmacology

Application of cAMP to the internal surface of an inside-out patch induces a reversible increase in the magnitude of the inward current during a step to –100 mV (**Figure 17.7b**). This effect of cAMP is due to a positive shift in

the steady-state activation curve of I_h current by 2 to 10 mV.

I_h is completely blocked in the presence of 1–3 mM of Cs^+ in the extracellular solution (**Figures 17.6c** and **17.7c**). A novel bradycardic agent ZM 227189 (10–100 µM; Zeneca), was recently shown to selectively block I_h. In contrast, I_h is insensitive to external Ba^{2+}, TTX, TEA and 4-AP that effectively block Na^+ or K^+ channels. To study I_h in isolation, Ca^{2+}, Na^+ and K^+ channels must be blocked by Cd^{2+} or Co^{2+} or Ni^{2+} (200 µM to 1 mM), TTX (1 µM), 4-AP (1 mM), TEA (10 mM), Ba^{2+} (1 mM).

In summary, I_h is carried by Na^+ and K^+ ions and is a voltage and time-dependent current. It has a slow time course of activation and is inactived at depolarized potentials where action potentials are firing. I_h is directly modulated by internal cyclic nucleotides such as cAMP or cGMP. It is reversibly decreased by 1–3 mM of extracellular Cs^+.

17.3 The subliminal voltage-gated currents that hyperpolarize the membrane

The common characteristic of these subliminal currents is to be outward, carried by K^+ ions and turned on at potentials more negative than the threshold for the opening of voltage-gated Na^+ channels of the action potential. Four types of outward K^+ currents will be explained: the early K^+ currents (I_A, I_D), the K^+ currents activated by intracellular Ca^{2+} (I_{KCa}), the muscarine-sensitive K^+ current (I_M) and the inward rectifier K^+ current (I_{KIR}).

17.3.1 The rapidly inactivating transient K^+ current: I_A or I_{Af}

I_A is a K^+ current which rapidly activates and inactivates in response to depolarizing steps from holding potentials negative to the resting membrane potential. It was originally described in 1971 by Connor and Stevens, in molluscan neurons, and termed 'A current'.

Structure of the main channel subunit

The I_A channel belongs to the family of *Shal* K^+ channels (or Kv4). They have the primary structure common to voltage-gated channels: six putative membrane spanning segments designated S1 to S6, flanked by intracellular domains of variable length and a pore domain P between S5 and S6.

Gating properties and ionic nature

The activity of medullary or hippocampal neurons in culture is recorded in voltage clamp mode in a medium containing TTX (to block Na^+ currents) and TEA (to block the K^+ currents of the delayed rectification), Cd^{2+} (200 μM) to depress Ca^{2+}-dependent currents, carbachol (50 μM) to block I_M (see Section 17.3.4) and Cs^+ (1–3 mM) to block I_h. When the membrane potential is maintained at –70 mV, depolarizing voltage steps (of 10 to 58 mV amplitude) evoke an outward current whose amplitude

increases with the amplitude of the depolarization (**Figure 17.8a**). This current activates rapidly (within milliseconds) and then inactivates rapidly and exponentially during the step. This is the 'A current', I_A. Inactivation of I_A is time- and voltage-dependent. It appears after a few milliseconds, which makes I_A short-lasting. In this respect I_A resembles more the I_{Na} of the action potential than the current of the delayed rectification, I_{KDR}. The current plateau which follows the peak of

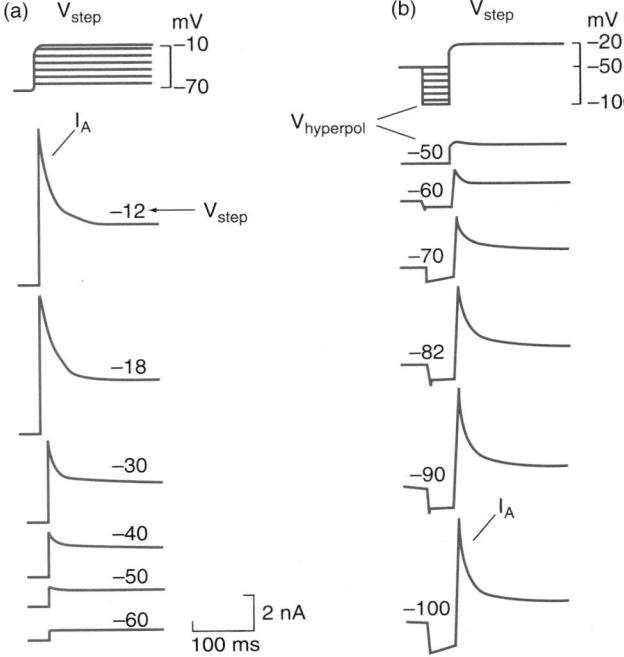

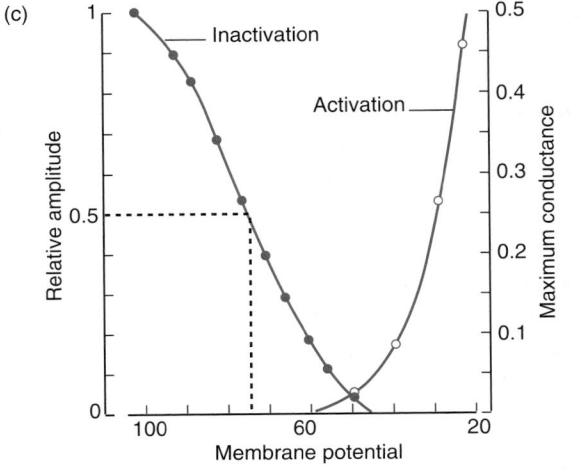

Figure 17.8 Activation–inactivation properties of I_A.
From Segal M, Rogawski MA, Barker JL (1984) A transient potassium conductance regulates the excitability of cultured hippocampal and spinal neurons, *J. Neurosci.* **4**, 604–609, with permission.

the I_A current represents the sum of the leakage current and of the outward currents which are not blocked by TEA.

When a hyperpolarizing voltage step ($V_{hyperpol}$) of varying amplitude is now applied during the 50 ms before the depolarizing voltage step (V_{step}) to –20 mV (**Figure 17.8b**), it can be seen that I_A is inactivated when the membrane potential is maintained at a value more positive than –50 mV; at these membrane potentials I_A cannot be activated by a depolarization. Also, I_A is de-inactivated when the membrane potential is maintained at a value more negative than –50 mV and can then be activated by depolarizations to membrane potentials positive to –50 mV and its amplitude increases with the difference $V_{hyperpol} - V_{step}$. Activation and inactivation curves (**Figure 17.8c**) have been constructed from the data in traces (a) and (b), respectively.

Pharmacology

I_A is blocked by application of 4-aminopyridine (4-AP, 1–3 mM) in the extracellular medium. It is insensitive to TEA, Cs^+ and Ba^{2+}. Thus there are two ways of blocking I_A, either by depolarizing the membrane above –50 mV, or by applying 4-aminopyridine. To study I_A, Na^+ and Ca^{2+} channels must be blocked by TTX (1 μM), Cd^{2+} or Co^{2+} or Ni^{2+} (200 μM to 1 mM).

In summary, I_A is a fast-inactivating (in the order of milliseconds) K^+ current. The threshold potential for its activation is situated at around –60 to –45 mV; i.e. at a value slightly more negative than the threshold potential for the inward Na^+ current of the action potential. I_A can be fully activated by a depolarization only when the membrane potential has been previously maintained at a potential more hyperpolarized than –60 mV (I_A is inactivated at resting membrane potential). It has characteristics which distinguish it from the K^+ currents of the delayed rectification: it is a rapidly activating and inactivating K^+ current and has pharmacological properties different from that of the delayed rectifier currents.

17.3.2 The slowly inactivating transient K^+ current, I_D or I_{As}

In addition to I_A, a K^+ current that also activates rapidly (within milliseconds) but slowly inactivates (over seconds) was first described by Storm (1988) in hippocampal pyramidal cells. It was termed 'D current' because it delays the cell firing.

Gating properties

The activity of the pyramidal cells of the hippocampus is intracellularly recorded in brain slices. Voltage clamp experiments are performed in the presence of external Cd^{2+} (200 μM) to depress Ca^{2+}-dependent currents, carbachol (50 μM) to block I_M (see Section 17.3.4) and Cs^+ (1–3 mM) to block I_h. When, in such conditions, a depolarizing voltage step to –26 mV is applied from a holding potential $V_H = -80$ mV, an outward current

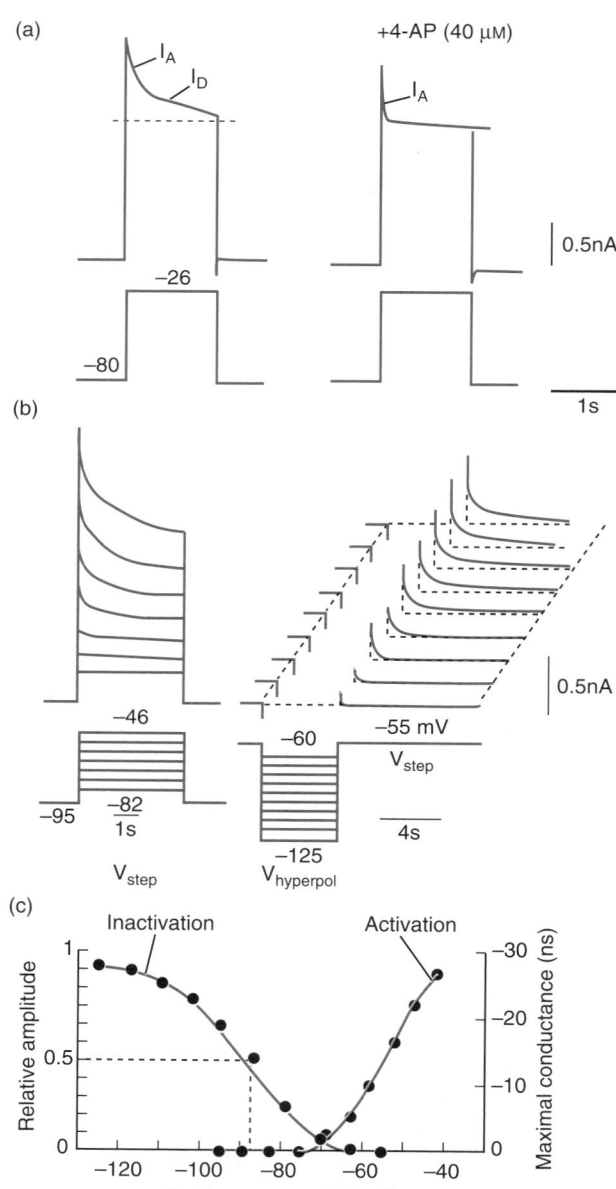

Figure 17.9 Activation–inactivation properties of I_D.
From Storm JF (1988) Temporal integration by a slowly inactivating K^+ current in hippocampal neurons, *Nature* **336**, 379–381, with permission.

consisting of two components is recorded: a fast inactivating component, sensitive to high doses of 4-aminopyridine (4-AP, 1–3 mM) and a slowly inactivating component sensitive to low doses (40 μM) of 4-AP (**Figure 17.9a**). The first component corresponds to I_A and the second one is termed I_D.

In order to construct the activation–inactivation curves of I_D, the same protocol as that explained for I_A is applied (**Figures 17.9b and c**). They show that I_D is half-inactivated at −88 mV, and is inactivated when the membrane potential is maintained at a value more positive than −50 mV (at these membrane potentials I_D cannot be activated by a depolarization). Further, I_D is de-inactivated when the membrane potential is maintained at a value more negative than −60 mV (it can then be activated by depolarizations to membrane potentials more positive than −70 mV). Therefore, I_D contrasts with I_A in having a threshold for both activation and inactivation 10–20 mV more negative (compare **Figures 17.8c** and **17.9c**).

Pharmacology

I_D is much more sensitive to 4-aminopyridine than I_A, the latter requiring 1–3 mM for a block and the former 30–40 μM. I_D is insensitive to TEA and Cs^+ ions. Thus there are two ways of blocking I_D, either by depolarizing the membrane above −70 mV or by applying 40 μM of 4-aminopyridine in the extracellular medium. To study I_D, Na^+ and Ca^{2+} channels must be blocked by TTX (1 μM), Cd^{2+} or Co^{2+} or Ni^{2+} (200 μM to 1 mM).

In summary, I_D has characteristics which distinguish it from the other K^+ currents. It inactivates more slowly (in the order of seconds) than the transient current I_A and activates more rapidly and at more negative potentials than the currents of the delayed rectification I_{KDR}. It has also different pharmacological properties.

17.3.3 The K⁺ currents activated by intracellular Ca²⁺ ions, I_{KCa}

I_{KCa} currents are outward K^+ currents sensitive to the intracellular concentration of Ca^{2+} ($[Ca^{2+}]_i$). In vertebrate neurons, these currents may be more or less sensitive to voltage, but for all of them an increase in the intracellular Ca^{2+} concentration is a necessary prerequisite to their activation. $[Ca^{2+}]_i$ increase may be the result of Ca^{2+} entry through voltage-dependent Ca^{2+} channels opened by depolarization, or Ca^{2+} entry through cationic receptor channels largely permeable to Ca^{2+} ions such as the NMDA-type glutamate receptors, or Ca^{2+} release from intracellular stores. I_{KCa} have been explained in Chapter 6.

17.3.4 The K⁺ current sensitive to muscarine, I_M

I_M is a depolarization-activated K^+ current originally described in frog sympathetic neurons by Brown and Adams in 1980, and studied since in a variety of other vertebrate neurons. I_M was so-called because it is inhibited by muscarinic acetylcholine receptor agonists such as the alkaloid muscarine. It is therefore under muscarinic cholinergic synaptic control.

Gating properties and ionic nature

I_M can be recorded in response to two types of voltage clamp protocols (in the presence of TTX). In the first protocol the membrane potential is stepped from −60 to −30 mV. At −60 mV, most of the M channels are closed. A step to −30 mV reveals, superimposed on the leak current (measured from the response to a symmetrical hyperpolarizing step to −90 mV), a slowly developing outward current due to the slow opening of M channels in response to membrane depolarization (**Figure 17.10a**).

The second type of protocol involves relaxation experiments (**Figure 17.10b**). The membrane is held at $V_H = -30$ mV, a potential at which M channels remain open and contribute a steady outward current. A negative step to −60 mV causes an instantaneous inward current (I_{leak}) followed by an inward current which slowly develops (I_M). When the membrane is repolarized to −30 mV, at the end of the voltage step, an instantaneous inward current (I'_{leak}) is recorded followed by a slow outward tail current (tail I_M).

The explanation of the recordings of **Figure 17.10b** is the following. When the membrane is stepped from −30 to −60 mV, all the M channels open at −30 mV do not close immediately nor at the same time. There is an instantaneous diminution of the outward current (recorded as an instantaneous inward current, I_{leak}). It represents the current through channels open at $V_H = -30$ mV; i.e. M channels and 'leak channels'. It therefore depends on the number of channels open at −30 mV. Then there appears an exponential diminution of outward current or slow inward relaxation (I_M) which reflects the kinetic of M channels closure in response to the hyperpolarizing step to −60 mV. When the membrane is stepped back to −30 mV, the M channels do not open instantaneously. There is a first instantaneous outward current (I'_{leak}) which represents the current through channels open at −60 mV ('leak channels' only since M channels are closed). This instantaneous outward current is smaller than the fast inward one recorded from −30 to −60 mV. It clearly indicates that M channels had closed in response to the preceding step from −30 to

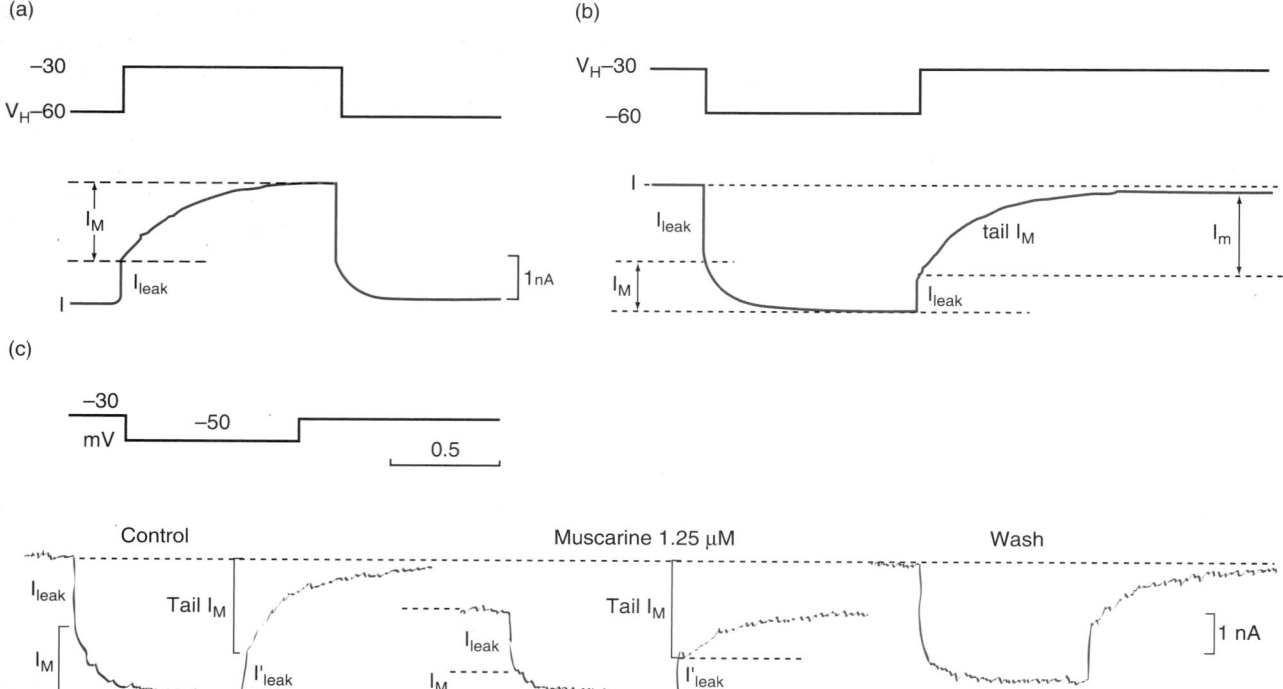

Figure 17.10 Characteristics of the M current, I_M.
Currents are recorded from a bullfrog sympathetic neuron in voltage clamp mode. **(a, b)** See text. **(c)** Effect of muscarine on I_M. The membrane is held at −30 mV and stepped to −50 mV. Muscarine evokes an inward current (the current trace is lower): it reduces the steady outward current through M channels open at −30 mV. In contrast, the baseline level attained at −60 mV, at the end of the command step, remains the same: muscarine does not produce an inward current at voltages where the M channels are normally shut. Inward and outward relaxations are largely depressed. Parts (a) and (b) adapted from Brown D, Adams PR (1980) Muscarinic suppression of a novel voltage sensitive K+ current in a vertebrate neuron, *Nature* **283**, 673–676; and Adams PR, Brown DA, Constanti A (1982) M-currents and other potassium currents in bullfrog sympathetic neurones, *J. Physiol* **330**, 537–572. Part (c) adapted from Adams PR, Brown DA, Constanti A (1982) Pharmacological inhibition of the M-current, *J. Physiol* **332**, 223–262; all with permission.

−60 mV (when the ohmic current is smaller in response to the same ΔV, it means that the membrane conductance is smaller). Then appears an outward tail current (tail I_M) through the M channels which slowly open again in response to the depolarization. The form of the outward current evoked by the return to the steady holding potential can be distorted by the presence of other K+ currents activated by this protocol (I_{KDR}, I_A, I_D and I_{KCa}), particularly when the membrane is stepped back to V_H from a potential more negative than −70 mV. The M channels seem to be fully closed at membrane potentials more negative than −60 mV, because in response to hyperpolarizing commands from −60 mV ($V_H = -60$ mV) only ohmic (passive) current is recorded (not shown).

With increasing step commands the inward relaxation reverses in direction at step potentials between −70 and −100 mV. This reversal potential shifts to a more positive value on raising external K+ concentration. Thus I_M is largely a K+ current.

Pharmacology

Muscarinic agonists decrease I_M as shown in **Figure 17.10c**. The consequent loss of the steady outward current under muscarine generates a steady inward current at −30 mV (difference between baseline control and muscarine) and a step to −50 mV now reveals mostly the leak current (I_{leak}) showing that most of M channels are already closed.

In summary, I_M is activated by depolarizations to membrane potentials positive to −60 mV. It activates slowly (within hundreds of milliseconds) and does not inactivate. I_M differs from the delayed rectifier current I_{KDR} involved in spike repolarization by having a 40 mV more negative activation threshold and slower kinetics. It differs from I_A and I_D transient K+ currents because it does not inactivate.

17.3.5 The inward rectifier K+ current, I_{Kir}

I_{Kir} is a K+ current that was originally described in skeletal muscle fibres by Sir Bernard Katz (1949). It is a Ba^{2+}-sensitive K+ current with an I/V relation showing rectification when the current is inward (at potentials more hyperpolarized than –90 mV). I_{Kir} is modulated by G proteins.

Structure of the main channel subunit

These channels form a new channel-gene superfamily: inwardly rectifying K+ channels possess only two putative transmembrane segments M1 and M2, which correspond to transmembrane regions S5 and S6 of voltage-gated K+ channels (see **Figure 3.11**).

Gating properties and ionic nature

The activity of the neurons of the accumbens nucleus is recorded intracellularly. The resting potential is very negative, around –85 mV. In single-electrode voltage clamp, when the current evoked by hyperpolarizing steps is recorded in the presence of varying concentrations of external K+, a series of I/V curves is obtained (**Figure 17.11a**). These curves increase in steepness between –50 and –120 mV. Thus the permeability to K+ is high when the current is inward ($V - E_K$ is negative) and low when the current is outward ($V - E_K$ is positive). In other words, inwardly rectifying channels conduct more efficiently when the membrane is negative to E_K.

Increasing the external K+ concentration increases the slope of the I/V curve (i.e. the conductance) and shifts the reversal potential to more positive values, thus showing that K+ ions participate in the current responsible for the inward rectification.

Rectification in native channels is due in part to voltage-dependent block by cytoplasmic Mg^{2+} ions and polyamines.

Pharmacology

Ba^{2+} (30–100 µM) causes an inward current at the resting potential (due to the blockade of the outward I_{Kir} present

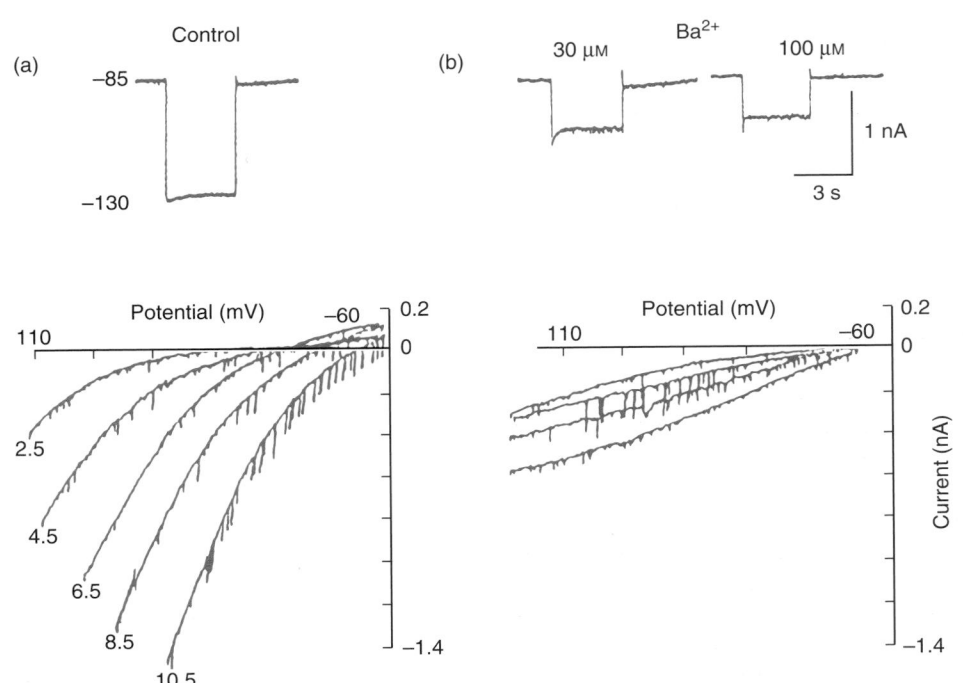

Figure 17.11 Characteristics of the inward rectifier current, I_{Kir}.
Currents are recorded from neurons of the nucleus accumbens, in single-electrode voltage clamp mode. **(a)** Inward current recorded in response to a hyperpolarizing step to –130 mV from a holding potential of –85 mV in control external K+ concentration (2.5 mM) (top trace). I/V relations in five different external K+ concentrations (bottom curves). The amplitude of the current has been measured at the end of 3–5 s steps, at steady state. **(b)** Same current as in (a) recorded in the presence of 30 and 100 µM of Ba^{2+} (top traces). I/V relations as in (a) but in the presence of 30 µM of Ba^{2+}. Adapted from Uchimura N, Cherubini E, North A (1989) Inward rectification in rat nucleus accumbens, *J. Neurophysiol.* **62**, 1280–1286, with permission.

at rest) and decreases I_{Kir} at all potentials tested. Ba^{2+} thus linearizes the I/V curves (**Figure 17.11b**).

In summary, I_{Kir} is activated at resting membrane potential and thus maintains potential close to E_K. Owing to rectification, I_{Kir} has a low amplitude in the outward direction. It is modulated by G proteins via the activation of synaptic metabotropic receptors.

17.4 Conclusions

Comparison between inward and outward voltage-gated currents is shown in **Figure 17.12**. Subliminal currents are on the left and supraliminal currents on the right. I_{CaT} has voltage properties similar to those of I_A and I_D but with opposite functions. I_h and I_M have symmetrical voltage properties and opposite functions.

Depending on their location, subliminal currents are activated by different signals. When located in dendrites they are activated by a depolarization (EPSP) or a hyperpolarization (IPSP) of synaptic origin. When located in the soma–initial segment membrane, they are activated by the first action potential generated or by the hyper-

polarization that follows an action potential (after spike hyperpolarization).

Depending on their location, subliminal voltage-gated currents also have different roles. When present in the dendritic membrane they boost or counteract EPSPs or IPSPs (see Chapter 18), but when present in the soma–initial segment membrane they underlie intrinsic firing patterns, modulate synaptically driven firing patterns or participate in network oscillations (see Chapters 20, 22 and 23). When present in the whole neuronal membrane, subliminal currents that are activated around rest and that do not rapidly inactivate (I_h, I_M, I_{KIR}) also determine resting membrane potential (see Chapter 4).

Further reading

Araki T, Ito M, Oshima T (1962) Potential changes produced by application of current steps in motoneurones. *Nature* **191**, 1104–1105.

Baldwin TJ, Tsaur ML, Lopez GA *et al.* (1991) Characterization of a mammalian cDNA for an inactivating voltage-sensitive K^+ channel. *Neuron* **7**, 471–483.

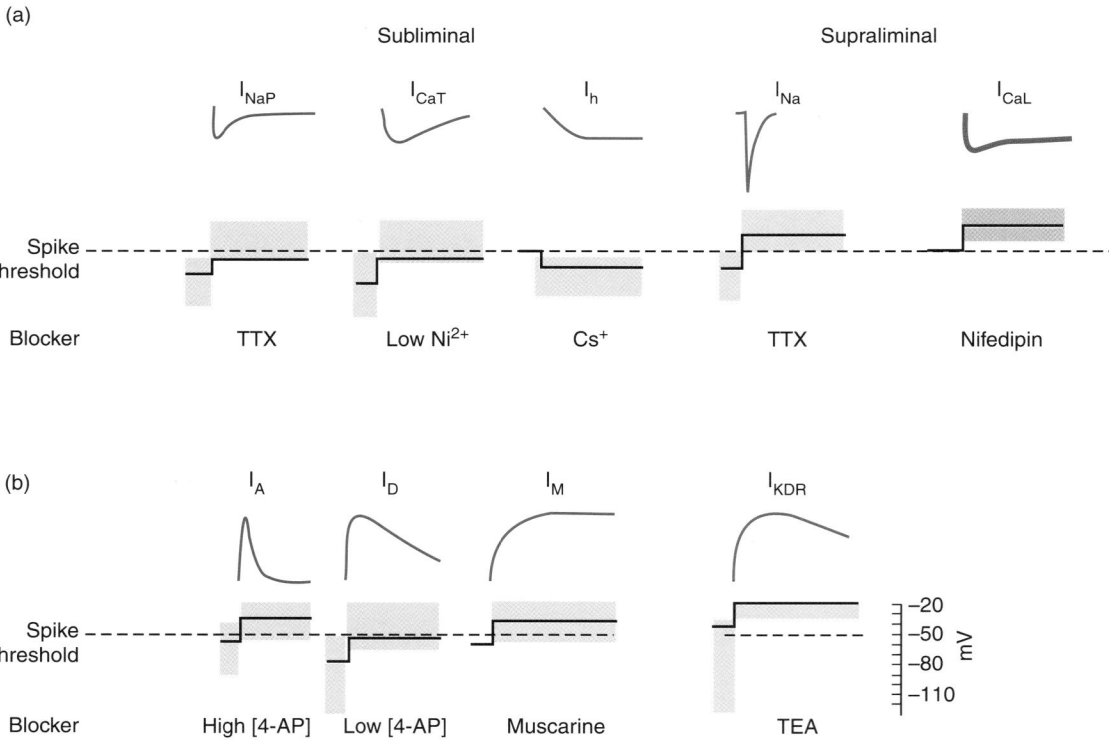

Figure 17.12 **Comparison between subliminal and supraliminal voltage-gated currents.**
(a) Inward and (b) outward voltage-gated currents. Subliminal currents are on the left and high threshold-activated currents are on the right. Currents (top traces) are shown in response to voltage steps (solid bottom traces). The voltage ranges of activation and inactivation are shown in shaded green. The effective blocking agents are indicated below. Part (b) adapted from Storm JF (1988) Temporal integration of a slowly inactivating K^+ current in hippocampal neurons, *Nature* **336**, 379–381, with permission.

Carbone E, Lux HD (1984) A low voltage-activated, fully inactivating Ca^{2+} channel in vertebrate sensory neurons. *Nature* **310**, 501–502.

Connor JA, Stevens CF (1971) Prediction of repetitive firing behaviour from voltage-clamp data on an isolated neurone soma. *J. Physiol.* **213**, 31–53.

Crill WE (1996) Persistent sodium current in mammalian central neurons. *Ann. Rev. Physiol.* **58**, 349–362.

Hotson JR, Prince DA, Schwartzkroin PA (1979) Anomalous inward rectification in hippocampal neurons. *J. Neurophysiol.* **42**, 889–895.

Huguenard JR (1996) Low-threshold calcium currents in central nervous system neurons. *Ann. Rev. Physiol.* **58**, 329–348.

Kay AR, Sugimori M, Llinas R (1998) Kinetic and stochastic nature of a persistent sodium current in mature guinea pig cerebellar Purkinje cells. *J. Neurophysiol.* **80**, 1167–1179.

Matsuda H, Saigusa A, Irisawa H (1987) Ohmic conductance through the inwardly rectifying K^+ channel and blocking by internal Mg^{2+}. *Nature* **325**, 156–158.

Miller AG, Aldrich RW (1996) Conversion of a delayed rectifier K^+ channel by three amino acids substitution. *Neuron* **16**, 853–858.

Pape HC (1996) Queer current and pacemaker: the hyperpolarization-activated cation current in neurons. *Ann. Rev. Physiol.* **58**, 299–327.

Perez-Reyes E, Cribbs LL, Daud A *et al.* (1998) Molecular characterization of a neuronal low-voltage-activated T-type calcium channel. *Nature* **391**, 896–900.

Standen NB, Stanfield PR (1978) A potential- and time-dependent blockade of inward rectification in frog skeletal muscle fibres by barium and strontium ions. *J. Physiol. (Lond.)* **280**, 169–191.

Somato-Dendritic Processing of Postsynaptic Potentials II. Role of Subliminal Depolarizing Voltage-Gated Currents

The preceding chapter showed that in a dendritic tree in which currents propagate passively, EPSPs are attenuated in amplitude and slowed in time course as they spread to the soma. As a consequence, excitatory or inhibitory synapses located on distal dendrites are less efficient in depolarizing or hyperpolarizing the soma–initial segment region threshold. Especially in the case of highly developed dendritic arbors and electrotonically remote synapses, the impact of elementary synaptic inputs on the somatic excitation–inhibition balance is predicted to be small on the sole basis of cable theory, unless major temporal and/or spatial summation occurs.

However, direct recordings from dendrites have demonstrated that some express voltage-gated channels that endow them with active membrane properties similar to the cell soma. In these neurons, dendrites do not behave as simple cables. We will consider here the *depolarizing* voltage-gated currents present in the dendritic or somatic membrane that operate at membrane potentials below action potential threshold (subliminal currents). One implication of these findings is that the amplitude and duration of EPSPs are modified as they spread to the axon initial segment. For this to occur, EPSPs must be of sufficient amplitude to activate dendritic or somatic voltage-gated currents. This modulation of postsynaptic potentials can occur locally, near their site of generation (i.e. in the dendritic spine or the adjacent dendrite) or in the proximal dendrites and soma, during their spread to the site of action potential initiation.

Modulation of postsynaptic potentials by voltage-gated currents has come under direct experimental scrutiny by the use of dendritic recordings and by the advent of imaging techniques with high spatial and temporal resolution. This permitted the design of experiments to answer the following three questions:

- Are subliminal voltage-gated currents present in the dendritic membrane?
- Are they distributed uniformly over soma–dendritic membranes, or are the electrogenic properties in dendrites fundamentally different from those in the soma?
- How do these dendritic or somatic currents shape excitatory postsynaptic potentials and affect input summation?

To address these questions, the models used are brain regions organized in layers such as the neocortex or the hippocampus. In such regions, dendritic recordings are much easier than in other structures since the dendritic layer is easily recognizable from the somatic layer.

To answer the above questions the activity of subliminal voltage-gated channels must be recorded in patches of dendritic membrane. Then, the amplitude of subliminal currents recorded from similar-sized patches of dendritic and somatic membranes must be compared. Experiments are thus performed in brain slices to allow outside-out, dendrite-attached or soma-attached recordings. For technical reasons, dendritic recording is limited to dendritic branches with a diameter greater than 1 μm.

18.1 Persistent Na$^+$ channels are present in soma and dendrites of neocortical neurons; I_{NaP} boosts EPSPs in amplitude and duration

The persistent Na$^+$ current I_{NaP} is a TTX-sensitive Na$^+$ current that activates below spike threshold and slowly inactivates (see Section 17.2.1). To record Na$^+$ current in isolation, the solution bathing the extracellular face of the patch contains NaCl. TEACl is added in the external solution or CsCl in the internal solution to strongly reduce outward K⁺ currents. Voltage-gated Ca²⁺ currents (and therefore Ca²⁺-activated currents) are blocked by substitution of Mn²⁺ for Ca²⁺ in the extracellular medium. Persistent Na⁺ current is identified by inward polarity, its low threshold of activation (10–15 mV negative to resting potential), and its blockade by TTX. It can be easily differentiated from the Na⁺ current of action potentials which activates at a higher threshold, has a much greater amplitude and inactivates much faster.

18.1.1 Persistent Na⁺ channels are present in the dendrites and soma of pyramidal neurons of the neocortex

Dendritic recordings

Single Na⁺ channel activity is recorded in patch clamp from dendrites of acutely isolated pyramidal neurons

of the neocortex (dendrite-attached recordings). Depolarizing voltage steps to –60/+10 mV are applied from a holding potential of –100/–120 mV. They evoke Na⁺ channel openings in all the recorded patches (**Figure 18.1a**). The most prominent activity in multi-channel patches consists of early, short-lived openings clustered within the first few milliseconds. In addition, a different Na⁺ channel activity consisting of prolonged or late openings is recorded. When many consecutive traces are averaged, this persistent channel activity is able to produce sizable net inward current even for 500 ms. The I/V relationship of the persistent component (**Figure 18.1b**) is not different from that of the macroscopic current recorded in the same cells.

Somatic recordings

Pyramidal neurons of the neocortex are loaded with the Na⁺-sensitive, membrane-impermeant, fluorescent dye SBFI (sodium benzofuram isophthalate; see Appendix

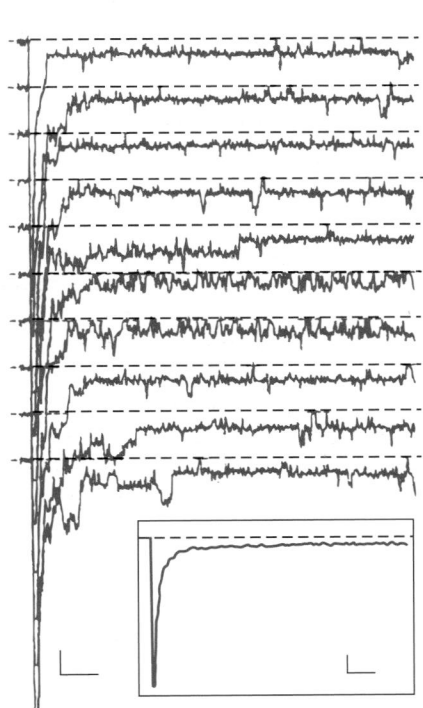

(a)

−20

−100

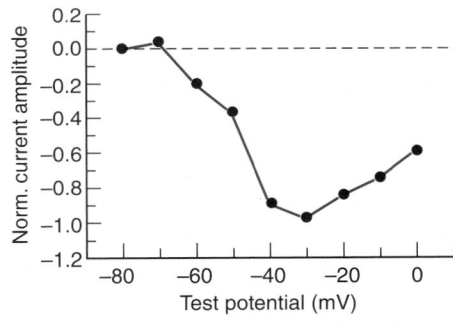

(b)

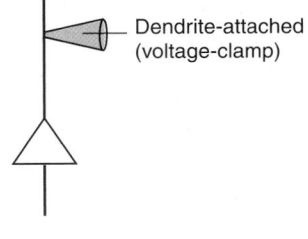

Dendrite-attached (voltage-clamp)

Figure 18.1 Persistent Na⁺ channel activity in dendrites of cortical pyramidal neurons.
(a) Na⁺ channel currents evoked by a 50 ms depolarizing pulse. The current traces shown are consecutive sweeps (scale bar 2 pA and 5 ms). *Insets*: Ensemble average current obtained from 20 consecutive sweeps (scale bar 2.5 pA and 5 ms). (b) Voltage-dependence of the persistent component of ensemble average currents obatined as in (a). The plot is normalized to the absolute value of its peak amplitude. Adapted from Magistretti J, Ragsdale DS, Alonso A (1999) Direct demonstration of persistent Na⁺ channel activity in dendritic processes of mammalian cortical neurones, *J. Physiol. (Lond.)* **521**, 629–636, with permission.

6.1). A slow depolarizing ramp is applied through the somatic intracellular electrode to a final depolarization (around −50 mV) that is known to activate I_{NaP} and is subthreshold for action potential initiation. **Figure 18.2a** (top trace) shows the subthreshold inward current evoked by the depolarizing ramp (middle trace), that totally disappears in the presence of TTX (**Figure 18.2b** top trace). During I_{NaP} activation, a TTX-sensitive increase of intracellular Na⁺ is observed in the soma (**Figure 18.2a and b**, bottom traces) as well as in the proximal part of the apical dendrite (not shown). Its activation results in a rise of intracellular Na⁺ in the soma and proximal dendrite. This strongly suggests that I_{NaP} channels are present in the somatic membrane. However, this experiment does not allow one to localize the exact site(s) of I_{NaP} generation since the rise of Na⁺ in the proximal dendrite can result from Na⁺ diffusion from the soma, and vice versa.

18.1.2 Dendritic persistent Na⁺ channels are activated by EPSPs; in turn, I_{NaP} boosts EPSP amplitude

Activation of dendritic I_{NaP} by local synaptic inputs is tested by simultaneous whole-cell dendritic and somatic recordings (in current clamp mode) made from the same pyramidal neuron of the neocortex. Dendritic EPSPs can be evoked either by (i) stimulation of afferents or by (ii) intradendritic current injection (simulated EPSP). These EPSPs must be subthreshold (they must not trigger Na⁺ action potentials), in order to only evoke the low threshold, TTX-sensitive, persistent Na⁺ current (I_{NaP}) and not the voltage-gated Na⁺ current of action potentials. The role of I_{NaP} on these EPSPs is then deduced by studying the effect of TTX on the amplitude and duration of EPSPs. However, since TTX affects postsynaptic Na⁺ channels as well as presynaptic ones, it affects synaptic

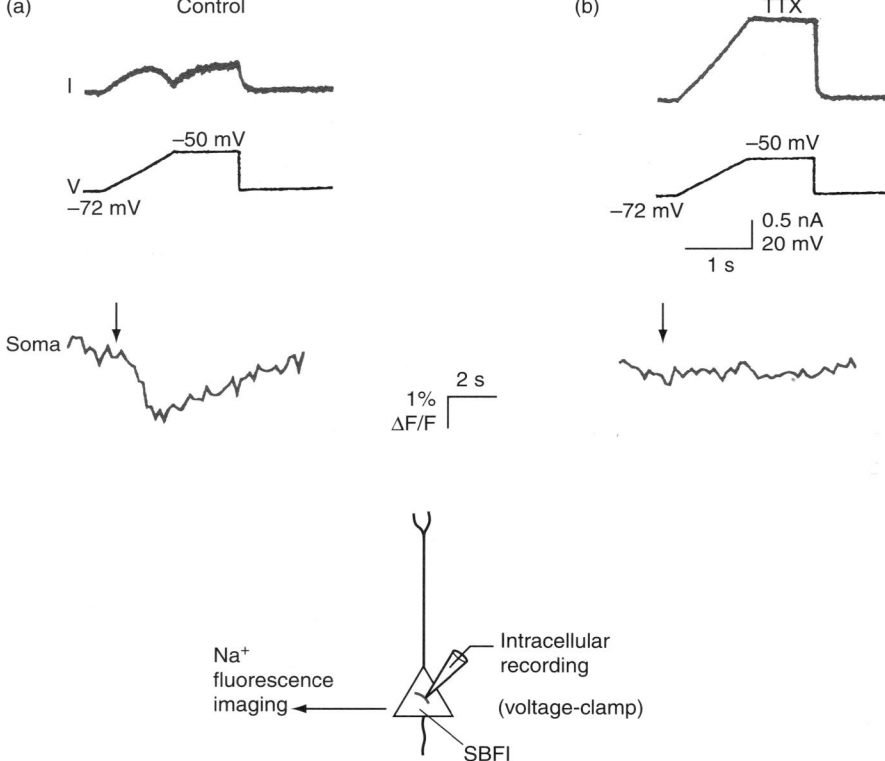

Figure 18.2 I_{NaP} activation and the resultant SBFI fluorescence changes in the soma of a pyramidal neuron of the neocortex.
(a) Intracellular recording (voltage clamp mode) of the current evoked by a depolarizing ramp from −72 mV to a 1 s constant step at −50 mV (top traces). The corresponding decrease of SBFI fluorescence in the soma is shown in the bottom trace. The arrow indicates time of voltage-clamp. A decrease of SBFI fluorescence reflects an increase of intracellular Na⁺ concentration. (b) The same experiment in the presence of 1 μM of TTX in the bath. Adapted from Mittman T, Linton SM, Schwindt P, Crill W (1997) Evidence of persistent Na⁺ current in apical dendrites of rat neocortical neurons from imaging of Na⁺-sensitive dye, *J. Neurophysiol.* **78**, 1188–1192, with permission.

transmission. Such a study therefore needs to bypass synaptic transmission by using only simulated EPSPs (protocol (ii)). Voltage change during an EPSP is simulated by dendritic current injection with a time course similar to that of an excitatory postsynaptic current (EPSC). With this aim, EPSCs are first recorded and then simulated. Simulated EPSPs generated by dendritic current injections are recorded both at their site of generation (dendritic site) and in the soma. Bath and local applications of TTX are used to determine whether I_{NaP} is involved in the amplification of simulated EPSPs and to localize where EPSPs are amplified, locally in dendrites or in the soma region.

When EPSPs recorded at the soma have an amplitude greater than 5 mV, bath application of TTX causes a substantial $29 \pm 2\%$ reduction in the peak amplitude and a $53 \pm 5\%$ reduction of the EPSPs surface (**Figure 18.3a**). At which site does a synaptic signal experience amplification while it travels from the dendrites to the axon

initial segment? The site of EPSP amplification is tested by local application of TTX to either the site of simulated EPSP generation in the dendrites or to the somatic region. Local application of TTX is achieved by pressure ejection of TTX from a patch pipette, the tip of which is placed close to either the dendritic recording site or the soma. To minimize the spread of TTX, a low concentration of TTX (100 nM) is used. That this TTX application does in fact block dendritic Na^+ channels is verified by its ability to reduce the amplitude of backpropagated Na^+ action potentials (see Chapter 19). I_{NaP} seems to be mostly located in the soma as shown in Figure 18.3b: local application of TTX to the dendritic recording site has little or no effect on the simulated EPSP, but when applied to the soma TTX reduced the somatic EPSP peak amplitude and integral. Therefore, in the neocortex, EPSPs activate I_{NaP} and in turn, I_{NaP} boosts EPSPs in amplitude and duration. This amplification occurs mainly in the somatic region.

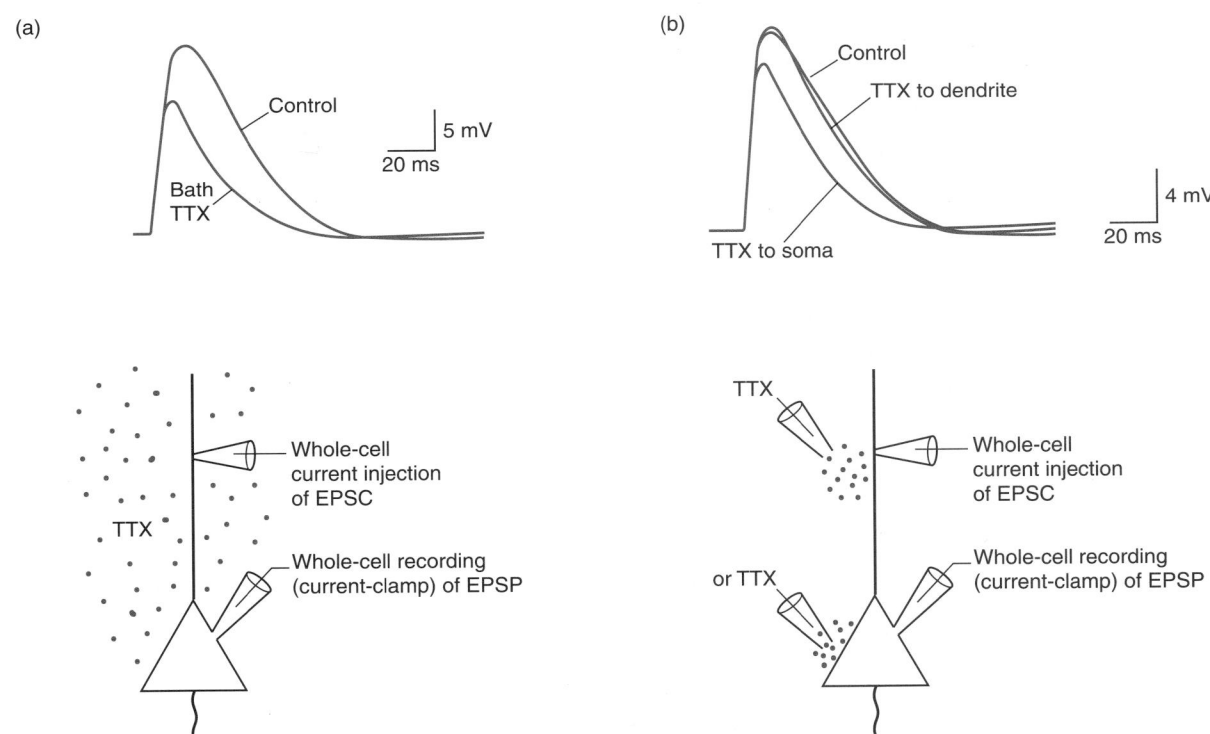

Figure 18.3 Effect of bath or local applications of TTX on the amplitude and duration of simulated dendritic EPSPs (pyramidal neurons of the neocortex).
EPSPs are generated (simulated EPSPs) by injection of an exponentially rising and falling voltage waveform into the current clamp input of the amplifier (dendritic current injections are performed 330 μm away from the soma). EPSPs are recorded from the soma (in whole-cell configuration and current clamp mode) after propagation in the dendritic tree. (a) Effect of bath application of TTX on the simulated EPSP recorded from the soma at resting membrane potential (–65 mV). (b) Effect of TTX locally applied near the dendritic or somatic recording sites, on simulated EPSPs recorded at resting membrane potential (–63 mV). Adapted from Stuart G, Sakmann B (1995) Amplification of EPSPs by axosomatic sodium channels in neocortical pyramidal neurons, *Neuron* **15**, 1065–1076, with permission.

18.2 T-type Ca²⁺ channels are present in dendrites of neocortical neurons; I_{CaT} boosts EPSPs in amplitude and duration

The T-type Ca²⁺ current is an amiloride- and Ni²⁺-sensitive Ca²⁺ current which activates below spike threshold, inactivates rapidly with time and is totally inactivated at –40 mV (see Section 17.2.2). In order to record Ca²⁺ current in isolation, the solution bathing the extracellular face of the patch contains Ba²⁺ (110–120 mM) as the charge carrier and TEACl and TTX for blocking K⁺ and Na⁺ currents, respectively. T-type Ca²⁺ current is identified by inward polarity, unitary current amplitude, activation–inactivation characteristics, sensitivity to Ni²⁺ or amiloride, and insensitivity to dihydropyridines (L-type blocker), ω-conotoxins or funnel web toxin (N-type and P-type blockers).

Are the pharmacological tools used in all the above experiments sufficiently selective to allow the conclusion that the observed Ca²⁺ current is I_{CaT}? The answer is no. These experiments do not exclude some partial contribution of a dendritic R-type Ca²⁺ current (I_{CaR}) which is also sensitive to Ni²⁺ and amiloride. However, since I_{CaR} is a high-threshold-activated current – it activates at higher depolarized potentials than I_{CaT} – it has been considered in the following experiments that the Ca²⁺ current activated in dendrites by step depolarizations or by EPSPs is I_{CaT}.

18.2.1 T-type Ca²⁺ channels are present in dendrites of pyramidal neurons of the hippocampus

The activity of a patch of apical dendritic membrane is recorded in the dendrite-attached configuration (voltage clamp mode). In response to depolarizing steps to –15 mV from a hyperpolarized potential (–85 mV, to de-inactivate T channels), channel openings are recorded. They occur mostly at the beginning of the depolarizing step, are of small unitary current amplitude (**Figure 18.4a**), and the i_T/V plot gives a unitary conductance γ_T of 7–11 pS (**Figure 18.4b**). They are sensitive to Ni²⁺ and amiloride (not shown). These data, together with the activation–inactivation characteristics (**Figure 18.4c**) reveal that T-type Ca²⁺ channels are present within the apical dendrite of pyramidal neurons. They are similar in basic characteristics to T-type Ca²⁺ channels recorded from many neuronal soma (compare with **Figure 17.4**).

18.2.2 Dendritic T-type Ca²⁺ channels are activated by EPSPs; in turn, I_{CaT} boosts EPSPs amplitude

Activation of dendritic I_{CaT} by local synaptic inputs is tested by simultaneous dendrite-attached and whole-cell somatic recordings from the same pyramidal neuron of the CA1 region. Subthreshold EPSPs are evoked by Schaffer collateral stimulation. These EPSPs must be subthreshold (they must not trigger Na⁺ action potentials), in order to evoke only the low-threshold, Ni²⁺-sensitive, Ca²⁺ current (I_{CaT}) and not the high-voltage-activated Ca²⁺ currents such as the L-, N- or P/Q-type currents. EPSPs are recorded from the soma (in current clamp mode) after propagation in the dendritic tree. Single-channel T-type Ca²⁺ currents are recorded from the patch of dendritic membrane (in voltage clamp mode). If channel openings only occur during EPSPs, they are considered to have been triggered by it.

In response to Schaffer collateral stimulation, the activity of single Ca²⁺ channels is recorded (**Figure 18.5a**). These single-channel currents are not recorded when the Ca²⁺ channel blocker CdCl₂ (0.5 mM) is present in the pipette (not shown). Single-channel openings are most often observed near the peak or falling phases of the EPSPs. EPSP-activated channel openings display small unitary current amplitude and slope conductance ($\gamma = 9 \pm 1.6$ pS) characteristic of T-type dendritic channels (see **Figure 18.4**). EPSPs with a peak amplitude of 10 mV (at the somatic recording site) are necessary for activation of T-type dendritic Ca²⁺ channels. When a 4 s hyperpolarizing prepulse is applied 400 ms before synaptic stimulation, the open probability (p_o) of T-type Ca²⁺ channels is increased in a voltage-dependent manner (**Figure 18.5b**). This suggests that a large proportion of the T-type Ca²⁺ channel population is inactivated at resting potential. Therefore, membrane hyperpolarization (as during IPSPs), by allowing channel de-inactivation, is necessary for maximal channel activation by EPSPs. Thus, the contribution of LVA Ca²⁺ channels to EPSP amplitude would be particularly enhanced for EPSPs occurring after hyperpolarizing IPSPs.

Another way to address the question of the activation of T-type Ca²⁺ current by EPSPs is to measure Ni²⁺-sensitive intradendritic [Ca²⁺] increase during subthreshold EPSPs. Whole-cell recordings in the soma are performed in conjunction with high-speed fluorescence imaging (FURA-2). To measure changes in intracellular Ca²⁺ concentration the fluorescent indicator FURA-2 is included in the pipette solution. Detectable increases in Ca²⁺ concentration are observed in response to as few as two consecutive synaptic stimulations (50 Hz) but a short train of five stimuli provides a very reproducible increase above baseline (2.2 ± 0.5% ΔF/F) (**Figure 18.6a**).

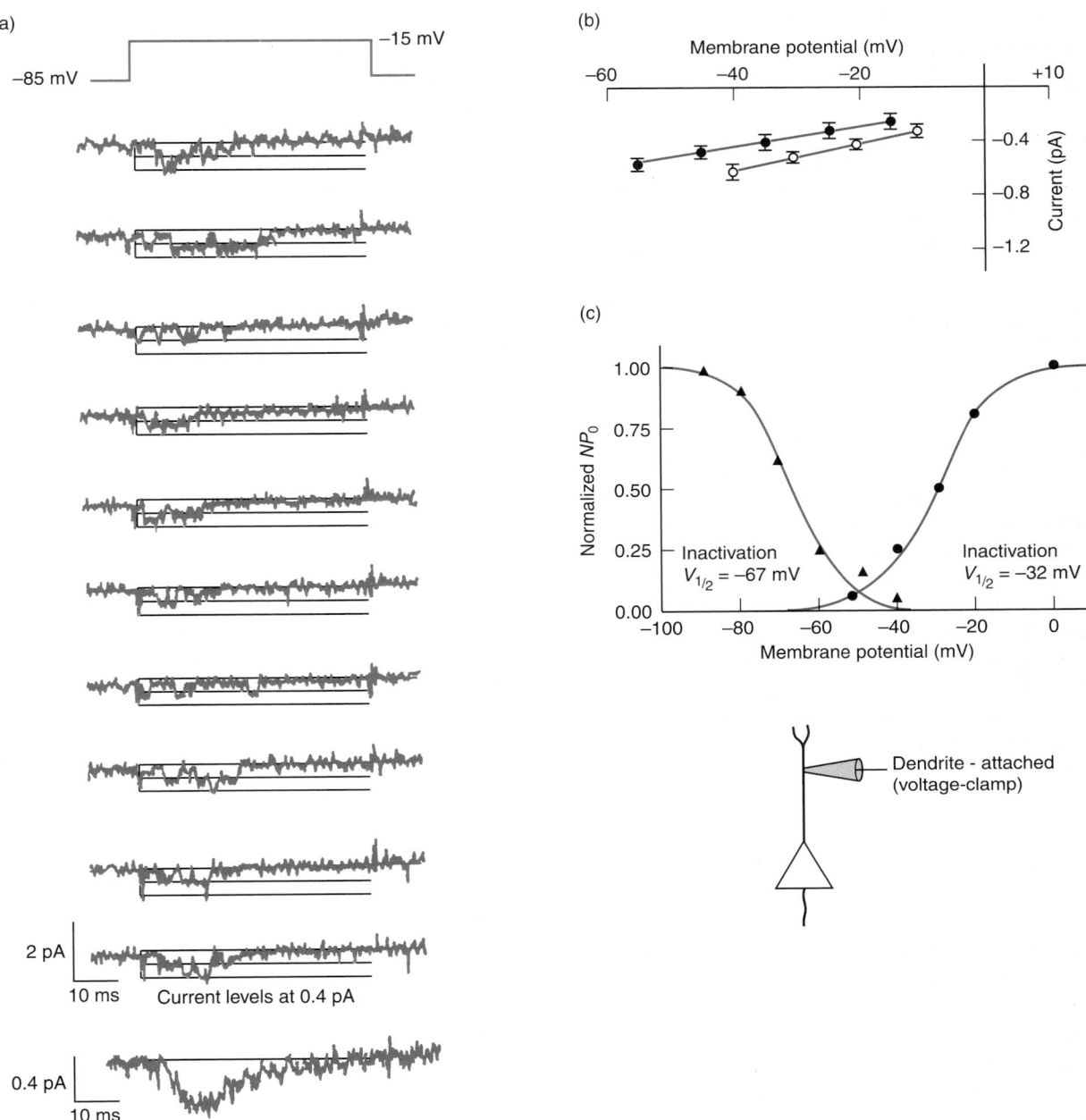

Figure 18.4 Dendritic low-voltage-activated Ca²⁺ channel activity in pyramidal neurons of the hippocampus.
(a) Consecutive sweeps of T-type Ca²⁺ channel activity recorded from a dendrite-attached patch (voltage clamp mode) in response to 60 ms depolarizing steps to –15 mV (V_H = –85 mV). Bottom trace is the ensemble average (104 sweeps) demonstrating significant inactivation during the 60 ms depolarizing step (110 mM of Ba²⁺ in the recording solution). (b) i_T/V plot of T-type Ca²⁺ channel activity. Unitary current amplitude is plotted as a function of membrane potential for patches recorded with either 20 mM (•) or 110 mM (o) Ba²⁺ as charge carrier. The slope (unitary conductance) γ_T is between 7 pS (20 mM of Ba²⁺) and 11 pS (110 mM of Ba²⁺). (c) Representative steady-state activation (•) and inactivation (▲) plots for dendritic LVA Ca²⁺ channels recorded in 20 mM of Ba²⁺. Adapted from Magee JC, Johnston D (1995) Characterization of single voltage-gated Na⁺ and Ca²⁺ channels in apical dendrites of rat CA1 pyramidal neurons, *J. Physiol. (Lond.)* **487**, 67–90, with permission.

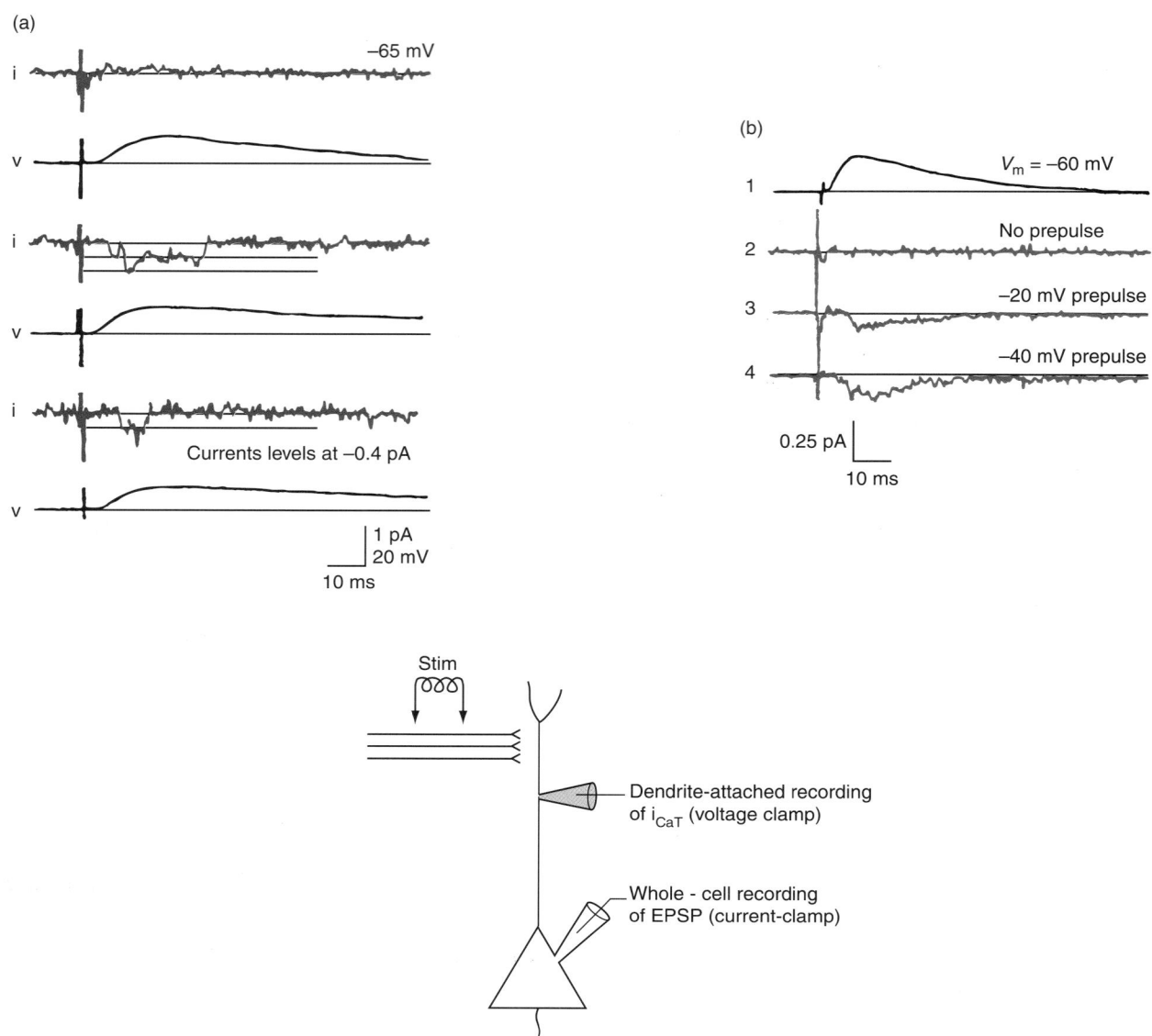

Figure 18.5 Synaptic activation of LVA Ca²⁺ channels in hippocampal CA1 pyramidal neurons.
Subthreshold EPSPs are evoked by Schaffer collateral stimulation and are recorded from the soma (in current clamp mode) after propagation in the dendritic tree. **(a)** Consecutive sweeps of dendrite-attached recordings (voltage clamp mode) with the patch held at −65 mV showing Ca²⁺ channel activity recorded at the dendritic site (*i*, top traces) and of subthreshold EPSPs (*V*, bottom traces) recorded at the somatic site (whole-cell configuration). **(b)** Hyperpolarizing prepulses (not shown) increase the activation of T-type Ca²⁺ channels by an EPSP. Ensemble average of 50 consecutive current traces without prepulse (2), ensemble average of 60 consecutive current traces after a 4 s prepulse of −20 mV (3), and ensemble average of 60 consecutive traces after a 4 s prepulse of −40 mV (4). The patch is returned to a holding potential that is 10 mV depolarized from resting potential 400 ms before synaptic stimulation in order to evoke an EPSP of similar amplitude (1) in all trials. Adapted from Magee JC, Johnston D (1995) Synaptic activation of voltage-gated channels in the dendrites of hippocampal pyramidal neurons, *Science* **268**, 301–304, with permission.

The rise in [Ca²⁺]$_i$ continues throughout the course of the synaptic stimulation and begins to decay back to baseline several milliseconds after the end of the EPSP train. It thus appears that subthreshold stimulations of sufficient amplitude result in a transient elevation of intradendritic [Ca²⁺].

[Ca²⁺]$_i$ transients are localized primarily to the area of the synaptic input (not shown). The localized nature of these [Ca²⁺]$_i$ signals implies that the largest changes in [Ca²⁺]$_i$ occur in the dendrites where the synaptic input is located and that this signal attenuates as it approaches the soma. Through which types of dendritic Ca²⁺

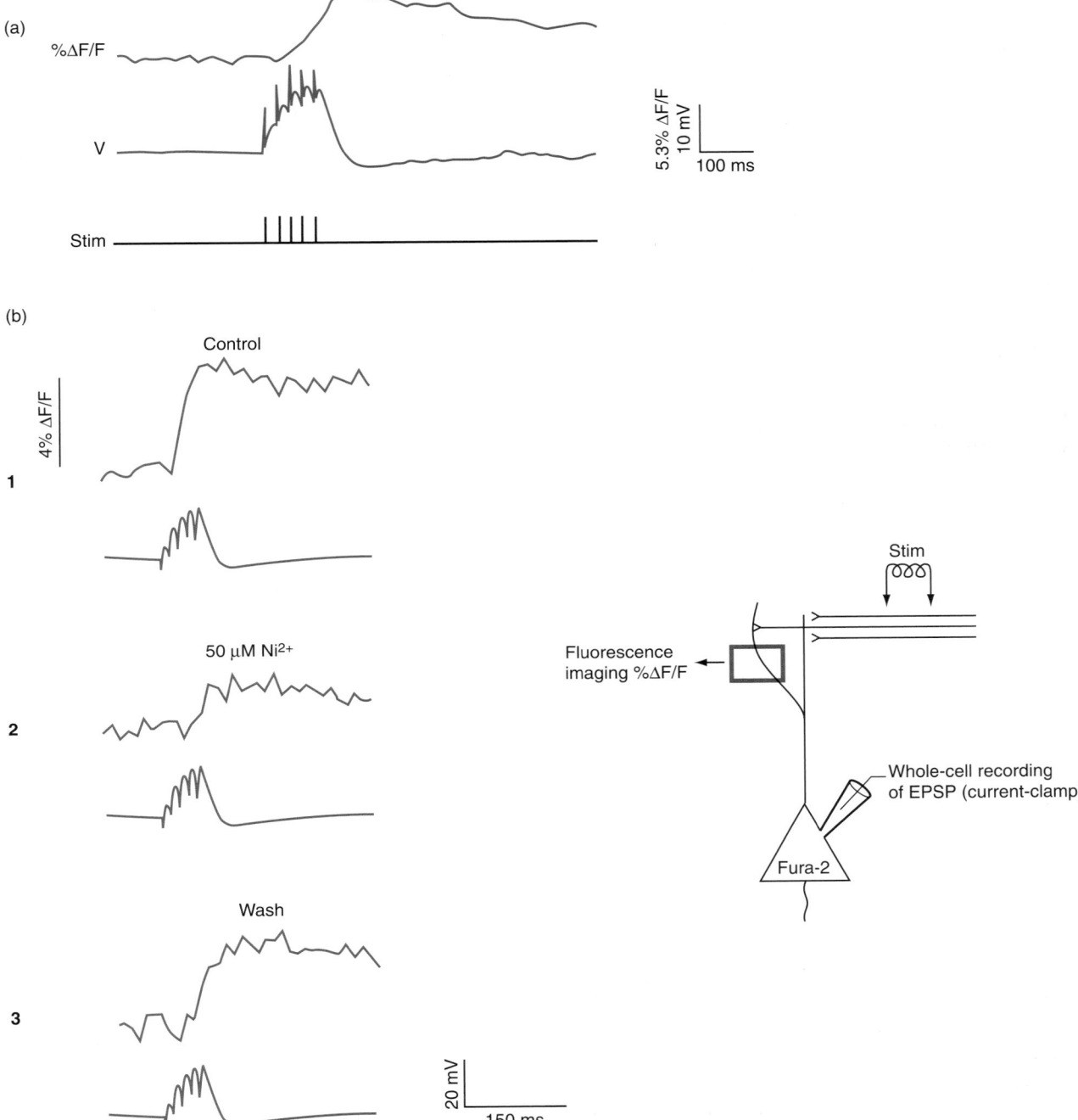

Figure 18.6 Subthreshold EPSPs cause a localized, Ni²⁺-sensitive elevation of intradendritic Ca²⁺ concentration.
Subthreshold EPSPs are evoked by stimulation of afferents close to the dendrite under study. **(a)** Time course of percentage change in FURA-2 fluorescence in a dendrite (%ΔF/F, top trace) evoked by a short train of five EPSPs and somatic voltage recordings (V) of the five EPSPs (whole-cell configuration, current clamp mode, bottom trace). The fluorescence trace is from the region delimited by the small green box on the schematic representation of the FURA-2 loaded neuron. **(b)** Localized percent change in FURA-2 fluorescence (%ΔF/F, top trace) induced by a short train of five EPSPs and somatic voltage recordings of the five EPSPs (bottom traces) in the absence (1), presence (2) and 20 min after washing (3) of 50 μM of NiCl₂. The somatic recording of EPSPs (bottom traces) is unaffected by Ni²⁺ application. All traces in the figure are averages of five consecutive sweeps. Adapted from Magee JC, Christofi G, Miyakawa H *et al.* (1995) Subthreshold synaptic activation of voltage-gated Ca²⁺ channels mediates a localized Ca²⁺ influx into the dendrites of hippocampal pyramidal neurons, *J. Neurophysiol.* **74**, 1335–1342, with permission.

channels are Ca^{2+} ions entering the cell; or does this $[Ca^{2+}]_i$ increase result from the release of intradendritic Ca^{2+} stores? For the first hypothesis, the candidates are Ca^{2+}-permeable receptor channels (NMDA or AMPA receptors; see Sections 11.2 and 11.4) and voltage-gated Ca^{2+} channels. Application of APV (50 µM), a specific antagonist of NMDA channels, has very little effect on the subthreshold Ca^{2+} signals as long as the EPSP amplitude is maintained constant. 50 µM of APV is therefore included in the bath solution for the remainder of the experiment. In contrast, membrane hyperpolarization to around −100 mV during synaptic stimulation prevents the synaptically induced rise in intradendritic Ca^{2+} concentration, indicating that Ca^{2+} entry is voltage-dependent. All these data demonstrate that $[Ca^{2+}]_i$ signals result from Ca^{2+} influx but not through NMDA or AMPA receptors (antagonists of AMPA receptors cannot be tested since they would cancel the EPSP which is an AMPA-mediated EPSP). This influx is then likely to occur through voltage-gated ion channels. The primary candidate is the T-type Ca^{2+} channel. The effect of 50 µM of Ni^{2+} is therefore tested. When bath applied, such a concentration of Ni^{2+} produces a 54 ± 5% block of the synaptically induced influx of Ca^{2+} and this block is completely reversible with washout of Ni^{2+} (**Figure 18.6b**).

What are the consequences of this local intradendritic Ca^{2+} increase? Does dendritic I_{CaT} boost EPSPs? To address this question, EPSPs are evoked far out on the apical dendrite and their shape is recorded at the soma with the dendritic I_{CaT} active or partially suppressed by local pressure application of I_{CaT} blockers such as Ni^{2+} or amiloride. EPSPs are evoked by afferent fibre stimulation at a frequency of 0.2 Hz and are recorded at the level of the soma (whole-cell configuration). To visualize the approximate spread of Ni^{2+} (5 µM) or amiloride (50 µM) in the tissue, both drugs are dissolved in 2% food colour solution. In control experiments, dendritic pressure application of food colour solution alone produces negligible reductions of EPSP amplitude. To study the role of dendritic I_{CaT} with minimum contamination by somatic I_{CaT}, the membrane potential is set to −70 mV at the soma and stimulation amplitude is adjusted to obtain EPSP peak amplitudes at the soma of 7 mV on average. Under these conditions somatic EPSP amplitude should be too small to activate LVA Ca^{2+} channels. Dendritic amiloride application reduces EPSP amplitude by 27 ± 2% and Ni^{2+} application reduces it by 33 ± 2.9% (**Figure 18.7**, top traces). The effects of both amiloride and Ni^{2+} reverse within 15–20 min of drug wash-out. Hyperpolarization of the membrane to −90 mV attenuates the effect of both antagonists (**Figure 18.7**, bottom traces). However, any of the observed effects can be due to a presynaptic action of Ni^{2+} or amiloride.

In order to check this, EPSPs are recorded extracellularly near the dendrite, at the level of afferent stimulation in control conditions and in the presence of blockers. Bath application of both drugs, at a concentration 10 times higher than that achieved during focal application around the apical dendrite, fails to impair synaptic transmission. Thereby this excludes any presynaptic action of Ni^{2+} or amiloride. Therefore, in CA1 pyramidal neurons, EPSPs activate a T-type Ca^{2+} current that can indeed alter the weight of EPSPs. This amplification occurs in dendritic regions.

18.3 The hyperpolarization-activated cationic current I_h is present in dendrites of hippocampal pyramidal neurons; for EPSPs, dendritic I_h decreases the current transmitted from the dendrites to the soma

The hyperpolarization-activated cation current I_h is a Cs^+-sensitive current that is turned on by hyperpolarization, is inward at potentials more hyperpolarized than its reversal potential (around −50 to −30 mV), and does not inactivate (see Section 17.2.3). To record I_h, the solution bathing the extracellular face of the membrane and the pipette solution contain control concentrations of Na^+, K^+ and Ca^{2+} ions.

18.3.1 H-type cationic channels are expressed in dendrites of pyramidal neurons of the hippocampus

The basic biophysical properties and the subcellular distribution of I_h are investigated in cell-attached configuration, voltage clamp mode. Long duration (1–3 s) hyperpolarizing steps evoke inward currents from cell-attached macropatches obtained from both the soma and apical dendritic regions but with different amplitudes (**Figure 18.8a**). These inward currents are slowly activating, non-inactivating and slowly deactivating (as seen on tail currents; see the inset of **Figure 18.8d** and Appendix 6.2). Currents begin to activate near −60 mV and steady-state current amplitude increases in an approximately linear manner with membrane hyperpolarization up to −140 mV (**Figure 18.8b**). Inclusion of 5 mM of Cs^+ in the external recording solution totally blocks the current, thus showing that it is an I_h current (**Figure 18.8c**).

The steady-state current amplitude at −130 mV progressively increases with distance away from the soma (soma: 8.9 ± 1.6 pA, $n = 21$; dendrite 300–350 µm away from the soma: 62.3 ± 8.5 pA, $n = 14$) (the mean dendritic length is 500 µm). The mean current can be

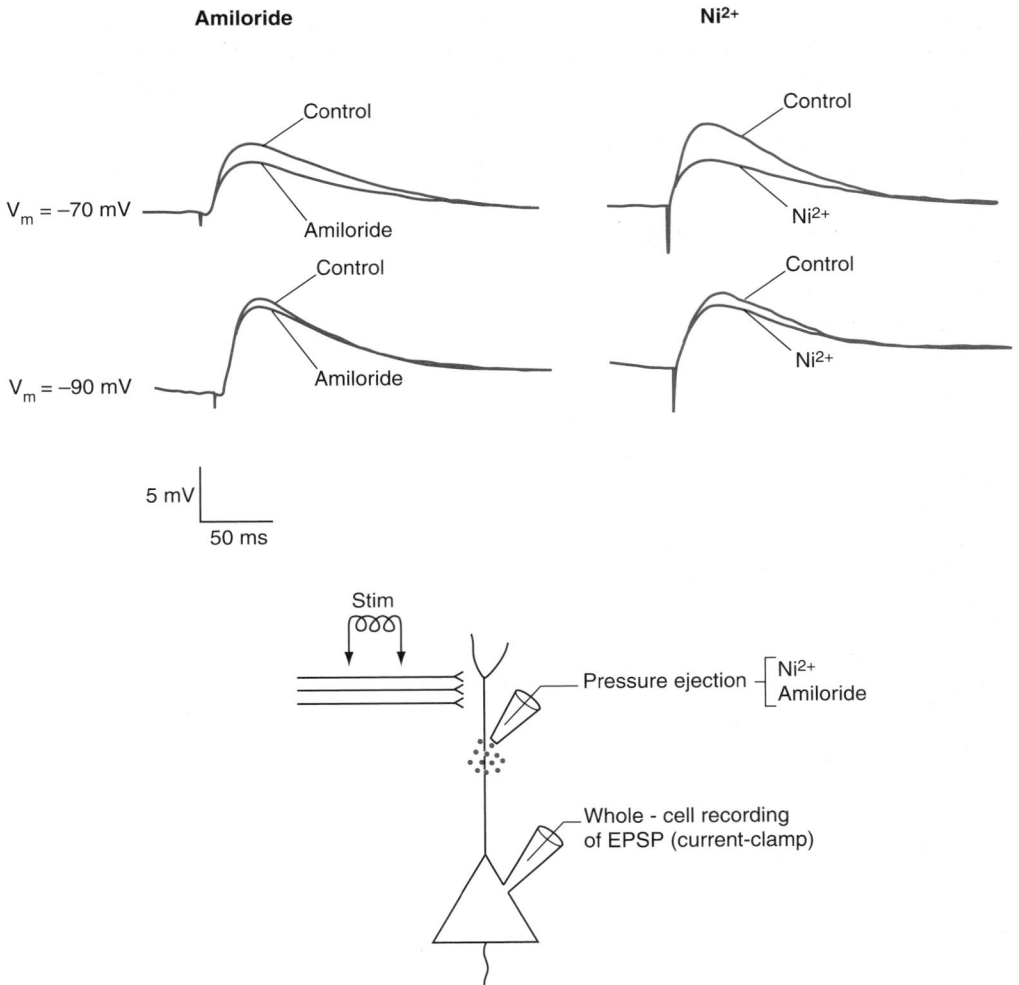

Figure 18.7 EPSPs in hippocampal pyramidal dendrites are amplified by an amiloride- and Ni²⁺-sensitive Ca²⁺ current.
EPSPs are evoked by stimulation of afferent fibres in the outer stratum radiatum. EPSPs are recorded from the soma (whole-cell configuration, current clamp mode) at two different membrane potentials (−70 and −90 mV) adjusted by current injection through the whole-cell pipette. Superimposed traces of averaged EPSPs ($n = 50$) recorded before and during local dendritic application of amiloride (50 μM, left) or Ni²⁺ (5 μM, right) show that both drugs reduce EPSPs recorded at −70 mV but do not significantly reduce them at −90 mV. Adapted from Gillessen T, Alzheimer C (1997) Amplification of EPSPs by low Ni²⁺ and amiloride-sensitive Ca²⁺ channels in apical dendrites of rat CA1 pyramidal neurons, *J. Neurophysiol.* **77**, 1639–1643, with permission.

converted to mean current density (per μm²) by normalizing to a 5 μm² patch area. It is 1.8 ± 0.3 pA μm⁻² at the soma as compared with a density of 12.5 ± 1.7 pA μm⁻² recorded from dendrites located 300–350 μm away from the soma. Therefore the density of I_h increases over 6-fold from soma to distal dendrites. Even with these elevated I_h densities, absolute I_h density is quite small compared with other dendritic channel densities, K⁺ channels in particular.

In conclusion, the ionic selectivity (data not shown), voltage ranges of activation and kinetics of activation and inactivation as well as the sensitivity to external Cs⁺ all fall within the ranges reported for a wide variety of

central and peripheral I_h in neurons as well as in cardiac cell types. Moreover, a 6-fold increase in I_h density is found across the somatodendritic axis.

18.3.2 Dendritic H-type cationic channels are activated by IPSPs; in turn, I_h decreases EPSPs amplitude

The impact of I_h channels on the shape and propagation of subthreshold voltage signals is determined by using simultaneous whole-cell current clamp recordings from both the soma and dendrites. EPSPs are simulated by

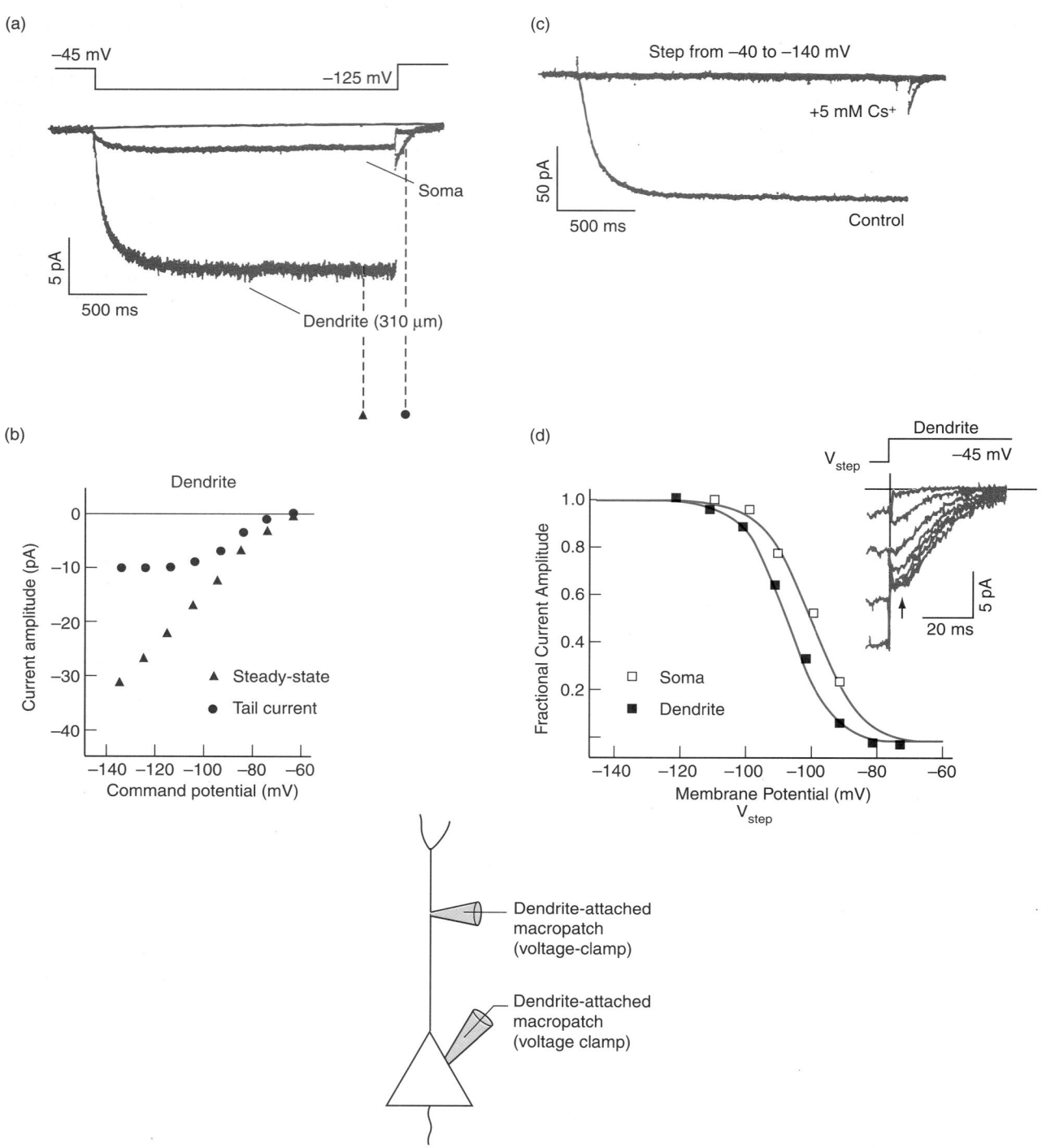

Figure 18.8 Dendritic and somatic hyperpolarization-activated cation current I_h in pyramidal neurons of the hippocampus.
(a) In a dendrite-attached macropatch located in the apical dendrite (310 μM from the soma), hyperpolarizing steps to –125 mV (V_H = –45 mV) evoke inward currents that are larger than those recorded from the soma with similar-sized pipettes. **(b)** I/V plots for steady-state inward current measured 900 ms after the start of the step (▲) and for inward tail current measured 5 ms after the end of the step (•). **(c)** Blockade by 5 mM of external Cs^+ of the inward current evoked by a hyperpolarizing step to –140 mV. **(d)** Activation curves generated from the tail currents (inset). The dendritic curve ($V_{1/2}$ = –89 mV) is shifted 6 mV hyperpolarized with respect to the somatic curve ($V_{1/2}$ = –83 mV). Command potentials (V_{step}) are given in 10 mV increments from –65 to –135 mV. Adapted from Magee JC (1998) Dendritic hyperpolarization-activated currents modify the integrative properties of hippocampal CA1 pyramidal neurons, *J. Neurosci.* **18**, 7613–7624, with permission.

dendritic current injection. Under control conditions, current injections in the dendritic compartment result in EPSP-shaped voltage transients, the amplitude and kinetics of which are filtered significantly as they propagate from the dendritic injection site to the recording somatic site (**Figure 18.9a**). When the amplitude of the simulated EPSP is 8.0 ± 0.5 mV at the dendritic recording site, it becomes 3.0 ± 0.2 mV at the somatic recording site. When the EPSP duration is 15 ± 0.8 ms at the dendritic site, it becomes 39 ± 2 ms at the somatic site. Repetitive dendritic current injections are also given to mimic repetitive synaptic inputs. These events are filtered similarly by dendritic arborizations (**Figure 18.9b**). When the peak amplitude is 24 ± 3 mV at the dendritic site, it becomes 8 ± 1 mV at the somatic site.

When the duration is 136 ± 1 ms at the dendritic site, it becomes 154 ± 2 ms at the somatic site.

I_h channel blockade with external Cs^+ increases single EPSP amplitude by $7 \pm 4\%$ at the dendritic site and by $10 \pm 2\%$ at the somatic site. It also increases EPSP duration by $10 \pm 2\%$ at the dendritic site and by $38 \pm 9\%$ at the somatic site (**Figure 18.9a**). For repetitive EPSPs, the presence of external Cs^+ increases the amplitude by $22 \pm 5\%$ at the dendritic site and by $42 \pm 8\%$ at the somatic site. For the duration the increase is $3 \pm 1\%$ at the dendritic site and $7 \pm 2\%$ at the somatic site (**Figure 18.9b**). Therefore, for single EPSPs, the amount of amplitude attenuation occurring between the dendrites and soma is the same in the presence or absence of I_h. In contrast, for repetitive EPSPs, the peak amplitude reached during

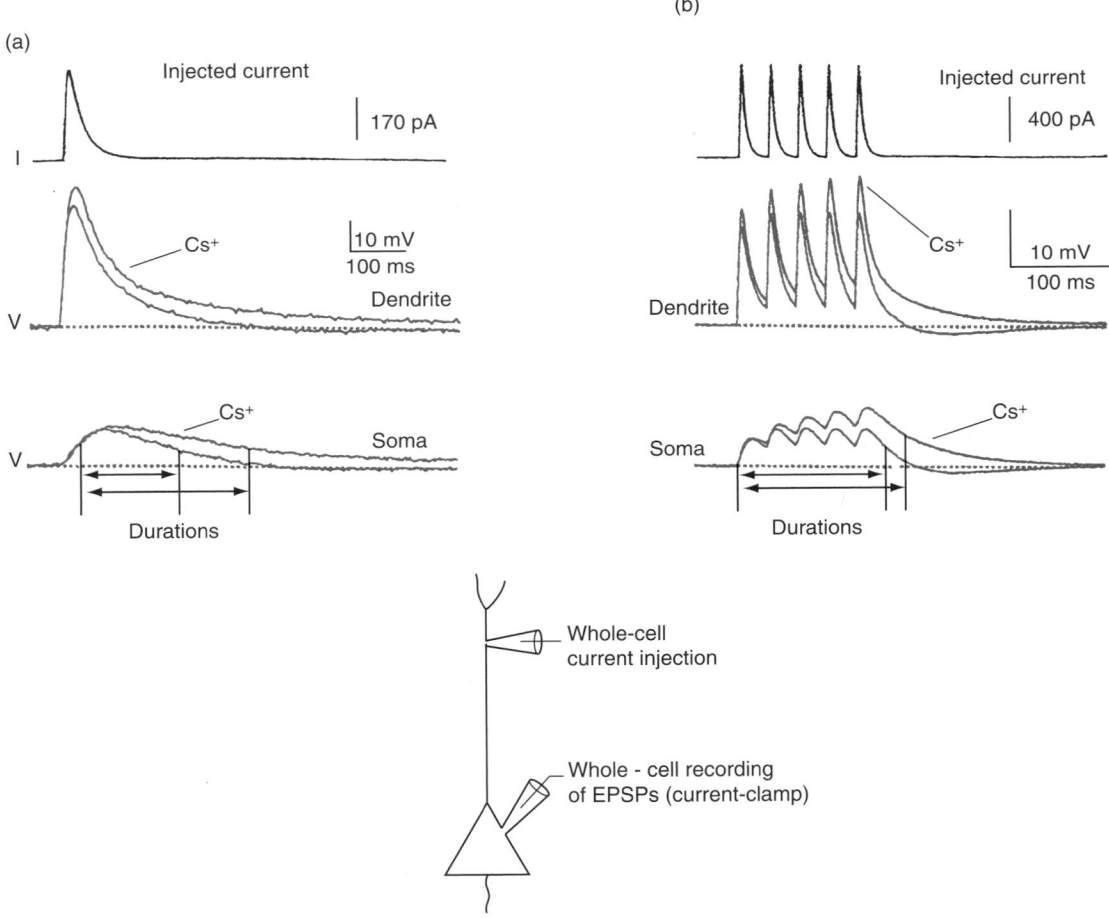

Figure 18.9 EPSP amplitude, duration and summation are all regulated by I_h in hippocampal pyramidal neurons.
EPSPs are generated by injection of an exponentially rising and falling voltage waveform into the current clamp input of the amplifier (dendritic current injections are performed 250 μm away from the soma). Simultaneous whole-cell recordings are performed from the dendrite and the soma of the same pyramidal neuron. (**a**) A single current injection into the dendritic electrode produces an EPSP-shape transient, the amplitude and duration of which is increased in the presence of 3 mM of external Cs^+. (**b**) Repetitive current injections produce a train of EPSP-shaped voltage transients, the peak amplitude and duration of which are also increased in the presence of 3 mM of external Cs^+. Adapted from Magee JC (1998) Dendritic hyperpolarization-activated currents modify the integrative properties of hippocampal CA1 pyramidal neurons, *J. Neurosci.* **18**, 7613–7624, with permission.

the train increases twice as much in the soma as in the dendrite. Thus for repetitive activity, the amount of attenuation occurring between the dendrites and the soma is reduced by I_h blockade.

The increase of amplitude of somatic EPSPs under conditions of I_h blockade is mostly the result of an elevation in effective input membrane resistance (due to I_h channels closure). In conclusion, dendritic I_h decreases the amount of current transmitted from the dendrites to the soma for EPSPs. Since I_h density is 6-fold more elevated in distal dendrites, the absolute effectiveness of more distal synaptic inputs (i.e. the total charge transferred from synapse to soma) is reduced by the increasingly large I_h conductance.

18.4 Functional consequences

18.4.1 Amplification of distal EPSPs by I_{NaP} and I_{CaT} counteracts their attenuation owing to passive propagation to the soma; it also favours temporal summation versus spatial summation

The subliminal voltage-gated I_{NaP} and I_{CaT} present in the dendrites of pyramidal neurons of the neocortex or the hippocampus boost the effects of local EPSPs by acting as either voltage or current amplifiers. This could be one solution to overcome the passive decay of EPSPs en route to the soma. This argument, however, is somewhat somatocentric; i.e. the emphasis on how dendrites amplify events so that they are bigger in the soma. An alternative viewpoint is that these channels are more important for dendritic interactions in the immediate vicinity of the synaptic inputs. For example, multiple EPSPs occurring on the same branch and within a narrow time should activate voltage-gated channels more strongly than a single EPSP and produce a much bigger response than would occur if EPSPs were on separate branches.

18.4.2 Activation of dendritic I_{CaT} generates a local dendritic $[Ca^{2+}]_i$ transient

Under physiological conditions, an EPSP-evoked $[Ca^{2+}]_i$ transient would occur mainly after the summation of a number of unitary EPSPs and thus would represent the integrated result of dendritic activity at a given moment and at a given location. A number of possible physiological functions for dendritic $[Ca^{2+}]_i$ transients exists. Intracellular Ca^{2+} may activate biochemical pathways,

Ca^{2+}-induced Ca^{2+} release as well as Ca^{2+}-activated K^+ currents present in the dendritic membrane. Such outward current would change the shape of the EPSP. Ca^{2+} is also implicated in postsynaptically induced forms of plasticity such as long-term potentiation or depression (see Chapter 21).

18.4.3 Activation of dendritic I_h, I_{NaP} and I_{CaT} alter the local membrane resistance and time constant

This in turn will influence both spatial and temporal summation of EPSPs. Moreover, I_h participates to resting potential, so that different densities of I_h from the soma could lead to different resting potentials in the dendrites. Moreover, I_h is deactivated by membrane depolarization as a result of EPSPs. This will produce an increase of membrane resistance. In contrast, activation of I_{NaP} and I_{CaT} by EPSPs will produce a decrease of membrane resistance.

18.5 Conclusions

We can now answer the three questions asked in the introduction:

- Subliminal depolarizing voltage-gated currents are present in the dendritic membrane of some CNS neurons. These are the depolarizing currents I_{NaP}, I_{CaT} and I_h.
- They are not distributed uniformly over somatodendritic membranes. In pyramidal neurons of the neocortex, I_{NaP} seems more efficient at the soma. In contrast, in pyramidal neurons of the hippocampus, I_h density increases from soma to distal dendrites.
- I_{NaP} and I_{CaT} activation boost EPSP amplitude and duration. In contrast, it is I_h deactivation that boosts EPSPs. Moreover I_{CaT} activation induces a transient and local increase of intradendritic Ca^{2+} concentration.

Finally, one must keep in mind that the state of voltage-gated channels, closed, open or inactivated, depends on the history of the membrane. If a segment of dendritic membrane has been previously depolarized before synaptic activity, the voltage-gated channels present in this segment of dendritic membrane will be already inactivated and will not play a role. There is therefore a dynamic aspect in the active properties of dendrites.

Further reading

Johnston D, Magee JC, Colbert CM, Christie BR (1996) Active properties of neuronal dendrites. *Annu. Rev. Neurosci.* **19**, 165-186.

Lipowsky R, Gillessen T, Alzheimer C (1996) Dendritic Na$^+$ channels amplify EPSPs in hippocampal CA1 pyramidal cells. *J. Neurophysiol.* **76**, 2181–2190.

Magee JC (1999) Dendritic I_h normalizes temporal summation in hippocampal CA1 neurons. *Nature Neurosci.* **2**, 508–514.

Markram H, Sakmann B (1994) Calcium transients in dendrites of neocortical neuron evoked by single subthreshold excitatory postsynaptic potentials via low-voltage-activated calcium channels. *Proc. Natl Acad. Sci. USA* **91**, 5207–5211.

Mouginot D, Bossu JL, Gähwiler BH (1997) Low-threshold Ca^{2+} currents in dendritic recordings from Purkinje cells in rat cerebellar slice cultures. *J. Neurosci.* **17**, 160–170.

Schwindt PC, Crill WE (1995) Amplification of synaptic current by persistent sodium conductance in apical dendrite of neocortical neurons. *J. Neurosci.* **74**, 2220–2224.

19
Somato-Dendritic Processing of Postsynaptic Potentials III. Role of High-Voltage-Activated Depolarizing Currents

Dendrites of neurons of the mammalian central nervous system (CNS) have long been considered as electrically passive structures which funnel postsynaptic potentials to the soma and axon initial segment, the site of action potential initiation. However, the recording of dendritic action potentials (at first with intracellular electrodes) from dendrites of pyramidal neurons of the neocortex, of pyramidal neurons of the hippocampus, of dopaminergic neurons of substantia nigra, and of Purkinje cells of the cerebellar cortex (**Figure 19.1**), strongly suggested that these dendrites express high-threshold-activated Na^+ or Ca^{2+} channels. This led to the suggestion that, in these neurons, synaptic integration is not solely governed by (passive) cable properties of dendrites. In the previous chapter we looked at the role of subliminal voltage-gated currents in the shaping of postsynaptic potentials. This chapter will examine the roles of high voltage-activated currents.

Dendritic events have recently come under direct experimental scrutiny by the use of dendritic patch recordings and by the advent of imaging techniques with high spatial and temporal resolution. This permitted the design of experiments to answer the following questions:

- Are high-voltage-activated (HVA) currents present in the dendritic membrane of some CNS neurons?
- Are they distributed uniformly over the soma-dendritic membrane so that electrogenic properties in dendrites are not fundamentally different from that in soma?
- How do the currents affect synaptic potentials and input summation?

This chapter looks at experiments performed on four types of central neurons, on pyramidal neurons of the neocortex or hippocampus, dopaminergic neurons of substantia nigra pars compacta, and Purkinje cells of the cerebellar cortex.

Figure 19.1 (Opposite) Examples of neurons of the mammalian central nervous system from which dendritic spikes are recorded.
Drawing of neurons (left) with the corresponding recording of dendritic spikes (right) evoked by afferent stimulation.
(a) Pyramidal neuron of the neocortex. **(b)** Pyramidal neuron of the hippocampus. **(c)** Dopaminergic neurons of the substantia nigra. **(d)** Purkinje cell of the cerebellar cortex. Part (a) adapted from Seamans JK, Gorelova N, Yang CR (1997) Contribution of voltage-gated Ca^{2+} channels in the proximal versus distal dendrites to synaptic integration in prefrontal cortical neurons, *J. Neurosci.* **17**, 5936–5948, with permission. Part (b) drawing by Taras Pankevitch and Roustem Khazipov and adapted from Tsubokawa H, Ross WN (1996) IPSPs modulate spike backpropagation and associated $[Ca^{2+}]_i$ changes in dendrites of hippocampal CA1 pyramidal neurons, *J. Neurophysiol* **76**, 2896–2906, with permission. Part (c) drawing by Jérôme Yelnik and adapted from Häusser M, Stuart G, Racca C, Sakman B (1995) Axonal initiation and active dendrite propagation of action potentials in substantia nigra neurons, *Neuron* **15**, 637–647, with permission. Part (d) adapted from Callaway JC, Lasser-Ross N, Ross WN (1995) IPSPs strongly inhibit climbing fiber-activated $[Ca^{2+}]_i$ increases in the dendrites of cerebellar Purkinje neurons, *J. Neurosci.* **15**, 2777–2787, with permission.

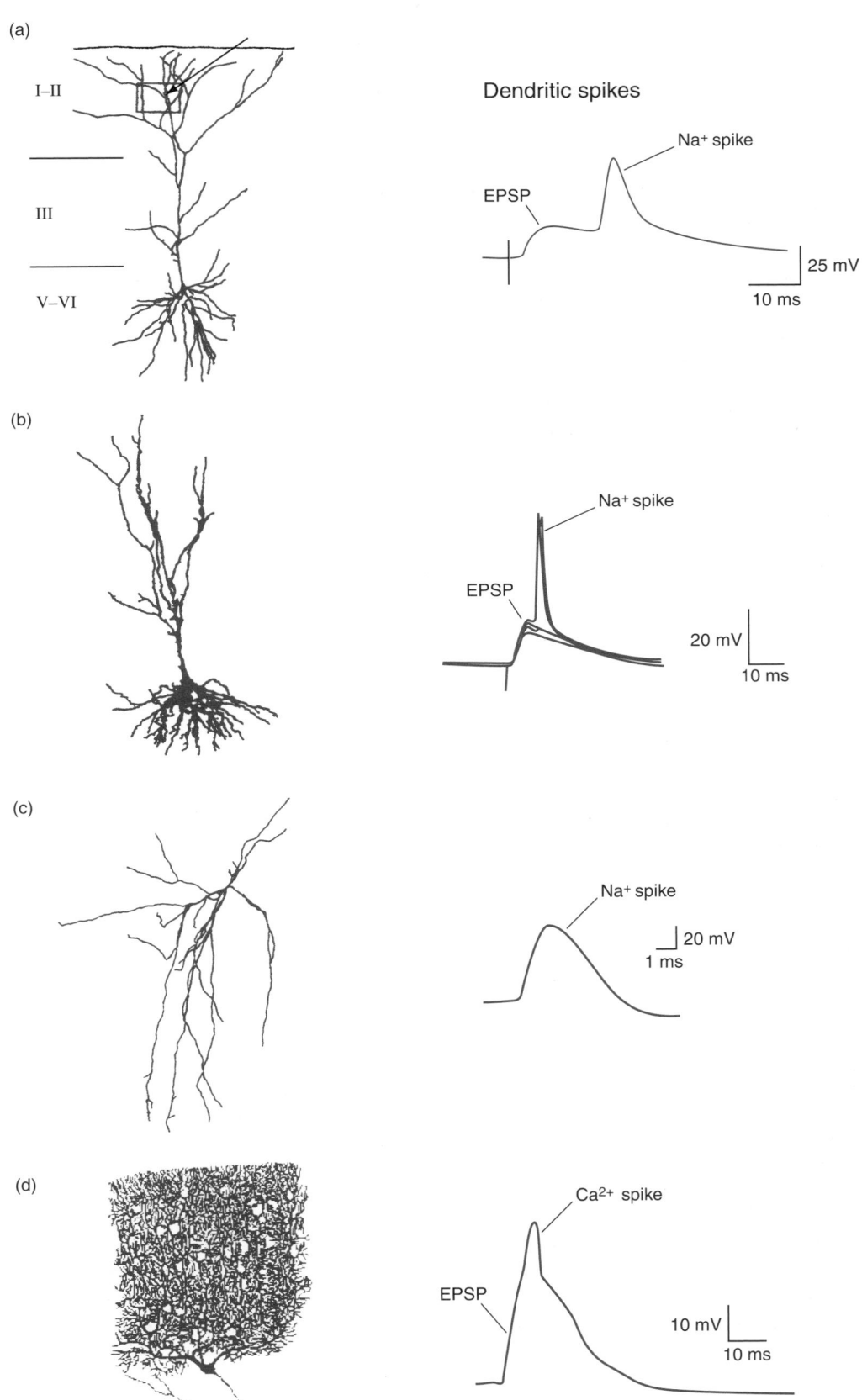

Dendritic spikes

19.1 High-voltage-activated Na⁺ and/or Ca²⁺ channels are present in the dendritic membrane of some CNS neurons, but are they distributed with comparable densities in soma and dendrites?

One way to answer the above questions is first to identify the activity of HVA channels in patches of dendritic membrane and then to compare the amplitude of the HVA current recorded from similar-sized patches of dendritic and somatic membranes. Experiments are performed in brain slices and recordings are either in the outside-out or dendrite-attached configuration. For technical reasons this type of patch recording is limited to dendritic branches with a diameter greater than 1 μm. In order to record Na⁺ channels, the solution bathing the extracellular face of the patch contains NaCl; and in order to strongly reduce outward K⁺ currents, TEACl is added in the external solution or CsCl in the internal solution. Na⁺ channel activity is identified by inward current polarity, voltage-dependent channel gating, unitary current amplitude, by its blockade by TTX and by the lack of effect of Cd²⁺.

19.1.1 High-voltage-activated Na⁺ channels are present in some dendrites

Pyramidal neurons of the hippocampus

In every dendrite-attached patch, Na⁺ channel activity is consistently found and more than a single channel is always recorded (**Figure 19.2a**). Na⁺ channels are opened by depolarizations of about 15 mV from rest. The i_{Na}/V relationship shows that Na⁺ channels have a unitary conductance γ_{Na} of 15 pS and a unitary current that reverses at E_{rev} = +54 mV (**Figure 19.2b**). This value is close to the calculated Nernst equilibrium potential assuming an intracellular Na⁺ concentration of 10 mM (extracellular concentration is 110 mM). These data, together with the activation–inactivation characteristics of dendritic i_{Na} (**Figure 19.2c**) reveal that HVA Na⁺ channels present in the apical dendrites of pyramidal neurons are similar in basic characteristics to HVA Na⁺ channels recorded in many neuronal somata (compare with **Figure 5.8**) with a difference concerning the inactivation properties (slow inactivation and slow recovery from inactivation for dendritic channels). This explains the decrease of amplitude of repetitive dendritic action potentials.

Pyramidal neurons of the neocortex

Outside-out macropatches of dendritic membrane are excised at different distances from the soma, up to 500 μm. In response to step depolarizations applied through the recording electrode, an inward current that rapidly inactivates and totally disappears in the presence of TTX (1 μM) in the bath is recorded (**Figure 19.3a**). This is observed whether patches are excised from proximal or more distal dendrites. Moreover, this TTX-sensitive Na⁺ current has a similar amplitude in patches taken from dendritic or somatic membranes, thus suggesting a similar somatic and dendritic density of Na⁺ channels in both membranes.

Dopaminergic neurons of the pars compacta of the substantia nigra

Outside-out patches are excised from somatic or dendritic membrane. In an attempt to maintain constant patch membrane area all recordings are made with pipettes of similar size. Multichannel TTX-sensitive sodium currents are recorded from both patches. The average peak Na⁺ current in somatic patches is 5.0 ± 1.3 pA and that in dendritic patches is 3.6 ± 1.6 pA. Again, in these neurons, there is a similar sodium-channel density in dendritic and somatic membranes.

Purkinje cells of the cerebellar cortex

The situation in these cells is fundamentally different. As suggested by the absence of large-amplitude Na⁺ action potentials in dendrites of Purkinje cells, there is an extremely low-amplitude, TTX-sensitive Na⁺ current in outside-out macropatches excised from dendrites (1.9 ± 0.4 pA) compared with that in patches excised from the soma (12.4 ± 1.5 pA) (**Figure 19.3b**). In fact, sodium-channel density steeply declines in dendrites with distance from the soma. These results were confirmed by experiments in Purkinje cells loaded with the Na⁺ indicator SBFI (sodium benzofuram isophthalate; see Appendix 6.1). During Na⁺ spikes, changes in the intracellular Na⁺ concentration were detected only in soma and not in dendrites. In these cells, Na⁺ channels are distributed non-uniformly over the somatic and dendritic membrane.

Conclusions

In pyramidal neurons of the neocortex or the hippocampus and in dopaminergic neurons of the substantia nigra there is a similar density of TTX-sensitive Na⁺

(a)

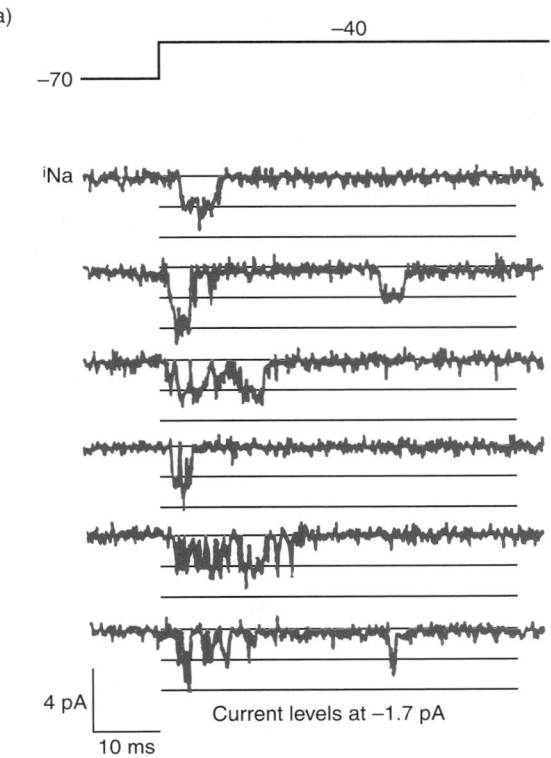

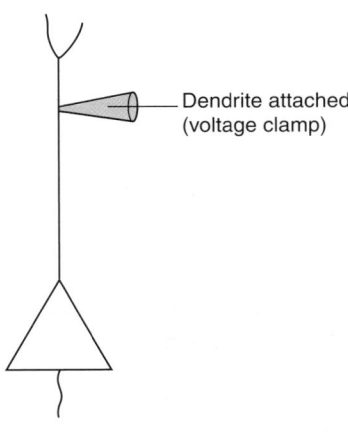

Dendrite attached
(voltage clamp)

(b)

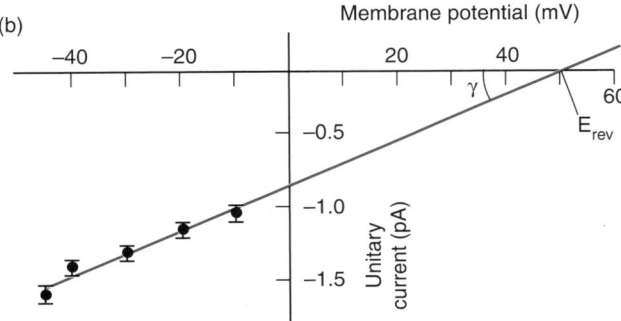

Membrane potential (mV)

Figure 19.2 Characteristics of dendritic Na⁺ channels in a pyramidal neuron of the hippocampus.
(a) Consecutive sweeps showing Na⁺ channel openings (dendrite-attached configuration, voltage clamp mode) in response to step depolarizations to −40 mV (V_H = −70 mV). Most of the channel openings occur at the beginning of the step but there are some late reopenings. (b) Current–voltage plot of Na⁺ channel activity. Unitary current amplitude from a total of 27 patches is plotted as a function of membrane potential. Bars are standard error of the mean (SEM). The slope indicates a unitary conductance γ of 15 pS and the extrapolated reversal potential E_{rev} is +54 mV.

channels in somatic and dendritic membranes up to several hundreds of μm from the soma. In contrast, there is a low density of Na⁺ channels in the dendritic membrane of Purkinje cells. It must be pointed out that most CNS dendrites contain a low density of HVA Na⁺ channels. Pyramidal neurons of the neocortex or hippocampus and substantia nigra neurons are exceptions.

(c)

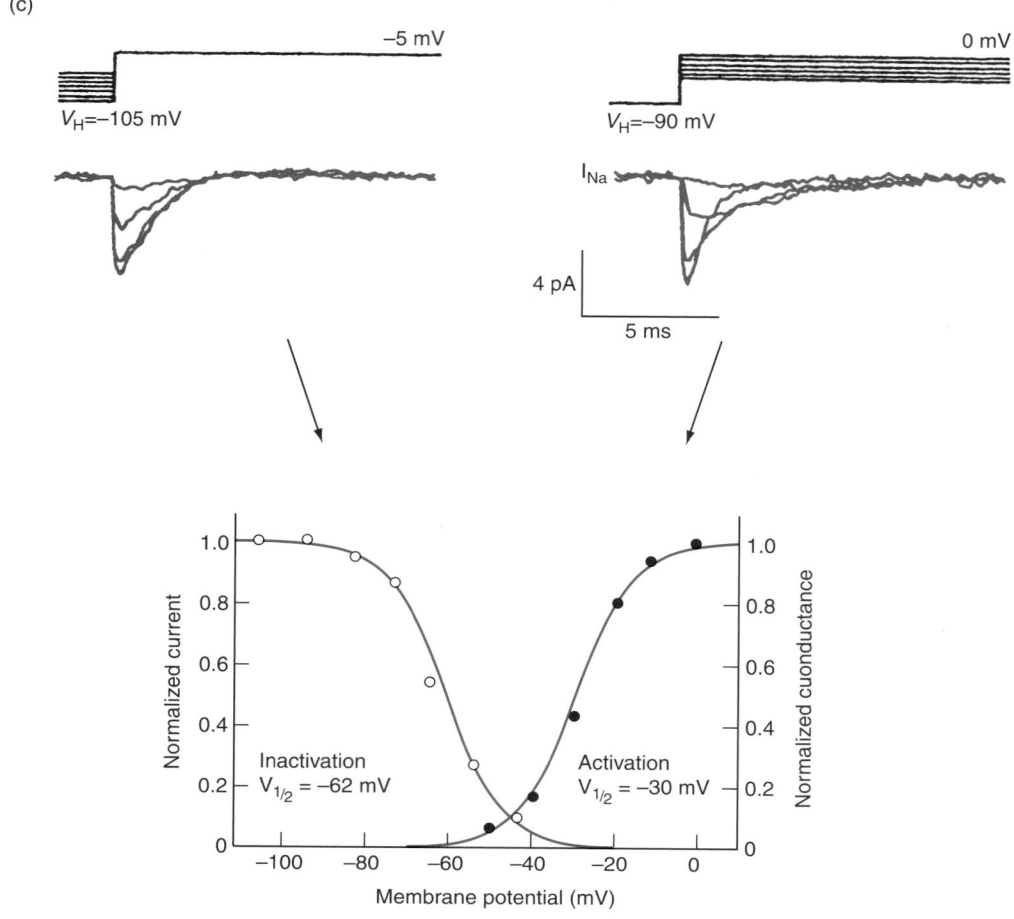

Figure 19.2

(c) Dendritic Na⁺ channel steady-state activation and inactivation characteristics. Activation is tested by applying depolarizing steps to −65 to 0 mV from $V_H = -90$ mV. Inactivation is tested by applying a depolarizing step to −5 mV from a V_H varying from −105 to −45 mV. The representative steady-state activation (black circle) and inactivation (open circle) plots for dendritic Na⁺ channels indicate that they are half-activated at $V_{1/2} = -30$ mV and half-inactivated at $V_{1/2} = -62$ mV. Adapted from Magee JC, Johnston D (1995) Characterization of single voltage-gated Na⁺ and Ca²⁺ channels in apical dendrites of rat CA1 pyramidal neurons, *J. Physiol. (Lond.)* **487**, 67–90, with permission.

19.1.2 Dendritic Na⁺ channels are opened by EPSPs and the resultant Na⁺ current boosts EPSPs in amplitude and duration

Pyramidal neurons of the hippocampus

Activation of dendritic voltage-gated channels by local synaptic inputs is tested by simultaneous dendrite-attached and whole-cell somatic recordings from the same pyramidal neuron of the CA1 region (**Figure 19.4**). Subthreshold EPSPs are evoked by Schaffer collateral stimulation (stim) and are recorded from the soma (in current clamp mode) after propagation in the dendritic tree. Single Na⁺ channel currents are recorded from the patch of dendritic membrane (in voltage clamp mode).

If channel openings occur only during EPSPs, they are considered to have been triggered by it.

When EPSPs of 15–20 mV amplitude and below action potential threshold are evoked, they consistently activate Na⁺ channels located within the CA1 dendrite-attached patch (**Figure 19.4a**). Most channel openings are near the peak of the EPSP, but occasional openings are encountered during either the rising or the falling phase of the EPSP. With TTX present in the pipette, there is no EPSP-associated channel activity in dendritic patches (not shown). Are these Na⁺ channels different from that opened by step depolarizations as shown in **Figure 19.2**? Plots of unitary current amplitude versus approximate membrane potential (in cell-attached recordings, membrane potential can only be evaluated

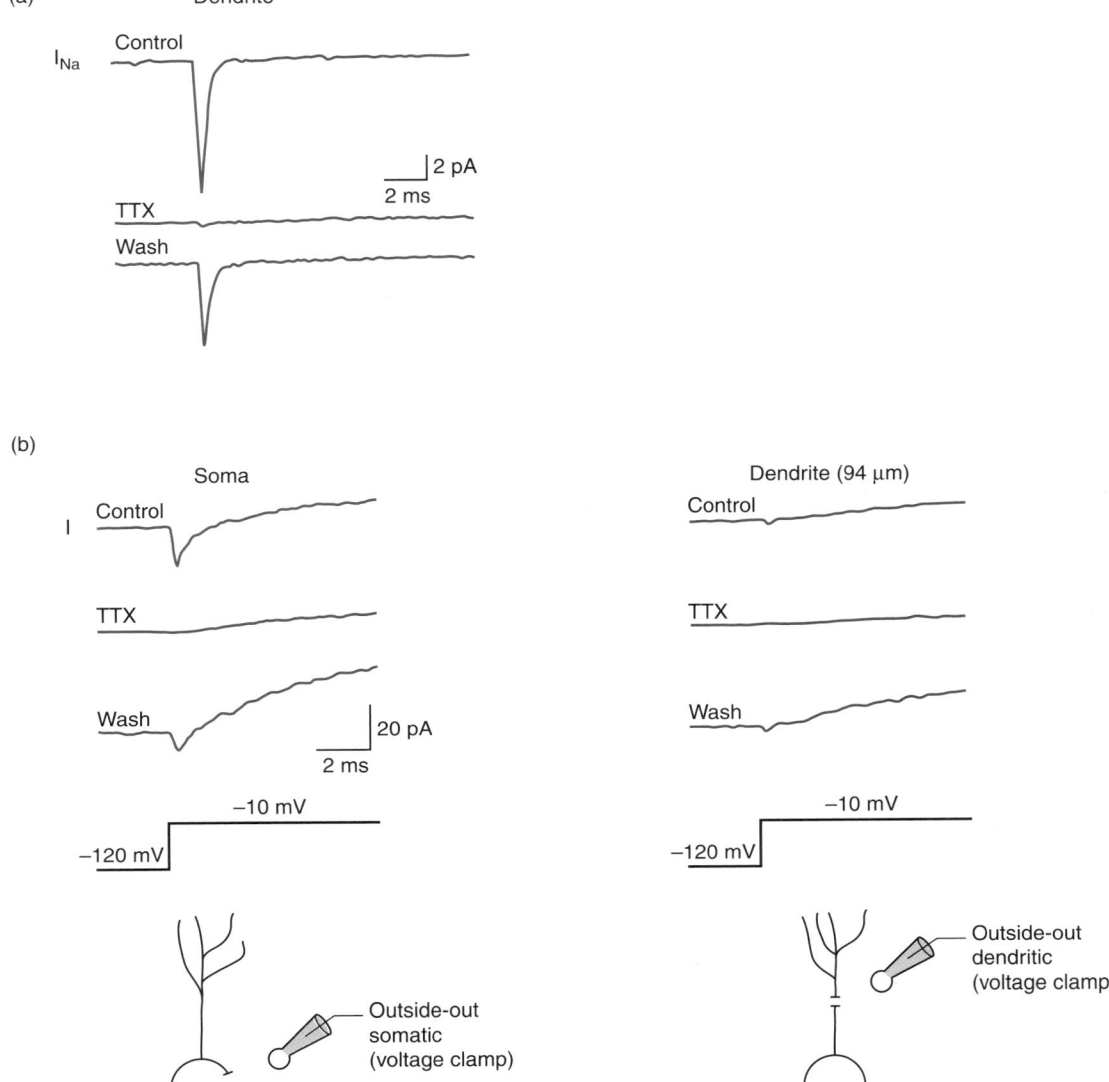

Figure 19.3 TTX-sensitive inward currents in dendrites of pyramidal neurons of the neocortex and Purkinje cells.
(a) Neocortex. Rapidly inactivating inward current evoked by a depolarizing step to -10 mV ($V_H = -90$ mV) in an outside-out dendritic macropatch excised from the apical dendrite of a layer V pyramidal neuron (439 µm from the soma) (control). This current is reversibly blocked in the presence of 500 nM of TTX in the external solution. **(b)** Purkinje cells. Voltage-activated currents evoked by a depolarizing step to -10 mV ($V_H = -120$ mV) in outside-out macropatches excised from either the soma (left) or dendrite (right, 94 µm from the soma) of Purkinje cells using similar-sized patch pipettes. A rapidly inactivating inward current followed by an outward current that is more prominent in the somatic membrane are recorded (control). Rapidly inactivating currents in both somatic and dendritic patches are reversibly blocked by the presence of 500 nM of TTX in the extracellular medium (TTX). Part (a) adapted from Stuart G, Sakmann B (1994) Active propagation of somatic action potentials into neocortical pyramidal cell dendrites, *Nature* **367**, 69–72, with permission. Part (b) adapted from Stuart GJ, Häusser M (1994) Initiation and spread of sodium action potentials in cerebellar Purkinje cells, *Neuron* **13**, 703–712, with permission.

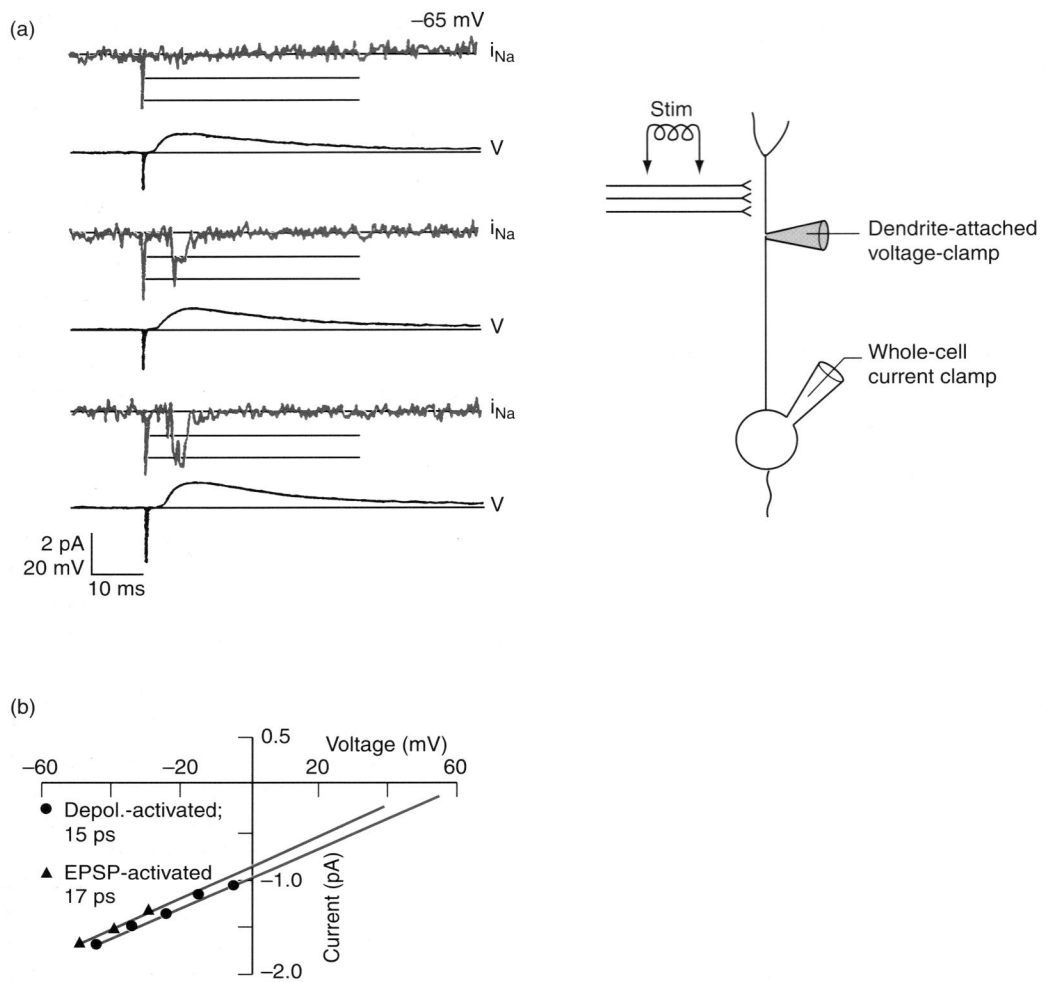

Figure 19.4 Na⁺ channel openings evoked by subthreshold EPSPs in dendrites of hippocampal pyramidal neurons.
(a) Consecutive sweeps of unitary Na⁺ currents recorded from a dendrite-attached patch (i_{Na}) and simultaneous whole-cell somatic recordings of the EPSPs (V) evoked by Schaffer collateral stimulation (bottom traces). **(b)** i_{Na}/V plots of unitary Na⁺ current evoked in the same patch by depolarizing steps (depol-activated) or by EPSPs (EPSP-activated). Adapted from Magee JC, Johnston D (1995) Synaptic activation of voltage-gated channels in the dendrites of hippocampal pyramidal neurons, *Science* **268**, 301–304, with permission.

approximately) show that the slope unitary conductance γ (16 ± 1 pS) and reversal potential E_{rev} (+56 ± 1 mV) of EPSP-activated channel openings are similar to those calculated from step depolarization in the same patches (**Figures 19.2b** and **19.4b**). This suggests that Na⁺ channels opened by EPSPs are the same as those opened by intracellular depolarization.

Activation of dendritic Na⁺ channels may elevate EPSP amplitude and prolong their duration. Dendritic Na⁺ channels are therefore capable of enhancing the efficacy of more distal and widely distributed synaptic contacts by increasing both the strength and duration of excitatory synaptic inputs.

19.1.3 Dendritic Na⁺ channels are opened by backpropagating Na⁺ action potentials

The question about the role of dendritic Na⁺ channels is the following: do dendritic Na⁺ channels allow the initiation of Na⁺ action potentials in dendrites in response to synaptic activity (**Figure 19.5a**), or do dendritic Na⁺ channels only allow active backpropagation of Na⁺ action potentials first initiated in the axon hillock region (**Figure 19.5b**)? To further explain the latter hypothesis it must be assumed that, in general, Na⁺ action potentials, once they have been initiated, actively (i.e. in a regenerative manner) propagate along the axon (orthodromic propagation; see Section 5.4) and at the same time passively propagate into the soma and

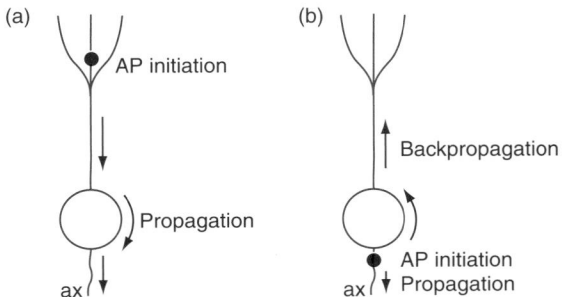

Figure 19.5 Schematic drawings of two hypotheses concerning the site of dendritic Na⁺ spike initiation.

(a) In response to dendritic EPSPs, Na⁺ action potential (AP) is locally initiated in dendrites (black point) and then actively propagates to the soma-initial segment and along the axon. (b) In response to dendritic EPSPs, Na⁺ action potential is first initiated at the soma-initial segment (black point) and then actively propagates along the axon and backpropagates (actively or passively) into the dendritic tree.

dendritic tree (passive backpropagation). Therefore the question is not 'do Na⁺ action potentials backpropagate in the dendritic tree? but rather 'do they backpropagate *actively* in the dendritic tree of neurons that contain HVA Na⁺ channels in their dendrites?'

Pyramidal neurons of the neocortex

Simultaneous whole-cell recordings (current clamp mode) are made from the soma and apical dendrite of the same pyramidal neuron in slices *in vitro*. To confirm that the recorded dendrite and soma belong to the same neuron, the cell is simultaneously filled from the somatic and the dendritic recording sites with different coloured fluorescent dyes present in the recording pipettes. In response to suprathreshold synaptic stimulation, action potential initiation occurs first at or near the soma (**Figure 19.6a**). Simultaneous recordings obtained from the soma and axon hillock of the same cell further show that initiation occurs first in the axon, possibly as a result of differences in geometry between soma and axon, as well as possible differences in the density, distribution and properties of voltage-activated channels in these structures.

Action potentials have also been observed to be generated in distal dendrites of neocortical pyramidal neurons in response to stimulation of afferents. However, these Na⁺ spikes attenuate as they spread to the soma and axon. As a consequence, Na⁺ action potentials are always initiated in the axon before the soma even when synaptic activation is intense enough to initiate dendritic regenerative potentials. Na⁺ action

potentials then actively propagate along the axon. Do they also actively backpropagate in the dendritic tree (**Figure 19.5b**)?

To investigate whether voltage-activated Na⁺ channels aid the backpropagation of somatic action potentials into the dendrites, the internal Na⁺ channel blocker QX-314 is included in the dendritic patch pipette during simultaneous somatic and dendritic recording. Following establishment of the dendritic patch, dendritic action potentials are observed to decrease progressively in amplitude before any change is observed in the amplitude or time course of the somatic action potential. This suggests that dendritic Na⁺ channels boost the amplitude of dendritic action potentials as they backpropagate into the dendritic tree.

To compare the expected attenuation of dendritic action potentials in the presence and absence of Na⁺ dendritic channels, TTX is applied in the bath. Since action potentials can no longer be evoked in this condition by current injection in the soma (Na⁺ channels are blocked), a voltage command simulating an action potential is applied at the soma. The amount of attenuation is compared with that of action potentials evoked in the soma in the absence of TTX in the extracellular medium (**Figure 19.6b**, 1,2). On average, from these experiments, the amplitude of evoked dendritic action potentials is 70% of that of somatic action potentials, whereas in the presence of TTX it represents only 30% (**Figure 19.6b**, 2,3). These results show unequivocally that there is a regenerative (active) backpropagation of somatic action potentials in the dendrites of layer-V pyramidal neurons via the activation of TTX-sensitive dendritic Na⁺ channels.

Dopaminergic neurons of the substantia nigra pars compacta

Simultaneous whole-cell recordings (current clamp mode) are made under visual control from the soma and dendrite of nigral dopaminergic neurons in slices. First, the site of action potential initiation is determined. In many dopaminergic cells, action potential is observed to occur first at the dendritic recording site (**Figure 19.7a**) and in some cases it is observed to occur first at the soma. To visualize the neuron recorded, the somatic pipette is filled with a biocytin-containing solution that is injected into the soma at the end of the recording session. Morphological examination of biocytin-filled neurons shows that in every case where the action potential is observed to occur first in the dendrite, the axon of the neuron is found to emerge from the dendrite from which the recording had been made (**Figure 19.7a**). In 76% of dopaminergic neurons, the axon is found to emerge from a dendrite sometimes as far as 240 μm from

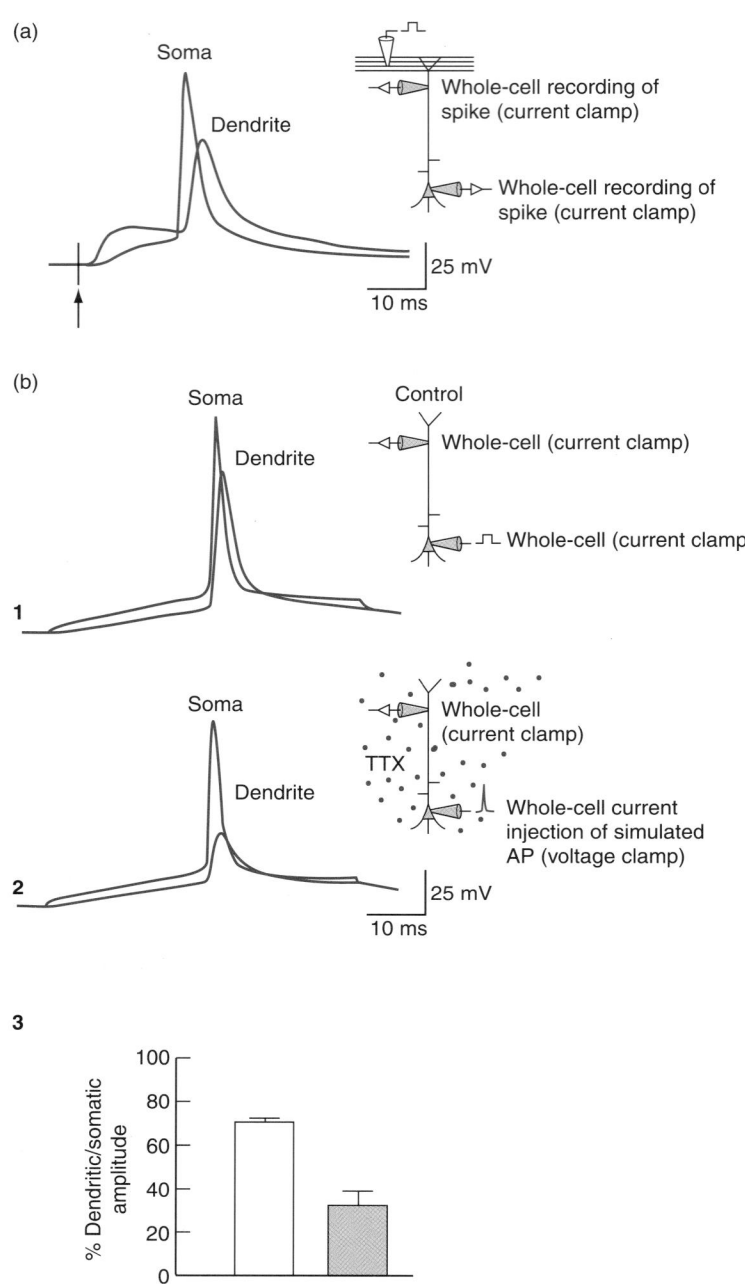

Figure 19.6 Site of initiation of Na⁺ action potential and its active backpropagation into the dendritic tree of pyramidal neurons of the neocortex.

(a) Na⁺ action potential evoked by distal synaptic stimulation in layer I and simultaneously recorded from the soma and a dendrite (dendritic recording is 525 μm from the soma). **(b)** Comparison of active and passive propagation of Na⁺ action potential in the apical dendrite studied with simultaneous somatic and dendritic recordings. b_1: An action potential is evoked in the soma by a depolarizing current pulse (200 pA, soma). It propagates in the apical dendrite where it is recorded (dendrite, 310 μm from the soma). b_2: A simulated action potential waveform is injected in the soma in the presence of 1 μM of TTX. The somatic voltage response (soma) propagates passively in the dendrites where it is recorded at the same location as in b_1 but in the presence of TTX (dendrite). The simulated somatic action potential is recorded later at the soma with a second somatic recording pipette (soma). b_3: Histogram of the average amplitude of dendritic action potentials recorded as in b_1 (open column) and of dendritic responses recorded as in b_2 (black column). Data are expressed as a percentage of the response recorded at the soma ± SEM; dendritic recordings 165–470 μm from the soma. Adapted from Stuart G, Sakmann B (1994) Active propagation of somatic action potentials into neocortical pyramidal cell dendrites, *Nature* **367**, 69–72, with permission.

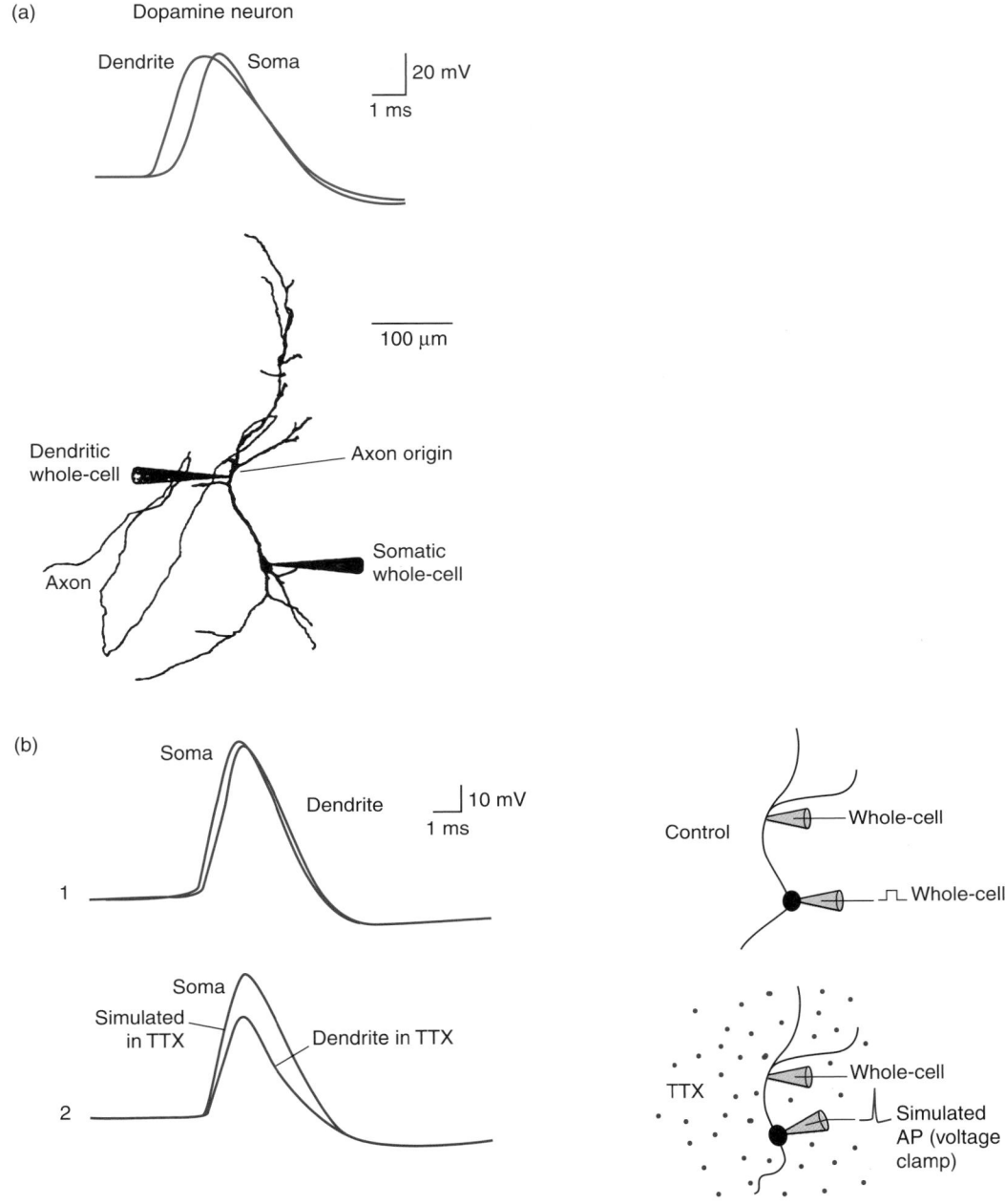

Figure 19.7 Site of initiation of Na⁺ action potential and its active backpropagation in the dendritic tree of dopaminergic neurons of the substantia nigra.

(a) Spontaneous Na⁺ action potential recorded simultaneously at the soma and dendrite (top) and the morphological reconstruction of the filled recorded neuron (below) with the location of the somatic and dendritic pipettes. The axon origin is indicated. The action potential is observed to occur first at the dendritic recording site, 195 μm from the soma; the axon of this cell emerges from the dendrite from which the dendritic recording is made (215 μm from the soma). (b) b_1: An action potential is evoked in the soma by a depolarizing current pulse (200 pA, soma). It propagates in the dendrite where it is recorded (dendrite, 100 μm from the soma). b_2: A simulated action potential waveform is injected in the soma in the presence of 1 μM of TTX. The somatic voltage response (soma) propagates passively in the dendrites where it is recorded at the same location as in b_1 but in the presence of TTX (dendrite). The simulated somatic action potential is recorded later at the soma with a second somatic recording pipette (soma). Adapted from Häusser M, Stuart G, Eacca C, Sakmann B (1995) Axonal initiation and active dendritic propagation of action potentials in substantia nigra neurons, *Neuron* **15**, 637–647, with permission.

the soma. When the action potential is observed to occur first in the soma, the axon is found to originate either from the soma or from a dendrite other that the one from which the dendritic recording had been made. Finally, in cases where the action potential appears to be simultaneous at the somatic and dendritic recording site, the axon is found to emerge from the dendrite in between the two recording pipettes. These findings indicate that the site of action potential initiation is always the axon hillock.

To determine whether Na$^+$ dendritic channels support the regenerative backpropagation of Na$^+$-dependent action potentials, the amplitude of action potentials evoked in control extracellular solution is compared with that of a voltage waveform (simulated action potential) injected in the soma in the presence of TTX in the bath. In all such experiments, the attenuation of a simulated action potential waveform injected in the soma in the presence of TTX is greater than that of the action potential evoked by somatic current injection in the absence of TTX (**Figure 19.7b**). These results suggest that dendritic Na$^+$ channels support the *active* backpropagation of Na$^+$ action potentials in the dendritic tree of nigral dopaminergic neurons.

The emergence of the axon from a dendrite rather than from the soma may have interesting consequences. It reverses the normal direction of propagation of the action potential in that the action potential will travel from the dendritic tree toward the soma. Consequently, the dendrite bearing the axon will experience the action potential before it spreads into the soma and other dendrites. In these neurons the final site of integration prior to the axon will not be at the soma but rather in the dendrites at the point where the axon emerges. This suggests that synapses made on the axon-bearing dendrite will be in an electrotonically privileged position (the concept of a 'privileged dendrite').

Purkinje cells

In these cells, Na$^+$ action potentials are initiated in the axon and decrease markedly with increasing distance from the soma, as shown with simultaneous somatic and dendritic recordings. On average, the amplitude of somatic Na$^+$ action potentials is 78.1 ± 7.6 mV whereas that of dendritic Na$^+$ action potentials is only a few millivolts at distances greater than 100 μm from the soma (**Figure 19.8a**). This strongly suggests that, in these neurons, Na$^+$ action potentials spread *passively* into the dendritic tree. In fact, in the presence of TTX, a simulated somatic action potential waveform attenuates in a similar manner as the synaptically evoked action potential (**Figure 19.8b**). This represents a striking contrast with neocortical layer-V pyramidal cells or nigral dopaminer-

gic neurons in which somatic Na$^+$ action potentials *actively* backpropagate into the dendrites. This marked attenuation of Na$^+$ action potentials is consistent with the observed low Na$^+$ current density in the dendrites of Purkinje cells compared with that found in the soma.

Conclusions

When TTX-sensitive voltage-gated Na$^+$ channels are present in high density in the dendritic membrane, they allow *active* backpropagation of Na$^+$ action potentials in the dendritic tree. This is, for example, the case with dendrites of pyramidal neurons of the neocortex and hippocampus and of dopaminergic neurons of the substantia nigra. In contrast, the active backpropagation of Na$^+$ action potentials does not exist in dendrites that have in their membrane a low density of Na$^+$ channels, like Purkinje cells of the cerebellum. In this latter case, which is in fact the general case, Na$^+$ action potentials backpropagate *passively* (with decrement) in the dendritic tree.

19.2 High-voltage-activated Ca^{2+} channels are present in the dendritic membrane of some CNS neurons, but are they distributed with comparable densities in soma and dendrites?

19.2.1 High-voltage-activated Ca^{2+} channels are present in some dendrites

In order to record Ca^{2+} channels in isolation, the solution bathing the extracellular face of the patch contains Ba^{2+} as the charge carrier and TEACl and TTX for blocking K$^+$ and Na$^+$ currents, respectively. Ca^{2+} channel activity is identified by inward current polarity, voltage-dependent channel gating, unitary current amplitude, single-channel behaviour and its blockade by Cd^{2+}.

Purkinje cells of the cerebellar cortex

To determine whether the dendrites of Purkinje cells contain HVA Ca^{2+} channels, dendrite-attached patch recordings are performed in slices. Patches always show the activity of several channels, thus suggesting a tight clustering of Ca^{2+} channels in the dendritic membrane. **Figure 19.9a** shows the I/V relationship of a multichannel inward current carried by 10 mM of Ba^{2+} and evoked by a voltage ramp from -80 to $+80$ mV applied to a dendrite-attached macropatch. This dendritic Ba^{2+} current activates at -35 mV and is maximal around

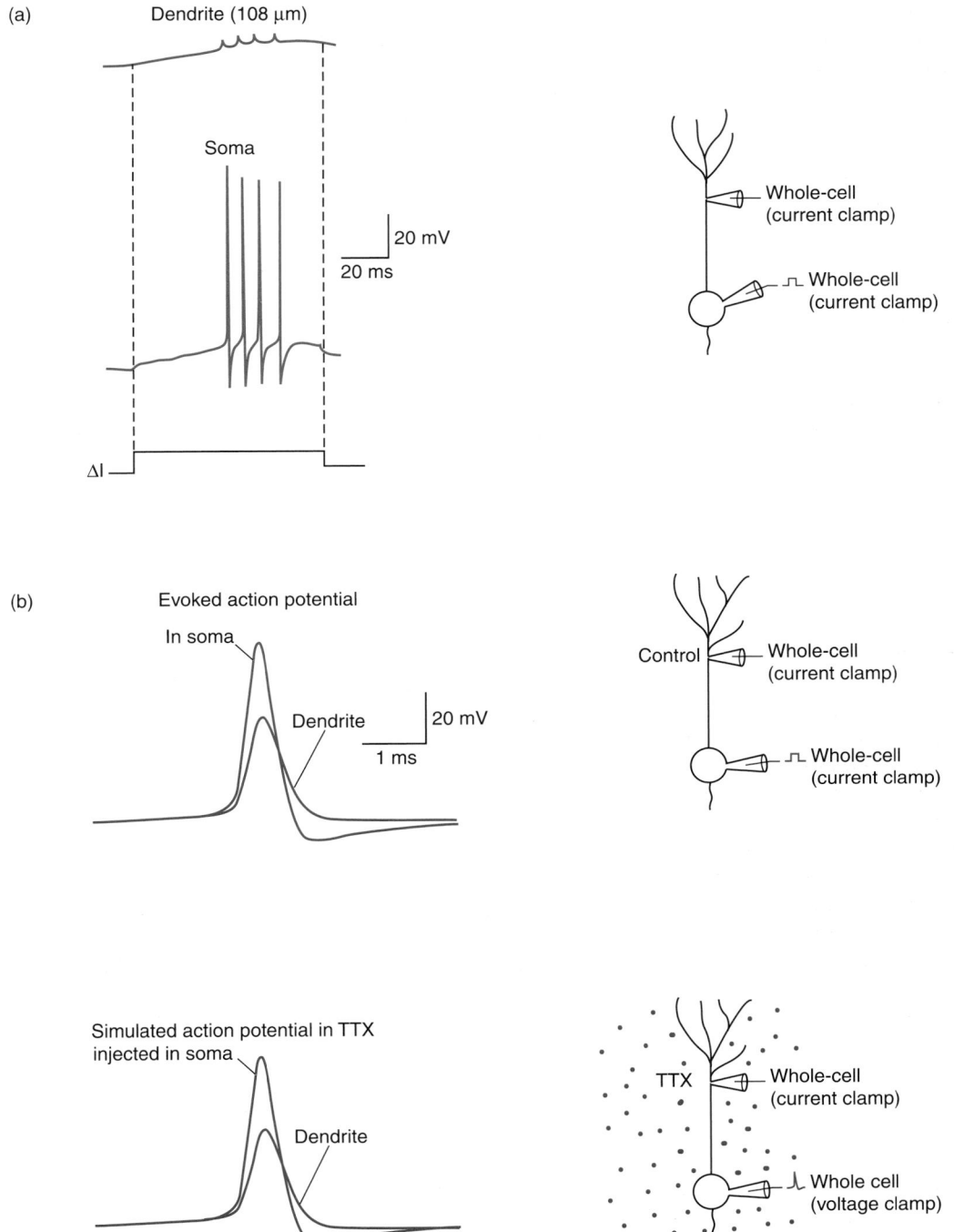

Figure 19.8 Passive propagation of Na⁺ action potentials in the dendritic tree of Purkinje cells.
(a) Simultaneous recordings at the soma and dendrite (108 μm from the soma) of a train of Na⁺ action potentials evoked by a somatic long depolarizing current pulse (100 pA). (b) b₁: An action potential is evoked in the soma by a depolarizing current pulse (soma). It propagates in the dendrite where it is recorded (dendrite, 47 μm from the soma). b₂: A simulated action potential waveform is injected in the soma in the presence of 1 μM of TTX. The somatic voltage response propagates passively in the dendrites where it is recorded at the same location as in b₁ but in the presence of TTX (dendrite). The simulated somatic action potential is recorded later at the soma with a second somatic recording pipette (soma). Adapted from Stuart GJ, Häusser M (1994) Initiation and spread of sodium action potentials in cerebellar Purkinje cells, *Neuron* **13**, 703–712, with permission.

0 mV. This HVA current is insensitive to the presence in the pipette solution of the specific blocker of N-type Ca^{2+} channels, ω-conotoxin GVIA (ωCgTx) and to the L-type channel opener (Bay K 8644). To test whether it is a P/Q-type Ca^{2+} current, a specific blocker, the funnel web spider toxin (FTX), is applied. Owing to the patch configuration, drugs must either be included in the pipette or be superfused over the cell before dendrite-attached recording, and a population of dendrite-attached recordings in control conditions is compared with the same number of recordings in the presence of the Ca^{2+} channel blocker. Funnel web toxin is the only drug that blocks the dendritic Ca^{2+} current (**Figure 19.9b**), thus showing that the dendritic Ba^{2+} current recorded is carried through P/Q-type Ca^{2+} channels. Their characteristics are close to that of P/Q-type channels recorded in Purkinje cells somata (see Section 6.1).

Pyramidal neurons of the hippocampus

In contrast to the above findings, in pyramidal neurons of the hippocampus there is a heterogeneous distribution of different types of Ca^{2+} channels within the soma-proximal dendritic trunks and more distal dendrites. Recordings of single Ca^{2+} channels in dendrite-attached patches show that L-type Ca^{2+} channels (sensitive to dihydropyridines) are observed at fairly high density only in the first 50 μm from the soma and at extremely low density in more distal dendritic patches where mainly Ni^{2+}-sensitive, T-type Ca^{2+} channels are present. Therefore HVA Ca^{2+} channels in these cells would be confined to the soma and very proximal dendrites.

Conclusions

Dendrites of Purkinje cells contain a high density of HVA Ca^{2+} channels of the P/Q type. In contrast, HVA Ca^{2+} channels are present at low density in dendrites of pyramidal neurons of the neocortex or the hippocampus. It must be pointed out that in most CNS dendrites there is a low density of HVA Ca^{2+} channels. Purkinje cells are exceptions.

19.2.2 High-voltage-activated Ca^{2+} channels of Purkinje cell dendrites are opened by climbing fibre EPSP; this initiates Ca^{2+} action potentials in the dendritic tree of Purkinje cells

The cerebellar Purkinje cells receive two kinds of excitatory inputs, a single powerful climbing fibre (CF) and many thousands of small parallel fibres (PF). The CF synapse arises from an axonal projection from the inferior olive, a brainstem nucleus. The CF synapse is composed of around 300 synaptic contacts located on the largest dendritic branches (thick and smooth dendrites) and on the smaller spiny dendrites (see **Figures 7.8** and **7.9**). The pioneering work of Llinas and Nicholson (1976) with intradendritic recordings showed that activation of this single distributed synapse evokes a large, all-or-none EPSP surmounted with one or two Ca^{2+}-dependent action potentials (complex spike; **Figure 19.10a**). They are Ca^{2+} spikes since they disappear in the presence of Cd^{2+}. They are characterized by a rather slow onset, but a large amplitude at dendritic level which fluctuates between 30 and 60 mV. Their time course is much longer than that of Na^{+} spikes. Their threshold is lower at the dendritic level: depolarizations at around 10 mV are sufficient to generate Ca^{2+} dendritic spikes at the dendritic level while 20 mV depolarizations are required at the somatic level to evoke them. This complex spike then evokes bursts of Na^{+} action potentials in the axon.

The climbing fibre-evoked EPSP underlying this complex spike can be uncovered in dendritic recordings by evoking a simultaneous IPSP by stimulation of interneurons (**Figure 19.10b**). Climbing fibre EPSP has a lower amplitude and a longer duration than the complex spike. This suggests that activation of a dendritic voltage-gated depolarizing current(s) amplifies the CF EPSP. Many data suggest that this dendritic depolarizing current is a P-type Ca^{2+} current. First, P channels are present in the dendritic membrane (see Section 19.2.1). Second, the complex spike is accompanied by a transient rise in intracellular Ca^{2+} concentration which is most prominent at dendritic locations (**Figure 19.10c**).

Modelling of the complex spike shows the currents underlying the CF-evoked complex spike and their sequence of activation (**Figure 19.11**). These currents are the large CF synaptic inward current (resulting from the summation of the around 300 unitary synaptic currents through glutamate AMPA receptors). CF-induced synaptic inward current depolarizes the dendritic membrane and thus activates P-type Ca^{2+} channels over large regions of the dendrites. The resulting Ca^{2+} current is responsible for almost all of the resulting additional depolarization and for dendritic Ca^{2+} spikes. Ca^{2+} spikes are generated at multiple sites along the dendritic tree, which explains why the CF EPSP recorded in a dendrite is sometimes surmounted by more than one Ca^{2+} spike. In turn, Ca^{2+} entry increases intradendritic Ca^{2+} concentration and thus activates the Ca^{2+}-activated K^{+} outward current in the whole dendritic tree. This repolarizes the complex spike. In conclusion, activation of the dendritic P-type Ca^{2+} current boosts the amplitude of the CF EPSP, and by activating K^{+} current leads to a faster repolarization of the EPSP (**Figure 19.10b**).

(a)

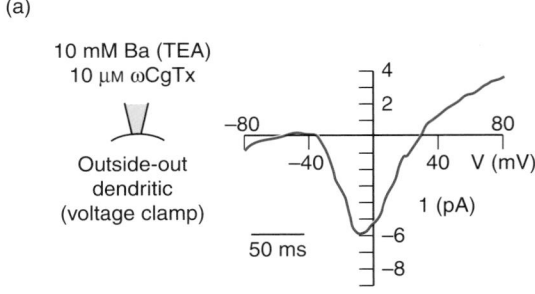

(b)

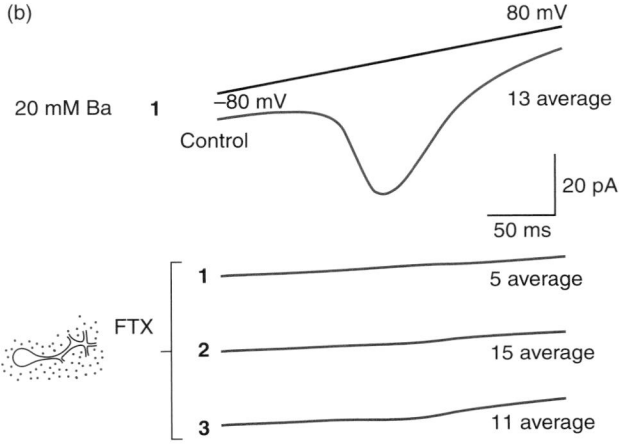

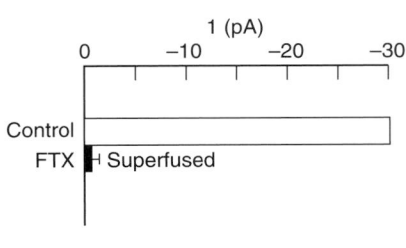

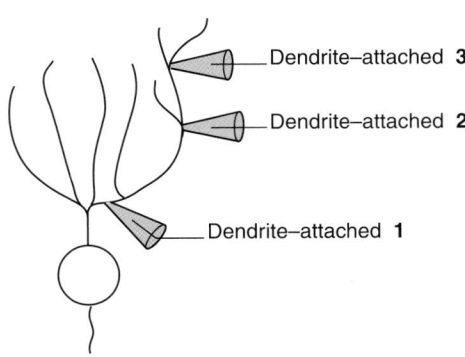

Figure 19.9 P-type Ca²⁺ channel current in dendrites of Purkinje cells.
(a) In the presence of 10 μM of ω-CgTx added to the 10 mM of Ba²⁺ pipette solution, currents are evoked in an outside-out macropatch of dendritic membrane by a depolarizing voltage ramp from −80 to +80 mV. The *I/V* plot shows that the evoked inward current peaks at −9 mV and activates at −44 mV. **(b)** Currents carried by 20 mM of Ba²⁺ evoked by voltage ramps (from −80 to +80 mV) in dendrite-attached macropatches in different conditions (left). *Top*: Averaged current in control conditions. *Lower traces*: Funnel web toxin (FTX) is first applied in the extracellular medium, then the patch is performed. Three different dendrite-attached patch recordings are shown (the approximate positions of the recording pipettes are indicated). The averaged currents recorded show the absence of inward Ba²⁺ current (right). Adapted from Usowicz MM, Sugimori M, Cherksey B, Llinas R (1992) P-type calcium channels in the somata and dendrites of adult cerebellar Purkinje cells, *Neuron* **9**, 1185–1199, with permission.

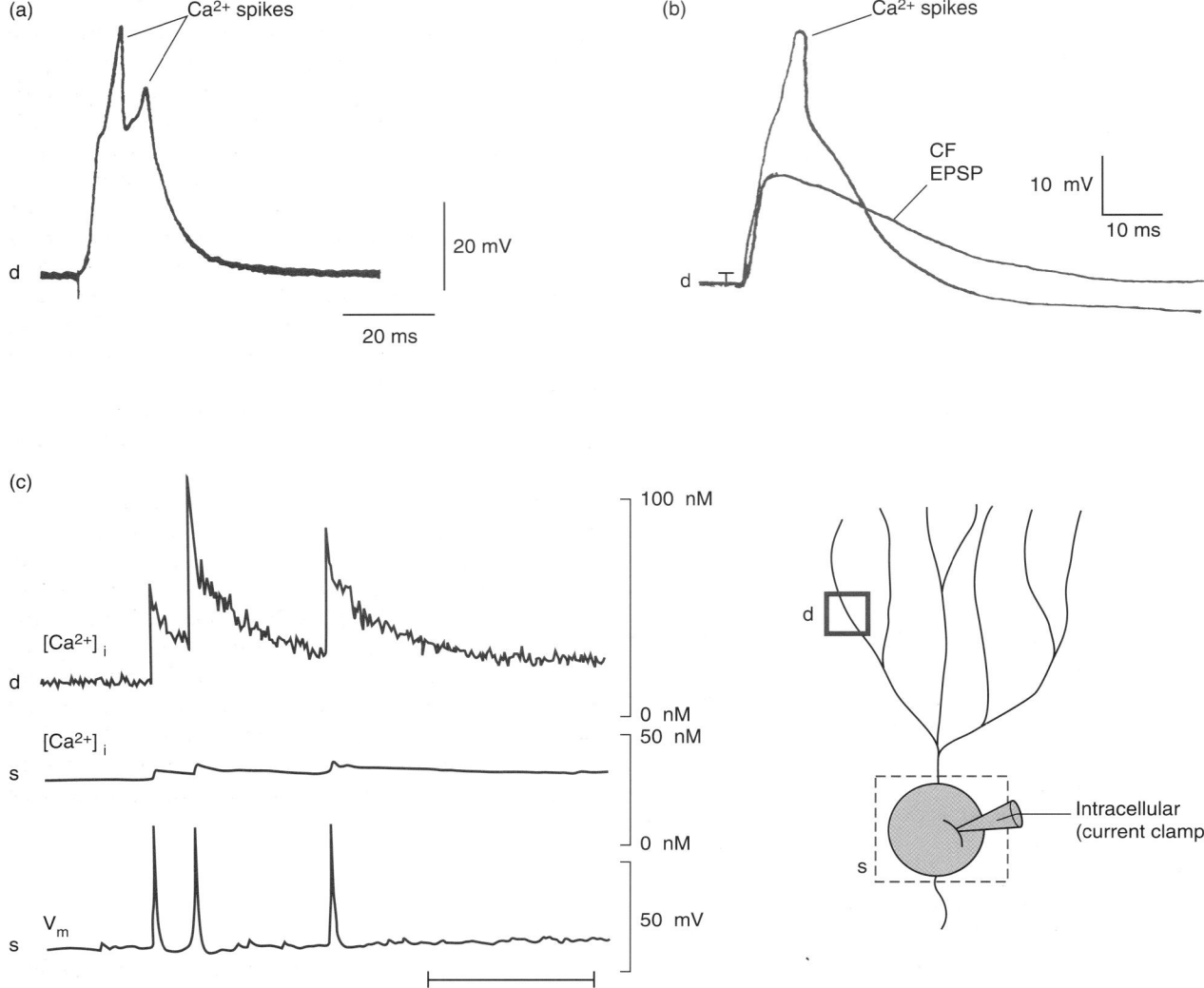

Figure 19.10 P-type Ca²⁺ current activated by climbing fibre EPSP in dendrites of Purkinje cells.
(a) Intradendritic recording of the synaptically evoked climbing fibre response that is surmounted by two Ca²⁺ spikes (intracellular recording in current clamp mode). (b) Intradendritic recording at resting potential of the climbing fibre EPSP showing a 2–3 ms wide Ca²⁺ spike and of the climbing fibre EPSP recorded during a concomitant IPSP (CF EPSP) (intracellular recording in current clamp mode). (c) Time course of [Ca²⁺]ᵢ recorded at a dendritic (d, top trace) and somatic (s, middle trace) site during spontaneous climbing fibre responses (s, bottom trace) recorded with simultaneous microfluorometric measurements of cytosolic free calcium concentration and intracellular (intrasomatic) electrophysiological recordings (current clamp mode). Part (a) adapted from Llinas R, Sugimori M (1980) Electrophysiological properties of *in vitro* Purkinje cell dendrites in mammalian cerebellar slices, *J. Physiol. (Lond.)* **305**, 197–213, with permission. Part (b) adapted from Callaway JC, Lasser-Ross N, Ross WN (1995) IPSPs strongly inhibit climbing fiber-activated [Ca²⁺]ᵢ increases in the dendrites of cerebellar Purkinje neurons, *J. Neurosci.* **15**, 2777–2787, with permission. Part (c) adapted from Knöpfel T, Vranesic I, Staub C, Gähwiler BH (1991) Climbing fiber response in olivo-cerebellar slice cultures: II. Dynamics of cytosolic calcium in Purkinje cells. *Eur. J. Neurophysiol.* **3**, 343–348, with permission.

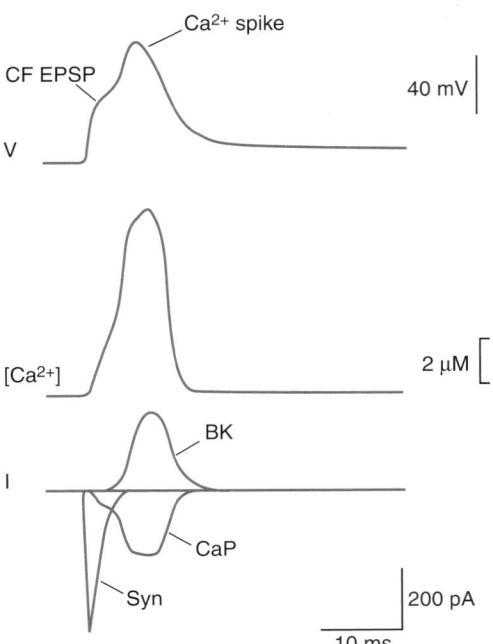

Figure 19.11 Dendritic currents underlying the climbing fibre-evoked EPSP in Purkinje cells.
Modelling of the CF response recorded in current clamp mode in a dendrite (top trace) and the underlying $[Ca^{2+}]_i$ transient (middle trace) and currents (I, bottom traces). The underlying currents are the synaptic glutamatergic current (Syn) which generates the climbing fibre EPSP, depolarizes the dendritic membrane and thus activates the dendritic P-type Ca^{2+} current (CaP) which further depolarizes the dendritic membrane, amplifies the EPSP and generates a Ca^{2+} spike (shown in top trace). The resultant $[Ca^{2+}]_i$ increase (middle trace) activates the BK current (BK, bottom trace) which rapidly repolarizes the membrane. Adapted from De Schutter E, Bower JM (1994) An active membrane model of the cerebellar Purkinje cell: II. Simulation of synaptic response, *J. Neurophysiol.* **71**, 401–419, with permission.

19.2.3 Dendritic high-voltage-activated Ca²⁺ channels are opened by backpropagating Na⁺ action potentials

Pyramidal neurons of the hippocampus

To test whether dendritic HVA Ca^{2+} channels are activated by subthreshold EPSPs or by higher amplitude depolarizations such as backpropagating Na^+ action potentials, simultaneous dendrite-attached (voltage clamp mode) and whole-cell somatic (current clamp mode) recordings are performed in the same neuron (**Figure 19.12a**). Excitatory postsynaptic potentials are evoked by Schaffer collateral stimulation. Na^+ spikes are evoked by intrasomatic injection of a depolarizing

current pulse. EPSPs and spikes are recorded from the soma while channel openings are recorded from the dendritic patch of membrane. Ca^{2+} channel activity present in the dendritic patch is first recorded and Ca^{2+} channels are classified as HVA or LVA (low-voltage-activated, also called 'subliminal') channels. Two types of Ca^{2+} channels are encountered regularly on dendrites greater than 100 μm from the soma, essentially the LVA T-type Ca^{2+} channels and less frequently the HVA L-type Ca^{2+} channels. Only the T-type channels are opened in response to subthreshold EPSPs. Instead, somatically generated action potentials or trains of suprathreshold synaptic stimulation are required for HVA channel activation (**Figure 19.12a**).

Dendritic HVA channel openings are observed during and after the repolarization phase of somatically generated Na^+ action potentials. This strongly suggests that dendritic HVA Ca^{2+} channels are opened by Na^+ action potentials backpropagating into the dendrites. Openings occur tens of milliseconds after the action potential. This provides an influx of Ca^{2+} throughout an extended portion of the dendritic tree (defined by the extent of action potential propagation). The spatial domain of the effects of these HVA Ca^{2+} channels will therefore be much more extensive compared with a local opening of Ca^{2+} channels by EPSPs. Thus, the HVA Ca^{2+} channels in the CA1 apical dendrites may modify synaptic strength over broad areas of the dendrites (see Chapter 21).

Conclusions

When HVA Ca^{2+} channels are present with a high density in the dendritic membrane, they allow *generation and propagation* of Ca^{2+} action potentials in dendrites. This is, for example, the case with dendrites of Purkinje cells. In contrast, Ca^{2+} action potentials do not exist in dendrites that contain in their membrane a low density of HVA Ca^{2+} channels, such as pyramidal neurons of the hippocampus.

19.3 Functional consequences

19.3.1 Amplification of distal synaptic responses by dendritic HVA currents counteracts their attenuation due to passive propagation to the soma

High-voltage-activated Na^+ and Ca^{2+} channels opened by EPSPs boost the effect of local synaptic inputs by acting as either voltage or current amplifiers. This could be one solution to overcome the passive decay of EPSPs, en route to the soma. This argument is somewhat

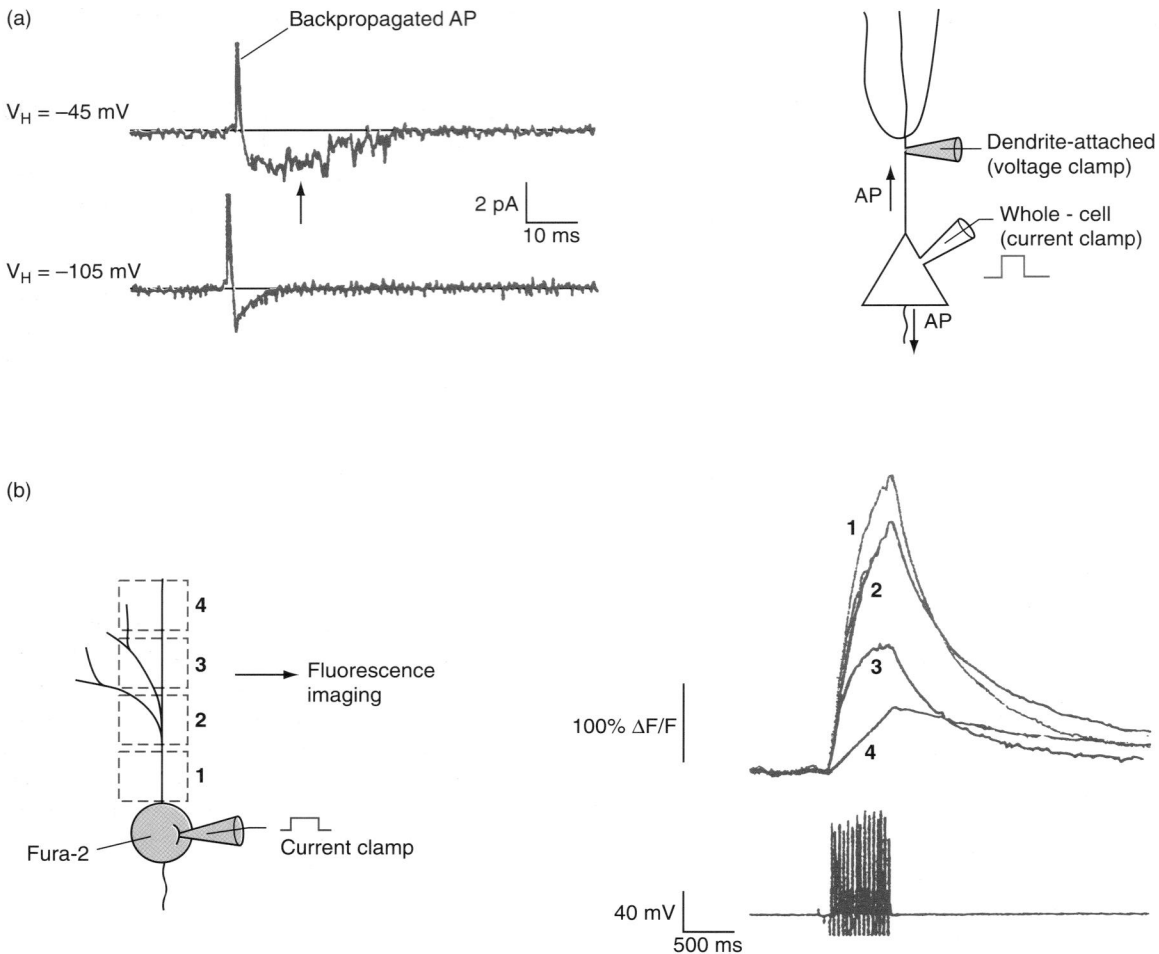

Figure 19.12 Activation of dendritic HVA Ca²⁺ channels by backpropagated Na⁺ action potential in hippocampal pyramidal neurons.

(a) An action potential is evoked in the soma by a depolarizing current pulse. It backpropagates in the dendrites and is recorded at a dendritic site as a capacitative current at two different holding potentials (backpropagated AP). When the dendritic patch is held 20 mV more depolarized than resting potential (−45 mV) numerous openings of channels are observed following the action potential. In contrast, when the dendritic membrane is held at −105 mV, the backpropagated action potential does not evoke channel openings. (b) Spike-induced [Ca²⁺]ᵢ transients in a FURA-2 loaded neuron. Normalized changes in dendritic fluorescence triggered by a train of 15 action potentials (elicited by a 15 ms depolarizing current pulse delivered at 25 Hz), are reversibly inhibited by 50 μM of Ni²⁺. Part (a) adapted from Magee JC, Johnston D (1995) Synaptic activation of voltage-gated channels in the dendrites of hippocampal pyramidal neurons, *Science* **268**, 301–304, with permission. Part (b) adapted from Christie BR, Eliot L, Ito KI *et al.* (1995) Different Ca²⁺ channels in soma and dendrites of hippocampal pyramidal neurons mediate-spike-induced Ca²⁺ influx, *J. Neurophysiol.* **73**, 2553–2557, with permission.

somatocentric; i.e. the emphasis is on how dendrites might amplify events so that they are bigger in the soma. An alternative viewpoint is that these channels are more important for dendritic interactions in the immediate vicinity of synaptic inputs. For example, multiple EPSPs occurring on the same branch and within a narrow time should activate voltage-gated channels more strongly than a single EPSP and produce a much bigger response than would occur if EPSPs were on separate branches.

19.3.2 Active backpropagation of Na⁺ spikes in the dendritic tree depolarizes the dendritic membrane, with multiple consequences

Most of the consequences of the presence of Na⁺ spikes (large amplitude depolarizations) in the dendrites are still hypotheses. The only well demonstrated one is the opening of dendritic Ca²⁺ channels and the consequent increase in intradendritic Ca²⁺ concentration. Such an increase will have by itself other consequences.

A retrograde signal that activates voltage-sensitive dendritic Ca²⁺ channels

In the hippocampus, Na⁺ action potentials open dendritic Ca²⁺ channels, leading to a widespread influx of Ca²⁺ in the dendrites. In order to localize and quantify the increase in intradendritic Ca²⁺ concentration resulting from backpropagated Na⁺ action potentials, pyramidal neurons of the hippocampus are loaded with FURA-2 and a train of action potentials is evoked by somatic depolarization through the whole-cell recording electrode. The evoked Ca²⁺ influx is thus visualized in the dendrite under fluorescence observation. Then to identify the type of Ca²⁺ channel involved and its localization along the dendrite, the same experiment is repeated in the presence of specific Ca²⁺ channel blockers. Finally a control experiment is performed in the absence of extracellular Ca²⁺. Results show that [Ca²⁺]ᵢ transients are largest in the proximal dendrites and smaller changes occur in more distal dendritic regions (**Figure 19.12b**).

One particular role for an intradendritic increase of Ca²⁺ concentration is found in dopaminergic neurons of the substantia nigra. [Ca²⁺]ᵢ increase triggers transmitter release from dendrites (the *presynaptic* effect). In these cells, clusters of synaptic vesicles containing dopamine are present in dendrites that behave in certain sites as presynaptic elements. Dendritic release of dopamine is Ca²⁺-dependent and TTX-sensitive. Backpropagated action potentials may thus provide the stimulus (i.e. intradendritic [Ca²⁺]ᵢ increase) to trigger dopamine release and evoke synaptic transmission from nigral dendrites to postsynaptic sites.

Apart from this very particular case, intradendritic [Ca²⁺]ᵢ increase will have a *postsynaptic* effect. Intracellular Ca²⁺ activates biochemical pathways, Ca²⁺-induced Ca²⁺ release as well as Ca²⁺-activated K⁺ currents present in the dendritic membrane. Such outward current changes the shape of EPSPs. Intracellular Ca²⁺ is also implicated in postsynaptically induced forms of plasticity such as long-term potentiation or depression (see Chapter 21).

A retrograde signal that amplifies NMDA-mediated synaptic currents

The transient depolarization due to backpropagated Na⁺ spikes may relieve the voltage-dependent Mg²⁺ block of NMDA receptor channels and amplify the signal mediated by these channels (see Section 11.4).

A retrograde signal that shunts ongoing synaptic integration

Backpropagated Na⁺ action potentials act as a signal to the dendritic tree that the axon has fired. This transient depolarization, by reducing the electrochemical gradient for cations, will diminish ongoing postsynaptic excitatory currents. Moreover, dendritic action potentials will open voltage-sensitive channels and thus diminish the resistance of the dendritic membrane and shunt ongoing synaptic integration. Finally, the rise in dendritic Ca²⁺ concentration could also transiently shunt out parts of the dendritic tree by opening Ca²⁺-activated K⁺ currents.

19.3.3 Initiation of Ca²⁺ spikes in the dendritic tree of Purkinje cells evokes a widespread intradendritic [Ca²⁺] increase

As seen above, intradendritic [Ca²⁺] increase will have a *postsynaptic* effect in Purkinje cells. It activates biochemical pathways, Ca²⁺-induced Ca²⁺ release as well as Ca²⁺-activated K⁺ currents present in the dendritic membrane. Such outward currents change the shape of EPSPs. Intracellular Ca²⁺ is also implicated in postsynaptically induced forms of plasticity such as long-term depression which has been extensively studied in Purkinje cells (see Chapter 21).

19.4 Conclusions

High-voltage-activated channels have been shown in the dendritic membrane of some CNS neurons such as pyramidal neurons of the neocortex and hippocampus, dopaminergic neurons of the substantia nigra pars compacta, and Purkinje cells of the cerebellar cortex. To answer the questions asked in the introduction:

■ High voltage-gated currents are present in the dendritic membrane of some CNS neurons. These are the depolarizing currents I_{Na}, I_{CaP} and I_{CaL}.

■ They are not all distributed equally over somato-dendritic membranes. I_{Na} is present at the same density in the somatic and dendritic membranes in pyramidal neurons of the neocortex or hippocampus and in dopaminergic neurons of the substantia nigra but is nearly absent in dendrites of Purkinje cells. I_{CaP} is present at the same density in the somatic and dendritic membranes in Purkinje cells. In contrast, I_{CaL} is mostly present in the somatic and very proximal dendritic membranes of pyramidal neurons of the hippocampus.

■ Since I_{Na}, I_{CaP} and I_{CaL} are activated at high voltage, they can be activated only by already large EPSPs or by Na^+ action potentials (for I_{CaP} and I_{CaL}).

I_{Na} may in theory boost EPSPs but it mostly supports the active backpropagation of Na^+ action potentials in pyramidal neurons of the neocortex or hippocampus and in dopaminergic neurons of the substantia nigra in response to suprathreshold EPSPs (these Na^+ action potentials are first initiated at the axon initial segment). I_{CaP} boosts climbing fibre EPSP and supports the initiation and active propagation of Ca^{2+} action potentials in dendrites of Purkinje cells. Direct (by EPSPs) or indirect (via dendritic Na^+ action potentials) activation of I_{CaP} and I_{CaL} induces a transient increase of intradendritic Ca^{2+} concentration that is more or less localized depending on the neuron considered.

Further reading

Callaway JC, Ross WN (1997) Spatial distribution of synaptically activated sodium concentration changes in cerebellar Purkinje neurons. *J. Neurophysiol.* **77**, 145–152.

Christie BR, Eliot LS, Ito K *et al.* (1995) Different Ca^{2+} channels in soma and dendrites of hippocampal pyramidal neurons mediate spike-induced Ca^{2+} influx. *J. Neurophysiol.* **73**, 2553–2557.

Colbert CM, Magee JC, Hoffman DA, Johnston D (1997) Slow recovery from inactivation of Na^+ channels underlies the activity-dependent attenuation of dendritic action potentials in hippocampal CA1 pyramidal neurons. *J Neurosci.* **17**, 6512–6521.

Eilers J, Konnerth A (1997) Dendritic signal integration. *Curr. Opin. Neurobiol.* **7**, 385–390.

Johnston D, Magee JC, Colbert CM, Christie BR (1996) Active properties of neuronal dendrites. *Annu. Rev. Neurosci.* **19**, 165–186.

Lüscher HR, Larkum ME (1998) Modeling action potential initiation and back-propagation in dendrites of cultured rat motoneurons. *J. Neurophysiol.* **80**, 715–729.

Markram H, Helm PJ, Sakmann B (1995) Dendritic calcium transients evoked by single back-propagating action potentials in rat neocortical pyramidal neurons. *J. Physiol. (Lond.)* **485**, 1–20.

Markram H, Lubke J, Frotscher M, Sakmann B (1997) Regulation of synaptic efficacy by coincidence of postsynaptic APs and EPSPs. *Science* **275**, 213–215.

Mitgaard J (1994) Processing of information from different sources: spatial synaptic integration in the dendrites of vertebrate CNS neurons. *Trend. Neurosci.* **17**, 166–172.

Miyakawa H, Lev-Ram V, Lasser-Ross N, Ross WN (1992) Calcium transients evoked by climbing fiber and parallel fiber synaptic inputs in guinea pig cerebellar Purkinje neurons. *J. Neurophysiol.* **68**, 1178–1188.

Schiller J, Schiller Y, Stuart G, Sakmann B (1997) Calcium action potentials restricted to distal apical dendrites of rat neocortical pyramidal neurons. *J. Physiol. (Lond.)* **505**, 605–616.

Stuart G, Schiller J, Sakmann B (1997) Action potential initiation and propagation in rat neocortical pyramidal neurons. *J. Physiol. (Lond.)* **505**, 617–632.

Stuart G, Spruston N, Sakmann B, Hausser M (1997) Action potential initiation and backpropagation in neurons of the mammalian CNS. *Trend. Neurosci.* **20**, 125–131.

Yuste R, Tank DW (1996) Dendritic integration in mammalian neurons, a century after Cajal. *Neuron* **16**, 701–716.

Firing Patterns of Neurons

The electrical activity of a neuron is related not only to the excitatory and inhibitory synaptic inputs that it receives, but also to its intrinsic electrophysiological membrane properties; i.e. the subliminal voltage-gated channels present in its dendritic, somatic and initial segment membranes and activated in the near-threshold range of membrane potential. As a result, the same postsynaptic depolarizing current will trigger different firing patterns according to the neuronal cell type recorded. In brief, the firing pattern (output) of a neuron results from the integration of synaptic currents (input) and subliminal voltage-gated currents present in the somatic and dendritic membrane. This concept was stated simply by Rodolpho Llinas in 1990: 'Nerve cells are not interchangeable: a neuron of a given kind cannot be functionally replaced by one of another type even if their synaptic connectivity and the type of neurotransmitter outputs are identical.'

In this chapter we shall consider the mammalian central nervous system to demonstrate how these intrinsic electrophysiological properties determine the firing patterns of neurons. We shall study the mechanisms underlying the firing patterns of medium spiny neurons of the striatum, of inferior olivary neurons, of Purkinje cells of the cerebellar cortex, and of thalamic and subthalamic neurons.

20.1 Medium spiny neurons of the neostriatum are silent neurons that respond with a long latency

The neostriatum belongs to basal ganglia. It contains several types of neurons among which medium spiny neurons are the most numerous. Medium spiny neurons are Golgi type I neurons that use GABA as a neurotransmitter. They project to globus pallidus and substantia nigra. They receive numerous inputs. Excitatory glutamatergic inputs come from neocortical and thalamic neurons. Several thousands of these, from nearly as many different afferent neurons, impinge on medium spiny neurons. Inhibitory GABAergic inputs come from local interneurons and from neurons of other basal ganglia nuclei. *In vivo*, medium spiny neurons are silent or exhibit a low level of spontaneous activity.

20.1.1 Medium spiny neurons are silent at rest owing to the activation of an inward rectifier K^+ current

When spontaneous synaptic transmission is intact, medium spiny neurons are silent or show brief episodes (0.1–3 s) of firing separated by long periods of silence. Intracellular recordings show that even during cell silence, membrane potential abruptly shifts between two preferred levels: a hyperpolarized level (–80 to –95 mV), called the *down state*, and a near-threshold depolarized level (–40 to –50 mV) called the *up state*. In the down state, neurons are silent; in the up state, neurons are either silent or generate intermittent action potentials on top of the largest membrane fluctuations (**Figures 20.1a and b**). These two states can last from several hundred milliseconds to seconds.

The down state

This does not result from a tonic inhibitory afferent synaptic activity since it is still observed when bicuculline (the $GABA_A$ receptor antagonist) is iontophoretically applied near the recording electrode. Moreover, in the presence of blockers of synaptic transmission, such as Ca^{2+} channel blockers, membrane fluctuations disappear and membrane potential remains stable in the down state (**Figure 20.1c**). Therefore, the down state does not depend on afferent activity. The down state is attributable to the presence of a strong and rapidly activating inwardly rectifying potassium-selective current (I_{KIR}; see Section 17.3.5) (**Figure 20.2**). Therefore, the membrane of these cells is 'clamped' near the K^+ equilibrium potential by the K^+-selective inward rectifier current, that is open at rest, in the absence of afferent synaptic activity. In brief, during the down state the

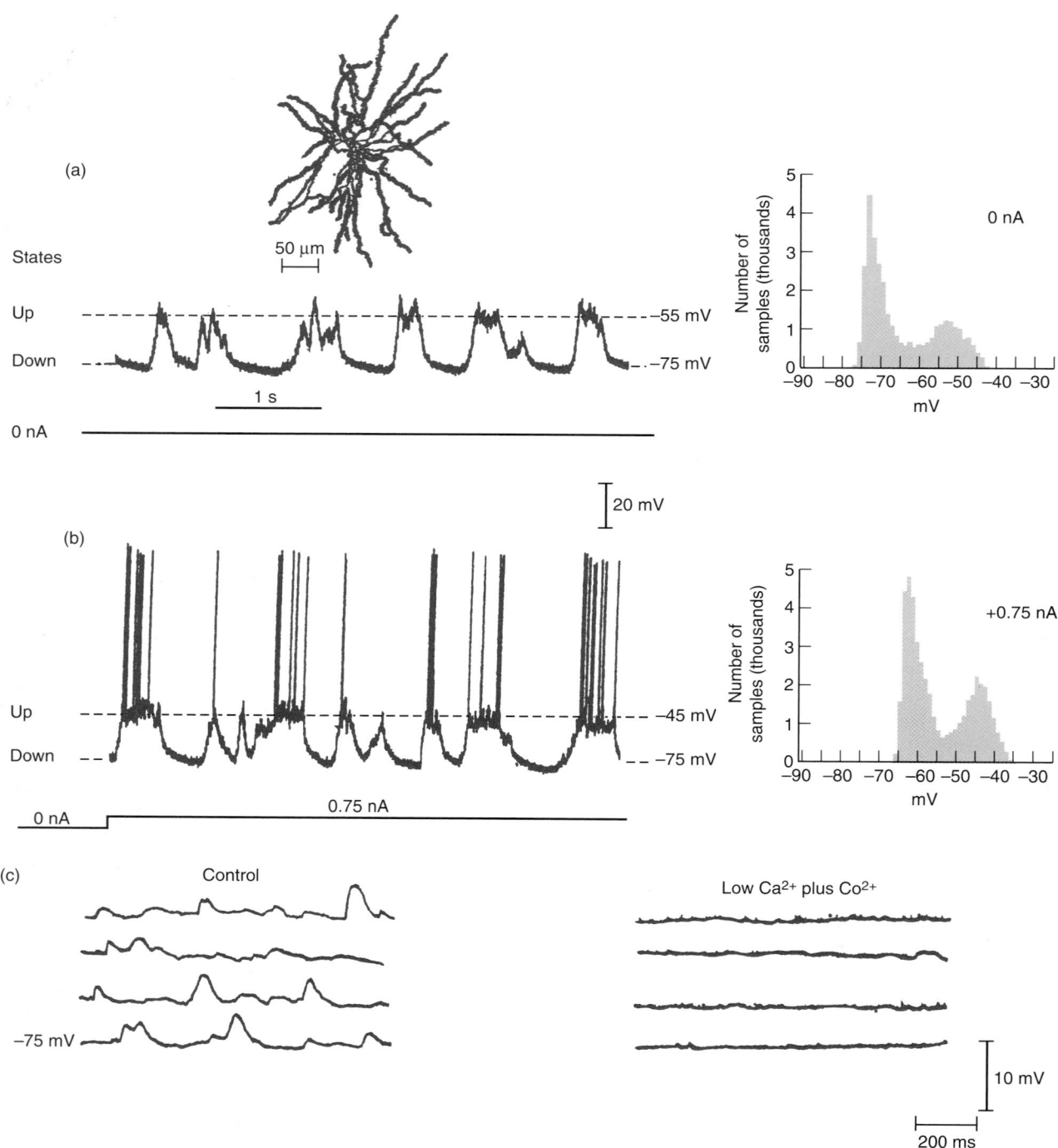

Figure 20.1 Spontaneous membrane potential fluctuations in medium spiny neurons of the neostriatum.
In vivo intracellular recordings of 'up' and 'down' states **(a)** at resting membrane potential and **(b)** during the continuous injection of a depolarizing current, of a medium spiny neuron (inset, calibration bar 50 μm). Histograms represent the time spent at various membrane potentials. The two peaks of each histogram represent the down and up states of the membrane potential. The proportion of the area of the histogram under each of the peaks represents the proportion of time spent in each state. The depolarizing current moves the peaks to the right. **(c)** *In vitro* intracellular recordings of up- and down-state transitions in control conditions and in the presence of a low external Ca^{2+} concentration (0.5 mM) and Co^{2+} (0.5 mM). In (a) and (b), intracellular electrodes are filled with 1 M of K acetate and in (c) with 2 M of KCl. Parts (a) and (b) adapted from Wilson CJ, Kawaguchi Y (1996) The origins of two state spontaneous membrane potential fluctuations of neostriatal spiny neurons, *J. Neurosci.* **16**, 2397–2410, with permission. Part (c) adapted from Calabresi P, Mercuri NB, Bernardi G (1990) Synaptic and intrinsic control of membrane excitability of neostriatal neurons: II. An *in vitro* analysis, *J. Neurophysiol.* **63**, 663–675, with permission. Drawing by Jérôme Yelnik.

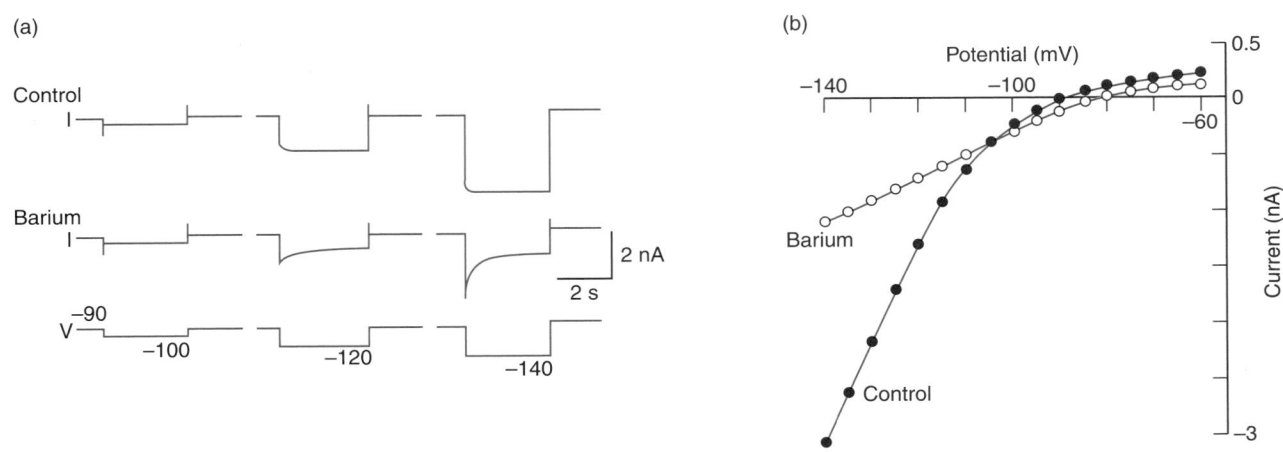

Figure 20.2 The inward rectification K⁺ current of medium spiny neurons.
(a) Membrane current (*I*) evoked by hyperpolarizing steps (*V*) to the indicated potentials (in mV), in control and in the presence of barium (10 μM). **(b)** *I/V* relations constructed from the steady-state *I* currents recorded in (a). Note the reversal potential at around −100 mV. Adapted from Uchimura N, Cherubini E, North RA (1989) Inward rectification in rat nucleus accumbens neurons, *J. Neurophysiol.* **62**, 1280–1286, with permission.

membrane potential is determined by I_{KIR} which dominates the other currents in the absence of strong depolarizing synaptic currents. As a result, these neurons are characterized by a low input resistance at resting membrane potential.

The up state

The up state, in contrast, absolutely requires the integrity of excitatory synaptic inputs to the neostriatal neurons. When the cortex is removed or temporarily inactivated, or when blockers of synaptic transmission are iontophoretically applied near the recording electrode, up-state transitions are abolished (**Figure 20.1c**). Similarly, up-state transitions are not recorded in neostriatal slices in which afferent input is interrupted. Up-state transitions depend on the synchronous activity of excitatory afferents arising from the cortico- and/or thalamo-striatal pathways. In brief, during the up state the membrane potential results from the interaction between strong depolarizing synaptic currents and intrinsic voltage-dependent subliminal currents, as explained below.

20.1.2 When activated, the response of medium spiny neurons is a long-latency regular discharge

The long-latency response of medium spiny neurons can be observed in response to an intracellular current pulse that mimics a depolarizing synaptic input (**Figure 20.3**). In the presence of a low dose of 4-aminopyridine

(4-AP, 30–100 μM), known to preferentially block the slowly inactivating transient K⁺ current (called I_{As} or I_D) (see Section 17.3.2), the latency of the first spike in response to a 400 ms depolarizing current pulse is largely reduced.

Voltage clamp recordings have shown that neostriatal medium spiny neurons possess at least three types of depolarization-activated K⁺ currents. There are the two types of transient A currents; i.e. the fast- (I_{Af} or I_A) and slow- (I_{As} or I_D) inactivating, activated at subthreshold membrane potentials (around −65 mV) and both sensitive to 4-AP (see Sections 17.3.1 and 17.3.2). There is also a non-inactivating current (I_{KDR}) available at more depolarized potentials (−20 to −30 mV) and relatively resistant to 4-AP but blocked by TEA (see Section 5.3). The importance of these voltage-dependent K⁺ currents in opposing depolarization and firing is also indicated by the large increase in the amplitude of the up state after such currents are poisoned by intracellular injection of caesium (cells depolarize to a mean potential of −30 mV instead of −55 mV in control solution). Moreover, caesium greatly enhances their frequency of occurrence and extends their duration.

Why does the response consist of a regular discharge with no adaptation? Adaptation (slowing of spike frequency inside a train) results from the progressive summation of the Ca²⁺-activated K⁺ current that underlies the slow AHP. In medium spiny neurons, this current is weak or absent.

Why do medium spiny neurons have a unique firing pattern? Rhythmic bursting currents are either suppressed in these neurons by the presence of K⁺ currents at both hyperpolarized and depolarized potentials, or are absent.

Summary

In the absence of afferent synaptic activity, medium spiny neurons are in the *down state* and silent. Transition from the down state to the *up state* is determined by excitatory synaptic inputs; but the level of depolarization during up states – which in turn deter-

mines the triggering or not of action potentials as well as the latency of this discharge – results from the interaction between the depolarizing glutamatergic synaptic current (mediated by AMPA receptors) and the intrinsic subliminal voltage-gated K⁺ currents that oppose depolarization.

20.2 Inferior olivary cells are silent neurons that can oscillate

The inferior olive is a brainstem nucleus whose neurons innervate and monosynaptically excite cerebellar Purkinje cells through characteristic axonal terminations known as *climbing fibres* (see **Figures 7.8** and **7.9**). They use an excitatory amino acid as a neurotransmitter, most probably glutamate.

20.2.1 Inferior olivary cells are silent at rest in the absence of afferent activity

In slices *in vitro*, extracellular and intracellular recordings reveal that inferior olivary neurons are generally silent at the resting membrane potential but can spontaneously display sequences of membrane oscillations in response to afferent synaptic activity (**Figure 20.4a**). Non-oscillating inferior olive cells have a resting membrane potential of –55 to –60 mV.

In response to stimulation of afferents or to intracellular current pulses, a typical rhythmic bursting activity is recorded with a frequency varying from 3 to 12 Hz, depending on membrane potential. Intracellular recordings in slices *in vitro* revealed that these cells have the intrinsic properties necessary to oscillate endogenously.

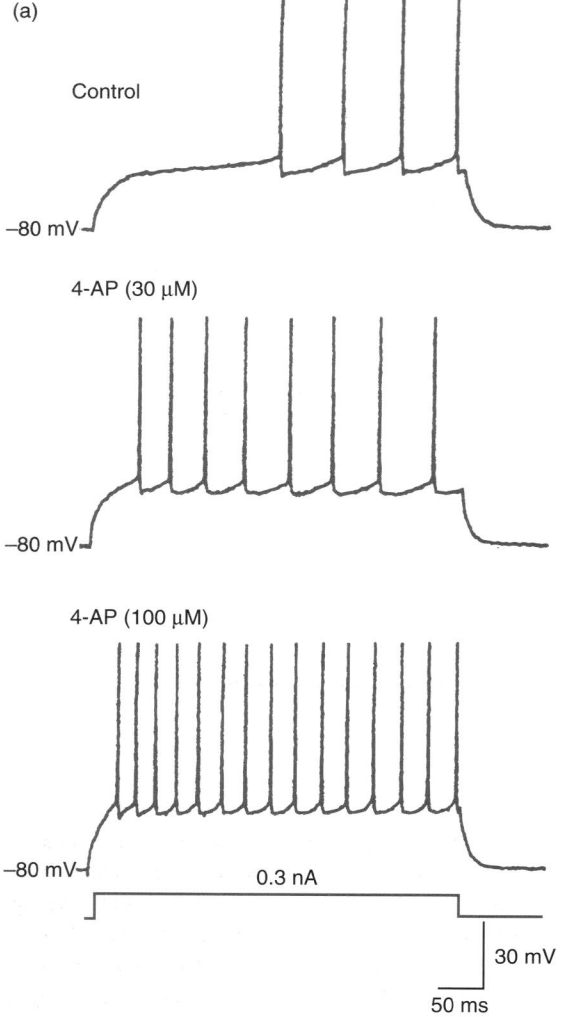
(a)

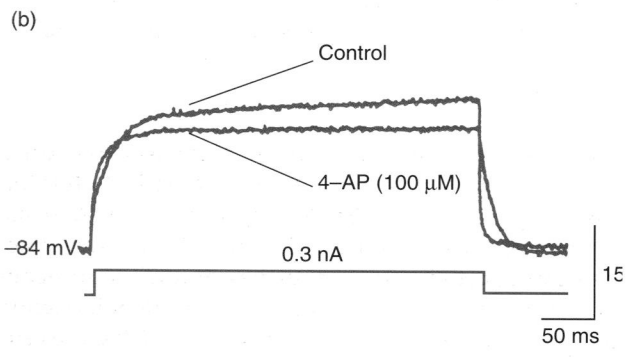
(b)

Figure 20.3 (Left) The long latency discharge of medium spiny neurons.

(a) A suprathreshold current pulse is delivered in control conditions and in the presence of 4-AP. Between pulses, the cell membrane is hyperpolarized back to the original resting membrane potential (–80 mV). 4-AP decreases the first spike latency and increases the frequency of discharge. (b) Comparison of the voltage deflections produced by a subthreshold 0.5 nA current pulse (400 ms duration) in the presence of TTX shows that 4-AP reduces the slope of the ramp potential and decreases the apparent time constant of the membrane (average of four responses). Adapted from Nisenbaum ES, Xu ZC, Wilson CJ (1994) Contribution of a slowly inactivating potassium current to the transition to firing of neostriatal spiny projection neurons, *J. Neurophysiol.* **71**, 1174–1189, with permission.

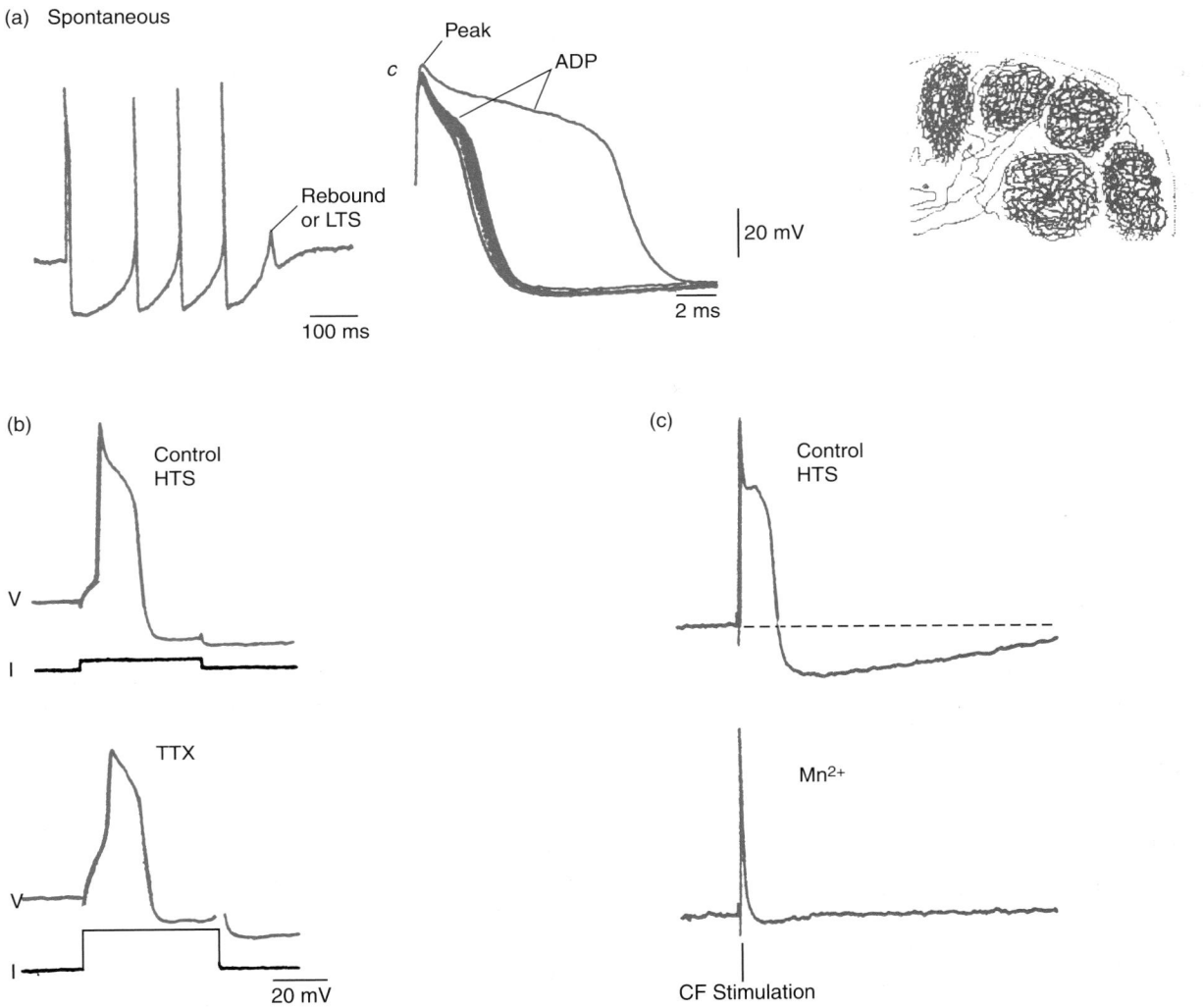

Figure 20.4 Complex spikes of inferior olivary neurons.
The activity of olivary neuron is intracellularly recorded under current clamp in cerebellar slices (inset represent five of these neurons).
(a) Spontaneous low-frequency train of spikes from an olivary neuron, displayed at two different sweep speeds. The action potentials shown at left are displayed superimposed at right at a faster sweep speed at right. The first action potential which arises from the resting membrane potential level has a slightly higher amplitude at the peak and a rather prolonged plateau (after-spike depolarization, ADP) which is followed by an after hyperpolarization (AHP). The rest of the spikes in the train become progressively shorter until failure of spike generation occurs (arrow, left) and the train terminates. **(b)** Effect of TTX (left) and Mn^{2+} (right) on the different parts of the complex spike evoked in two olivary neurons either by a depolarizing intracellular current pulse (left) or climbing fibre stimulation (CF, right). Part (a) adapted from Llinas R, Yarom Y (1986) Oscillatory properties of guinea-pig inferior olivary neurones and their pharmacological modulation: an *in vitro* study, *J. Physiol. (Lond.)* **376**, 163–182, with permission. Part (b) adapted from Llinas R, Yarom Y (1981) Electrophysiology of mammalian olivary neurones *in vitro*: different types of voltage-dependent ionic conductances, *J. Physiol. (Lond.)* **315**, 549–567, with permission. Drawing by Ramon Y Cajal, 1911.

20.2.2 When depolarized, inferior olivary cells oscillate at a low frequency (3–6 Hz)

When inferior olivary cells are slightly depolarized, their response to a depolarizing current pulse is characterized by an initial fast-rising spike (1 ms duration) which is prolonged to 10–15 ms by a plateau (ADP: after-spike depolarization) on which small action potentials are sometimes superimposed (**Figure 20.4**). It is followed by a large-amplitude long-lasting (150–200 ms) after-hyperpolarization (AHP) which silences the spike-generating activity and terminates in a rebound depolarization (arrowhead). The rebound depolarization may evoke another complex action potential: these cells have oscillatory membrane properties. Owing to their difference of threshold potential of initiation, the peak and plateau are called *high-threshold spike* (HTS), whereas the rebound depolarization is called *low-threshold spike* (LTS).

Pioneering *in vitro* studies by Llinas and Yarom in 1981 described the ionic currents that underlie the endogenous oscillatory properties of single inferior olivary neurons. The analysis of the currents responsible for this discharge configuration gives the following description. To record the low- and high-threshold spikes together or the low-threshold spike in isolation, the membrane potential is respectively maintained at a depolarized potential (**Figures 20.4b** and **20.5a**) or a hyperpolarized potential (**Figure 20.5b**).

- ■ TTX abolishes the peak of the action potential, showing that it results from the activation of the voltage-dependent I_{Na} (**Figures 20.4b** and **20.5a**).
- ■ Ca^{2+} channel blockers decrease the after-depolarization (ADP), the small superimposed action potentials, the AHP and the rebound depolarization, but leave intact the early Na$^+$-dependent

spike (**Figures 20.4c** and **20.5b**). This shows that ADP, AHP and rebound depolarization are all Ca^{2+}-dependent. The plateau is the result of the activation of a high-threshold Ca^{2+} current since the depolarization required to evoke it in the presence of TTX is high (see current trace I in **Figure 20.4b**, compare control and TTX). This current, localized in the dendrites is activated by the fast Na$^+$-dependent action potential.

- ■ The after-hyperpolarization (AHP) is dependent on the amplitude of the ADP (**Figure 20.5a**, compare a$_1$ and a$_2$) and is blocked by external Ba^{2+} ions. It results from the activation of the Ca^{2+}-sensitive K$^+$ currents (I_{KCa}).
- ■ The rebound depolarization or low-threshold spike (LTS) is suppressed by Ca^{2+} channel blockers (**Figure 20.5b**) and is activated at subthreshold potentials. It is due to the activation of a low-threshold Ca^{2+} current (I_{CaT}) localized at the level of the soma. This current is de-inactivated during the period of after-hyperpolarization and activated when the hyperpolarization decreases.

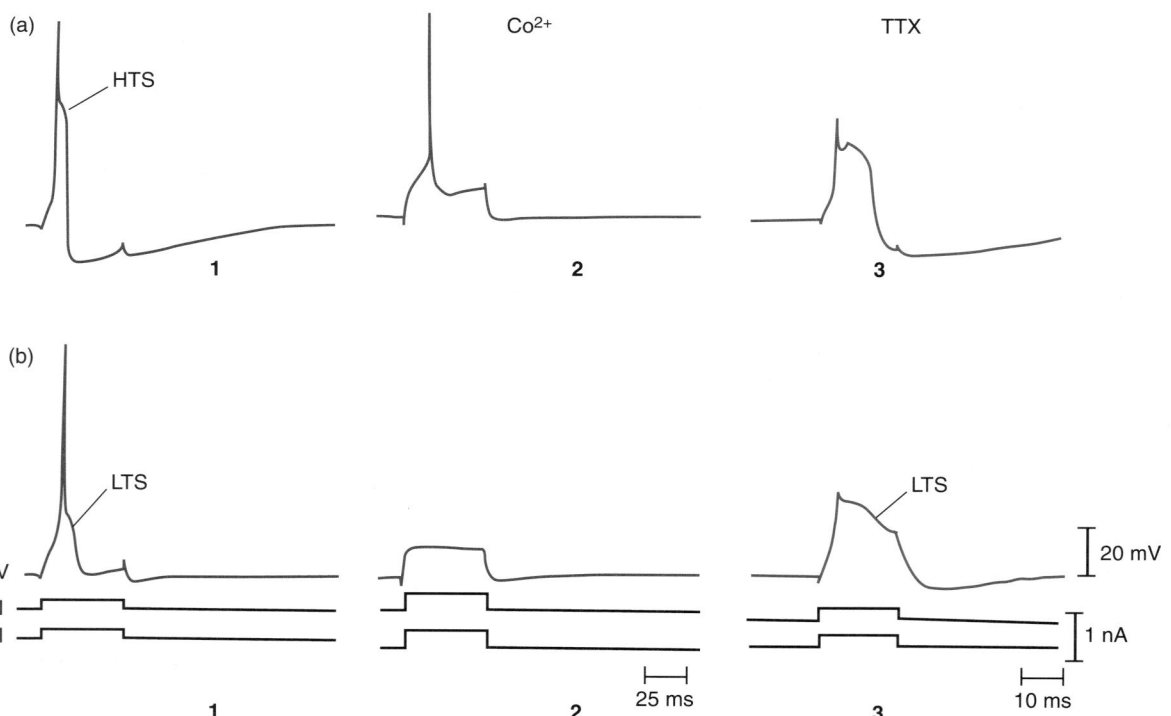

Figure 20.5 The high- and low-threshold Ca^{2+} spikes of inferior olivary neurons.
Effect of membrane potential on excitability. A depolarizing current pulse of constant amplitude evokes (**a**, 1) a high-threshold Ca^{2+} spike (HTS) at resting membrane potential and (**b**, 1) a low-threshold Ca^{2+} spike (LTS) at a more hyperpolarized potential. Note that the ADP and AHP are smaller in (b) than in (a). From left to right, effect of Co^{2+} and TTX in the same conditions. Adapted from Llinas R, Yarom Y (1981) Electrophysiology of mammalian olivary neurones *in vitro*: different types of voltage-dependent ionic conductances, *J. Physiol. (Lond.)* **315**, 549–567, with permission.

Summary

Inferior olivary neurons are silent at rest. When depolarized to the threshold potential of the voltage-sensitive Na$^+$ channels, a sodium action potential is generated in the soma–initial segment region and the dendritic membrane is depolarized up to the level of activation of the high-threshold Ca^{2+} channels. The entry of Ca^{2+} ions through these channels causes a dendritic calcium plateau (ADP) and then the activation of Ca^{2+}-sensitive K$^+$ channels. The resulting I_{KCa} hyperpolarizes the membrane (AHP). This after-spike hyperpolarization allows the de-inactivation of the T-type Ca^{2+} channels. As the amplitude of the AHP diminishes and the membrane potentials return to baseline, the low-threshold Ca^{2+} current (I_{CaT}) is activated, generates a 'low-threshold' Ca^{2+}-dependent spike, which reinitiates the cycle by activating again the Na$^+$/Ca^{2+} action potential (sodium spike–ADP sequence). The cycle can thus repeat itself at 3–6 Hz without any external intervention (**Figure 20.6a**).

20.2.3 When hyperpolarized, inferior olivary cells oscillate at a higher frequency (9–12 Hz)

When inferior olivary cells are slightly hyperpolarized, their response to a depolarizing current pulse is characterized by cycles of low-threshold Ca^{2+} spikes activating one or two fast Na$^+$ spikes and followed by a pronounced after-hyperpolarization, at a frequency of 9–12 Hz

(**Figure 20.6b**). The enhancement of rhythmic oscillations with hyperpolarization suggests that a depolarizing current such as I_h may contribute to these oscillations. I_h is activated upon membrane hyperpolarization, is carried by both Na$^+$ and K$^+$ ions and has a reversal potential around −30 to −40 mV. Therefore, at hyperpolarized potentials, I_h is inward and depolarizing.

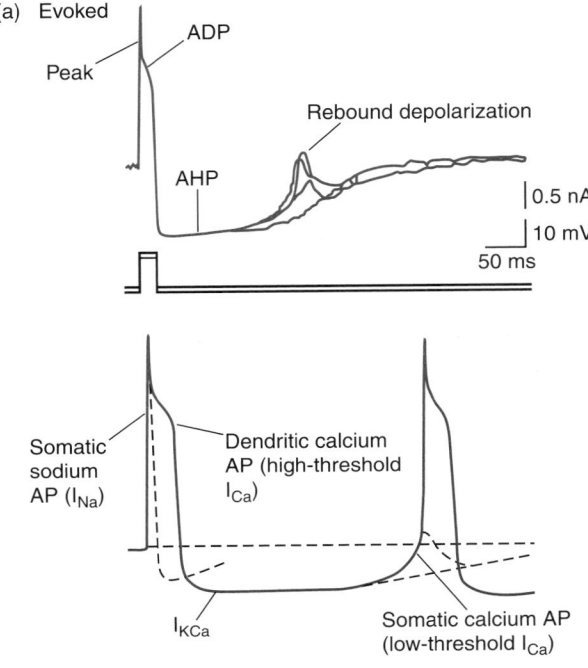

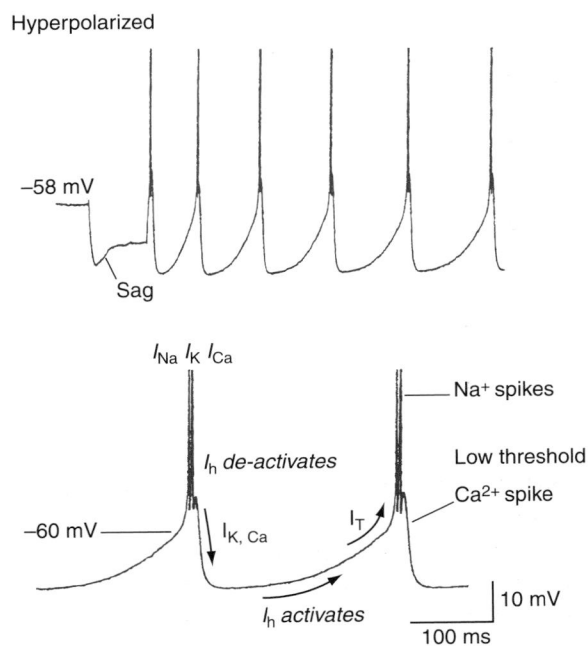

Figure 20.6 (Right) Ionic currents underlying the discharge configuration of inferior olivary neurons.

(a) In slightly depolarized cells, direct stimulation of the neuron by injecting a depolarizing current step evokes a sequence consisting of a TTX-sensitive action potential, followed by Ca^{2+}-dependent events, a plateau (ADP), a period of after-hyperpolarization (AHP) and a depolarizing rebound of variable amplitude (four superimposed top traces). Schematic of this discharge configuration and indication of the different currents sequentially activated (see text for explanation) (bottom trace). **(b)** Direct intracellular injection of a hyperpolarizing current pulse is associated with a depolarizing sag and the generation of a rhythmic sequence of low-threshold Ca^{2+} spikes (top trace). Schematic of this discharge configuration and indication of the different currents sequentially activated (see text for explanation) (bottom trace). Part (a) adapted from Llinas R, Yarom Y (1981) Properties and distribution of ionic conductances generating electroresponsiveness of mammalian inferior olive neurons *in vitro*, *J. Physiol. (Lond.)* **315**, 569–584, with permission. Part (b) adapted from Bal T, McCormick D (1997) Synchronized oscillations in the inferior olive are controlled by the hyperpolarization-activated cation current I_h, *J. Neurophysiol.* **77**, 3145–3156, with permission.

On the basis of pharmacological experiments, the following sequence of events is proposed to explain oscillations at hyperpolarized potentials. Activation of a somatic low-threshold Ca^{2+} spike which generates one or two Na^{+} spikes is followed by an AHP, mediated largely by the activation of an apamin-sensitive Ca^{2+}-activated K^{+} current. In addition, during the low-threshold Ca^{2+} spike, a portion of I_h is deactivated; this facilitates the generation of the AHP by allowing it to reach more negative potentials. The AHP subsequently results in two important effects: removal of inactivation of I_T and the activation of I_h. Activation of I_h depolarizes the membrane toward the threshold of activation of I_T and subsequently promotes the generation of a low-threshold Ca^{2+} spike and associated Na^{+} action potentials and therefore reinitiates the oscillation (**Figure 20.6b**). In hyperpolarized olivary cells, 9–12 Hz oscillations are recorded owing to a decrease of the involvement of the high-threshold Ca^{2+} current, resulting in a shortening of the duration of the AHP.

When the membrane potential is in a region between rhythmic oscillations at hyperpolarized and depolarized membrane potentials, inferior olivary cells are silent.

20.3 Purkinje cells are pacemaker neurons that respond by a complex spike followed by a period of silence

Purkinje cells are located in the cerebellar cortex in the so-called Purkinje cell layer (see **Figure 7.8**). The dendritic tree of Purkinje cells in the rat receive about 175 000 excitatory glutamatergic synaptic contacts from parallel fibres of granule cells and around 300 from a single climbing fibre of an inferior olivary neuron. They also receive about 1500 GABAergic inputs from local interneurons. However, even when deconnected from these inputs, Purkinje cells present a tonic, single-spike, spontaneous activity – thus called *intrinsic*.

20.3.1 Purkinje cells present an intrinsic tonic firing that depends on a persistent Na^{+} current

Cerebellar Purkinje neurons *in vivo* show high-frequency, regular spontaneous firing that is independent of synaptic activity since it is still recorded in cerebellar slice preparations or cultured Purkinje neurons when synaptic activity is blocked or in isolated Purkinje neurons (**Figure 20.7a**). TTX abolishes this intrinsic firing in all cells tested (**Figure 20.7b**), whereas Ca^{2+} channel blockers did not suppress it (not shown), suggesting that it consists of Na^{+}-dependent spikes.

How are these spikes generated in the absence of synaptic activity?

Spikes are generated by the spontaneous depolarization that, between consecutive spikes, depolarizes the membrane from the peak of the AHP to the threshold potential of the following spike. This phase of slow depolarization is called *pacemaker potential* or *pacemaker depolarization*, by analogy with pacemaker activity of cardiac cells. To identify the ionic currents that flow during spontaneous activity, previously recorded action potentials are used as voltage commands, and ionic currents during these voltage commands are recorded in voltage clamp (**Figure 20.7c**). This shows that pacemaker depolarization depends mainly on a persistent TTX-sensitive Na^{+} current (I_{NaP}) (see Section 17.2.1) present in the cell body of Purkinje cells.

Another key factor allowing spontaneous firing is the lack of active K^{+} currents between −70 and −50 mV which allows a high input membrane resistance during the pacemaker depolarization (note that these membrane properties are just the opposite of that of striatal medium spiny neurons; see Section 20.1.1). Thus, initially a small Na^{+} current can depolarize the membrane to the threshold potential of Na^{+} spikes. Moreover, the cationic I_h present in these cells may also play a role at the beginning of the pacemaker depolarization. The K^{+} currents that repolarize the spikes in Purkinje neurons are notable for their very fast deactivation so that the membrane does not hyperpolarize very deeply (there is not a prominent AHP). The rapid deactivation of K^{+} current also returns the input resistance to a high value within milliseconds so that the small interspike I_h and I_{NaP} can effectively depolarize the membrane for another action potential. These Na^{+} spikes then passively propagate in the dendritic tree (see **Figure 20.9**).

20.3.2 Purkinje cells respond to climbing fibre activation by a complex spike

We will study the response of Purkinje cells to one of its excitatory afferents, the climbing fibres that are the axons of inferior olivary neurons. In the adult, a single climbing fibre innervates each Purkinje cell. This innervation has the following particular characteristic. The climbing fibre winds itself around the dendrites making a great number of 'en passant' boutons along its course (see **Figures 7.8** and **7.9**). These synapses are excitatory and the neurotransmitter is an excitatory amino acid, probably glutamate. The activation of a climbing fibre thus causes a massive all-or-none depolarization of the dendritic arborization and an activation of the high-threshold Ca^{2+} channels present at different points along the dendrites (see **Figures 19.10** and **20.9**). Thus, in response to the activation of a climbing fibre, several

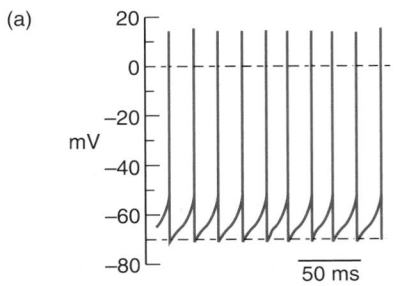
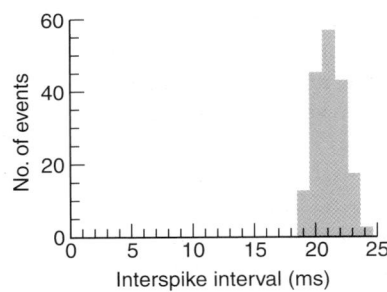

(a)

(b)

Control   3 nM TTX   10 nM TTX   10 nM TTX
                                      early   late

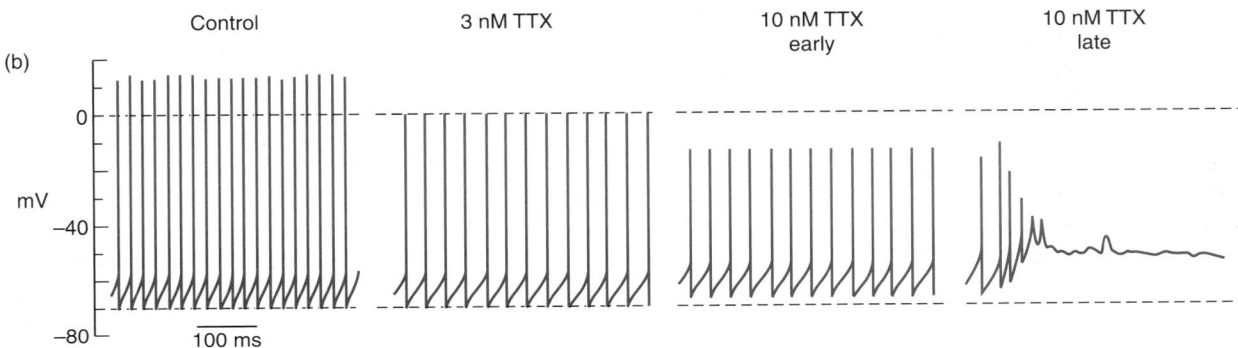

(c)

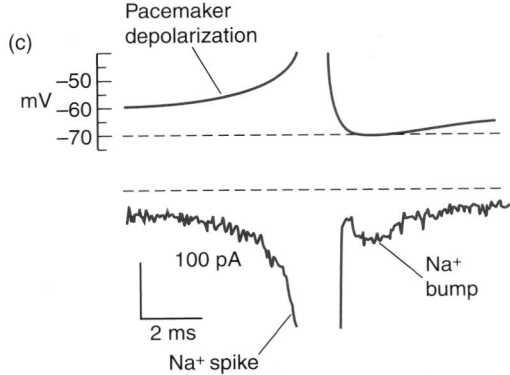

Figure 20.7 The intrinsic tonic firing of isolated Purkinje cells.

(a) Spontaneous action potentials recorded from an isolated Purkinje neuron in control conditions (left) and interspike interval histogram for the same cell (right). Dotted lines indicate –70 and 0 mV. (b) Spontaneous firing in control extracellular medium and in the presence of TTX as indicated. This cell continues to fire for some time in 10 nM of TTX (early) before silencing and resting at –51 mV (late). (c) Kinetics of Na^+ currents evoked by the spike train protocol. The spike train in (a) is used as a command voltage (top trace) and the currents evoked are recorded in voltage clamp (bottom trace). The first 13 ms are shown. The arrow indicates the bump of Na^+ current that occurs when the action potential command reaches its trough. Spike and bump Na^+ currents are sensitive to TTX (not shown). Adapted from Raman IM, Bean BP (1999) Ionic currents underlying spontaneous action potentials in isolated Purkinje neurons, *J. Neurosci.* **19**, 1663–1674, with permission.

Ca²⁺ action potentials are generated in the dendrites. These Ca²⁺ action potentials propagate passively along the dendrites, summing together and depolarizing the axon initial segment to the threshold for triggering sodium action potentials (**Figure 20.8a**). Ca²⁺ spikes force the cell to respond with a high-frequency burst of Na⁺ spikes at the level of the soma and axon. Afferent information coming from the inferior olive is thus amplified.

The climbing fibre response is followed by a long-lasting hyperpolarization (**Figure 20.8b**) that is abolished in the presence of TEA, but unaffected by TTX, thus suggesting that it is mediated by a voltage-sensitive, Ca²⁺-dependent K⁺ current. Repeated activation of the climbing fibre gradually induces an additional hyperpolarization with a much longer time course that is accompanied by a reduction of the frequency of Na⁺ spikes (**Figure 20.8c**). Therefore, climbing fibre

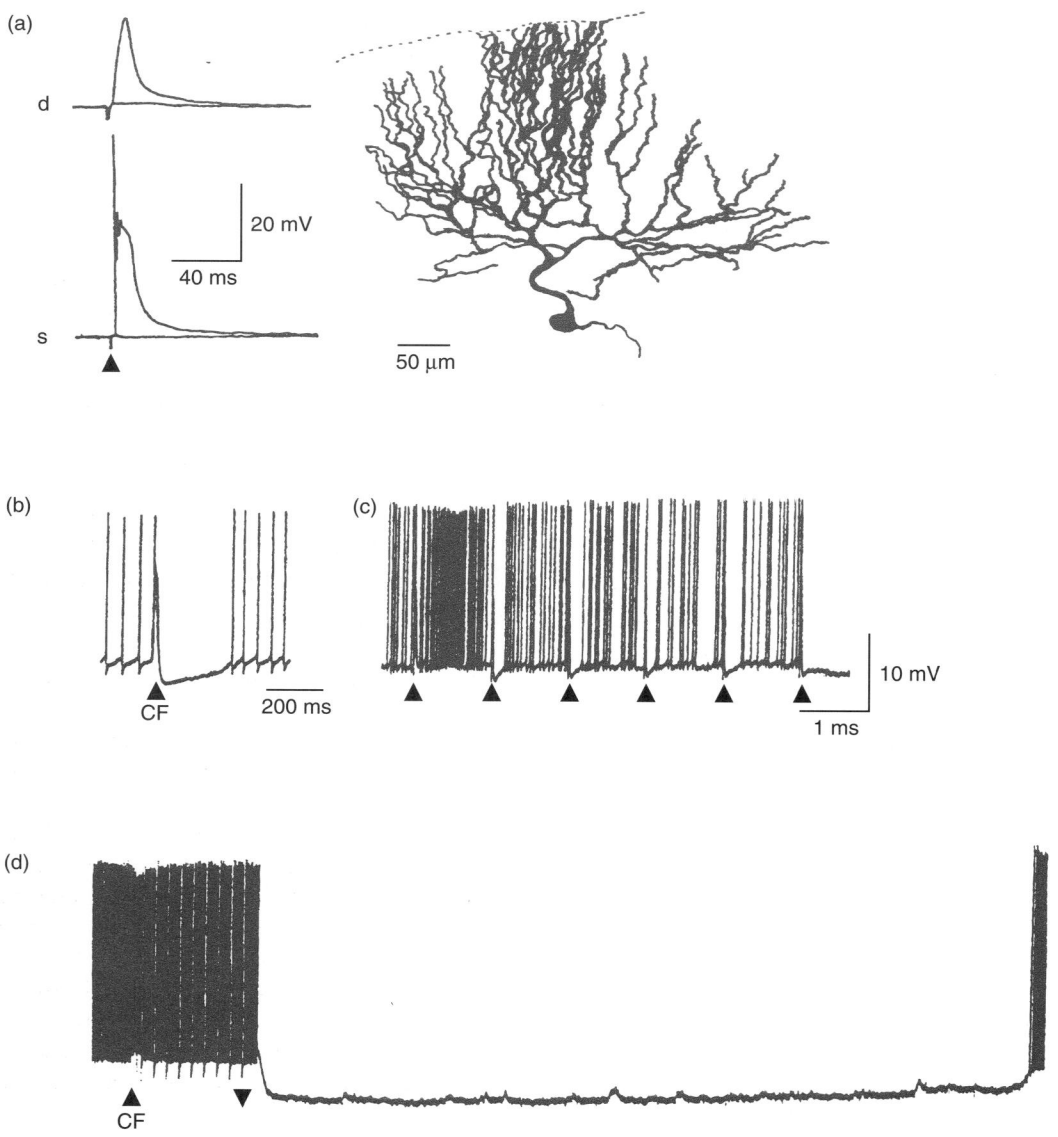

Figure 20.8 Climbing fibre response of Purkinje cells and its after effect.
(a) All-or-none dendritic (d, top) and somatic (s, bottom) climbing fibre response. The position of the traces relative to the drawing of the recorded Purkinje cell indicates the recording sites. **(b)** Climbing fibre (CF) response followed by a transient inactivation of spontaneous firing. **(c)** Climbing fibre stimulation at 1 Hz (arrowheads). **(d)** At a slower sweep speed, the long-lasting hyperpolarization following a train of climbing fibre stimulation at 1 Hz is shown. Adapted from Hounsgaard J, Mitgaard J (1989) Synaptic control of excitability in turtle cerebellar Purkinje cells, *J. Physiol. (Lond.)* **409**, 157–170, with permission.

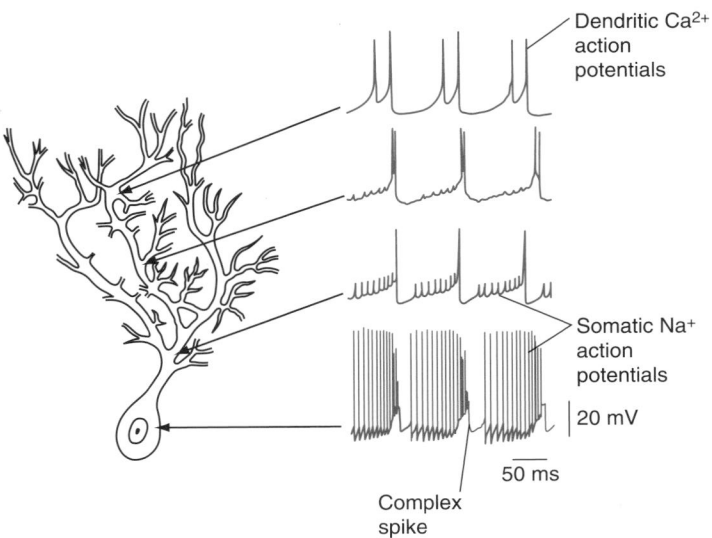

Figure 20.9 **Integration of Na⁺ and Ca²⁺ action potentials in Purkinje cells.**
The activity of Purkinje cells is recorded intracellularly in the soma and in three different regions of the dendritic tree (current clamp mode) in cerebellar slices. Na⁺-dependent action potentials are spontaneously evoked at the soma-axon hillock region. They passively backpropagate in the dendritic tree (note their rapid and strong diminution in amplitude). Ca²⁺-dependent action potentials evoked at different points of the dendritic tree (in response to climbing fibre activation) propagate passively to the axon hillock region where they evoke the complex response followed by a period of cell silence. Adapted from Llinas R, Sugimori M (1980) Electrophysiological properties of *in vitro* Purkinje cell dendrites in mammalian cerebellar slices, *J. Physiol. (Lond.)* **305**, 197–213, with permission.

responses are potent regulators of Purkinje cell excitability. For example, in cells with a high spontaneous firing rate, climbing fibre responses evoked at 10 Hz shift the membrane potential by 10–15 mV, to a level well below the threshold for Na⁺ spikes (**Figure 20.8d**). The nonlinear membrane properties of the soma–dendritic membrane of Purkinje cells are such that only small changes in current are needed to shift the membrane potential in the depolarizing or hyperpolarizing direction.

Summary

Purkinje cells are not silent at rest, they display a tonic firing mode of Na⁺-dependent action potentials that depends on the depolarizing drive of an intrinsic persistent Na⁺ current. These action potentials passively backpropagate in the dendritic tree. In response to climbing fibre activation, a Na⁺–Ca²⁺ spike is evoked (resulting from the activation of the high-threshold dendritic Ca²⁺ current and of the somatic Na⁺ current). It is followed by a long-lasting inhibition of intrinsic tonic firing due to the activation of Ca²⁺-activated K⁺ currents. Therefore, repetitive activation of an excitatory input (climbing fibre) can lead to a long-lasting inhibition of Purkinje cells, as a result of the activation of intrinsic outward currents.

20.4 Thalamic and subthalamic neurons are pacemaker neurons with two intrinsic firing modes: a tonic and a bursting mode

The *thalamus* relays and integrates information destined for the cerebral cortex (see **Figure 1.14**). It is formed from many nuclei which are classically separated into two groups: the specific nuclei and the non-specific nuclei, according to whether they project to a localized area of the cerebral cortex or to several functionally different areas. When recorded in brain slices *in vitro*, the thalamocortical and thalamic reticular neurons have complex intrinsic properties that allow them to display two firing patterns, a tonic one and a bursting one, depending on membrane potential (**Figure 20.10a**). Similarly, *in vivo*, during periods of slow-wave sleep, rhythmic burst firing is prevalent, whereas waking activity is dominated by the occurrence of trains of action potentials.

The *subthalamic nucleus* (STN) is part of basal ganglia. Its name comes from its localization ventral to the thalamus. STN controls the output of basal ganglia to the thalamus. It contains a homogeneous population of Golgi type I neurons that use glutamate as a neurotransmitter and project to both substantia nigra and the internal pallidal segment. Like thalamo-cortical

(a)

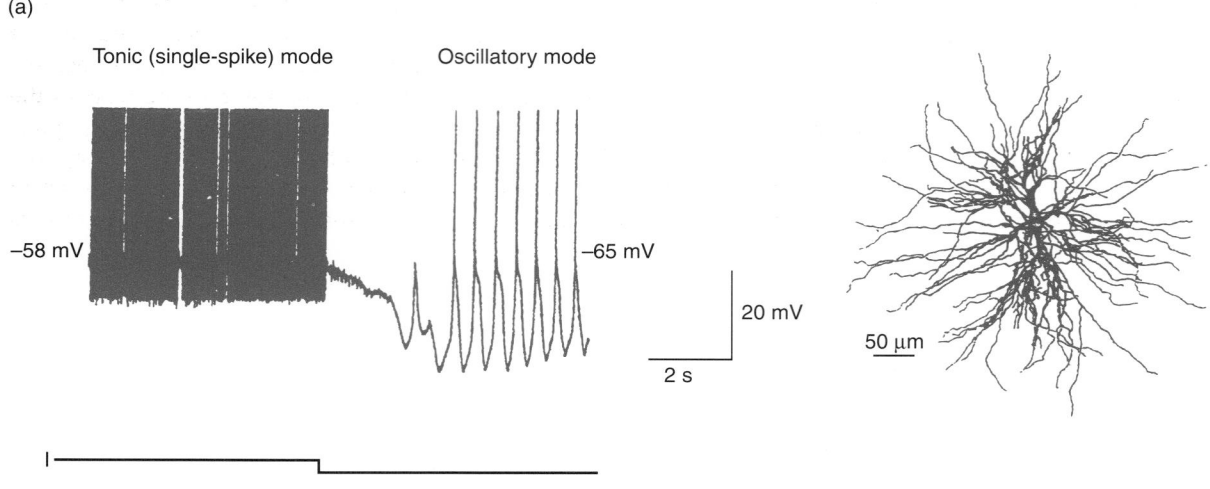

(b)

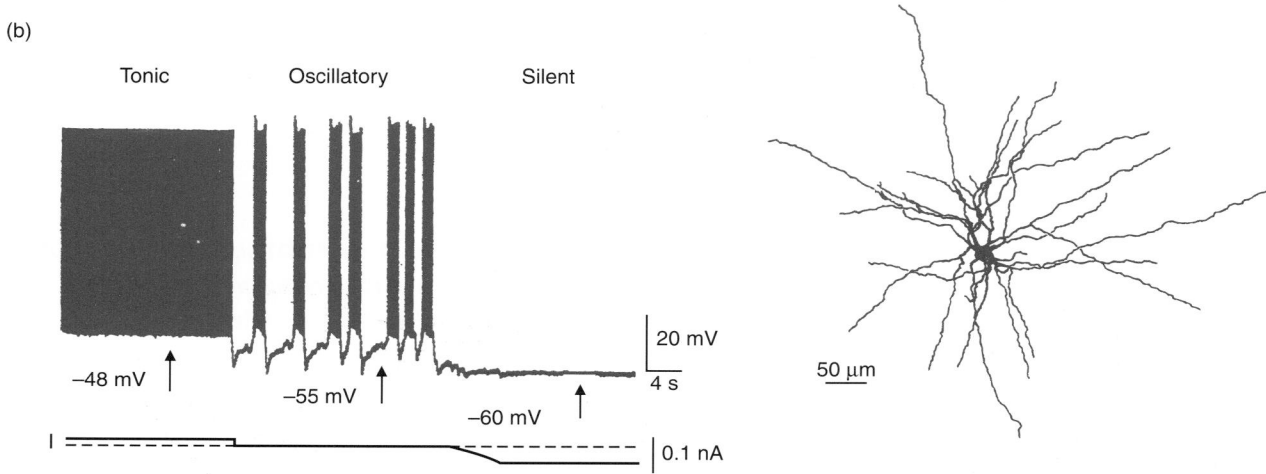

Figure 20.10 The two states of activity of thalamic and subthalamic neurons.
(a) The activity of a thalamocortical neuron (inset) is recorded in current clamp. When depolarized to –58 mV with intracellular injection of current, the neuron displays the tonic firing mode and switches to the oscillatory bursting mode when hyperpolarized. **(b)** The same protocol applied to a subthalamic neuron (inset) allows one to record the two firing modes. When the membrane is further hyperpolarized, the cell becomes silent. Part (a) adapted from McCormick DA, Pape HC (1990) Properties of a hyperpolarization-activated cation current and its role in rhythmic oscillation in thalamic relay neurones, *J. Physiol. (Lond.)* **431**, 291–318, with permission. Part (b) adapted from Beurrier C, Congar P, Bioulac B, Hammond C (1999) Subthalamic neurons switch from single-spike activity to burst-firing mode, *J. Neurosci.* **19**, 599–609, with permission. Drawings by Jérôme Yelnik.

neurons, when recorded in brain slices *in vitro*, STN neurons display two firing patterns, a tonic one and a bursting one, depending on the membrane potential (**Figure 20.10b**). In awake resting animals, STN neurons have a tonic mode of discharge; whereas during and after limb and eye movements as well as in a parkinsonian state, STN neurons discharge bursts of high-frequency spikes.

In both neuronal types, tonic firing is recorded at more depolarized potential than burst firing (**Figure 20.10**). Modulation of the membrane potential by the activity of afferents thus plays an important role in the triggering of either one of the discharge configurations.

20.4.1 The intrinsic tonic (single-spike) mode depends on a persistent Na⁺ current

Tonic activity of STN neurons recorded in slices *in vitro* is still present when blockers of synaptic transmission are added in the external medium, such as the Ca^{2+} channel blockers Co^{2+}, Cd^{2+} or Mn^{2+} (**Figure 20.11a**). This shows that the single-spike mode results from a cascade of voltage-gated currents intrinsic to the membrane. As in Purkinje neurons, spikes are generated by the spontaneous depolarization that, between consecutive spikes, depolarizes the membrane from the peak of the AHP to the threshold potential of the following spike. TTX (1 μM) abolishes spontaneous firing, indicating that it consists of Na⁺ spikes. Interestingly, at the onset of action of TTX, a few subthreshold slow depolarizations

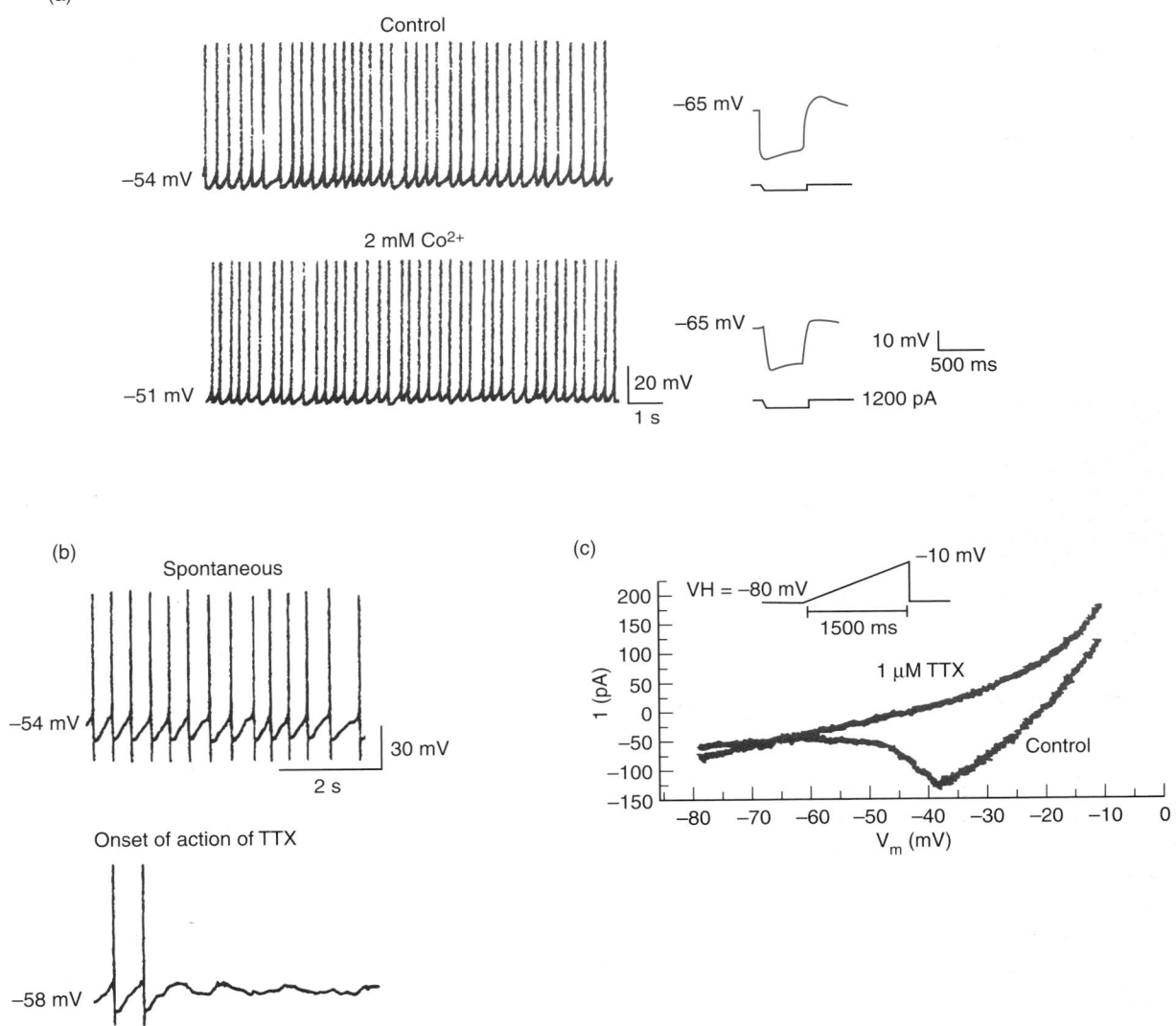

Figure 20.11 Na⁺ currents are critical for intrinsic tonic firing mode of subthalamic neurons.
(a) Tonic activity of a STN neuron recorded in control medium and during application of Co^{2+} (left). Right traces show that the low-threshold Ca^{2+} spike evoked at the break of a hyperpolarization pulse is strongly decreased in Co^{2+} to attest that Ca^{2+} channels are effectively blocked in these conditions. (b) Tonic activity recorded in control medium and at the onset of TTX (1 μM) application.
(c) Persistent Na⁺ current recorded in whole-cell patch clamp in response to a depolarizing ramp (5 mV s⁻¹) in the absence (control) and presence of TTX. Parts (a) and (c) adapted from Beurrier C, Bioulac B, Hammond C (2000) Slowly inactivating sodium current (I_{NaP}) underlies single-spike activity in rat subthalamic nucleus, *J. Neurophysiol.* **83**, 1951–1957, with permission. Part (b) adapted from Bevan MD, Wilson CJ (1999) Mechanisms underlying spontaneous oscillation and rhythmic firing in rat subthalamic neurons, *J. Neurosci.* **19**, 7617–7628, with permission.

that normally lead to spike firing are still observed (**Figure 20.11b**). As in Purkinje cells, this phase of slow depolarization, the pacemaker depolarization, depends mainly on the activation of a persistent TTX-sensitive Na+ current (I_{NaP}) present in these neurons and which presents a voltage-dependency that allows it to be activated in the pacemaker range (**Figure 20.11c**).

The same ionic mechanism underlies tonic firing in thalamic neurons (see **Figure 20.14a**). It is important to note that in both cells the other key factor that allows spontaneous firing is the weak presence of active K+ currents between −70 and −50 mV which allows a high input membrane resistance. Thus, a small Na+ current can depolarize the membrane to the threshold potential of Na+ spikes. Moreover, in thalamic and subthalamic neurons, there is a significant contribution of I_h (see Section 17.2.3) to the resting membrane potential as shown by the hyperpolarizing effect of external Cs+. This hyperpolarization is in general large enough to move the cell into the burst mode of action potential generation (see **Figure 20.14c**), suggesting that the fraction of I_h open at rest depolarizes the membrane and maintains it in a stable state where the neuron discharges in the single-spike mode.

20.4.2 The bursting mode depends on a cascade of subliminal inward currents: I_h, I_{CaT}, I_{CaN}

The burst of action potentials which rise from the peak of each slow depolarization or low-threshold spike (LTS) disappear in the presence of TTX. In contrast, LTS is not affected by TTX but disappears in the presence of Ca2+ channel blockers (**Figure 20.12**). This demonstrates that the fast action potentials are sodium spikes and that LTS results from a Ca2+ current. This slow depolarization appears only when the membrane has been previously hyperpolarized for at least 150 ms, suggesting that it results from a low-threshold-activated T-type

Ca2+ current (I_{CaT}). This current is normally inactivated at resting membrane potential (or at potentials more depolarized than resting potential) and is de-inactivated by a transient hyperpolarization of the membrane. The low-threshold spike leads to the activation of a high-threshold Ca2+ current, the entry of Ca2+ ions (probably in the dendrites) and the activation of Ca2+-sensitive K+ currents (I_{KCa}). Each action potential is followed by a phase of after-hyperpolarization (see **Figure 20.14b**).

The hyperpolarization-activated cationic current (I_h) known to be present and activated in the oscillatory range in thalamic neurons also plays a role. For example, application of small amounts of Cs+ hyperpolarizes the membrane and reduces the AHP. As already said, a fraction of I_h is open at rest and depolarizes the membrane. In addition, during the low-threshold Ca2+ spike and the generation of action potentials, a portion of I_h is deactivated (owing to the depolarization). This deactivation of I_h facilitates the generation of the AHP by allowing it to reach more negative potentials (see **Figure 20.14b**). This pronounced AHP subsequently results in two important effects: removal of inactivation of I_{CaT} and the activation of I_h. The latter in turn depolarizes the membrane potential toward the threshold for activation of I_{CaT} and subsequently promotes the generation of a low-threshold Ca2+ spike and associated Na+-dependent action potentials.

20.4.3 The transition from one mode to the other in response to synaptic inputs

When do thalamic and STN neurons discharge in a single spike? At resting membrane potential or at potentials more positive than rest, I_{CaT} (see Section 17.2.2) is inactivated and the regular frequency firing pattern can thus occur. In this state, an EPSP evokes a regular train of discharge.

When do thalamic and STN neurons discharge in bursting mode? Bursting mode requires that the

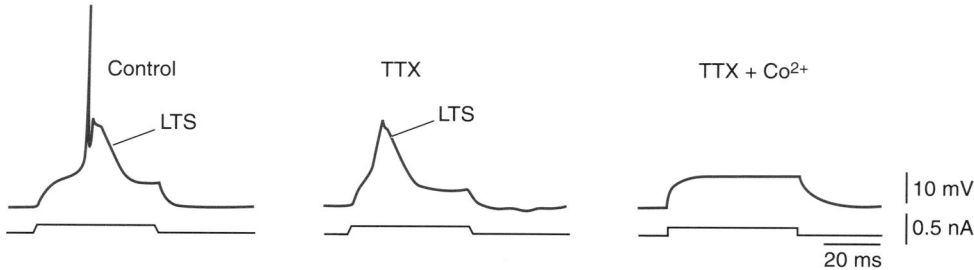

Figure 20.12 Thalamic oscillations depend on a low-threshold Ca2+ spike (LTS).
When the membrane of a thalamocortical neuron is hyperpolarized to −65 mV, a depolarizing current pulse evokes a LTS that is insensitive to TTX and abolished by Co2+ (1 mM). Note the presence of a TTX-sensitive Na+ spike in control conditions. Adapted from Llinas R, Jahnsen H (1982) Electrophysiology of thalamic neurones *in vitro*, *Nature* **297**, 406–408, with permission.

(a)

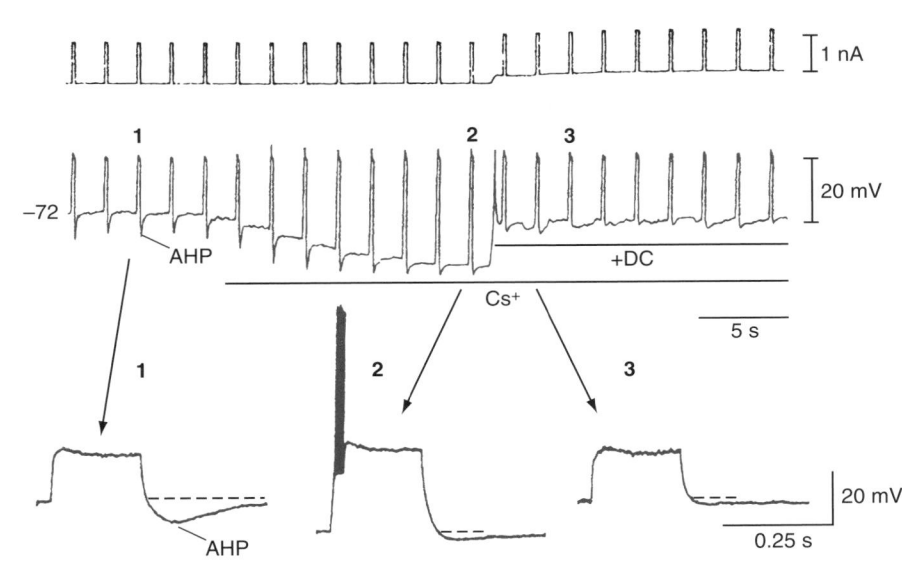

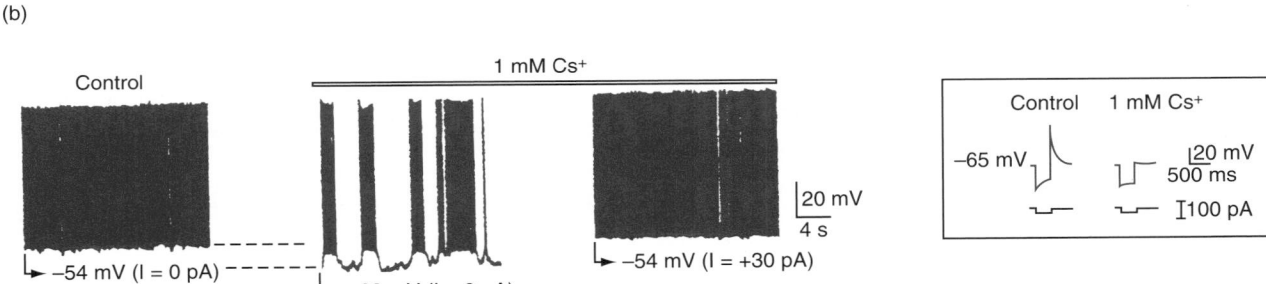

Figure 20.13 Contribution of I_h to resting potential and firing mode.
(a) Thalamocortical neuron. A depolarizing current pulse from resting potential (–72 mV) which does not result in a LTS (1) or the generation of action potential is applied. Cs application results in a substantial hyperpolarization of the membrane that de-inactivates the LTS thereby activating a burst of spikes (2). Compensation for the hyperpolarization with intracellular injection of current (+DC) reveals that the AHP is nearly abolished during Cs+ (3). (b) Subthalamic (STN) neuron. In control conditions, at rest, a STN neuron discharges in the single-spike mode. Bath application of Cs+ hyperpolarizes the membrane by 8 mV and shifts STN activity to burst firing mode. Continuous injection of positive current shifts the membrane potential back to the control value and to single-spike activity, though Cs+ is still present. Concomitantly, the depolarizing sag in response to negative current pulse is strongly decreased as well as the depolarizing rebound seen at the break of pulse, to attest that I_h is strongly reduced (insets). Part (a) adapted from McCormick DA, Pape HC (1990) Properties of a hyperpolarization-activated cation current and its role in rhythmic oscillation in thalamic relay neurones, *J. Physiol. (Lond.)* **431**, 291–318, with permission. Part (b) adapted from Beurrier C, Bioulac B, Hammond C (2000) Slowly inactivating sodium current (I_{NaP}) underlies single-spike activity in rat subthalamic nucleus, *J. Neurophysiol.* **83**, 1951–1957, with permission.

membrane is at a potential more negative than the resting potential, so that I_{CaT} is de-inactivated and thus may be activated. Bursting state is present as long as the membrane is hyperpolarized. For example, at the break of an IPSP or in response to an EPSP evoked during or after an IPSP, a short sequence of bursts is recorded. In this case the bursting mode is transient; it is not a stable state. Unless hyperpolarized, thalamic and STN neurons

discharge in single-spike mode. We see here that IPSP does not always mean inhibition of the postsynaptic neuron: when neurons have the ability to oscillate, an IPSP can evoke a burst of spikes (i.e. an excitation). This is observed for example in STN neurons, during and after the execution of a conditioned movement.

In vivo, thalamocortical neurons discharge in the single-spike or bursting mode, depending on the

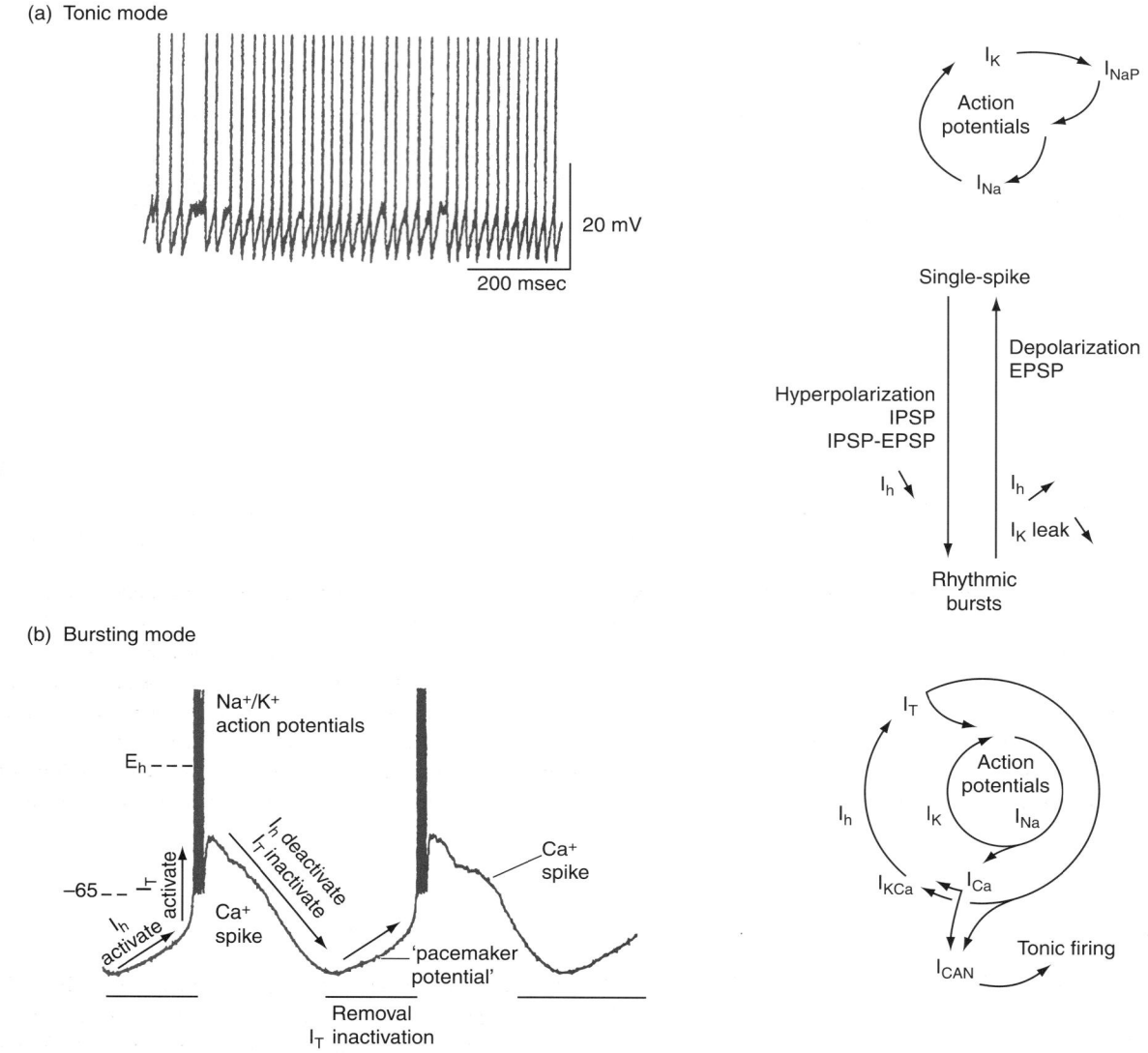

Figure 20.14 Currents underlying the tonic and burst firing modes.
Recordings and scheme of the ionic basis of **(a)** the tonic mode and **(b)** the bursting mode of thalamic neurons. Adapted from McCormick DA, Pape HC (1990) Properties of a hyperpolarization-activated cation current and its role in rhythmic oscillation in thalamic relay neurones, *J. Physiol. (Lond.)* **431**, 291–318; and Bal T, McCormick DA (1993) Ionic mechanisms of rhythmic burst firing and tonic activity in the nucleus reticularis thalami, a mammalian pacemaker, *J. Physiol. (Lond.)* **468**, 669–691, with permission.

waking state of the animal: a stable bursting mode is observed during slow-wave sleep, a stable single-spike mode during waking or paradoxical sleep (see **Figure 20.15**). The transition from the electroencephalogram (EEG)-synchronized sleep to the waking or rapid-eye-movement (REM)-sleep state (paradoxical sleep) occurs with a progressive depolarization of thalamocortical cells and the abolition of intracellular slow oscillations (LTS) and burst firing, and the appearance of tonic activity. Such changes can be mimicked by the activation of muscarinic or glutamatergic metabotropic receptors

that reduce a resting leak K⁺ current in thalamocortical neurons (see **Figure 20.14**). The modulation of I_h can also play a role as seen in **Figure 20.13**. For example, activation of serotoninergic and β-adrenergic metabotropic receptors shifts the voltage-dependence of I_h to more positive membrane potentials. This reduces the ability of cells to oscillate. Together these results suggest that the release of acetylcholine, glutamate, serotonin and norepinephrine abolishes sleep-related activity in thalamocortical networks and facilitates the single-spike activity typical of the waking state.

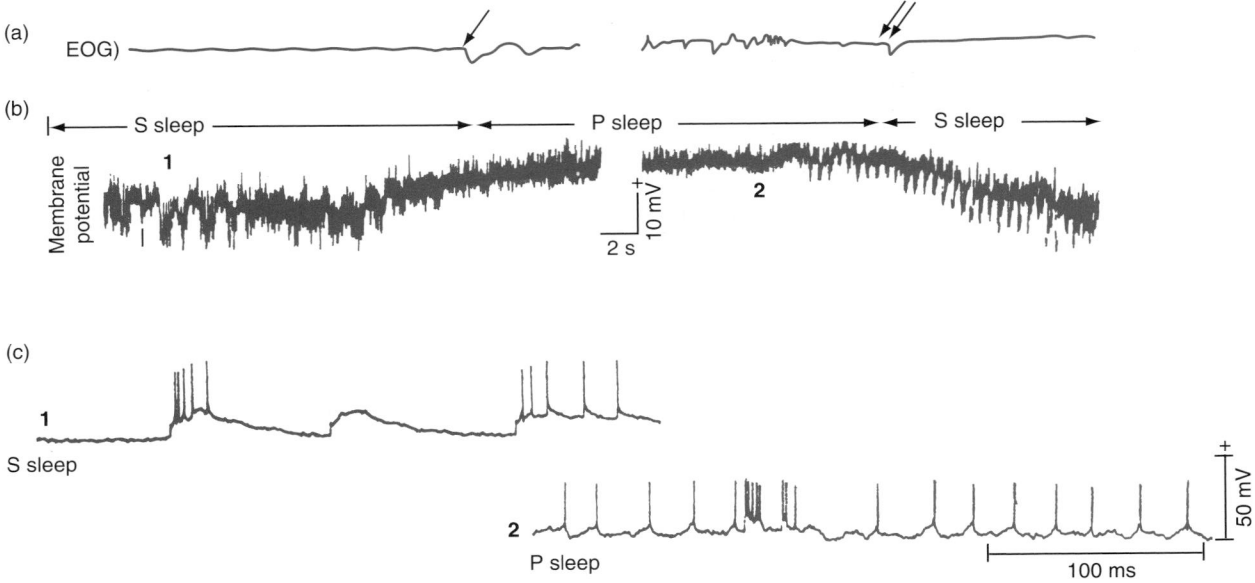

Figure 20.15 *In vivo*, **thalamic neurons display the single-spike or bursting mode, in relation to behavioural state.**
Simultaneous display of **(a)** eye movements (electro-oculogram, EOG) and **(b)** membrane potential of an intracellularly recorded thalamic neuron during slow-wave sleep (S sleep) and paradoxical sleep (P sleep) in an intact animal. **(b)** The neuron is already depolarized by 8 mV, when the animal enters P sleep (first eye movement, arrow). Depolarization is maintained throughout P sleep. Upon last eye movement (double arrow), membrane potential repolarizes as the animal goes back to S sleep (the trace is filtered at 0–75 Hz). **(c)** Enlarged sequences (labelled 1 and 2 under trace (b)) of spontaneous activities: 1, bursting mode during S sleep (hyperpolarized resting potential); 2, single-spike mode during P sleep (depolarized resting potential). Adapted from Hirsch J, Fourment A, Marc ME (1983) Sleep-related variations of membrane potential in the lateral geniculate body relay neurons of the cat, *Brain Res.* **259**, 308–312, with permission.

Summary

Thalamic and subthalamic neurons can function either as relay systems or as oscillators. During oscillations afferent informations have a low probability of evoking a response. For example, when thalamic neurons are oscillating during slow-wave sleep, there is a marked diminution of responsiveness of thalamic neurons to activation of their receptive fields, 'presumably owing to the hyperpolarized state of these neurons, the interrupting effects of spontaneous thalamocortical rhythms and the frequency limitations of the burst firing mode'. Oscillations are also recorded in pathological conditions: in the STN of parkinsonian patients and in the thalamocortical networks during absence epileptic seizures. Noteworthy, during these oscillations, motor or sensory processing is unpaired.

Further reading

Bal T, Von Krosigk M, McCormick DA (1994) From cellular to network mechanisms of a thalamic synchronized oscillation. In: Buzski G (ed.) *Temporal Coding in the Brain*, Berlin: Springer-Verlag.

Byrne JH (1980) Analysis of ionic conductance mechanisms in motor cells mediating inking behavior in *Aplysia californica. J. Neurophysiol.* **43**, 630–650.

Crépel F, Pénit-Soria J (1986) Inward rectification and low threshold calcium conductance in rat cerebellar Purkinje cells: an *in vitro* study. *J. Physiol. (Lond.)* **372**, 1–23.

Llinas RR (1988) The intrinsic electrophysiological properties of mammalian neurons: insights into central nervous system function. *Science* **242**, 1654–1664.

Llinas RR, Jahnsen H (1982) Electrophysiology of mammalian thalamic neurons. *Nature* **297**, 406–408.

McCormick DA, Bal T (1997) Sleep and arousal: thalamocortical mechanisms. *Ann. Rev. Neurosci.* **20**, 185–215.

Synaptic Plasticity

Synaptic responses undergo short- and long-term modifications. This chapter examines the mechanisms underlying plasticity in adult synapses. Developmental forms of plasticity are not covered here.

21.1 Short-term potentiation (STP) of a cholinergic synaptic response as an example of short-term plasticity: the cholinergic response of muscle cells to motoneuron stimulation

Repetitive high-frequency (>15 Hz) stimulation of the presynaptic element (motoneuron) leads to a short-term potentiation (STP) of the postsynaptic response of the muscle cell. As shown in **Figure 21.1**, successive stimulations produce in these conditions excitatory postsynaptic currents (EPSC) of greater and greater amplitudes. This phenomenon, first discovered at the

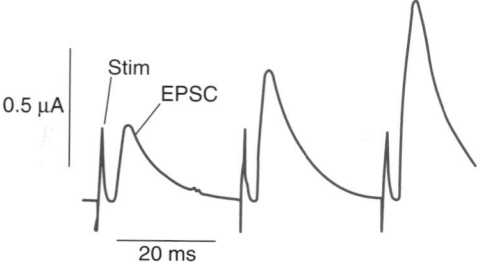

Figure 21.1 Presynaptic facilitation at the frog neuromuscular junction.
The activity of a frog sartorius muscle cell is recorded in normal Ringer solution ($V_m = -90$ mV). The motor endplate currents are evoked by repetitive stimulations (stim) of the motor nerve (2 µA intensity, 5 ms duration). The average current intensity (EPSC) in response to the first stimulation is 0.5 µA. This amplitude gradually rises following second and third stimulations. The inward currents are represented upwardly, which is unusual. Adapted from Katz B, Miledi R (1979) Estimates of quantal content during chemical potentiation of transmitter release, *Proc. R. Soc. Lond.* **B205**, 369–378, with permission.

neuromuscular junction, is also observed at the squid giant synapse and in mammalian afferent synapses to motoneurons.

In the squid giant synapse, synaptic facilitation has the following characteristics. When the presynaptic element repeatedly fires, an increase of the postsynaptic response amplitude is observed. This increase diminishes with a time constant of the order of tens of milliseconds. Simultaneous recordings of presynaptic action potentials, presynaptic Ca^{2+} current (I_{Ca}), variations of the intracellular Ca^{2+} concentration and postsynaptic depolarization shows that the postsynaptic response amplitude increases when:

- the amplitude and length of presynaptic spikes are unchanged;
- the amplitude of the presynaptic I_{Ca} evoked by each presynaptic depolarizing pulse or action potential is constant;
- the increase of the presynaptic intracellular Ca^{2+} concentration is identical in response to each depolarizing pulse or action potential.

The increase of intracellular Ca^{2+} concentration ($[Ca^{2+}]_i$) in the presynaptic element slowly disappears, in about one second, whereas the Ca^{2+} current and the release of the neurotransmitter both last about 1 ms. Katz and Miledi, in 1965, were the first to propose that STP is due to residual Ca^{2+} ions still present in the presynaptic active zone when the second presynaptic spike occurs. The following hypothesis was proposed. Ca^{2+} ions enter the presynaptic element through voltage-gated Ca^{2+} channels opened by the depolarization. The intracellular Ca^{2+} concentration is very high at active zones at the end of the action potential. These Ca^{2+} ions act rapidly and locally on target molecules to trigger the exocytosis of synaptic vesicles with a probability p. At the same time, the Ca^{2+} ions are also buffered in the cytoplasm and are actively transported to the extracellular medium or inside the organelles (see Section 8.2.4). But a residual and quite high $[Ca^{2+}]_i$ is still present close to the presynaptic membrane for some time. This $[Ca^{2+}]_i$ value is not high enough to trigger neurotransmitter release, but added to the incoming increase of $[Ca^{2+}]_i$ accompanying the arrival of the second action potential (when the delay between the two action potentials is short) it increases neurotransmitter release probability to the second action potential, and thus causes potentiation of the postsynaptic response.

STP can also be induced by high-frequency stimulation (conditioning tetanus) of the afferent motoneuron (model of the crayfish neuromuscular junction) (**Figure 21.2a**). In that case, the postsynaptic response (EPSP) that is recorded at regular intervals after the tetanus is potentiated, and then decays to control amplitude within 1.5 s (**Figure 21.2b**, 1). In order to test the hypothesis of Katz and Miledi, a photolabile Ca^{2+} chelator, diazo-2, is injected into the presynaptic terminals. The motoneuron is penetrated at the level of an axon branch with a microelectrode containing KCl (to record presynaptic activity), the photolabile Ca^{2+} chelator diazo-2 (to chelate Ca^{2+} ions with an affinity of 150 nM after photolysis) and fluorescein (to monitor the progress of injection). First, the control STP is recorded (**Figure 21.2b**, 1). Then diazo-2 is injected into the presynaptic axon in order to test that before photolysis diazo-2 has little effect on STP since the unphotolysed chelator has a low power to chelate Ca^{2+} ions (**Figure 21.2b**, 2). An ultraviolet flash is given after the tetanus in order to produce a chelator with 150 nM Ca^{2+} affinity: the STP of the postsynaptic response is prevented (**Figure 21.2b**, 3).

NB These results show that STP is due to residual free Ca^{2+} ions following presynaptic activity. What are the molecular targets of Ca^{2+} action in short-term plasticity? Many candidates exist among vesicular, plasma membrane and cytoplasmic proteins of the presynaptic element (see Section 8.3). This identification awaits further experiments.

21.2 Long-term potentiation (LTP) of a glutamatergic synaptic response: example of the glutamatergic synaptic response of pyramidal neurons of the CA1 region of the hippocampus to Schaffer collaterals activation

21.2.1 The Schaffer collaterals are axon collaterals of CA3 pyramidal neurons which form glutamatergic excitatory synapses with dendrites of CA1 pyramidal neurons

The hippocampus is a telencephalic structure with a rostrocaudal extension in the rat. It is composed of two closely interconnected crescent-like regions, Ammon's horn and the dentate gyrus (**Figure 21.3a**). Ammon's

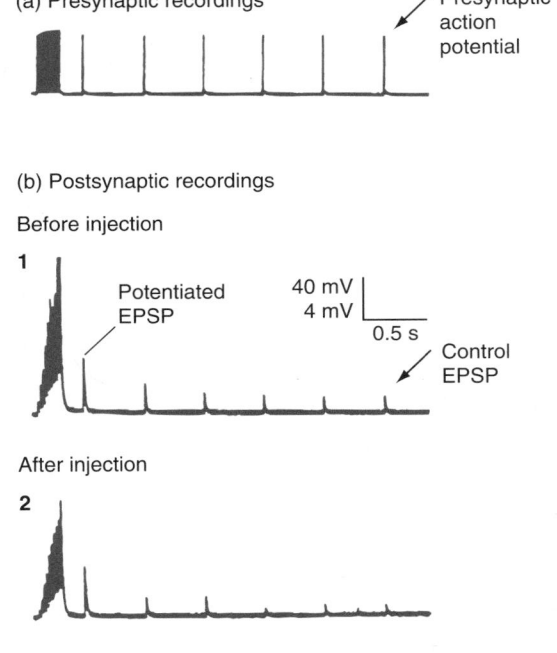

Figure 21.2 Rapid reduction of residual Ca^{2+} ions quickly eliminates STP.
The activity of the crayfish dactyl opener muscle cell is intracellularly recorded in current clamp mode in response to the stimulation of an axonal branch of the presynaptic motoneuron. The electrode positioned inside the presynaptic axon is filled with diazo-2 (50 mM) and fluorescein (10 mM) in KCl (3 M) in order to both stimulate the presynaptic axon and to fill it with the Ca^{2+} chelator. A conditioning tetanus (10 stimuli at 50 Hz) followed by a single stimulus at 2 Hz is applied to the axon.
(a) Action potentials recorded from the preterminal axon branch.
(b) The response (EPSP) of the postsynaptic muscle cell is recorded in control conditions (1), after the intracellular injection of diazo-2 (2) and after photolysis of diazo-2 by an ultraviolet flash given after the tetanus (3). Adapted from Kamiya H, Zucker RS (1994) Residual Ca^{2+} and short-term synaptic plasticity, *Nature* **371**, 603–606, with permission.

horn is formed by a layer of principal neurons, the pyramidal neurons, and is subdivided in three regions called CA1, CA2 and CA3 (CA for *cornu ammonis*). The dentate gyrus is formed by a layer of principal neurons called *granular cells*. Numerous interneurons are present in each region (see also Chapter 22).

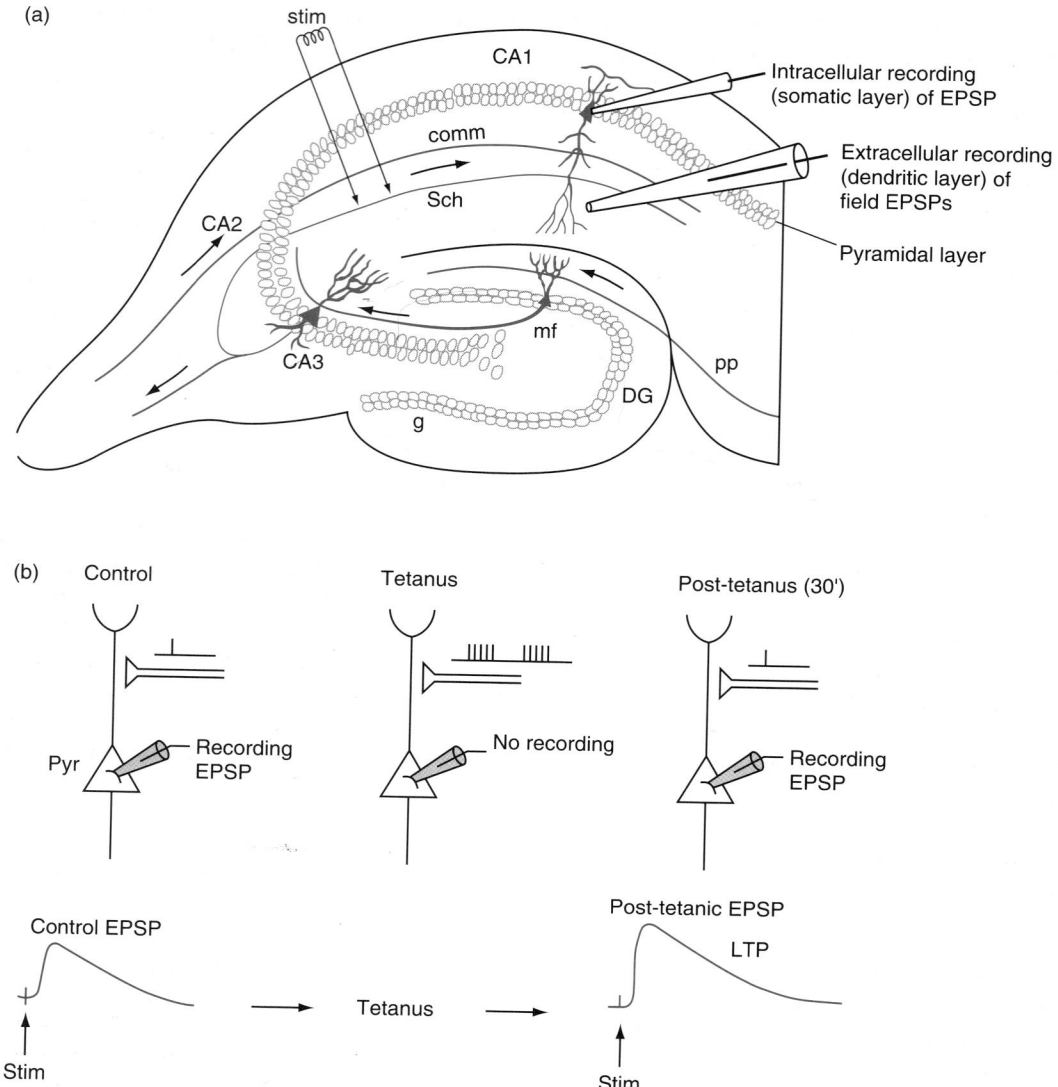

Figure 21.3. Tetanic LTP in the hippocampus is induced by high-frequency stimulation of afferent fibres.
(a) Coronal section of the rat hippocampus showing the major excitatory connections. CA1, CA2, CA3 regions of the hippocampus; DG, dentate gyrus layer composed of granular cells (g) which send their axons (mossy fibres, mf) to CA3 pyramidal dendrites. CA3 pyramidal cells send axon collaterals, called Schaffer collaterals (Sch), to CA1 pyramidal apical dendrites. The tetanic stimulation (stim, for example 1–4 trains of 10 stimulations at 100 Hz applied every 1 s) is applied to Schaffer collaterals and the AMPA-mediated postsynaptic response is recorded intracellularly in the soma of a pyramidal cell (EPSP or EPSC) and/or extracellularly in the layer of CA1 pyramidal dendrites. comm, commissural fibres; pp, perforant path. (b) A CA1 pyramidal neuron represented upside down compared with its position in the coronal section and the afferent Schaffer collaterals. The AMPA-mediated EPSP evoked by a single stimulation of Schaffer collateral (one vertical bar) is intracellularly recorded in the presence of bicuculline. After a tetanic stimulation of the Schaffer collaterals (shown as high-frequency bars), a potentiation of the glutamatergic EPSP evoked by a single stimulation is recorded. Adapted from Kauer JA, Malenka RC, Nicoll RA (1988) Persistent postsynaptic modification mediates long-term potentiation in the hippocampus, *Neuron* **1**, 911–917, with permission.

The pyramidal cells of CA3 have branched axons. One branch leaves the hippocampus and projects to other structures. The other branches are recurrent collaterals that form synapses with dendrites of CA1 pyramidal neurons. These collaterals run in bundles and form the Schaffer collateral pathway; and their terminals form asymmetrical synapses with the numerous spines of CA1 dendrites. These synapses are excitatory and the neurotransmitter is glutamate. Owing to the laminar organization of the hippocampal structure, it is possible to stimulate selectively the Schaffer collateral pathway (stim) and to record the evoked excitatory postsynaptic potential (EPSP) in a CA1 pyramidal soma either *in vivo* or *in vitro* (**Figure 21.3a**). EPSPs can be recorded from a single neuron (intracellular or whole-cell somatic recording) or extracellularly in the dendritic layer from a population of neurons (field EPSPs).

We shall restrict our study of long-term potentiation (LTP) to the synaptic response of CA1 pyramidal neurons to Schaffer collateral stimulation in hippocampal slices, recorded in the presence of bicuculline (an antagonist at GABA$_A$ receptors) in order to prevent the participation of GABAergic inhibitory responses resulting from interneuron activation.

21.2.2 Observation of the long-term potentiation of the Schaffer collateral-mediated EPSP

The pioneering observation was made by Bliss and Lomo, in 1973, that high-frequency stimulation of Schaffer collaterals in the rat hippocampus *in vivo* produces an increase of the amplitude of the Shaffer collateral-mediated EPSP recorded from the postsynaptic pyramidal neuron (**Figure 21.3b**). The exact protocol is the following. A single stimulus applied repeatedly at a very low frequency (0.02–0.03 Hz) to Schaffer collaterals evokes stable control EPSPs in the postsynaptic pyramidal neuron. These control responses can be averaged to give a mean control EPSP. Control EPSPs are largely mediated by non-NMDA receptors since they are nearly completely abolished by CNQX (not shown). A tetanic stimulation is then applied to the Schaffer collateral pathway through the same stimulating electrode (one train of 1 s duration, composed of 50–100 stimuli at 100 Hz). After this tetanus, the same single stimulus applied repeatedly at the same very low frequency, through the same stimulating electrode, now evokes 'post-tetanic' EPSPs of larger amplitude: the EPSP is potentiated. Since this potentiation lasts from minutes to hours it is a long-term potentiation (LTP).

Is LTP restricted to the synapses that have been tetanized?

Two EPSPs evoked in one pyramidal neuron in response to the stimulation of two different Schaffer collaterals inputs are recorded (**Figure 21.4a**). When only one input (S_1) is tetanized, the response evoked by a single shock at S_1 is potentiated (LTP of EPSP$_1$) whereas the response evoked in the same pyramidal neuron at S_2 (EPSP$_2$) is not potentiated: LTP is synapse-specific. In other words, when generated at one set of synapses by repetitive

activation, LTP does not normally occur in other synapses on the same cell.

21.2.3 Long-term potentiation (LTP) of the glutamatergic EPSP recorded in CA1 pyramidal neurons results from an increase of synaptic efficacy (or synaptic strength)

LTP of the Schaffer collateral-mediated EPSP can have several origins. We shall study some of the hypotheses one by one.

Does LTP result from a non-specific change of postsynaptic cell excitability?

To test this hypothesis, a pulse of depolarizing current is injected directly into the pyramidal cell. The response of the membrane is the same before and after the tetanus, at all potentials tested. Therefore, LTP does not result from a change of the total resistance of the postsynaptic membrane. It is also not due to a persistent reduction of the inhibitory GABAergic responses since it is still observed in the presence of bicuculline, a GABA$_A$ receptor antagonist.

Does LTP result from an increase in the number of stimulated axons?

One way to answer this question is to record simultaneously the presynaptic action potentials (afferent volley) and the postsynaptic response. This is possible with extracellular recordings at the level of apical dendrites of pyramidal cells. A single stimulus applied repeatedly at a low frequency (0.02–0.03 Hz) to the Schaffer collaterals evokes a stable 'control' field EPSP recorded by an extracellular electrode placed in the dendritic field of CA1 pyramidal neurons (**Figures 21.3a** and **21.4b**, left and middle). A field EPSP corresponds to the response of a population of pyramidal neurons situated close to the recording electrode and connected to the stimulated axons. Its slope is proportional to the amplitude of the currents generated in the postsynaptic neurons. After the stimulating artefact, before the field EPSP develops, the afferent volley is recorded (inset).

As a control intracellular EPSP, the control field EPSP is mediated predominantly by non-NMDA receptors since it is nearly completely abolished by the bath application of CNQX (not shown), a selective antagonist of AMPA receptors. A tetanic stimulation (one train of 1 s duration, composed of 50–100 stimuli at 100 Hz) is then applied to the Schaffer collateral pathway through the stimulating electrode. After this tetanus, the same single stimulus,

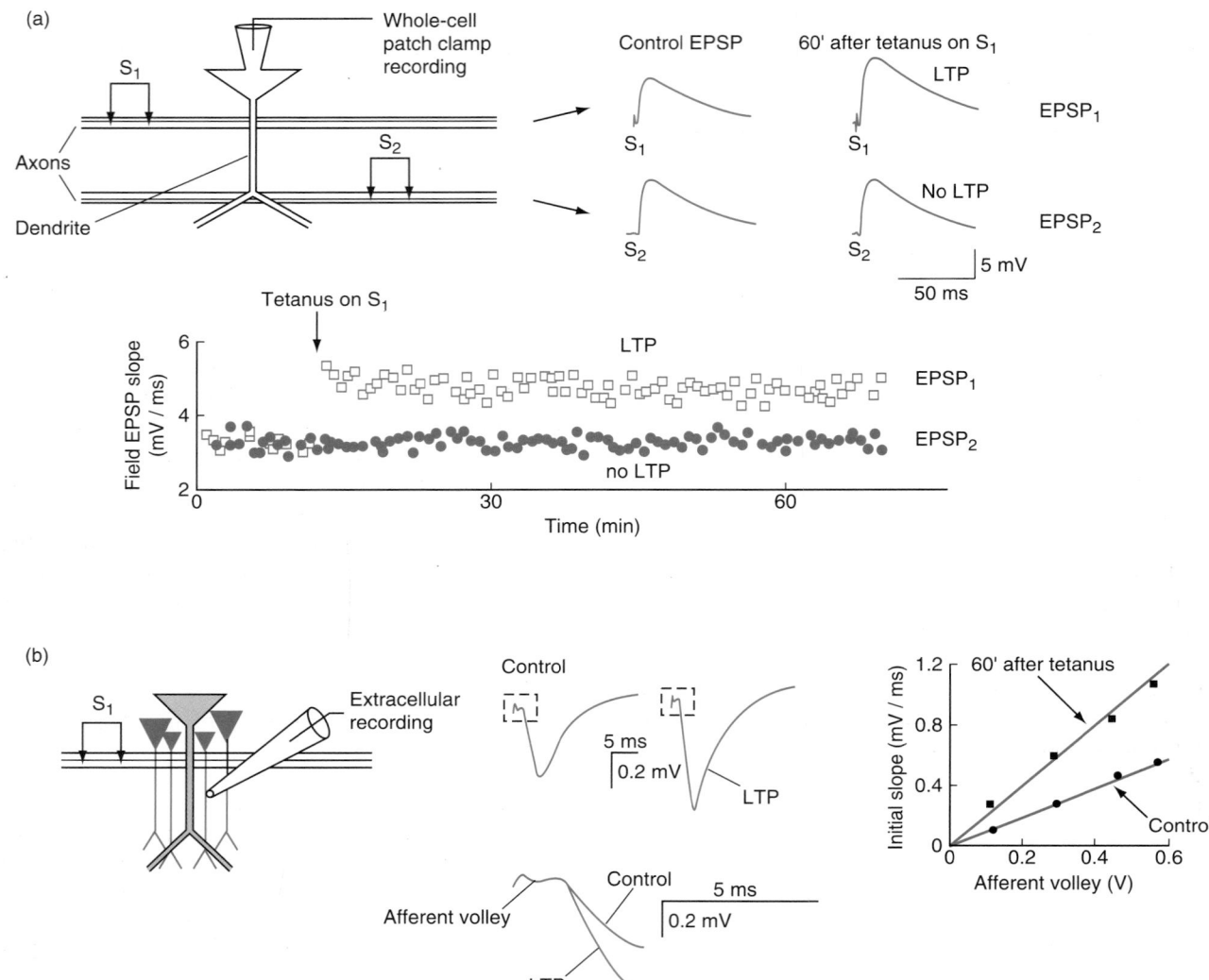

Figure 21.4 Tetanic LTP is synapse specific.
(a) The postsynaptic responses (control EPSP$_1$ and EPSP$_2$) of a single pyramidal neuron are intracellularly recorded in current clamp mode (whole-cell patch) in response to stimulations S$_1$ and S$_2$. Then, stimulus S$_1$ is tetanized but not stimulus S$_2$. Sixty minutes after the tetanus on S$_1$, EPSP$_1$ and EPSP$_2$ are recorded again. The diagram illustrates the time course of the initial slope of EPSP$_1$ and EPSP$_2$ before and after the tetanus on S$_1$. (b) Extracellular recording of the response of a population of CA1 pyramidal neurons to stimulation (S$_1$) of afferent Schaffer collaterals. The stimulation S$_1$ evokes an afferent volley (the extracellular recording of presynaptic action potentials in all stimulated afferent axons) and a field EPSP (the extracellular recording of the postsynaptic response of pyramidal neurons). Sixty minutes after a tetanus (two trains of 100 Hz, 1 s duration, 30 s interval) applied through the same stimulating electrode, the field EPSP is recorded. Note the increased initial slope 60 min after the tetanus (enlarged dotted squares). The input/output curves depict the amplitude of the afferent volley versus the initial slope of the field EPSP. Part (a) from L. Aniksztejn and (b) from H. Gozlan, personal communications.

again through the same stimulating electrode, now evokes a 'post-tetanic' field EPSP of larger amplitude and with a steeper initial slope than the control one: the field EPSP is potentiated (LTP). The value of the initial slope of a field EPSP (or of an intracellular EPSP) is an accurate index of the changes of the monosynaptically evoked postsynaptic excitatory response since the field EPSP (as well as the intracellular EPSP) can be composed of monosynaptic as well as polysynaptic unitary EPSPs. This potentiation of EPSP amplitude and slope is persistent: it lasts hours when recorded in the *in vitro* hippocampal slice preparation and days when induced in the freely moving animal. However, the afferent volley (the presynaptic component) is unchanged.

LTP is an increase of synaptic strength

Following a tetanic stimulation, the presynaptic component (the afferent volley) is unchanged whereas the peak amplitude and the initial slope of the postsynaptic one (field EPSPs) are potentiated (by 30% and 200%, respectively). The input/output curve depicting the initial slope of the field EPSPs versus afferent volley amplitude has a different slope before (control) and 60 minutes after the tetanus (**Figure 21.4b**, right). This result shows that potentiation of the postsynaptic response does not result from an increase of the number of stimulated axons but from a genuine increase in synaptic efficacy: the same input evokes an enhanced output.

LTP consists of two phases: induction and maintenance

LTP-generating mechanisms are classically separated into two phases: a brief induction phase (1–20 s) which occurs during tetanus, and a following expression phase; i.e. the mechanisms sustaining the persistent enhancement of synaptic efficacy. Therefore LTP is triggered rapidly (within seconds) whereas it is maintained for long periods of time (for hours in *in vitro* preparations and days *in vivo*). We will now analyse these two phases.

21.2.4 Induction of LTP results from a transient enhancement of glutamate release and a rise in postsynaptic intracellular Ca²⁺ concentration

Why is tetanic stimulation necessary to induce LTP? What does tetanic stimulation add to a single shock stimulation?

Tetanic stimulation evokes a large release of glutamate from Schaffer collateral terminals compared with a single shock. Glutamate released in synaptic clefts during tetanus binds to non-NMDA and NMDA receptor-channels but also to the metabotropic glutamate receptors (receptors linked to G proteins) present in the postsynaptic membrane (see **Figure 21.7**). The fact that tetanic stimulation can be replaced by a pairing diagram consisting of low-frequency stimulation of Schaffer collaterals combined with the intracellular depolarization of the postsynaptic neuron suggests that one of the roles of the tetanus is to depolarize the postsynaptic membrane. This is confirmed by the following experiment. When the postsynaptic potential is hyperpolarized during the tetanic stimulation, LTP is not induced. The tetanus-induced depolarization is the large EPSP

recorded during the tetanus and which results from the strong activation of AMPA receptors (see **Figures 21.5(2) and (4)** and **21.7**).

What does induce postsynaptic depolarization?

Several observations led to the conclusion that in CA1, induction of LTP is not just depolarization-dependent but also NMDA receptor-dependent: the application of APV, the selective antagonist of NMDA receptors, during the tetanic simulation prevents the induction of LTP (**Figure 21.5**). In contrast, antagonists of non-NMDA receptors such as CNQX, applied during the tetanus, do not prevent the induction of LTP. Therefore, induction of LTP is voltage- and NMDA receptor-dependent. These results confirm that, in the CA1 region of the hippocampus, tetanus induces a postsynaptic *depolarization* generated by the enhancement of glutamate release. This postsynaptic depolarization is a necessary perequisite for LTP induction, because it allows the activation of NMDA receptors.

What is the role of postsynaptic NMDA receptor activation?

To explain that LTP is APV-sensitive, the following hypothesis is proposed. The postsynaptic depolarization evoked by the tetanic stimulation allows the activation of postsynaptic NMDA receptors and the subsequent Ca²⁺ entry into the postsynaptic element. In fact, during tetanic stimulation an increase of $[Ca^{2+}]_i$ is observed in the dendrites of the postsynaptic pyramidal cells as visualized with a fluorescent calcium-sensitive dye. When this transient elevation of $[Ca^{2+}]_i$ is prevented by the intracellular injection of a Ca²⁺ chelator agent (BAPTA) in the recorded pyramidal cell before the tetanus or by a strong postsynaptic depolarization which decreases the driving force for Ca²⁺ entry, LTP is not observed or is reduced. A simultaneous extracellular recording of the field EPSP shows that LTP is, however, generated in the other stimulated cells (which were not injected with BAPTA or depolarized). These results indicate that an increase of $[Ca^{2+}]_i$ is essential for the induction of LTP.

For how long must $[Ca^{2+}]_i$ remain increased in the postsynaptic element to trigger LTP?

The duration for which $[Ca^{2+}]_i$ must remain elevated to induce LTP was tested by injecting into the recorded neuron a photosensitive Ca²⁺ chelator. This compound, diazo-4, has a low affinity for Ca²⁺ ($K_D = 89\ \mu M$) which

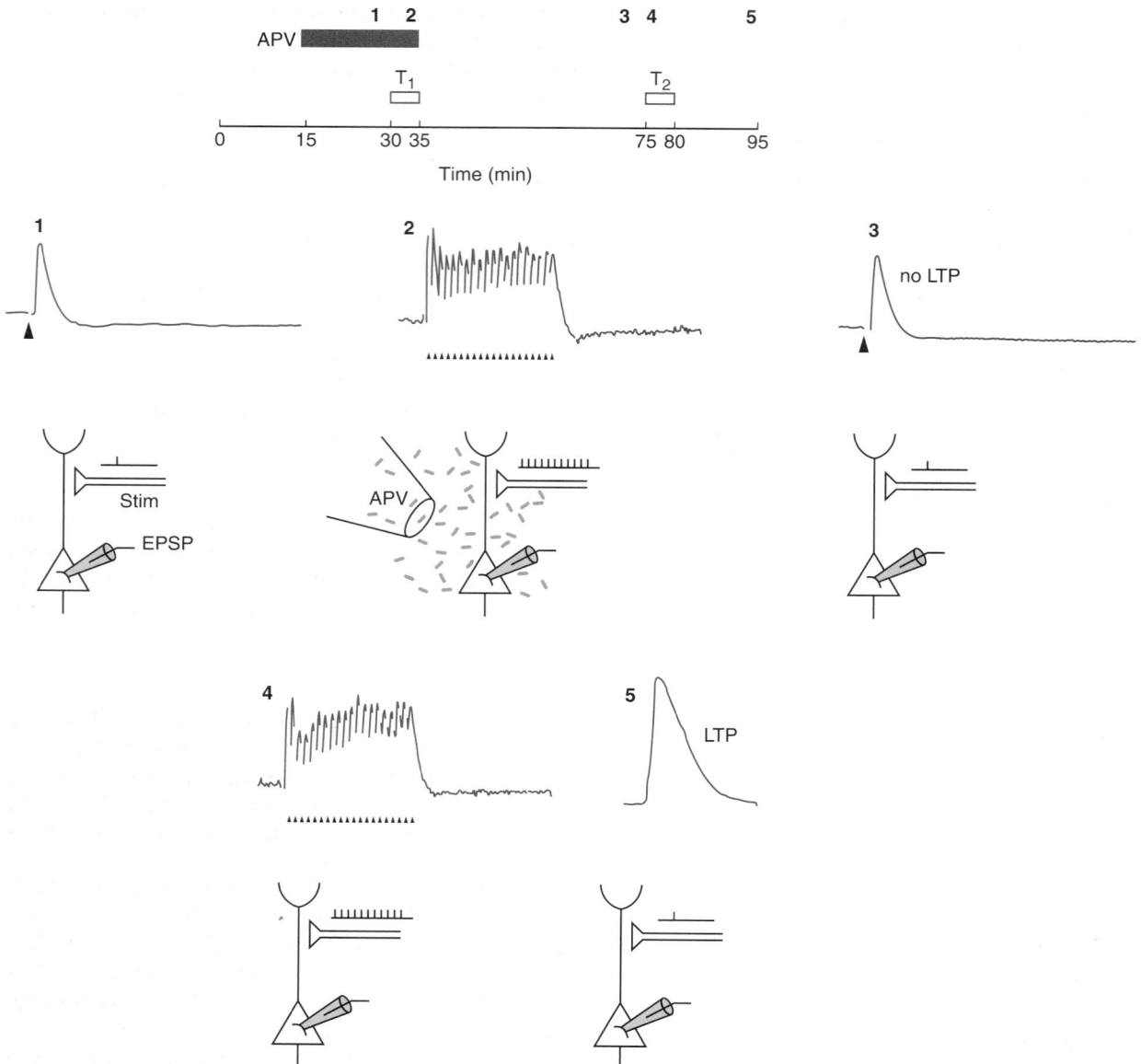

Figure 21.5 NMDA receptor activation is required for LTP induction.
An intracellular glutamatergic EPSP is evoked by Schaffer collateral stimulation (1). D-APV (20 μM, black bar) is applied before and during the tetanus (T₁, 2). LTP is not induced since the EPSP recorded one hour after wash of APV (3) has the same peak amplitude as the control one (1). A second tetanus (T₂, 4) is applied in the absence of D-APV; the EPSP is now potentiated (LTP, 5). Note that APV evokes only a small change of the depolarization of the membrane during the tetanus (compare 2 and 4). T₁ and T₂ are identical periods of tetanic stimulation composed of 10–12 high-frequency trains at 30 s interval. Each train comprised 20 stimulations at 100 Hz.
Adapted from Collingridge GL, Herron CE, Lester RAJ (1988) Frequency-dependent N-methyl-D-aspartate receptor-mediated synaptic transmission in rat hippocampus, *J. Physiol.* **399**, 301–312, with permission.

can be suddenly (in 100–400 μs) increased ($K_D = 0.55$ μm) when a UV flash inducing the photolysis of its diazo-acetyl groups is applied to the cell (**Figure 21.6a**). Thus, introduction of diazo-4 into a cell does not affect ambient Ca^{2+} levels before the application of UV light. The manipulation of the delay between the LTP-inducing tetanus and photolysis of diazo-4 allows one to determine the minimum duration of postsynaptic $[Ca^{2+}]_i$ increase necessary to induce LTP. When Ca^{2+} is chelated by diazo-4 photolysis 2.5 s or more after the tetanus, LTP is still induced (**Figure 21.6b**). In contrast, if the UV flash follows the 1 s duration tetanus without

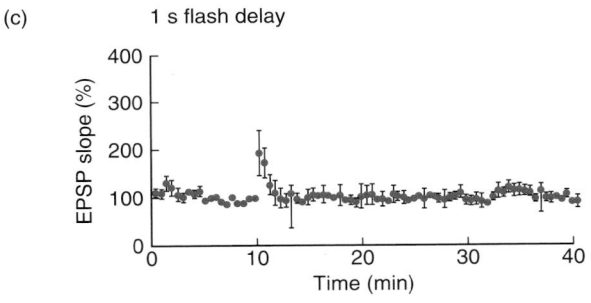

(a)

$K_d = 89\ \mu M$ $K_d = 0.55\ \mu M$

(b) 2.5 – 4 s flash delay

(c) 1 s flash delay

Figure 21.6 (Left) Photolysis of diazo-4, 1 s after the start of the tetanus, prevents LTP.
The activity of CA1 pyramidal cells is recorded in current clamp mode (whole-cell configuration) in hippocampal slices. The whole-cell electrode contains diazo-4, a Ca^{2+} chelator (1–2.5 mM). **(a)** Structure of diazo-4 before and after photolysis. **(b)** diazo-4 is photolysed 2.5 s or 4 s following the start of the tetanus (stimuli given at 100–200 Hz for 1 s, from time 10 min). Even after this short delay, LTP of the glutamatergic EPSP is induced ($n = 8$). **(c)** Photolysis of diazo-4 immediately at the end of the 1 s duration tetanus (given at time 10 minutes) prevents the induction of LTP of the glutamatergic EPSP ($n = 5$). In the same experiments, LTP of the field (extracellular) EPSP is observed (not shown). Adapted from Malenka RC, Lancaster B, Zucker RS (1992) Temporal limits on the rise in postsynaptic calcium required for the induction of long term potentiation, *Neuron* **9**, 121–128, with permission.

stimulated terminal. Glutamate activates postsynaptic non-NMDA and metabotropic glutamate receptors. NMDA receptors, owing to Mg^{2+} block, are weakly activated and contribute little to the basal EPSP (**Figure 21.7a**).

During tetanus

The high-frequency stimulation (tetanus) activates a certain number of afferent axons (**Figure 21.7b**). This enhances the release of glutamate from the stimulated terminals, thus evoking a postsynaptic depolarization due to the inward current through postsynaptic non-NMDA (AMPA) receptors and probably also the activation of metabotropic glutamate receptors (mGluR). Activation of AMPA receptors depolarizes the postsynaptic elements (spines) to the point where the Mg^{2+} blockade of the NMDA receptors is removed, thus allowing the influx of Ca^{2+} ions into the spines through NMDA channels and a further depolarization of the membrane. The depolarization of synaptic origin can also bring the postsynaptic membrane to the threshold for dendritic voltage-gated Ca^{2+} channel activation allowing an additional Ca^{2+} entry. The short-lasting (few seconds) rise in $[Ca^{2+}]_i$ resulting from NMDA and Ca^{2+} channel activation provides the necessary trigger for the subsequent events: activation of Ca^{2+}-dependent protein kinases and other Ca^{2+}-dependent processes, which lead to the expression of LTP; i.e. a persistent increase in synaptic efficacy (see maintenance or expression, Section 21.2.5).

delay, the induction of LTP is prevented (**Figure 21.6c**). Therefore an increase of $[Ca^{2+}]_i$ lasting at most 2.5 s (1 s during the tetanus plus 1.5 s after) is sufficient for LTP induction.

The hypothetical model for LTP induction

The following model is proposed to explain the induction of LTP in the CA1 region of the hippocampus.

Before tetanus

A single shock evokes the release of glutamate from the

Metabotropic glutamate receptors regulate the threshold of LTP induction

In the presence of t-ACPD, a selective agonist of metabotropic glutamate receptors (mGluRs), a

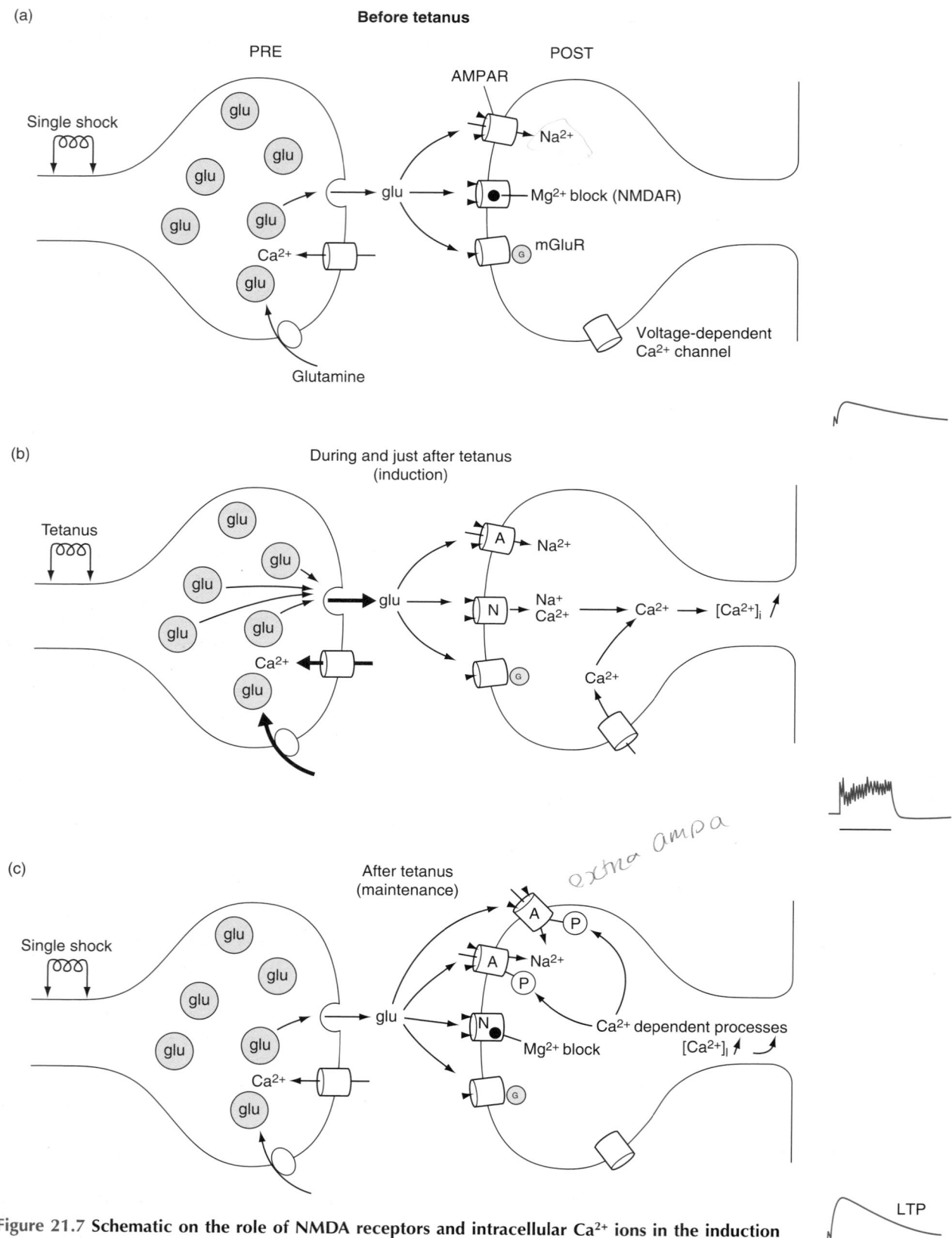

Figure 21.7 Schematic on the role of NMDA receptors and intracellular Ca²⁺ ions in the induction and maintenance of LTP.

See text for explanation.

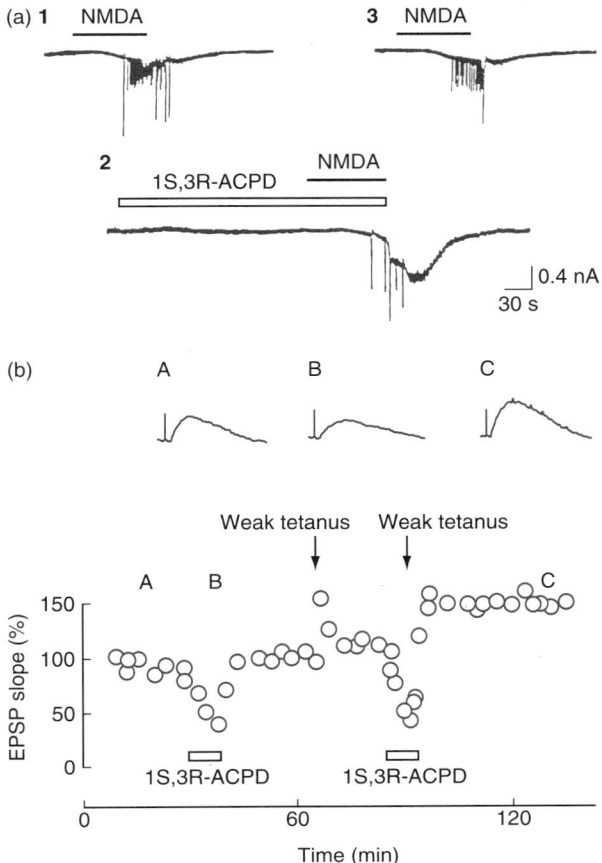

(a) 1

(b)

A   B   C

Weak tetanus   Weak tetanus

Figure 21.8 mGluRs activation potentiates NMDA-mediated currents and facilitates LTP induction of AMPA-mediated EPSP.

(a) The activity of a CA1 pyramidal neuron is intracellularly recorded in single-electrode voltage clamp mode in slices. The external solution contains TTX to block synaptic activity and K⁺ channel blockers and the intracellular electrode is filled with CsCl. Bath application of NMDA (10 μM, 90 s) evokes an inward current (1) with rapid inward voltage-gated Ca^{2+} currents evoked in unclamped regions of the neuronal membrane. Bath application of 1S,3R-ACPD (50 μM, 4 min), a mGluR agonist, before and during NMDA application (10 μM, 90 s) potentiates the NMDA-evoked current (2). This effect is reversible since 5 minutes after washing NMDA (10 μM, 90 s) evokes an inward current (3) of similar amplitude to the one observed in control (1). (b) The activity of a CA1 pyramidal neuron is intracellularly recorded in current clamp mode in slices. The diagram shows the amplitude of the initial slope of the AMPA-mediated EPSP recorded in response to Schaffer collaterals stimulation. Bath application of 1S,3R-ACPD (50 μM, 2 min) reversibly depresses the EPSP (compare B with A). A subthreshold tetanic stimulation of Schaffer collaterals (weak tetanus: stimuli at 50 Hz for 0.5 s) induces a short-term potentiation of the EPSP (trace not shown). The same weak tetanus given during bath application of 1S,3R-ACPD (50 μM, 2 min) now induces a long-term potentiation of the EPSP (C). Part (a) adapted from Ben Ari Y, Aniksztejn L (1995) Role of glutamate metabotropic receptors in long term potentiation in the hippocampus, *Sem. Neurosci.* **7**, 127–135, with permission. Part (b) adapted from Aniksztejn L, Otani S, Ben Ari Y (1992) Quisqualate metabotropic receptors modulate NMDA currents and facilitates induction of LTP through protein kinase C, *Eur. J. Neurosci.* **4**, 500–505, with permission.

subthreshold tetanus (which alone triggers only short-term potentiation), now generates a LTP (**Figure 21.8**). This effect is blocked by APV, a selective antagonist of NMDA receptors and by protein kinase C (PKC) inhibitors. It indicates that activation of metabotropic glutamate receptors reduces the threshold of LTP induction, an effect mediated by NMDA receptors and protein kinase C. This effect is specific to mGluRs since application in similar conditions of agonists of iGluRs, AMPA or NMDA, in addition to the subthreshold tetanus fails to trigger LTP.

In control situations (in the absence of tetanus) a link between mGluRs, protein kinase C and NMDA receptors is suggested by numerous experiments:

■ In intracellular recordings of pyramidal neurons of the CA1 region of the hippocampus, the mGluR agonist t-ACPD enhances the current generated by NMDA but not by AMPA applications, in the presence of TTX (to block action potentials and therefore network activity) and K⁺ channels blockers.

■ This effect is blocked by the intracellular injection of a protein kinase C inhibitor.
■ The intracellular injection of protein kinase C enhances the NMDA receptor-mediated current.
■ Protein kinase C phosphorylation sites are present on NMDA receptors.
■ In oocytes transfected with cDNAs coding for mGluRs and NMDA receptors, the mGluR agonist t-ACPD increases NMDA currents, an effect blocked by protein kinase C inhibitors.
■ In a wide range of cell types, kinases and phosphatases modulate rapidly and reversibly NMDA receptor activity.

These results suggest that the activation of postsynaptic mGluRs enhances (via protein kinase C) the postsynaptic NMDA receptor-mediated current (activated by the release of glutamate evoked by a subthreshold tetanus applied to the afferents). This enhancement of NMDA receptor-mediated response, together with the activation of AMPA receptors, induces LTP of the glutamatergic AMPA receptor-mediated response.

21.2.5 Expression of LTP (also called maintenance) involves a persistent enhancement of the AMPA component of the EPSP

Owing to the Mg^{2+} block of NMDA receptors, the control glutamatergic EPSP recorded in CA1 pyramidal neurons (in the presence of physiological concentrations of Mg^{2+}) is mainly mediated by non-NMDA receptors (**Figure 21.7a**) since it is negligibly affected by APV (the selective antagonist at NMDA receptors) and nearly completely blocked by CNQX. The same analysis of the relative contribution of NMDA and non-NMDA receptors was applied to the potentiated EPSP after a tetanus.

The EPSC (postsynaptic excitatory current) evoked in CA1 pyramidal neurons in response to Schaffer collaterals stimulation is recorded with patch clamp techniques (whole-cell patch) at two different holding potentials. At $V_H = -80$ mV, the EPSC is mainly mediated by AMPA receptors owing to the Mg^{2+} block of NMDA receptors at this hyperpolarized potential. In contrast, at $V_H = +30$ mV the control EPSC (which is inverted since the reversal potential of the glutamate response is 0 mV) is mixed and mainly mediated by NMDA receptors as shown by the small effect of CNQX (**Figure 21.9a**). The early rising phase of the EPSC is mainly mediated by AMPA receptors, while the current measured 100 ms after the stimulation is mainly mediated by NMDA receptors.

The recorded cell is subjected to a procedure which induces LTP. After the tetanus, the membrane potential is returned to -80 mV and the test stimulation of Schaffer collaterals is regularly applied to verify that the EPSC is now potentiated (LTP has been induced) (**Figure 21.9b**). This potentiated EPSC is also recorded at +30 mV in order to evaluate the amplitudes of the early AMPA and the late NMDA components. The early component (AMPA-mediated) approximately doubles while the late component (NMDA-mediated) remains rather stable (**Figure 21.9c**). Therefore LTP of the glutamatergic response, in this experiment, is primarily mediated by an enhancement of the AMPA component of the synaptic current.

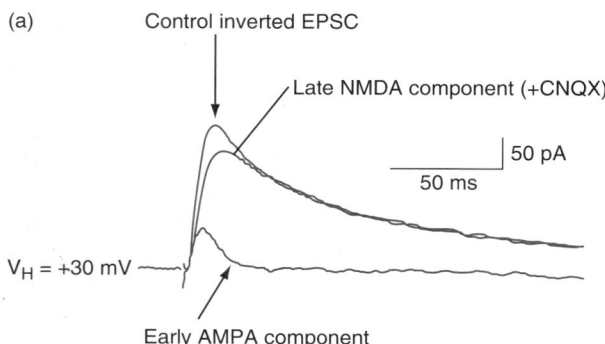

(a)

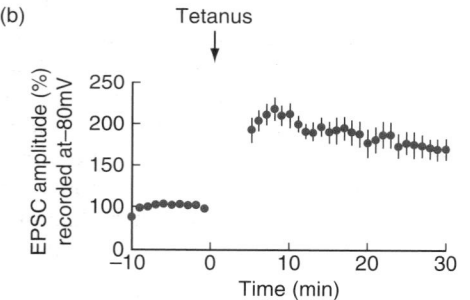

(b)

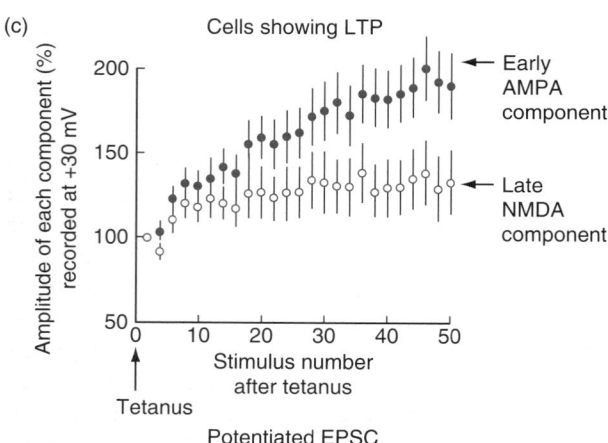

(c)

Figure 21.9 (Left) Differential enhancement of the non-NMDA and NMDA components in LTP.

The excitatory postsynaptic current (EPSC) evoked by Schaffer collaterals stimulation is recorded in a CA1 pyramidal neuron in hippocampal slices with patch clamp techniques (whole-cell patch). **(a)** At $V_H = +30$ mV, the EPSC is inverted (control). Application of the non-NMDA selective antagonist (CNQX) selectively reduces the early component of the current, leaving the late component (NMDA receptor-mediated) unaffected. The subtracted record (sub = control – CNQX insensitive) illustrates the time course of the AMPA receptor-mediated component (CNQX-sensitive). **(b)** The EPSC peak amplitude (expressed as a percentage of the control) is plotted against time, before and after the tetanus applied to evoke LTP ($V_H = -80$ mV, except during the tetanus). The total EPSC is clearly potentiated by the procedure. **(c)** The EPSC peak amplitude, expressed as a percentage of the control, is measured from just after the induction of LTP to 30 min after ($V_H = +30$ mV). The early (CNQX-sensitive) AMPA receptor-mediated component is clearly potentiated while the late (CNQX-insensitive) NMDA receptor-mediated component is not significantly potentiated. Recordings in (b) and (c) are from the same cell; to obtain the curves in (b) and (c), the membrane potential is continuously shifted from -80 to +30 mV. Adapted from Perkel DJ, Nicoll RA (1993) Evidence for all or none regulation of neurotransmitter release: implications for long term potentiation, *J. Physiol.* **471**, 481–500, with permission.

This differential effect of the tetanus can be explained by:

- an increase in the density of AMPA receptors in the synaptic cleft (clustering);
- a change in the properties of AMPA receptors (affinity, unitary current amplitude);
- an increase in the effective spread of synaptic current from dendritic spines into dendrites (a change of diameter of the neck of the spines for example).

This differential enhancement of the two components of the EPSC favours the hypothesis that *expression* of LTP requires postsynaptic mechanisms and does not result exclusively from a presynaptic mechanism, such as a persistent enhancement of glutamate release. If the expression of LTP resulted only from a presynaptic mechanism, a similar increase of both components of the EPSC should have been observed (assuming that AMPA and NMDA receptors are co-localized in the same postsynaptic membrane). However, not all investigators agree on the mechanisms of LTP expression and in particular on the postsynaptic origin of these mechanisms. As shown above, LTP *induction* clearly requires postsynaptic events (activation of NMDA receptors, increase of postsynaptic $[Ca^{2+}]_i$. Therefore, if LTP expression were presynaptic, that would imply that some message must be sent from the postsynaptic spines to the presynaptic elements. This retrograde messenger would be generated postsynaptically and would trigger a sustained enhanced release of glutamate by the presynaptic element.

The Ca^{2+} signal is translated into an increase in synaptic strength by biochemical pathways

What are the biochemical pathways activated by intradendritic Ca^{2+} increase that are key components absolutely required for translating the Ca^{2+} signal into an increase in synaptic strength? Amongst the kinases, the Ca^{2+} calmodulin-dependent protein kinase II (CaMKII) plays a crucial role:

- CaMKII is found in high concentrations in the postsynaptic density in spines, near postsynaptic glutamate receptors.
- Injection of inhibitors of CaMKII in the postsynaptic cell, or genetic deletion of a critical CaMKII subunit, block the ability to generate LTP.
- When autophosphorylated on Thr(286), the activity of CaMKII is no longer dependent on Ca^{2+}-calmodulin. This allows its activity to continue long after the Ca^{2+} signal has returned to baseline.
- Replacement of endogenous CaMKII by a form of

CaMKII containing a Thr286 point mutation (by the use of genetic techniques) block LTP.
- Finally, CaMKII directly phosphorylates the AMPA receptor in situ.

Several other protein kinases have been suggested to contribute to LTP, including protein kinase C (PKC) since its selective inhibition by intracellular injection of a PKC inhibitory peptide (PKCI) prevents LTP induction.

Expression of LTP involves the phosphorylation and persistent upregulation of AMPA receptors

A persistent enhancement of the AMPA component of the EPSP could result from a persistent modification in the function or the number of postsynaptic AMPA receptors (see Figure 21.7c). The former hypothesis implies either an increase in unitary current amplitude or an increase in the probability of opening of the channel. Such a change in receptor function generally involves a phosphorylation by a serine or a threonine kinase. In fact, induction of LTP specifically increases the phosphorylation of Ser831 of the GluR1 subunit, an effect that is blocked by a CaMKII inhibitor (AMPA receptors in CA1 pyramidal cells are heteromers composed primarily of GluR1 and GluR2 subunits). Moreover, genetic deletion of GluR1 subunit prevents the generation of LTP in CA1 pyramidal cells.

In agreement with the second hypothesis is the physiological and anatomical evidence of a rapid and selective upregulation of AMPA receptors after the induction of LTP. For example, when the GluR1 subunit of AMPA receptors is tagged with green fluorescent protein (GFP) and transiently expressed in hippocampal CA1 neurons, its distribution can be observed with a two photon laser scanning microscope (see Appendix 6.1). After a tetanus, a rapid delivery of tagged receptors to dendritic spines is observed.

21.2.6 Multiple ways to induce LTP, multiple forms of LTP and multiple ways to block LTP induction

Although synchronous activation of a number of presynaptic fibres by high-frequency stimulation is the most reliable way to evoke LTP (**Figure 21.10a**), LTP can be also evoked *in vitro* by a combination of low-frequency stimulation of presynaptic afferents and postsynaptic injection of a depolarizing current pulse to activate NMDA receptors and voltage-gated Ca^{2+} channels (**Figure 21.10b**); and by a combination of low-frequency stimulation of presynaptic afferents and bath application of a selective agonist at metabotropic glutamate

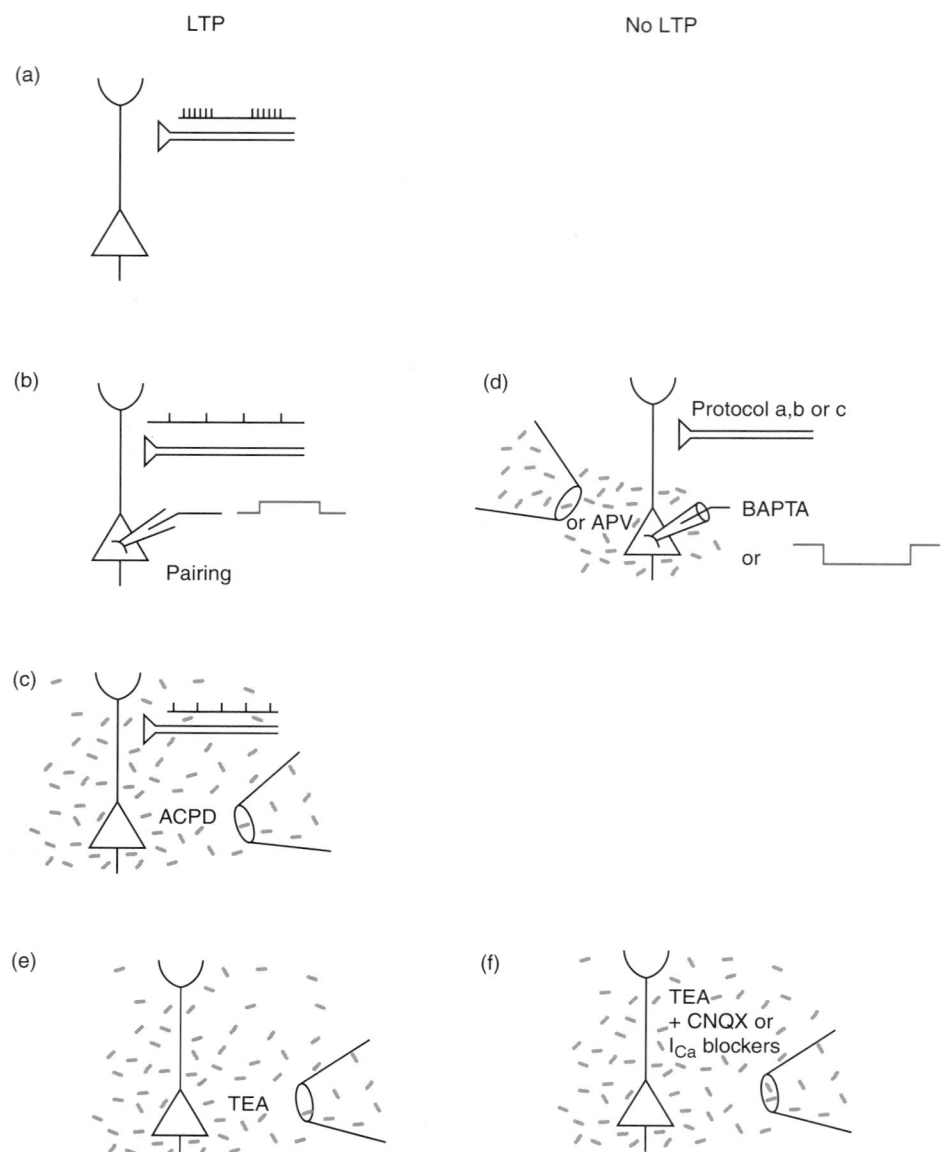

Figure 21.10 Hippocampal LTP.

(a)–(d) Tetanic LTP and **(e, f)** TEA-induced LTP. The multiple ways of induction are shown in (a)–(c) and (e), and blockade of induction in (d) and (f).

receptors (**Figure 21.10c**). All these forms of LTP induction are blocked by bath application of APV, an antagonist at NMDA receptors, by intracellular injection of a Ca^{2+} chelator (BAPTA), or by intracellular injection of a hyperpolarizing current pulse during tetanic stimulation (**Figure 21.10d**).

Another form of LTP is induced by bath application of K^+ channel blockers such as tetraethylammonium chloride (TEA) that depolarizes the presynaptic elements and enhances transmitter release (**Figure 21.10e**). This form of LTP also requires a rise of the postsynaptic intracellular Ca^{2+} concentration. This rise is produced by the

entry of Ca^{2+} ions through voltage-gated Ca^{2+} channels activated by the depolarization resulting from the closure of K^+ channels by TEA. In contrast to tetanus LTP, TEA-induced LTP is not synapse-specific since all the synapses are activated by bath application of TEA. Moreover, TEA-induced LTP is NMDA receptor-independent. It is blocked by bath application of CNQX (an antagonist at AMPA receptors) or of Ca^{2+} channel blockers, or by intracellular injection of a Ca^{2+} chelator (**Figure 21.10f**).

The observation that a rise of the intracellular Ca^{2+} concentration is a necessary prerequisite for LTP induction raises the possibility that a wide range of physiological or pathological processes known to evoke a rise of [Ca²⁺]ᵢ would trigger long-lasting changes of synaptic efficacy. Both seizures, which generate synchronized giant paroxysmal activity, and anoxic–ischaemic episodes which generate LTP of *NMDA receptor*-mediated EPSPs (anoxic LTP), are in fact associated with [Ca²⁺]ᵢ rises and long-lasting changes of synaptic efficacy. In such cases, LTP of excitatory synaptic transmission may participate in the pathological consequences of these insults.

21.2.7 Summary: principal features of LTP in the Schaffer collateral–pyramidal cell glutamatergic transmission

- LTP is a long-lasting phenomenon, persisting for hours *in vitro* and days or weeks in the intact animal.
- LTP is synapse-specific.
- LTP results from an increase in the synaptic response without changes in the number of stimulated presynaptic axons.
- LTP does not result from a persistent change of postsynaptic cell excitability.
- LTP does not result from a persistent reduction of the inhibitory GABAergic responses.
- LTP consists of two phases: a brief induction phase (1–20 s) followed by the expression phase; i.e. the mechanisms sustaining the persistent enhancement of synaptic efficacy.
- *Induction* of LTP is voltage- and NMDA-dependent. It requires depolarization of the postsynaptic membrane (resulting from AMPA receptors activation) *and* activation of NMDA receptors which leads to Ca²⁺ entry into the postsynaptic spine and postsynaptic [Ca²⁺]ᵢ increase; the localized [Ca²⁺]ᵢ increase in the dendritic spines activated by the tetanized afferents accounts for the input specificity of LTP.
- *Maintenance* of LTP, at least during the initial phase, results from the triggering of a Ca²⁺-dependent cascade of events leading to postsynaptic modifications of AMPA receptor function and localization, and to persistent enhancement of the synaptic glutamatergic response (LTP).

21.3 The long-term depression (LTD) of a glutamatergic response: example of the response of Purkinje cells of the cerebellum to parallel fibre stimulation

Purkinje cells represent the single output neurons of the cerebellar cortex. Each of them receives two distinct excitatory inputs, one from parallel fibres (axons of granule cells) and the other from a climbing fibre (axons of the contralateral inferior olive cells). These two types of inputs display distinct characteristics. A single climbing fibre terminates on each Purkinje cell. This powerful one-to-one excitatory input makes multiple synapses on the soma and proximal dendrites of the Purkinje cell (**Figure 21.11**; see also **Figures 7.8** and **7.9**). In contrast, many parallel fibres converge on each Purkinje cell but each fibre makes few synapses on each Purkinje cell.

The putative neurotransmitter at parallel-fibre and climbing-fibre synapses is glutamate. Fast excitatory synaptic transmission at these synapses is mediated entirely by non-NMDA ionotropic glutamatergic receptors, since both synapses lack NMDA receptors in the adult – in marked contrast to most other neurons in the brain (**Figure 21.11**, inset). In addition, parallel-fibre/Purkinje-cell synapses also bear mGluR1 receptors known to be coupled to phospholipase C, activation of which leads to production of inositol trisphosphate (IP₃) and diacylglycerol (DAG).

The dual arrangement of the two excitatory synaptic inputs raises the question of the role of the powerful input (climbing fibre) on the weaker input (parallel fibres). The coactivation of climbing fibre and parallel fibre inputs induces a persistent decrease in the efficacy of the parallel-fibre/Purkinje-cell synapse. This decrease of efficacy is called *long-term depression* (LTD). With the experimental advantages of *in vitro* brain slices and culture preparations, cerebellar LTD constitutes a simple model to study activity-dependent changes confined to excitatory synapses.

21.3.1 The long-term depression of a postsynaptic response (EPSC or EPSP) is a decrease of synaptic efficacy

Ito and coworkers (1982) were the first to demonstrate in the rabbit cerebellum *in vivo* that conjunctive stimulation of the afferent climbing and parallel fibres leads to an LTD of synaptic transmission at parallel-fibre/Purkinje-cell synapses. In other terms, LTD is the attenuation of the Purkinje cell response to parallel fibres after the conjunctive stimulation of parallel and climbing fibres.

The activity of a Purkinje cell is intracellularly recorded in current clamp mode in rat cerebellar slices. The stimulation of parallel fibres evokes an EPSP resulting from the activation of postsynaptic AMPA receptors by glutamate released from the stimulated terminals since it is totally blocked by CNQX, a selective AMPA receptor antagonist. After recording this control parallel-fibre-mediated EPSP for several minutes, parallel fibres are then stimulated in conjunction with the

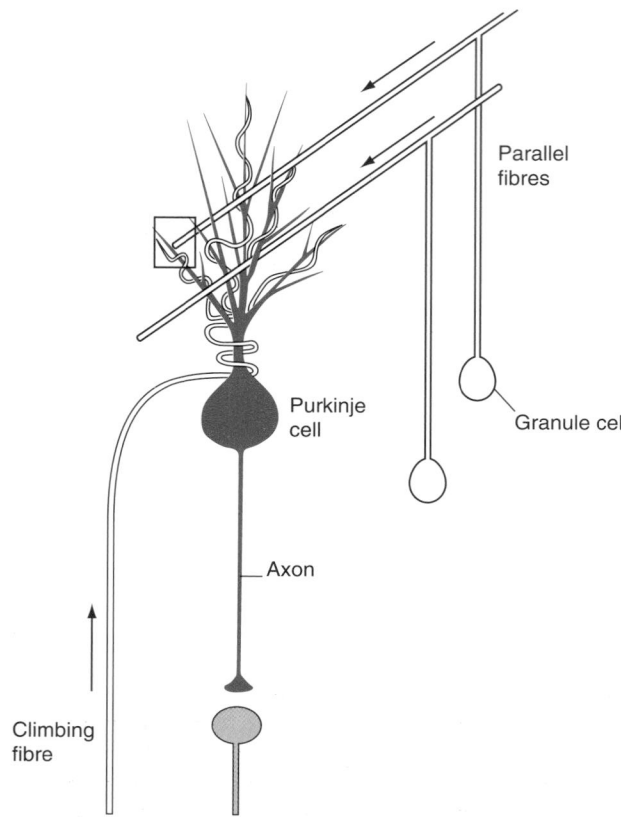

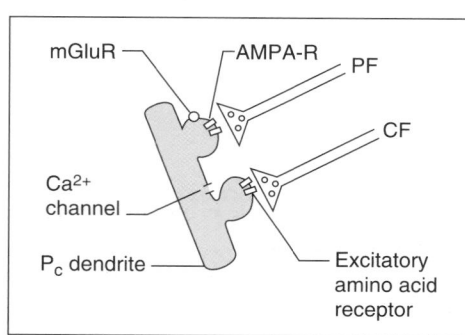

Figure 21.11 Simplified neural circuit in the cerebellar cortex.

Inset shows a more detailed view of the synaptic contacts between a parallel or a climbing fibre terminal and the Purkinje cell dendrite. AMPA-R, AMPA receptor; mGluR, metabotropic glutamate receptors; VDCC, voltage-dependent calcium channels; CF, climbing fibre; PF, parallel fibre; Pc, Purkinje cell. Adapted from Daniel H, Levenes C, Crépel F (1998) Cellular mechanisms of cerebellar LTD, *Trend. Neurosci.* **9**, 401–407, with permission.

climbing fibre at low frequency, 4 Hz for 25 s. After this conjunctive stimulation, the same stimulation of parallel fibres as in the control now evokes a smaller EPSP (**Figure 21.12**). The parallel-fibre-mediated EPSP stays

attenuated for the rest of the recording session. It is a long-term depression (LTD).

The persistent decrease of the parallel-fibre-mediated synaptic response can be also studied in another *in vitro* preparation, a culture of Purkinje cells, granule cells and an inferior olivary explant (**Figure 21.13a**). The parallel-fibre-mediated postsynaptic excitatory current (EPSC) is first recorded in voltage clamp (**Figure 21.13b**). The repetitive conjunctive stimulation of a single granule cell (whose axon is a parallel fibre) and the inferior olivary explant (which sends an axon, the climbing fibre, to the recorded Purkinje cell) is then applied while the Purkinje cell activity is recorded in current clamp mode. When switching back to voltage clamp mode, the parallel fibre-mediated EPSC (in response to granule cell stimulation) is persistently decreased. This *in vitro* preparation allows the stimulation of a single presynaptic granule cell before and after LTD induction. Therefore, it can be demonstrated that LTD is observed though the number of parallel fibres stimulated before and after the conditioning stimulation is identical (a depressed EPSC or EPSP could in fact result from a decrease in the number of stimulated axons).

21.3.2 Induction of LTD requires a rise in postsynaptic intracellular Ca²⁺ concentration and the activation of postsynaptic AMPA receptors

As already studied in Sections 19.2.2 and 20.3, the response of a Purkinje cell to the activation of its afferent climbing fibre is an all-or-none response composed of an initial depolarization, an overshooting action potential and following depolarizing humps. Since the activation of the afferent climbing fibre potently activates the voltage-gated Ca²⁺ channels present in the membrane of Purkinje dendrites (**Figure 21.11**, inset), it was supposed that the consequent rise in intradendritic Ca²⁺ concentration played a role in LTD. In fact, *in vivo* experiments have shown that hyperpolarization of the membrane by the activation of stellate cells during co-stimulation of parallel and climbing fibres prevents the occurrence of LTD.

[Ca²⁺]ᵢ rises during co-stimulation

In order to simultaneously record the synaptic responses and the intracellular Ca²⁺ concentration, the activity of a Purkinje cell is recorded in patch clamp (whole-cell patch) in the presence of a fluorescent calcium dye, FURA-2, injected into the cell (**Figure 21.14**; see also Appendix 6.1). First, the control EPSC in response to parallel fibre stimulation is recorded in the

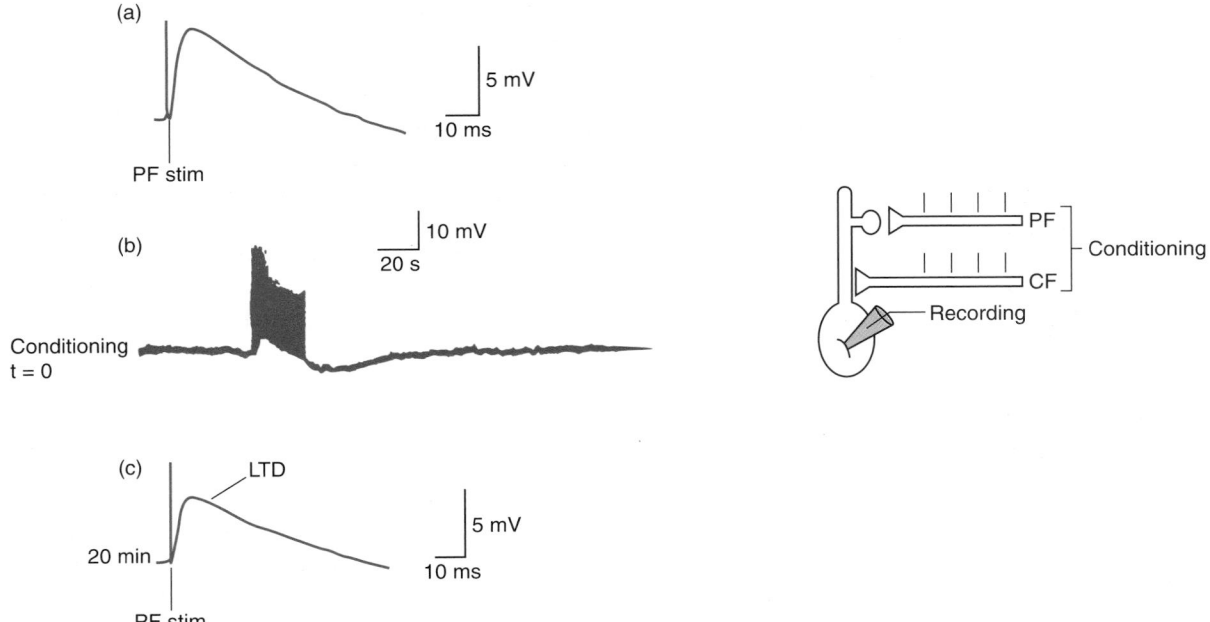

Figure 21.12 LTD of the parallel-fibre-mediated EPSP.
The activity of a Purkinje cell is intracellularly recorded in current clamp mode in a cerebellar slice. (a) The EPSP in response to PF stimulation (the stimulating electrode is placed in the superficial molecular layer) is recorded in the presence of picrotoxin (40 µM) to block IPSPs mediated by local interneurons. (b) CF and PF are then stimulated conjointly at 4 Hz for 25 s. To stimulate climbing fibres, a second electrode is placed in the white matter. (c) Twenty minutes after the end of conditioning stimulation, the EPSP recorded in response to PF stimulation is still depressed in amplitude. Adapted from Sakurai M (1990) Calcium is an intracellular mediator of the climbing fiber in induction of cerebellar long term depression, *Proc. Natl Acad. Sci. USA* **87**, 3383–3385, with permission.

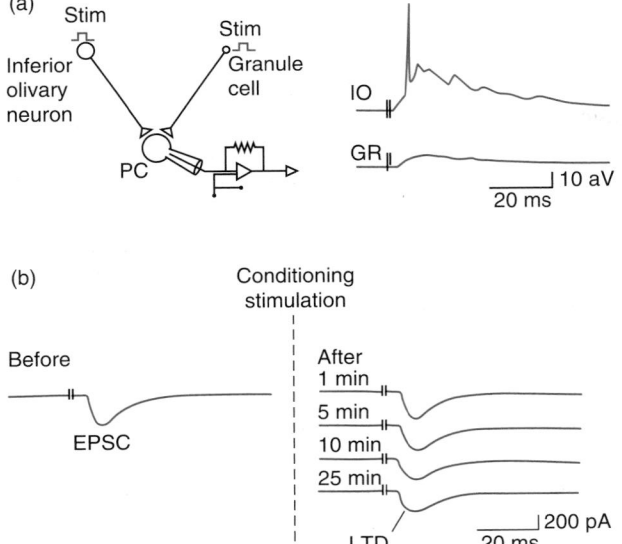

Figure 21.13 (Left) Cerebellar LTD is observed when a single parallel fibre is stimulated.
(a) The activity of a Purkinje cell is recorded in patch clamp (whole-cell patch) in co-cultures of rat cerebellar Purkinje cells (PC), granule cells and an explant of inferior olivary neurons, to record the evoked postsynaptic current (EPSC). The conditioning stimulation consists of the conjunctive stimulation of a single granule cell (GR) and the inferior olivary explant (IO) at 2 Hz for 20 s while the Purkinje cell membrane is recorded in current clamp mode. (b) The Purkinje cell membrane is held at $V_H = -50$ mV in voltage clamp mode and the response (EPSC) to the activation of a single granule cell is recorded before and 1, 5, 10 and 25 min after the conditioning stimulation. Adapted from Hirano T (1990) Depression and potentiation of the synaptic transmission between a granule cell and a Purkinje cell in rat cerebellar culture, *Neurosci. Lett.* **119**, 141–144, with permission.

Purkinje cell. Then, parallel fibres and climbing fibres are co-stimulated in phase at a low frequency (1–4 Hz; dotted line). Five minutes after this conditioning stimulation, the response to the same parallel fibre stimulation recorded from the same Purkinje cell begins to decrease and stays attenuated thereafter. Cerebellar LTD is associated with an increase of Ca^{2+} concentration in Purkinje cell dendrites during the conditioning stimulation.

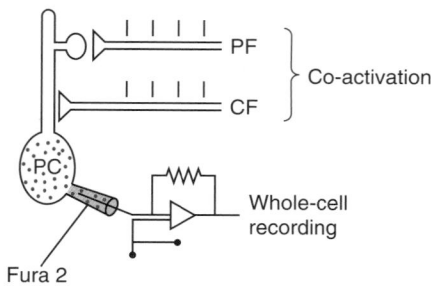

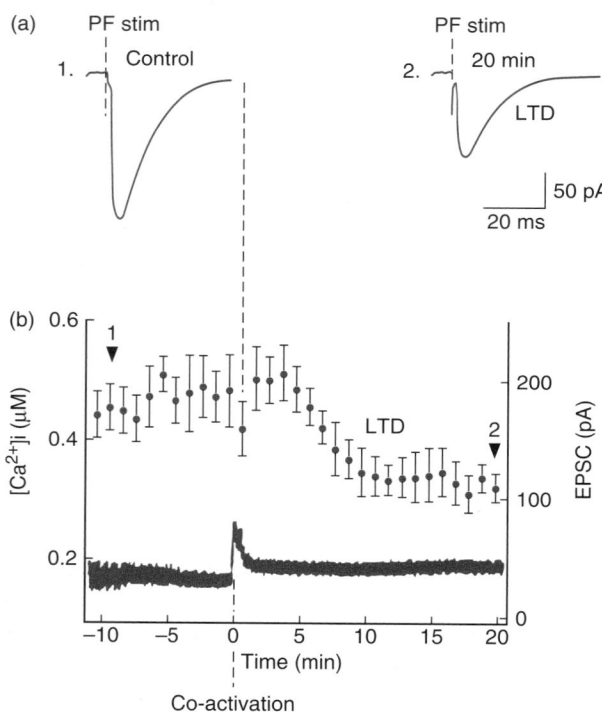

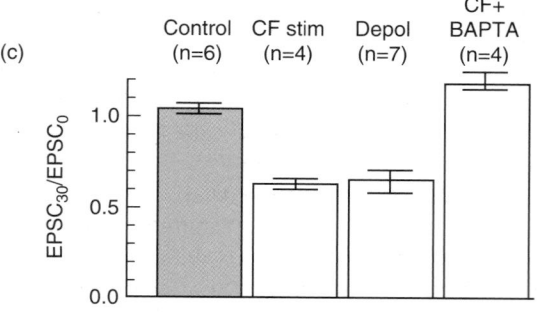

LTD of the response to parallel fibre is not observed when the parallel fibres are stimulated alone at 1–4 Hz; what adds the climbing fibre stimulation?

Voltage-gated Ca^{2+} channels located in the membrane of Purkinje cell dendrites are activated by the climbing-fibre-mediated EPSP. This suggests that the resulting increase of intradendritic Ca^{2+} concentration is a necessary prerequisite for LTD induction. This hypothesis is tested by hyperpolarizing the Purkinje cell membrane during the co-stimulation or by injecting of a Ca^{2+} chelator into the Purkinje cell before the co-stimulation (**Figure 21.15**), or by removing the external Ca^{2+} ions, in order to prevent the rise of intradendritic Ca^{2+} concentration: all these procedures block LTD induction. Along the same lines, climbing fibre stimulation can be replaced by direct intracellular depolarization of the Purkinje cell which evokes Ca^{2+} spikes. This is called the 'pairing protocol' (**Figure 21.16a**).

In conclusion, LTD of synaptic transmission at parallel-Purkinje cell synapses is triggered by a rise of intracellular Ca^{2+} concentration resulting from Ca^{2+} entry in Purkinje cell dendrites through voltage-gated Ca^{2+} channels opened by the membrane depolarization during co-stimulation of climbing and parallel fibres.

Figure 21.14 (Left) An increase of intracellular Ca^{2+} concentration is observed during LTD induction.
The activity of a Purkinje cell is recorded in patch clamp (whole-cell patch) in a thin slice of rat cerebellum. The patch pipette also contains FURA-2 in order to record on-line the intracellular Ca^{2+} concentration. **(a)** The excitatory postsynaptic current (EPSC) recorded in voltage clamp in response to parallel fibre stimulation (PF stim, 1 Hz) is recorded before (control) and 20 min after the conditioning stimulation (co-activation: conjunctive stimulation of parallel and climbing fibres while the Pc membrane is recorded in current clamp mode). **(b)** Time course of changes in parallel-fibre-mediated EPSC amplitude (top curve) and in [Ca^{2+}]$_i$ (bottom curve). The conditioning stimulation (given at time 0) induces a LTD of the EPSC (with a delay) and an immediate transient rise of [Ca^{2+}]$_i$. Note that the stimulation of parallel fibres before the conditioning stimulation does not induce significant changes of [Ca^{2+}]$_i$. **(c)** Average changes in PF-mediated EPSC expressed as the ratio of EPSC amplitude before (EPSC$_0$) and 30 min (EPSC$_{30}$) after co-activation, in four different conditions: no co-activation (control), co-activation (CF stim), pairing (depol) and co-activation in the presence of BAPTA (CF + BAPTA) in the patch electrode. From Konnerth A, Dreessen J, Augustine GJ (1992) Brief dendritic calcium signals initiate long lasting synaptic depression in cerebellar Purkinje cells, *Proc. Natl Acad. Sci. USA* **89**, 7051–7055, with permission.

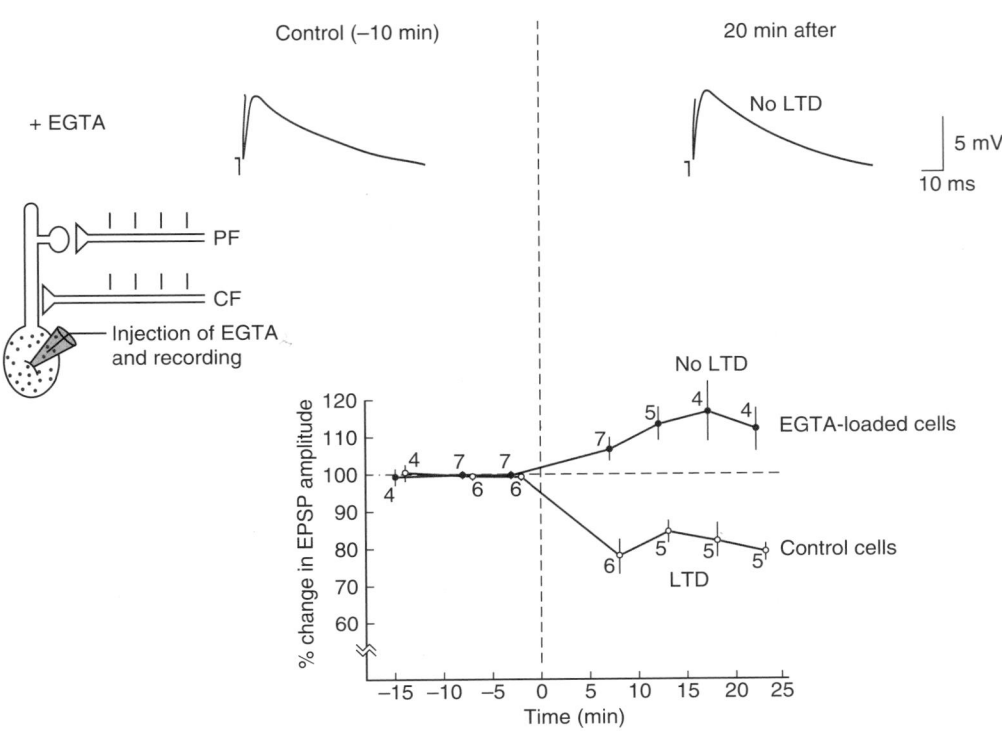

Figure 21.15 The induction of cerebellar LTD requires an increase of intracellular Ca²⁺ concentration.
The activity of a Purkinje cell is intracellularly recorded (current clamp mode) in a guinea pig cerebellar slice. The amplitude of the EPSP recorded in response to parallel fibre stimulation is recorded before and after the conditioning stimulation (conjunctive stimulation of PF and CF at 4 Hz for 25 s) in control cells (white circles). The same experiment is performed after intracellular injection of the Ca²⁺ chelator EGTA into the recorded Purkinje cells (black circles). The respective averaged EPSPs recorded in the presence of EGTA are shown in the insets. The time 0 represents the end of conjunctive stimulation. The values at each plotted point represent the number of cells recorded. Adapted from Sakurai M (1990) Calcium is an intracellular mediator of the climbing fiber in induction of cerebellar long term depression, *Proc. Natl Acad. Sci. USA* **87**, 3383–3385, with permission.

LTD of the response to parallel fibre is not observed when the climbing fibre is stimulated alone at 1–4 Hz; what adds the parallel fibre stimulation?

The glutamate released from parallel fibre terminals activates the non-NMDA receptors present in the postsynaptic membrane (ionotropic AMPA receptors and metabotropic glutamate receptors, mGluR1; **Figure 21.11**, inset). AMPA receptors mediate the excitatory response (EPSP or EPSC) evoked by parallel fibre stimulation since it is totally blocked by the application of CNQX, a selective antagonist of this class of receptors. In order to test the role of non-NMDA receptors in LTD induction, CNQX is bath applied during or after a pairing protocol (direct Purkinje cell depolarization with parallel fibre stimulation). The blockade of non-NMDA receptors during the pairing protocol prevents LTD induction while it has no effect after the pairing protocol (once LTD is induced) (**Figures 21.16b and c**).

In order to test the role of the non-NMDA receptors in LTD induction, parallel fibre stimulation can also be replaced by external application of agonists at non-NMDA receptors. Parallel fibre stimulation during the conditioning stimulus can be replaced by the application on the Purkinje cell dendrites of glutamate or quisqualate (agonists on *both* AMPA and metabotropic receptors, or a solution containing *both* AMPA and an agonist of metabotropic receptors) (see **Figures 21.21c and d**). The activation of AMPA receptors alone by AMPA or the application of NMDA are ineffective. This is in keeping with the recent demonstration that antibodies directed against mGluR1 subunit blocks LTD induction in cultured Purkinje cells. The final demonstration of the participation of mGluR to LTD induction in acute cerebellar slices has been given recently by showing that LTD of the parallel fibre-mediated EPSP is markedly impaired in knockout mice lacking mGluR1 (see **Figure 21.21f** and Section 14.4).

In conclusion, the activation of the parallel fibres during the conjunctive or pairing stimulation allows the release of glutamate and the activation of both AMPA and metabotropic glutamatergic postsynaptic receptors.

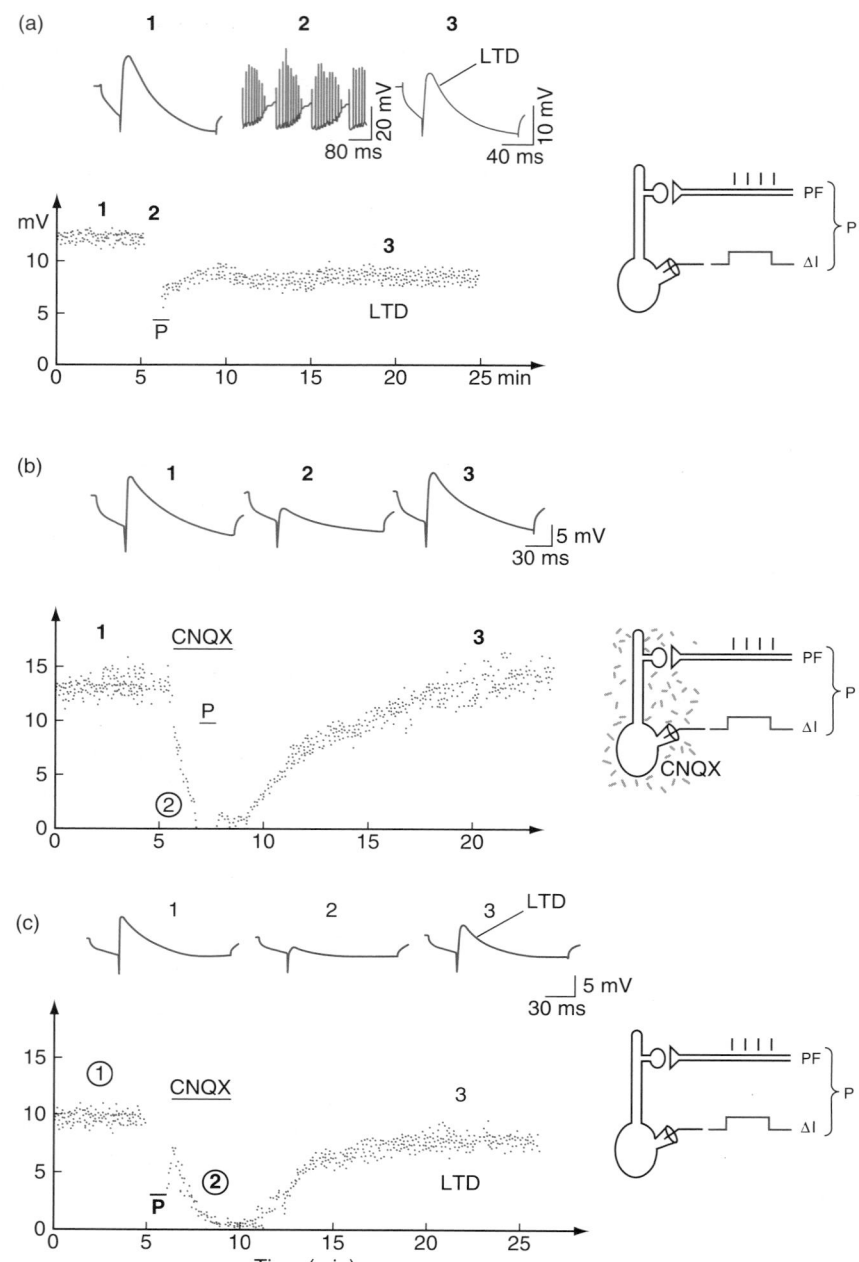

Figure 21.16 Induction of cerebellar LTD requires the activation of postsynaptic AMPA receptors.
The activity of a Purkinje cell is recorded in patch clamp (whole-cell patch, current clamp mode) in cerebellar thin slices. The PF-mediated EPSP is evoked during a hyperpolarizing current pulse before and after the pairing in order to test the variation of membrane resistance during the experiment. (**a**, top traces) A control EPSP is recorded in response to parallel fibre stimulation (1). After the pairing (P) – i.e. intracellular depolarizing pulses to evoke Ca^{2+} spikes in conjunction with parallel fibre stimulation (2) – a LTD of the parallel-fibre-mediated EPSP is observed (3). Note the change in calibrations between 1, 3 and 2. (**a**, bottom trace) Plot of the EPSP amplitude against time. (**b**) The same experiment as in (a) but in the presence of CNQX (4 µM) in the bath before, during and after pairing (P). During CNQX application the parallel-fibre-mediated EPSP (2) is completely blocked since it is mediated by AMPA receptors. (**c**) The same experiment as in (b) but CNQX is bath applied after pairing (P). Part (a) adapted from Hémart N, Daniel H, Jaillard D *et al.* (1995) Receptors and second messengers involved in long term depression in rat cerebellar slices *in vitro*: a reappraisal, *Eur. J. Neurosci.* **7**, 45–53, with permission.

These, with the concomitant rise in intracellular calcium concentration, are possibly the necessary and sufficient processes for LTD induction, since the conditioning stimulation can be replaced by a direct depolarization of the Purkinje cell membrane to activate voltage-dependent Ca^{2+} channels (to mimic climbing fibre stimulation) and the concomitant application of agonists of AMPA and metabotropic receptors (to mimic parallel fibre stimulation) (see **Figure 21.21d**).

21.3.3 The expression of LTD involves a persistent desensitization of postsynaptic AMPA receptors

The fact that co-activation of Purkinje cells by climbing fibre stimulation and iontophoretic application of glutamate on Purkinje cell dendrites induces a long-lasting decrease of the response to this agonist led Masao Ito to postulate that LTD of parallel-fibre-mediated EPSP or EPSC is due to a long-term desensitization of ionotropic glutamate receptors of Purkinje cells (a desensitized state is a state where the probability of the channel opening is very low). This would explain the decrease in synaptic efficacy.

In Purkinje cells in cerebellar slices, a pairing procedure known to induce LTD of the synaptic response induces a long-lasting decrease of the response to iontophoretic application of glutamate (or quisqualate, not shown) but not of aspartate (**Figure 21.17**). This suggests that LTD of synaptic transmission between parallel fibres and Purkinje cells is accompanied by LTD of the responsiveness of Purkinje cells to glutamate or quisqualate, whereas that to aspartate is unaffected. The observed decrease in efficacy of glutamate or quisqualate in activating Purkinje cells could involve a desensitization of AMPA receptors. What are the mediators between Ca^{2+} entry and the long-term changes of AMPA receptors?

21.3.4 Second messengers are required for LTD induction: examples of protein kinases C and nitric oxide (NO)

Activation of PKC

The metabotropic receptors mGluR1 are abundantly expressed in Purkinje cells. These receptors are coupled to phospholipase C and their activation leads to the formation of inositol trisphosphate (IP_3) and diacylglycerol (DAG). Moreover, Ca^{2+}-dependent PKC is also expressed abundantly in Purkinje cells. Therefore,

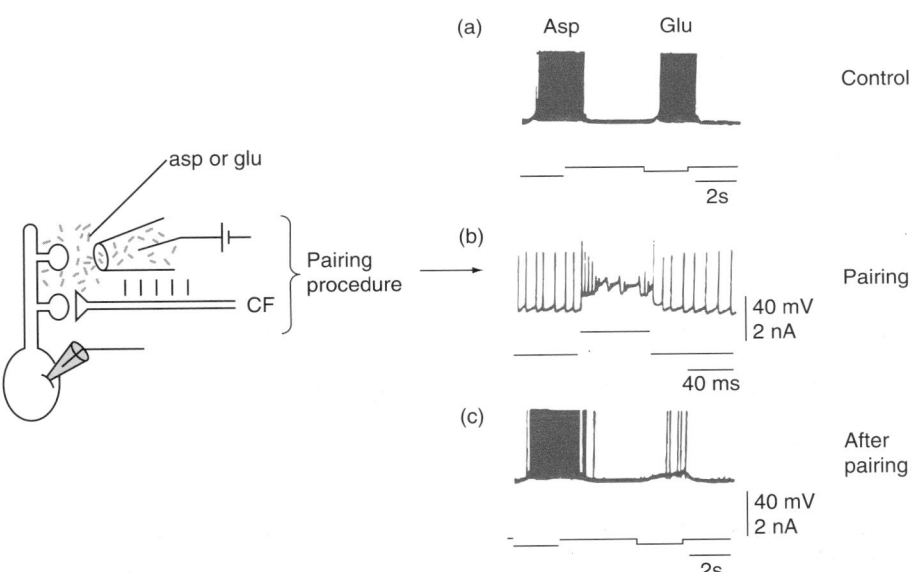

Figure 21.17 The postsynaptic glutamate response is selectively depressed.
The response of a Purkinje cell to iontophoretic application of glutamate (glu) or aspartate (asp) is intracellularly recorded (current clamp mode, $V_m = -65$ mV) in cerebellar slices. **(a)** Glutamate or aspartate are alternatively ejected in the dendritic field of the recorded Purkinje cell. They both evoke a transient membrane depolarization which reaches the firing level. **(b)** The conditioning stimulation used to induce LTD consists of climbing fibre stimulation (2–4 Hz) paired for 1 min with the ejections of glutamate and aspartate at 2 min intervals. **(c)** Twenty minutes after the pairing procedure, the response to glutamate is selectively depressed (the response to aspartate is left unaffected). Adapted from Crépel F, Krupa M (1988) Activation of protein kinase C induces a long term depression of glutamate sensitivity of cerebellar Purkinje cells: an *in vitro* study, *Brain Res.* **458**, 397–401, with permission.

during the conditioning stimulus, the Ca^{2+}-dependent kinases such as protein kinase C can be activated by both the increase of intracellular Ca^{2+} concentration due to climbing fibre activation (see **Figure 21.14b**) and the activation of mGluR1 by glutamate released from parallel fibres. The role of protein kinase C in LTD is tested by injecting into the recorded Purkinje cell a selective inhibitor of protein kinase C (PKC 19-36) before the conditioning stimulus (**Figure 21.18**). In such conditions, LTD is not induced. Moreover, selective expression of a PKC inhibitor in Purkinje cells in transgenic mice leads to a complete blockade of LTD induction, supporting the hypothesis that activation of PKC is necessary for LTD induction.

Antibodies directed against mGluR1 as well as mGluR1 knockout mice were used to demonstrate the role of these metabotropic receptors in LTD induction: in

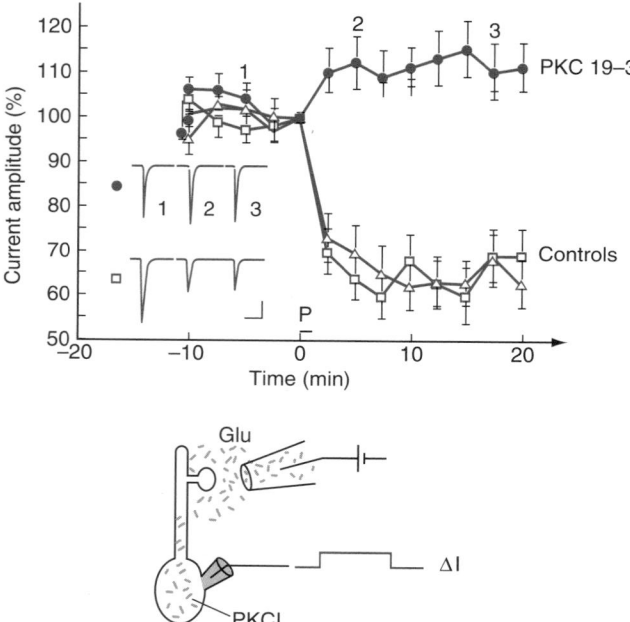

Figure 21.18 Protein kinase C inhibition prevents LTD induction.

The activity of a Purkinje cell is recorded in patch clamp (whole-cell patch) in the presence of the selective PKC inhibitor, PKC 19-36 (black circles) or a non-inhibitory control peptide (triangle) or the intracellular solution only (square) in the patch pipette. The control EPSC evoked by parallel fibre stimulation is recorded for 10 min and the conditioning stimulation is applied at $t = 0$. It consists of the conjunctive application of glutamate and intracellular depolarization. LTD of the EPSC is not observed in cells dialysed with PKC 19-36. Scale bars: 100 pA, 2 s. Adapted from Linden DJ, Connor JA (1991) Participation of postsynaptic PKC in cerebellar long term depression in culture, *Science* **254**, 1656–1659, with permission.

both preparations long-term depression at the parallel-fibre/Purkinje-cell synapse is absent. These preparations also permitted testing of the possible role of internal Ca^{2+} stores: Is the combination of direct activation of IP_3-sensitive Ca^{2+} stores in Purkinje cell dendrites and a conventional pairing protocol in mGluR1-deficient mice (mGluR1-/-), sufficient to rescue LTD in the cerebellum of these animals by bypassing the disrupted mGluR1 (**Figure 21.19**)? Caged-IP_3 and the fluorescent Ca^{2+}-sensitive dye fluo-3 are present in the whole-cell pipette. The recording session starts 30–45 minutes after whole-cell 'break in' to allow diffusion of the compounds in the dendrites of the recorded Purkinje cell *in vitro* (in cerebellar slices). Control parallel-fibre EPSPs are recorded in control conditions (trace 1). Pairing (simultaneous depolarization of the Purkinje cell and parallel-fibre stimulation) is first performed in the absence of photolysis of caged-IP_3. It induces only a transient depression of the EPSP (trace 2). A second pairing is then performed with concomitant photolysis of caged-IP_3. The transient intracellular Ca^{2+} increase in response to UV flash is visualized by the change of fluorescence of fluo-3 (bottom inset, $\Delta F/F$). After such pairing, parallel-fibre EPSPs are depressed by 76.2 ± 8.2% even 20 minutes after the pairing period (trace 3). The same protocol in the presence of the inhibitory PKC 19-36 peptide fails to induce LTD (not shown). This demonstrates that the impairment of LTD in mGluR1-deficient Purkinje cells is caused by the lack of functional mGluR1 preventing the second-messenger cascade activation. It also suggests that the combination of Ca^{2+} influx through voltage-gated Ca^{2+} channels (in response to Purkinje cell membrane depolarization) and Ca^{2+} release from IP_3-sensitive Ca^{2+} stores is capable of restoring LTD in mGluR1 knockout mice.

The hypothesis is the following. During the conditioning stimulus, the formation of diacylglycerol (DAG) following activation of mGluR1, together with the cytosolic Ca^{2+} increase due to the activation of voltage-gated channels (and perhaps the release of Ca^{2+} ions from internal stores due to the formation of IP_3), leads to the activation of protein kinase C. This, with other second-messenger cascades, would lead directly or indirectly to phosphorylation of AMPA receptors and activation of their transition to a stable desensitized state and thus to LTD (**Figure 21.20**).

NO formation and cGMP

Nitric oxide (NO) is a gas that is highly diffusible through the lipidic membranes. It is synthesized from arginine in the presence of the NO synthase, with one form sensitive to Ca^{2+} ions. NO synthase is absent in Purkinje cells but is expressed at high levels in

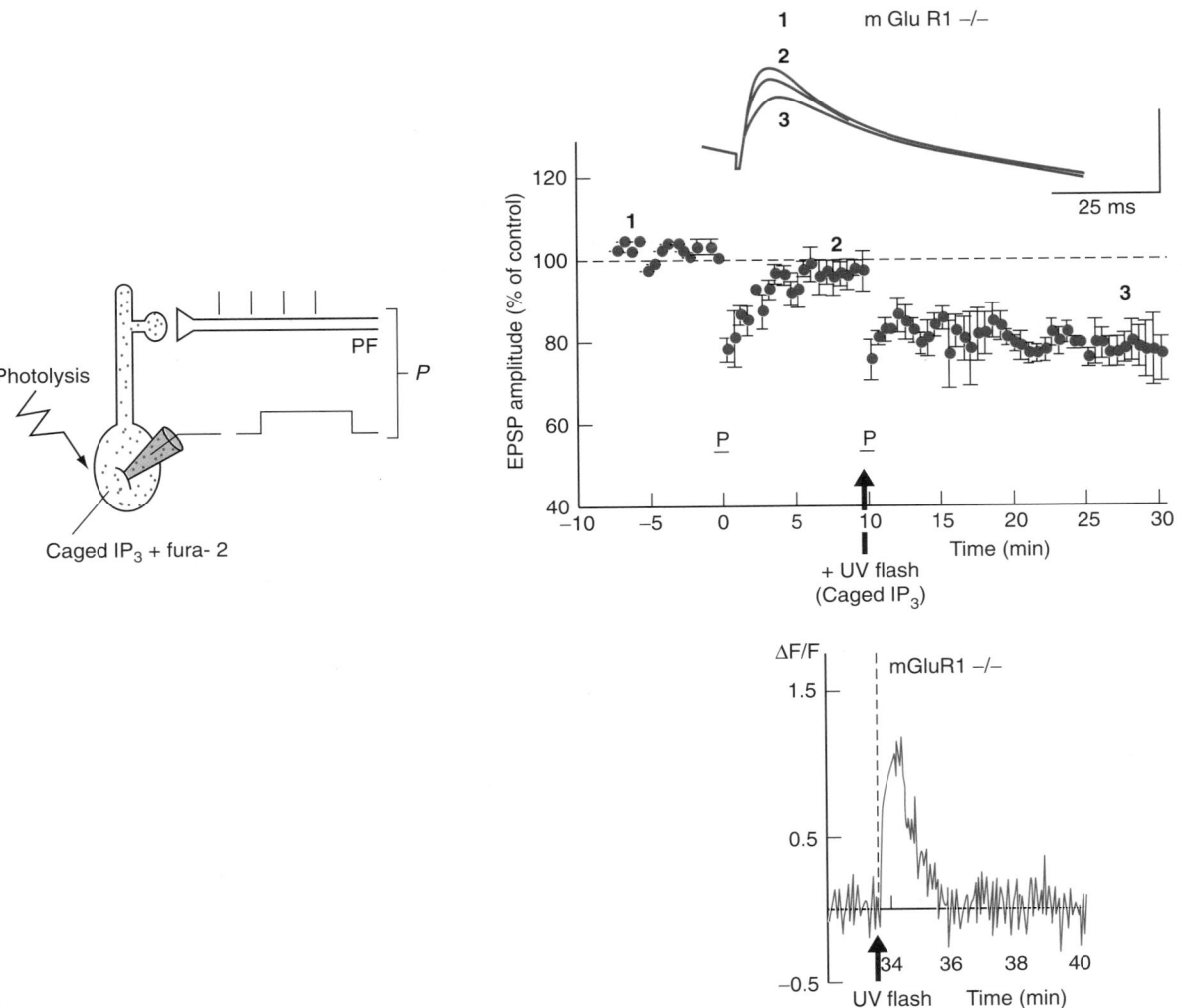

Figure 21.19 LTD in mGluR1-deficient Purkinje cells.
The central plot represents the normalized amplitude of PF-mediated EPSPs against time before and after two successive pairing protocols (P), first at $t = 0$ in the control condition and then at $t = 10$ minutes, combined with photolysis of caged IP3. Each point is the mean ± SEM of separate experiments in four cells. The top inset represents superimposed averaged EPSPs recorded at the indicated times. The bottom inset represents the Ca-induced fluorescence change evoked by photorelease of caged IP3 in a FURA-2-loaded cell. Adapted from Daniel H, Levenes C, Fagni L *et al.* (1999) Inositol-1,4,5-trisphosphate-mediated rescue of cerebellar long-term depression in subtype 1 metabotropic glutamate receptor mutant mouse, *Neuroscience* **91**, 1–6, with permission.

neighbouring neural elements such as parallel fibres and basket cells. The target of NO is probably the soluble (cytoplasmic) guanylate cyclase in cells where it is produced as well as in neighbouring cells. NO, by activating guanylate cyclase, would lead to the formation of cGMP.

In order to test a possible role of NO in LTD induction in cerebellar slices, a potent NO synthase inhibitor, *N*-methylarginine, is bath applied during the experiment. It totally prevents the induction of LTD in response to a classic pairing protocol. Moreover, bath application of a NO donor (sodium nitroprusside), or the injection of cGMP into Purkinje cells, both durably depress the par-allel-fibre-mediated EPSP (they mimic LTD). Finally, LTD is totally inhibited by intracellular injection into Purkinje cells of the selective and potent inhibitor of soluble guanylate cyclase, 1H-(1,2,4)oxadiazolo(4,3-a)quinoxalin-1-one (ODQ). All these results suggest that NO and cGMP participate in the events leading to LTD.

Pathways leading to NO synthase activation and increase of cGMP concentration in Purkinje cells are not yet fully understood. The hypothesis is the following. After a large entry of Ca^{2+} into Purkinje cells during a conventional pairing protocol, a resulting K^+ efflux through Ca^{2+}-activated K^+ conductances depolarizes neighbouring presynaptic cellular elements to such an

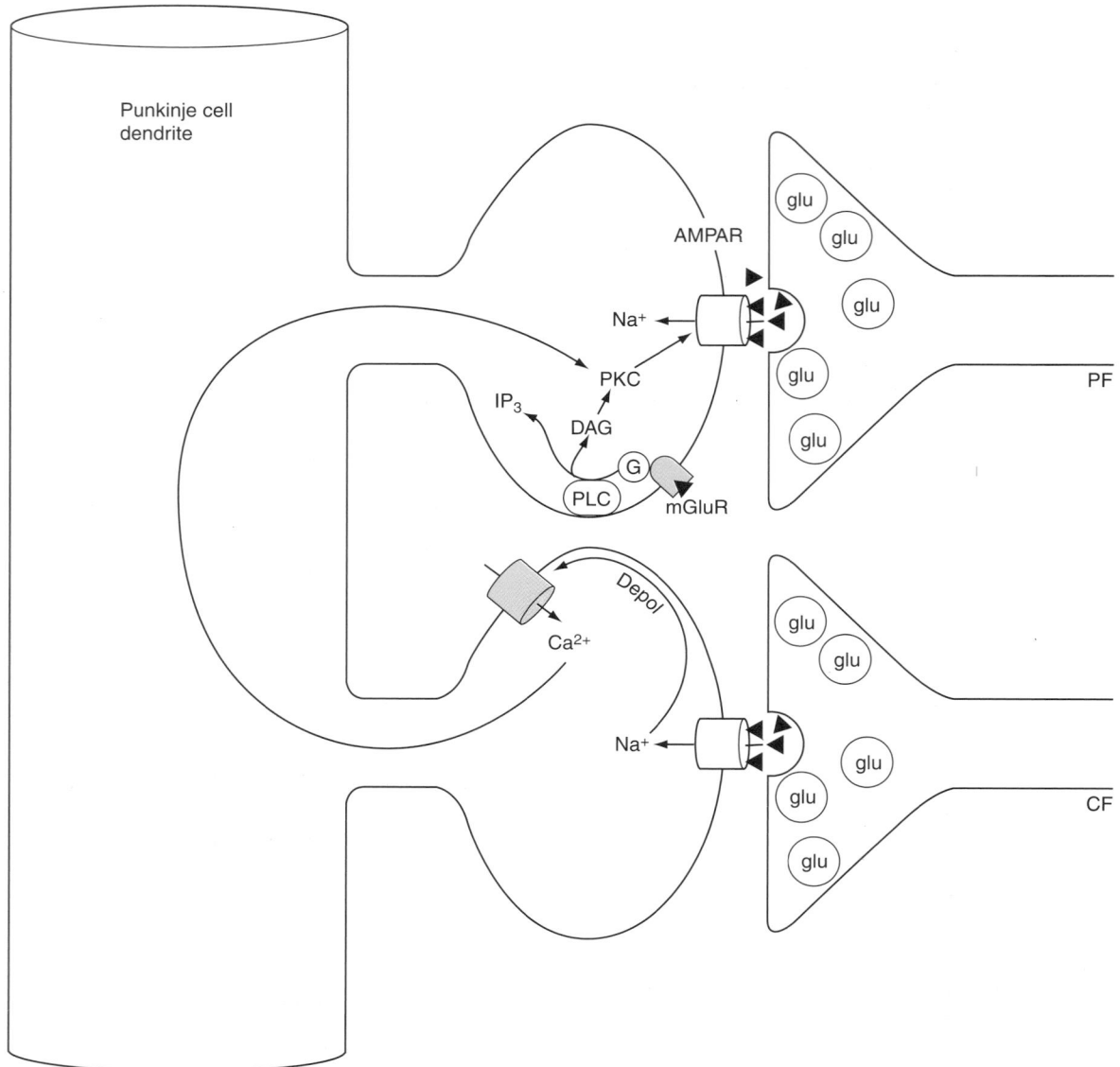

Figure 21.20 Schematic of some of the putative mechanisms of cerebellar LTD induction.

extent that they can produce a sufficient amount of NO to activate soluble guanylate cyclase in nearby Purkinje cells by a paracrine effect. Then, cGMP would in turn activate a cGMP-dependent protein kinase (PKG). The resulting phosphorylations would lead directly or indirectly to phosphorylation of AMPA receptors and activate their transition to a stable desensitized state and thus to LTD.

21.3.5 The different ways to induce or block cerebellar LTD

Long-term depression of the response of a Purkinje cell

to parallel fibre activation can be *induced* by (**Figures 21.21a–d**):

- conjunctive stimulation of the afferent parallel and climbing fibres;
- conjunctive stimulation of the parallel fibres and intracellular injection of a depolarizing current (which evokes Ca^{2+} spikes) into the Purkinje cell;
- conjunctive iontophoretic application of glutamate, quisqualate or AMPA + t-ACPD to the Purkinje cell dendrites and stimulation of its afferent climbing fibre;
- conjunctive iontophoretic application of glutamate or quisqualate or AMPA + t-ACPD to the Purkinje

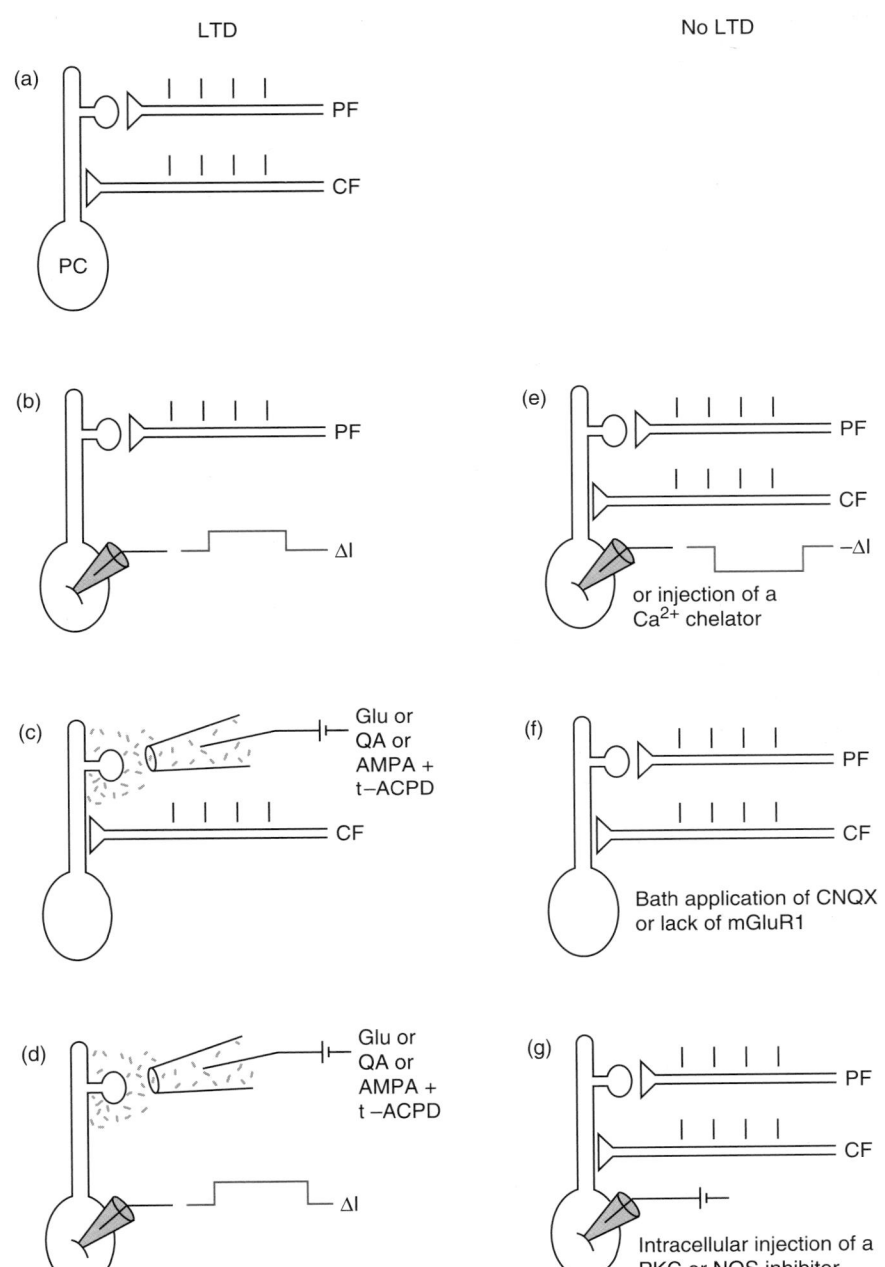

Figure 21.21 Cerebellar LTD.
The different ways of **(a)** induction or **(b)** blockade of induction.

cell dendrites and intracellular injection of depolarizing current (which evokes Ca²⁺ spikes) into the Purkinje cell.

Long-term depression of the response of a Purkinje cell to parallel fibre activation can be *blocked* by (**Figures 21.21e–g**):

- intracellular injection of a Ca²⁺ chelator into the Purkinje cell or injection of a hyperpolarizing current

into the Purkinje cell during the conjunctive stimulation or the pairing protocol;

- bath application of CNQX or the lack of mGluR1 in the cerebellum and notably in Purkinje cell membrane (mGluR1 gene-deficient mice are obtained by disrupting the mGluR1 gene);

- intracellular injection in the Purkinje cell or bath application of an inhibitor of protein kinase C or NO synthase before the conditioning stimulus.

21.3.6 Summary: Principal features of LTD in parallel-fibre/Purkinje cell glutamatergic transmission

■ LTD results from a decrease of the parallel-fibre-mediated EPSC or EPSP without changes in the number of afferent axons stimulated: it is a depression of the synaptic efficacy.

■ LTD is a very long-lasting phenomenon since it persists for the duration of the experiment, up to several hours.

■ LTD is input specific: it is restricted to those parallel fibre synapses activated at the same time as climbing fibres.

■ LTD is associated with a large increase of Ca^{2+} concentration in Purkinje cell dendrites which occurs during the conjunctive stimulation of parallel and climbing fibres.

■ LTD is expressed as a depression of AMPA-mediated current at the parallel-fibre/Purkinje cell synapses activated at the same time as climbing fibres. It results from the long-term desensitization of AMPA receptors which requires the activation of protein kinase C and the production of NO (at least in intact tissues).

Further reading

Carroll RC, Lissin DV, Zastrow von M et al. (1999) Rapid redistribution of glutamate receptors contributes to long-term depression in hippocampal cultures. Nature Neurosci. 2, 454–460.

Conquet F, Bashir ZI, Davies CH et al. (1994) Motor deficit and impairment of synaptic plasticity in mice lacking mGluR1. Nature 372, 237–243.

Crépel F, Audinat E, Daniel H et al. (1994) Cellular locus of the nitric oxide-synthase involved in cerebellar long-term depression induced by high external potassium concentration. Neuropharmacology 33, 1399–1405.

De Zeeuw CI, Hansel C, Bian F et al. (1998) Expression of a protein kinase C inhibitor in Purkinje cells blocks cerebellar LTD and adaptation of the vestibulo-ocular reflex. Neuron 20, 495–508.

Galarreta M, Hestrin S (1999) Frequency-dependent synaptic depression and the balance of excitation and inhibition in the neocortex. Nature Neurosci. 1, 587–594.

Levenes C, Daniel H, Crépel F (1998) Long term depression of synaptic transpission in the cerebellum: cellular and molecular mechanisms revisited. Prog. Neurobiol. 55, 79–91.

Lev-Ram V, Makings LR, Keitz PF et al. (1995) Long-term depression in cerebellar Purkinje neurons results from coincidence of nitric oxide and depolarization-induced Ca^{2+} transients. Neuron 15, 407–415.

Magee JC, Johnston D (1997) A synaptically controlled, associative signal for Hebbian plasticity in hippocampal neurons. Science 275, 209–213.

Malenka RC, Nicoll RA (1999) Long term potentiation: a decade of progress? Science 285, 1870–1874.

Sanes JR, Lichtman JW (1999) Can molecules explain long term potentiation? Nature Neurosci. 2, 597–604.

Shi SH, Hayashi Y, Petralia RS et al. (1999) Rapid spine delivery and redistribution of AMPA receptors after synaptic NMDA receptors activation. Science 284, 1811–1816.

Yeckel MF, Kapur A, Johnston D (1999) Multiple forms of LTP in hippocampal CA3 neurons use a common postsynaptic mechanism. Nature Neurosci. 2, 625–630.

Part 4

Activity and Development of Networks: The Hippocampus as an Example

The Adult Hippocampal Network

The hippocampus is part of the limbic system which mediates emotions and aspects of learning and memory. In the rat, it is a rostro-caudal structure (**Figure 22.1**) whereas in primates it is strictly localized in the temporal lobe.

The hippocampus is composed of two interconnected crescent-like regions (**Figures 22.2a and b**): the Ammon's horn (cornu ammonis) and the dentate gyrus (DG, also called fascia dentata). On a coronal section, Ammon's horn of the rat can be further subdivided into two regions, CA1 and CA3 (CA for cornu ammonis) (**Figure 22.2b**). In humans, two other subdivisions exist, CA2 and CA4. CA2 lies between CA1 and CA3 whereas CA4 is inserted in the dentate gyrus. Ammon's horn and dentate gyrus both contain a layer of principal neurons that are projection neurons (Golgi type I): the pyramidal cells and the granular cells, respectively. Numerous local interneurons (Golgi type II) are present in each region. Principal cells use an excitatory amino acid as a neurotransmitter whereas interneurons use GABA.

22.1 Observations and questions

What is a network?

In nuclei of the central nervous system, various types of neurons are generally present: projection neurons (Golgi type I) whose axons project to neurons located outside the nucleus, and local interneurons (Golgi type II) whose axons project to neurons located inside the nucleus. These neuronal types are connected to each other (intrinsic connections): they form a network. Each network receives afferents from neurons located in other nuclei (extrinsic connections).

Are networks completely different from one nucleus to another or are there some fundamental principles of organization?

In the neocortex and hippocampus, Golgi type I neurons

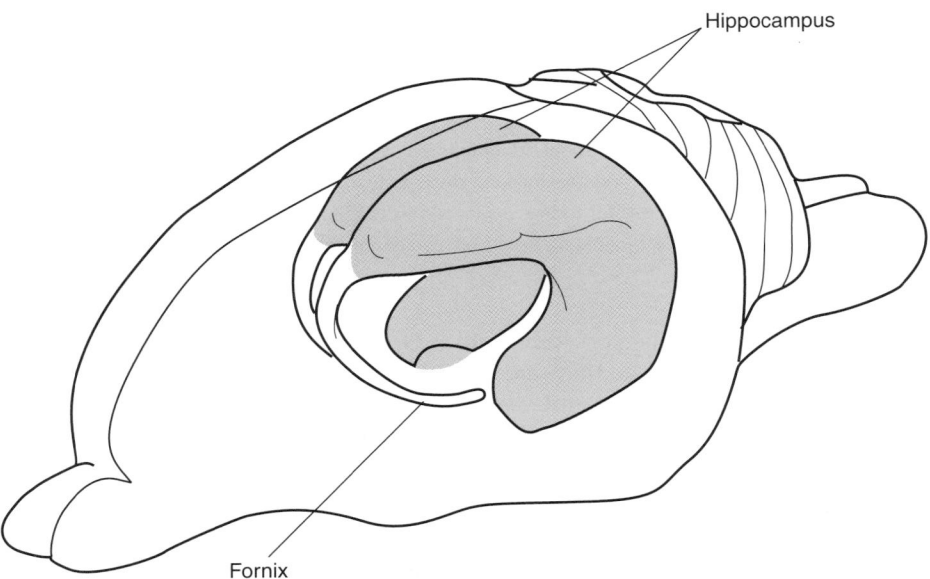

Figure 22.1 **Schematic of the localization of the two hippocampi inside a rat brain.**

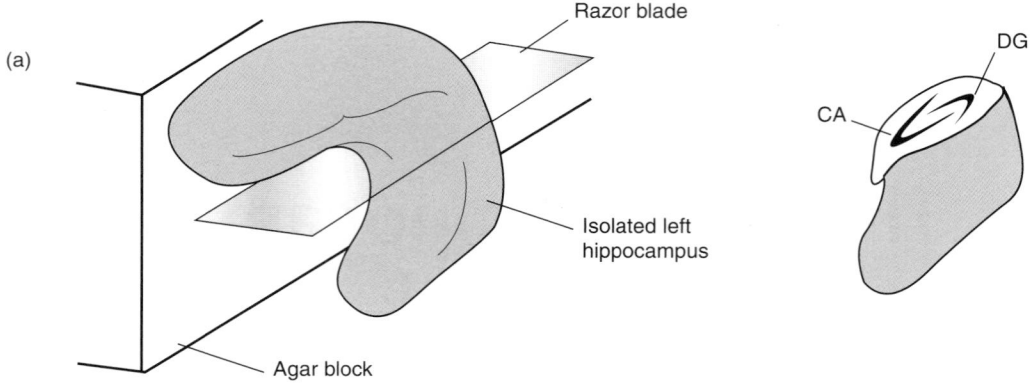

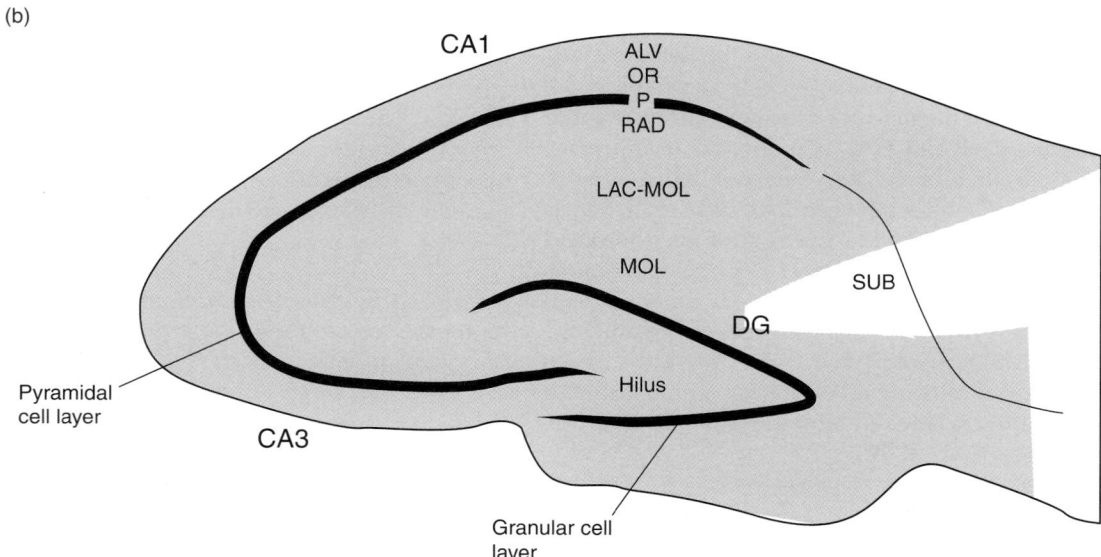

Figure 22.2 Structure of the rat hippocampus.

(a) Schematic of the slice preparation protocol. **(b)** Bright-field photomicrograph of a transverse section of the hippocampus stained with the Nissl method which stains neuronal somata and proximal dendrites (due to the presence of the Golgi apparatus). gr, granular cell; pyr, pyramidal cell; SUB, subiculum. See the text for further explanations. Adapted from Ishizuka N, Weber J, Amaral DG (1990) Organization of intrahippocampal projections originating from CA3 pyramidal cells in the rat, *J. Comp. Neurol.* **295**, 580–623, with permission.

are the pyramidal cells, in the cerebellar cortex they are the Purkinje cells, and in the striatum they are the medium spiny neurons. Pyramidal cells are glutamatergic whereas Purkinje cells and medium spiny neurons are GABAergic. Aside from these principal cells, a large variety of local GABAergic interneurons are present in all these nuclei.

Does the precise knowledge of intrinsic and extrinsic connections as well as the firing patterns of neurons allow us to explain how network oscillations are generated?

In the hippocampus of the freely moving rat, several types of oscillations are recorded from populations of neurons *in vivo* (extracellular recordings). For example, a rhythmic slow activity called 'theta' (5–10 Hz) is recorded during exploratory behaviour, such as sniffing,

(a)

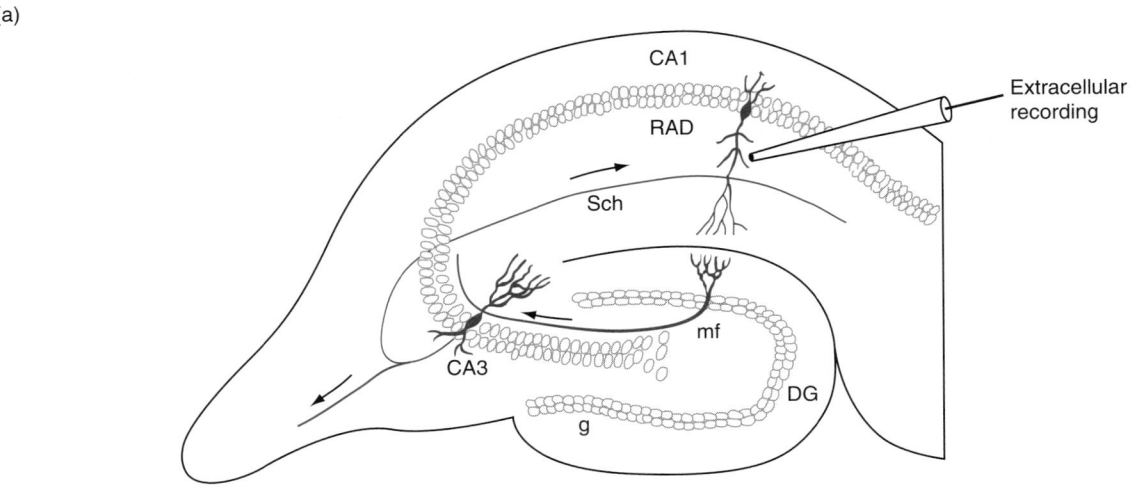

(b)

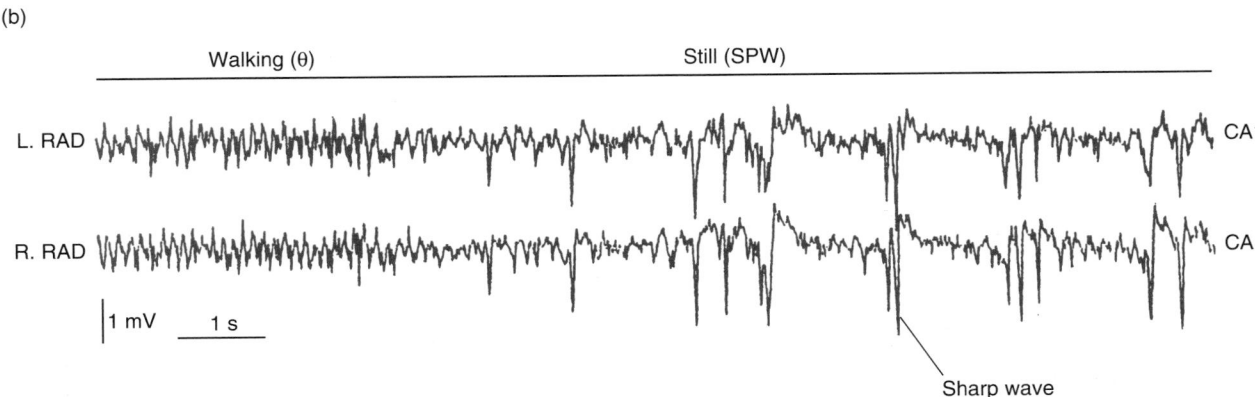

Figure 22.3 Extracellular field recordings of hippocampal oscillations in a freely moving rat.
An extracellular recording electrode is implanted in the stratum radiatum of the CA1 region of each hippocampus, the left (L) and the right (R). During exploratory activity (walking), regular theta waves are recorded (θ); during immobility, large monophasic sharp waves (SPW) are recorded. Note the bilaterally synchronous nature of SPW. Adapted from Buzsàki G (1989) Two-stage model of memory trace formation: a role for 'noisy' brain states, *Neuroscience* **31**, 551–570, with permission.

rearing and walking, and the paradoxical phase of sleep; once the animal stays still, or during consummatory behaviours or slow-wave sleep, intermittent sharp waves (SPW) are recorded in the dendritic layer of CA1–CA3 (**Figure 22.3**). These oscillations are network oscillations.

Neuronal oscillations have two main origins. They can be *intrinsic* to the neuron when they result from the activation of a cascade of currents intrinsic to the membrane, as described for thalamic and subthalamic neurons in Section 20.4. They can be *extrinsic* when they result from the activity of a group of interconnected neurons, from the activity of their synapses, as is the case for hippocampal neurons.

The aim of the present chapter is to give a description

of the adult hippocampal network and to explain how it can generate oscillations.

22.2 The hippocampal circuitry

22.2.1 Ammon's horn

Ammon's horn is a curved structure. It has a laminar organization with five layers. Owing to its U-shape, the layers (and pyramidal cells) are upside down in CA1 compared with CA3 (**Figures 22.2b** and **22.6b**).

Principal cells are called the pyramidal cells; they use an excitatory amino acid, probably glutamate, as a neurotransmitter

The principal cells, the pyramidal cells, have their soma aligned in a thin layer called the *pyramidal cell layer* (**Figure 22.2b**). The name of these cells comes from the clear pyramidal shape of their dendritic tree (**Figure 22.4a**). The cell body has a diameter of 20 µm. Three main dendritic trunks emerge from the cell body, one apical and two basal. Apical dendrites extend in the stratum radiatum (so called because of the radial organization of apical dendrites from all pyramidal cells) and arborize in stratum lacunosum moleculare. Basal dendrites ramify in stratum oriens. Dendrites have numerous spines. In CA3, the proximal part of apical dendrites of pyramidal cells present giant spines (thorny excrescences; **Figure 22.4b**) that are the postsynaptic elements of the synapses with granular cells of dentate gyrus (see below). Axons of pyramidal cells run in stratum alveus where they emit numerous collaterals before leaving the hippocampus.

Several types of inhibitory interneurons innervate pyramidal neurons; they use GABA as a neurotransmitter, and their cell body is located in the four more internal layers of CA

The activity of pyramidal cells is modulated not only by extrinsic afferences but also by intrinsic ones coming from local inhibitory interneurons. Four main types of inhibitory interneurons have been described in Ammon's horn, all GABAergic. They have their cell bodies in the five layers of the CA regions which are from the external to the internal part of the hippocampus (**Figures 22.2b** and **22.5a**, left): stratum alveole (ALV), stratum oriens (OR), stratum pyramidale (p), stratum radiatum (RAD) and stratum lacunosum moleculare (LAC-MOL). Interneurons are classified according to their site(s) of termination on pyramidal neurons (**Figure 22.5a**, right):

- Basket cells (BC) innervate the soma and proximal dendrites located in stratum pyramidale and radiatum. Cell bodies of basket cells are located in stratum pyramidale.
- Bistratified cells (BiC) innervate both apical and basal dendrites on their proximal part located in stratum radiatum and oriens. Cell bodies of bistratified cells are located in stratum oriens/radiatum.
- Oriens-lacunosum moleculare cells (O-LMC)

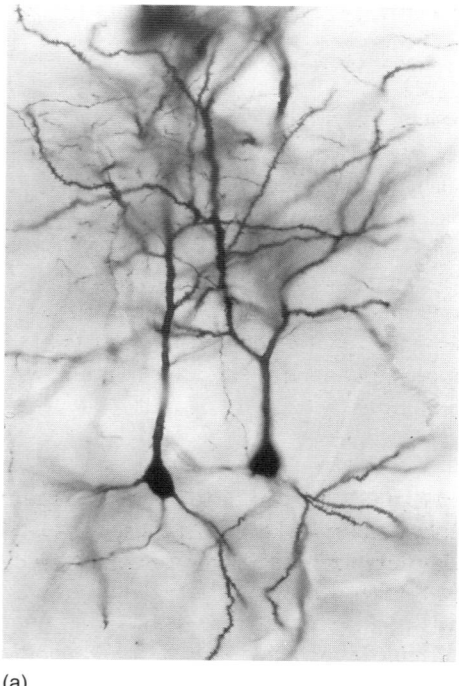

(a)

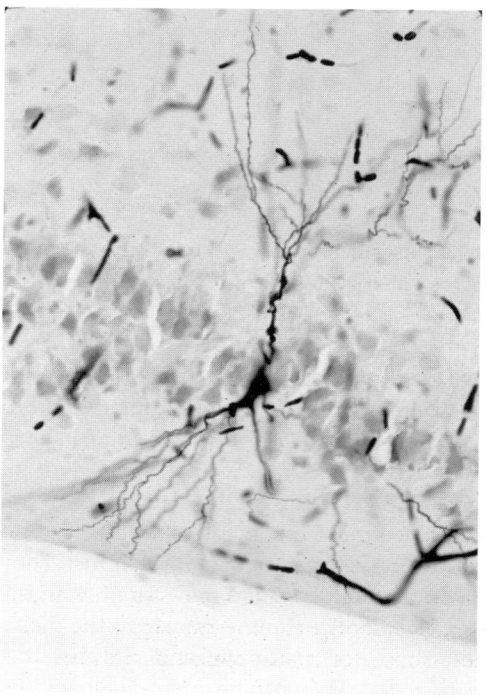

(b)

Figure 22.4 Photomicrographs of stained Golgi CA1 and CA3 pyramidal neurons.
(a) CA1; (b) CA3. In (b) a Nissl colouration shows the density of neuronal cell bodies in the pyramidal layer. Photographs: (a) by Olivier Robain; (b) by Jean Luc Gaiarsa.

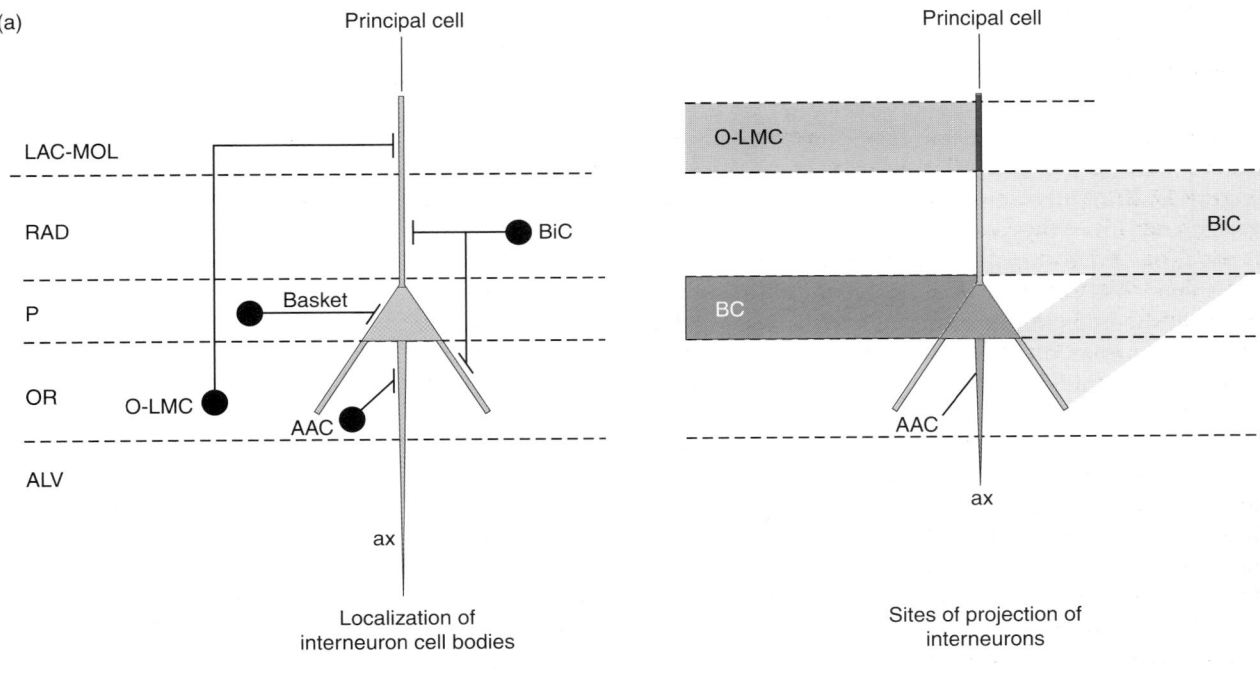

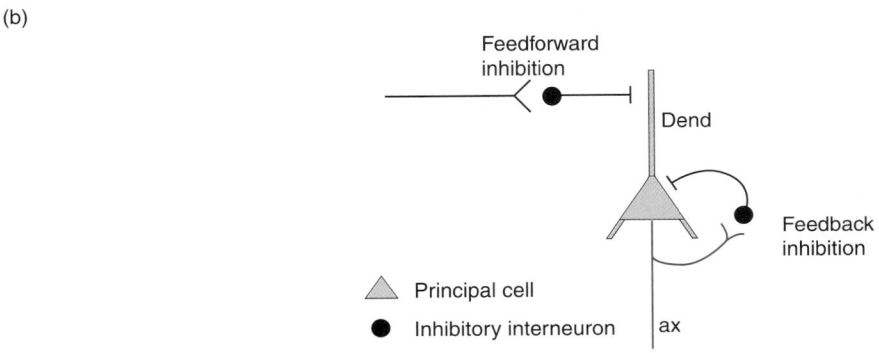

Figure 22.5 Intrinsic connections in CA1 and CA3.

(a) Schematic of a pyramidal cell indicating the localization of the cell bodies of the different interneurons (left) and the segregated postsynaptic domains innervated by the distinct presynaptic interneurons (right). **(b)** Illustration of feedforward and feedback inhibition. Part (a) adapted from Maccaferri G, Roberts DB, Szucs P *et al.* (2000) Cell surface domain specific postsynaptic currents evoked by identified GABAergic neurones in rat hippocampus *in vitro*, *J. Physiol.* **524**, 91–116, with permission.

innervate distal apical dendrites located in stratum lacunosum moleculare. Cell bodies of O-LMC are located in stratum oriens.

■ Axo-axonic cells (AAC), also called chandelier cells, innervate exclusively the axon initial segment. Cell bodies of axo-axonic cells are located in stratum oriens.

When interneurons are activated by extrinsic afferences they participate in feedforward inhibition; when they are activated by recurrent axon collaterals of pyramidal cells they participate in feedback inhibition (**Figure 22.5b**). Some interneurons like O-LMC are involved only in feedback inhibition since they are activated only by axon collaterals from principal cells.

22.2.2 The dentate gyrus

The dentate gyrus is also a curved structure, with a U-shape and a three-layer organization (see **Figure 22.2b**).

Principal cells called the granular cells use an excitatory amino acid as a neurotransmitter

The principal cells called the granular cells have their soma densely packed in a thin layer, the granular cell layer. Somas have a small diameter (14–18 μm) and are ovoid. Dendritic trees emerge from the apical pole of somas and form the molecular layer. Axons, called mossy fibres, have a small diameter (0.5 μm) and are not myelinated. They emerge from the basal pole of somas, divide in the hilus in numerous collaterals that contact local interneurons, and cross the hilus to make synapses with CA3 pyramidal cells.

Several types of inhibitory interneurons innervate granular cells; they use GABA as a neurotransmitter and their cell body is located in the three layers of DG

The same four types of interneurons as those found in Ammon's horn have been described in the dentate gyrus (DG). Interneurons located in stratum pyramidale in CA are located in the granular layer in DG. Similarly, interneurons located in stratum oriens of CA are in the hilus of DG and those in stratum radiatum of CA are in stratum moleculare of DG.

22.2.3 Principal cells form a tri-neural excitatory circuit

The main circuit inside the hippocampal formation involves the principal cells: granular cells of DG, pyramidal cells of CA1 and pyramidal cells of CA3. All these cells use an excitatory amino acid as a neurotransmitter. First, granular cells project on to CA3 pyramidal cells (**Figure 22.6a**). Their axon (called mossy fibres) terminates on the proximal portion of CA3 apical dendrites, on to giant spines. This restricted zone of projection forms the stratum lucidum (LUC), a sublayer of the radiatum that exists only in the CA3 region. Synapses between mossy fibres and dendritic spines of CA3 pyramidal cells are giant synapses (see **Figure 7.3**). In turn, CA3 pyramidal cells send axon collaterals, called the Schaffer collaterals, to CA1 pyramidal cells, on the distal part of their apical dendrites, at the level of stratum lacunosum moleculare. In coronal slices *in vitro*, all these circuits are present since they are organized in the transverse plane (**Figure 22.6b**).

In addition, pyramidal cells of the CA3 and CA1 regions emit local axon collaterals that contact local interneurons. Similarly, granular cells emit axon collaterals that locally innervate interneurons. Moreover, in CA3, pyramidal cells are connected to each other by

excitatory recurrent collaterals (**Figure 22.6c**). Therefore, local circuits superimpose on the main tri-neuronal excitatory circuit (**Figure 22.7**). Local circuits are detailed below in Sections 22.3 and 22.4.

22.2.4 Extrinsic afferences to principal cells and interneurons

The two major pathways that convey afferent information to the hippocampus are the *perforant* pathway coming from entorhinal cortex and the *fornix* coming from the medial septum and anterior thalamus. Moreover, the two hippocampi are interconnected by the *commissural* pathway. These connections and their functions will not be studied here.

22.3 Activation of interneurons evoke inhibitory GABAergic responses in post-synaptic pyramidal cells

To study the response of a postsynaptic pyramidal neuron to a presynaptic interneuron, the activity of these connected neurons is recorded concomitantly. Two neurons that are connected are called a pair.

22.3.1 Experimental protocol to study pairs of neurons

The hippocampus is an adequate structure to study pairs of neurons. Thanks to its laminar organization, the localization of the cell bodies of the different neurons is strictly organized. For example, in slices of the rat hippocampus, when an electrode is inserted in the pyramidal layer of the CA1 region, the probability of impaling or patching the cell body of a pyramidal neuron is high and that of an interneuron (a basket cell for example) around ten times less (**Figure 22.5a**, left). Conversely, when the electrode is inserted in stratum oriens or radiatum, the probability of impaling or patching a pyramidal cell is close to 0 whereas that for an interneuron (O-LMC, AAC, BiC) it is very high, close to 1.

To record the activity of an interneuron–pyramidal cell pair, one electrode (electrode 1) is placed in stratum oriens or radiatum or pyramidale to patch or impale an interneuron, and the other electrode (electrode 2) is placed in the stratum pyramidale to patch or impale a pyramidal cell (**Figure 22.8**). The activity of the interneuron is always recorded in current clamp mode and the activity of the pyramidal cell is recorded either in voltage clamp (to record the inhibitory postsynaptic current or IPSC) or current clamp (to record the inhibitory postsynaptic potential or IPSP). Recordings

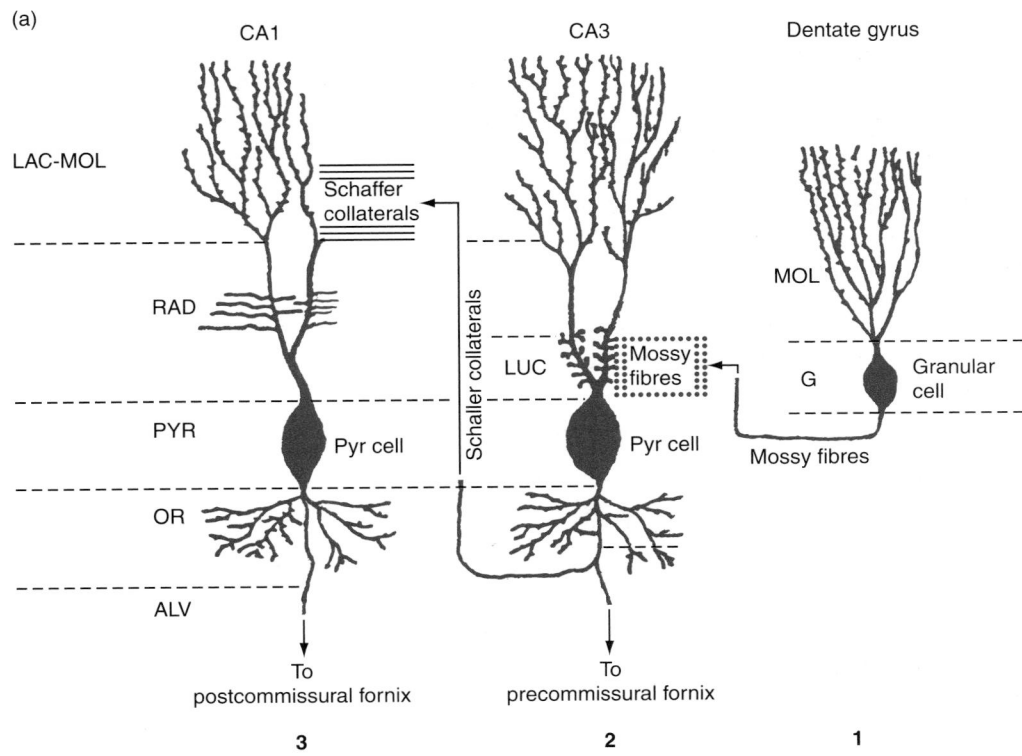

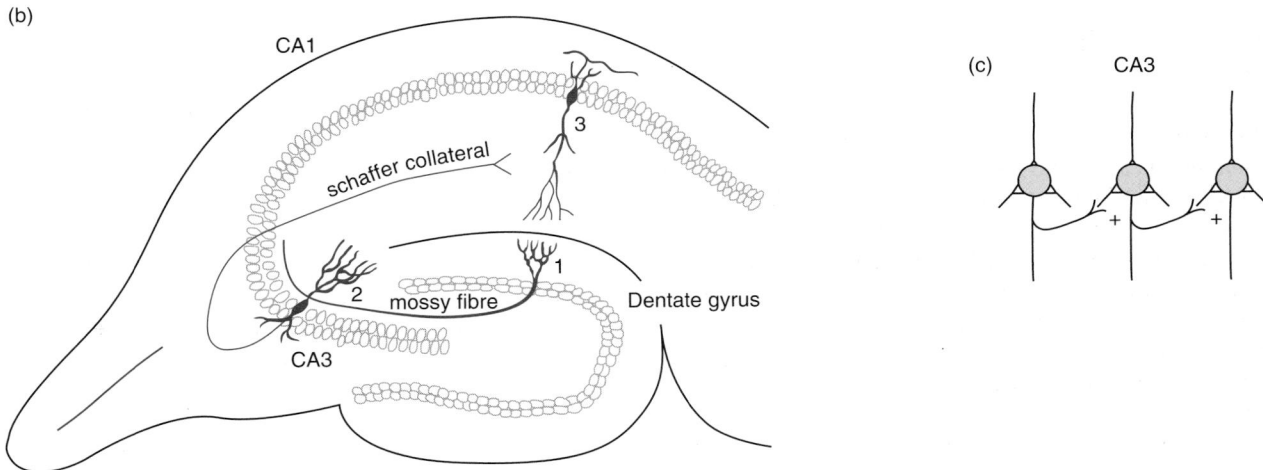

Figure 22.6 The tri-neuronal circuit between principal cells.

(a) Sites of termination of axons of principal cells on target principal cells (which are CA1 and CA3 pyramidal cells). Axons of granular cells are called mossy fibres. Axonal collaterals of CA3 pyramidal cells are called Schaffer collaterals. (b) The tri-neuronal circuit is organized in the transverse plane. LUC, stratum lucidum of CA3; pyr cell, pyramidal cell. (c) Illustration of recurrent excitation. Part (a) adapted from Altman J, Brunner RL, Bayer SA (1973) The hippocampus and behavioral maturation, *Behav. Biol.* **8**, 557–596, with permission.

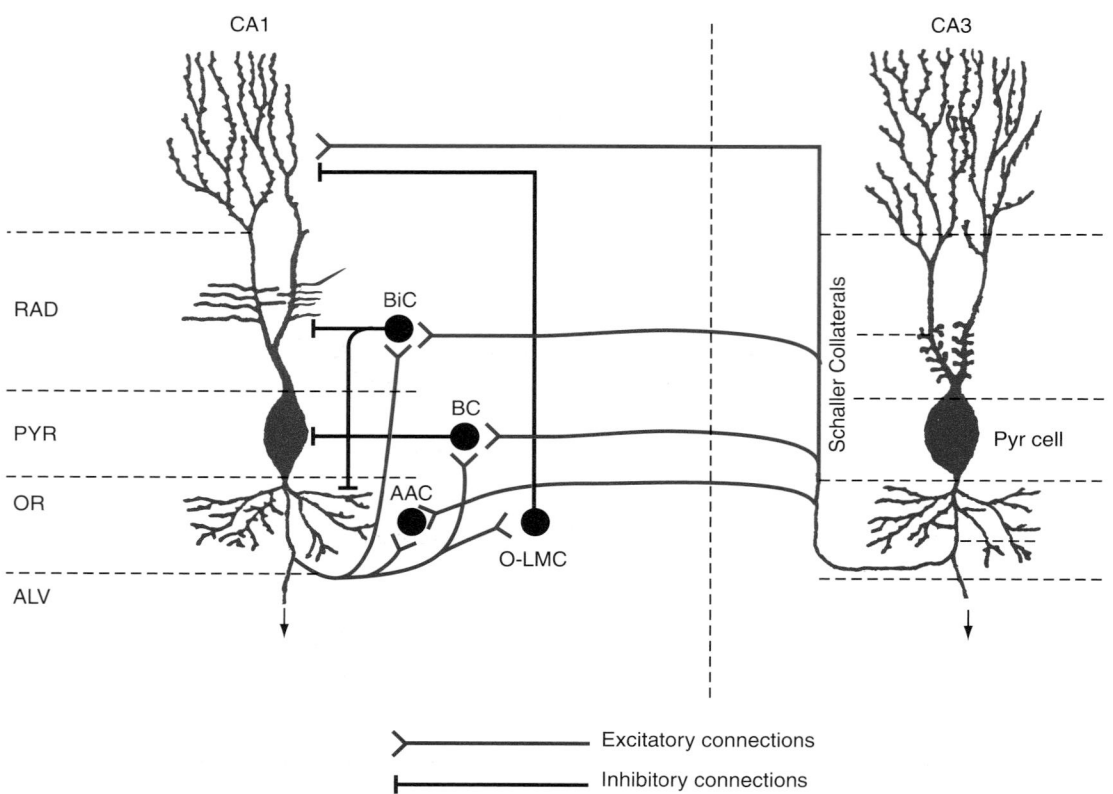

CA1

CA3

RAD

BiC

BC

PYR

OR

AAC

O-LMC

ALV

Schaffer Collaterals

Pyr cell

Excitatory connections

Inhibitory connections

Figure 22.7 Schematic of the synaptic circuitry in the CA1 region of the hippocampus and afferent connections from Schaffer collaterals of CA3 pyramidal cells.

Adapted from Altman J, Brunner RL, Bayer SA (1973) The hippocampus and behavioral maturation, *Behav. Biol.* **8**, 557–596, with permission.

are performed with either intracellular or whole-cell electrodes. Interneurons and pyramidal cells are identified during the recording session. To do so, spontaneous action potentials and evoked responses are recorded. Interneurons are characterized by the presence of an after-hyperpolarization following their action potentials and by their response to a long-lasting depolarizing current pulse which lacks spike frequency accommodation (**Figure 22.8** – compare recordings in (a) and (b)).

To check a connection between the interneuron and the pyramidal cell, electrode 1 is used as the stimulatory electrode and electrode 2 as the recording one. Spontaneous firing of the recorded interneuron is prevented by the continuous injection of a hyperpolarizing current. A suprathreshold square current pulse is injected into the interneuron to evoke action potentials (an example is given in **Figure 22.9**). If an IPSC or IPSP is evoked in the pyramidal cell in response to interneuron stimulation, the two neurons are thus identified as a pair of synaptically coupled neurons. If no synaptic response is recorded, electrode 1 is left in place and electrode 2 is changed (or the reverse). Another interneuron or pyramidal cell is patched (or impaled) and stimu-

lated. When a pair is found, the study of the synaptic response can begin.

After the recording session, the type of interneurons recorded are identified on morphological criteria. To do this, electrodes 1 and 2 are filled with biocytin which diffuses or is injected into the cell. Slices are then fixed and biocytin-filled cells are visualized by the avidin-biotinylated horseradish peroxidase method. The dendritic tree and axonal arborization of the recorded neurons are drawn by reconstruction from serial 60 μm thick sections under a light microscope. This also allows one to check that the two neurons are connected and to count the number of contacts. Then, under electron microscopy, the type of synapses between the two neurons and the number of active zones can be precisely analysed.

In summary, the basis for the selection of pairs of connected neurons are: (i) the presence of a short latency (monosynaptic) IPSC or IPSP in the pyramidal cell following an action potential in the putative interneuron; (ii) stable recordings from both cells for sufficient time to obtain an averaged IPSC or IPSP; and (iii) recovery of at least part of the biocytin-labelled interneuron to allow its identification.

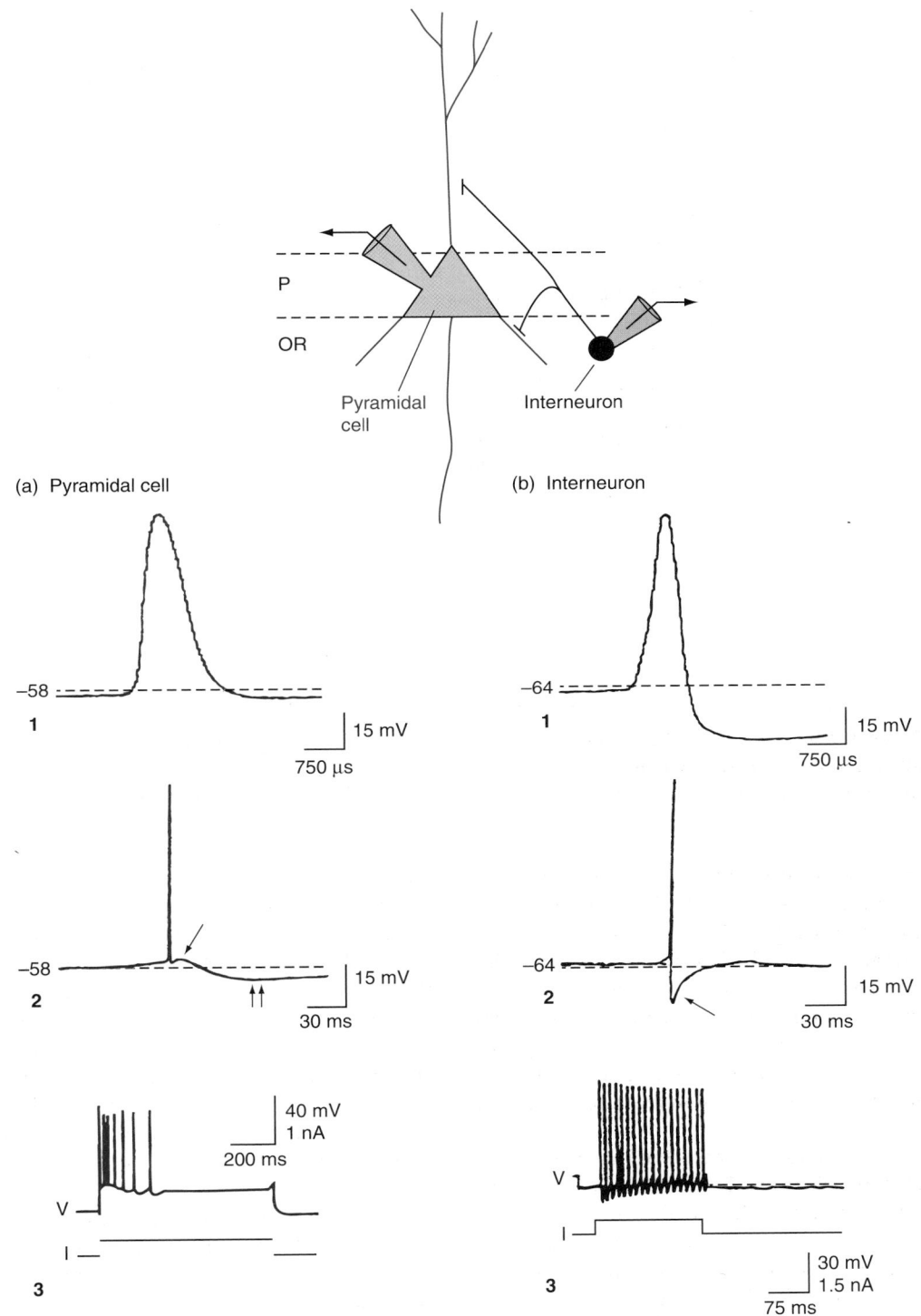

Figure 22.8 Physiological characteristics that differentiate pyramidal neurons from interneurons.
(a) Action potential of a pyramidal neuron at a fast (1) and a slow (2) timebase to show the presence of an after-spike depolarization (arrow) followed by a slow after-spike hyperpolarization (double arrow). The bottom trace (3) shows the response of a pyramidal neuron to a depolarizing current pulse. **(b)** Action potential of an interneuron recorded in the stratum oriens (OR) at a fast (1) and a slow (2) timebase to show the presence of a fast after-hyperpolarization (arrow). The bottom trace (3) shows the response of an interneuron to a depolarizing current pulse. Adapted from Lacaille JC, Williams S (1990) Membrane properties of interneurons in stratum oriens-alveus of the CA1 region of rat hippocampus *in vitro*, *Neuroscience* **36**, 349–359, with permission.

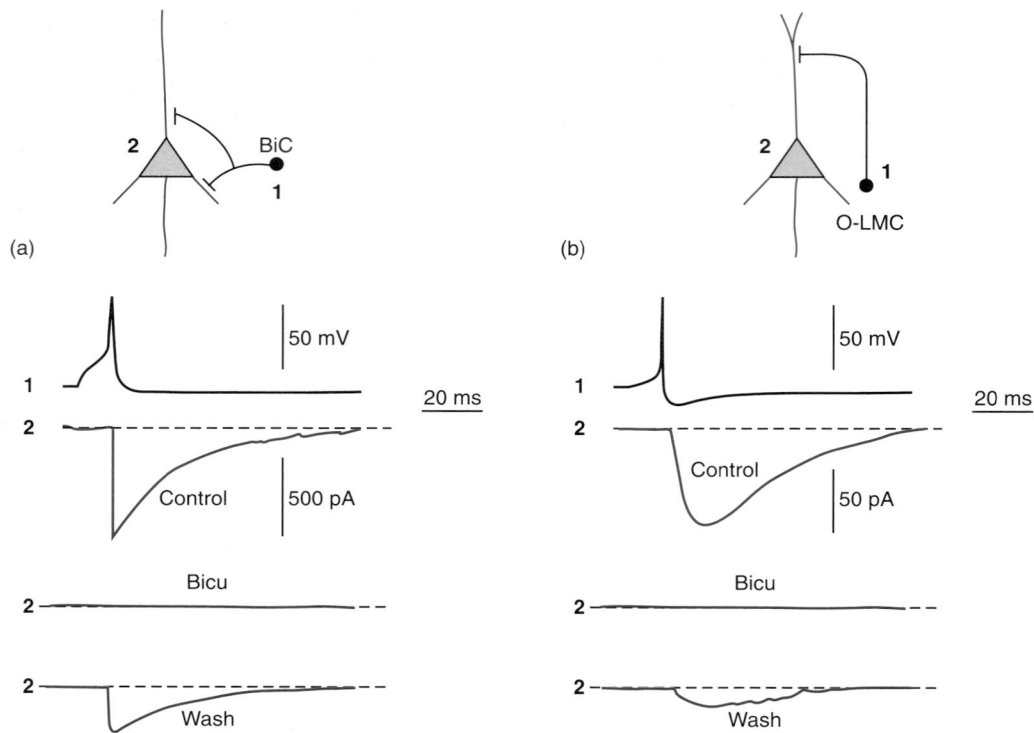

Figure 22.9 Unitary IPSCs (uIPSCs) evoked in pyramidal cells in response to different types of interneurons are all mediated by GABA$_A$ receptors.

Averaged uIPSC evoked in a pyramidal neuron (2) in response to a single spike in a bistratified interneuron (1a, BiC) or an oriens lacunosum moleculare interneuron (1b, O-LMC) in control conditions, in the presence of bicuculline (Bicu, 10 μM) and after partial wash-out of the drug (Wash). Adapted from Maccaferri G, Roberts DB, Szucs P et al. (2000) Cell surface domain specific postsynaptic currents evoked by identified GABAergic neurones in rat hippocampus in vitro, J. Physiol. **524**, 91–116, with permission.

22.3.2 Unitary inhibitory postsynaptic currents (IPSCs) evoked by different types of interneurons are all GABA$_A$-mediated but have different kinetics when recorded at the level of the soma

To study the synaptic current evoked in a pyramidal neuron in response to a single action potential in the presynaptic interneuron, the activity of both neurons is recorded in whole-cell configuration.

Whole-cell patch recordings

The intrapipette solution of electrode 1 (interneuron) is designed to allow the recording of action potentials (in mM): 130 K gluconate, 2 MgCl$_2$, 0.1 EGTA, 2 ATP, 0.3 GTP, 10 Hepes and 0.5% biocytin. Action potentials are generated in the interneuron by injection of a suprathreshold square current pulse at 0.1–1 Hz.

The intrapipette solution of electrode 2 (pyramidal cell) is designed to record GABA$_A$-mediated currents in

isolation (in mM): 100 CsCl, 2 MgCl$_2$, 0.1 EGTA, 2 ATP, 0.3 GTP, 40 Hepes, 5 QX-314 and 0.5% biocytin, at a pH of 7.2. QX-314 and Cs$^+$ strongly reduce voltage-gated Na$^+$ and K$^+$ currents, respectively. Ionotropic glutamate receptors are blocked by DNQX 20 μM and D-AP5 50 μM in the bath. The synaptic current is recorded in voltage clamp mode (V_H = –70 mV). Internal Cl$^-$ concentration is 104 mM and the external concentration is 135 mM, which gives a reversal potential for Cl$^-$ ions close to 0 mV (recall that in physiological conditions E_{Cl} is around –70 mV; see Section 10.3.4). Therefore, at V_H = –70 mV, when GABA$_A$ receptors open, there is an outflow of Cl$^-$ through channels permeable to Cl$^-$ ions; it is recorded as an inward current (an inward current is by convention an inward movement of positive charges; see Section 3.3.3).

Unitary IPSCs evoked by different types of interneurons are all mediated by GABA$_A$ receptors

When a single action potential is evoked in the presynaptic interneuron, an inward current is recorded in the postsynaptic pyramidal cell (**Figure 22.9**). This inward current is totally blocked by bicuculline (Bicu, an antagonist of GABA$_A$ receptors), thus showing that it is mediated by GABA$_A$ receptors. This holds true for all the following pairs: BiC–pyr, O-LMC–pyr, BC–pyr and AAC–pyr.

These GABA$_A$-mediated currents are called *inhibitory postsynaptic currents* (IPSCs), though they are inward, because in control Cl⁻ conditions they would be outward and thus inhibitory. An IPSC which results from a single action potential in the presynaptic neuron is called a *unitary IPSC* (uIPSC).

Proximally and distally generated unitary IPSCs have different kinetic parameters

The unitary IPSCs of **Figure 22.9** are recorded at the level of the soma of pyramidal cells. When evoked in distal dendrites by O-LMC, unitary IPSCs are passively conducted along the apical dendrite before being recorded in the soma. In contrast, unitary IPSCs evoked at the level of the soma by basket cells (BC) or at the axon initial segment by axo-axonic cells (AAC) are generated at sites close to the recording electrode. As shown in **Figure 22.10**, distally evoked unitary IPSCs have a slower time to peak (also called the risetime) than those evoked in proximal dendrites and soma. Unitary IPSCs evoked by axo-axonic cells have a fast risetime (0.8 ± 0.1 ms) whereas those evoked by basket cells have a slower risetime; and those evoked in the most distal pyramidal dendrites by oriens lacunosum moleculare cells have a very slow risetime (6.2 ± 0.6 ms). The kinetics of unitary IPSCs recorded in the soma of pyramidal cells reflect the domain of innervation: this can result from electrotonic dendritic filtering (see Section 16.1) and/or the lack of voltage clamp of the more distal locations and/or site-specific subunit composition of GABA$_A$ receptors.

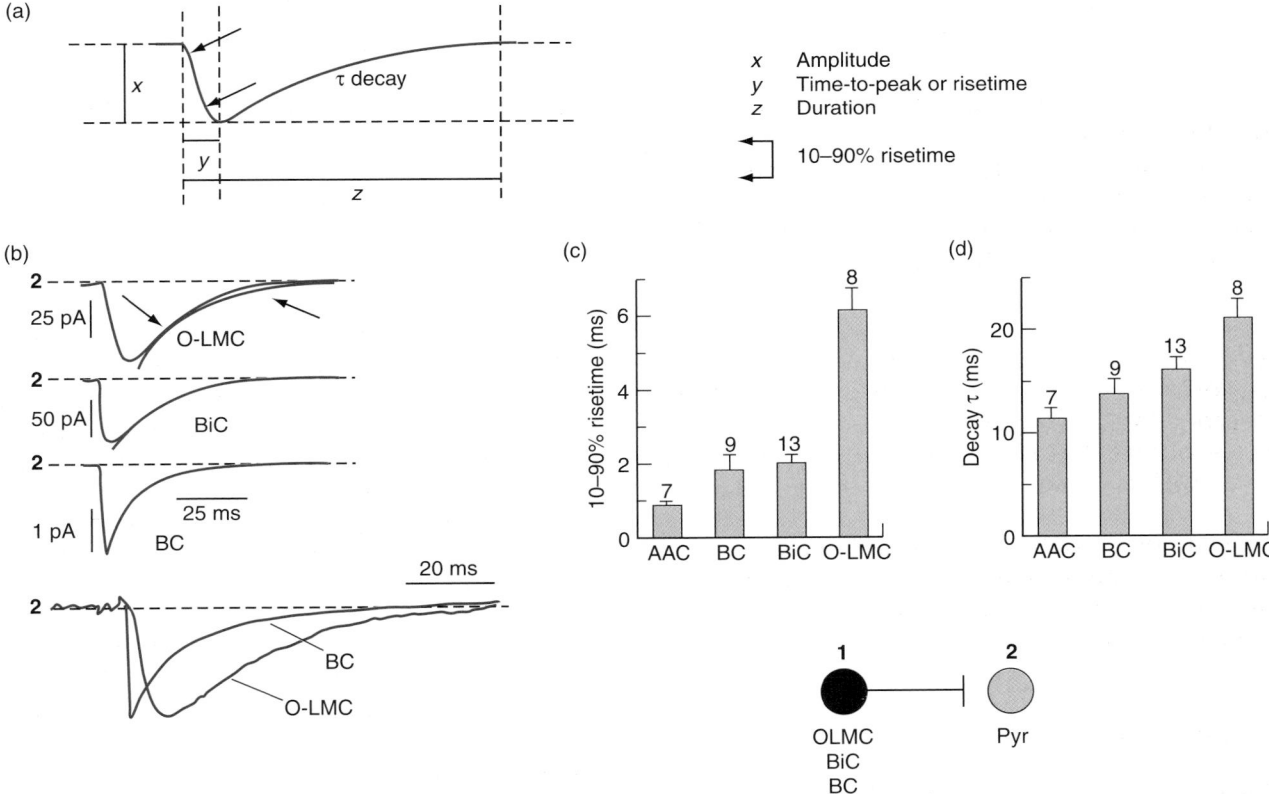

Figure 22.10 Kinetic parameters of unitary IPSCs evoked in a pyramidal cell in response to different types of interneurons.
(a) Definition of the parameters of postsynaptic currents. (b) Comparison of the risetime (or time to peak) and decay phase of three different uIPSCs. Bottom trace shows superimposed averaged uIPSCs generated by a presynaptic basket cell (BC) or oriens lacunosum moleculare cell (O-LMC). (c) Histogram of the risetimes (10–90%) and (d) of the decay (τ, time to 63% of decay) of the uIPSCs generated by different classes of presynaptic interneurons. Adapted from Maccaferri G, Roberts DB, Szucs P *et al.* (2000) Cell surface domain specific postsynaptic currents evoked by identified GABAergic neurones in rat hippocampus *in vitro*, *J. Physiol.* **524**, 91–116, with permission.

In summary, in Ammon's horn, the synapses established by interneurons on the soma (BC), on proximal or distal dendrites (BiC, O-LMC) or the axon initial segment (AAC) of pyramidal cells are all inhibitory and GABA$_A$-mediated. This means that GABA$_A$ synapses are present all along the somato-dendritic tree and axon initial segment of pyramidal cells. Depending where they are generated on the dendritic tree, GABA$_A$-mediated IPSCs have different risetimes.

22.3.3 GABA$_A$-mediated IPSCs generate IPSPs in postsynaptic pyramidal cells

IPSCs generate transient hyperpolarizations of the postsynaptic membrane, called *inhibitory postsynaptic potentials* (IPSPs). To study the IPSPs evoked in a pyramidal neuron in response to a presynaptic interneuron in physiological conditions, the activity of both neurons is recorded with intracellular electrodes filled with 1.5 M of KCH$_3$SO$_4$ (and 2% biocytin) so as not to change the internal Cl$^-$ concentration. In these conditions, the reversal potential for Cl$^-$ ions is around -70 mV, which is close to that *in vivo*.

In **Figure 22.11**, a single spike in the presynaptic interneuron (bistratified cell) evokes a transient hyperpolarization in the postsynaptic pyramidal neuron; this is called inhibitory (IPSP) because it hyperpolarizes the membrane to a potential far from the threshold of spike initiation. It is unitary (uIPSP) since it is evoked by a single presynaptic spike. To evoke this uIPSP, the presynaptic action potential first propagates to the numerous synaptic terminals of the interneuron and evokes the release of GABA from all or some of these terminals. Therefore, a unitary IPSC or IPSP can result from the activation of one or more release sites, depending on the number of synapses established by the presynaptic interneuron on the recorded postsynaptic pyramidal neuron and on the number of active zones per synapse (see **Figure 8.2**). A study under electron microscopy then reveals the exact number of synaptic complexes since a single synaptic bouton may establish multiple synaptic complexes.

In the example of **Figure 22.11**, there are six synaptic contacts between the axon of the presynaptic basket cell and the postsynaptic pyramidal neuron. Electron microscopy shows that these six synaptic contacts correspond to six synaptic complexes (there is a single active zone per bouton). Therefore, a maximum of six release sites is responsible for this unitary IPSP. This allows one to calculate the average amplitude of an IPSP evoked by the activity of one release site only: it is around 30 µV (220 µV divided by 6) which is a very small hyperpolarization. In **Figure 22.12**, the IPSP evoked by an axoaxonic cell corresponds to the activity of eight synaptic contacts between a presynaptic axo-axonic cell and a

pyramidal neuron. This GABA$_A$-mediated IPSP reverses at -78 mV (range -65 to -78 mV), which is close to E_{Cl}. Morphological studies show that inhibitory interneurons establish an average of 5–30 synaptic contacts with a single postsynaptic pyramidal cell.

22.3.4 GABA$_B$-mediated IPSPs are also recorded in pyramidal neurons in reponse to strong interneuron stimulation

The activity of a CA3 pyramidal cell is intracellularly recorded with electrodes filled with 2 M of KMeSO$_4$ so as not to change the intracellular concentration of Cl$^-$. A stimulating electrode is placed in the hilus (it stimulates local interneurons and excitatory afferents from granular cells of the dentate gyrus). In response to the stimulation, a complex synaptic response is recorded (**Figure 22.13**): a prior EPSP (inset) followed by a biphasic IPSP (early and late). When QX-314, a derivative of lidocaine that blocks voltage-gated Na$^+$ currents (fast and persistent) and GABA$_B$ receptor-activated K$^+$ current (see Chapter 13), the late component disappears. In contrast, in the presence of bicuculline in the bath the early component disappears (not shown). This shows that the early IPSP is mediated by GABA$_A$ receptors whereas the late phase is mediated by GABA$_B$ receptors.

Postsynaptic GABA$_B$ receptor-mediated IPSPs are recorded only in response to a strong activation of interneurons. This effect is absent in the response to a single spike in interneurons, suggesting that a larger release of GABA in the synaptic cleft is necessary to activate postsynaptic GABA$_B$ receptors. This late IPSP prolongs the inhibition of pyramidal cells by GABAergic interneurons.

22.4 Activation of principal cells evokes excitatory glutamatergic responses in postsynaptic interneurons and other principal cells (synchronization in CA3)

To study the physiological response of a postsynaptic neuron to an action potential in the presynaptic pyramidal neuron, the activity of these connected neurons is recorded concomitantly with intracellular or whole-cell electrodes. Electrodes 1 and 2 are filled with 4% biocytin in 0.5 M of potassium acetate. In these conditions the reversal potential for Cl$^-$ ions is around -70 mV, which is close to that *in vivo*.

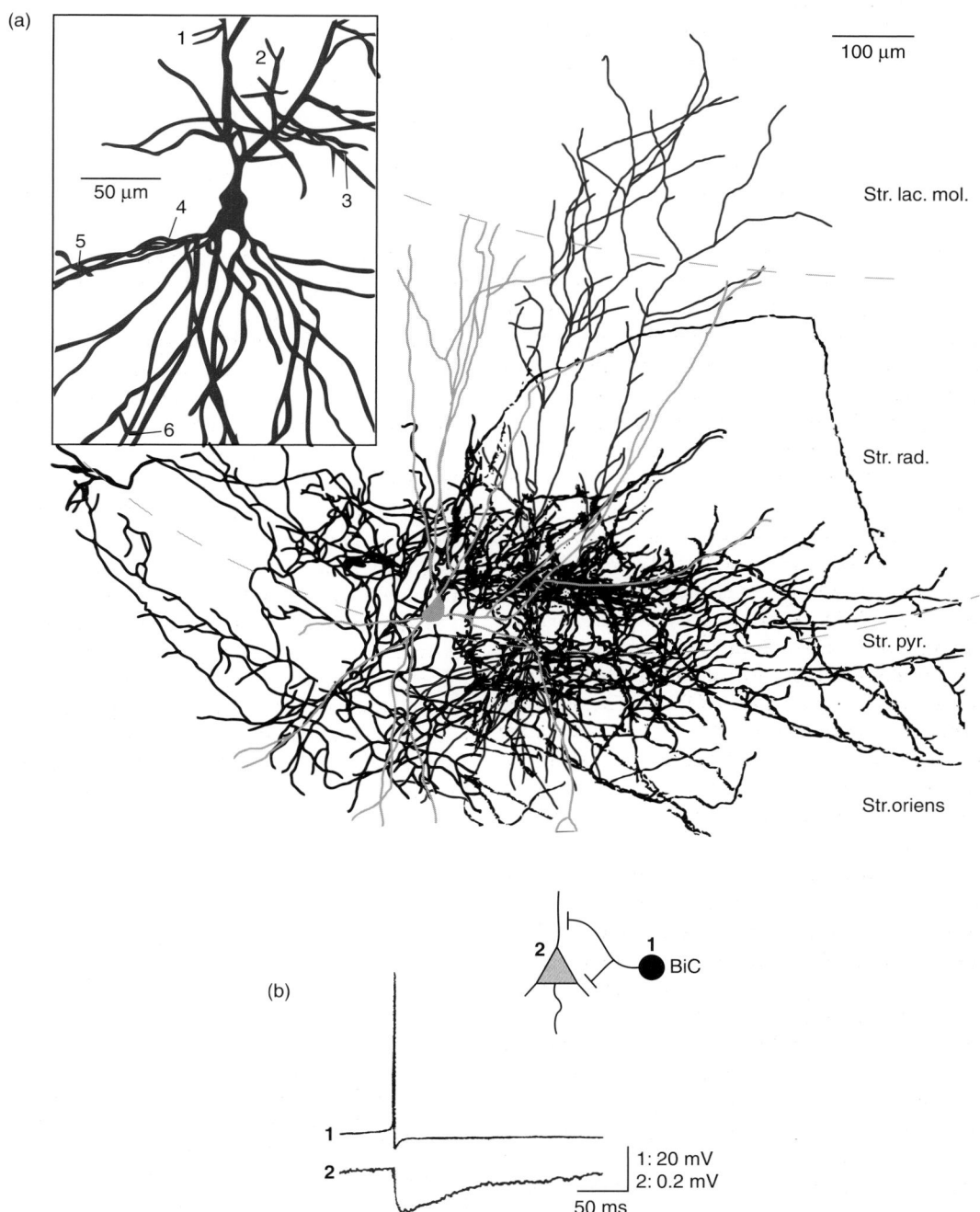

Figure 22.11 Unitary IPSP evoked in a CA1 pyramidal cell in response to a bistratified cell (BiC) and location of contact sites.
(a) Reconstruction of the biocytin-filled presynaptic interneuron (somato-dendritic tree in grey, axon in black) and postsynaptic pyramidal dendrites (green). The inset shows the location of the six contact sites between the GABAergic axon (black) and the postsynaptic pyramidal cell (green). (b) An action potential in BiC (1) elicits a small-amplitude, short-latency unitary IPSP in the postsynaptic pyramidal cell (2). (Trace 2 is an averaged unitary IPSP.) Adapted from Buhl EH, Halasy K, Somogyi P (1994) Diverse sources of hippocampal unitary inhibitory postsynaptic potentials and the number of synaptic release sites, *Nature* **368**, 823–828, with permission.

22.4.1 Pyramidal neurons evoke AMPA-mediated EPSPs in interneurons

EPSPs elicited in interneurons in response to a single action potential in the presynaptic pyramidal cell have a mean amplitude of 1–4 mV and a time to peak of 1.5–4 ms. They are totally blocked by CNQX, the selective blocker of AMPA receptors (not shown). They fluctuate in amplitude at all synapses examined and sometimes fail (**Figure 22.14a**). This latter observation suggests that there is a low probability of release or the existence of a few release sites. In fact, under light microscopy, in all pairs studied, a single synaptic contact is identified between the filled pyramidal cell and interneuron.

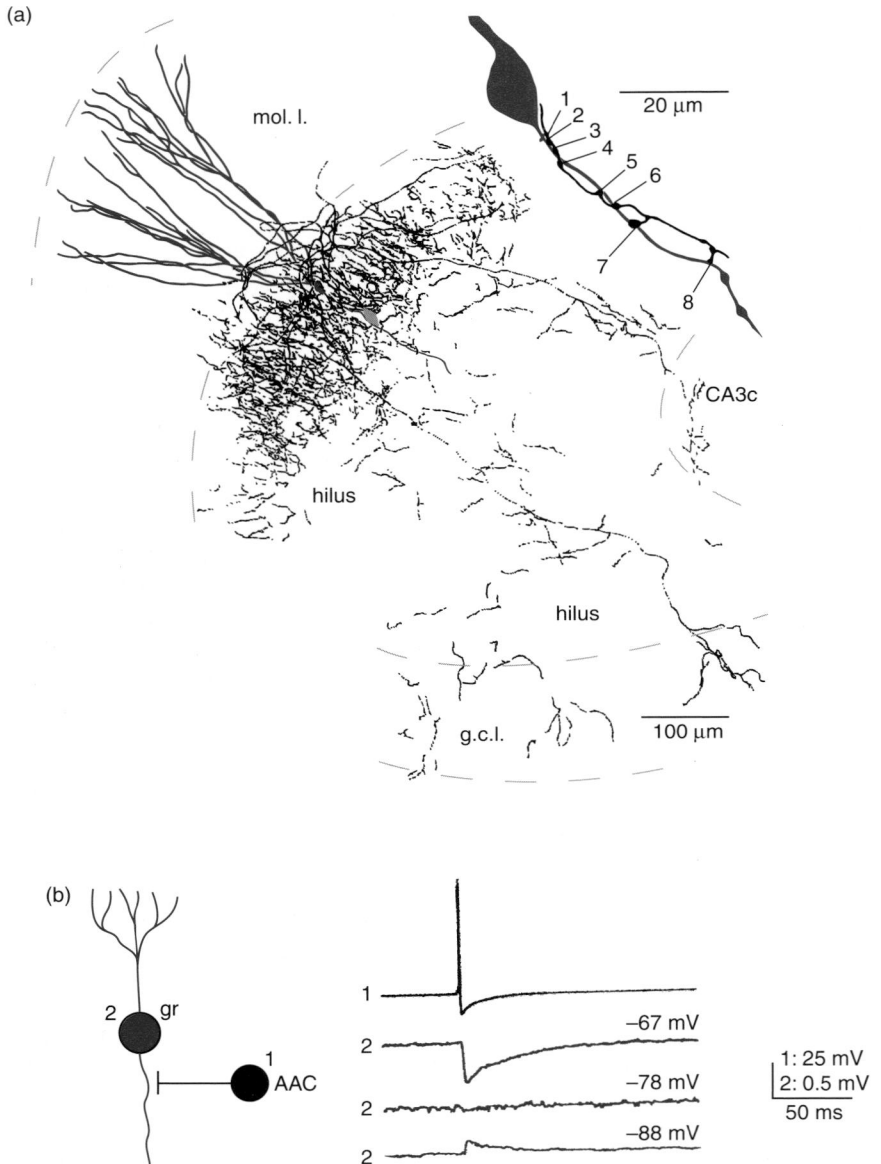

Figure 22.12 Unitary IPSP evoked in a CA3 pyramidal cell in response to an axo-axonic cell (AAC) and location of contact sites.

(a) Reconstruction of the biocytin-filled presynaptic interneuron (soma in grey, axon in black) and postsynaptic granular cell (green). The top right shows the location of the eight contact sites between the GABAergic axon (black) and the axon initial segment of the postsynaptic granular cell (green). **(b)** An action potential in AAC (1) elicits a small-amplitude, short-latency unitary IPSP in the postsynaptic granular cell (2) that reverses at around –78 mV (traces 2 show averaged EPSPs). Adapted from Buhl EH, Halasy K, Somogyi P (1994) Diverse sources of hippocampal unitary inhibitory postsynaptic potentials and the number of synaptic release sites, *Nature* **368**, 823–828, with permission.

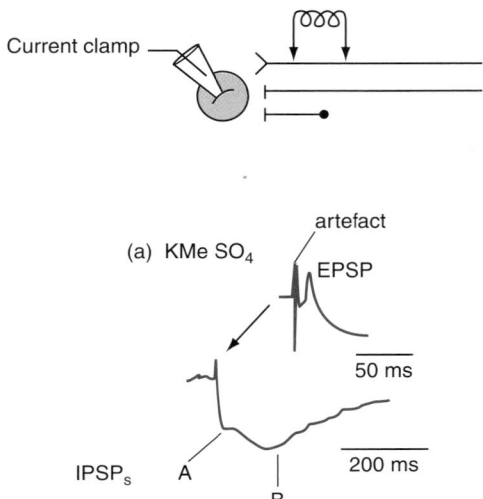

(a) KMe SO$_4$

artefact

EPSP

50 ms

200 ms

IPSP$_s$ A

B

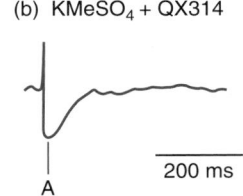

(b) KMeSO$_4$ + QX314

A

200 ms

Figure 22.13 GABA$_A$ and GABA$_B$ receptor-mediated IPSPs in pyramidal cells.
(a) CA3 pyramidal cells respond to a hilar stimulation by a biphasic IPSP preceded by an EPSP (inset). The biphasic IPSP consist of an early (A) and a late (B) IPSP. **(b)** In the presence of QX 314 (50 mM) in the pipette solution, stimulation no longer evokes the late IPSP whereas the early one (A) is spared (as well as the EPSP, not shown). The pipette is filled with potassium methyl sulphate (KMeSO$_4$). Adapted from McLean HA, Ben Ari Y, Gaiarsa JL (1995) NMDA-dependent GABA$_A$-mediated polysynaptic potentials in the neonatal rat hippocampal CA3 region, *Eur. J. Neurosci.* **7**, 1442–1448, with permission.

Electron microscopy shows that each contact has a single active zone.

Studies are performed in the hippocampus on a large number of cells in order to obtain quantitative data: pyramidal cells are filled *in vivo* with neurobiotin, and parvalbumine-containing interneurons (basket and axo-axonic cells) are revealed by immunocytochemistry. This study confirms that each filled pyramidal axon establishes a single contact with parvalbumine-containing interneurons. By counting the boutons terminating on interneurons, it has been shown that as over 1000 excitatory synapses terminate on a single inhibitory cell, suggesting that more than 1000 pyrami-

dal cells converge on to one interneuron. This excitatory drive presumably contributes to the high frequency of the spontaneous firing of hippocampal interneurons.

Interestingly, single pyramidal cell action potentials cause inhibitory cells to fire at resting membrane potential with a probability of 0.4 (**Figure 22.15**). The mean interval between pre- and postsynaptic spikes is 2.9 ± 0.7 ms. Factors contributing to spike-to-spike transmission are the low firing threshold of inhibitory interneurons, their depolarized resting membrane potential and the large EPSCs elicited by pyramidal cells leading to large EPSPs (of the order of the millivolts) owing to the high input membrane resistance of interneurons (**Figure 22.14b**). Moreover, CA3 pyramidal cells have a tendency to discharge in bursts of several action potentials (with 5–10 ms intervals). This has as a consequence that the security of transmission is enhanced and temporal summation occurs when the interval between presynaptic spikes is shorter than the time course of EPSPs (**Figure 22.14b**).

22.4.2 EPSPs in interneurons lead to feedback inhibition of pyramidal neurons

When two pyramidal cells of the CA3 region are recorded simultaneously, firing in one pyramidal cell can evoke an IPSP in the other pyramidal cell (**Figure 22.16a**). The mean IPSP latency is 3.5 ± 0.7 ms and the mean amplitude 1.9 ± 0.6 mV. Bicuculline (a GABA$_A$ receptor antagonist) as well as CNQX (an AMPA receptor antagonist) completely suppresses these evoked IPSPs. This experiment excludes the possibility that pyramidal cells establish monosynaptic inhibitory connections. It shows in contrast that these IPSPs result from a bisynaptic connection between pyramidal cells: the first synapse is glutamatergic and the second one GABAergic. There are two ways to block this IPSP: to block synaptic transmission at the first synapse with CNQX or at the second synapse with bicuculline.

22.4.3 CA3 pyramidal neurons are monosynaptically connected via glutamatergic synapses

Neighbouring pyramidal cells of CA3 are monosynaptically connected via axon collaterals (see **Figure 22.6c**). In pairs of pyramidal neurons, presynaptic pyramidal action potentials evoke EPSPs in the postsynaptic pyramidal cell (**Figure 22.17**) that are sensitive to CNQX. These EPSPs are considered to be monosynaptic on the basis of their mean latency (range 0.8–1.2 ms) and the proportion of transmission failures (small in monosynaptic connections).

22.4.4 Overview of intrinsic hippocampal circuits

The main circuit is the tri-neuronal circuit between the excitatory principal cells (see **Figures 22.6a and b**). In each region, dentate gyrus, CA1 or CA3, axon collaterals of principal cells excite inhibitory interneurons which in turn inhibit other principal cells (feedback inhibition). Interneurons are also directly activated by extrinsic excitatory afferences (feedforward inhibition). In CA3, principal cells (pyramidal cells) are monosynaptically connected via excitatory axon collaterals (see **Figure 22.6c**).

22.5 Oscillations in the hippocampal network: example of sharp waves (SPW)

Gyorgy Buzsaki discovered sharp waves (SPW) in 1983 when recording from CA1 stratum radiatum and a pyramidal cell layer simultaneously in the freely moving rat. When the rat is exploring, typical theta waves are present. When the animal becomes immobile or goes to sleep (slow wave stage), large-amplitude intermittent sharp waves of 40–120 ms replace theta oscillations (see **Figure 22.3**). The frequency of the intermittent sharp

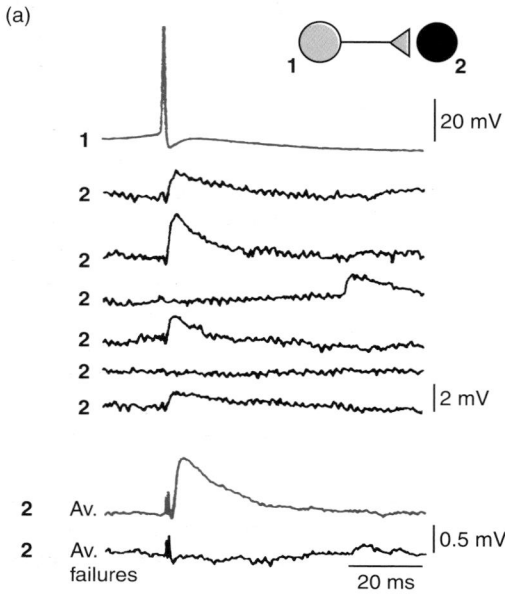

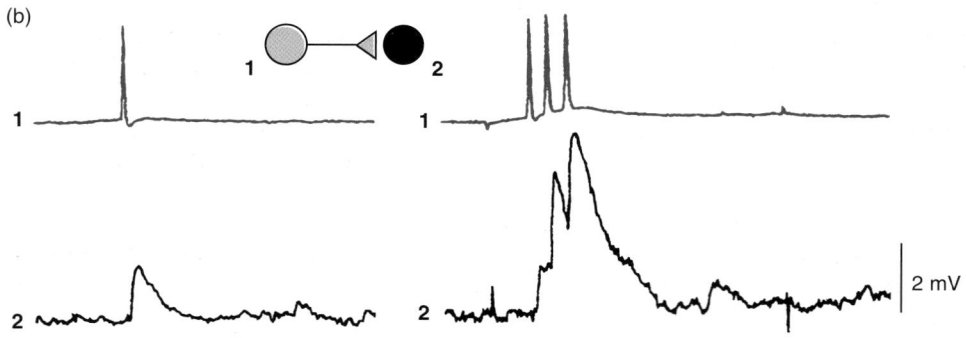

Figure 22.14 Unitary EPSP evoked in an inhibitory interneuron in response to a CA3 pyramidal cell.
(a) A single spike in the presynaptic pyramidal cell (1) evokes a unitary EPSP in the postsynaptic interneuron (2) that fluctuates in amplitude and sometimes fails. An averaged EPSP and an averaged trace of failures ($n = 38$) are shown below. Av: average. **(b)** EPSPs initiated in an inhibitory interneuron in response to a single spike (left) or a train of three spikes (right) in the presynaptic pyramidal cell (1). On the right there is a temporal summation of the EPSPs. Adapted from Miles R (1990) Synaptic excitation of inhibitory cells by single CA3 hippocampal pyramidal cells of the guinea pig *in vitro*, *J. Physiol.* **428**, 61–77, with permission.

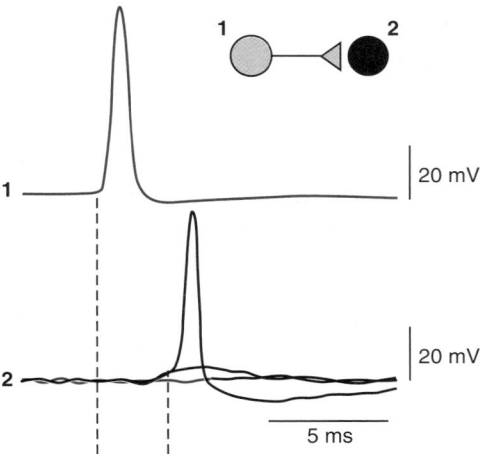

Figure 22.15 Spike to spike transmission at an excitatory synapse between a CA3 pyramidal neuron and a postsynaptic inhibitory interneuron.

In response to successive single spikes in a presynaptic pyramidal cell (1, only one spike is displayed), one transmission failure, one unitary EPSP and one unitary EPSP that causes postsynaptic firing are recorded in the postsynaptic interneuron (2, three superimposed traces). Adapted from Miles R (1990) Synaptic excitation of inhibitory cells by single CA3 hippocampal pyramidal cells of the guinea pig *in vitro*, *J. Physiol.* **428**, 61–77, with permission.

waves ranges from 0.02 to 3 Hz. Recordings in layers of the CA1 region with extracellular electrodes show that sharp wave amplitude is maximal in stratum radiatum, the layer where apical dendrites of CA1 pyramidal neurons extend (**Figure 22.18a and b**). The immediate cause of sharp waves in the CA1 region is the synchronous discharge of a large number of CA3 pyramidal neurons. This results in the near-simultaneous depolarization of CA1 pyramidal cells via Schaffer collaterals which terminate dominantly on apical CA1 dendrites (see **Figure 22.6**) (recall that the extracellular recording of EPSPs from a population of neurons, called field EPSP, appears as a downward deflection in extracellular recordings; see **Figure 21.4b**). In brief, sharp waves represent a coherent depolarization of the apical dendrites of CA1 pyramidal neurons.

However, the synchronous discharge of a large number of CA3 pyramidal neurons also directly activates interneurons (see **Figure 22.7**). Therefore, concurrent with sharp waves, pyramidal cells and interneurons are activated synchronously (interneurons are even activated earlier than target pyramidal cells, because of their lower spike threshold). As a result, dendrites of CA1 pyramidal cells respond by summed EPSPs (see **Figure 22.14b**) to bursts of action potentials in Schaffer collaterals and by summed IPSPs in response to bursts of action potentials in axons of interneurons. How do CA1 pyramidal cells finally respond?

Whenever a sharp wave is present in the radiatum, a 140–200 Hz field oscillation is present in the pyramidal cell layer (**Figures 22.18b and c**). This is best shown by filtering the field potential below 50 Hz (to suppress oscillations at a frequency under 50 Hz). This reveals high-frequency oscillations that form a ripple. These oscillations are most prominent in the pyramidal layer (**Figure 22.18**, trace 5). The fast field oscillation is believed to represent summed fast IPSPs in the somata of pyramidal cells brought about by the activated interneurons.

The explanation is the following. Interneurons, including basket and axo-axonic (chandelier) cells, fire together (perhaps coupled by gap junctions) at around 200 Hz and impose a series of IPSPs on the somata of pyramidal cells. Some pyramidal cells are excited through their dendrites strongly enough so that excitation can overcome somato-axonal inhibition. However, because of these series of IPSPs in the soma and axon initial segment membrane, the spike(s) emerge at the periods where inhibition is least (i.e. out of phase with the spikes of the interneurons; **Figure 22.19**). In short, inhibition does not necessarily prevent firing but serves to time the occurrence of spikes.

Sharp waves are envisaged as an endogenous mechanism for consolidating synaptic changes and transferring information from the hippocampus to neocortex during sleep. The strong depolarization of pyramidal cell dendrites during a sharp wave burst enhances the size of fast dendritic spikes (see Section 19.3.2). The large membrane depolarization also triggers Ca^{2+} spikes which, in turn, may alter the weights of the simultaneously active nearby synapses (see Section 19.3.3).

22.6 Summary

What is a neuronal network?

A neuronal network is formed by neurons from the same nucleus. It is described by the connections between these neurons, the type of synapse (glutamatergic, GABAergic, etc.), and the arrangement of the synapses on somato-dendritic trees.

Are networks completely different from one nucleus to another or are there some fundamental principles of organization?

Networks have in common a basic organization. There are always principal cells and most often interneurons (the subthalamic nucleus is, for example, devoid of interneurons whereas striatum contains many differents types of these). Interneurons are always connected so as to provide feedforward and feedback inhibitions.

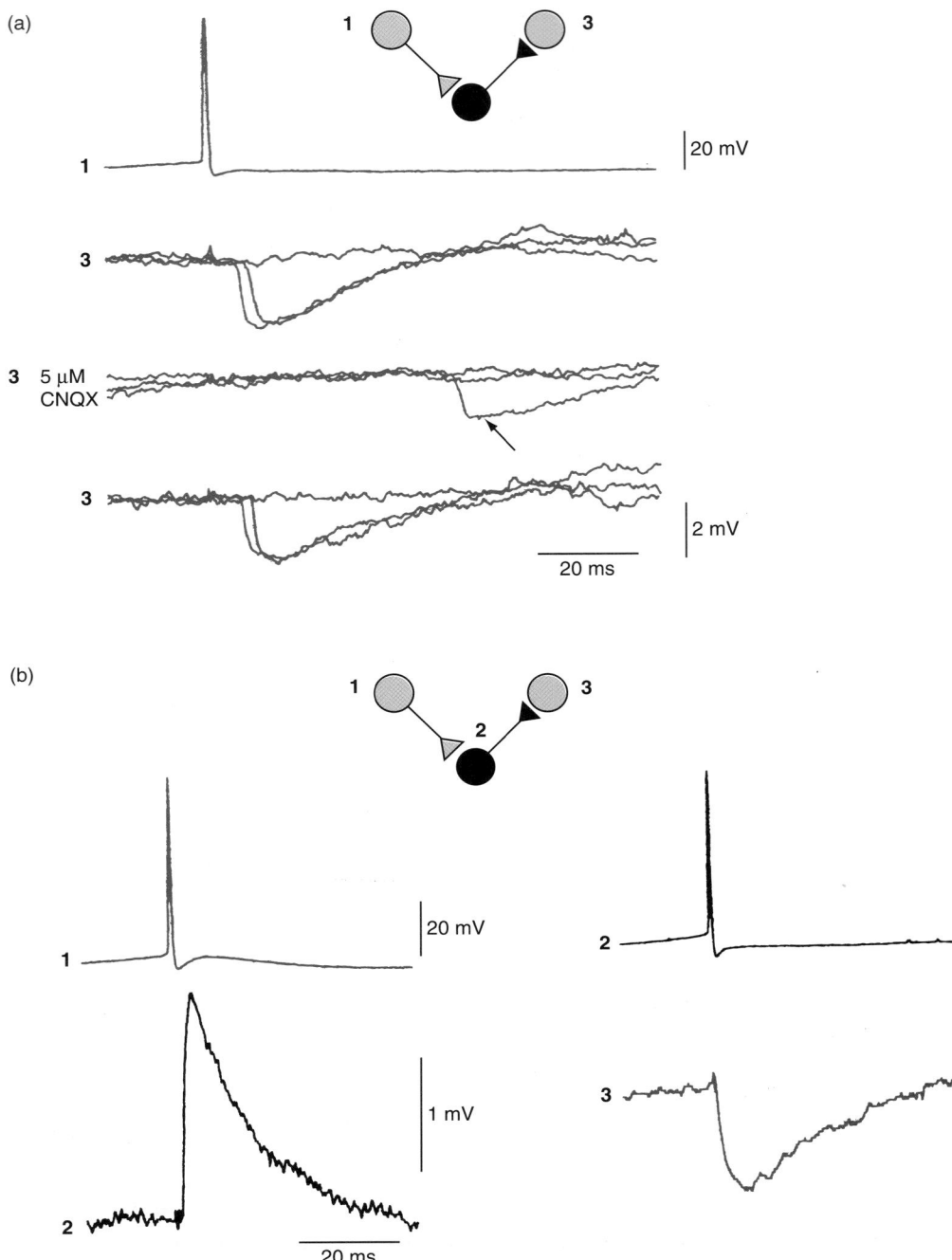

Figure 22.16 Feedback inhibition between two CA3 pyramidal cells.
(a) In response to a single spike in one pyramidal cell (1), an IPSP is recorded in a neighbouring pyramidal cell (3). Upper trace 2 s
three superimposed responses to three presynaptic action potentials (trace 1, only one spike is displayed). There is one transmission
failure and two IPSPs. Middle trace 3 shows the effect of CNQX in the bath: the evoked IPSPs is suppressed but spontaneous ones
still present (arrow). Bottom trace 3 shows the return to control solution. **(b)** Sequential recordings of the three connected cells.
Pyramidal cell 1 activates interneuron 2 (average of uEPSP, $n = 40$) and interneuron 2 inhibits cell 3 (average of uIPSP, $n = 40$). Ada
from Miles R (1990) Synaptic excitation of inhibitory cells by single CA3 hippocampal pyramidal cells of the guinea pig *in vitro*, *J.*
Physiol. **428**, 61–77, with permission.

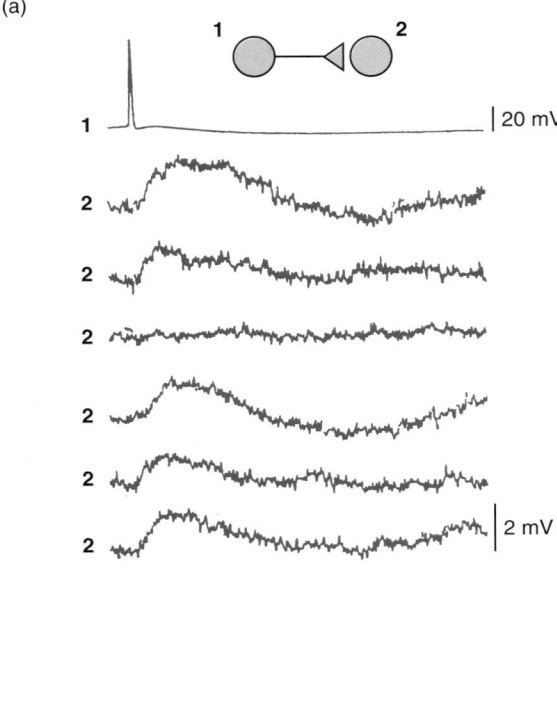

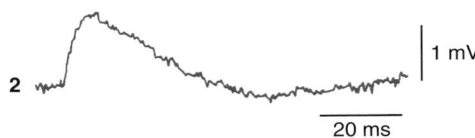

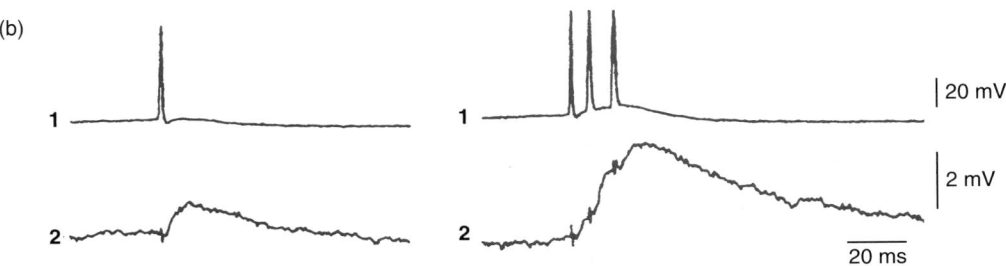

Figure 22.17 Unitary EPSP evoked in a CA3 pyramidal cell in response to a CA3 pyramidal cell.
Ionosynaptic unitary EPSP evoked in a postsynaptic pyramidal cell (2) in response to a single spike in the presynaptic pyramidal cell
he EPSP fluctuates in amplitude and sometimes fails. Bottom trace shows an averaged EPSP. **(b)** EPSPs initiated in a postsynaptic
nidal cell (2) in response to a single spike (left) or a train of three spikes (right) in the presynaptic pyramidal cell (1). On the right
is a temporal summation of the EPSPs. Part (a) adapted from Miles R, Wong RKS (1986) Excitatory synaptic interactions between
neurones in the guinea pig hippocampus, *J. Physiol.* **373**, 397–418, with permission. Part (b) adapted from Miles R (1990) Synaptic
ation of inhibitory cells by single CA3 hippocampal pyramidal cells of the guinea pig *in vitro*, *J. Physiol.* **428**, 61–77, with
ission.

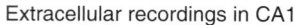

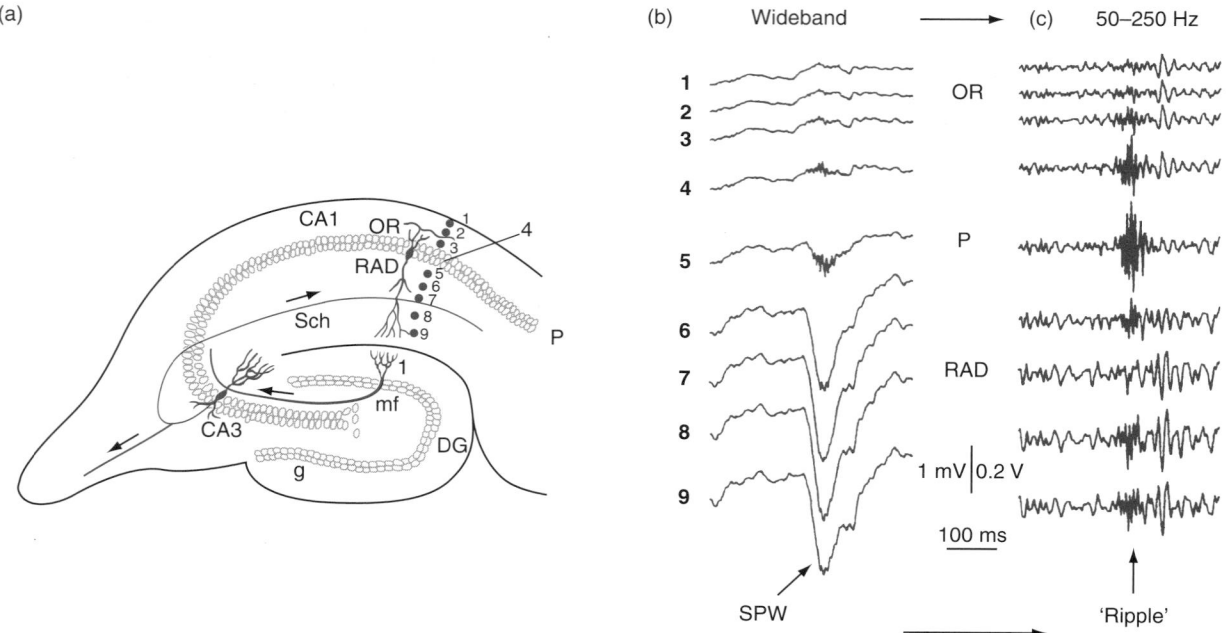

Figure 22.18 Sharp waves (SPW) in CA1 of the awake immobile rat and the high-frequency oscillations (ripples).
(a) The extracellular activity of a population of neurons is recorded with nine extracellular electrodes in the CA1 region. **(b)** Extracellular recordings show that the sharp waves are the most pronounced in the apical dendritic layer (stratum radiatum, RAD). **(c)** When the recordings in (b) are filtered in order to leave only the events with a frequency between 50–250 Hz, high-frequency oscillations that form a ripple are revealed. Ripples are particularly prominent in the pyramidal layer (p). Note that the amplitude scale is increased 5-fold between (b) and (c). Adapted from Ylinen A, Bragin A, Nadasdy Z *et al.* (1995) Sharp wave-associated high frequency oscillation (200 Hz) in the intact hippocampus: network and intracellular mechanisms, *J. Neurosci.* **15**, 30–46, with permission.

Afferent extrinsic connections impinge on to principal cells and interneurons.

Does the precise knowledge of intrinsic and extrinsic connections as well as the firing patterns of neurons allow us to explain how network oscillations are generated?

Yes, it does, if the pattern of afferent activity in extrinsic afferent axons is known.

Further reading

Buzsaki G, Horvath Z, Urioste R *et al.* (1992) High-frequency network oscillation in the hippocampus. *Science* **256**, 1025–1027.

Csicsvari J, Hirase H, Czurko A *et al.* (1999) Oscillatory coupling of hippocampal pyramidal cells and interneurons in the behaving rat. *J. Neurosci.* **19**, 274–287.

Kamondi A, Acsady L, Buzsaki G (1998) Dendritic spikes are enhanced by cooperative network activity in the intact hippocampus. *J Neurosci.* **18**, 3919–3928.

Nadasdy Z, Hirase H, Czurko A *et al.* (1999) Replay and time compression of recurring spike sequences in the hippocampus. *J Neurosci.* **19**, 9497–9507.

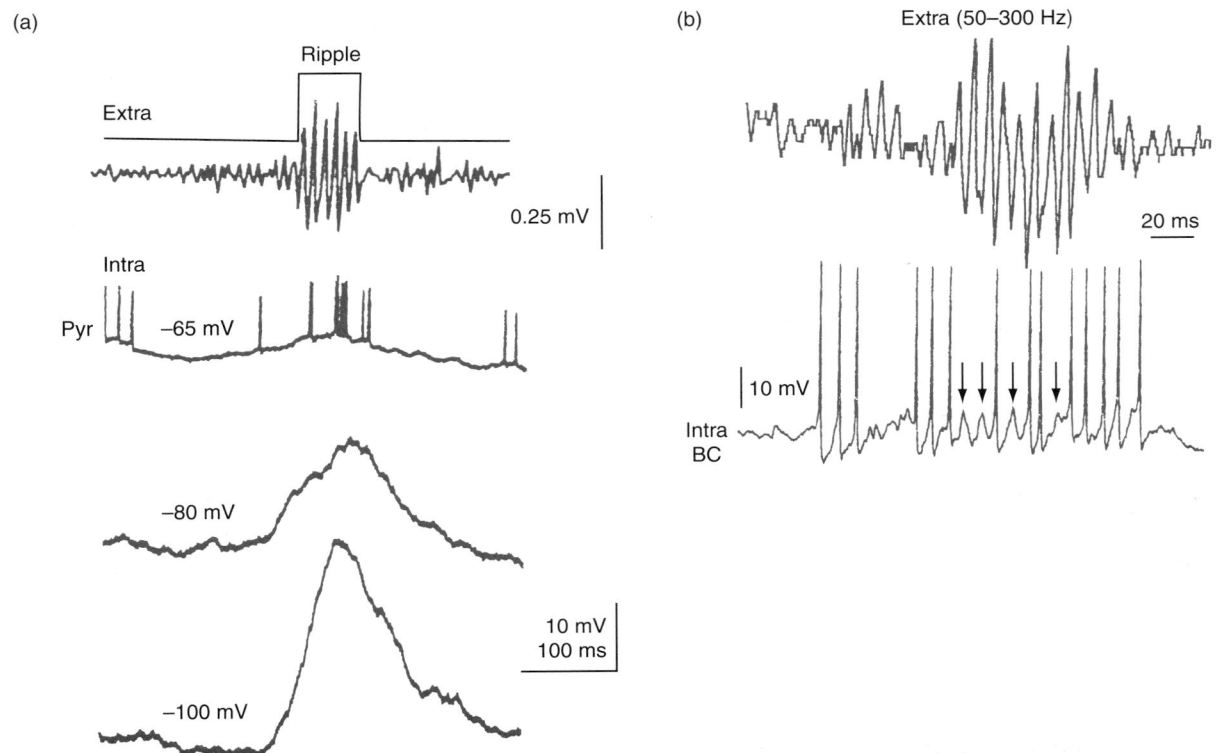

Figure 22.19 Intracellular activity of a pyramidal neuron and an interneuron during high-frequency oscillations (ripples). Intracellular recording **(a)** from a CA1 pyramidal neuron and **(b)** from a CA1 basket cell (BC) during a single ripple event. In (a), membrane hyperpolarization of the pyramidal cell from −65 to −100 mV reveals a strong depolarization force during the ripple. Part (a) adapted from Ylinen A, Bragin A, Nadasdy Z *et al.* (1995) Sharp wave-associated high frequency oscillation (200 Hz) in the intact hippocampus: network and intracellular mechanisms, *J. Neurosci.* **15**, 30–46, with permission. Part (b) adapted from Freund TF, Buzsaki G (1996) Interneurons in the hippocampus, *Hippocampus* **6**, 347–470, with permission.

Maturation of the Hippocampal Network

Developing neurons and circuits have several unique features and mechanisms that differ from those in adults. Firstly, several processes and cascades occur in the developing but seldom in the adult brain – including cell migration, differentiation, programmed cell death etc. Also, the subunit composition of ionotropic and metabotropic receptor channels or of voltage-gated ionic channels are often different in developing neurons, some are expressed only during development, others only in more adult stages. This chapter describes some of the sequential events that take place during the construction of the hippocampal network. It concentrates on the maturation of the main neuronal elements of the hippocampus, pyramidal neurons and interneurons, and their transmitters glutamate and GABA, which in the adult provide most of the inhibitory and excitatory drives, respectively. The properties of electrical activity that result from this maturation are described and compared with what is observed in the adult hippocampus.

23.1 GABAergic neurons and GABAergic synapses develop prior to glutamatergic ones

23.1.1 GABAergic interneurons divide and arborize prior to pyramidal neurons and granular cells

One question that emerges when analysing the maturation of the circuit is that of the parallel or sequential formation of its main neuronal components. Do interneurons and pyramidal neurons become functional at the same developmental stage or are they sequentially functional? To determine that, the Bromodeoxyuridine (BrdU) technique can be used. This consists of injecting BrdU systemically to be incorporated in the DNA of neurons in the process of dividing. When this agent is labelled, it becomes possible to determine in a structure which neurons are dividing and at which age of gestation. Such studies have so far suggested that GABAergic interneurons divide prior to the

principal neurons (CA1–CA3 pyramidal neurons and granular cells of the dentate gyrus) (**Figure 23.1**). Thus, in the rat, interneurons divide between E13 (embryonic age, 13 days) and E17 whereas pyramidal neurons divide between E16 and E21 (there is an additional difference between CA3 and CA1 pyramidal neurons, the former reaching maturity earlier). The granule cells of the fascia dentata have a primarily postnatal division; it is estimated that over 85% of the granule cells in the rat will divide in the three-week period following birth.

Therefore, interneurons are mature at an earlier stage than the bulk of principal cells. To determine if this is also manifested by a sequential maturation of the axonal and dendritic arbors, it is possible to patch-clamp interneurons and pyramidal neurons and inject them with dyes. Such studies suggest that interneurons indeed mature and arborize at an earlier stage than pyramidal neurons. Therefore, the interneuronal circuit is in a situation to exert an important modulatory role

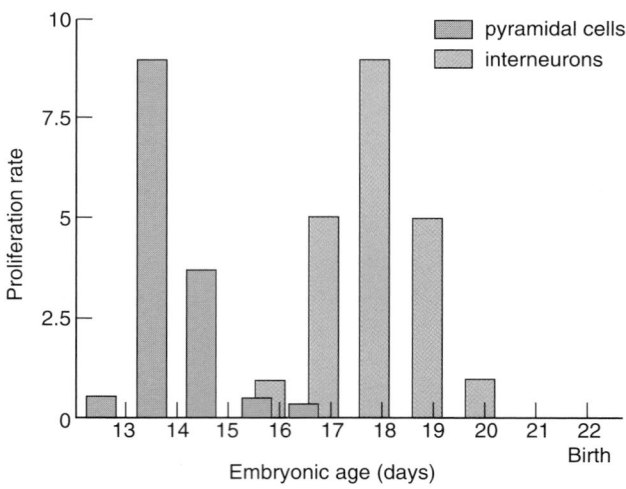

Figure 23.1 Histogram showing the proliferation rate of pyramidal cells (green) and interneurons (black) according to the embryonic age of the rat.
Adapted from Bayer SA (1980) Development of the hippocampal region in the rat: I. Neurogenesis examined with ^{3}H-thymidine autoradiography, *J. Comp. Neurol.* **190**, 87–114, with permission.

on the growth of pyramidal cells and the formation of the hippocampal network.

This observation raises the following question: *Since GABAergic interneurons are mature before glutamatergic pyramidal neurons, do these interneurons establish synapses before the glutamatergic ones on to target pyramidal neurons?*

23.1.2 GABAergic synapses are the first synapses established on to pyramidal cells

To determine the formation of GABA and glutamate synapses, the activity of pyramidal neurons is recorded in the whole-cell configuration (voltage clamp mode) in slices at an early stage – say at birth – and the properties of the postsynaptic currents (PSCs) that occur spontaneously or in response to electrical stimulation are determined. This is followed by morphological reconstruction of the recorded neurons (marked by intracellular injection of biocytin). At birth (P0, postnatal day 0), pyramidal neurons in the rat are composed of three populations (**Figure 23.2**):

■ Eighty percent of the neurons have a soma and an axon but essentially no apical or basal dendrites. These neurons are 'silent' in that no spontaneous or evoked synaptic current is recorded from them even in response to strong electrical stimuli (**Figure 23.2a**). These neurons do, however, express extrasynaptic receptors since bath applications of GABA or glutamate agonists evoke the usual currents (not shown) observed in more adult neurons, suggesting that the expression of receptors precedes that of functional synapses. They are identified as neurons (and not glia) by their ability to generate spikes in response to an intracellular depolarization.

■ Ten percent of the pyramidal neurons have a bigger soma, an axon and a small apical dendrite restricted to the initial part of the stratum radiatum and no basal dendrite. In these neurons, GABA$_A$-receptor-mediated PSCs are recorded but glutamate-receptor-mediated EPSCs are absent (the synaptic response is fully abolished in the presence of bicuculline) (**Figure 23.2b**). There are only GABAergic synapses

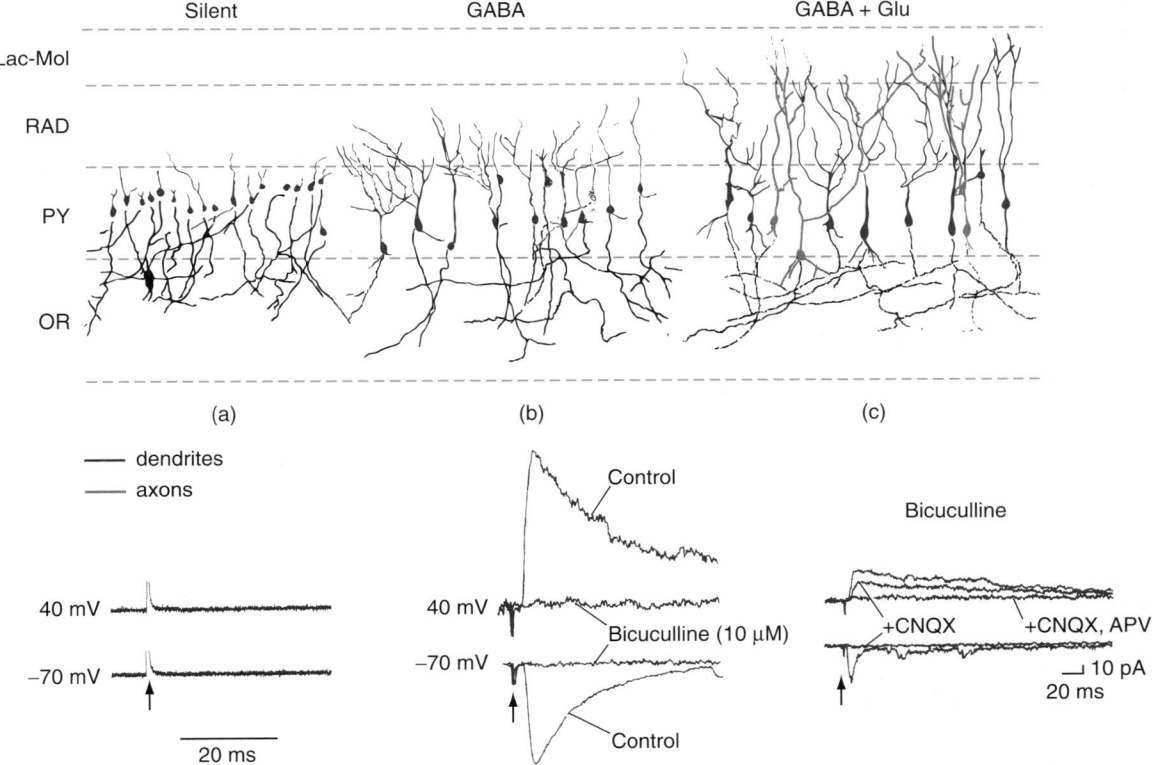

Figure 23.2 Pyramidal cells at P0, grouped accordingly to their synaptic properties.
The activity of pyramidal cells is recorded at P0 in whole-cell configuration (voltage clamp mode) in response to stratum radiatum stimulation. Recorded cells are injected with biocytin and reconstructed with a camera lucida. (a) Silent cells displaying no synaptic current. (b) Cells displaying a bicuculline-sensitive (GABA$_A$-mediated) synaptic current only. (c) Cells displaying bicuculline- (GABA$_A$), CNQX- (AMPA) and APV- (NMDA) sensitive synaptic currents. Arrow indicates the stimulating artefact. Adapted from Tyzio R, Represa A, Jorquera I *et al.* (1999) The establishment of GABAergic and glutamatergic synapses on CA1 pyramidal neurons is sequential and correlates with the development of the apical dendrite, *J. Neurosci.* **19**, 10372–10382, with permission.

established on these neurons: they are thus of the 'GABA only' type. In these whole-cell experiments, the reversal potential of Cl⁻ is 0 mV, which explains why we speak of PSC rather than IPSC.

■ Ten percent of the neurons have an extensively arborized apical dendrite that penetrates to the most distal part of the apical dendrite (lacunosum moleculare) and a more developed basal dendrite. In these neurons, GABA$_A$- *and* glutamate-receptor-mediated PSCs are recorded as shown by the sequential use of selective antagonists (**Figure 23.2c**). Thus, there are GABA and Glu synapses established on these neurons: they are of the 'GABA + Glu' type.

Similar recordings in embryonic slices (E19) indicate that, at this age, all pyramidal neurons (100%) are 'silent', instead of 80% at P0.

All these results show that GABAergic synapses are established prior to glutamatergic ones on pyramidal neurons. Moreover, GABAergic synapses are formed only when the pyramidal neurons have an apical dendrite (glutamatergic synapses are established on the pyramidal neurons when the apical dendrite reaches the stratum lacunosum moleculare).

Parallel immunocytochemical data confirm that synaptic markers such as synaptophysin (**Figure 23.3**) or synapsin or markers of GABAergic terminals are first observed at birth at the level of the apical dendrites of pyramidal neurons. They are observed neither in the pyramidal layer nor in stratum oriens at this early stage.

23.1.3 Sequential expression of GABA and glutamate synapses is also observed in the hippocampus of subhuman primates *in utero*

Similar studies have been performed in fetal and embryonic macaque rhesus hippocampus during the second part of gestation (birth takes place around E165 in this species) in order to understand whether the GABA–Glu sequence of innervation applies also to other species, and in particular to non-human primates. The monkey embryos are removed by caesarian intervention (between E85 and E154) and hippocampal slices obtained. The activity of pyramidal cells is recorded in voltage clamp (whole-cell configuration) and neurons are filled with biocytin and reconstructed. As for the postnatal rat, fetal pyramidal neurons of the macaque can be divided into three populations (**Figure 23.4**):

■ 'Silent' neurons, that have an axon but no dendrites, are silent in that they express no spontaneous or evoked synaptic activity (**Figure 23.4a**). 'Silent' neurons generate sodium action potentials when depolarized (they are neurons, not glia). Bath-applied GABA or glutamate agonists evoke currents (not shown), indicating that the receptors are functional but not the synapses.

■ Neurons that have axons and small apical dendrites express only GABA$_A$-mediated PSCs (**Figure 23.4b**).

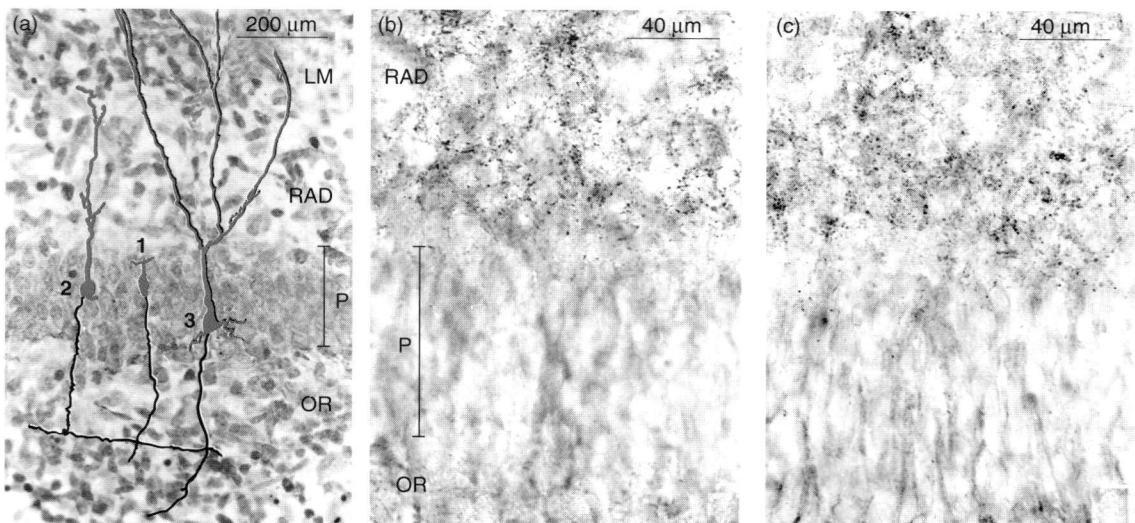

Figure 23.3 Presence of synaptic boutons in stratum radiatum but not in stratum pyramidale at P0.

(a) CA1 hippocampal section stained with cresyl violet (shown here as grey). Three pyramidal cells are shown: silent (middle), GABA only (left) and GABA + Glu (right), to demonstrate the distribution of the dendrites within all the layers. Other sections from the same hippocampus depict immunolabelling with (b) synaptophysin and (c) synapsin (see also Figure 23.2). The labelling is observed in stratum radiatum but not pyramidale.

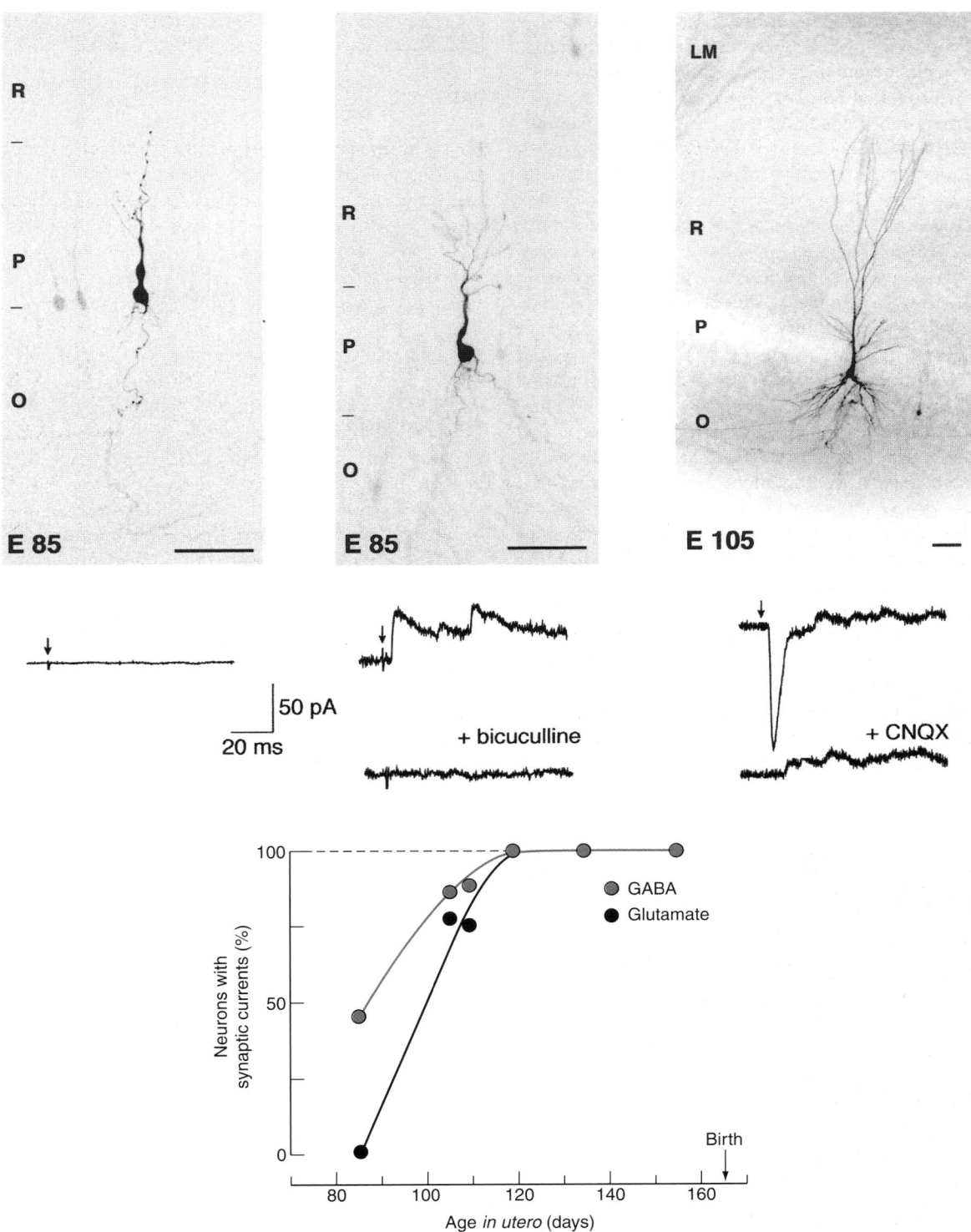

Figure 23.4 Monkey pyramidal cells at embryonic ages.
The activity of pyramidal cells is recorded in whole-cell configuration (voltage clamp mode) in response to stratum radiatum stimulation. Recorded cells are injected with biocytin and reconstructed with a camera lucida. **(a)** *From left to right:* Silent cells at E85 displaying no synaptic current, cells at E85 displaying bicuculline-sensitive (GABA$_A$-mediated) synaptic currents only, and cells at E105 displaying CNQX- (AMPA) sensitive synaptic current. Arrows indicate the stimulating artefact. **(b)** Developmental curve to depict the progressive expression at the embryonic stage of GABA and glutamate synapses. M. Esclapez and R. Khazipov, personal communication.

There are only GABAergic synapses established on these neurons; they are thus of the 'GABA only' type.

■ Neurons that have an arborized apical dendrite as well as basal dendrites exhibit both GABA_A- and glutamate-mediated PSCs (**Figure 23.4c**). Thus, there are GABA and Glu synapses established on these neurons; they are of the 'GABA + Glu' type.

This sequence is observed in both CA1 and CA3, with the only difference that the latter matures earlier. Quantification of the percentage of neurons expressing GABAergic synapses and glutamatergic synapses indicates that in the beginning of mid-gestation over 50% of CA1 pyramidal neurons have functional GABAergic but not glutamatergic synapses (**Figure 23.4d**). In contrast, a few weeks later, one month before birth, all pyramidal neurons have both GABA and glutamate synapses. This results from the high speed of establishment of glutamatergic synapses during this period. Therefore, the sequence described for the rat hippocampus applies also to that of monkeys and probably of humans too. However, the gestation period during which the sequence is established is different: the first week postnatal in the rat, and the beginning of the second part of the gestation period in the rhesus monkey.

23.1.4 Questions about the sequential maturation of GABA and glutamate synapses

To summarize, the first synapses to be established on pyramidal neurons of the hipppocampus are the GABAergic synapses between interneurons and the dendrites of pyramidal neurons (**Figure 23.5**). Glutamatergic synapses are formed at a later stage (such as synapses between two pyramidal cells or between extrinsic glutamatergic fibre tracts and pyramidal cells). This sequential expression suggests that the developmental stage of the target determines whether or not synapses will be established with presynaptic axons. This also suggests that the rules governing the formation of GABA and glutamate synapses differ, the latter requiring more mature postsynaptic targets.

These observations in turn raise the following questions:

■ Does the activation of GABA_A receptors in immature neurons evoke a current and a potential change identical to that in adults, or does the neonatal GABA_A synaptic response have different properties?
■ Is the other major inhibitory response, the metabotropic GABA_B-receptor-mediated IPSP, functional in immature neurons?
■ What are the consequences of these developmentally

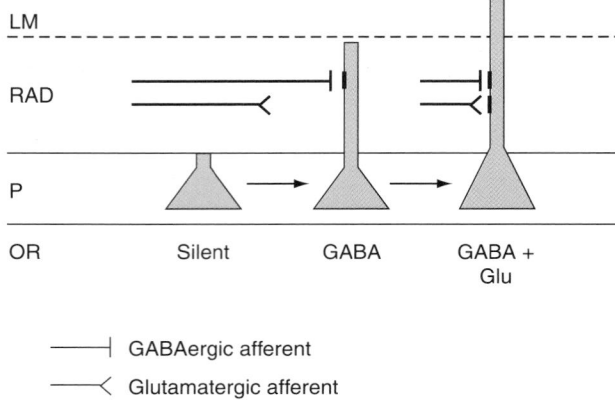

Figure 23.5 Schematic of the different stages of maturation of CA1 pyramidal cells at P0.
See the caption to Figure 23.2.

regulated features on the electrical properties of the immature network? How does the immature network discharge?

23.2 GABA_A- and GABA_B-mediated responses differ in developing and mature brains

23.2.1 Activation of GABA_A receptors is depolarizing and excitatory in immature networks because of a high intracellular concentration of chloride

In the adult hippocampus, activation of GABA_A receptors at rest evokes an inward flow of Cl⁻ ions across the postsynaptic membrane (i.e. an outward current) which results in membrane hyperpolarization (see **Figures 10.17** and **22.9**), a decrease in membrane resistance and a shunt effect (see **Figure 10.18** and Section 10.5.3). GABA_A-mediated inhibition is the key element that provides the basis for the coordinated synchronized neuronal activity. Removal of this inhibition leads in the adult hippocampus to the generation of epileptiform activities. In contrast in the immature hippocampus, GABA_A receptors have a totally different function – they mediate excitation (EPSPs).

GABA_A receptor activation evokes a depolarization and bursts of action potentials in the immature hippocampus

To determine the properties of the GABA_A-mediated response in immature neurons, the activity of pyramidal cells is recorded in embryonic or early neonatal slices. One puzzling observation is that the GABA$_A$ receptor antagonist bicuculline, which in the adult generates epileptiform activity, in contrast produces a full blockade of spontaneous activity in slices at an early developmental stage (**Figure 23.6a**), suggesting that GABA exerts an excitatory action at this stage. In keeping with this, intracellular and whole-cell recordings (current clamp mode) show that GABA$_A$ receptor activation leads to a depolarization of the membrane and the

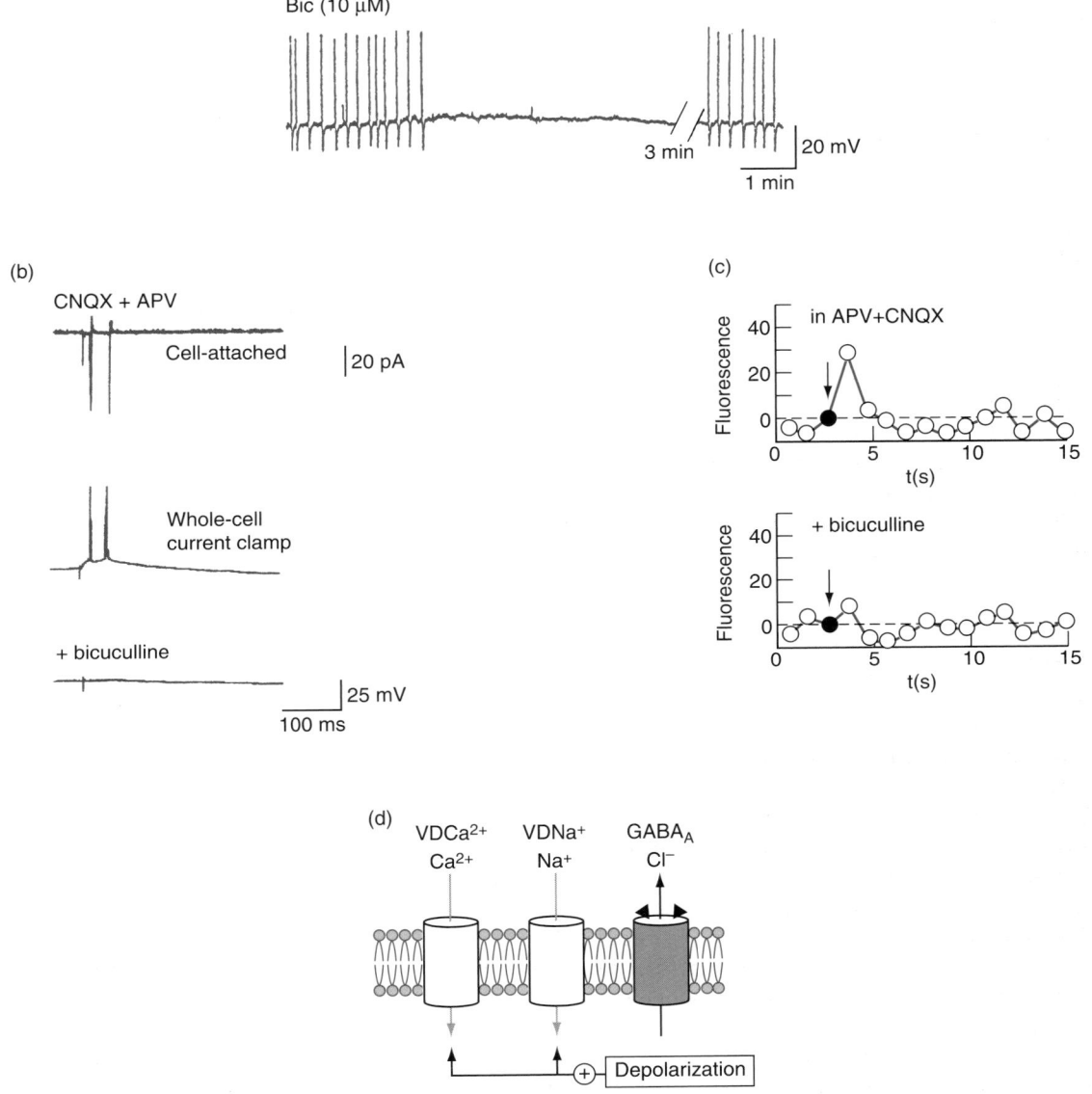

Figure 23.6 Synaptic activation of GABA$_A$ receptors is depolarizing in neonatal rat hippocampus.
The activity of CA3 hippocampal neurons recorded in slices *in vitro*. **(a)** Effect of bicuculline on the spontaneous activity of a pyramidal cell recorded with K methyl sulphate intracellular electrodes at –70 mV. **(b)** Response of an interneuron to stimulation in stratum radiatum in the continuous presence of CNQX (10 μM) and APV (50 μM). The excitatory response is recorded from the same interneuron in the cell-attached and whole-cell configuration (current clamp mode). It is totally abolished by bicuculline (10 μM). **(c)** In the same conditions, electrical stimulation also evokes an increase of [Ca^{2+}]$_i$ that is abolished by bicuculline, in a pyramidal neuron loaded with fluo-3. **(d)** GABA$_A$ receptor activation leads to membrane depolarizing and thus opening of voltage-dependent (VD) Na$^+$ and Ca^{2+} channels. Part (a) adapted from Gaïarsa JL, Coradetti R, Ben-Ari Y, Cherubini E (1990) GABA mediated synaptic events in neonatal rat CA3 pyramidal neurons *in vitro*: modulation by NMDA and non-NMDA receptors, In: Ben Ari Y (ed.) *Excitatory Amino Acids and Neuronal Plasticity*, New York: Plenum Press. Part (b) adapted from Ben-Ari Y, Khazipov R, Leinekugel X *et al.* (1997) GABA$_A$, NMDA and AMPA receptors: a developmentally regulated 'ménage à trois', *Trend. Neurosci.* **20**, 523–529. Part (c) adapted from Khazipov R, Leinekugel X, Khalilov I *et al.* (1997) Synchronization of GABAergic interneuronal network in CA3 subfield of neonatal rat hippocampal slices, *J. Physiol. (Lond.)* **498**, 763–772; all with permission.

generation of sodium action potential(s). This is also observed in cell-attached recordings in which the intracellular concentration of Cl⁻ is not altered (**Figure 23.6b**). Therefore, the GABA$_A$ response of immature pyramidal neurons is depolarizing and excitatory: it depolarizes the membrane of immature neurons up to the threshold potential of action potential generation!

This excitatory effect of GABA results from an elevated concentration of intracellular Cl⁻ in immature neurons owing to a delayed maturation of the Cl⁻-extruding mechanism (transporters) or of Cl⁻ channels that participate in the control of intracellular Cl⁻ concentrations. Similar depolarizing actions of GABA have now been observed in a wide range of structures and animal species, suggesting that it is a general property of developing central networks (see below).

GABA$_A$-receptor-mediated depolarization evokes Ca^{2+} entry through both the voltage-gated Ca^{2+} and NMDA channels

Activation of GABA$_A$ synapses in immature neurons leads to an increase of intracellular Ca^{2+} concentration ([Ca^{2+}]$_i$), as shown by Ca^{2+} imaging techniques (**Figure 23.6c**). In order to understand the underlying mecha-

nism (recall that GABA$_A$ receptor channels are not permeable to Ca^{2+} ions), two main hypotheses can be tested: the [Ca^{2+}]$_i$ increase results either from the activation of voltage-gated Ca^{2+} channels or from the activation of NMDA receptor channels.

To test the first hypothesis, synaptic GABA$_A$ receptors are activated by stimulation of afferents in the presence of CNQX + APV, the blockers of ionotropic glutamate receptors. An increase of intracellular Ca^{2+} concentration is still observed and is blocked by the subsequent application of bicuculline (**Figure 23.6c**) or of antagonists of Ca^{2+} channels such as nifedipin or D-600 (not shown). Therefore, the activation of neonatal GABA$_A$ receptors results in a [Ca^{2+}]$_i$ increase due, at least partly, to Ca^{2+} entry through voltage-gated Ca^{2+} channels (**Figure 23.6d**).

Conversely, in the presence of antagonists of voltage-gated Ca^{2+} channels, synaptic GABA$_A$ receptor activation still induces a small increase of [Ca^{2+}]$_i$ that is abolished by APV, the selective antagonist of NMDA receptor channels (not shown). This suggests that the GABA$_A$-mediated depolarization is sufficient to remove the voltage-dependent Mg^{2+} block of NMDA channels (see **Figure 23.8a**). This is further confirmed by recordings of single NMDA-channel activity and cell-attached recordings of the synaptic responses evoked in the presence of AMPA receptor antagonist.

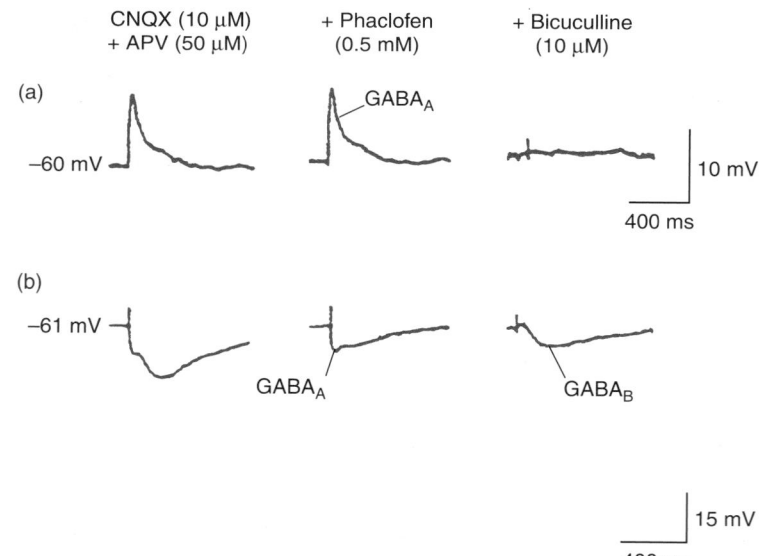

Figure 23.7 GABA$_B$-mediated response is absent in neonate and present in adult pyramidal cells.
The activity of CA3 pyramidal cells recorded with an intracellular electrode filled with K methyl sulphate in the continuous presence of blockers of ionotropic glutamate receptors (CNQX + APV). **(a)** In the neonate: In response to electrical stimulation of stratum radiatum, a depolarizing response is recorded in the neonatal pyramidal cell. This response is mediated by GABA$_A$ receptors since it is unaffected by application of the GABA$_B$ antagonist phaclofen but is totally abolished by the GABA$_A$ antagonist bicuculline. **(b)** In the adult: In contrast, stimulation induces a biphasic hyperpolarization. Phaclofen reduces the late component (GABA$_B$) and leaves intact the early one (GABA$_A$) whereas bicuculline suppresses the early one and leaves intact the late one. Adapted from Gaiarsa JL, Tseeb V, Ben-Ari Y (1995) Postnatal development of pre- and postsynaptic GABA$_B$-mediated inhibitions in the CA3 hippocampal region of the rat, *J. Neurophysiol.* **73**, 246–255, with permission.

Synergy between GABA$_A$ receptors and NMDA receptor channels in the immature hippocampus

Therefore, in immature neurons, there is a synergistic action between GABA$_A$ and NMDA receptors. This stands in contrast with the adult situation. In the neonatal hippocampus, GABAergic synapses act much like AMPA-receptor-mediated synapses at a later developmental stage: they provide the excitatory drive required to generate sodium and calcium action potentials as well as to activate NMDA receptors (see **Figure 23.8**).

There are however, additional factors to take into account to fully comprehend the operative mode of the immature circuit. Even when the effects of GABA are depolarizing and excitatory, there is an inhibitory component due to a shunt mechanism. Also, at a given age of the rat, owing to the heterogeneity of hippocampal neurons, GABA will exert different actions in different neurons – excitatory in one and inhibitory in the other – presumably because they are in a different developmental stage. Thus, recording from different neurons in the same slice can reveal a cocktail of effects, including in some a net excitatory action, in others a dual effect (excitatory and inhibitory).

23.2.2 GABA$_B$-receptor-mediated IPSCs have a delayed expression in immature neurons

Maturation is also associated with alterations in the development of inhibition mediated by GABA$_B$ (as well as adenosine or serotonin) receptors. In adults, activation of these receptors exerts a powerful control at both postsynaptic and presynaptic levels: at the postsynaptic level it generates a large hyperpolarization due to the activation of K$^+$ channels via a G protein (it reverses at E_K). At the presynaptic level, activation of these receptors reduces the release of GABA and the amplitude of the GABAergic synaptic currents via a reduction of a presynaptic Ca^{2+} current and/or the activation of K$^+$ channels in axon terminals. During maturation, the postsynaptic GABA$_B$ receptors are not functional at an early stage (at birth and until P5–P6 in pyramidal neurons) (**Figure 23.7**). Binding studies show that the receptors are present, but intracellular injection of GTPγS to activate G proteins fails to activate GABA$_B$-receptor-mediated currents. Therefore the absence of GABA$_B$-mediated currents is not due to a delayed expression of the receptors but more likely to a delayed coupling of the GABA$_B$ receptors to G proteins and K$^+$

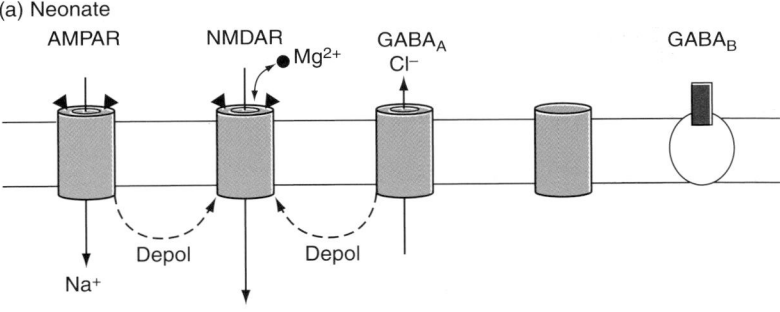

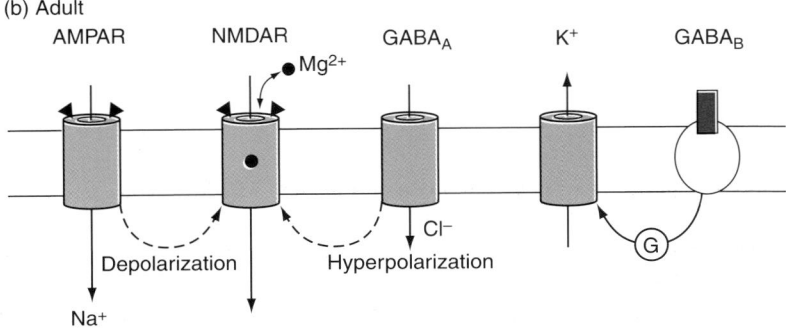

Figure 23.8 Major developmental changes in the GABA–glutamate interactions.
See text for explanations. Adapted from Leinekugel X, Medina I, Khalilov I *et al.* (1997) Ca^{2+} oscillations mediated by the synergistic excitatory actions of GABA$_A$ and NMDA receptors in the neonatal hippocampus, *Neuron* **18**, 243–255, with permission.

channels (**Figure 23.8a**). In keeping with this, the other members of this family (metabotropic receptors) are also not operative at birth.

In contrast, the presynaptic mechanisms are operational already before birth in pyramidal neurons; the activation of GABA$_B$ (or adenosine and serotonin receptors) leads to a reduction of the PSCs in pyramidal neurons or interneurons (not shown). Therefore, the developing circuit operates with the two main postsynaptic receptor-mediated inhibitory mechanisms, GABA$_A$ and GABA$_B$, being poorly developed or acting in a reversed manner. In neonatal hippocampus, the principal mode of operation of transmitter-gated inhibition relies on a presynaptic control of transmitter release.

23.3 Network-driven giant depolarizing potentials (GDPs) provide most of the synaptic activity in the neonatal hippocampus

Electrical activity in neonatal rats (postnatal days P0 to P8) is characterized by the presence of spontaneous network-driven *giant depolarizing potentials* (GDPs) that provide most of the synaptic activity. GDPs are large and long-lasting (several hundreds of milliseconds) synaptic potentials giving rise to bursts of spikes, that occur repetitively at a frequency varying between 0.05 and 0.2 Hz (**Figure 23.9a**). Studies in hippocampal slices show that GDPs are recorded in the vast majority of neurons (both pyramidal neurons and interneurons) in slices obtained from the brain of rats aged between birth and a week postnatally (**Figure 23.9c**). GDPs also prevail prenatally in the monkey during the second half of gestation (E85 to E135).

(a)

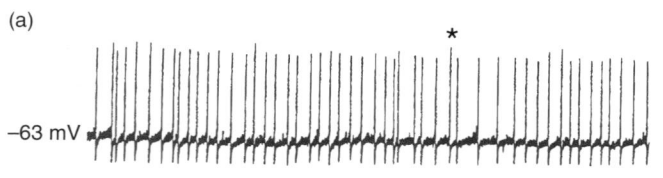

−63 mV

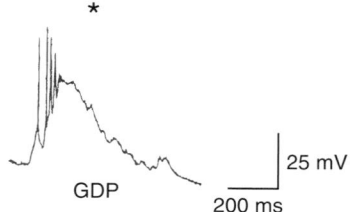

GDP

25 mV

200 ms

(b)

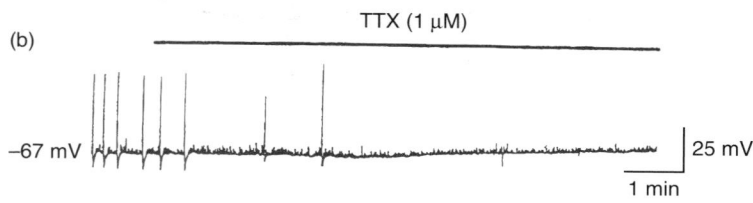

TTX (1 µM)

−67 mV

25 mV

1 min

(c)

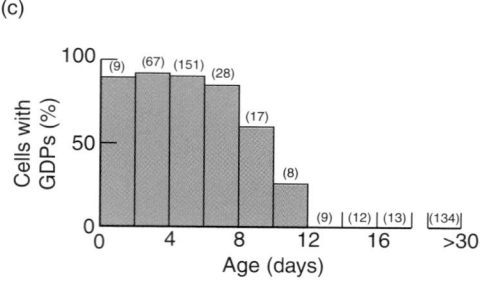

Figure 23.9 Spontaneous giant depolarizing potentials (GDPs) are generated in a polysynaptic circuit in neonatal hippocampus.

(a) Spontaneous GDPs are recorded from a CA3 pyramidal neuron with an intracellular electrode filled with K methyl sulphate. The inset shows a GDP on an extended timescale. **(b)** Spontaneous GDPs are blocked by TTX. **(c)** Histogram of the number of pyramidal cells with GDPs as a function of the age of the rat. The number of recorded cells is in parentheses. Part (a): JL Gaïarsa, personal communication. Parts (b) and (c) adapted from Ben-Ari Y, Cherubini E, Corradetti, Gaïarsa JL (1989) Giant synaptic potentials in immature rat CA3 hippocampal neurones, *J. Physiol. (Lond.)* **416**, 303–325, with permission.

23.3.1 Giant depolarizing potentials result from GABAergic and glutamatergic synaptic activity

GDPs are network-driven (in contrast to pacemaker patterns that are generated by the recorded neuron independently of its synaptic inputs), since (i) they are blocked by TTX (**Figure 23.9b**); (ii) their amplitude but not their frequency is modified by alterations of the resting membrane potential as expected from a synaptic current in contrast to an endogenous pacemaker oscillation; and (iii) they are often blocked by the GABA$_A$-receptor antagonist bicuculline (see **Figure 23.6a**) but also by ionotropic glutamate receptor antagonists (CNQX and APV), suggesting that both GABA and glutamate participate in their generation.

Determination of the currents underlying GDPs with patch-clamp recordings (voltage clamp mode) reveals that GABA$_A$ currents are present either alone or in conjunction with AMPA and NMDA receptor-mediated currents (**Figures 23.10a and b**). The relative participation of GABA and glutamate most likely depends on the maturational stage of the recorded neuron, reflecting the heterogeneity of the neuronal population.

The mechanism underlying the generation of GDPs therefore includes a network-driven barrage of depolarizing GABA and glutamate postsynaptic currents impinging on to pyramidal neurons and in turn leading to a recurrent GABAergic excitation from the GABAergic interneurons. This is also suggested by paired recordings from a pyramidal neuron and an interneuron, which show that GDPs are synchronous in connected neurons and that there are very few action potentials generated outside the GDPs (**Figure 23.10a**). Therefore, GDPs are triggered by the combined depolarizing effects of GABA- and glutamate-mediated currents and by a basic circuit that includes feedforward excitation of pyramidal neurons and interneurons

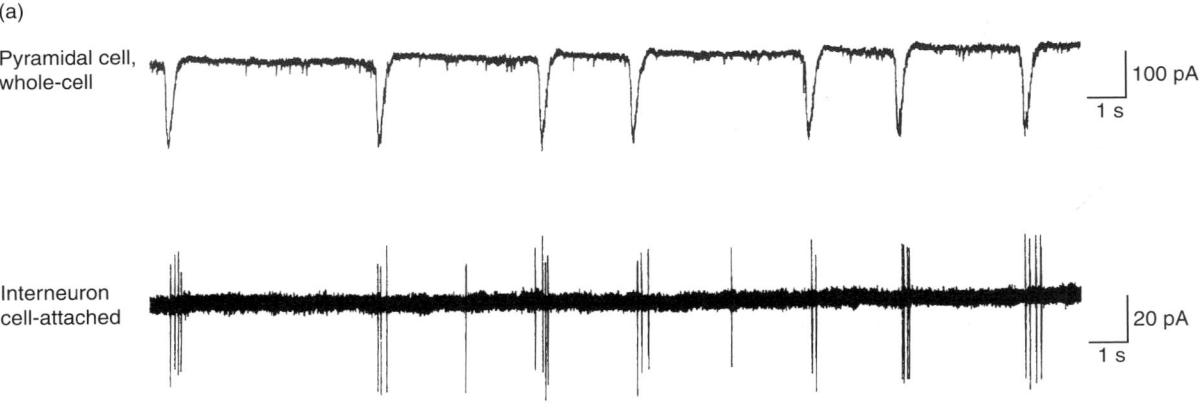

(a)

Pyramidal cell, whole-cell

100 pA

1 s

Interneuron cell-attached

20 pA

1 s

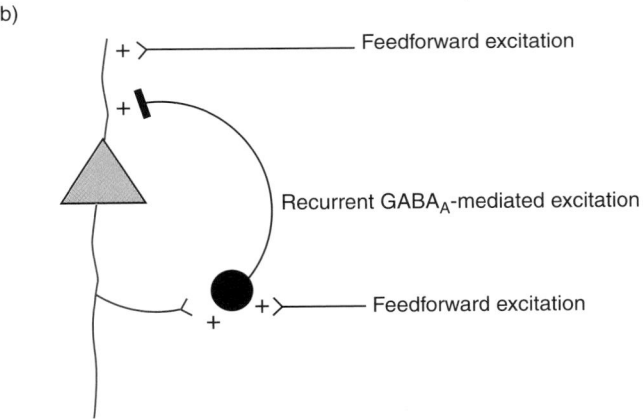

(b)

+)——————— Feedforward excitation

Recurrent GABA$_A$-mediated excitation

+)——————— Feedforward excitation

Figure 23.10 GDPs are synchronous in pyramidal cells and interneurons.
(a) Dual recordings of spontaneous currents (voltage clamp mode) in a CA3 pyramidal neuron (whole-cell configuration, upper trace) and a neighbouring interneuron (cell-attached configuration, lower trace). Note that bursts of currents of action potentials in the interneuron are synchronous with currents of GDPs in the pyramidal cell. (b) Schematic explaining the generation of GDPs. Part (a) adapted from Khazipov R, Leinekugel X, Khalilov I et al. (1997) Synchronization of GABAergic interneuronal network in CA3 subfield of neonatal rat hippocampal slices, *J. Physiol. (Lond.)* **498**, 763–772, with permission.

followed by the recurrent depolarization produced by the recurrent collaterals of GABAergic interneurons (**Figure 23.10b**).

23.3.2 Giant depolarizing potentials are generated in the septal pole of the immature hippocampus and then propagate to the entire structure

Paired recordings in slices show that virtually all neurons have GDPs and that these are fully synchronous with neurons that are not too distant. To study the mechanism of the generation and propagation of GDPs, it is possible to record from an intact hippocampus superfused *in vitro*. In this preparation, the entire hippocampi are dissected and placed in a conventional *in vitro* chamber (**Figure 23.11**). With multiple whole-cell (and extracellular field recordings) it is shown that *GDPs propagate with a septo-temporal gradient of automaticity.* This is directly shown by recordings with multiple electrodes along the rostro-caudal axis. This type of experiment shows that there is a rostro-caudal latency (**Figure 23.11a**). In addition, transection of the hippocampus in two along the longitudinal axis reveals that in both hemisected hippocampi there is a rostro-caudal latency (**Figures 23.11b and c**). Therefore, the rostral pole of the hippocampus, being the most active, paces the rhythm of the entire structure. Since GDPs are present in isolated portions of hippocampus, including mini-slices of CA3 or dentate gyrus subfields, the neuronal elements required for their generation are present in local neuronal circuits. However, the anterior parts of the hippocampus have a higher frequency of GDPs than the caudal ones.

This situation has some similarities with the generation of rhythmic activity in the cardiac muscle in which different parts, including sinoatrial node, atrioventricular node, His bundle and Purkinje fibres, have autorhythmic potentials that allow them to discharge periodically. However, the sinoatrial node is the normal pacemaker owing to a higher rhythm of activity. The mechanisms underlying the role of the anterior parts are not presently known but are likely to be due to a rostro-caudal gradient of maturation.

Using the two interconnected hippocampi *in vitro* it is also possible to determine the hemispheric propagation of GDPs. Paired whole-cell recordings from two neurons in each hippocampus reveal that, even during the first few days after birth, GDPs can propagate from one hippocampus to the other and back, suggesting that the commissural connections are mature. This also suggests that the two hippocampi can synchronize each other at an early developmental stage.

In contrast, structures connected to the hippocampus such as the septum or the entorhinal cortex do not

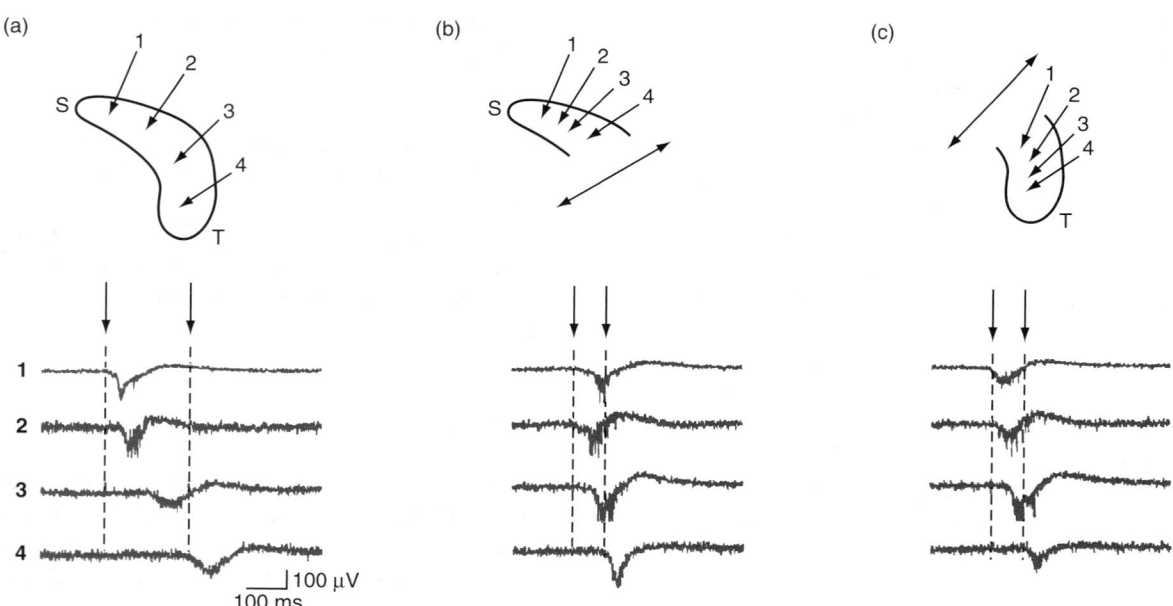

Figure 23.11 GDPs propagate in the rostrocaudal direction in immature hippocampus.
The spontaneous GDPs of four populations of hippocampal neurons are simultaneously recorded with four extracellular electrodes in **(a)** the intact hippocampus, or in **(b)** the isolated rostral or **(c)** caudal halves of the hippocampus of neonatal rats. In extracellular recordings, GDPs are recorded as inward field potentials. Adapted from Leinekugel X, Khalilov I, Ben-Ari Y, Khazipov R (1998) Giant depolarizing potentials: the septal pole of the hippocampus paces the activity of the developing intact septohippocampal complex *in vitro*, *J. Neurosci.* **18**, 6349–6357, with permission.

generate GDPs if they are disconnected from the hippocampus, but they do express GDPs originating in and propagating from the hippocampus. Therefore, the hippocampus must constitute a major source of network-driven synaptic activity that can modulate the electrical activity of brain structures with which it is connected.

23.4 Hypotheses on the role of the sequential expression of GABA- and glutamate-mediated currents and of giant depolarizing potentials

The earlier expression of GABAergic currents, its depolarizing action and the resulting GDPs are key properties of developing networks. Similar effects of GABA have been described in several brain and peripheral structures, and GDP-like events also predominate in virtually all the structures studied so far, including spinal cord, retina and neocortex. This raises the question of the role of this sequential expression of synapses, of the depolarizing actions of GABA, and of the GDPs. The following considerations should be taken into account:

- Owing to their long durations, $GABA_A$-mediated PSCs are highly suitable for summation (tens of milliseconds, in contrast to the milliseconds duration of AMPA-mediated PSCs). This is of importance in immature neurons that possess very few synapses initially, so that there are few spontaneous PSCs to summate if the excitatory drive is provided only by the brief AMPA-mediated PSCs. Furthermore, even if more depolarized than the resting potential, the reversal potential for GABAergic currents is closer to rest than that of glutamatergic PSCs. This and the shunting mechanism, which is inherent to the operation of GABAergic currents, prevent the occurrence of too strong depolarizations and of excitotoxic stimuli that occur when glutamatergic receptors are repetitively stimulated.
- The combined actions of GABA and glutamate facilitate the generation of a large increase of $[Ca^{2+}]_i$ as a result of the activation of voltage-gated Ca^{2+} channels and the removal of the Mg^{2+} blockade from NMDA channels (**Figure 23.8**). In keeping with this, studies in neonatal slices using Ca^{2+} imaging techniques indicate that GDPs are associated with important $[Ca^{2+}]_i$ oscillations (**Figure 23.12**). Other observations suggest that a rise of $[Ca^{2+}]_i$ is needed for dendritic growth and synapse formation.
- Network-driven oscillations like the GDPs may participate in the formation of functional neuronal units like the formation of visual columns. This may follow the Hebbian rule 'neurons that fire together wire together'. Network-driven oscillations provide

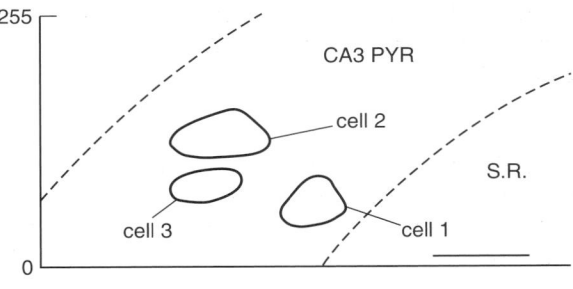

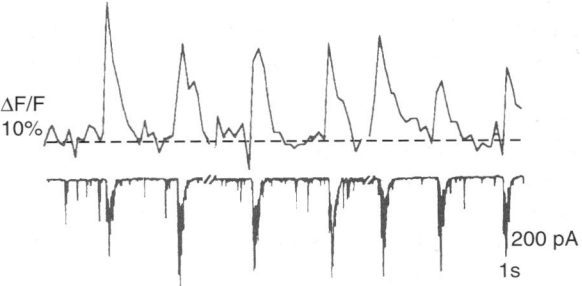

Figure 23.12 Synchronous spontaneous Ca^{2+} oscillations in CA3 pyramidal neurons.

CA3 pyramidal neurons in slices are loaded with fluo-3 and their activity is simultaneously recorded in whole-cell configuration (voltage clamp mode). Each spontaneous GDP current is concomitant to a transient increase of intracellular Ca^{2+} concentration. Adapted from Leinekugel X, Medina I, Khalilov I *et al.* (1997) Ca^{2+} oscillations mediated by the synergistic excitatory actions of $GABA_A$ and NMDA receptors in the neonatal hippocampus, *Neuron* **18**, 243–255, with permission.

a suitable way of organizing these units as both presynaptic and postsynaptic neurons will be excited in a synchronized manner. It is likely that these immature patterns of oscillations play an important role in electrically interconnecting neurons that will become part of an ensemble of neurons subsequently.

23.5 Conclusions

The first synapses to be established in the hippocampus are the GABAergic synapses between interneurons and pyramidal cells or between two interneurons. In these synapses, transmission is mediated by $GABA_A$ receptors.

Activation of $GABA_A$ receptors induces a depolarization of the postsynaptic membrane, in contrast to what is observed in mature neurons where $GABA_A$ receptors mediate inhibition (i.e. membrane hyperpolarization or silent inhibition). This $GABA_A$-mediated depolarization is strong enough to activate voltage-gated channels such as Na$^+$, Ca^{2+} or NMDA channels and thus to evoke action potentials and Ca^{2+} entry.

GABA$_B$ receptors are not active in the postsynaptic membrane of immature GABAergic synapses owing to uncoupling to G proteins and target K$^+$ channels. GABA$_B$ receptors are functional in the presynaptic membrane where they mediate presynaptic inhibition of GABA release.

As a consequence, GABA$_A$ receptors in the immature hippocampus play the role of AMPA receptors in adult networks, and the only transmitter-mediated synaptic inhibition present in immature hippocampal neurons is a GABA$_B$-mediated presynaptic one. The immature hippocampal network displays spontaneous discharges, owing to GABA$_A$-mediated giant depolarizations, which periodically allow Ca^{2+} entry and transient increases of intracellular Ca^{2+} concentration in hippocampal neurons.

Further reading

Garaschuk O, Hanse E, Konnerth A (1998) Developmental profile and synaptic origin of early network oscillations in the CA1 region of rat neonatal hippocampus. *J. Physiol. (Lond.)* **507**, 219–236.

Hollrigel GS, Ross ST, Soltesz I (1998) Temporal patterns and depolarizing actions of spontaneous GABA$_A$ receptor activation in granule cells of the early postnatal dentate gyrus. *J. Neurophysiol.* **80**, 2340–2351.

LoTurco JJ, Owens DF, Heath MJ *et al.* (1995). GABA and glutamate depolarize cortical progenitor cells and inhibit DNA synthesis. *Neuron* **15**, 1287–1298.

Menendez de la Prida L, Bolea S, Sanchez-Andres JV (1998) Origin of the synchronized network activity in the rabbit developing hippocampus. *Eur. J. Neurosci.* **10**, 899–906.

Obrietan K, van den Pol AN (1998) GABA$_B$ receptor-mediated inhibition of GABA$_A$ receptor calcium elevations in developing hypothalamic neurons. *J. Neurophysiol.* **79**, 1360–1370.

Owens DF, Boyce LH, Davis MB, Kriegstein AR (1996) Excitatory GABA responses in embryonic and neonatal cortical slices demonstrated by gramicidin perforated-patch recordings and calcium imaging. *J. Neurosci.* **16**, 6414–6423.

Reichling DB, Kyrozis A, Wang J, MacDermott AB (1994) Mechanisms of GABA and glycine depolarization-induced calcium transients in rat dorsal horn neurons. *J. Physiol. (Lond.)* **476**, 411–421.

Rivera C, Voipio J, Payne JA *et al.* (1999) The K$^+$/Cl$^-$ cotransporter KCC2 renders GABA hyperpolarizing during neuronal maturation. *Nature* **397**, 251–255.

Rohrbough J, Spitzer NC (1996) Regulation of intracellular Cl$^-$ levels by Na$^+$-dependent Cl$^-$ cotransport distinguishes depolarizing from hyperpolarizing GABA$_A$ receptor-mediated responses in spinal neurons. *J. Neurosci.* **16**, 82–91.

Index